A TEXT BOOK OF ANIMAL HUSBANDRY

Eighth Edition

A Textbook of Animal Husbandry

G. C. Banerjee
Ph.D. (Animal Sc.) Cornell, U.S.A
Ex DEAN of Post-Graduate Studies
Bidhan Chandra Krishi Viswavidyalaya

Oxford & IBH Publishing Co. Pvt. Ltd.
New Delhi

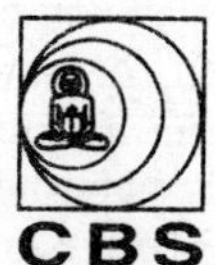

(A Unit of CBS Publishers & Distributors Pvt Ltd)

New Delhi • Bengaluru • Chennai • Kochi • Kolkata • Mumbai
Hyderabad • Jharkhand • Nagpur • Patna • Pune • Uttarakhand

A TEXTBOOK OF ANIMAL HUSBANDRY

OXFORD & IBH
(A Unit of CBS Publishers & Distributors Pvt
204 FIE, Patparganj Industrial Area, Delhi-110 092
E-mail: delhi@cbspd.com, cbspubs@airtelmail.in

Reprint: 2016, 2017, 2018, 2019, 2020

ISBN 978-81-204-1260-6

Printed at Mudrak, Noida, UP, India

To The Divine Mother
Your blessings could alone inspired me for completion of the job you desired.

To my Family
Your love and understanding helped shape this book. I am home again.

To the Student
Hope this text helps you grow and discover the thrill of exploring domestic animals.

PREFACE TO THE EIGHTH EDITION

For nearly 35 years I have had the privilege of teaching various aspects of Animal Husbandry to students of Veterinary and Agricultural Sciences, as also some professionals. This has made it possible to revise this book seven times since its first publication in 1964 while retaining its primary objective—to present an update in the science and art of husbandry of domestic animals in simple and meaningful language.

This endeavour resulted in, I sincerely believe, a concise documentation and collation of components of Animal Husbandry into a comprehensive whole in a simple and lucid language, understandable to both students and professionals. My aim has been to tell a scientific and technically sound precise story instead of presenting a data base encyclopedia on the subject.

The bulk of this edition has increased as with earlier editions, resulting primarily from addition of new chapters, one on Yak and the other on Rabbits and an introduction to microbiology. Several chapters have been extensively revised and enlarged. These include those on elementary anatomy and physiology, artificial insemination, animal blood, animal nutrition, camel and mammary glands & lactation. The rest of the chapters also received comprehensive brush up to accomodate recent developments in their respective areas. To foster a better understanding of the materials presented, a glossary has been incorporated initially in chapter 1.

I sincerely hope that the wider coverage presented in all the chapters in this edition will prove of singular utility not only to the graduate students, researchers and teachers but also to progressive farmers and professionals-cum-technologists of all Asian Countries.

Deep apreciation is extended to Dr. John Edwin M. of Tamil Nadu Veterinary & Animal Science University for allowing me to incorporate some materials including some of the photographs as appeared in his manual "Deep freezing of semen".

In preparing this latest revision I have been greately aided by suggestions received from many of the teachers and of my former students including Dr. D.K. Basu, Principal, Eastern Regional Demonstration & Training centre, NDDB (Siliguri) in West Bengal, Dr. Manojit Biswas of National Bank for Agricultural & Rural Development Hyderabad, Dr. Lalmohan Mandal, Professor and Head, Department of Animal Science, Bidhan Ch. Krishi Viswavidyalaya, West Bengal, Dr. S.K. Dasgupta, Asst. Commissioner (CD) Ministry of Agriculture, Gov't of India, Dr. R.C. Saha, Senior Scientist, NDRI, Kalyani, Nadia are noteworthy. I am sincerely grateful to all of them individually.

Appreciation is also expressed to Shri Sudin Das for his remarkable art work.

My sincere appeciation to Miss Jhinuk Chatterjee, M.Sc. (Zoology), University of Kalyani, for her splendid assistance which contributed enormously to the successful publication of this edition.

Finally, I would like to extend my sincere appreciation to my wife, Mrs. Arati Banerjee for the strains she was subjected to and tolerated so patiently while I burnt the midnight oil, day after day, month after month and year after year. During this period she took the load of my shoulders—responsibilities that could well have diverted my attention from this gigantic academic endeavour. I spared neither time nor expense as I honed this book to a level of perfection I dreamt of achieving. If it serves its primary objectives, I will be gratified and satisfied and will know my labours were not lost in the sands of time.

26th January 1998

G.C. Banerjee

B-8/122, Kalyani (Nadia) Pin: 741235
West Bengal. Phone: (033) 828 700

PREFACE TO THE FIRST EDITION

While I was a student I felt the need of a suitable textbook on Animal Husbandry to meet the requirements of graduate students. As a teacher also I feel the necessity no less when I find my students getting lost in the larger volumes of the standard books on different aspects of Animal Husbandry. This inspired me to write a textbook on the subject especially meant for the students of B.Sc. (Ag.), B.V.Sc. (A.H.), B.Sc. (Dairy Husbandry) and I.D.D. (Dairy Husbandry) classes.

In this book I do not pretend to claim credit for any original contributions on the subject. Rather it should be viewed as a concise collection of various important topics—which I prepared as a teacher of the subject.

The book has been divided into six chapters dealing respectively with Mechanisms of heredity; Mechanisms of reproduction; Artificial insemination; Animal breeding; Animal nutrition and Dairy farm management.

In writing these chapters every endeavour has been made to represent the topics in as simple and classified a manner as could be, so that students with elementary knowledge in Mathematics, Chemistry and Physics will be able to grasp the ideas conveyed in the book.

My acknowledgements are due to Dr. P.K. Bose, Research Officer, Eastern Regional Animal Nutrition Centre and my colleague Shri Bibekananda Ray for their helpful criticism and valuable suggestions.

I am also indebted to Shri Sukumar Dana of Kalyani University and Shri Mahendra Narayan Chowdhury of the Veterinary Extension Section of this Institute for their generous and sincere help and advice for the chapters on Mechanisms of heredity and Artificial insemination respectively.

My thanks are also due to Shri Himanka Prodhan, one of my students of B.Sc. (Ag.), Hons. Class in the University of Kalyani, for preparing quite a large number of diagrams for this book.

I shall be failing in my duties if I do not mention the name of Dr. S.B. Chattopadhyay, Principal, College of Agriculture, Kalyani University and Dr. S. N. Singh, Head of the Department of A.H. & Dairying, B. R. College, Agra, without whose encouragement and help this work could not have been possible.

I am also indebted to Shri Manoranjan Roy, Librarian, Faculty of Agriculture, Kalyani University, for placing the entire library resources at my disposal.

Finally my sincere thanks are also due to my wife Srimati Arati Banerjee, who spared no pains to go through the manuscript several times and helped me greatly in proof-reading, editing and preparing the Bibliography.

Any suggestions for the improvement of the book will be thankfully received.

15th July, 1964
Faculty of Agriculture
Kalyani University, West Bengal

G. C. BANERJEE

CONTENTS

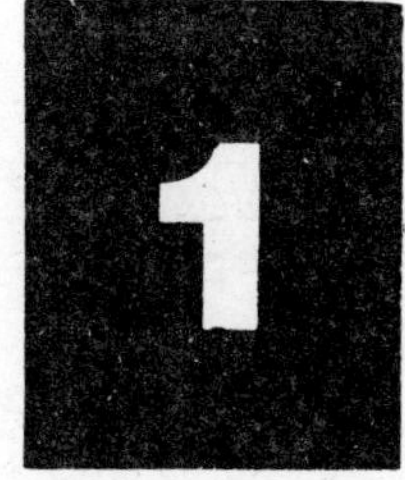

TAXONOMY, DOMESTICATION AND ANIMAL HUSBANDRY IN INDIA

What is Animal Husbandry ?

By the word "Animal" although it includes any of the various organisms belonging to the kingdom *Animalia*,distinguished from plant kindgom by their non-photosynthetic methods of nutrition, non-cellulosic cell membrane and centralised nervous system but yet when we talk of animal husbandry, we mean only those domesticated animals which are reared mostly for economic or for recreation purposes in any particular region. such as Cattle, buffalo, sheep, goat, yak, camel, pig, horse, dog, poultry etc.

The word "Husbandry" comes from the management of domestic affair, but at present the word is also used in management of farming such as Crop husbandry and Animal husbandry. The term used in connection with animal husbandry includes proper feeding, breeding, health care, housing and many other activities.

Thus "Animal Husbandry" may be defined as a science as well as an art of management including scientific feeding, breeding, housing, health care of common domestic animals aiming for maximum returns.

Taxonomy

Taxonomy is the science of classification applied to living things and it involves their identification, naming and arrangement. The system of classification devised by Linnaeus (1707-1798), a Swedish botainist, has now been accepted universally as a means of reference. In this system each individual type of organism is called a *species.* Species or organism having close similarities are arranged in a group known as a genus (pl. genera). Genera with similar characteristics are put in the same family, simil lar families into orders and orders into classes. This system uses two Latin names to describe each organism. The generic name refers to its genus and is written with a capital letter and the specific names indicate its species and is written with a small letter. For example, the name *Homo sapiens* referes to species known as *sapiens* beonging to the genus *Homo* in case of a human being. The generic name is often abbreviated to one or two letters, e.g.B. for Bos, C. for *Capra*, E. for *Equus.* Most animals and plants can be classified according to their morphology, i.e. according to their shape, in conjunction with evidence obtained from fossils.

Zoological Classification (Taxonomy) of Common domestic animals

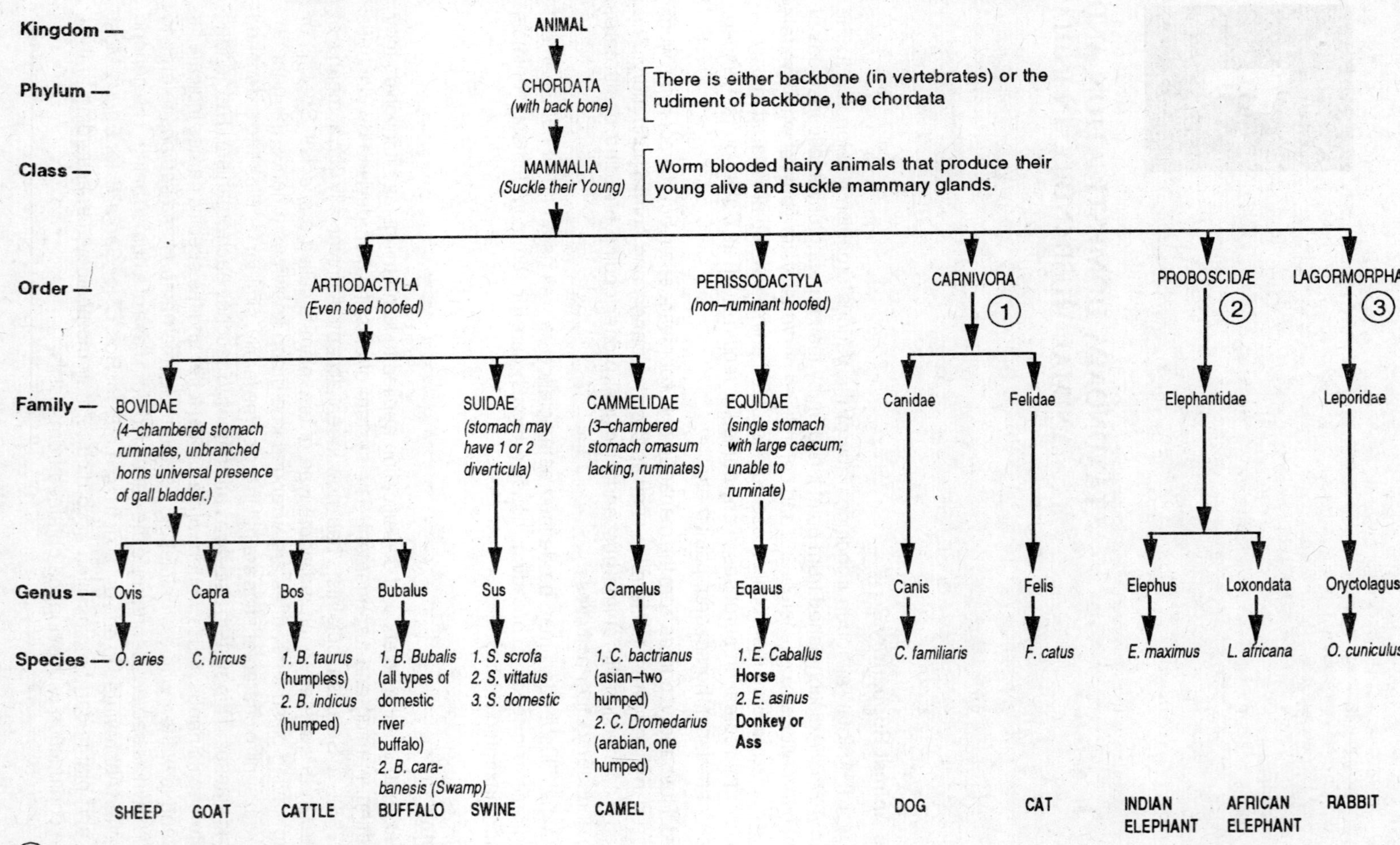

(1) Flesh eating mammals, powerful jaws and claws.

(2) Thick skin with scant hair, skull bones are thick with air passage (sinuses). Testis abdominal.

(3) Continually growing incisors are present. Locomotion by jumping method.

In general the taxonomic system is constructed according to the plan developed by Karl Von Linne in the middle part of 18th century:

1. Kingdom
2. Phylum
3. Class
4. Order
5. Family
6. Genus
7. Species

For example, a human being belongs to the Kingdom *Animal,* Phylum *Chordata,* Class *Mammalia,* Order *Primate,* Family *Hominidae,* Genus *Homo,* Species *spaiens.*

Table 1.1

FAO Statistics on Livestock Population

The Table below is the latest FAO Statistics on Livestock Population of the countries in Asia-Pacific Region, 1988.

(Unit: 1,000 heads)

Country	Cattle	Buffalo	Pig	Sheep	Goat	Chicken	Duck
Bangladesh	23,500	1,964	—	1,123	10,700	64,000	32,000
Bhutan	409	7	63	27	32	—	—
China	73,946	20,860	335,116	102,650	77,932	1,850,000	323,000
India	201,401	75,605	10,519	56,980	108,493	206,000	9,000*
Indonesia	6,470	3,049	6,500*	5,488	13,704	434,000	29,000
Iran**	8,350	230	—	34,500	13,600	105,000	—
Japan	4,667*	—	11,725*	29	48	351,000	—
Kampuchea	1,950	700	1,500	1	1	7,000	3,000
Korea DPR	1,250	—	3,100	372	285	20,000	—
Korea REP	2,386	—	4,281	3	166	59,000	1,000
Laos	590	1,000	1,520	—	76	9,000	—
Malaysia	636	245	2,258	102	347	58,000	4,000
Mongolia	2,600	—	140	13,200	4,450	—	—
Myarmar (Burma)	10,000	2,200	3,000	295	1,100	34,000	6,000
Nepal	6,374	2,890	479	833	5,125	10,000	—
Pakistan	17,300	13,900	—	27,000	32,300	152,000	1,000
Philippines	1,600	2,890	7,580	30	2,130	60,000	5,000
Sri Lanka	1,831	1,029	101	28	510	9,000	—
Thailand	5,034	6,403	4,268	95	80	83,000	19,000
Vietnam	2,800	2,680	11,800	23	455	75,000	34,000
Australia	23,500	—	2,720	164,00	600	56,000	—
Fiji	160	—	30	—	60	2,000	—
New Zealand	7,999*	—	428*	64,800*	1,000	9,000	—
Papua New Guinea	123	—	1,523	2	17	4,000	—
Samoa, W.**	27	—	65	—	—	1,000	—
Tonga	8	—	65	—	11	—	—
Vanuatu	105	—	79	—	12	—	—
Asia-Pacific total	**405,114**	**135,654**	**408,860**	**471,697**	**273,250**	**3,663,000**	**466,000**
World	**1,265,976**	**140,648**	**889,141**	**1,171,403**	**521,974**	**9,661,000**	**528,000**
Indian livestock population as (%) percent of world	15.90	53,75	1.25	4.86	20.78	2.13	1.70

Note: * = Unofficial. ** = 1987 Figures.

Animals are also classified on the basis of their nature of rumination (regurgitation). Some of them are listed below :

List of common domestic animals classified on the basis of whether they are

Non-ruminants or Ruminants

Non-ruminants (having single stomach)	Ruminants (All ruminates; number of stomach may vary from usual of Four)
1. Elephant	1. Cattle
Asian	Humped
African	Humpless
2. Rhinocerus	2. Buffalo
Indian	Asian
White	African
Black	Indian
3. Hippopotamus	3. Sheep
4. Horse	4. Goat
Domestic	5. Nilgai
Wild	6. Giraffe
Pony	7. Deer
5. Zebra	8. Bison
Grevy	9. Llama (3 chambered stomach)
Plains	10. Camels (3 chambered stomah)
Mountain	
6. Ass	Among species of the family *camelidae* which includes camels, vicunas, alpacas, llamas, the omasum is missing as it has been anatomically modified into small tubular and is structurally a part of the abomasum. Surprisingly enough, the reticulum contains glandular cells.
7. Pig	
8. Man	
9. Dog	
10. Monkey	
11. Rabbit	
12. Hamster	

THE BEGINNING OF ANIMAL HUSBANDRY

Man in the Old Stone Age (1,000 – 8,000 B. C.) made no attempt to domesticate animals but used to ate those animals that he was lucky to hunt. In the New Stone Age (8,000—6,000 B. C.)

Table 1.2 Mature Body Weights and Ages of Selected Species

Common Name	Species Name	Mature Body Weight (kg)	Mature Age	Longevity (year)	Maximum Recorded Lifespan (yr)	Birth Weight (kg)
Dairy cattle	*Bos taurus/indicus*	464–653	5 yr	20–25	30	25–45
Horse	*Equus caballus*	450	3–5 yr	20–25	50	45–55
Goat	*Capra hircus*	26–102	2 yr	10–15	18	2.5–3.5
Swine	*Sus scrofa*	70–128	—	16–18	27	1.0–2.0
Sheep	*Ovis aries*	34–80	2 yr	10–18	20	2.0–4.0
Rabbit	*Oryctolagus cuniculus*	3.0–4.9	1 yr	5–8	>13	.04–.08
Chicken	*Gallus domesticus*	1.5–3.3	20–30 weeks	2–5	30	.049–.065
Turkey	*Meleagris gallopavo*	5.0–14.8	28–35 weeks	—	12.3	0.52–.056

Altman and Dittmer, 1964, Fox ett al. 1984. Blakely and Bade, 1982. Cole and Garrettt, 1980; Acker, 1983

Table 1.3

Common Names for the Sexes, Young, Groups and Birthing of Various Animals

Animal	Male	Female	Young	Group	Name for giving birth
Antelope	buck	doe	kid	herd	kidding
Bear	boar	sow	cub	sleuth	cubbing
Beaver	boar	sow	pup	colony	—
Bird	cock/stag	hen	fledgling/ nestling	flock	hatch
Bison	bull	cow	calf	herd	calve
Bobcat	tom	lioness/queen	kitten	litter	—
Cat	tom	pussy/queen	kitten	clowder	queening
Cattle	bull	cow/heifer	calf	herd/drove	calve
Chicken	rooster/cock	hen/pullet	chick	flock	hatch
Deer	buck/stag	doe	fawn	herd	—
Dog	dog	bitch	pup/puppy	kennel	whelp
Donkey	jackass	jennet/ jenneyass	colt	herd	foal
Duck	drake	duck	duckling	flock	hatch
Elephant	bull	cow	calf	herd	calve
Fox	reynard	vixen	cub/pup	earth/skulk	pupping
Giraffe	bull	cow	calf	herd	calve
Goat	billy/buck	nanny	kid	trip	kidding
Goose	gander	goose	gosling	gaggle/flock	hatch
Hog	boar	sow/gilt	piglet/shoat	herd/drove	farrow
Horse	stallion/stud	mare/dam	foal colt (male) filly (female)	stable/herd	foal
Kangaroo	buck/boomer	doe/flyer	joey	troop/herd	—
Lion	lion/tom	lioness/she lion	cub	pride/flock	whelp
Ostrich	cock	hen	chick	flock	hatch
Owl	owl	jenny/ howlet	howlet/owlet	flock	—
Ox	steer	cow	stot	herd/drove	calve
Rabbit	buck	doe	kitten	colony	—
Rat	buck	doe	—	colony	—
Seal	bull	cow	pup	herd/harem/ rookery	—
Sheep	buck/ram	ewe/dam	lamb/ lambkin	flock/hurtle	lamb
Swine – see hog					
Turkey	tom	hen	poult	flock	hatch
Walrus	bull	cow	cub	herd	—
Whale	bull	cow	calf/cub/pup	herd/pod	pupping
Wolf	he-wolf	she-wolf	cub/pup	pack	whelp
Zebra	stallion	mare	colt	herd	foal

man changed from hunter to husbandman of animals by domestication. Domestication came after food cultivation. The first animals to be domesticated may have been the dog and goat probably 8,500 to 9,000 years ago from to-day. The place was the hills of South Western Asia in the Lebanese and Palestinian mountains.

Table 1.4 **Gestation Periods***

Species	(days)	Species	(days)	(months)
Livestock		**Wild Animals**		
Ass	365	Ape, Barbary	210	
Cattle:		Bear, black		7
Angus	281	Bison		9
Ayrshire	279	Camel	410	
Brown Swiss	290	Coyote	60–64	
Charolais	289	Deer, Virginia	197–220	
Guernsey	283	Elephant		20–22
Hereford	285	Elk, Wapiti		8½
Holstein	279	Giraffe		14–15
Jersey	279	Hare	88	
Red Poll	285	Hippopotamus	225–250	
Shorthorn	282	Kangaroo, red	32–34**	
INDIAN	282	Leopard	92–95	
Goat	148–156	Lion	108	
Horse, heavy	333–345	Llama		11
Horse, light	330–337	Marmoset	140–150	
Pig	112–120	Monkey, macaque	150–180	
Sheep:		Moose	240–250	
Mutton breeds	144–147	Musk ox		9
Wool breeds	148–151	Opossum	12–13	
Pets		Panther	90–93	
Cat	59–68	Porcupine	112	
Dog	56–68	Pronghorn	230–240	
Guinea pig	58–75	Raccoon	63	
Hamster	15–18	Reindeer		7–8
Mouse	19–31	Rhinoceros, African	530–550	
Rabbit	30–35	Seal		11
Rat	21–30	Shrew	20	
Fur Animals		Skunk	62–65	
Chinchilla	105–115	Squirrel, grey	44	
Ferret	42	Tapir	390–400	
Fisher	338–358	Tiger	105–113	
Fox	49–55	Walrus		12
Marten, European	236–274	Whale, sperm		16
Pine Marten	220–265	Wolf	60–63	
Mink	40–75	Woodchuck	31–32	
Muskrat	28–30			
Nutria (coypu)	120–134			
Otter	270–300			

*Adapted from *Merck Veterinary Manual*, 5th edition

**Delayed development as long as a "joey" is in the pouch

Table 1.5

Visual Parameters of Selected Species

Common Name	Species Name	Visual field (Degrees)	Binocular Vision (Degrees)	Colour Perception[a]
Dairy cattle	*Bos indicus*	330—360[b]	25—50[b]	Yes
Horse	*Equus caballus*	330—350[b]	30—70[b]	Yes
Goat	*Capra hircus*	320-340[b]	20—60[b]	Yes
Swine	*Sus scrofa*	310[b]	30—50[b]	Yes
Sheep	*Ovis aries*	330—360[b]	20—50[b]	Yes
Rabbit	*Oryctolagus cuniculus*	330[b]	10—35[b]	Yes
Chicken	*Gallus domesticus*	300[c]	10—35[c]	Yes
Turkey	*Melearis gallopavo*	300[c]	10—35[c]	Yes

a Based upon presence of cone cells.

b Fedde, M.R. (1976) Respiration in "*Avian Physiology*", 3rd edn Springer Verlag, New York, U.S.A.

c Kare, M.R., and Rogers, J.G. Jr. (1976) *Sense organs . In Avian Physiology*, 3rd edn, Springer Verlag, New York, U.S.A.

Table 1.6

Average Rectal Temperatures of Various Species

	Average		Range	
Animal	°C	°F	°C	°F
Stallion	37.6	99.7	37.2–38.1	99.0–100.6
Mare	37.8	100	37.3–38.2	99.1–100.8
Donkey	37.4	99.3	36.4–38.4	97.5–101.1
Camel	37.5	99.5	34.2–40.7	93.6-105.3
Beef cow	38.3	101	36.7–39.1	98.0–102.4
Dairy cow	38.6	101.5	38.0–39.3	100.4–102.8
Sheep	39.1	102.3	38.3–39.9	100.9–103.8
Goat	39.1	102.3	38.5–39.7	101.3–103.5
Pig	39.2	102.5	38.7–39.8	101.6–103.6
Dog	38.9	102	37.9–39.9	100.2–103.8
Cat	38.6	101.5	38.1–39.2	100.5–102.5
Rabbit	39.5	103.1	38.6–40.1	101.5–104.2
Chicken (daylight)	41.7	107.1	40.6–43.0	105.0–109.4

From Andersson, B.E. : Temperature regulation and environmental phisiology. In Dukes' Physiology of Domestic Animals, 10th Ed. Edited by M. J. Swenson. Ithaca, NY, Cornell University Press, 1984.

Table 1.7

Table of Norms

Features of the Reproductive Cycle (Pets)*

	Cats	Dogs	Guinea pigs	Hamsters	Mice	Rabbits
Age at puberty	6–15 months	6–12 months**	55–70 days	5–8 weeks	35 days	5½–8½ months
Cycle type	Provoked ovulation, seasonally polyestrous, spring & early fall	Monestrous, all year, but mostly late winter & summer	Polyestrous	Polyestrous	Polyestrous	Polyestrous, induced ovulation
Cycle Length	15–21 days	6–7 months	16 days	4 days	4 days	1 month or more
Duration of heat	9–10 days in absence of male, 4–6 days if mated	4–14 days standing heat	6–11 hours	10–20 hours	9–20 hours	1 month or more
Best time for breeding	Daily from day 2 of heat	On alternate days from day 2 to end of heat	10 hours after start of heat	At start of heat, 8–10 p.m.	At start of heat	Anytime
First heat after birth	4–6 weeks	3–5 months	6–8 hours	1–2 weeks after litter removed	2–4 days after litter removed	Immediate
Number of young	1–10	1–22	1–8	1–12	1–12	3–13

*Adapted from *Merck Veterinary Manual*, 5th edition

** Earlier in smaller breeds, later in larger breeds

ANIMAL HUSBANDRY IN INDIA—PRESENT AND FUTURE

India has basically been an agricultural country and it is likely to continue to be so for a long time to come. At present 70 per cent of Indians are dependent for their livelihood on agriculture. Thirty per cent of the total land holdings are held by 70 per cent of small and marginal farmers who held 80 per cent of the total livestock in the country. Crop agriculture in India depends mainly on bullocks which contribute approximately 40,000 MW of power to agricultural operations.

In spite of this the country has been unable to be assured of needed supplies of food grains and of animal products including milk till the middle of 1960s. During the period of last 25 years, however, it has been possible to achieve substantial progress and build up a buffer stock of few million tonnes of food grain every year. The indepth analysis carried out some 10 years back about the progress and prospects of Indian agriculture has shown the existence of potentialities. It is necessary to make everyone in the country aware of these potentials as also the tasks to be performed to realise these potentials for the good of the country in particular and the world in general.

The production and use of animal products in the human diet is receiving tremendous attention. With this object in view the need for developing Animal Husbandry is recognised very well. The other objectives are to provide animal power for farmings, adoptation of better land use pattern—the land which is not suited for arable cropping should be put under grass or trees—so much needed for protection to soil. Among other objectives of Animal Husbandry, the utilisation of agro-industrial by-products for converting those into valuable animal products so much needed by all of us. The creation of thousands of employment opportunities through out the year by adopting animal industry on large scale shall also be a part of the objectives of Animal Husbandry in India.

According to FAO statistics on livestock (1988), there are 201.4 million cattle, 75.6 million buffaloes, 56.98 million sheep, 108.49 million goat, 10.5 million pigs, 206 million chickens and 9.0 million ducks.

Cattle and Buffaloes

India has 14 per cent of the world's cattle and 50 per cent of the world's buffalo population. Cattle alone produces about 42 per cent (13.8 MMT) of the total milk produced (32.75 MMT) in the country during 1982. During the year 1987-88 the country produced 46.1 MMT, thus exceeding the target of 45.9 MMT, according to the annual report of the Department of Agriculture and Co-operation. Thus India is now occupying first position regarding its milk production among the developing countries of the world. When compared with the world the country occupies third position in quantum of total milk production. The gross value of output of milk and milk products amounts to over Rs. 7,500 crores, compared to other agricultural outputs such as rice—Rs. 11,573 crores and wheat Rs. 5,225 crores.

Although there has been a substantial increase in milk production over the years, the corresponding increase in human population has brought the per capita availability of 144 g milk per day which is far lower than the recommended level of 210 g per head per day. The average milk production of a milking cow is only 173 kg and that of buffalo is about 500 kg milk in one lactation. Sixty five million Indian buffaloes contribute about 54 per cent of the total milk produced in our country. Regarding animal commodity cattle and buffalo contribute approximately 80 per cent of the total GNP (Gross National Product) of about Rs. 20,000 crores per annum.

Poultry

We also produced about 15 billion eggs per year and more than 75 million broilers in 1985 from a meagre figure of 4 million in 1971. Poultry meat coutributed to nearly 17 per cent of the total meat production value of one million tonnes in 1985.

The value of poultry production has risen from Rs. 65 crores in 1961 to Rs. 1,000 crores in 1985. When compared with per capita/year consumption it is only 20 eggs and 240 g poultry meat as against 260–300 eggs and 20–30 kg poultry meat consumption in some of the developed countries. Conservative industry projections place the turn of the century estimates at upwards of 30,000 million eggs and 400 million broilers thus raising the annual per capita availability of 30 eggs and 540 g poultry meat for an estimated human population of approximately one billion by that year. Such a fast expansion in egg and poultry meat production would require about 135 million improved laying stock, 450 million broiler chicks with feed requirement going upto about 7.5 million tonnes per year. The Five Year Plan allocation has now increased substantially to Rs. 602 million in the Seventh Plan from a figure of Rs. 28 million in the Second Plan.

Table 1.8

Meat production from slaughtered animals and poultry

(000 MT)

Species of animals	Meat Production in India				
	1974-76	1980	1981	1982	1983
Beef and veal	61	74	78	80	80
Buffalo meat	98	120	127	130	132
Mutton and lamb	102	120	125	127	132
Goat meat	228	270	277	288	288
Pig meat	54	70	75	80	80
Poultry meat	88	113	120	130	136
Total meat	714	870	916	945	958

Sheep

The country has around 45.03 million sheep in 1982 producing around 132 million kg of mutton comprising about 14 per cent of the total meat production from all species in the country. Although the sheep population remained almost static at around 48 million between 1951–1977, it registered a substantial increase between 1977–1982. The current wool production is around 39.8 million kg, most of which is in the form of variable carpet quality and only around 5 million kg is useable in the worsted sector. The country is exporting handknotted carpets and hosiery worth Rs. 150 crore and is importing around 14 million kg of apparel wool.

Goats

According to 1982 census, the country has around 90 million goats. The species provide dependable source of income to 40 per cent of rural population below the poverty line in India and to many who do not possess any land. Inspite of 42 per cent annual slaughter of goats the population continues to increase at the rate of about 1.2 per cent per year. Its economic contribution to the national economy is to the tune of Rs. 350 crores annually through (i) the production of 9,55,000 MT of milk (comprising 2.9 per cent of the total milk production of the country), (ii) 305,000 MT of meat (which is obtained through sacrifice of 38.86 million goats annually and constitutes 40.7 per cent of the total meat produced in the country), (iii) 79,000 MT of fresh skin, (iv) 40 MT of pashmina, and (v) 340 million MT of manure. However, the average production of milk, meat and fibre per individual is much below the world average. In India a goat is primarily used as a meat animal. At present the internal demand is 20 times higher than the present production. It is thus apparent that an increase in individual production of the indigenous goat is essential to boost the natural production.

Livestock as National Economy

The present contribution of livestock to the national economy is estimated to be Rs. 15,000 crores mainly from milk and milk products (70 per cent); meat and meat products (11.5 per cent); poultry (8.8 per cent) and dung for fuel (7.8 per cent). In addition the value of other animal products as eggs, wool, leather goods etc., makes the total of Rs. 15,000 crores. Apart from above items, the value of draught power from 88 million bullocks including 8 million buffalo bullocks indispensable to agricultural operations is of the order of Rs. 5,000 crores. According to some other estimates, the market value of all the domesticated species in India is of the order of Rs. 40,000 crores.

Although there has been a substantial increase of cattle and buffalo population by about 32 per cent and 61 per cent respectively over the 1956 base and thereby increase in milk production both from cattle and buffaloes over the years, the corresponding increase in human population was 79 per cent. This has offset the gains made in milk production. Current trends of growth in human population suggest that since more and more land would be used for cereal production, the feed resources for livestock are likely to be further reduced.

The total human population by the year 2000 at the current growth rate would be around 997 million. To feed this population at the minimum recommended level (210 g per individual per day) we would need around 76 million tonnes of milk. The cattle and buffalo population by 2000 would be 246 (including 49 million cross-breds) and 109 million respectively, which together would produce around 68 million tonnes of milk including 4 million tonnes from goats and other species.

We are in deficit both in feed and fodder to a large extent. National Commission on Agriculture in 1976 indicated that India was short of 44 per cent concentrate, 38 per cent green fodder and 44 per cent dry fodder. The commission also estimated the requirement of feeds by the year 2000. Projections were made on the assumption that with the addition of more and more high yielding cross-breds, we shall be able to reduce the numbers. This assumption does not seem to hold true as there has been an increase in cattle and buffalo population by 32 per cent and 61 per cent respectively over the 1956 base.

The available feed and fodder situation, however, demands that we reduce the numbers of cattle and buffaloes by selection.

With the diminishing land resources for agriculture due to urbanisation and fast increasing human population, the total cropped area is likely to be further reduced and most of the land would be used for cereal production for human consumption. The feed resources for livestock are thus likely to be further reduced.

In order to increase the per capita consumption of milk, meat and eggs, we have to think in terms of increased production considering the ever increasing population in one hand and overall scarcity of quality animals and their feed on the other hand. The disproportionately small output has been attributed to a number of causes. Chief among them are:

Feeding: Inadequate feed and nutrition to support our vast livestock and poultry population.

Breeding: Low genetic potentiality for high production due to the absence of selection for milk, meat, eggs and wool. Disorganised breeding programme is another factor.

Management: Lack of efficient and scientific management. Poor uniformity in data collection in the country regarding livestock.

Disease control: Lack of application of modern techniques to control diseases.

Considerable pioneering work in some of these areas are now being carried out by all the National Research Institutes, viz., National Dairy Development Board, Indian Grassland and Fodder Research Institute, Indian Veterinary Research Institute, Central Institute for Research in Buffaloes, Central Avian Research Institute, Central Sheep and Wool Research Institute, Central Institute for Research on Goat, National Research Centre on Camel, Agricultural Universities of the country and others.

There is no doubt that major improvements in animal productivity will take place through the traditional methods of giving attention to feeding, breeding, management and disease control, but it is no longer possible to obtain the targets of achieving production by using only conventional technologies. Nevertheless, it may thus be worthwhile for achieving maximum exploitation of our livestock and poultry by applying new approach of recent biotechnology in the field of animal nutrition, reproduction, breeding and management. Researchers in molecular biology and immunology have made their most significant rank in helping us to achieve the aim.

What is Biotechnology?

Biotechnology is a new scientific field, has crystallized and developed rapidly during the past 15–20 years. It is the application of biological organisms, systems or processes to manufacturing and service industries. In 1981 the European Federation of Biotechnology defined it as "integrated use of biochemistry, microbiology and chemical engineering in order to achieve the technological application of the capacities of microbes and cultured tissue cells" Agriculture and medical technology (e.g. the construction of heart-lung mechanism) are thus excluded from this definition.

The role of biotechnology in upgrading animal production is largely one of supplying tools to assist animal producers with breeding, feeding, management and disease control.

Animal Health

For providing health cover, currently, there are 14,849 veterinary hospitals and dispensaries in the country, besides there are 19,286 veterinary first aid centres. It is envisaged to increase the number of hospital/dispensaries to 19,452 by the end of Seventh Plan. There will be at least one veterinarian for every 10,000 cattle units, 5 regional disease diagnostic laboratories and in addition disease surveillance centres in 12 states. A central authority, independent of the drug controller, would be established to ensure quality control of all veterinary immuno-biologicals. The IVRI has set up a centre for animal disease research and diagnosis and strengthened its regional disease and diagnosis facilities.

The production of veterinary immuno-biologicals is also being strengthened. It is expected that 50 million doses per annum will be produced by the end of the Seventh Plan programmes for control and eradication of nationally important diseases, viz. rinderpest and FMD, although contagious bovine pleuropneumonia in cattle, Marek's and pullorum diseases (Bacillary with diarrhoea) in poultry, swine fever in pigs and rabies in dogs will also receive attention. Efforts to develop disease free zones at least in three states are also in progress.

Veterinary, Dairy and Animal Science Education

There are 25 Veterinary Colleges and 8 dairy technology colleges preparing graduates in veterinary and animal sciences and dairy technology respectively. In addition the IVRI and NDRI have formal training programmes in Veterinary and Dairy Sciences. RBS College at Agra and Allahabad Agricultural Institute are producing Master's degree holders in Animal and Dairy Science since few decades in the country. IVRI and NDRI are now recognised as "deemed to be University" preparing candidates in various disciplines of Veterinary & Animal Sciences both at post-graduate and doctorate levels.

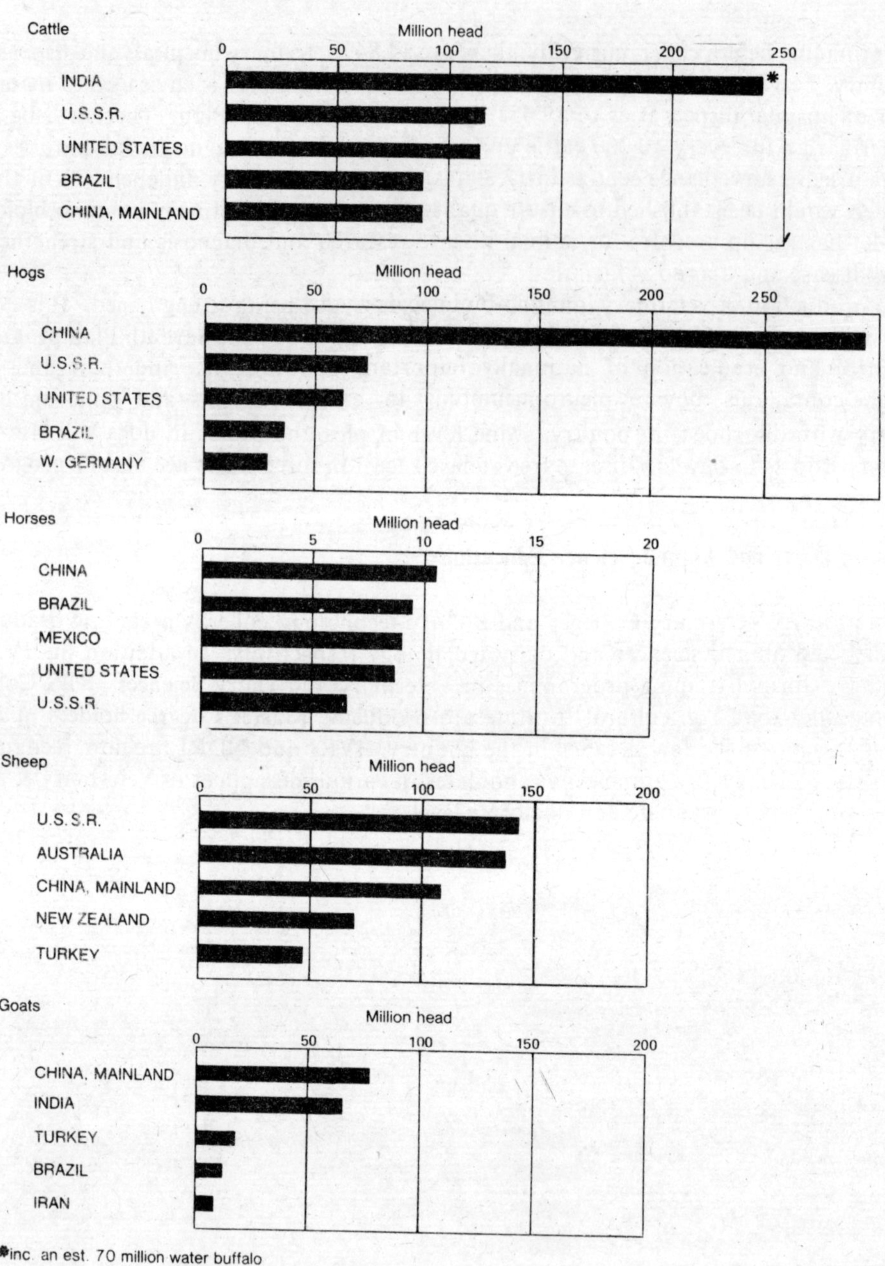
Countries that lead in the Production of Selected World Domestic Animals
Cattle
Million head
0
50
100
150
200
250
INDIA
U.S.S.R.
UNITED STATES
BRAZIL
CHINA, MAINLAND
Hogs
Million head
0
50
100
150
200
250
CHINA
U.S.S.R.
UNITED STATES
BRAZIL
W. GERMANY
Horses
Million head
0
5
10
15
20
CHINA
BRAZIL
MEXICO
UNITED STATES
U.S.S.R
Sheep
Million head
0
50
100
150
200
U.S.S.R.
AUSTRALIA
CHINA, MAINLAND
NEW ZEALAND
TURKEY
Goats
Million head
0
50
100
150
200
CHINA, MAINLAND
INDIA
TURKEY
BRAZIL
IRAN
*inc. an est. 70 million water buffalo

Countries that lead in the Production of Selected World Animal Products

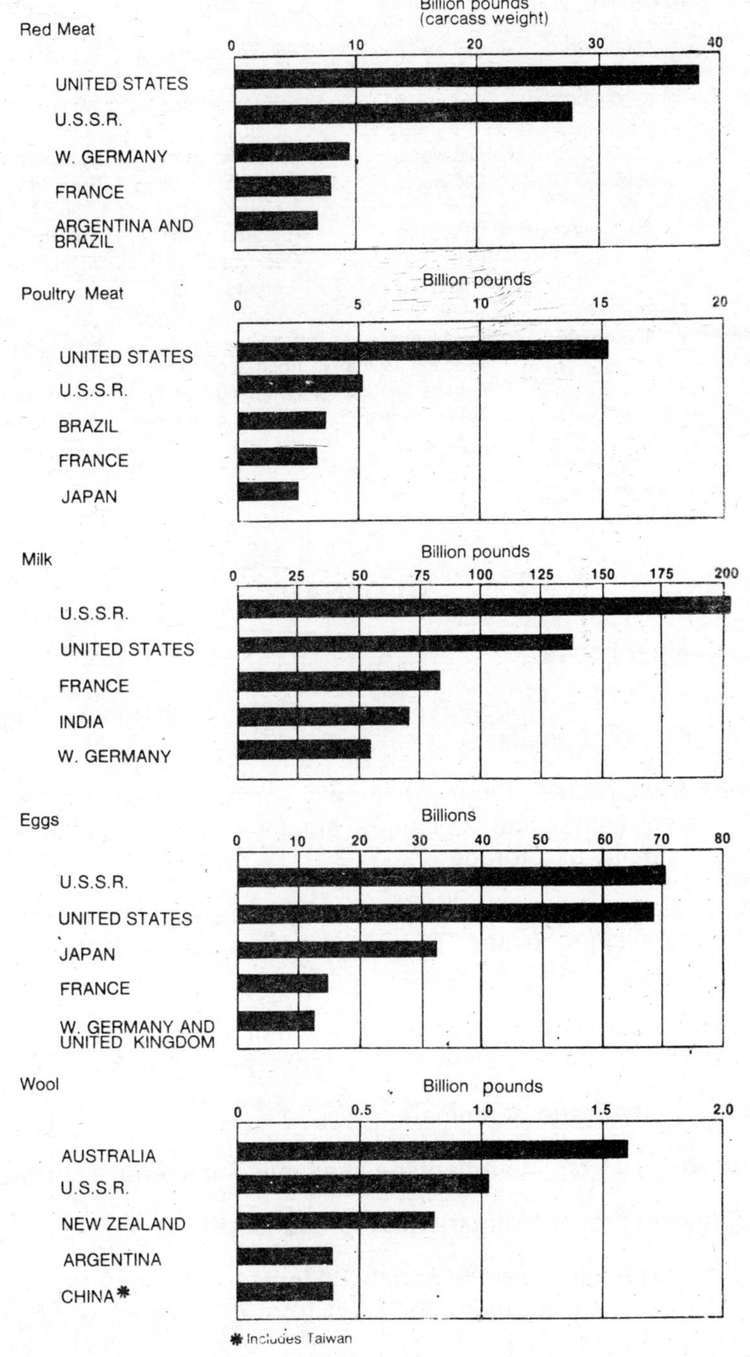

* Includes Taiwan

Table 1.9
THE DOMESTICATION OF ANIMALS

Species	When, B.P.,* years	Where	Why	How
Dog	8500–9000	Old and new worlds	Pet, companion	Wolf or jackal
Goat	8500–9000	Old world	Food, milk, and clothing	Wild goat
Pig	8000–9000	Old world	Food and sport	European wild boar
Sheep	6000–7000	Old world	Food, milk, and clothing	European mouflon and Asiatic urial
Cattle	6000–6500	Old world	Religious reasons	Aurochs
Chickens	5000–5500	India, Sumatra, and Java	Cockfights, shows, food, and religion	Jungle fowl
Horse	4000–5000	Old world	Transportation	Wild horse
Ducks	?	Probably China	Food and feathers	Wild duck
Geese	?	Greece and Italy	Food and feathers	Wild goose
Turkeys	?	Mexico or North America	Food and feathers	Wild turkey

*B.P. means *before present.*

GLOSSARY

Abattoir A slaughter house

Abomasum The fourth or true stomach of the cow, comparable in function to that of simple–stomached animals.

Acid detergent fiber (ADF) Fiber (principally lignin and cellulose) extracted from a feedstuff using a chemical technique employing an acidic detergent. Used to evaluate the quality of a forage.

Acidosis A condition of the blood which is brought about by an increase in acidity as a result of metabolic processes. There is a consequent reduction in the amount of alkali in the blood.

Active transport Energy–requiring translocation of a substance across a membrane, usually against its concentration or electrochemical gradient.

Adipose tissue Fatty tissue of animals

Ad libitum (ad lib) Term used to reflect the availability of a feed on a free–choice basis.

Aerobic A biological process requiring the presence of oxygen.

Afterbirth The fetal membranes that attach the fetus to the membranes of the pregnant female and which are normally expelled from the female within 3 to 6 hr after parturition.

Agalactia Failure to secrete milk following parturition.

Alimentary canal The tubulous passageway leading from the mouth to the anus. It includes the mouth, pharynx, esophagus, stomach, small intestines, large intestines, and rectum.

Alveolus A very small structure found in the mammary gland, almost spherical in shape, lined with a single layer of epithelial cells, in which milk is manufactured by the female.

Ambient That which surrounds (e.g., the temperature around us is the ambient temperature).

Amnion The innermost fetal membranes, which form a fluid–filled sac for the protection of the embryo.

Anarobe An organism able to live in the absence of free oxygen, or in greatly reduced concentrations of free oxygen.

Angstrom A unit of measurement : 1/10,000,000 of a millimeter (10^{-7}mm)

Anorexia Lack of appetite

Antibiotics Chemical compounds antagonistic to some forms of life produced by and obtained from certain living cells. Antibiotics are used in animal and human medicine to combat certain disease organisms and in animal feeding to enhance performance.

Antibody A substance produced in an animal as a protective mechanism to combat invasion by a foreign material (antigen).

Antigen A high–molecular–weight substance (usually protein) that, when foreign to the bloodstream of an animal, stimulates the formation of a specific antibody.

Apoenzyme The protein portion of an enzyme. The apoenzyme and coenzyme form the functioning holoenzyme.

ATP Adenosine triphosphate, a high energy organic phosphate of great importance in energy transfer in cellular reactions. Universal energy currency of cells.

Artificial insemination The injection of mechanically procured semen into the reproductive tract of the female without coition and with the aid of mechanical or surgical instruments.

Ataxia Failure of muscle coordination.

Atrophy A defect or failure of nutrition or physiological function manifested as a wasting away or diminution in size of cell, tissue, organ, or part.

Autopsy Examination, including dissection, of a carcass to learn the cause and nature of disease or cause of death. Also called Postmortem.

Backfat A term used in swine production that refers to the amount of fat deposited along the back in animals of either sex. Usually measured at typical market weights of 200–230 pound. An excessive amount of backfat is considered to be an undesirable trait.

Balanced ration The feed or combination of feeds that will supply the daily nutrient requirements of an animal.

Barrel That part of the animal's body between the fore and rear legs.

Barrow A male swine animal that was castrated at an early age before reaching sexual maturity and before developing the physical characteristics peculiar to boars.

Basal metabolism The chemical changes that occur in the cells of an animal in the fasting or resting state when it uses just enough energy to maintain vital cellular activity, respiration, and circulation.

Bedding Leaves or straw which is given to animals to lie on.

Biological Value The percent utilization of protein within the animal body, expressed by the formula

$$\%BV = \frac{\text{N intake}-[(\text{FaecalN}-\text{Metab.N}) + (\text{Urigenous N}-\text{Endogenous N})}{\text{N intake}-(\text{Faecal N}-\text{Metabolic N})}$$

Bleating The noise made by goats, specially females at œstrus.

Blind quarter In cattle, a mammary gland quarter that does not secrete milk or one that has an obstruction in the teat that prevents the removal of milk. A nonfunctional mammary gland.

Bloat A disorder of ruminants characterized by the accumulation of gas in the rumen.

Bolus A masticated morsel of food ready to be swallowed.

Bomb calorimeter An apparatus used to measure the heat of combustion of feeds, or feces.

Brainstem Made up of mid and hind brain. Coordinate automatic involuntary processes.

Breed Animal having a common origin and characteristics that distinguish them from other groups within the same species

Browse Feed taken from trees and shrubs (including leaves, twigs and bark).

Brush border A free epithelial cell surface bearing numerous microvilli.

Bull index (sire index) A measure of inheritance of milk and/or milk nutrient production that a bull tends to transmit to his daughters.

Calf starter A dry concentrate feed especially formulated for use with young calves from birth to 3 or 4 months of age.

Cannibalism Consists of one pig or chicken biting the tail or other body part of another. Most frequently observed in closely confined, growing–finishing pigsand chickens.

Carboxyhemoglobin The compound formed when carbon monoxide combines with hemoglobin. CO competes successfully with oxygen for combination with hemoglobin, producing tissue anoxia.

Centromere The point on the chromosome at which identical chromatids are joined and by which chromosomes are attached to a spindle fiber.

Chelating agent An organic compound that can bind cations (metallic ions) by forming a stable, inert complex that is soluble in water; used in softening hard water, in purifying sewage, and in eliminating high concentrations of undesirable metallic or radioactive elements in the blood or tissues.

Coenzyme A substance, usually non–protein and of low molecular weight, necessary for the action of some enzymes.

Colostrum The first milk produced by the female immediately after giving birth to young. It is highly nutritious and a rich source of antibodies.

Conception The fecundation of the ovum. The action of conceiving or becoming pregnant.

Coprophagy The ingestion of own faeces as in rabbit.

Cotyledon An area where the membranes of the fetus and the uterine lining are in close association such that the nutrients can pass to and wastes can pass from the circulation of the developing young.

Creep An area accessible to small calves, lambs, or pigs, but not to adult animals, to enable the young to consume additional feed to supplement nutrients obtained from nursing.

Critical temperature The atmospheric temperature below which vasomotor control of the body temperature (e.g., vasoconstriction, vasodilation, sweating, etc.) ceases to maintain body temperature.

Crude fiber The portion of feedstuffs identified by proximate chemical analysis that is composed of cellulose, hemicellulose, lignin, and other polysaccharides. These compounds make up the structural and protective parts of plants. Crude fiber level are high in forages and low in grains.

Crude protein In the proximate analysis of feedstuffs, a figure representing protein content arrived at by multiplying the total nitrogen in a feed by 6.25.

Cryptorchidism In the male, a condition where the testes are retained in the body rather than descend into the scrotum. Results in infertility.

Culling The process of eliminating nonproductive or undesirable animals.

Dentition Refers to the dental pattern in various species of animals. A dental formula includes both the numbers and types of teeth, temporary and permanent, in both the upper and lower jaw.

Dicoumarl A chemical compound found in spoiled sweet clover. It has an anticoagulant and can cause internal hemorrhages when eaten by cattle.

Diuretics Are substances which produce diuresis, that is, which cause a copious excretion of urine.

Docking Removal of the tail. A common practice in lambs.

Domesticate To bring a wild animal or fowl under control and to improve it through careful selection, mating and handling so that its products or services become more useful to humans.

Drenching A common method of administering medicine to an animal by mixing the medicine with water, elevating the animal's head, and giving the dose from a bottle.

Dressing percentage Carcass weight/live weight.

Dry cow A cow that is not producing milk

Drying off The act of causing a cow to cease lactation in preparation for her next lactation.

Dry period Nonlactating days between lactations.

Dual-purpose animal One which is kept for both milk and meat production.

Dysgenesis A defect in breeding so that hybrids cannot mate between themselves but may produce offspring with members of either family of their parents. Such offspring are sterile.

Dystocia Abnormal or difficult labor at parturition, causing difficulty in delivering the fetus and placenta.

Ear-notching A notch or series of notches made in the ear of animal as a means of identification

Edema The presence of abnormally large amounts of fluid in the intercellular tissue spaces of the body, as in swelling of mammary glands commonly accompanying parturition in many farm animals.

Efferent nerves The nerves that carry messages from the central nervous system to the effectors, the muscles and glands. They are divided into two systems : somatic and autonomic (automatic).

Efficacy Effectiveness. For e.g., the effectiveness of an antibiotic in the therapy of a certain disease.

Ejaculate Refers to the semen ejected from the male at the time of copulation or to the semen collected as a part of the procedure in artificial insemination.

Electron-transport Chain (Respiratory Chain) A series of enzymes that transfer electrons from substrate molecules to molecular oxygen.

Embryo A young organism in the early stages of development. In animals, the period from fertilization until life is noted.

Embryo transplant Artificial transfer of the embryo from the natural mother to a recipient female by mechanical means.

Encephalomalacia A Condition characterized by softening of the brain. A disease causing lesions of the brain in young poultry, caused by a deficiency of vitamin E in the diet.

Endemic (Enzootic) Pertaining to a disease commonly found with regularity in a particular locality.

Ensilage (silage) Plant material preserved in a wet state subsequent to fermentation ina silo.

Enteritis Any inflammatory condition of the intestinal linings of animals or humans.

Epizootic Designating a widely diffused disease of animals, that spreads rapidly and affects many individuals of a kind concurrently in any region, thus correspoding to an epidemic in humans.

Ergot A fungus found in feeds that is toxic to animals.

Eructation The act of belching or casting up gas from the stomach by mouth.

Escutcheon The area at the rear of a cow that extends upward just above and in back of the udder where the hair turns upward in contrast to the normal downward direction of hair.

Esophageal groove In ruminants, a semicanal providing passage for fluid materials from the esophagus to the abomasum in young animals. In mature animals the function of the esophageal groove is questionable.

Estrous cycle The period from one estrus, or heat period, to the next.

Estrus The period of heat or sexual excitement in the female.

Excrement Waste material discharged from the body, especially from the alimentary canal.

Exotic The term used to describe animals foreign to a region.

FAO Food and Agriculture Organisation. An agency of the United Nations that collects and disseminates information on the production, consumption and distribution of food throughout the world. It was organized in 1945 and has some 120 member nations; it is headquartered in Rome.

Farrowing pen A specially designed pen in which sows are placed at the time of farrowing. These pens contain gurd rails to prevent the sow from laying on newly born pigs.

Fauna Usually refers to the overall protozoal population present.

Fecundity Efficiency ot an individual in production of young. Animals that bring forth young frequently, regularly, and in the case of those that bear more than one offspring at a birth, in large numbers, are said to e fecund.

Feed efficiency The units of feed consumed per unit of weight increase or unit of production (milk, meat, eggs).

Fibrinogen A soluble protein present in the blood and body fluids of animals that is essential to the coagulation of blood.

Fistula A permanent opening made in the body wall of an animal through which there is communication between the animal's interior and the external environment. An example is a rumen fistula – a permanent opening created surgically between the interior of the rumen and the outside.

Fleece The entire coat of wool as it comes from the sheep or while still on the live animal.

Flora In nutrition it generally refers to the bacteria present in the digestive tract.

Flushing The practice of feeding female animals especially well, just previous to the breeding season, in order to stimulate their reproductive organs to the maximum activity. This is thought to result in a higher percentage of conceptions.

Forage Roughage of high feeding value. Grasses and legumes fed at the proper stage of maturity and quality are forages.

Foster mother A doe or ewe that raises a kid or lamb of which she is not the natural mother.

Free-martin A heifer, usually sterile, born twin with a bull.

Friedman test A test for pregnancy in which a small amount of urine of the tested animal is injected into the bloodstream of a virgin rabbit. Pregnancy is indicated by certain changes in the ovaries of the rabbit.

Fungi (singular, Fungus) Plants that contain no chlorophyll, flowers or leaves. They get their nourishment from dead or living organic matter.

Gametes Reproductive cells. Sperm produced by the male and ova (or eggs) by the female.

Gluconeogenesis Formation of glucose from protein or fat.

Glycogenesis Conversion of glucose into glycogen

Glycogenolysis Conversion of glycogen into glucose

Glycolysis Conversion of carbohydrate into lactate by a series of catalysts. The breaking down of sugars into simpler compounds.

Ham The rear quarter of a pig or of a pork carcass.

Haylage Forage ensiled at a relatively low moisture content (usually 40 to 50%).

Heat increment (HI) The increase in heat production following consumption on food when an animal is in a thermoneutral environment. It consists of increased heats of fermentation and of nutrient metabolism. There is also a slight expenditure of energy in masticating and digesting food. This heat is not wasted when the environmental temperature is below the critical temperature. This heat may then be used to keep the body warm.

Hematopoietic An agent that promotes the formation of blood cells.

Herbivorous animals Animals that habitually rely upon plants and plant products for their food.

Heterosis The increased stimulus for growth, vigor, or performance often shown by a crossbred individual. Hybrid vigor.

Holocellulose Total structural carbohydrate in a plant. It excludes soluble sugars, starch, and pectins.

Homeotherm A "warm–blooded" animal. An animal that maintains its characteristic body temperature even though environmental temperature varies.

Horn–buds Small bumps on a young's head where horns are starting to grow.

Hulls The outer protective covering seeds.

Husks Refers to the fibrous covering of the grain after removal of hulls.

Impregnate To make pregnant; to fertilize.

Intrinsic factor A chemical substance in normal stomach juice necessary for the absorption of vitamin B_{12}.

In vitro Within artificial environment, as within a test tube.

In vivo Within the living body.

Iodinated casein (thyroprotein) A product produced when casein, a milk protein, is treated with iodine. The resulting product possesses thyroactivity and is sometimes fed to milk cows to stimulate milk production.

Ion An atom bearing a net charge due to loss or gain of electrons.

Lactation period The number of days a cow secretes milk following each parturition.

Legumes A family of plants which are usually high in protein and which naturally improve the nitrogen content of the soil.

Lethal characters Presence of hereditary factors in the germ plasm that produce an effect so serious as to cause the death of the individual either at birth or later in life.

Lignin A polymer of phenolic substances impregnating the cellulose frame work of certain plant cell wall resulting poor digestibility of Cellulose. Lignin is essentially indigestible.

Limiting amino acid The essential amino acid of a protein that shows the greatest percentage deficit in comparison with the amino acids contained in the same quantity of another protein selected as a standard.

Lipid Any of a group of biologically important substances that are insoluble in water and soluble in fat solvents such as ether, chloroform, and benzene. Principal chemical components of lipids are fatty acids and glycerol.

Loose housing A housing system for cattle whereby animals are untied and unstanchioned in a shelter and are free to move at will from the inside to the outside and from a feeding area to a resting area.

Lysozyme A substance present in human nasal secretions, tears and certain mucus. It is also present in egg whites, in which it hydrolyzes polysaccharidic acids. It is bactericidal for only a few saprophytic bacteria and is inactive against pathogens and organisms of the normal flora.

Mammary veins (milk veins) Blood veins visible on the underside of the cow and extending forward from the fore udder.

Marbling Fat deposits in the lean tissue in meat.

Mastectomy Removal of the mammary gland.

Micelle A microscopic particle made from an aggregation of amphipathic molecules in solution

Milk letdown The squeezing of milk out of the udder tissue into the gland and teat cisterns.

Milk replacer A feed material for young animals which has many of the nutritive characteristics of milk, is fed in a fluid form, and contains an appreciable level of nonfat dry milk solids.

Milk vein A large blood vessel which runs under the center of the animals belly towards the udder.

Milk well Opening in the cow's abdomen through which the mammary vein passes on its way to the heart from the udder.

Mohair The wool of Angora goats; a soft white wool in great demand for clothing.

Molt (Molting) The shedding and replacing of feathers of poultry birds. Snakes and certain arthropods also shed their outer coverings and develop a new one.

Monogastric Having only one stomach or only one compartment in the stomach. Examples of monogastric animals are swine, mink and rabbits.

Monoparous A term designating animals that usually produce only one offspring at each pregnancy. Horses and cattle are monoparous.

Needle teeth The small, tusklike teeth on each side of the upper and lower jaws in swine. In good swine management, the tops of these teeth are removed shortly after birth to avoid damage to the sow's udder by the nursing pig.

Negative balance A term used in animal nutrition or physiology that describes a situation where an animal is excreting or secreting more of a specific nutrient than it is ingesting.

Nondescript An animal of inferior quality that can not be identified as belonging to a specific breed.

Nonreturns The conventional method of measuring "fertility" in artificial breeding. If, after an original insemination, a cow is not reported for reinsemination within a certain designated period, she is considered a "nonreturn" and is assumed to be pregnant.

Nymphomania An abnormal reproductive condition in cattle in which the female is in more or less constant estrus.

Offal The parts of a butchered animal that are removed in dressing it. Generally has reference to the inedible parts.

Oxidation The loss of electrons by an atom or molecule.

Parous A term referring to females having produced one or more young.

Pashmina The undercoat of Cashmere goats, a soft wool in great demand for clothing.

Pasture Grassland used for animals to graze.

Pens Small enclosed areas inside a building which are used for keeping animals separately.

Persistency The quality of being persistent, as in the ability of lactating animals to maintain milk production over a period of time.

pH A numerical value that expresses degree of acidity or alkalinity of a material as the negative logarithm (to the base 10) of the hydrogen ion concentration.

Phagocytes White blood cells that destroy bacteria in the bloodstream.

Pheromone A substance secreted externally by certain animal species to affect sexual behaviour of the species.

Pica An appetite for materials not usually considered to be food such as isobserved in phosphorus–deficient animals; a depraved appetite.

Pinning Collection of dung around the vent of very young lambs that has dried to the point of interfering with normal bowel movements.

Pork The meat that comes from swine.

Prolificacy Ability to give birth to a large number of young. This term can refer to individual animals, groups of animals, or species.

Proven sire A dairy bull whose genetic transmitting ability has been measured by comparing the milk production performance of his daughters with that of the daughter's dam and/or herd mates under similar conditions.

Proximate analysis A chemical analysis that represents the gross composition of a feed. The feed components identified by this procedure include nitrogen (crude protein), nitrogen–free extract, ether extract, ash, and dry matter.

Puberty The period of life at which the reproductive organs first became functional. This is characterized by estrus and ovulation in the female and semen production in the male.

Purebred Any animal that traces back through all its lines to the foundation stock of the breed it represents. In some breeds, animals resulting from four or five generations of crossing to purebred sires are recognized as purebreds.

Putrefaction The decomposition of proteins by microorganisms under anaerobic condition.

Regurgitate To cast up undigsted feed from the stomach to the mouth as done by ruminants.

Repeatability The tendency of an animal to repeat its performance (e.g., a dairy cow in successive lactations, a sheep in successive wool clips, etc.). In dairy bulls, this term is used to indicate certainty with which predicted difference reflects true transmitting ability.

Reproductive cycle The sexual cycle of the nonpregnant female. Characterizd by the occurrence of estrus (heat) at regular intervals (e.g., in the cow, every 21 days).

Respiratory quotient (RQ) The RQ is used to indicate the type of food being metabolized. This is possible because carbohydrates, fats and proteins differ in the relative amounts of oxygen and carbon contained in their molecules. Also the relative volumes of O_2 consumed and CO_2 produced during metabolism of each type of food vary. RQ is calculated as follows :

$$RQ = \frac{\text{Volume } CO_2 \text{ produced}}{\text{Volume } O_2 \text{ consumed}}$$

Respiration calorimeter An apparatus for measuring the gaseous exchange between an animal and the surrounding atmosphere. With this apparatus it is possible to measure the energy required for the various body functions and activities and the energy content of feeds.

Retained placenta Placental membranes not expelled at parturition.

Regor mortis The stiftness of body muscles that is observed shortly after the death of an animal. It is caused by an accumulation of metabolic products, specially lactic acid in the muscles.

Rumination ("chewing the cud") The process of regurgitating and rechewing food; unique to ruminants.

Selection Biologically, any process, natural or artificial, that permits certain individuals to leave a disproportionately large (or small) number of offspring in a group or population.

Selection index In animal breeding, a single overall numerical value derived by weighting values for several traits based on heritability and economic importance. Index values are used in determining which animals are selected for breeding and which are culled.

Serum therapy The treatment of clinical cases of disease with serum of immunized animals.

Sire Index A figure that is indicative of the transmitting ability of a sire. In dairy cattle this figure is expressed in terms of quantity of milk or a milk component such as fat or protein.

Slop-feeding A system of feeding animals (usually pigs) that involves mixing dry feed with a fluid, usually water or skim milk. Thus the animal consumes its feed in the form of a slurry.

Springer A term commonly associated with female cattle showing signs of advanced pregnancy.

Staple-length The length of the cut hair or wool of a goat or sheep.

Steer A male bovine castrated before development of secondary sex characteristics.

Sternum The breastbone

Stillborn Born lifeless; dead at birth.

Stover Fodder; mature cured stalks of grain from which seeds have been removed, such as stalks of corn without ears.

Strippings Towards the end of milking, the last bit of milk is harder to milk out; the removal of this last bit is called stripping.

Stud A unit or herd of selected animals kept for breeding purposes. Often referred to as a seedstock herd.

Succulence A condition of plants characterized by juiciness, freshness, and tenderness, making them appetizing to animals.

Supernumerary teats Extra teats (more than four) in a bovine. In good dairy herd management, supernumerary teats are removed at an early age before they become highly vascularized.

Superovulation The production by the ovaries of more than the usual number of eggs at the time of estrus. Usually induced by hormone treatment.

Symbiosis An association of two different kinds of living organisms with mutual benefit.

Syndrome A group of signs and symptoms that occur together and characterize a disease.

Tassel Cartilaginous outgrowth at the base of the throat in some goats and sheep.

Teaser A male (bull or ram) made incapable, by vasectomy or by use of an apron to prevent copulation, of impregnating a female.

Tethering A way of controlling the movement of animals by means of a rope or chain.

Total digestible nutrients (TDN) A term used in animal feeding that designates the sum of all the digestible organic nutrients. (Digestible fat is multiplied by 2.25 because of its higher energy content.) TDN is a way of expressing the energy content of a feed.

Uremia A toxic accumulation of urinary constituents in the blood.

Villi Numberous fingerlike projections extending from the intestinal wall into the lumen of the small intestine. Nutrients are absorbed from the intestine into the bloodstream through the villi.

Viscera The large internal organs of the thoracic and abdominal and pelvic cavitis of the body.

Volatile fatty acids Short chain organic acids that are volatile upon stream distillation. These compounds are formed in the rumen as a result of bacterial degradation of cellulose and other carbohydrates. Examples are acetic, propionic, and butyric acid.

Weaning Taking the nursing young away from the mother and depriving it of the opportunity to nurse. This term is also used when calves are removed from diets containing fluid milk or milk replacer.

X chromosome A sex chromosome found in mammals. All of the eggs produced by the female contain X chromosomes. When two X chromosomes are present in the fertilized egg, a female develops.

Y chromosome A sex chromosome found only in male mammals. When a fertilized egg contains an X chromosome and a Y chromosome, a male develops. About 50% of the sperm produced by the male contain Y chromosomes.

Zero–grazing A system of feeding in which animals are kept in buildings and yards and fodder is taken to them.

2

AN INTRODUCTION TO MICROBIOLOGY

Microbiology is the study of microorganism (microbes). Microorganisms are very small, usually single-celled, organisms which are not individually visible to the naked eye. They can only be seen with the aid of a microscope. They are widely distributed in the environment and are found in foods. Certain of them, if present in food in large enough numbers, can cause food poisoning. Microorganisms are the main cause of food 'going off', i.e. food spoilage. However, not all microorganisms are undesirable. In fact they are essential to all forms of life since they break down complex organic matter and return nutrients to the soil. Microorganisms are used by man in the production of certain foods, e.g. bread and yoghurt.

Although some of the effects of microorganisms have been known and utilised for thousands of years, these microscopic organisms were first seen and studied only 300 years ago. In 1675 a Dutch lens grinder, van Leewenhoek, made a microscope with lenses of sufficiently good quality that he was able to observe microorganisms in a variety of materials such as teeth scrapings and pond water. The significance of his findings was not appreciated at the time. It was nearly 200 years later that a Frenchman, Louis Pasteur, studied fermentation processes and demonstrated that it was microorganisms which caused an undesirable sour taste in some wines. He developed a process of heating wine to kill the microorganisms which caused the souring. This process is still used today to kill undesirable organisms in many food products and is known as pasteurisation. While Pasteur was working in France, Robert Koch, in Germany, demonstrated that anthrax, a fatal disease of sheep and cattle, was caused by a bacterium. From this time onwards great advances were made in the field of microbiology. The organisms responsible for a large number of diseases were identified. In Scotland, Joseph Lister introduced the idea of antiseptic surgery and greatly reduced the incidence of infection in patients during and after surgery.

Classification of Microorganisms

Microorganisms can be classified into five biological types:

1. Protozoa
2. Algae
3. Viruses
4. Microscopic fungi—moulds and yeasts
5. Bacteria

This list classifies microorganisms according to their structure. It is sometimes more convenient to classify them according to their role in relation to human beings. In this functional classification there are four groups:

1. Pathogens

These are microorganisms which cause disease. All viruses are pathogenic but only some are pathogenic to man. Certain bacteria also cause disease in man. Some of these diseases can be transmitted by food, e.g. food poisoning, cholera and typhoid.

2. Spoilage Organisms

These microorganisms do not cause disease but they spoil food by growing in the food and producing substances which alter the colour, texture and odour of the food, making it unfit for human consumption. Examples of food spoilage including the souring of milk, the growth of mould on bread and the rotting of fruits and vegetables.

3. Beneficial Organisms

Many microorganisms have a beneficial effect and can be used in the service of man. Few people realise the important part they play in everyday life.

(a) Microorganisms are essential to life since they are responsible for the rotting or decay of organic matter. The complex organic components of dead plants and animals are broken down by microbial activity into simpler, inorganic compounds which are made available for new plant growth, and the whole cycle of life is able to continue.

In the treatment of sewage, microorganisms are used to break down complex organic compounds.

(b) Microorganisms are used at various stages during the manufacture of certain foods. Their activities are essential in the production of foods such as bread, beer, wine, cheese and yoghurt.

(c) Antibiotics, such as penicillin, are substances used to destroy pathogens in the body. Many are produced as a result of microbial activity. For example, penicillin is obtained from a mould called *Penicillium*.

(d) Certain microorganisms may be used as a concentrated protein foods in the future.

4. Inert Organisms

This group includes those organisms which are neither harmful nor beneficial to man. *Commensals* are organisms which live in human but which do not cause disease in the part of the body where they are normally present. For example, *Streptococcus faecalis* is a bacterium which is harmless in its normal habitat, the large intestine. However, some commensals can be pathogenic if they spread to areas of the body where they are not normally found. *Streptococcus faecalis*, for example, causes disease if it infects the kidneys.

Although it is convenient to use a functional classification, it must be emphasised that this is not a hard and fast division. An individual organism may, in differing circumstances, fall into each of the four groups. For example, the bacterium *Escherichia coli* is generally considered to be inert. However, in some cases it may be pathogenic since it can cause food poisoning. Certain strains can cause food spoilage without causing illness. It has been used for removing glucose from egg white prior to drying, so may therefore be considered useful.

Protozoa

Protozoa are small single-celled animals. They are motile, i.e. capable of independent movement. They mostly live in water, for example in ponds, rivers and the sea and in the water in soil. A common example is *Amoeba*.

They feed by engulfing tiny food particles and reproduce by binary fission i.e. dividing into two halves.

The majority of protozoa are non-pathogenic but there are a few pathogenic species of some importance. For example, *Entamoeba histolytica* causes amoebic dysentery, a type of dysentery common in the tropics. Malaria is caused by the protozoan *Plasmodium* which is transmitted by mosquitoes. Toxoplasma gondii is an organism sometimes found in animals which may be transmitted to man during the handling of raw meat (particularly pork and mutton). It is estimated that there are one million people in the world infected with the organism but the disease (known as toxoplasmosis) is relatively harmless.

Algae

Algae are simple plants. Some are macroscopic (large), e.g. seaweeds, but many are microscopic. They contain chlorophyll or a similar pigment which enables them to photosynthesis. This means that they do not require complex organic substances as food but can utilise carbon dioxide and water. Microscopic algae usually live in water. Although each cell is capable of an independent existence they tend to grow in a mass and are often visible as green slime on the surface of ponds. Some types of algae, such as *Chlorella*, can be grown on the surface of water, harvested and used as a source of protein.

Viruses

These are the smallest of all microorganisms, varying in size from 10 to 300 nanometer (1 nm = 10^{-9} metre). Most viruses are not visible under the light microscope. Viruses are acellular, i.e. they do not have a cellular structure. They are made up of a central core of nucleic acid surrounded by a protein coat. They cannot feed, grow or multiply in isolation; they must always live as parasites in larger living cells. A virus particle attaches itself to a cell and the core of the virus penetrates and directs the life of the cell so that many more virus particles are formed. These new particles are then set free to attack other cells. The host cell is injured or even destroyed by the invading virus. Therefore viruses are always pathogenic; they cause disease in man, animals, plants and other microorganisms.

Some examples of virus diseases

Host	Virus disease
Man	Common cold, Influenza, Measles, Mumps, Chickenpox, Smallpox, Poliomyelitis
Animals	Foot-and-mouth disease, Rabies, Distemper, Myxomatosis, Psittacosis
Plants	Mosaic diseases

Most virus diseases in man are transmitted by contact but some are known to be transmitted by contaminated food or water, e.g. infectious hepatitis and poliomyelitis. Some diseases may be transmitted to man from animals, for example rabies from dogs and psittacosis from parrots.

Most virus diseases of man confer immunity, i.e. an attack of the disease confers resistance to a subsequent attack. This is due to the production of antibodies, substances formed in the body in response to infection. Artificial immunity may be conferred by means of vaccination. A vaccine consists of a weakened or dead form of a pathogen and when it is injected into the body it is practically harmless yet it induces antibody production.

Many virus diseases of animals and plants are of economic importance. Millions of rupees are lost annually due to destruction of crops and livestock by virus diseases.

Microscopic fungi

Fungi are plants but, unlike green plants, they do not possess any chlorophyll. They are therefore unable to photosynthesise and require complex organic compounds as food. Those that grow and feed on dead organic material are termed *saprophytes,* while those feeding on living plants and animals are *parasites.*

1. Moulds

Moulds are usually multicellular, i.e. each mould growth consists of more than one cell. However, each cell is capable of independent growth and therefore moulds may be classified as microorganisms. Moulds consist of thin thread-like strands called hyphae (sing. hypha). The hyphae grow in a mass on or through the medium on which the mould is growing. This mass of hyphae is known as the mycelium. There are basically two types of mould:

(a) *Non-septate moulds.* These do not possess cross walls (septae). The hyphae are continuous tubes containing many nuclei dispersed throughout the cytoplasm and are therefore considered to be multicellular.

(b) *Septate moulds.* These possess septae or cross walls which divide the hyphae into separate cells, each cell containing a nucleus.

Reproduction

Reproduction in moulds is chiefly by means of asexual spores. In non-septate moulds the spores are normally formed within a spore case or sporangium, at the tip of a fertile hypha. Most septate moulds reproduce by forming unprotected spores known as conidia. Conidia are cut off, either singly or in chains, from the tip of a fertile hypha.

When ripe the spores are released into the air. If they find their way to a suitable substrate (food) they germinate and produce a new growth of mould. Some moulds also produce sexual spores, by the fusion of two hyphae.

Many moulds cause food spoilage. Spoilage may occur even in refrigerated foods. However, certain moulds are used in food production particularly in cheese making; Danish blue, Roquefort and Camembert are mould-ripened. Moulds are also used in the manufacture of soya sauce and some products used in the food industry, e.g. citric acid.

A few moulds are pathogenic causing diseases in plants such as potato blight, and skin infections in man such as 'athlete's foot' and ringworm. Ergot, a fungus that attacks rye, can produce a serious illness (known as ergotism) in animal and human who eat products made from the infected grain.

One of the most spectacular developments in medicine in this century was the discovery of penicillin and other antibiotics produced by moulds.

2. Yeasts

Yeasts are simple single-celled fungi, they are mainly saprophytic and usually grow on plant foods. Yeast cells may be oval, rod-shaped or spherical. They are larger than bacteria and under a high-power microscope a distinct nucleus is visible.

Reproduction

Most yeasts reproduce asexually by a simple process known as 'budding'. In one part of the cell the cytoplasm bulges out of the cell wall. The bulge or 'bud' grows in size and finally separates as a new yeast cell. This process is shown below.

Yeasts may cause spoilage in certain foods, e.g. fruit juices, jams and meat. These yeasts are normally referred to as 'wild yeasts' in order to distinguish them from those used commercially in the production of alcoholic drinks and bread.

The economic importance of yeast lies in its ability to break down carbohydrate foods into alcohol and carbon dioxide. This process, known as *alcoholic fermentation*, is anaerobic, i.e. takes place in the absence of oxygen. Yeast contains a collection of enzymes known as zymase which is responsible for the fermentation of sugars, such as glucose, into ethanol (ethyl alcohol) and carbon dioxide. Alcoholic fermentation may be represented by the following equation:

Under anaerobic Condition

$$\underset{\text{glucose}}{C_6H_{12}O_6} \longrightarrow \underset{\substack{\text{ethanol}\\\text{(ethyl alcohol)}}}{2C_2H_5OH} + \underset{\substack{\text{carbon}\\\text{dioxide}}}{2CO_2}$$

If a plentiful supply of oxygen is available, yeast cells will respire aerobically. In this case yeast enzymes are able to break down sugars more completely, and carbon dioxide and water are produced.

Under aerobic Condition

$$\underset{\text{glucose}}{C_6H_{12}O_6} + \underset{\text{oxygen}}{6O_2} \longrightarrow \underset{\substack{\text{carbon}\\\text{dioxide}}}{6CO_2} + \underset{\text{water}}{6H_2O}$$

More energy is obtained from aerobic than from anaerobic respiration. It is important when yeast is being grown commercially that it is supplied with plenty of air so that sufficient energy is available for growth.

The two most important industrial uses of yeast are in breadmaking and for the production of alcohol. The species generally used in these processes is *Saccharomyces cerevisiae*.

Production of alcoholic beverages

All alcoholic beverages, such as beers, wines and spirits, are produced by the anaerobic fermentation of a carbohydrate material by yeast. A large range of starting materials can be used; the carbohydrate may be in the form of starch, e.g. in wheat, barley, rice or potatoes, or in the form of sugars, e.g. in fruits, molasses or added sugar (sucrose). In addition the following substances may be added.

1. *Diastase.* Yeast cells are not able to produce enzymes capable of breaking down starch. Therefore, if starch is used, a substance containing amylase (diastase) must be added. Amylase is an enzyme which catalyses the breakdown of starch into maltose. Malt (germinating barely) has a high amylase content and is used in the brewing of beer.

2. *Available nitrogen.* This is necessary for the synthesis of protein during the growth and multiplication of the yeast cell. This nitrogen may be provided by protein present in the carbohydrate-containing food used, e.g. by the wheat, or it may be added in the form of ammonium salts, or nitrates.

3. *Water.* Water is necessary for the growth of the yeast and also to increase the volume of the mixture.

The mixture is enclosed in a container and oxygen is excluded; this ensures that respiration is anaerobic rather than aerobic. It is then held at a warm temperature in order to encourage the yeast cells to grow and multiply. Fermentation is allowed to continue until the desired concentration of alcohol is obtained. The maximum concentration which can be achieved by fermentation is 16%, since if it increases further the yeast cannot grow. The alcohol content of fortified wines, spirits and liqueurs is increased by distillation.

Breadmaking

The main ingredients used in breadmaking are flour, water, yeast and salt. These are made into a dough and fat, milk and sugar may also be added. The flour provides starch, amylase and protein and is an excellent food for the yeast. The bread dough is allowed to ferment prior to baking and the carbon dioxide produced causes the dough to rise. During baking the carbon dioxide expands causing the loaf to rise further.

Bacteria

Bacteria (sing. bacterium) are a very important group of microorganisms because of both their harmful and their beneficial effects. They are widely distributed in the environment. They are found in air, water and soil, in the intestines of animals, on the moist linings of the mouth, nose and throat, on the surface of all animal and plant body.

Bacteria are the smallest single-celled organisms, some being only 0.4 μm (micrometre) in diameter. The cell contains a mass of cytoplasm and some nuclear material (it does not have a distinct nucleus). The cell is enclosed by a cell wall and in some bacteria this is surrounded by a capsule or slime layer. The capsule consists of a mixture of polysaccharides and polypeptides.

Bacteria are classified into four basic groups depending on the shape of the cells.

1. Coccus (pl. cocci)—spherical.
2. Bacillus (pl. bacilli)—rod-shaped.
3. Vibrio— short, curved rods.
4. Spirillum (pl. spirilli)—long, coiled threads.

When bacteria are grown on a culture medium in the laboratory the cells may be grouped together. Cocci, for example, may be joined in chains (Streptococci) or arranged in clusters (Staphylococci).

Motility

Some bacteria are motile, i.e. capable of movement. These bacteria posses long thread-like structures called flagella (sing. flagellum) which originate from inside the cell membrane. The flagella move in a whip-like manner and help to propel the bacteria through liquid, such as water. Bacteria can be classified further according to the number of flagella they possess and the position of the flagella on the bacterial cell.

Reproduction

Bacteria reproduced by a process known as binary fission. The nuclear material reproduces itself and divides into separate parts and then the rest of the cell divides, producing two daughter cells which are equal in size. This process is shown hereunder.

Spore Formation

Spores are hard resistant bodies which are formed by some types of bacteria when conditions become adverse, i.e. when they are unable to survive in their environment and to obtain the materials necessary for growth. The spore is formed within the bacterial cell and then the rest of the cell disintegrates. Spores can survive adverse conditions for very long periods of time. When conditions become favourable the spore germinates producing a new bacterial cell. Spore formation occurs in only certain type of bacteria. The two groups of bacteria which form spores (*Bacillus* and *Clostridium*) are both rod-shaped.

Bacterial spores are resistant to heat and can survive in food when food is cooked. They are also resistant to cold (e.g. refrigeration) and to many chemical products designed to kill bacteria, such as disinfectants.

The normal cells of bacteria are described as *vegetative cells* to distinguish them from spores.

Toxins

Bacteria produce a variety of substances as a result of their metabolism. Some of these substances are harmful to man and animals and are known as toxins (i.e. poisons). There are two types of toxins:

1. Endotoxins

Endotoxins are produced within the bacterial cell and are not released into the body until the cell dies. Therefore, they tend to have a localised effect and usually cause harm in the region of the body where the bacteria are living. The symptoms of diseases caused by bacteria producing endotoxins usually do not appear untill some time after the living bacteria enter the body, since it is some time before the bacterial cells disintegrate. It should be noted that living bacteria must enter the body in order to cause this type of illness.

2. Exotoxins

Exotoxins are produced by bacteria and secreted into the surroundings. The toxin may act in the area around the bacteria but often it is carried by the bloodstream to produce its harmful effect in another part of the body. It is not necessary to ingest living bacteria; the illness is caused by the toxin alone. Some types of food poisoning illnesses are caused by eating a food containing an exotoxin, which has survived even though the bacteria which produced it have died. The symptoms of the illness may appear very soon after the exotoxin enters the body, although this is not always the case. Exotoxins tend to be more sensitive to destruction by heat.

Both types of toxins may be enterotoxins, i.e. substances which have a harmful effect on the digestive system. There is some confusion about the use of all three words to describe toxins and some texts give alternative definitions. This confusion may be due to the fact that some bacteria produce both types of toxins. Also in some cases it is not known exactly which type of toxin the bacteria produces.

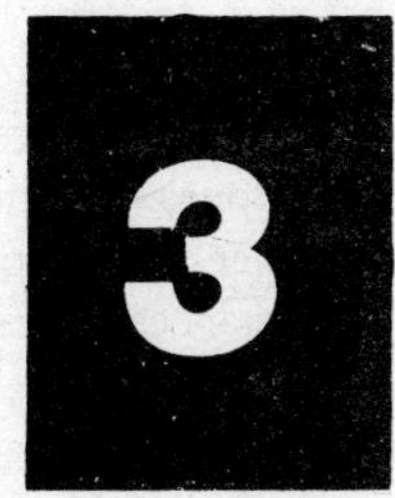

ELEMENTARY ANATOMY AND PHYSIOLOGY

Anatomy

Anatomy is the study of the structure of the body. A knowledge of how the animal's body functions, helps with the understanding of animal husbandry and the reasoning of many management decisions concerned with feeding, growth and health of animals.

Table 3.1

Nomenclature for Systematic Anatomy

System	*Name of Study*	*Chief Structures*
Skeletal system	Osteology	Bones
Articular system	Arthrology	Joints
Muscular system	Myology	Muscles
Digestive system	Splanchnology	Stomach and intestines
Respiratory system	"	Lungs and air passages
Urinary system	"	Kidneys and bladder
Reproductive system	"	Ovaries and testes
Endocrine system	Endocrinology	Ductless glands
Nervous system	Neurology	Brain, spinal cord, nerves
Circulatory system	Angiology	Heart, vessels
Integumentary system	Dermatology	Skin
Sensory system	Esthesiology	Eye, ear

THE SKELETON SYSTEM

The animal's skeleton is living tissue. It has nerves and blood vessels, it can be damaged by disease, can break and repair and can adjust to changes in stress. The skeleton consists mainly of bone. Areas of cartilage are also present.

Functions of the Skeleton

1. To give shape to the body.
2. To provide anchor points for muscles and therefore movement.
3. As a reserve for minerals, mainly calcium, phosphorus and magnesium.

4. For the production of red blood cells in the marrow of some long bones.
5. For the protection of vital organs, for example the rib cage protects the heart and lungs.

Bones of young animals are composed of about 60 per cent fibrous tissue while in old animals 60 per cent is composed of lime salts and thus it is more brittle than the former. Among inorganic substances, calcium, phosphorus and magnesium are the major elements which are never permanently retained by the bones. On the outside, bone is hard and compact but inside there is often a cavity, the medullary cavity, containing marrow (especially in long bones like those that form the limbs). Near the ends there is a type of bone known as 'spongy bone' although it is actually quite hard. Marrow is a soft tissue richly supplied with blood and is involved in the formation of blood cells. The outside of the bone is covered by a thin membrane, the *periosteum*, which is supplied with blood vessels and nerves.

The vertebrate skeleton has an axial and an appendicular (limb) part. The axial skeleton consists of the vertebrate, the ribs and sternum, and the skull; on the other hand the appendicular skeleton, includes the bones of both forelimb and hindlimb.

Axial Skeleton

The vertebra are arranged into a vertebral column or backbone extending from the base of the skull all the way caudally into the tail. There are fine distinct sections of the vertebrate column. The vertebra from each are specialized to perform their different functions.

Cervical Region

The cervical vertebrae are specialised to allow movement of the head in all directions.

Thoracic Region

The thoracic vertebrae are specialised for the attachment of the ribs. In mammals, each rib articulates with two thoracic vertebrae. The thorax provides bony protection for the thoracic and abdominal organs inside and attachment for the very important muscles of breathing and the extrinsic muscles of the forelimb. In Zebu (*Bos indius*) Indian Cattle, the spines of the last six thoracic and first three lumber vertebrae are divided dorsally. This bifidity is not seen in European cattle (*Bos taurus*).

Lumber Region

The lumber vertebrae can be distinguished by their well developed transverse processes. These are in some respects analogous to the ribs in that they serve as attachment for muscles of breathing. However, they also provide attachment for epaxial muscle as well.

Sacral Region

The sacral vertebrae are fused into a composite bone called the *sacrum*. On each side the sacrum bears a large flattened process for articulation to the ilium of the pelvic girdle.

Coccygeal Region

The caudal vertebrae are progressively reduced. These serve as sites for insertion of the muscles used in moving the tail.

Axial Skeleton of Fowl

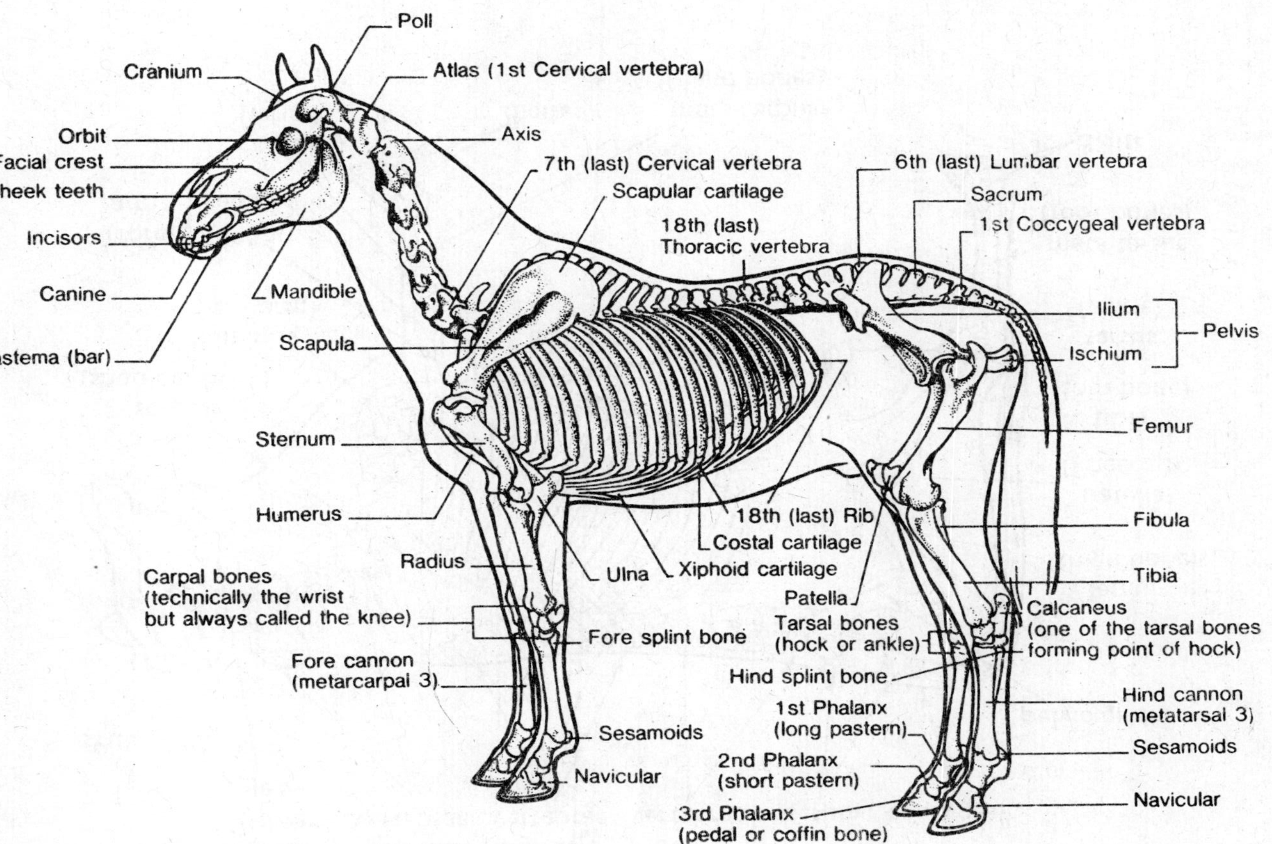
Poll
Cranium
Atlas (1st Cervical vertebra)
Orbit
Axis
Facial crest
Cheek teeth
Incisors
Canine
Diastema (bar)
Mandible
7th (last) Cervical vertebra
Scapular cartilage
18th (last)
Thoracic vertebra
6th (last) Lumbar vertebra
Sacrum
1st Coccygeal vertebra
Ilium
Ischium
Pelvis
Scapula
Sternum
Humerus
Radius
Ulna
Carpal bones
(technically the wrist
but always called the knee)
Fore splint bone
Fore cannon
(metarcarpal 3)
Sesamoids
Navicular
18th (last) Rib
Costal cartilage
Xiphoid cartilage
Patella
Tarsal bones
(hock or ankle)
Hind splint bone
1st Phalanx
(long pastern)
2nd Phalanx
(short pastern)
3rd Phalanx
(pedal or coffin bone)
Femur
Fibula
Tibia
Calcaneus
(one of the tarsal bones
forming point of hock)
Hind cannon
(metatarsal 3)
Sesamoids
Navicular

Fig. 3.1 Anatomy of the Horse.

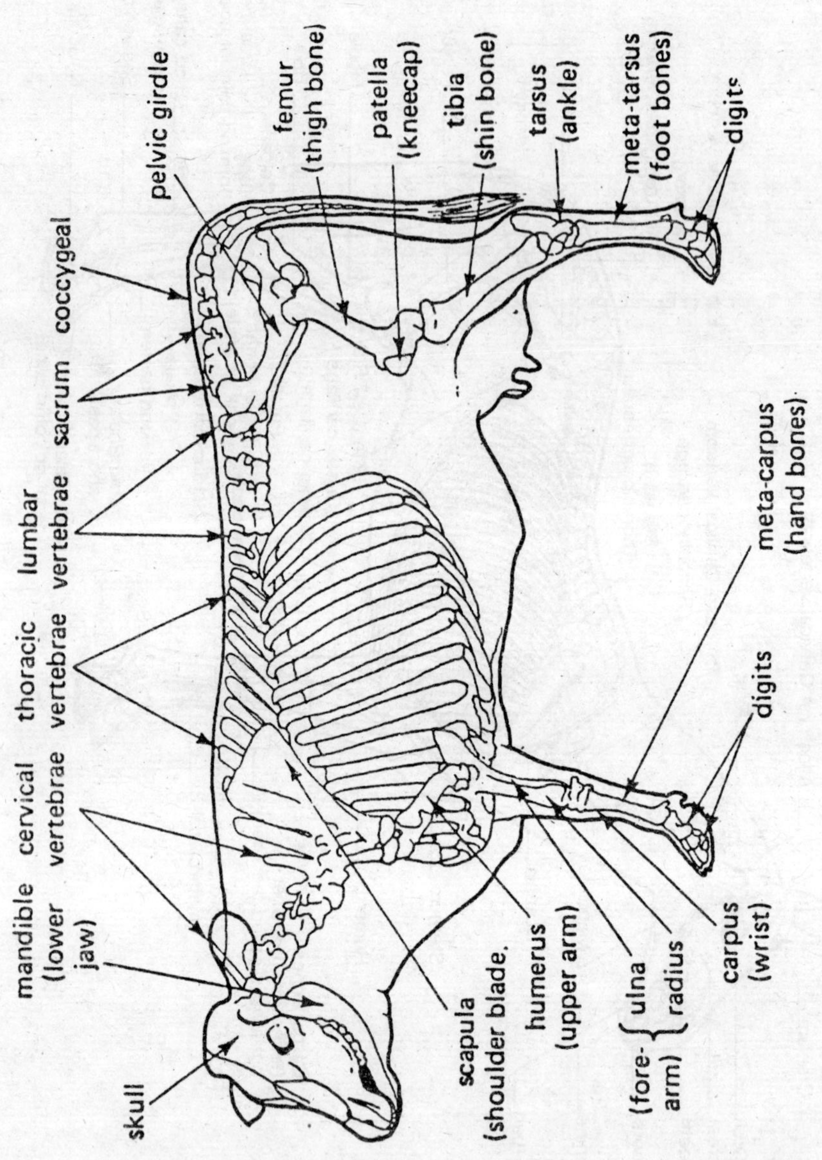

Fig. 3.2 Anatomy of the Cow.

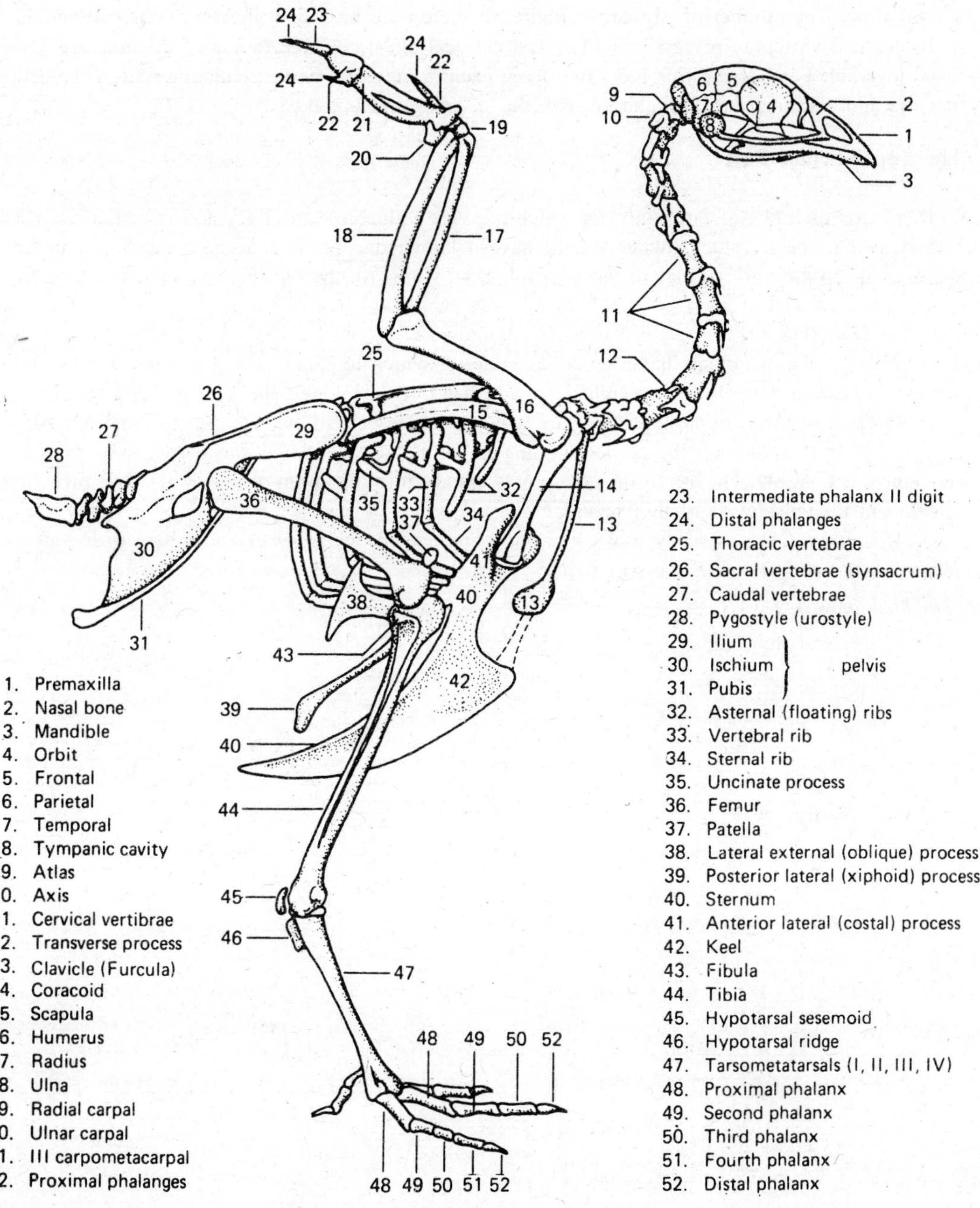
24 23
24
22
24
22 21
19
20
18
17
9
10
6 5
7 4
8
2
1
3
11
12
25
26
27
28
29
15
16
14
32
36
35
33
37
34
13
30
41
38
40
31
43
42
39
40
44
45
46
47
48 49 50 52
48 49 50 51 52
1. Premaxilla
2. Nasal bone
3. Mandible
4. Orbit
5. Frontal
6. Parietal
7. Temporal
8. Tympanic cavity
9. Atlas
10. Axis
11. Cervical vertibrae
12. Transverse process
13. Clavicle (Furcula)
14. Coracoid
15. Scapula
16. Humerus
17. Radius
18. Ulna
19. Radial carpal
20. Ulnar carpal
21. III carpometacarpal
22. Proximal phalanges
23. Intermediate phalanx II digit
24. Distal phalanges
25. Thoracic vertebrae
26. Sacral vertebrae (synsacrum)
27. Caudal vertebrae
28. Pygostyle (urostyle)
29. Ilium
30. Ischium
31. Pubis
pelvis
32. Asternal (floating) ribs
33. Vertebral rib
34. Sternal rib
35. Uncinate process
36. Femur
37. Patella
38. Lateral external (oblique) process
39. Posterior lateral (xiphoid) process
40. Sternum
41. Anterior lateral (costal) process
42. Keel
43. Fibula
44. Tibia
45. Hypotarsal sesemoid
46. Hypotarsal ridge
47. Tarsometatarsals (I, II, III, IV)
48. Proximal phalanx
49. Second phalanx
50. Third phalanx
51. Fourth phalanx
52. Distal phalanx

Fig.3.3 Anatomy of the Chicken

In the fowl the axial skeleton shows some differences from that of the mammal. In the coccygeal region there is only one bone, the *pygostyle.* The avian lumber and sacral vertebrae are fused into a *synsacrum.* The number of ribs are variable, so there may be 5 or 6 thoracic vertebrae and 17 to 16 cervical vertebrae respectively. The last cervical and first three thoracic vertebrae are also fused together. Four of the ribs have two parts each: a vertebral part articulating with a thoracic vertebra and a sternal part articulating with the *sternum* or *breastbone.*

The Appendicular Part

It consists of limbs of farm animals which are very vulnerable to injury and infection, so it is important that the livestock owner should have a knowledge of its anatomy. The bones in the limbs of sheep are very similar to those of the cow, whilst, in the pig there is a slight variation.

The Fore Limb (Fig. 3.4)

1. *Scapula.* Farm animals have no collar bone on which to 'hang' the fore limb. Instead the scapula is held in place by being embedded in a band of very tough shoulder muscle.

2. *Radius and Ulna.* In humans these are two separate bones (in the forearm) to enable twisting at the wrist. In farm animals the radius and ulna are bound together by fibrous tissue, so on twisting movement is possible. The top of the ulna points upto to form the point of the elbow. This provides attachment for muscles and better leverage.

3. *Metacarpus.* In cows this looks like one bone, except at its lower end where it divides to form the start of the cow's two-part foot.

The hind limbs (Fig. 3.4)

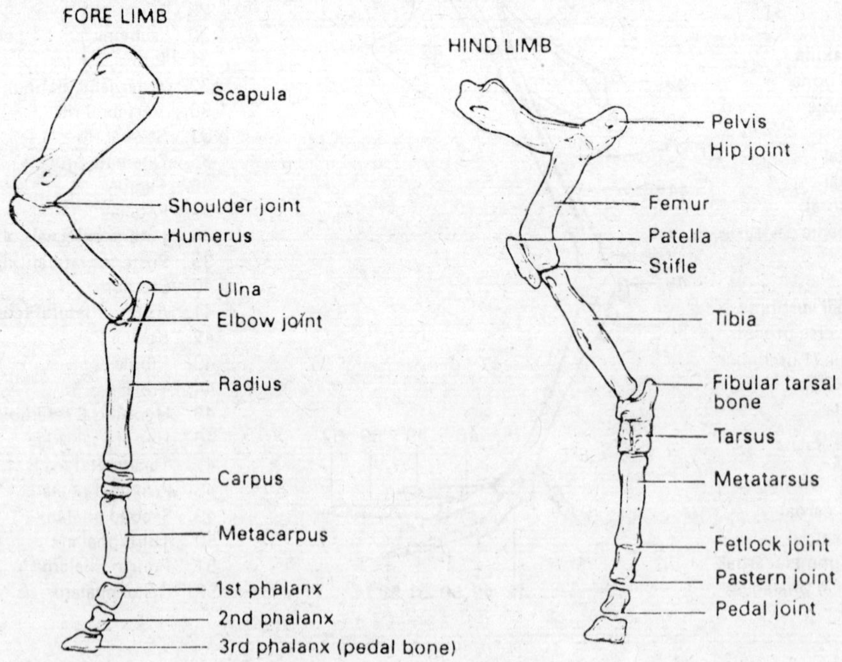

Fig. 3.4 The fore limb and the hind limb of a cow.

1. *Pelvis.* Three bones fused together to form the pelvic girdle. It is through this ring of bone that the young animal must pass at birth. In the case of the sow there are usually no problems as the piglets are so small, but problems can arise for the ewe and the cow. A common misconception is that the pelvic 'bones slacken for calving'. This is not so, it is the slacking of ligaments in the pelvic that gives the feeling of slackness.

2. *Femur.* One of the biggest bones in the body, heavily muscled, running downward and forward.

3. *Patella.* The equivalent of the kneecap in man.

4. *Fibular tarsal bone.* This projects upwards and backwards to form a lever for attachment of the *Achilles tendon.*

5. *Metatarsus.* As the metacarpus of the fore limb.

Foot/Hoof

Below the metacarpus (fore limb) and metatarsus (hind limb), all four feet have the same structure.

In cow's and buffalo's two-part foot (Fig. 3.5) each part is known as a digit and each digit is composed of three bones known as *phalanges* (singular : phalanx). The third phalanx, which has the same shape as the outer hoof, is commonly referred to as the *pedal bone.*

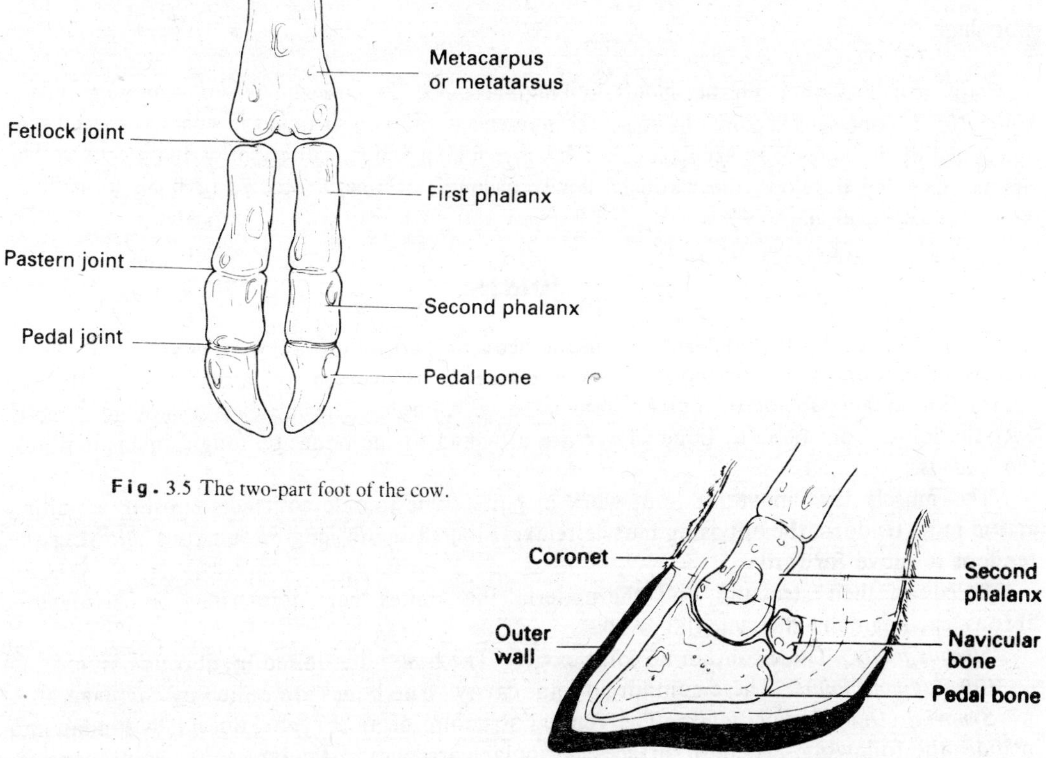

Fig. 3.5 The two-part foot of the cow.

Fig. 3.6 Cross-section through a cow's foot.

In Fig(3.6) it can be seen that the outer hoof (horn) comes up to almost the centre of the second phalanx, so little movement is allowed in the pedal joint. The area where the outer wall joins the skin of the leg is known as the *coronet.* The *navicular* bone is a small bone situated at the rear of the pedal bone.

The pedal bone is covered with a substance known as laminae or 'quick'. The laminae is very sensitive and is richly supplied with blood vessels. It has specialised cells which produce the hard outer wall of the hoof.

Growth and Repair of Bone

In the young animal there is a layer of cartilage within the bone that acts as a growing point. The bone will lengthen and thicken. This process is brought about by two specialised cells:

Osteoclasts — Which break down the cartilage.

Osteoblasts — Which deposit minerals onto bone to build a rigid material.

These two cells are also involved in the repair of bone; oesteoclasts dissolve any splinters of bone and osteoblasts build up new bone. The speed of any repair depends to a large extent on the blood supply to the bone. As the bone of young animals has a better blood supply than the bone of older animals, breaks in young bone will normally heal more quickly. The broken ends must be touching and immobilized for fibrous tissues to form in the break and so start the process of repair.

Cartilage

Cartilage is a flexible, elastic, glossy-looking substance composed mainly of a protein called *Chondrin.* It is present in joints to help with movement and is also found in noses, ears and the lower end of rib bones. The skeleton of a fetus is made up almost entirely of cartilage, but as the animal ages and develops, the cartilage slowly changes to bone, a process of bone formation, known as *ossification.*

JOINTS

These are the site of junctions or unions between two or more bones, especially one that admits of motion of one or more of the components. Movement in joints is caused by the contraction and expansion of muscles associated with joints. The muscles do not go directly over the joints from bone to bone. They are attached to the bones by tough, inelastic fibres, the *tendons.*

The muscle that move the joint work in pairs. One muscle contracts causing a pulling action in its tendons, the opposing muscle relaxes, increasing in length, and thus allowing the tendons to move forward.

Based on their structure and the material that unites them, joints may be classified as fibrous, cartilaginous and synovial joints.

Fibrous joints. These contain no joint cavity. The bones are united by fibrous tissue.

Cartilaginous joints. These contain no joint cavity. The bones are united by cartilage.

Synovial (Diarthrodial) joints. The general structure of most synovial joints is similar and includes the following: articular surfaces, articular cartilages, articular cavity, joint capsule, and ligaments.

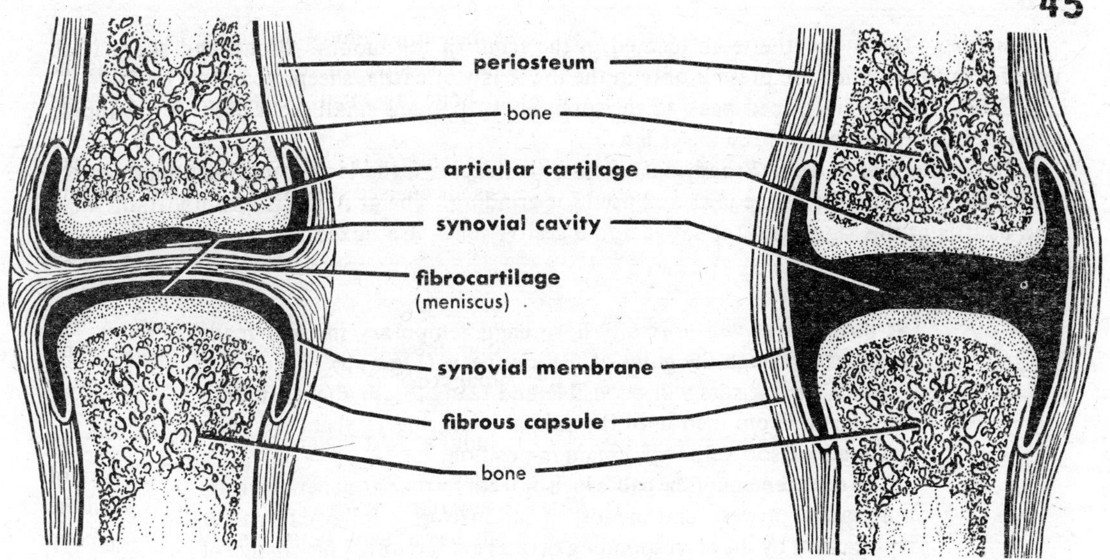

Fig. 3.7 Types of Synivial articulations.

DENTITION

Teeth can be considered as part of the skeleton, but they are really a modified form of skin. They contain the hardest substance in the animal's body, the enamel. There are three types of teeth in mammals:

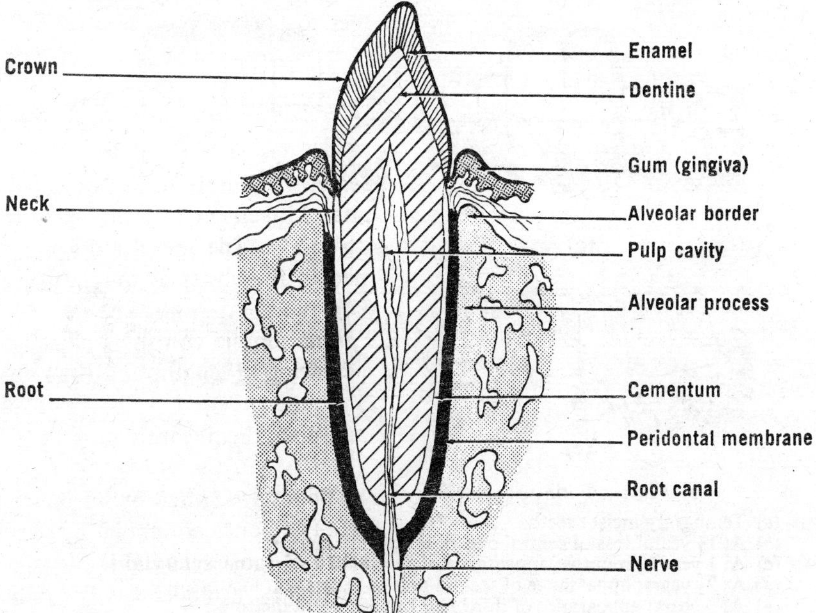

Fig. 3.8 Structure of a tooth.

Incisors. These are the teeth located in the front of the mouth. Broad and sharp teeth used for cutting. They are present only in the lower jaw of cattle, sheep, goat and buffalo.

Canine. These are placed back to incisors. Sharp pointed small teeth used for gripping and ripping; present only in the lower jaw.

Pre-molars and molars. Broad, flat teeth with ridges are the largest and strongest of all teeth, found in the sides of the jaws and used for grinding. The grinding is an important function as it is at this stage that the saliva and digestive juices are mixed into the mass of chewed food.

Cattle

At birth calves will normally have eight temporary incisors ready to appear through the gums of the lower jaw (Fig. 3.9 *a*).

All of the incisors will be visible and ready to use about 1 month after birth. From then until the animal is nearing 1½ years old these calfhood incisor teeth will remain in position.

The replacement of the calf's incisor teeth by the permanent incisors is a gradual process, and the loss of calf incisors is followed by their replacement by the corresponding permanent incisors. This change of calf to adult teeth follows a definite and fairly regular pattern (Fig. 3.9 *b–f*)

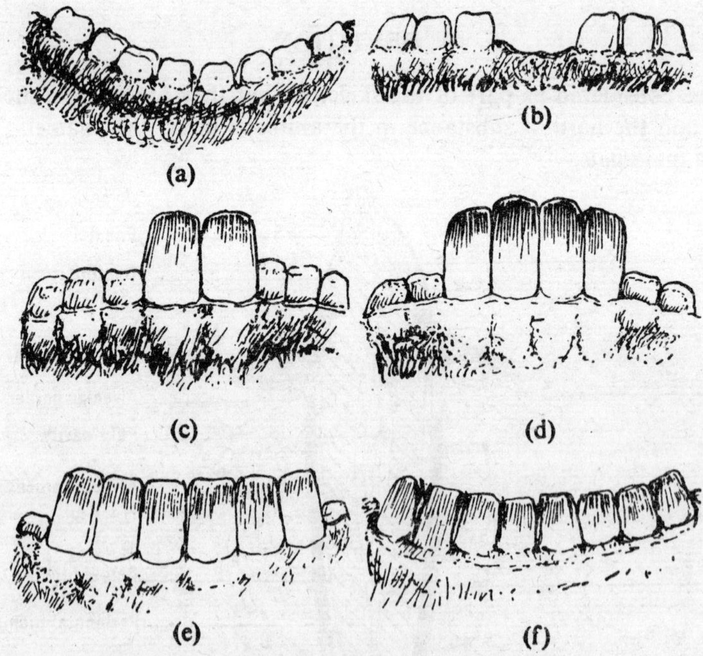

Fig. 3.9 Development of teeth in Cattle

(*a*) Temporary incisor teeth.
(*b*) At 1½ years: loss of central pair of temporary incisors.
(*c*) At 1 year 10 months: appearance of central pair of permanent incisors.
(*d*) At 2½ years: appearance of second pair of permanent incisors.
(*e*) At 3 years: appearance of third pair of permanent incisors.
(*f*) At 3½ years: appearance of fourth pair of permanent incisors—'full mouth'.

Sheep

A similar, but much speeded-up, pattern of change of teeth takes place with sheep (Fig. 20).

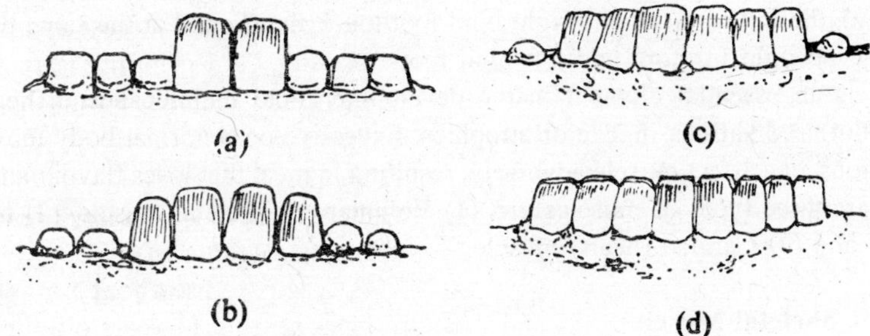

Fig. 3.10 Development of teeth in Sheep.
(*a*) At 1 year: appearance of first pair of permanent incisors.
(*b*) At 1 year 10 months: appearance of second pair of permanent incisors.
(*c*) At 2 years 3 months: appearance of third pair of permanent incisors.
(*d*) At 3 years: appearance of fourth pair of permanent incisors—'full mouth'.

Number and type of permanent teeth

	Incisors	Canine	Pre-molar	Molar	Total
Cattle upper jaw	0	0	6	6	32
Cattle lower jaw	8	0	6	6	
Sheep upper jaw	0	0	6	6	32
Sheep lower jaw	8	0	6	6	
Pigs upp:r jaw	6	2	8	6	44
Pigs lower jaw	6	2	8	6	

Animals are born with a temporary set of 'milk teeth'. These are later replaced by 'permanent teeth'. In cattle, buffaloes, seep and goat the incisors of the upper jaw are replaced by a hard dental pad.

THE MUSCLE SYSTEM

The selling of muscle (meat) is a major part of animal husbandry man. Indeed, the goat, sheep, pig and beef industries depend on it. Approximately 48% of the body is muscle mass.

Muscles are composed of bundles of muscle cells (muscle fibres), which are contractile. The main function of the muscular system is *locomotion* defined as progressive movement. Types of locomotion or gaits used by four-legged land vertebrates include the following:

1. In walking only one foot in four leaves the ground at a time.
2. In running only one foot touches the ground at a time.
3. In pacing, the natural gait of camels, the fore and hind feet on the same side.
4. In trotting (a pace between walking and running as found in horse with legs moving together diagonally), the left forefoot and right hind foot touch the ground at the same time, followed in turn by the right forefoot and left hind foot.

Locomotion is an essential element in the development and maintenance of healthy muscle. Muscle that is not used shrinks in size or atrophies. Excessive or abnormal body movement under stressful conditions, can affect muscle adversely, resulting in meat that loses flavour and deteriorates rapidly. There are three types of muscles viz. (1) Voluntary or skeletal muscle, (2) Involuntary or smooth muscle and (3) Cardiac (heart) muscle.

1. Voluntary or Skeletal Muscle

This forms the bulk of body muscle, and therefore, of 'meat'. The typical voluntary muscle has a tendon at each end, usually, fixed to a bone, with the muscle block in between. The muscle is composed of fibres grouped together in bundles (Fig. 3.11)

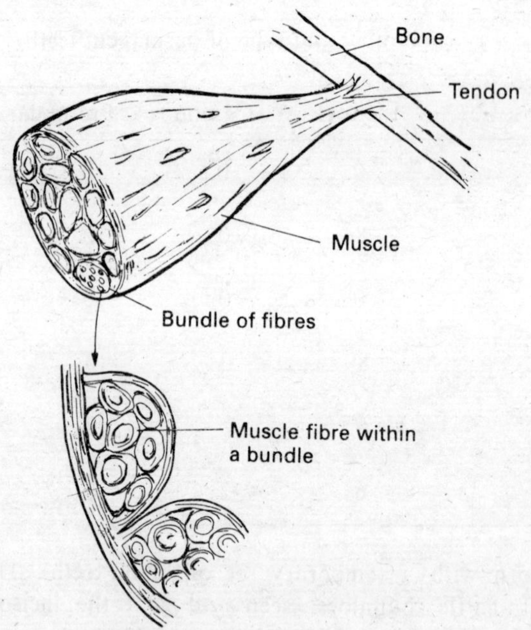

Fig. 3.11 Structure of voluntary muscle.

Each fibre is supplied with a nerve and a blood vessel. When the nerve is stimulated, the fibre contracts. The stronger the nerve impulse, more powerful the contraction. This can result in a reduction in the oxygen content of myoglobin (There are 2 major heme containing proteins, *myoglobin* and *haemoglobin* responsible for holding and transporting oxygen in the body). In the absence of oxidative metabolism, acidity of the muscle increases. Reduced oxygen content darkens meat as myoglobin, like hemoglobin, is darker when deoxygenated.

In the presence of high acidity, meat deteriorates rapidly even when adequately refrigerated.

Careful attention to humane (having the kind feelings proper to man) slaughter can thus save money for the butcher and is obviously a practice to be encouraged everywhere.

Voluntary muscle is under the direct control of the animal's will.

2. Involuntary or Smooth Muscle

This type of muscle, which has a different structure from voluntary muscle, is found around internal organs, e.g. the gut and blood vessels.

This means that food can be moved along the gut by wave-like contractions of the muscle (peristalsis) and that blood vessels can expand and contract when necessary. These muscles work independently of the animal's will and are controlled by the central nervous system.

3. Cardiac (heart) Muscle

This is an involuntary muscle with a different structure to both voluntary and smooth muscle. It has a short but very strong contraction followed by a period of rest, thus the beating action of the heart. One side of the heart contracts whilst the other rests. It acts independently of the body, but hormones can alter the speed of the beat such as adrenalin.

PHYSIOLOGY

Physiology deals with the science that states the function of various parts and organs of living organism i.e., it is concerned with how the body works.

THE DIGESTIVE ORGANS

This consists of the organs directly concerned in the reception, digestion and absorption of the food, its passage through the body and the expulsion of the unabsorbed portion. The system can be divided as (*A*) *Alimentary canal*—It runs from the lips to the anus. It has mouth, pharynx, oesophagus, stomach, small intestine, large intestine and rectum. (*B*) *Accessory digestive organs*—It includes teeth, tongue, salivary, liver glands and pancreas.

Digestive Organs of Ruminants

A. ALIMENTARY CANAL

The alimentary canal of the ruminants is much more complex than that of the non-ruminants. It has four compartments in the stomach namely, (*i*) the *Rumen*, or paunch; (*ii*) the *Reticulum*, or honey comb; (*iii*) the *Omasum*, or many plies; and (*iv*) the *Abomasum*, or the true stomach. The intestine represents a long tubule approximately 180 feet long in average dairy cattle. The first three compartments of the compound stomach are considered to be the enlargements of the oesophagus or gullet. This peculiar feature of the stomach in ruminants seems to have developed under the stimulus of coarse feeds and feeding on them in a hurry without proper mastication.

The Mouth

It is the organ of prehension, mastication, insalivation and rumination The prehension (food gathering) is assisted by the rough tongue and teeth of a ruminant. It is followed by a preliminary chewing called mastication and mixing of the saliva. Enormous amount of saliva (100-200 lit. per day in a cow) is secreted by the three pairs of salivary glands located in the mouth region. It is rich in sodium bicarbonate and its amount increases with dry and acidic feeds like hay and silage. It lubricates the bolus and facilitates its passage through the pharynx and the oesophagus to the rumen. There is no ptyalin (a digestive enzyme present in some other species) in the saliva of the ruminants, therefore, no digestion takes place in the mouth of the ruminants.

After prehension is complete, the cow starts chewing her cud called rumination. The rough materials which escaped through grinding during preliminary mastication, and are stored and exposed to bacterial action in the rumen, are forced back into the mouth (regurgitation) for further mastication. This is also known as rumination. The regurgitated bolus weighing from 90–120 gm requires 3 seconds to ascend, about 50 seconds for rechewing and 105 seconds to descend. Rumination is therefore, a long process and occupies about 8 hours. If the animal is alarmed or disturbed or goes sick it ceases to ruminate.

After the bolus is thoroughly masticated and mixed with saliva it is swallowed again with the help of the throat muscle. This time it remains almost semisolid and goes into the ventral sac of the rumen wherefrom it finally passes to abomasum tnrough reticulum and omasum. Water and other liquid drinks reach the omasum and/or abomasum directly. This is made possible by the oesophageal groove.

The Oesophagus

The oesophagus, a direct continuation of the pharynx, is a muscular tube extending from the pharynx to the upper most part of the stomach known as *cardia* just caudal to the diaphragm. From the pharynx the oesophagus passes dorsal to the trachea and usually Inclines somewhat to the left in the neck.

The muscular wall of the oesophagus consists of two layers that cross obliquely, then spiral and finally form an inner circular and outer longitudinal layer. The cardia is ordinarily tightly closed by contraction of a ring of muscle tissue, the *Cardiac sphincter*, but this muscle relaxes and the cardia relaxes and then cardia opens wide when boli are passing into or out of the rumen and when gas escapes.

The Rumen

It is the largest compartment of the stomach and has a very great significance in ruminant digestion and has several functions to perform. Even fifty years ago, the rumen action was a deep dark mystery. Today, thanks to scientific research, much more is known about the rumen processes than were known, 60 years ago.

This large voluminous sac which extends from the diaphragm to the pelvis almost entirely fills the left side of the abdominal cavity. The rumen is subdivided into sacs by thick muscular boundaries known as pillars, which appear from the exterior of the rumen as grooves. The dorsal and ventral sacs are separated by a nearly complete circle. The dorsal sac is the largest compartment. The dorsal sac overlaps the ventral sac and is continuous cranially with the reticulum over the *ruminoreticular* fold, which separates the floor of the rumen from the floor of the reticulum.

Caudally the dorsal sac is further subdivided by the dorsal coronary pillars, which form as incomplete circle bounding the dorsal blind sac. The caudal part of the ventral sac is a

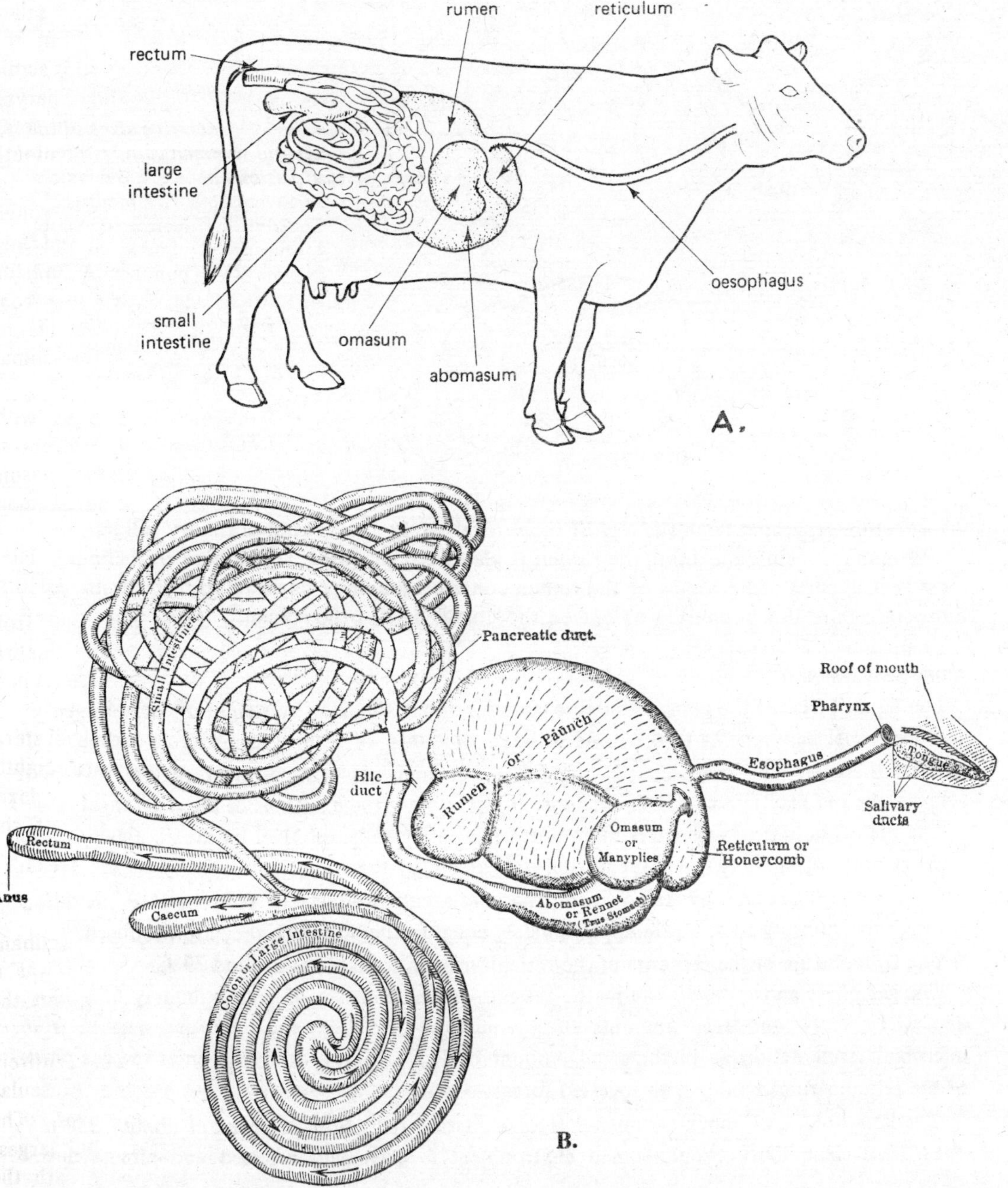

Fig. 3.12 (A) Digestive tract inside a Cow. (B) The same schematic tract in more details.

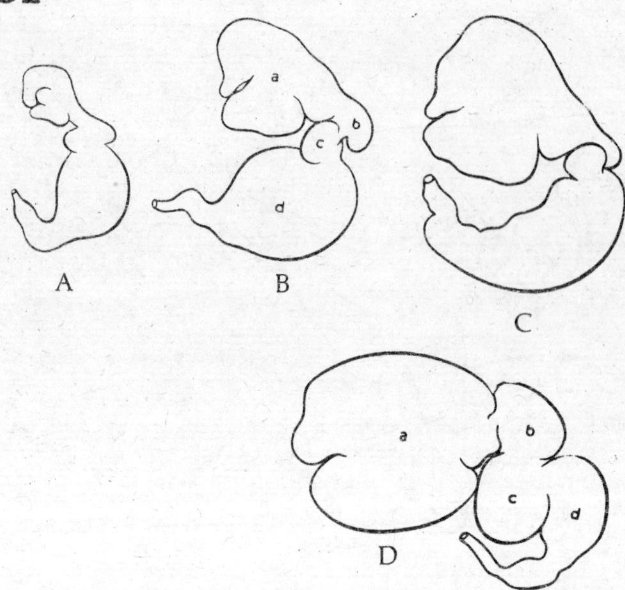

Fig. 3.13 ***Relative sizes of the bovine stomach compartments at various ages.*** A. 3 days old. B. 4 weeks old. C. 3 months old. D. Adult. *a*, rumen; *b*, reticulum; *c*, omasum; *d*, abomasum. From Nickel, R., Schummer, A., and Seiferle, E.: The Viscera of the Domestic Mammals. 2nd Ed. Berlin, Verlag Paul Parey, 1979.

diverticulum separated from the rest of the ventral sac by the ventral coronary pillars.

The mucous membrane lining the rumen is glandless stratified squamous epithelium. The most ventral parts of both sacs of the rumen contain numerous papillae up to 1 cm. in length, but papillae are almost entirely absent on the dorsal part of the rumen.

Rumen environment

The liquid phase of the rumen contents contains about 10 – 20% by weight of organic matter and has a pH between 5.8 to 6.8. With large amounts of readily fermentable carbohydrate entering the rumen, however, the pH may fall to around pH 4.0. Conversely, on very poor forages, the pH may rise to pH 7.5 or more, but these are the extremes of the pH range.

The pH of the reticulo-rumen is maintained at a fairly constant level by the alkalanity of the large volumes of saliva (pH = 8.0) entering the rumen, by the buffering capacity of the HCO_3 content of the saliva and by removal of the acidic end products of microbial fermentation through the rumen wall at a rate approximately equal to that at which they are produced.

The temperature of the contents of the reticulo-rumen is stable at around 39°C.

The gas phase above the digesta in the reticulo-rumen consists of approximately 65% CO_2, 25% CH_4, 7% N_2 and trace amounts of H_2 and O_2. The CO_2 and CH_4 are derived from microbial fermentation as in the small amount of H_2. The N_2 and O_2 enter the gas phase of the reticulo-rumen along with ingested forage.

The liquid phase of reticulo-rumen has an oxidation-reduction potential of about – 350 mV, thus it is clear that reticulo-rumen environment is extremely reduced and almost devoid of oxygen.

The inorganic solutes present in the reticulo-rumen are derived from the saliva. Of the cations present in the rumen, only Na^+ is transported across reticulo-ruminal wall in gradient

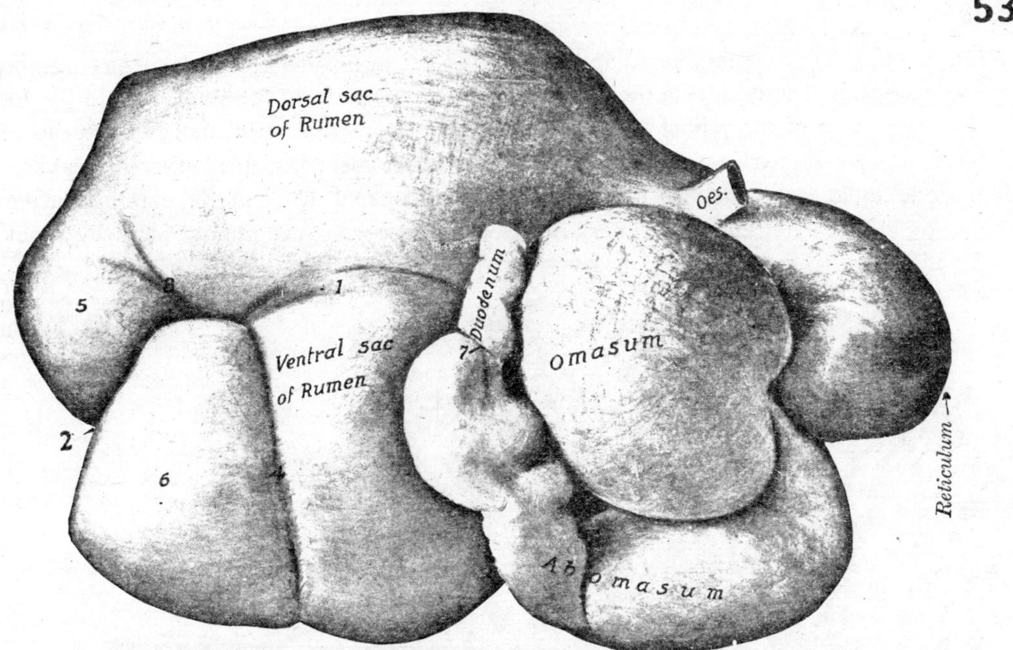

Fig. 3.14 Stomach of a Cow, right view. Oes., oesophagus; 1, right longitudinal groove of rumen; 2, posterior groove of rumen; 3, 4, coronary grooves; 5, 6, posterior blind sacs of rumen; 7, pylorus.

which occurs between the rumen and the blood stream. As a consequence of this, the ionic content of the rumen closely reflects that of the saliva.

The Reticulum

The reticulum is the most cranial compartment. It is also called the honey comb, and as the names imply, it is lined with mucous membrane containing many intersecting ridges which subdivide the surface into honey comb like compartments. The surface is stratified squamous epithelium. The location of the reticulum immediately behind the diaphragm places it almost in opposition to heart, so any foreign objects such as wire or nails that may be swallowed tend to lodge in the reticulum and are in a very good position to penetrate into the heart. The reticular groove commonly referred to as the oesophageal groove, extend from the cardia to the omasum, and is formed by two muscular folds which can close to direct materials from the oesophagus into the omasum directly, or open and permit the materials to enter the rumen. The groove appears to be less functional in adult ruminants than in suckling animals. However, it has been demonstrated that in drenching sheep, the drench enters the abomasum directly.

The Omasum

The omasum is a spherical organ filled with muscular laminae, bearing pointed papillae arranged in such a manner that food is moved from the *reticulo-omasal* orifice between the laminae, and on to the *omaso-abomasal* orifice. Each lamina contains three layers of muscle, including a central layer continuous with the muscle wall of the omasum.

The floor of the omasum as well as the leaves are covered with stratified squamous epithelium.

At the junction of the omasum and abomasum is an arrangement of folds of mucous membrane, the *vela terminalia*, derived from the omasum in the cow, but from the abomasum in the sheep.

The large size of the reticulo-rumen has already been mentioned and, as the turnover rate of the reticulo-rumen is of the order of 1-1.5 volumes per day, it is clear that a very large volume of liquid enters the omasum from the reticulo-rumen. The material entering the omasum contains 90-95% water and the primary function of this organ is to remove water by about 50%.

In addition to removing water, the omasum also absorbs VFA.

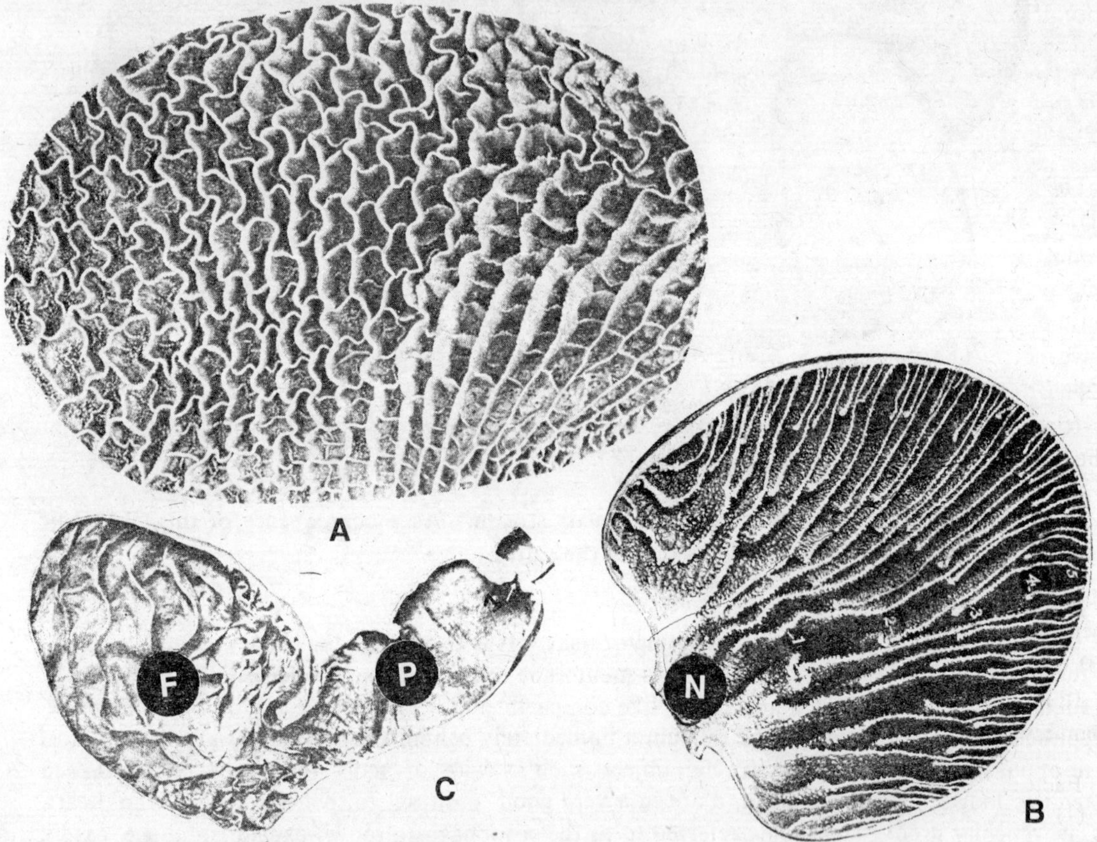

Fig. 3.15 (A) The interior of bovine reticulum. Note typical 'honey combed' cell structure; (B) Cross section of bovine omasum with the ingesta washed out. 1, 2, 3, 4, 5, are laminae of different sizes. N, is the neck of the omasum; (C) The interior of bovine abomasum; (F) The Fundus gland region; (P) The pyloric region; (I) The pylorus.

The Abomasum

The abomasum (true stomach) is the first glandular portion of the ruminant digestive system. It is located ventral to the omasum and extends caudally on the right side of the rumen. The pylorus (terminal part of the abomasum) is a sphincter (thickening of circular smooth muscle fibres) at the junction of the stomach and small intestine.

The epithelium of the abomasum changes abruptly from the stratified squamous epithelium of the omasum to a tall simple columnar epithelium capable of producing mucus. Presumably the mucus covering the stomach epithelium prevents the digestive juices from digesting the stomach cells.

The abomasum corresponds in structure and function to the fundic region of the stomach of non-ruminants. The abomasal epithelium possesses cells which secrete electrolytes, specially HCl, pepsin and mucus. The pH of this section is in the range of pH 1.0 – 1.3 and overall pH of abomasal contents is about pH 2.0. The low pH of abomasal contents is responsible for the death of the microbes entering the abomasum ; it also provides optimum conditions for activity of the peptic enzymes responsible for the digestion of microbial protein in the abomasum.

The acidity of stomach contents varies among the domestic animals, being highest in carnivores (pH 1 or less in dogs), and lowest in monogastric herbivores (pH 1.1-6.8 in horses). In carnivores the stomach will virtually empty it-self between each meal. In herbivores ingesta may remain within the stomach for several days.

The control of gastric secretion involves several regulatory phases as follows :

(1) *Cephalic or Reflex phase*

Gastric secretion may be initiated by such things as the sight, smell or taste of food which may not enter the stomach. Stimuli reach the stomach by way of the vagus nerves to the myenteric plexus. (the nerve net work of the stomach wall). Herbivorous animals do not appear to have a cephalic phase of gastric stimulation.

(2) *Gastric phase*

It accounts for about 75% of the total gastric juice secretion and occurs when food reaches the stomach. The distension of the stomach also results in a vasovagal reflex by which impulses are sent to the brain and then back to the stomach by way of the vagus nerves to stimulate the flow of gastric juice and also release of the hormone gastrin.

The hormone is synthesised and released by the "G" cells in the antrum of the stomach. It causes the parietal cells to secrete HCl and intrinsic factor (IF), and the chief cell to secrete pepsinogen and stimulates gastric motility.

(3) *Intestinal phase*

It involves small amount of gastric juice that continue to be secreted as long as chyme remains in the small intestine, even though no food remains in the stomach.

Factors that inhibit gastric secretion are as follows :

(1) Feedback mechanism depends on the distention of the duodenum, fluidity of the chyme in the duodenum, and the concentration of amino acids and chyme acidity in the duodenum. As any of these substances increase in the duodenum, it also decreases the release of gastrin from the G cells, which in turn decreases the HCl secretion from the parietal cells.

(2) A second factor is involved in the control of gastric secretion. Two hormones, *secretin* and *cholecystokinin* (CCK) are synthesised by and secreted from mucosal cells in the duodenum in response to the same stimuli (i.e. chyme, pH, fluidity, digestive state). These hormones are secreted directly in the blood and are carried back to the stomach by the vascular system. In the stomach they decrease motility, inhibit the release of gastrin and thus inhibits HC secretion.

(3) The stomach has a direct mechanism also, when the pH becomes low due to a high HC concentration, this will inhibit the release of gastrin from the antral G cells, which in turn will inhibit the further secretion of HCl.

The Small Intestine

The small intestine is divided into three parts, duodenum, jejunum and ileum, because of histological or microscopic structural difference.

The *doudenum* is the first part of the small intestine. It is closely attached to the body wall by a short mesentery, the mesoduodenum. Ducts from the pancreas and liver enter the first part of the duodenum.

The *jejunum* is indistinctly separated from the duodenum. It begins approximately where the mesentery starts to become rather long. The jejunum and ileum are continuous, and there is no gross demarcation between them.

The *ileum* is the last part of the small intestine. It enters the large intestine at the *ileo-ceco-colic junction.*

It is impossible to give a definite location for the jejunum and ileum, but they tend to be located toward the left ventral portion of the abdominal cavity in non-ruminants. The terminal part of the ileum, however, joins the *cecum* (horse) or cecum and colon (other animals) in the right caudal part of the abdominal cavity.

The small intestine is the chief site of absorption in most of the domestic animals. The mucus membrane of only the small intestine consists of numerous tiny finger like projections known as *villi.* Animals with the most rapid digestive and absorptive processes have a more highly developed system of villi to provide a greater surface area for absorption. Each villus is further surrounded by innumerable fingerlike projections known as *microvilli* for the sake of unimaginable greater surface area for the absorption of nutrients. Villi undergo rhythmic (pumping) contractions, pendulum movements and tonic contractions and is controlled by a hormone, *villikinin* and thus aids in absorption.

The duodenum receives both bile from the gall-bladder and pancreatic secretions from the pancreas via a duct which at the point of entry into the duodenum is common to both organs since the bile duct and pancreatic duct fuse some 2-3 cm from this point.

Bile consists largely of bile acids and bile pigments, with small amounts of cholesterol, lecithin, electrolytes and protein. Bile acids before entering the duodenum conjugated of either glycine, giving glycocholic acid salt or taurine, giving taurocholic acid salts. Esterification takes place at the terminal carboxyl group of the parent acid.

The secretions of the pancreas include the proteolytic enzymes trypsinogen (converted to the active form, trypsin, by enterokinase secreted by the duodenum), chymotrypsinogens and procarboxypeptidases (both activated by trypsin) and carboxypeptidase. Proteolytic enzymes constitute some 70% of the total protein secreted by bovine pancreas. Also present in the pancreatic secretions are DNA ase, RNA ase, pancreatic lipase and an alpha amylase similar to that present in the saliva. These enzymes together with the pepsin secreted by the abomasum are responsible for the degradation of the microbial cells entering the region of the gastrointestinal tract posterior to the reticulo-rumen and also of the feed protein which have escaped reticulo-ruminal degradation (bypass amount).

The secretions present in the small intestine appear to consist largely of electrolytes, particularly Na^+ and Cl^-. The pH of the small intestine differs along its length, ranging from pH 7.1 in the region of jejunum to approximately pH 8.0 at the ileum. These pH values are maintained through the presence of HCO_3^- ions.

Extensive degradation of microbial cells takes place in the small intestine as is evidenced by the presence of fatty acids with odd numbers of carbon atoms and of double bond positional isomers characteristic of bacterial fatty acids. However, degradation of carbohydrate polymers (other than starch) which have escaped microbial degradation in the reticulo-rumen does not take place to any large extent. The feed lipids which have escaped reticulo-rumino fermentation (bypass portion) also gets digested at small intestine.

The Large Intestine

In the ruminant the large intestine consists of the cecum and colon. This cecum has one blind end that projects caudally. Cranially, it is continuous with the colon. This junction is marked by the entrance of the ileum at the ileo-ceco-colic orifice.

The colon passes forward between the two layers of mesentary which support the small intestine. Here it is arranged in coils, the *ansa spiralis*. The first portion spirals toward the

Table 3.2 LARGE INTESTINES

	Horse	*Cow*	*Sheep*	*Pig*	*Dog*
Size	(a) Large colon: 10 to 12 ft. (3 to 3.5 m.) long, 10 in. (25 cm.) diameter, (average) (b) Small colon: 10 to 12 ft. (3 to 3.5 m.) long, 3 in. (7.5 cm.) diameter	35 ft. (10.5 m.) long, 3 in. (7.5 cm.) average diameter	15 ft. (4.5 m.) long, 2 in. (5 cm.) average diameter	10 to 15 ft. (3 to 4.5 m.) long, 2 in. (5 cm.) average diameter	2 ft. (0.6 m.) long, 1 in. (2.5 cm.) diameter. Size varies with breed
Specific characters	Sacculated with longitudinal bands. Vary in number from 1 to 4 on large colon, to 2 on small colon	Tubular, no bands or sacculations. Part is coiled in two directions (ansa spiralis). No differentiation into large and small colon	As cow	Coiled like cow Cecum 3 bands and 3 sacculations. First part of colon 2 bands and 2 sacculations extending to coils. Remainder has no bands	Short and like shepherd's crook. In 3 parts: (i) ascending, (ii) transverse, and (iii) descending. No bands
Position	Large colon: Mainly in ventral abdominal cavity as dorsal and ventral coils. Extends from sternum to pelvic brim. Origin and termination situated dorsally caudal to stomach. Small colon: Lies dorsal to large colon and mingled with small intestines	In dorsal abdominal cavity, to right of median plane with small intestines. Coiled part in lower right flank	As cow	On each side of median plane, mainly to the left caudal to the stomach. Coiled part in ventral part of abdominal cavity, dorsal to umbilicus	Short ascending part lies along right flank, with long descending part on left of median plane extending to the pelvic cavity

centre of the coils (centripetally) and the next part spirals away from the centre (centrifugally). After leaving the *ansa spiralis* the colon crosses to the left side and continues caudally to the rectum and the anus, the terminal part of the digestive tract.

The environmental conditions in the large intestine and caecum are not dissimilar to these in the rumen, both having redox potentials of the order of—350 mV and a typical pH range of the order of 6.5—7.0

The VFA which occur as the major end products of microbial fermentation in the rumen are also found in large intestine and caecum due to microbial degradation of polysaccharides as well as other carbohydrates which have escaped digestion at a lower total concentration. (Rumen, 100—150mM ; Caecum, 60 mM and in large intestine 7 mM).

An important aspect of microbial fermentation in the large intestine and caecum from the host animal's point of view is that the microbial cells synthesised in these regions of the intestinal tract are not subjected to subsequent digestion, and therefore, are not available as potential sources of protein to the host animal.

Table 3.3 CECUM

	Horse	*Cow*	*Sheep*	*Pig*	*Dog*
Capacity	4 to 5 gal. (18 to 22 liters)	1 to 1.25 gal. (4.5 to 5.5 liters)	1 quart (1 liter)	3 pints to 1 gal. (1.5 to 4.5 liters)	Less than 0.5 pint (0.25 liters)
Size	4 ft. long, 8 to 10 in. diameter (1.25 m. × 20 to 25 cm.)	30 in. long, 5 in. diameter (75 × 12 cm.)	10 in. long, 2 in. diameter (25 × 5 cm.)	8 to 12 in. long, 3 to 4 in. diameter (20 to 30 cm. × 7.5 to 10 cm.)	5 to 6 in. long, 1 to 1.5 in. diameter (12 to 15 cm. × 2.5 to 4 cm.)
Shape	Comma-shaped. Sacculated with four longitudinal bands. Two extremities, one rounded (base), other pointed (apex)	Tubular with rounded free extremity	As cow	Tubular and sacculated with three longitudinal bands. Extremity rounded	Tubular and coiled
Position	Base extends from 15th rib to tuber coxae on right of median plane. Longitudinal axis extends ventrally over right flank to xiphoid region generally. Cranial border lies parallel with and 5 to 6 in. (12.5 to 15 cm.) ventral to costal arch	Extends along right flank from near the ventral end of the last rib to the pelvic inlet	As cow	A vertical position in the left or right flank, reaching the abdominal floor between the umbilicus and the pubis	On the right, midway between flank and median plane, dorsal to the umbilical region
Openings	The ileum and large colon enter at lesser curvature of the base. Openings are 2 in. (5 cm.) apart	Colon and cecum continuous. Ileum joins obliquely	As cow	As cow	Ileum and colon continuous and cecum joins obliquely

It would not be unreasonable to suggest that the volatile fatty acids of hind gut and caecal origin contribute about 30% of the total VFA entering ruminant bloodstream, the remaining 70% being largely of ruminal origin. Water is also absorbed from the large intestine and caecum to the extent of 1.0—1.25 liters per day in sheep. Amino nitrogen @0.5—1.6 gram/day are also absorbed in sheep in the region of large intestine.

B. ACCESSORY DIGESTIVE ORGANS

The Salivary Glands

The main salivary glands consist of three pairs of well defined glands viz., *parotid*, *mandibular*, and *sublingual*. The other salivary glands include *labial*, *buccal*, *lingual* and *palatine* glands. The dog has also a zygomatic salivary gland near the eye. *The parotid salivary gland* is located ventral to each ear in relation to the caudal border of the mandible. The duct penetrates the mucous membrane of the cheek near the upper third or fourth cheek tooth. The *mandibular* or *submaxillary salivary gland* is located ventral to the parotid gland just caudal to the mandible. The mandibular salivary duct opens ventral to the tongue on a little papilla located in the fold that holds the tongue to the floor of the mouth. The *sublingual salivary gland* is located deep to the mucous membrane along the ventral side of the lateral surface of the tongue near the floor of the mouth. With the exception of the horse, the gland has a monostomatic portion that empties on to the floor of the mouth by way of major sublingual duct.

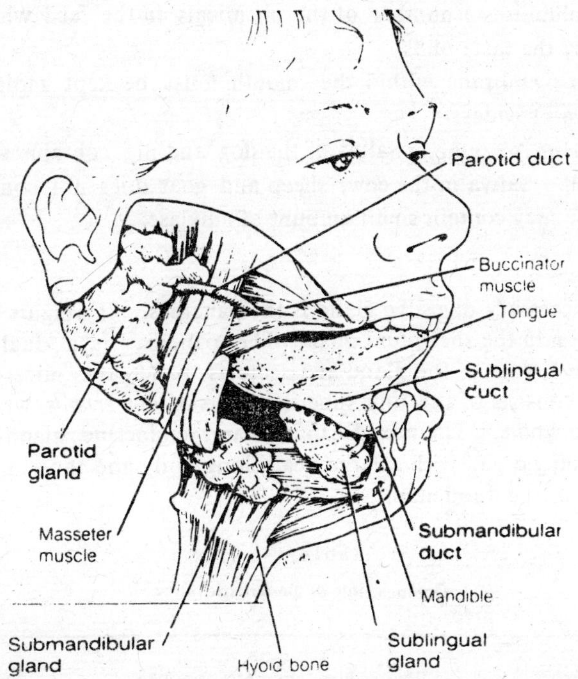

Fig.3.16 The salivary glands. Glandular secretions are carried to the mouth through ducts.

The secretion of the saliva in ruminants is continuous, but the rate is greatly increased by stimuli associated with feeding, rumination and the presence of coarse feeds. An adult human may produce about 1.5—2 liters of saliva daily. In cattle total volume may range from 100—200 liters per day or sometimes equivalent to the volume of the rumen.

Paired parotid, inferior molar and buccal salivary glands produce thin watery secretions, highly alkaline having high concentration of HCO_3^- ions with very little mucoprotein. Saliva from the paired submaxillary, sublingual, and labial salivary glands as well as the unpaired pharyngeal gland secrete a glycoprotein, mucin. The saliva of ruminants tends to be slightly alkaline (pH about 8). The uses of saliva in digestion are manyfold, including the following :

1. **Lubricant.** These secretions act as aids in mastication, formation of the bolus and swallowing.
2. **Buffering capacity.** A large quantity of bicarbonate is secreted in saliva, serving as a buffer in the ingesta.
3. **Nutrients for rumen microorganisms.** Saliva contains considerable amounts of urea, mucin, phosphorus, magnesium and chloride which all are utilised by rumen microbes.
4. **Prevention of frothing.** Gas can accumulate in the rumen and may cause bloat condition when eruction process is impaired. Saliva—acting as a surfactant—helps to prevent this problem.
5. **Taste.** Saliva solubilises a number of the chemicals in the feed which, once in solution, can be detected by the taste buds.
6. **Protection.** The membrane within the mouth must be kept moist in order to remain viable which saliva provides.
7. **Source of digesting enzyme.** Saliva of the dog and pig contains some amylase capable of digesting starch. Saliva in the cow, sheep and goat does not contain amylase, but the saliva of the horse may contain small amount of amylase.

2. The Pancreas

The second main accessary digestive gland is the pancreas. It weights 350 to 500 gram in the ox, and 50-70 gram in the sheep and goat. The pancreas is a dual organ. Its exocrine portion forms the great mass of the gland and secretes pancreatic juice into the duodenum. The endocrine tissue consists of the tiny spherical *islets of langerhans* which account for less than 1 per cent of the whole. The mixed exocrine and endocrine glands is elongated. The pancreas is a soft, lumpy organ with a large head, long body and tapering tail. The head lies within the concavity of the duodenum.

Table 3.4

Composition of pancreatic juice

Enzyme precursors	—	Trypsinogen, chymotrypsinogen
Active enzymes	—	Elastase, amylase, lipase
Cations	—	Sodium, potassium, calcium
Anions	—	Chloride, bicarbonate
pH	—	7.5–8.0

N.B. : The inactive enzyme precursor *trypsinogen* is converted to the active *trypsin* by the enzyme *enterokinase*, which is liberated from unidentified cells of the duodenal mucosa. Trypsin also acts on the precursor *Chymotrypsinogen* to form the active chymotrypsin.

Exocrine pancreas: This is a compound tubulo-acinar gland, the acini are composed of cells which contain granules of the digestive enzymes (Zymogen granules) The acini are connected with excretory ducts which finally coalesce into a single duct which enters the duodenum.

FUNCTIONS OF PANCREATIC JUICE. (1) The alkalinity of the juice aids in the neutralisation of the acid chyme passing into the duodenum from the stomach. This is an important function, since the enzymes of the pancreatic juice act optimally in an alkaline medium.

(2) Trypsin is formed from its precursor trypsinogen which hydrolyses the protein ingested to polypeptides and amino acids. The enzyme has its optimum pH at 8.0—9.7.

(3) Chymotrypsin, when formed from chymotrypsinogen has the action of curdling milk.

(4) The α-amylase converts all forms of starch rapidly into maltose.

(5) The pancreatic lipase converts neutral triglycerides to di-and monoglycerides and free fatty acids.

Regulation of Pancreatic Secretion

The exocrine secretory activities of the pancreas are controlled both hormonally and neurally. Two hormones, *secretin* and *cholecystokinin,* are released into the blood-stream from the mucosa of the duodenal and jejunal portions of the small intestine when gastric acid or chyme enters the intestine. Secretin which is released primarily in response to the presence of HCl, stimulates the release from the pancreas of a watery fluid that contains large amounts of bicarbonate ions. Secretin has little effect on the release of pancreatic enzymes.

Cholecystokinin (also known as pancreozymin), which is released principally in response to the presence of breakdown products of digestion protein of fats and carbohydrates in the duodenum mainly promotes the release of digestive enzymes from the pancreas—by circulating through blood. These two duodenal hormones also feed back to the stomach, as explained earlier, by decreasing secretion in the stomach and slowing the process of peristalsis.

Neurally, pancreatic secretion may be stimulated by way of the vagus nerves and the effect is mostly on enzymatic secretion. The response is specially evident during the cephalic and gastric phases of stomach secretion.

3. The Liver and Biliary System

The liver is the largest gland in the body. It is an important organ of intermediate metabolism. It has also an exocrine section, the bile, which is conveyed to the duodenum by the ducts of the liver, which convey bile from and within the liver to duodenum, and the gall bladder which stores and concentrates bile. All domestic animals except the horse have this gall bladder. Bile leaves the liver through the *hepatic duct*, which joins the *cystic duct* coming from the gall bladder to form the *common bile duct*, which then passes to the first part of the duodenum.

The composition and the role of bile will further be explained in connection with the digestion and absorption of lipids in non-ruminants in the later part of this chapter.

Regulation of Bile secretion

The rate of bile-secretion is chemically, neurally and hormonally controlled.

Chemical substances that increase bile flow are called *Choleretics*. Bile salts present in the

Table 3.5 Functions of Gastrointestinal Secretions

Organ	Secretion (Secreted by)	Principal Components and enzymes	Action of components including end products of digestion
MOUTH AND PHARYNX	Saliva (Salivary glands)	Water, Mucus, Salts, SALIVARY AMYLASE (ptyalin),MALTASE	Softens food, Makes food slippery, Provide neutral medium for action of salivary amylase and help to preserve teeth,against acids formed by bacteria, Splits cooked starch into dextrin and maltose or some glucose.
RUMEN		Various enzymes from microorganisms	Enzymes act on carbohydrates yield VFA; splits protein and non-protein nitrogenous compounds into ammonia, Hydrolyzes the triglyceride and galactolipid, releasing free falty acids (FFA) and allowing the glycerol and galactose to be fermented to volatile falty acids (VFA), Enough microbial protein (dead) will pass out to stomach and so on; vitamins B and K are also produced.
STOMACH (abomasum)	Gastric Juice (HCl acid & Mucus) from glands of the stomach walls	Water, Mucus, Hydrochloric acid, PEPSIN (secreted as pepsinogen), RENIN	Further softens food; Prevents gastric juice from damaging the stomach wall; Stops the action of salivary amylase and allows pepsin to work. Kills many germs. Splits certain proteins into proteoses and peptones, i.e. shorter chain polypeptides, Curdles milk in adults (when rennin scare or absent and in any case ineffective). Curdles milk in many young mammals. Presence in man doubtful. Regulate emptying of dissolved food into small intestine; solubilyze food particles.
DUODENUM (small intestine)	Pancreatic juice (pancreas)	Water, Alkaline salts PANCREATIC LIPASE, PANCREATIC AMYLASE, TRYPSIN (secreted as trypsinogen) CHYMO-TRYPSIN (secreted as chymotrypsinogen), CARBOXYPEPTIDASE, CHOLESTEROLESTERASE	Help to increase alkalinity in intestine and combine with fatty acids to form soaps ; Splits fats into fatty acids and glycerol (Acts more effectively than gastric lipase). Splits all forms of starch and dextrin into maltose. Split certain proteins, proteoses and peptones into shorter polypeptide chains and liberate some amino-acids. cholesterol esterifies with falty acids.
	Bile (stored in the gall bladder of liver)	Water, Bile pigments, Bile salts	Waste materials–excreted with faeces or absorbed and re-excreted later, Alkaline therefore , neutralise acidity of chyme and stop action of pepsin but allow action of intestinal enzymes. Emulsify fats.
SMALL INTESTINE	Intestinal juice from Duodenal glands and Goblet cells throughout the small intestine	Water, Mucus ENTERO-KINASE, PEPTIDASES (Carboxypeptidase, Aminopeptidase, Dipeptidase) MALTASE, SUCRASE, LACTASE) PLOYNUCLEOTIDASE	Protects intestinal mucosa, Activates trypsinogen forming trypsin; trypsin then activates chymotrypsinogen, Split amino-acids, one at a time, from the acid and amino ends, respectively, of the polypeptide chains. Splits the final dipeptide residues, Splits maltose into glucose, splits sucrose into glucose and fructose, splits lactose into glucose and galactose. In ruminants glucose and fructose formation is extremely low. Galactose formation is high in young mammals.
LARGE INTESTINE		Cellulase from microorganisms	Storage and concentration of undigested matter by absorption of salt and water; mixing and propulsion of contents. Cellulose and other undigested polysaccharides gets digested to form VFA.. Microbial protein, B-vitamins and vitamin K are formed.

plasma as a result of enterohepatic circulation act as powerfull choleretics that stimulate bile flow.

Stimulation of the vagus nerves can also increase the rate of hepatic bile secretion.

In response to the presence of fat and protein breakdown products in the chyme, the hormone *Cholecystokinin* (CCK) previously known as *pancreozymin* is released from the duodenal mucosa which strongly stimulates gall bladder to contract. Secretin apart from its effect as stimulator for pancreatic bicarbonate also causes secretion of bile (not the rate of bile acid production).

Digestive Organs of Non-ruminants

The digestive organs of non-ruminants are much simpler. They differ from ruminant system mainly, in the structure of stomach and large intestine, and hence these two sections of the alimentary canal will be discussed here. The general description of other parts may be at present taken as more or less like ruminants.

The Non-ruminant stomach

The simple stomach is divided into three regions : *Cardiac, fundic* and *pyloric*. These vary considerably in size and shape between species. The fundic and pyloric regions are the principal centers of glandular activity.

The cardiac region is closest to the oesopageal region and contains the cardiac glands. They are mucous glands, and do not produce enzymes.

The body of the stomach is called the fundic region and contains the *fundic* or *gastric glands.* These are composed of three types of cells, (1) *body chief cells,* (2) *neck chief cells* and (3) *parietal cells.* Body chief cells are found in the body and deeper parts of the gastric

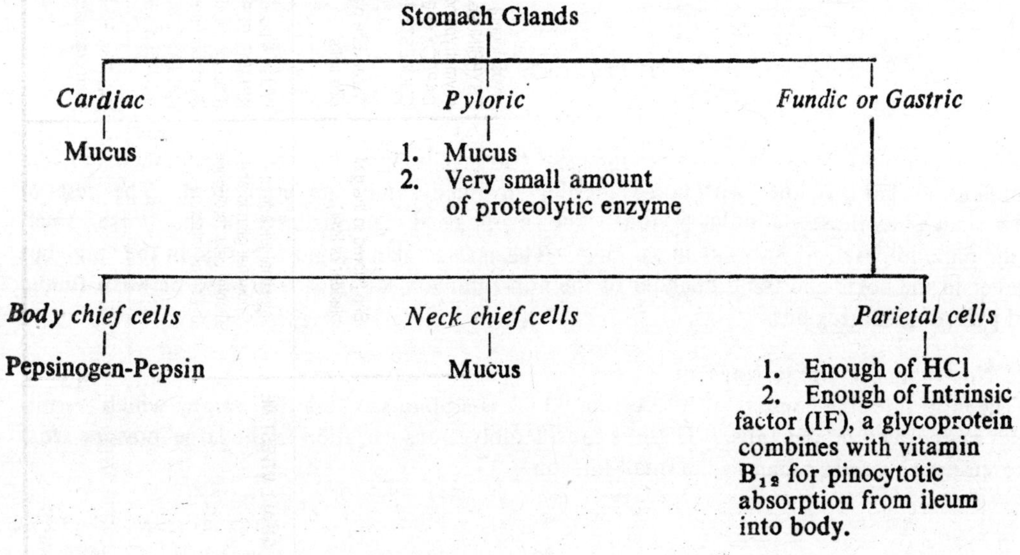

glands. They are enzyme producers and contain so called *zymogen granules* (substances from which gastric enzymes are derived), Neck chief cells line the gastric glands near their openings and are mucus secreting cells. Parietal or border cells produce HCl and "intrinsic factor".

The posterior part of the stomach is called the pyloric region and contains the pyloric glands. The products of their secretion are mucus and small amounts of proteolytic enzymes.

Gastric juice = All substances contributed to the stomach lumen by the mucosal cells. It includes H_2O, cations, anions, HCl, IF, pepsinogen, rennin etc.

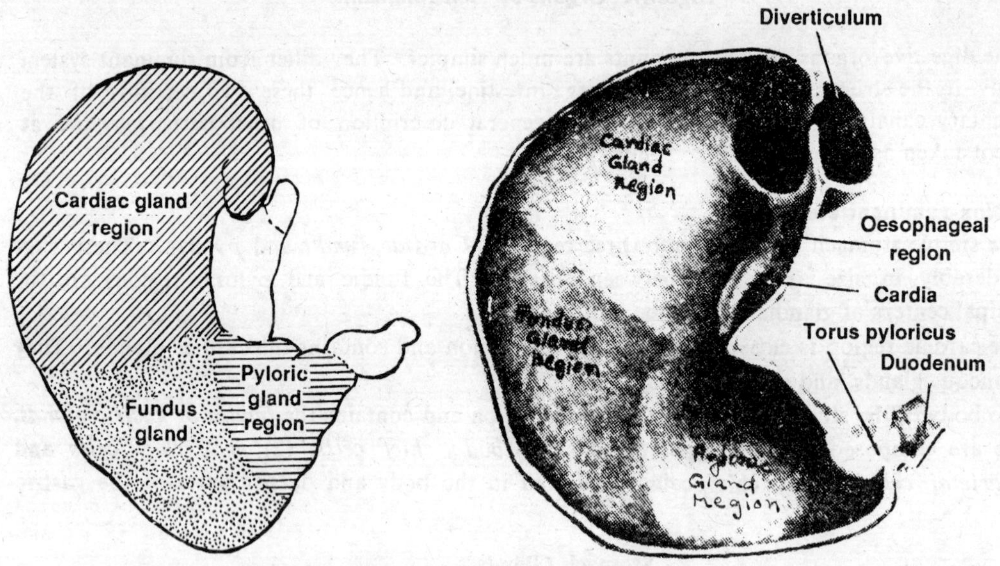

Fig. 3.17 Stomach of a Pig.

In the non-ruminant stomach the esophageal region compares to the forestomachs of the ruminant, in that it is lined with non-glandular stratified squamous epithelium. The rest of the stomach has those glandular region. The esophageal region is large in the horse, small in the pig and practically absent in the dog. The cardiac gland region is large in the pig but smaller in the horse and the remainder of the non-ruminant stomach is divided between fundic and pyloric gland regions.

The Non-ruminant Large Intestine

The large intestine consists of the cecum, which is a blind sac and the colon, which terminates as the rectum and anus. There is considerably more variation in the large intestine from one species to another than in the small intestine

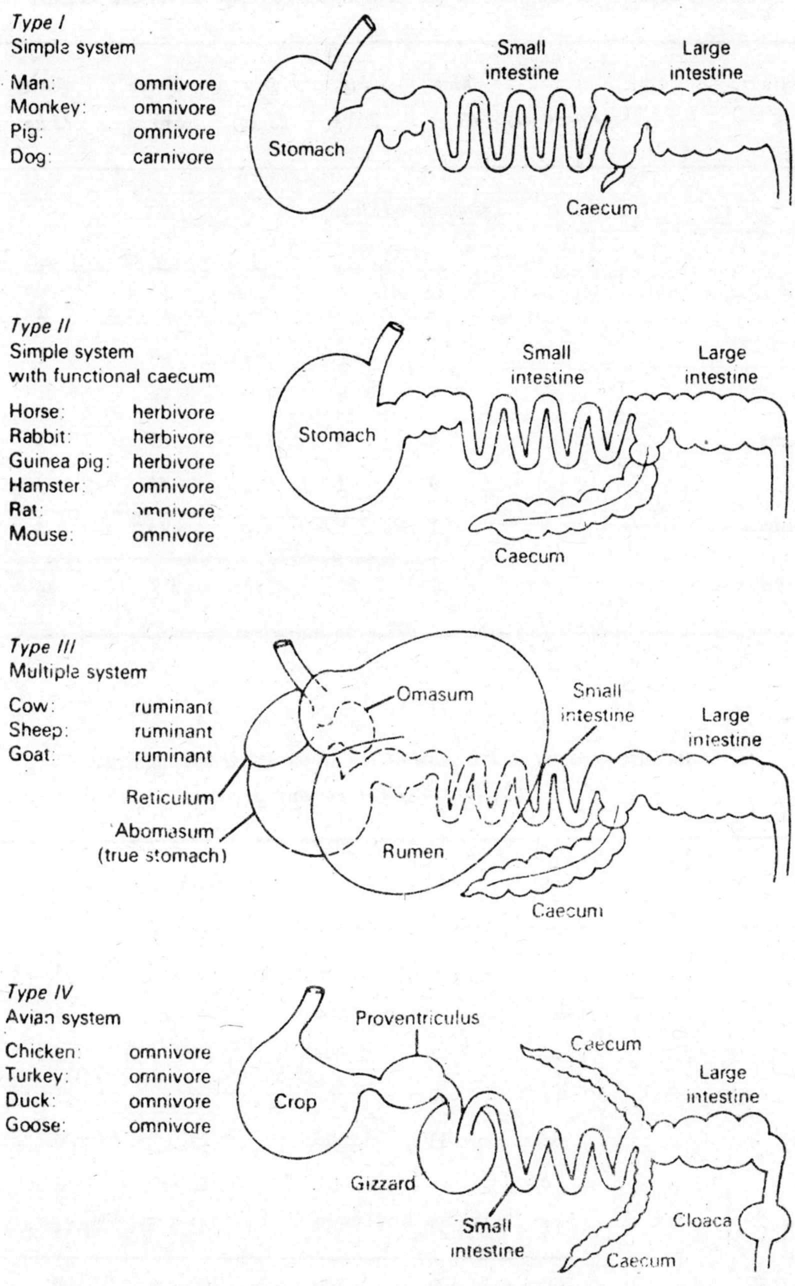

Fig. 3.18 Classification of animals according to type of digestive systems.

Table 3.6

Absolute capacity of the parts of the gastrointestinal tract of various animals

Parts of digestive tract		*Man*	*Pig*	*Dog*	*Horse*	*Sheep*	*Cattle*
	Average body wt.	*68 kg*	*200 kg*	*18 kg*	*680 kg*	*75 kg*	*450 kg*
			Capacity (Litres)				
Rumen		—	—	—	—	23	202
Reticulum		—	—	—	—	2	8
Omasum		—	—	—	—	1	19
Abomasum		1	8	4.3	18	3	23
Small Intestine		4	9	1.6	53	9	66
Cecum		0	1	0.1	44	1	10
Large Intestine		1	9	1.0	96	5	28
Total G.I. Tract		6	27	7.0	211	44	356

Table 3.7

Relative capacity of the parts of G.I. tract of various mammals
(% Total digestive system)

Parts of digestive tract	*Man*	*Pig*	*Dog*	*Horse*	*Sheep*	*Cattle*
Rumen	—	—	—	—	53	53
Reticulum	—	—	—	—	5	3
Omasum	—	—	—	—	2	5
Abomasum	17	30	61	9	7	6
Small Intestine	66	33	24	25	20	20
Cecum	0	4	1	21	2	2
Large Intestine	17	33	14	45	11	11
Total G.I. Tract	100	100	100	100	100	100

THE RESPIRATORY SYSTEM

This is the process of breathing. Air is *inspired* through the nasal passages, via the wind pipe on trachea, into the lungs, and later *expired.* There is a general rhythm to respiration.

The purpose of respiration is to supply oxygen, through lungs, to the blood as a vital need to the the life of the animal, and to rid the system of unwanted CO_2 and water vapour

All domestic animals have a pair of lungs suspended in the thoracic body cavity one on either side of the chest. They are extremely elastic and spongy. The heart is considerably smaller and lies between the lungs.

Table 3.8

	Air inhaled %	*Air exhaled* %
Nitrogen	79.04	79.04
Oxygen	20.93	16.02
Carbon dioxide	00.03	4.38

Atmospheric air inspired through the larynx and long cartilaginous tube called trachea and then through the two major *bronchi* (bronchial tube), one going to each lung; smaller bronchioles; until the terminal, dead end, sac like structures, the *alveoli* are reached.

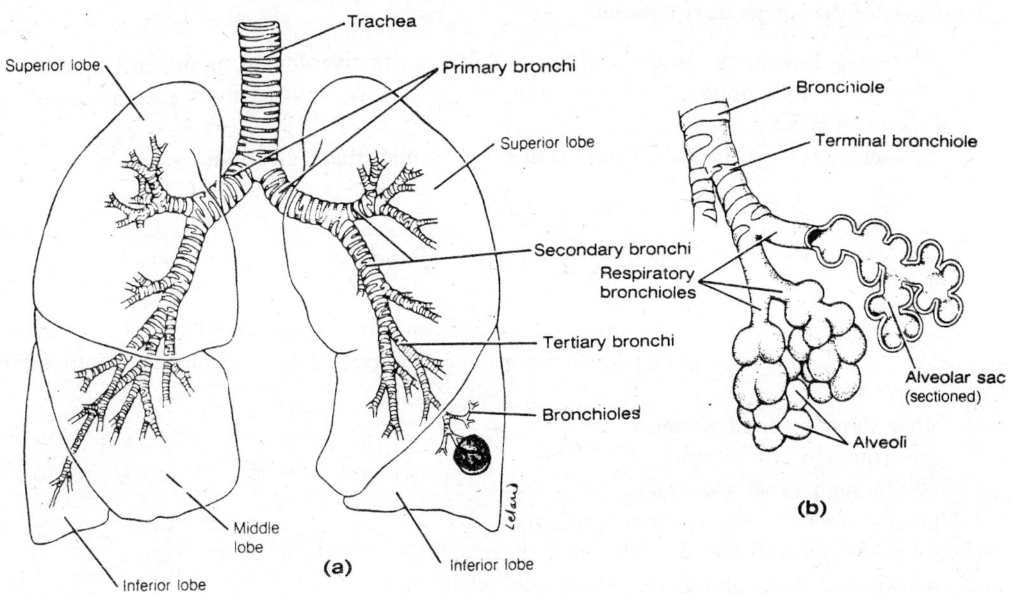

Fig. 3.19 (a) The trachea, the bronchi and the lungs.
(b) The termination of bronchioles into alveoli.

The actual exchange of the respiratory gases takes place between the alveoli and the blood which flows through very fine neighbouring capillaries.

Rate of respiration

The speed of the respirations varies with many internal and external factors. It is faster during fever, after exercise, during powerful emotions, such as fear, anger, sexual excitement, etc.; during very cold or very hot weather, when the body condition is very fat, or when radiation is obstructed through too thick a covering of wool, fur etc., or too much clothing.

It is slower than normal during resting, either when lying or when sleeping.

Normal rates in adult domesticated animals are as follows:

Table 3.9

Horse	8–12 per minute
Ox	12–16 per minute
Sheep and Goat	12–20 per minute
Pig	10–16 per minute
Dog	15–30 per minute

With poor ventilation there lies great danger that some diseases of the lungs, e.g. tuberculosis and virus pneumonia will spread, through the expired breath of diseased animals, and set up the trouble in those which are still healthy.

Malfunctions of the Respiratory System

1. *Pneumonia* has many causes resulting in fluids in the alveoli causing difficult breathing:
2. *Pleurisy* is inflammation of the lining of the thorax, causing fluid accumulation and difficult breathing.
3. *Tuberculosis* results in loss of lung tissue due to microbial infection.

THE EXCRETORY SYSTEM

Normal cellular activity (metabolism) results in the formation of waste products. In large quantities some of these products can be toxic and need to be excreted. The waste products that require excretion are:

1. Carbon dioxide (through lungs)
2. Water (through sweat glands)
3. Salts (through sweat and urine)
4. Nitrogen products (mostly through urine)

These are transported in the blood system to the organs which make up the excretory system—the lungs, the skin and the main excretory organ, the kidneys.

The Lungs

These have been dealt with in previous section "The Respiratory System". Carbon dioxide and some water diffuse from the blood stream and are excreted by the lungs.

The Skin

The skin is a protective outer layer to the body. It has many nerve endings which transmit the sensations of heat, cold and touch to the brain. The outer layer, the *epidermis*, is a mass of cells with no blood supply or nerve endings. Its main function is protection and it varies in thickness according to the area that needs protection. Below the epidermis is the true skin, the *dermis*, with a blood supply and nerve endings. It contains hair follicles and sebaceous or grease glands which produce a protective film or oil. This oil, such as the oil lanolin in sheep's wool, protects the coat from water penetration.

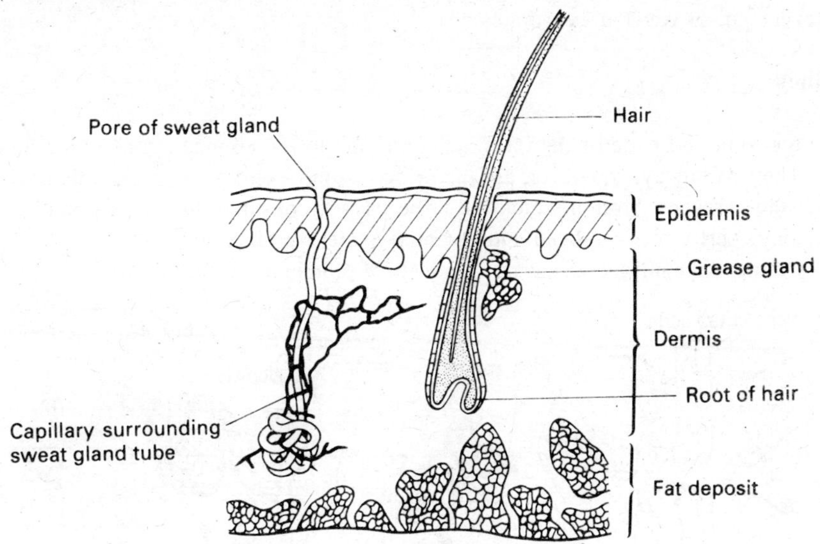

Fig. 3.20 Cross-section through skin.

The skin also contains many sweat glands. Each gland consists of a tube with one end opening as a pore on the skin surface, the other end being blind. The tube is surrounded by blood capillaries. *Water and salts diffuse out from the capillaries and into the sweat tube*. This travels to the skin surface where it evaporates to aid cooling of the body.

Sweat glands are present in the skin of all livestock except the goat. Cattle and pigs sweat only from the nose and snout, whilst a sheep has a thin supply of sweat glands all over its body. So much for the saying 'sweating like a pig'.

Excretion of Water and Salt through Skin

During the period when environmental temperature increases, then also the animal cannot avoid generating heat, except by taking rest, this may be reduced to a minimum. At high temperature the arterioles of the skin are then dilated. Blood flows freely and the skin is kept at a high temperature. The sweat glands will then start secreting. Most farm animals, however, are not efficient sweaters, but they have a technique which results in the evaporation of water. They breathe very rapidly, causing a lot of air to pass rapidly in an out of the mouth. Sheep and cattle pant in this way, but the dog is the most efficient because it has a relatively large, wide opening mouth and a highly mobile tongue which is allowed to flop out. The mouth and tongue are kept very moist.

This is a technique which man cannot imitate, for he always over-ventilates the lungs, removes carbon dioxide too rapidly and becomes dizzy.

The pig is not an efficient sweater, nor has it the power of effectively disposing heat by panting. Its method of cooling is to wallow in water or mud. When it is in a very hot building and cannot follow this instinct it will urinate on the floor and wallow in its own urine, first on one side then the other, thus continuously exposing a wet side to the air.

It may be noted that water has got the highest latent heat of evaporation, 589 cal. per gram which means that to change 1 gm of liquid water to 1 gm. of water vapour without any change in temperature, 589 cal. are required. By this means the body is able to rid itself of 589 cal. of heat for every gm of water it evaporates.

The Kidney

The lungs, skin and parts of the intestine contribute to the elimination of waste products from the body. The two kidneys, however, are the primary adult excretory organs in the mammal. They along with the passages through which the urine passes, constitute the urinary tract.

The kidneys perform two related and essential excretory functions:

1. They remove the nitrogenous waste products of protein metabolism such as *urea* in mammals,

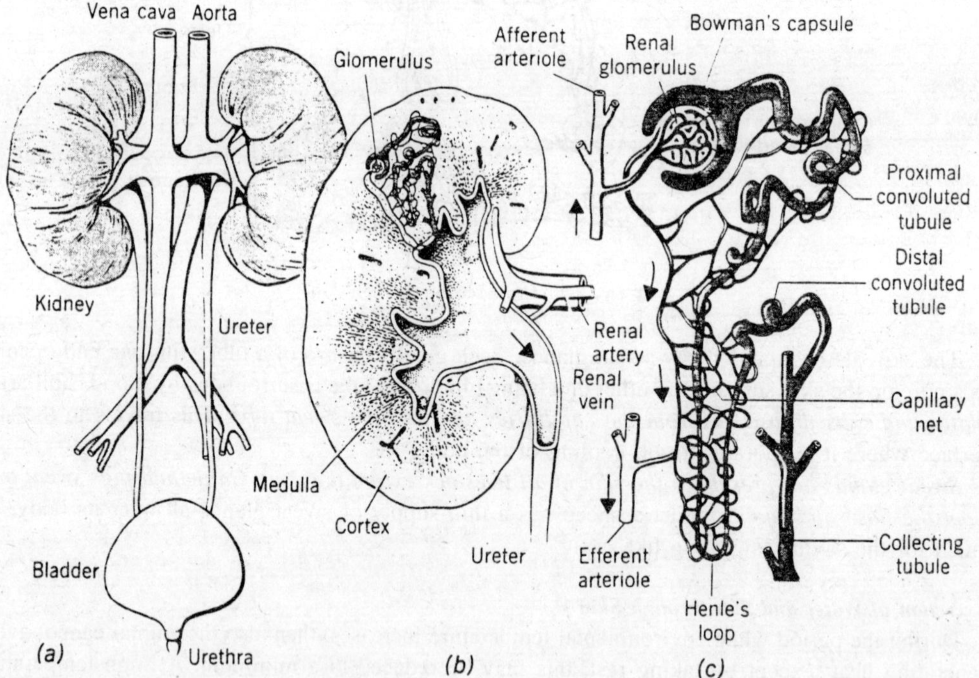

Fig. 3.21 The kidneys. (*a*) Principal parts. (*b*) Location of nephrons. (*c*) Details of nephron and associated capillary bed. Each kidney has about 1 million nephrons. Fluids and solutes (but not colloids, lipids, or cells) leave the blood in the glomerulus and selectively return in the promixal and distal tubules. Final electrolyte adjustments are made primarily in the distal tubules.

and amphibians; uric acid in birds, reptiles and in some insects and many mammals, ammonium ion in most aquatic invertebrates, thus kidney filters waste products from blood.

2. They regulate the acid-base balance (pH) of the animal's internal environment by eliminating controlled amounts of water and inorganic salts.

Blood from all parts of the body carries nutrient molecules, water and waste products of tissue metabolism to the kidney. The structure of the kidney is such that it is able to filter out some of these and to reabsorb the useful ones.

Gross Anatomy of the Urinary Tract

The gross location and appearance of kidneys in all warm blooded animals is similar. The left and right kidneys are located on the dorsal wall of the abdominal cavity. In sheep and pigs they are the normal 'bean' shape. In cattle and birds, the kidneys have distinct subunits or lobes. In cattle and buffaloes the left kidney being able to 'float' in order to accommodate the changes in shape of the rumen.

If the kidney is cut mid-sagittally, two regions, are readily apparent. In the uni-lobed kidneys (in sheep, pig, horse, human etc.) the entire, outer region, the *cortex*, appears lighter than the inner region, the medulla. In other animals like in cattle, buffaloes and birds each subunit or lobe is subdivided into cortical and medullary areas. Each kidney is supplied with blood from the *renal artery*, wih the *renal vein* taking blood away (Fig.3.22)There is also a tube called the *ureter* which takes the mixture of excretory products, the urine to the bladder.

The arrangement of the remaining excretory passages, the *ureters*, the *urinary bladder* and *urethra*, varies somewhat between species. In birds, the ureters empty into the cloaca. In mammals, however, the ureters carry urine to the urinary bladder for storage.

Each kidney has many urine collecting tubules arranged radially. A cup-shaped structure called *Bowman's capsule* (Fig3.22)forms one end of the tubule, the other end opening into the ureter.

The renal artery supplies each kidney with blood that contains water, salts and urea which need to be removed. Inside the kidney the renal artery divides into smaller branches, with each branch

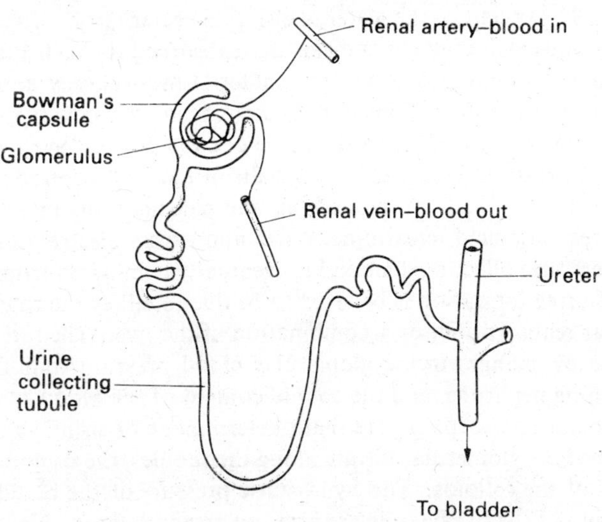

Fig. 3.22 The urine excretory system.

forming a small bunch of capillaries inside the Bowman's Capsule. This bunch of capillaries is called the *glomerulus.* Waste products in the blood diffuse out of the capillary walls into the capsule, with the resulting urine passing into the ureter.

The kidneys are responsible for maintaining the balance of water under the overall control of hormones, in the body. As urine passes down the tubule the required amount of water is absorbed back into the body. The Capillaries from each Bowman's capsule rejoin to form the renal vein which now carries blood that is cleaned of excess salts, water and urea.

Mechanism of Kidney Function

The kidney's two main functions are the excretion of waste (and excess) materials from the bloodstream; and, secondly, the maintenance of the correct proportions of water in the blood, the correct levels of its chemical constituents, and the correct pH.

Blood is supplied to the kidney by the renal artery. It enters the nephron through the afferent arteriole which leads to a filtration chamber known as Bowman's capsule. This capsule contains a conglomeration of capillary blood vessels known as the glomerulus, which filters the blood. The heart supplies the energy to run this efficient "filtration pump."

The unfiltered blood consists of cellular and plasma constituents. It passes out of the glomerulus by way of the efferent arteriole which ramifies around the tubules after breaking up into a second set of capillaries.

The filtrate passes into Bowman's capsule before going into the tubules. The filtered components are water, electrolytes, such as NaCl, (NH_2) HPO_4, KCl, $NaHCO_3$, and low molecular weight organic substances such as glucose, essential nutrients, and urea. These must be reabsorbed (urea 30-40%) to a great degree to maintain the volume and composition of extracellular fluid. Glomerular filtration separates a large amount of fluid; however, during its passage through the proximal tubule, the loop of Henle, and the distal tubule, a considerable amount of filtrate must be reabsorbed to maintain homeostasis. In the process of tubular reabsorption, 98 to 99 per cent of the water of the glomerular filtrate, together with electrolytes and organic compounds including glucose etc. are reabsorbed through the cell walls and back into the bloodstream. The composition of this material must closely approximate that of the extracellular fluid to prevent distortions in fluid composition. The kidney cells provide energy for the reabsorption process which has a dual role of controlling electrolyte balance and maintaining a constant hydrostatic pressure. This results in the reabsorption of the necessary physiological amounts of water, sodium, potassium, and chloride ions into the bloodstream, and the excretion of urea, uric acid, creatinine, water and excess electrolytes in the filtrate. The filtrate residue enters the collecting duct and is eventually eliminated from the kidney as urine.

The control of urine formation is believed to be due to either the rate of glomerular filtration, rate of tubular reabsorption, or a combination of the two. The rate of glomerular filtration may be varied by changes in the glomerular blood pressure and flow, changes in the number of functioning nephrons, and the colloid content of the blood plasma.

The rate of tubular reabsorption, the main determinant of urine volume, is influenced by the rate of passage of the glomerular filtrate along the tubules, the osmotic pressure of the fluid in the tubules, and of the colloids. The hydrostatic pressure of the blood in the tubule capillaries and the activity of the tubule cells are also important factors. Neural factors have little effect on the kidney.

Hormonal Effects on Kidndy Function

The adrenal cortex and the posterior lobe of the pituitary influence the reabsorption of sodium, chloride, potassium, and water. The antidiuretic hormone, vasopressin from the posterior pituitary inhibits the reabsorption of sodium and chloride but increases the absorption of water in the distal convoluted tubule. Hormones from the adrenal cortex (desoxycorticosterone and aldosterone) are essential for the reabsorption of normal amounts of sodium and chloride in the same part of the tubule.

Regulation of Acid-base Balance

In normal metabolism, the acid-base balance is maintained as follows:

1. $CO_2 + H_2O \xrightarrow{\text{carbonic anhydrase}} H_2CO_3 \rightleftharpoons H^+ + HCO_3^-$
2. $NaHPO_4 \rightarrow Na^+ + NaHPO_4^- \rightarrow$ glomerular filtrate
3. $NaHPO_4^- + H^+ + NaH_2PO_4 \rightarrow$ urine
4. $HCO_3^- + Na^+ \rightarrow NaHCO_3 \rightarrow$ plasma and urine

The bicarbonate ions which pass the glomeruli and enter the filtrate are all reabsorbed. This occurs by means of an exchange of hydrogen ions secreted by the tubule cells in exchange for sodium ions which are present in the filtrate.

Hydrogen ions are made available in the tubule cells (Equation 1) due to the action of carbonic anhydrase, a zinc-protein enzyme.

In the glomerular filtrate, the hydrogen ions combine with the bicarbonate ions to form carbonic acid, which then reverts to water which is excreted and carbon dioxide which is reabsorbed by the tubule cells. During this time, sodium ions pass from the tubular urine into the tubule cells where they unite with bicarbonate ior s to form sodium bicarbonate (Equation 4). The sodium bicarbonate then passes into the plasma and extracellular water where its concentraiion is maintained.

A similar exchange mechanism occurs between hydrogen ions of the renal tubule cells and disodium phosphate (Na_2HPO_4) which dissociates into sodium ions (Na^+) and monohydrogen phosphate ions ($NaHPO^-_4$) (Equation 2). The sodium ion moves into the tubule cells and a hydrogen ion (H^+) moves from the tubule cells to unite with the monohydrogen phosphate ($NaHPO^-_4$) ion to form a dihydrogen phosphate salt (NaH_2PO_4), removing a hydrogen ion from the body (Equation 3).

CIRCULATORY SYSTEM

The system includes the *heart*, the *blood vessels* and *blood*.

The heart

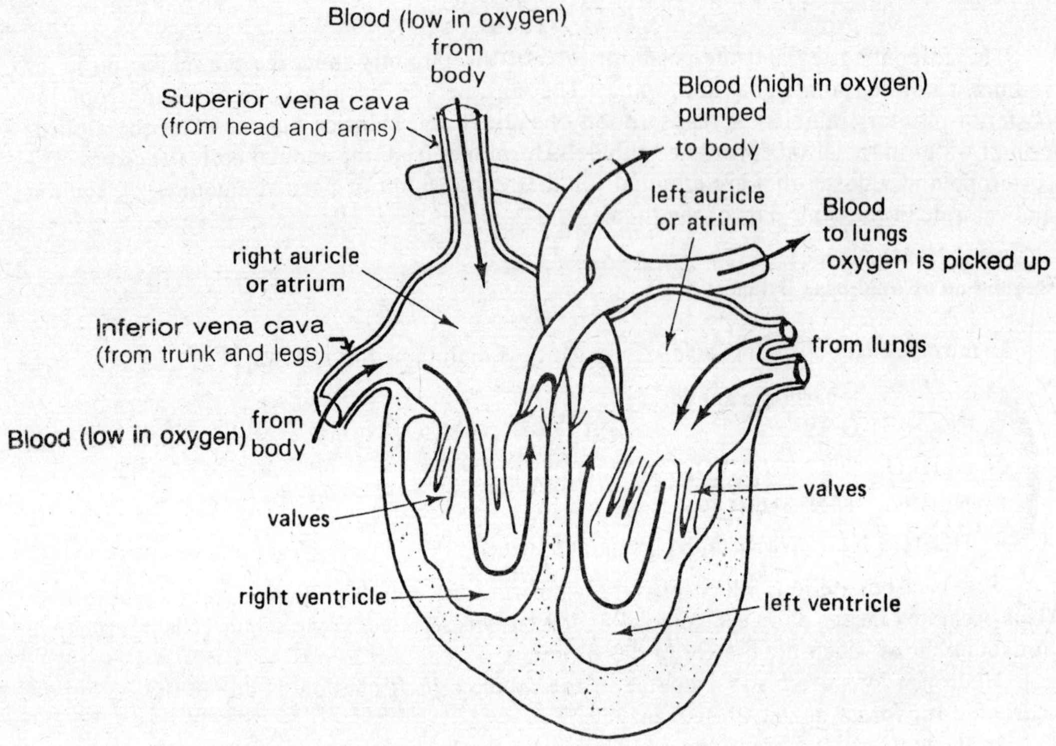

Fig. 3.23 Structure of the Heart. Arrows indicate direction of blood flow.

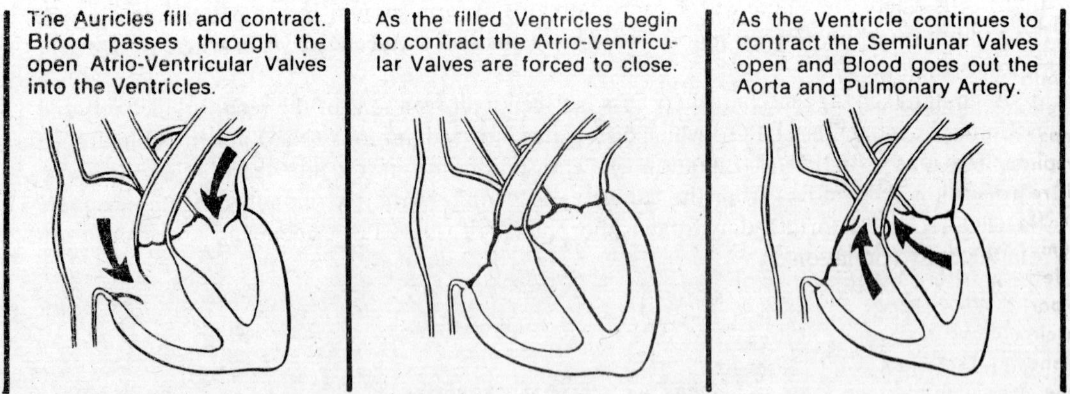

The Auricles fill and contract. Blood passes through the open Atrio-Ventricular Valves into the Ventricles.
As the filled Ventricles begin to contract the Atrio-Ventricular Valves are forced to close.
As the Ventricle continues to contract the Semilunar Valves open and Blood goes out the Aorta and Pulmonary Artery.

Heart—Blood in the heart's right side returns from the body depleted of oxygen. That in the left chambers has just been cleansed and oxygenated in the lungs. With each heartbeat the two sides simultaneously eject blood. From the right it goes to the lungs. From the left it enters the circulation. This cycle constantly returns clean, oxygen-rich blood to nourish the body.

Fig. 3.24 The cardiac cycle.

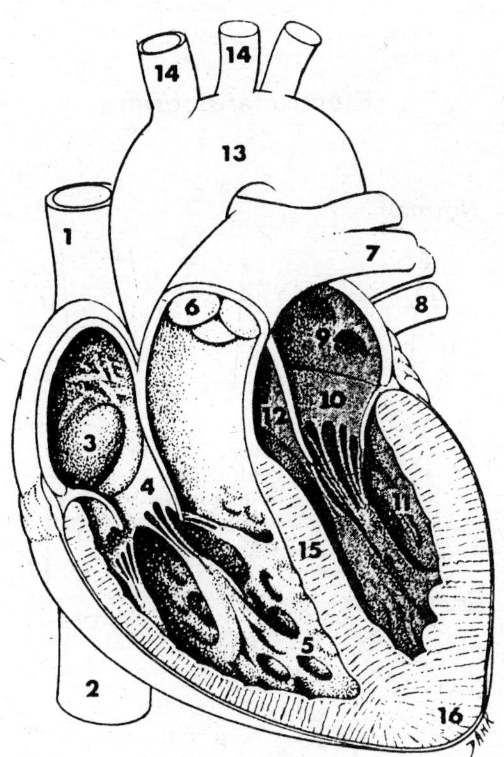

Fig. 3.25 Blood enters the heart by way of the superior vena cava (1) and inferior vena cava (2), into the right atrium (3). The tricuspid valve (4) releases it into the right ventricle (5), which pumps it through the pulmonary valve (6) and pulmonary artery (7) into the lungs for oxygen and release of carbon dioxide. The pulmonary vein (8) then carries the blood into the left atrium (9) and the mitral valve (10) feeds it to the left ventricle (11). Finally it is pumped past the aortic valve (12) into the aorta (13) and back into circulation via branch arteries (14 and others not shown). Dividing the two sides of the heart is the muscular septum (15). The point of the heart (16) is called the apex.

Conduction Pathway

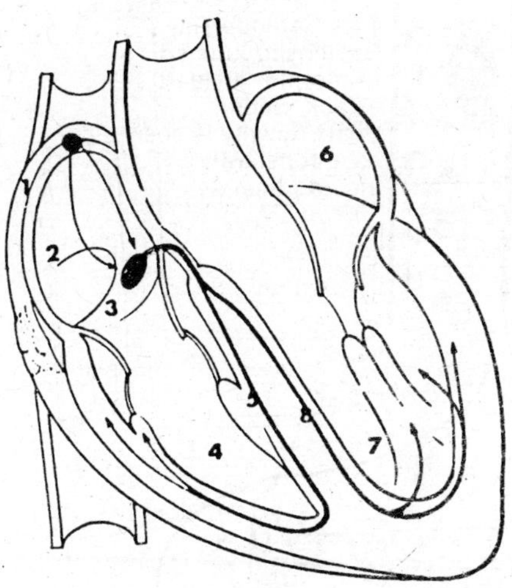

1 Sinoatrial Node (Pacemaker)
2 Right Atrium
3 Atrioventricular Node
4 Right Ventricle
5 Right "Nerve" Branch
6 Left Atrium
7 Left Ventricle
8 Left "Nerve" Branch

This is the pattern of the heartbeat that pumps and circulates the blood. The rhythm of the contractions is established by the sinoatrial node, a mass of specialized muscle fibers in the wall of the right atrium. That impulse travels through both atria, which contract, to the atrioventricular node. These fibers then transmit the impulse via the right and left "nerve" branches causing contraction of the two ventricles. The impulses of the heart increase during activity and diminish during rest.

Fig. 3.26 Conduction system of the Heart. The beat is initiated by the Sinoatrial Node

The Electrocardiogram ECG

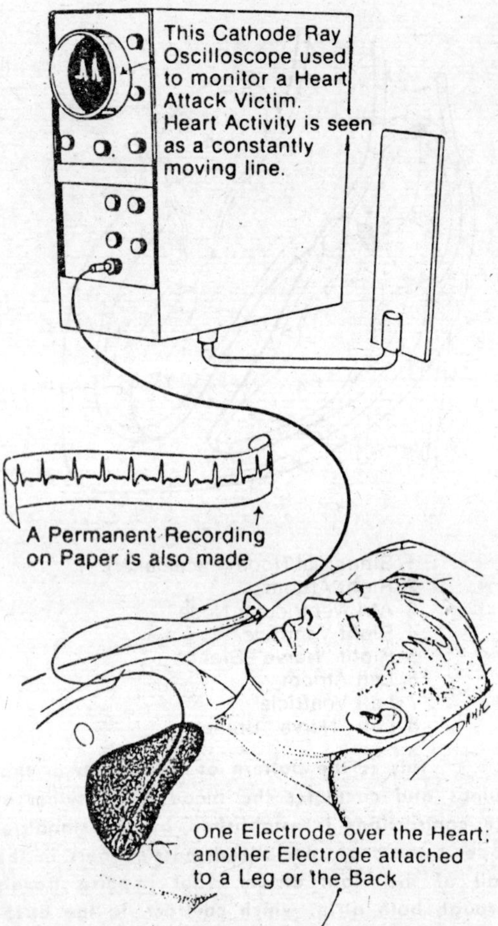
A Recording of the Electrical Activity of the Heart
This Cathode Ray Oscilloscope used to monitor a Heart Attack Victim. Heart Activity is seen as a constantly moving line.
A Permanent Recording on Paper is also made
One Electrode over the Heart; another Electrode attached to a Leg or the Back

ECG—With electrodes in place on the person's body, the irregular waves produced by the electrical impulses of the beating heart register on the electrocardiograph. Simultaneously the waves' patterns are reproduced by a writing device on moving paper. When read by a physician, these patterns can indicate irregularities of the heart.

Fig. 3.27 The Electrocardiogram.

Electrocardiograms

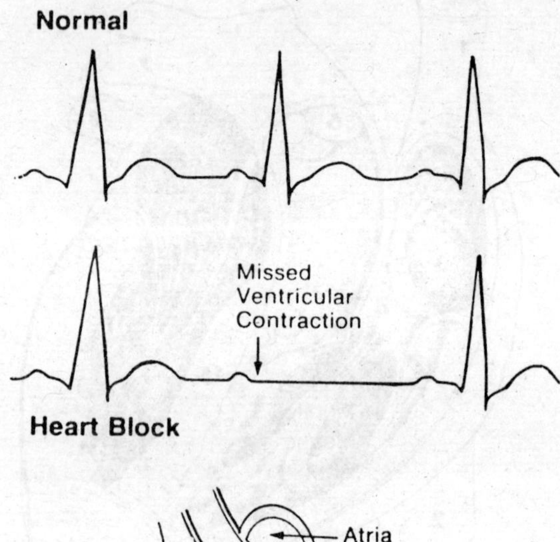
Normal
Missed Ventricular Contraction
Heart Block
Atria
Ventricles
Interruption in Conduction System

Heart Block—An electrocardiogram reveals the existence of a heart block. The condition results when the signal for the rhythmical heartbeat fails to reach the ventricles, the lower chambers of the heart. Without this electrical impulse, they contract more slowly than the two atria, the upper chambers, and miss a contraction.

Fig. 3.28

The heart is located in the thoracic cavity between the lobes of the lungs. It is a strong muscular pump, consisting of two distinct sides. The right side accepts blood from the body into the right auricle. The blood then passes through the valves into the right ventricle when

Table 3.10

Heart Rates (beats/minute)*

Animal	Average	Range
Human	70	58–104
Ass	50	40–56
Bat	750	100–970
Camel	30	25–32
Cat	120	110–140
Cow	55	45–70
Dog	–	100–130
Elephant	35	22–53
Giraffe	66	–
Goat	90	70–135
Guinea pig	280	260–400
Horse	44	23–70
Lion	40	–
Monkey	192	165–240
Mouse	534	324–858
Rabbit	205	123–304
Rat	328	261–600
Sheep	75	60–120
Skunk	166	144–192
Squirrel	249	96–378
Swine	–	58–86
Chicken (adult)	–	250–300
Chicken (baby)	–	350–450

*Adapted from *Merck Veterinary Manual*, 5th edition

the heart relaxes. As it contracts, the blood is circulated to the lungs through pulmonary artery to be enriched with oxygen.

The oxygeneted blood then returns from the lungs to the left side of the heart through pulmonary vein into left auricle. From this chamber it passes into the left ventricle, and thence to the dorsal aorta, the main artery of the body. From this numerous arteries convey blood to the capillary systems in the organs and tissues. The closing of the valves between the chambers (auricles and ventricles) is the heart beat. The heart beat can indicate the state of health of the animal. In normal adults it is for cattle: 45 to 60 per minute and for pigs and sheep: 70 to 80 per minute. If excited or stressed, the animals heart rate will rise. The heart undergoes contraction (systole) and relaxation (diastole) rhythmically throughout the animal's life.

Blood vessels

Blood circulates around the body in a network of tubes which vary in diameter from 0.0001 mm to 10.0 mm and form a continuous system. *Arteries* are blood vessels that carries

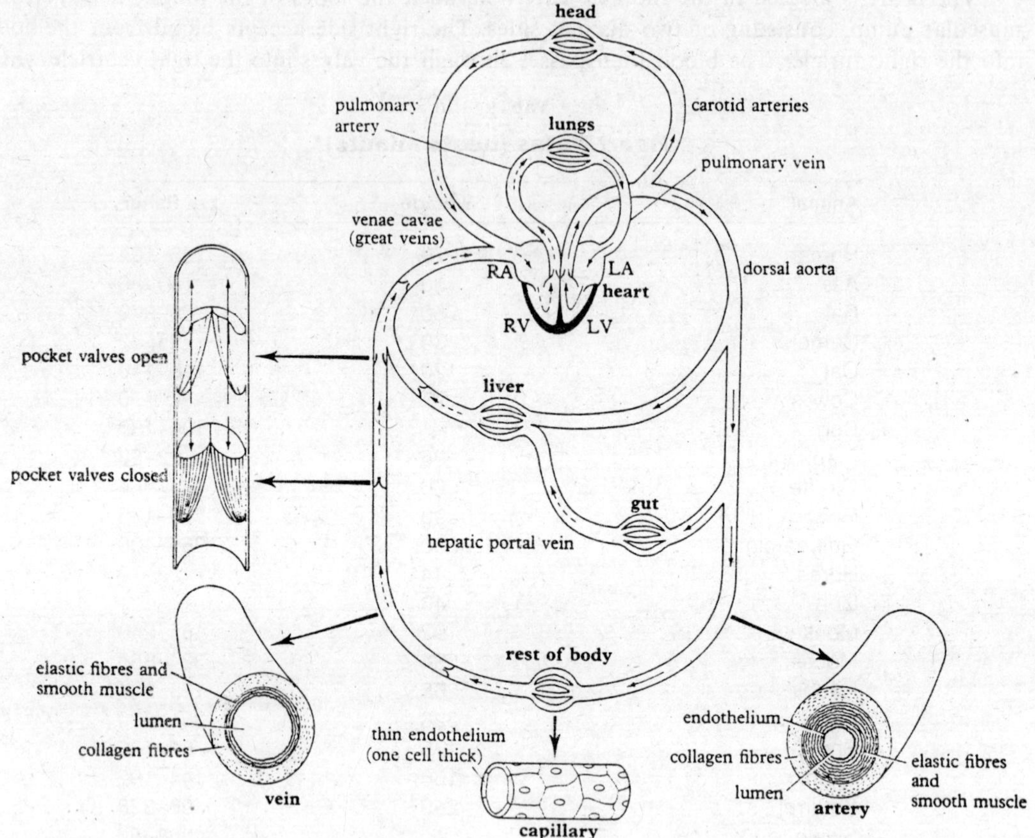

Fig. 3.29 General plan of the mammalian circulation and the detailed structure of some of its component structures. The thick tough walls of the arteries, well endowed with smooth muscle and connective tissue, are admirably suited to withstanding the pressures resulting from the pumping of the heart. The thinner-walled veins, equipped with pocket valves, minimize resistance to the flow of blood back to the heart after it has been through the narrow capillaries. The capillary walls are only one cell thick, thereby facilitating rapid diffusion of respiratory gases and soluble food materials between blood and tissues. **RA**, right atrium; **LA**, left atrium; **RV**, right ventricle; **LV**, left ventricle. Solid arrows, oxygenated blood; broken arrows, deoxygenated blood.

oxygen rich blood from the heart (except Pulmonary artery) to various body tissues. Walls are thick and contain heavy muscle layer that can withstand the blood pressure produced by heart. They branch into smaller and smaller tubes known as arterioles and then capillaries.

Capillaries are minute blood vessels that lie between the arterioles and the beginning of venules and veins. They are very tiny and thin walled (one cell thick) and widely distributed in all tissues. Transfer of nutrients from blood to tissue, and waste products from tissues to blood, occurs in capillaries.

The Veins. These are blood vessels that return blood from throughout the body to the heart and that convey it to the lungs, where carbon dioxide collected from the body and oxygen of the atmosphere are exchanged. Both arteries and veins have valves which prevent 'back flow'.

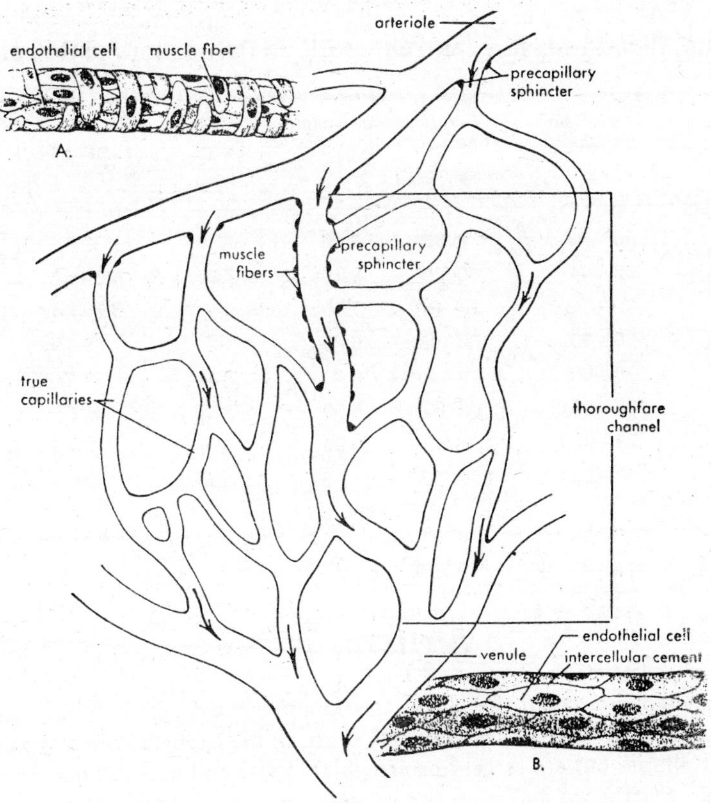

Fig. 3.30 Schematic representation of a capillary bed. Insert A shows some of the muscle fibers of the proximal part of a thoroughfare channel. Insert B shows a part of a true capillary.

Table 3.11 **Metabolic Parameters of Selected Species**

Common Name	Respiratory Rate (br/min)	Lung Tidal Volume (ml)	Body Temp (°C)	Lower Critical Temperature (°C)	Upper Critical Temperature (°C)	Basal Metabolic Rate (KCal)[a]	Pulse rate per mnt.
Beef cattle	12—20	3450.0	38.5	—21	27	8220	—
Dairy cattle	18—28	3450.0	38.5	—21	27	8220	45—55
Horse	8—16	9000.0	38.0	—	—	6840	30—40
Goat	10—20	310.0	39.0	20	28	—	70—80
Swine	8—18	—	39.0	18	32	3580	70—80
Sheep	10—20	—	39.5	—3	29	1875	70—80
Rabbit	36—56	15.8	38.9	—	—	190	—
Chicken	15—30	40.0	41.7	18	26	110	300
Turkey	25—35	—	—	—	—	—	—

a Calculated as 70 x BW $^{.75}$

Source : *Handbook of Animal Sc.* (1991), Putman, P.A. (ed)., Academic Press, Inc.

Table 3.12

Heart Rate, Blood Pressure, and Other Blood Parameters of Selected Species

Common Name	Heart Rate (Beats/Min)	Blood Pressure (sys/dias mm Hg)	Blood Volume (% live bw)	Blood pH	Hematocrit	Erythrocyte Diameter (µm)	Haemoglobin (g/dl)
Dairy cattle	60—70	134/88	7.70	7.38	32.4	5.6	11.0
Horse	32—44	80/50	9.70	7.35	28—42	5.6	14.5
Goat	70—135	120—84	7.00	—	27—34	4.1	10.0
Swine	60—80	169/108	6.75	—	39.1	6.2	13.0
Sheep	70—80	114/68	8.00	7.44	31.7	5.0	11.5
Rabbit	123—304	110/80	5.50	7.35	41.5	7.5	—
Chicken	178—458	131/95	5.00	7.54	32—45	7.0x12.0	9.0
Turkey	160—288	270/167 235/141	6.00—8.00	7.50	38	15.5x7.5	—

Source : *Handbook of Animal Sc.* (1991), Putman, P.A. (ed)., Academic Press, Inc.

LYMPHATIC SYSTEM

In parallel to blood circulatory system, the mammals have got another lymphatic system. It consists of (a) Lymph vessels—the channels begin in the tissue as blind lymph capillaries like that of blood capillaries but are larger and irregular in size and are situated throughout the body except the brain, spinal cord and eyes, (b) Lymph nodes also called lymph glands are discrete nodular structures scattered along the course of lymphatic vessels, and (c) Lymph, the tissue fluid.

How Lymph Is Produced?

The process of lymph formation is connected with the metabolic interchange between the blood and the tissues. As blood flows through the blood capillaries, part of the plasma nutrients and oxygen passes from the vessels into the surrounding tissues and forms the tissue fluid. The tissue fluid bathes the cells, and a continuous metabolic interchange takes place between the fluid and the cells; nutrients and oxygen enter the cell, and the waste products pass into the fluid. Part of the tissue fluid containing waste products returns to the blood through the walls of the blood capillaries. At the same time some tissue fluid passes not into the blood capillaries, but into the lymph capillaries and forms the lymph. The process of formation and outflow of lymph intensifies during increased activity of the organs.

Main Roles of the System

The system represents an accessory route by which fluids can flow from the interstitial spaces into the blood. And, most important of all, the lymphatics can carry proteins and even large particulate matter away from the tissue spaces, neither of which can be removed by absorption directly into the blood capillary. It also plays an important role in absorption and transportation of long chain fatty acids and vitamin K from the intestine to the blood. It also acts as a defence mechanism against noxious materials by filtering them out of tissue fluid and phagocytising them, thereby assisting in the control of infection and antibody formation.

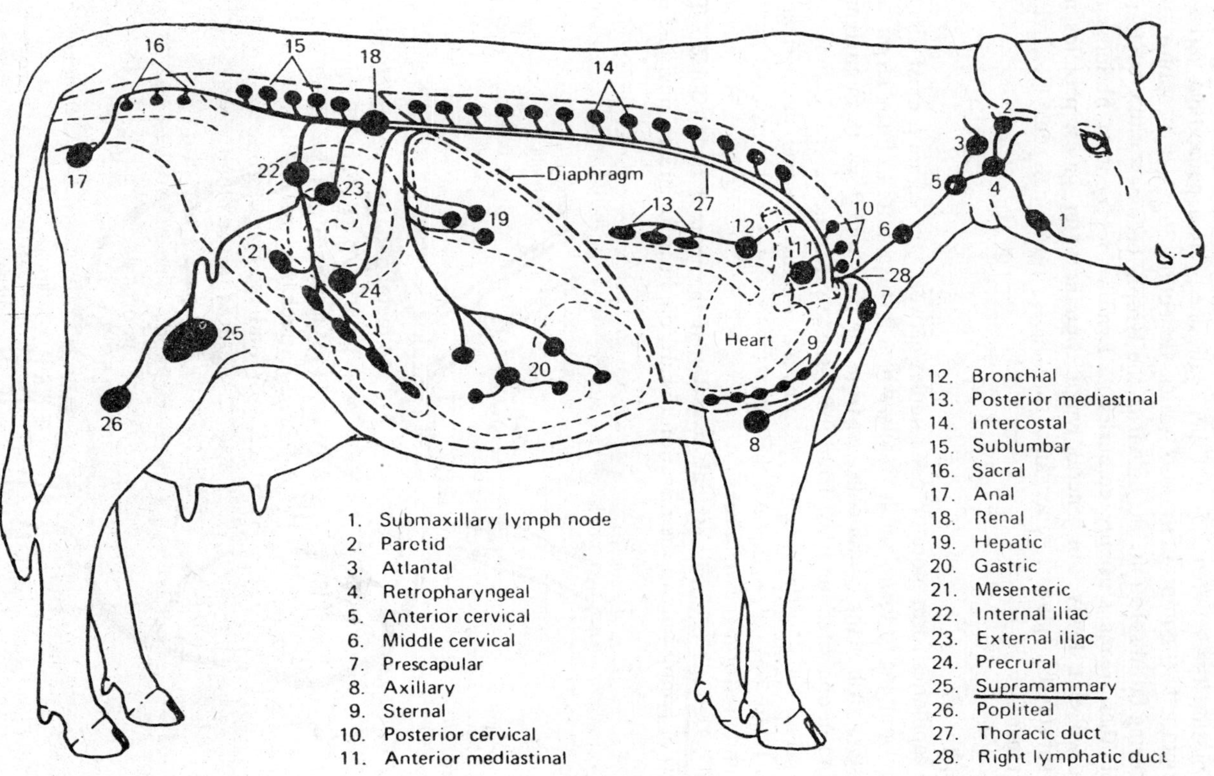

16
15
18
14
17
22
23
Diaphragm
13
27
12
10
19
21
24
11
28
25
7
Heart
9
20
26
8
2
3
5
4
6
1
1. Submaxillary lymph node
2. Parotid
3. Atlantal
4. Retropharyngeal
5. Anterior cervical
6. Middle cervical
7. Prescapular
8. Axillary
9. Sternal
10. Posterior cervical
11. Anterior mediastinal
12. Bronchial
13. Posterior mediastinal
14. Intercostal
15. Sublumbar
16. Sacral
17. Anal
18. Renal
19. Hepatic
20. Gastric
21. Mesenteric
22. Internal iliac
23. External iliac
24. Precrural
25. Supramammary
26. Popliteal
27. Thoracic duct
28. Right lymphatic duct

Fig. 3.31 Schematic drawing of the lymphatics of the Cow.

Composition of Lymph

Lymph is a mixture of capillary filtrate and tissue fluid which has entered lymph capillaries. The fluid resembles blood plasma except for a lower concentration of plasma proteins (2.2–3.4 per cent). In plasma it is between 5.5—6.7 per cent. The protein percentage varies depending upon the origin. The composition also varies depending upon the nature of nutrients absorbed. During fat absorption, the colour of the lymph becomes milky-white (the lymph flowing out of other organs is usually colourless). Lymph does contain fibrinogen and prothrombin, and will clot slowly. In general, lymph contains water, gases, proteins, non-protein nitrogenous substances, glucose, inorganic substances, hormones, enzymes, vitamins and immune substances.

Flow of Lymph

The lymph capillaries form more or less complex network throughout most tissues. These network finally combine to form lymph vessels, which in turn unite to form larger and larger lymphatic vessels. All of the lymph collected from the body and flows through lymph vessels are sluggish and in one direction only, from the tissue towards the heart. Ultimate object of the flow is to get an entry to the venous system by way of the *thoracic duct*, *right lymphatic duct* (if present) and *tracheal ducts*. All these ducts enter the cranial vena cava or the jugular veins as they unite to form the vena cava.

The lymph vessels have numerous valves scattered throughout their course. The valves permit the flow of lymph only in the direction toward the heart or great veins just cranial to the heart.

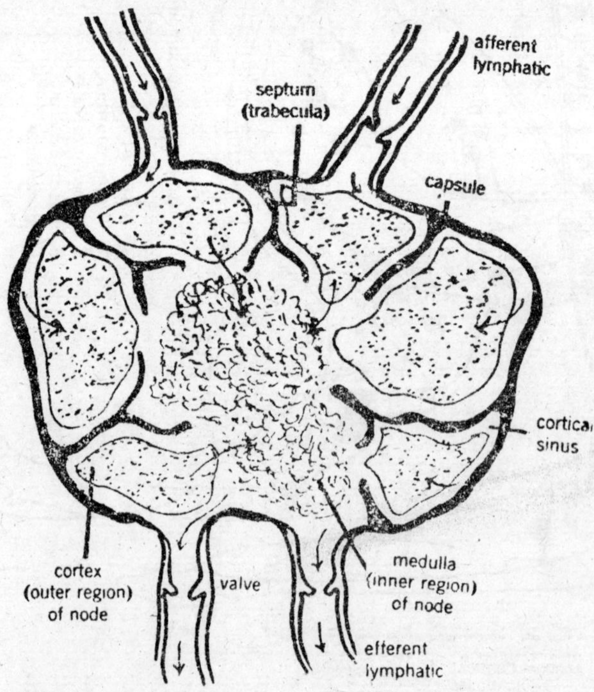

Fig. 3.32 Diagrammatic sketch of lymph node.

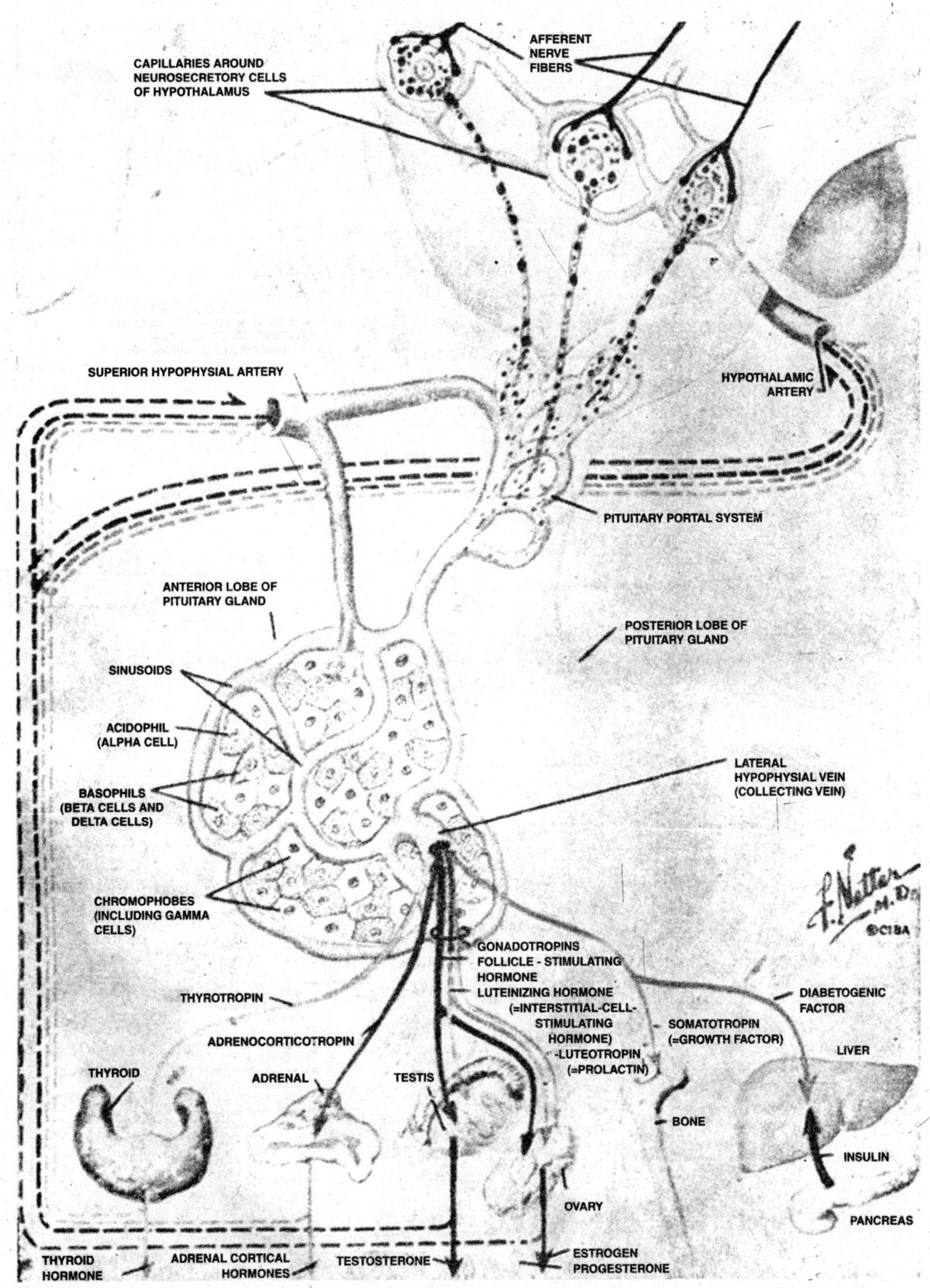

Plate 1. Relation of the hypothalamus to the anterior lobe of the pituitary gland. Note that the humoral substances from neurosecretory cells in the hypothalamus pass to the anterior lobe of the pituitary gland through the portal system (Copyright by CIBA Pharmaceutical Products Inc.).

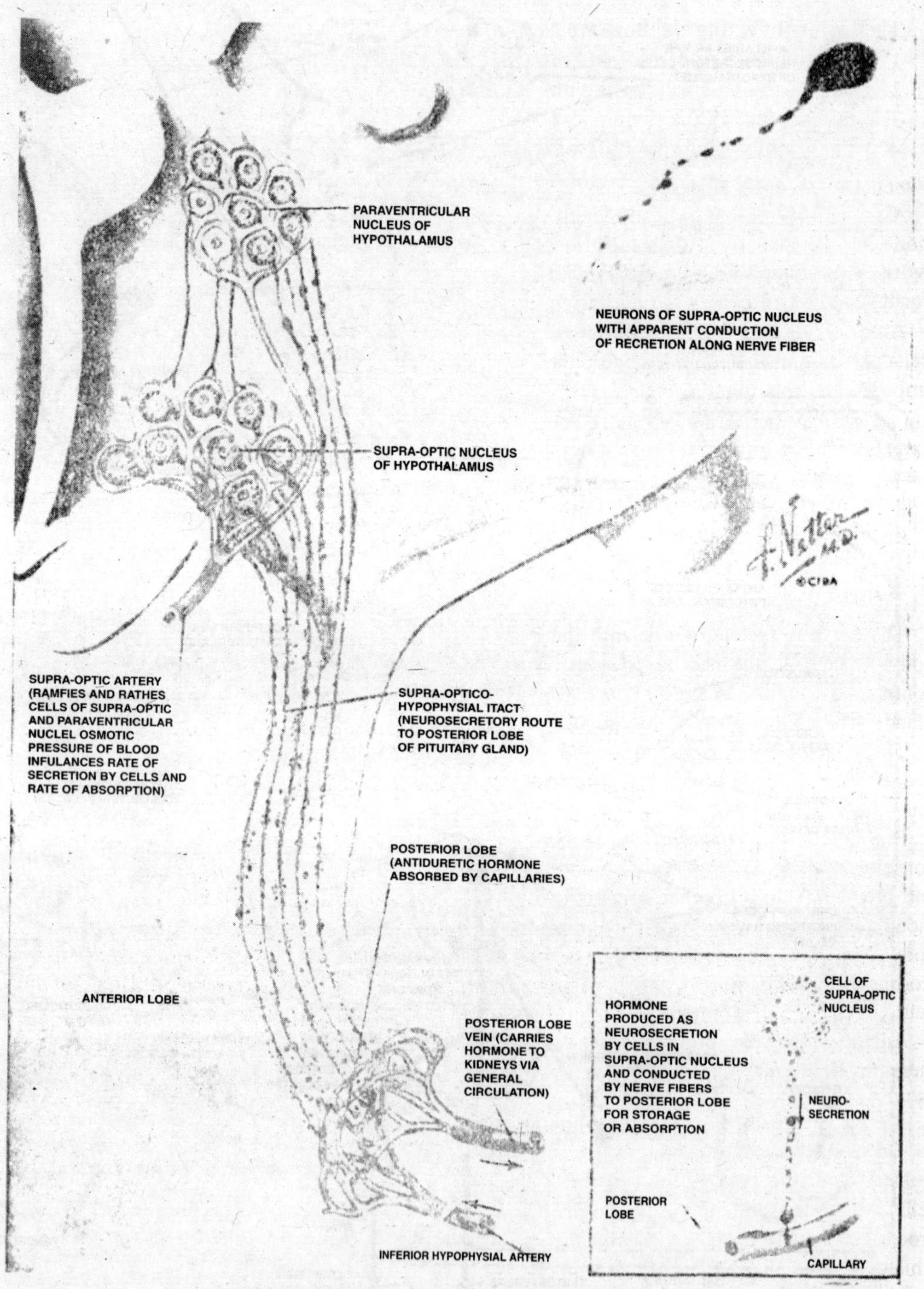

Plate 2. Relation of the hypothalamus to the posterior lobe of the pituitary gland. In contrast to the anterior lobe, the posterior lobe is innervated by the supraopticohypophyseal tract. The secretion products are conducted along the nerve fibers from the hypothalamus to the capillaries.
(Copyright by CIBA Pharmaceutical Products Inc.) Modified.

The factors affecting the flow are as follows:

1. the difference in pressure at the two ends of the lymph system,
2. the massaging effects of the muscular movements,
3. the presence in the lymph vessels of valves which permit flow in one direction only,
4. the propulsive contractility of lymphatic vessels.

Function of Lymph Nodes

Also called lymph glands, are small roundish or elongated masses of lymphatic tissue. Each node has a connective tissue capsule which gives off trabeculae into the interior. The framework of the lymph nodes consists of reticular tissue. Between the trabeculae are nodules which form lymphocytes. Consequently lymph nodes are haematopoietic organs.

Among functions of lymph nodes, is the production of lymphocytes which are phagocytic cells capable of ingesting foreign particles, thereby removing them from the lymph before it is implied into the blood.

In addition to filtering the lymph, the nodes have the ability to form antibodies. Thus when bacteria and protein antigens arrives at lymph nodes, they are first phagocytised, and then during the following week or more specific antibodies are formed against them and emptied into the circulating body fluids to destroy additional bacteria or bacterial toxins.

NERVOUS SYSTEM

The nervous system, along with the endocrine system, provides the control functions for the body. In general, the nervous system controls the rapid activities of the body, such as muscular contractions, rapidly changing visceral events and even the rates of secretion of some endocrine glands. The endocrine system regulates principally the metabolic functions of the body.

The nervous system is unique in the vast complexity of the control reactions that it can perform. It can receive literally thousands of bits of information from the different sensory organs and then integrate all these to determine the response to be made by the body.

Brain is the supervisory centre of the nervous system in all vertebrates. The brain controls both conscious behaviour (e.g. walking and thinking, and most involuntary behaviour (e.g., heartbeat and breathing). In all higher animals it is also the site of emotions, memory, self awareness and thought. It functions by receiving information via nerve cells (neurons) from every part of the body, evaluating the data, and then sending directives to muscle and glands apart from simply storing the information. A single neuron may receive information from as many as 1,000 other neurons.

Anatomically, the brain occupies the skull cavity and is enveloped by three protective membranes.

Components of the Nervous System

Nervous tissue is composed of three functionally different types of cells: (1) *Neurons* (nerve cells), which transmit impulses; (2) *Schwann cells*, which form a segmented covering around the processes of many of the neurons of the peripheral nervous system; and (3) *Neuroglia* (glial cells), which are specialized to serve as supportive tissues between the neurons in the central nervous system.

Neurons

The neuron (nerve cell) is the basic anatomic and physiologic unit of the nervous system. It has the ability to respond to stimulation by initiating and conducting an impulse. Some other cells such as muscle fibres, are also capable of conducting impulses, but the unique shape of the nerve cell makes it specially well suited to serve as communicator. Neurons possess process that can be quite long. For example, in some cases a single neuron—that is, a single cell—extends from the spinal cord to the tip of a toe!

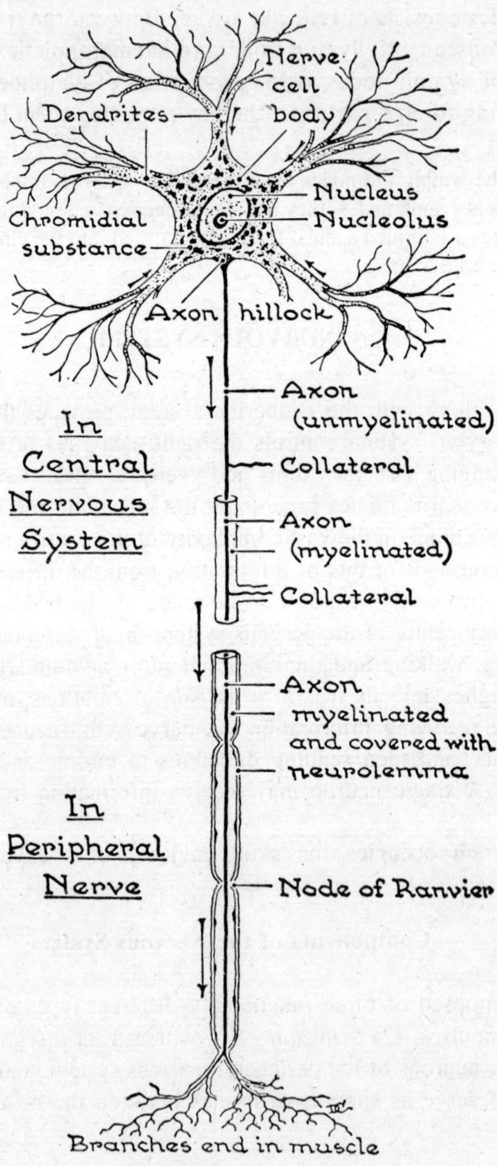

Fig. 3.33 Diagram of a multipolar neuron.

Schwann Cells

In some nerve fibres axons are surrounded by a type of satellite cell called Schwann cells.

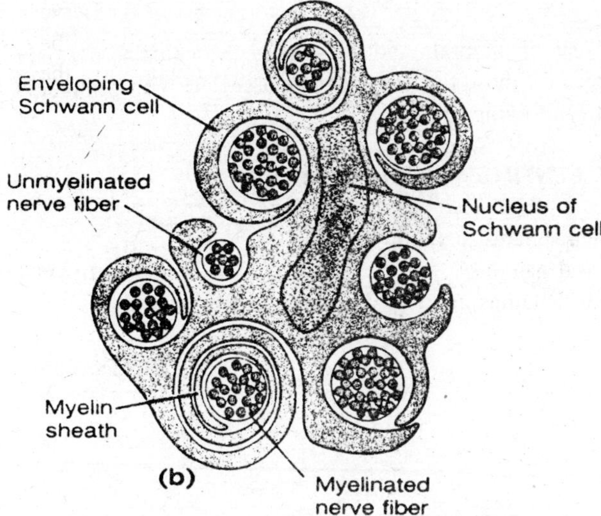

Fig. 3.34 The ultrastructure of myelinated and unmyelinated neurons. **(a)** Diagram of a myelinated nerve fiber. **(b)** A single Schwann cell encompassing eight neurons. The neurons around which the Schwann cell has coiled are myelinated; the neurons thar are simply engulfed by the Schwann cell are unmyelinated.

Neuroglia

There are billions of neurons within the central nervous system, there are even more supportive cells distributed among the neurons. These are neuroglia thought to provide structural support for the neurons, are involved in the transfer of nutrients and assist in the removal of waste products from the neurons.

Organization of Nervous System

Although there is actually only one nervons system, it can be thought of as being separated into various divisions based on either structural locations or unique functional characteristics. It should be kept in mind, however, that these divisions—which are themselves called *nervous systems*—are all integral parts of a single nervous system. Structurally, the nervous system may be

Table 3.13 **Organisation of the Nervous System**

According to location	*According to function*
Central Nervous System	**Scmatic Nervous System**
Brain	**Autonomic Nervous System**
Spinal cord	Sympathetic nervous system
Peripheral Nervous System	Parasympathetic nervous system
Cranial nerves and their associated receptors and ganglia	
Spinal nerves and their associated receptors and ganglia	

divided into two parts (1) *The Central Nervous System* and (2) *peripheral nervous system*. but according to function, (1) Somatic nervous system and (2) Autonomic nervous system as below:

Central Nervous System

The Central nervous system (CNS) consists of the brain and the spinal cord, contains not only components of transmission, but also provides for those functions that we associate with computors such as memory, a central processing unit for solving problems.

DIVISION OF THE CENTRAL NERVOUS SYSTEM

1. BRAIN	Cerebrum; Cerebral hemispheres including Cerebral cortex and basal ganglia Diencephalon including thalamus and hypothalamus	**FOREBRAIN**
	Mid brain Pons Medulla	**BRAINSTEM**
	Cerebellum	

2. SPINAL CORD

The brain is completely encased within 10 bony structures, the cranial cavity of the skull and the spinal cord within the Vertebrate canal of the spinal column.

The Brain

The brain is the part of the CNS that is situated in the cranial cavity. It is developed from three primary vesicles: the prosencephalon (forebrain), mesencephalon (midbrain) and rhombencephalon (hindbrain). By further growth, elongation and bending, the primary vesicles become divided into

Table 3.14

Subdivisions of the Neural Tube and the Major Adult Structures Derived from Each

Primary division	*Subdivision*	*Adult brain structures*	*Neural canal region*
Prosencephalon (forebrain)	Telencephalon	Cerebral hemispheres (cerebrum) Cerebral cortex Basal ganglia Olfactory bulbs and tracts	Lateral ventricles and upper portion of the third ventricle
	Diencephalon	Epithalamus Thalamus Hypothalamus	Most of the third ventricle
Mesencephalon (midbrain)	Mesencephalon	Corpora quadrigemina Cerebral peduncles	Cerebral aqueduct
Rhombencephalon (hindbrain)	Metencephalon	Cerebellum Pons	Fourth ventricle
	Myelencephalon	Medulla oblongata	Part of the fourth ventricle
Spinal cord	Spinal cord	Spinal cord	Central canal

5 secondary vesicles. Further details of the major adult derivatives of the secondary five vesicles as well as the cavities that drain them are given below:

Short description about some major brain structures are given below:

1. *Brainstem*: The brainstem is literally the stalk of the brain: through it passes all the nerve fibres relaying signals of affarent input and efferent output between the spinal cord and higher brain centres. In addition brainstem gives rise to a number of pairs of cranial nerves. It is composed of (i) Midbrain, (ii) Pons, (iii) Medulla oblongata.

Running through the entire brainstem is a core of tissue called the reticular formation, which is composed of small, highly branched neurons.

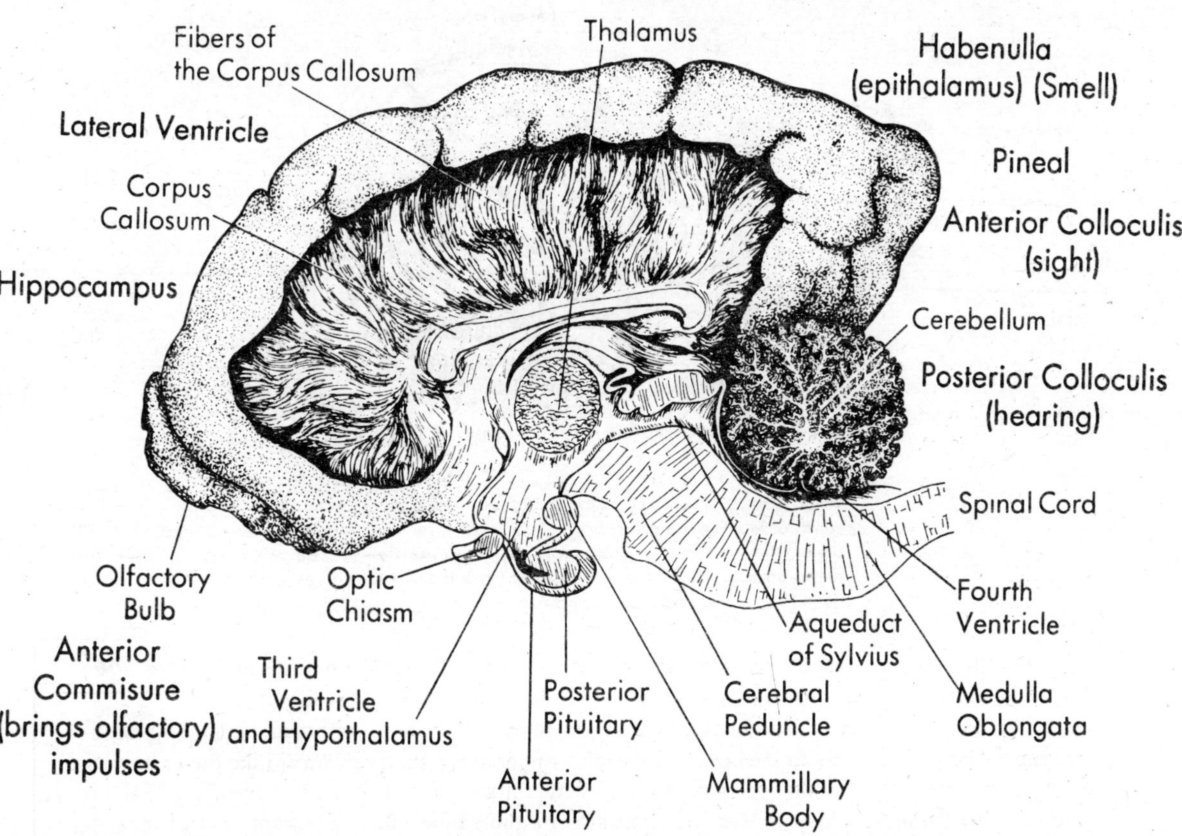

Fig. 3.35 Sagittal section of the brain partially excavated. (After Meyer in Miller, Christensen, and Evans, Anatomy of the Dog, courtesy of W. B. Saunders Co.)

2. *Cerebellum*: The *Cerebellum* functions as a coordinator (maintaining balance) of the brain's other centres and is a mediator between them and the body. It functions chiefly as a coordinator of *muscular activity* in eating, talking, running and walking. Damage to the cerebellum results in incoordination, which interferes with voluntary muscular action, but it does not cause paralysis. Farm animals have a large cerebellum, although elephants and whales probably have the largest

to body size. The location of the cerebellum relative to the brainstem and forebrain can be seen (Fig.3.36).

3. *Forebrain*: The large part of the brain remaining when the brainstem and cerebellum have been excluded in the forebrain. It consists of a central core (the diencephalon) and the right and left *cerebral hemisphere* (the cerebrum). The hemispheres, although largely separated by a longitudinal divisions are connected to each other by axon bundles known as *Commissures*, the *Corpus callosum* being the largest.

The outer part of the cerebral hemispheres, the cerebral cortex, is a cellular shell about 3 mm thick. The cortex is divided into several parts, or lobes (the frontal, parietal, occipital and temporal lobes. (Fig. 3.36).

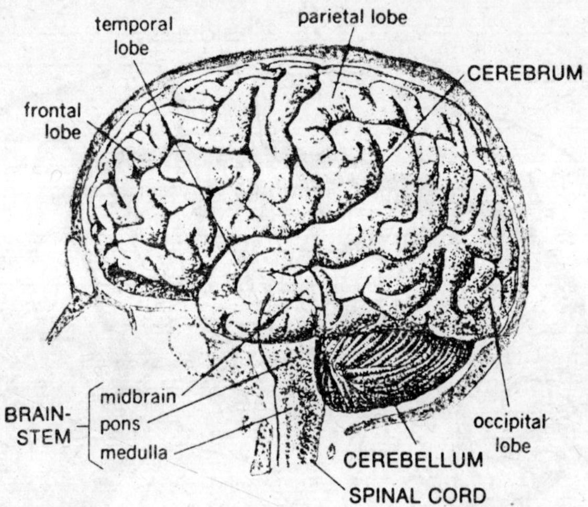

Fig.3.36 The three major divisions of the brain: the brainstem, cerebellum, and forebrain. The outer layer of the forebrain (the cerebrum) consists of four lobes, as shown. The diencephalon, which is an extension of the brainstem and lies deep within the brain, is not shown.

The cortex is an area of grey matter. In other parts of the forebrain, nerve fibre tracts predominate, their whitish myelin coating distinguishing them as white matter.

4. The *thalamus*, part of the diencephalon, is a relay station and important integrating centre for sensory input on its way to the cortex and is also important in motor control. Like the brainstem, it contains a central cone that is part of the reticular formation. The *hypothalamus*, which lies below the thalamus is a tiny region. It appears to be the single most important control area for the regulation of the internal environment.

5. The pons and *medulla oblongata* control reflex action such as breathing, swallowing, vomiting and blinking of the eyelids. They usually act independently of the cerebrum and cerebellum.

Spinal Cord

The spinal cord is a slender cylinder about as big around as the little figer in adult cattle and buffaloes.

Fig(3.37) shows the basic division of a cross section of the spinal cord. The central butterfly—

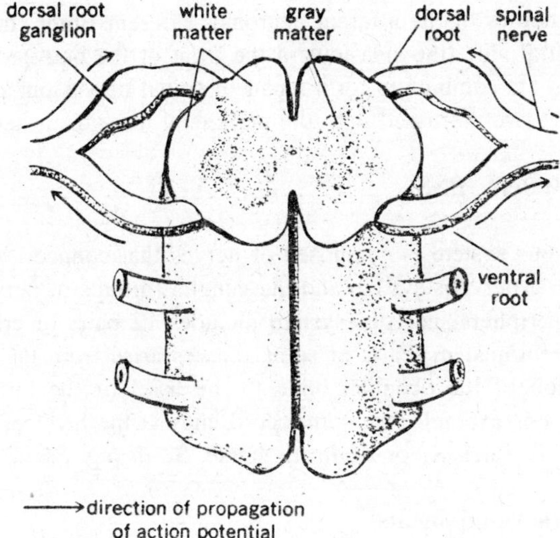

Fig. 3.37. Section of the spinal cord (ventral view i.e., fror the front).

shaped area is called the *grey matter*; it is filled with interneurons, the entering fibres of affarent neurons, and glial cells. The grey region is surrounded by *white matter*, which consists largely of myelinated axons. These axons are organized into groups called tracts and pathways, which run longitudinally through the cord, some descending to convey information from the brain to the spinal cord (or from upper to lower levels of the cord), other ascending to transmit in the opposite direction.

Groups of affarent fibres (from peripheral receptors) enter the spinal cord on the dorsal side (the side toward the back of the body); these groups form the *dorsal roots* and contain the *dorsal*

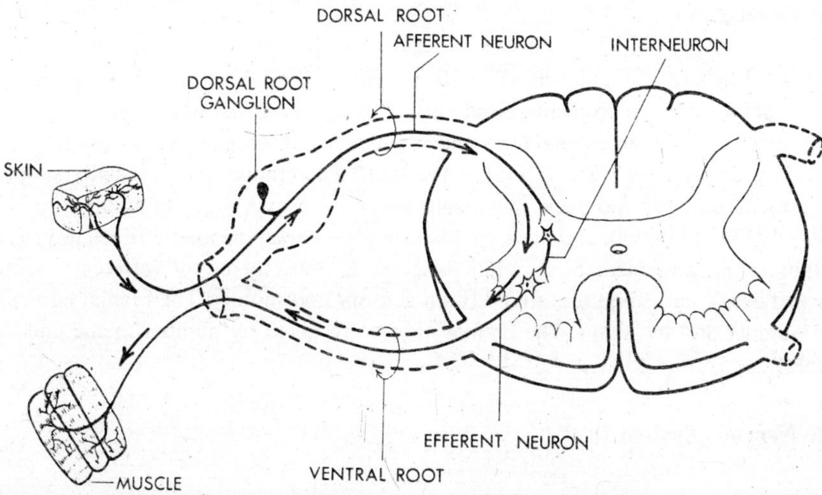

Fig. 3.38–Diagrammatic cross-section of the spinal cord. (Kitchell in Miller, Christensen, and Evans, *Anatomy of the Dog*, courtesy of W. B. Saunders Co.)

root ganglia (the cell bodies of the affarent neurons). Efferent fibres (to effector cells) leave the spinal cord on the ventral side (the side toward the front of the body) via the *ventral roots.*

Dorsal and ventral roots combine to form a pair of spinal nerves one on each side of the spinal cord. (The spinal nerves are discussed with the peripheral nervous system).

Peripheral Nervous System (PNS)

The peripheral nervous system is composed of nerves that connect the more outlying parts of the body with the central nervous system and the ganglia (groups of nerve cell bodies) associated with the nerves. The peripheral nervous system includes 12 pairs of cranial nerves, which arise from the brain and the brainstem. Pairs of spinal nerves arise from the spinal cord, which itself extends from the region of the occipital bone to the level of the lumber and sacral vertebra, depending on species. For example, the spinal cord ends at the level of the first sacral vertebrae (S1) in the bovine (S3 in calf); S1 or S2 in the horse, S2 in pig, S1 in sheep and goat.

Spinal Nerves (Somatic Components)

The somatic division also known as voluntary nervous system and is made up of all the fibres going from the central nervous system to skeletal muscle cells. The cell bodies of these neurons are located in groups in the brain or spinal cord; their large diameter, myelinated axons leave the central nervous system and pass directly (i.e. without any synapse) to skeletal muscle cells. The neurotransmitter substance released by these neurons is *acetylcholine*.

With the exception of cervical nerves and coccygeal nerves, there is a pair of spinal nerves (one right and one left which emerge behind the vertebra of the same serial number and name).

Almost as soon as the spinal nerve emerges from the vertebral canal it divides into a dorsal branch and a ventral branch. Both of these branches are mixed nerves, because it contains both sensory and motor fibres.

Cranial Nerves

There are 12 pairs of cranial nerves with a right and left nerve comprising each pair. Most of the cranial nerves emerge from the basal surface of the brainstem and have their nuclei of origin in the brainstem. After emerging from the brainstem, the cranial nerves usually leave from the cranial cavity through holes (foramina) in the skull. The cranial nerves usually supply innervation to structures in the head and neck. The vagus nerve is an exception. In addition to its sensory and motor supply to the pharynx and larynx it also supplies parasympathetic fibres to visceral structures in the thorax and abdomen. Some cranial nerves are strictly motor (efferent), some are strictly sensory (affarent), and some are mixed (both sensory and motor). The cranial nerves are designed both by number and by name. The cranial nerves are listed by number, name and distribution as listed below.

Somatic Nervous System

It is also called the voluntary nervous system. It includes somatic *motor nerve* cells or efferent neurons that carry impulses from the central nervous system to the skeletal muscle, thus produces contraction of the skeletal muscle. This may be under the conscious control of the individual or

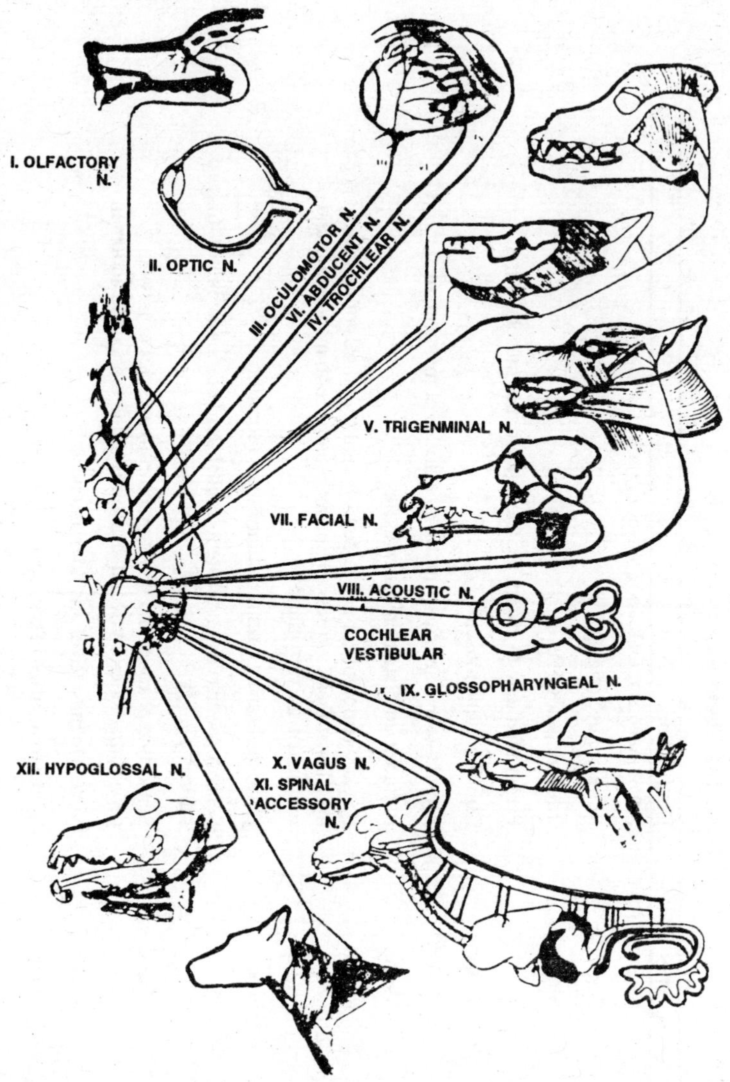

Fig. 3.39 Origin and distribution of cranial nerves in dog.

in the case of reflex response which may not be conciously controlled.

Somatic *sensory nerve cells* or *affarent neurons* carry impulses from the sense organs like skin, the fascia and around the joint to the central nervous system.

Autonomic Nervous System

The autonomic nervous system differs anatomically from the somatic motor mechanism. The chief difference lies in the fact that the autonomic fibres which originate in the spinal cord do not innervate muscle or gland directly. It may be seen that the fibre ends in synaptic union with a

Table 3.15

Cranial Nerves

No.	Name	Type	Distribution
I	Olfactory	Sensory	Nasal mucous membrane (sense of smell)
II	Optic	Sensory	Retina of eye (sight)
III	Oculomotor	Motor	Most muscles of eye
			Parasympathetic to ciliary muscle and circular muscle of iris
IV	Trochlear	Motor	Dorsal oblique muscle of eye
V	Trigeminal	Mixed	Sensory-to eye and face; motor-to muscles of mastication.
VI	Abducens	Motor	Retractor and lateral rectus muscles of eye
VII	Facial	Mixed	Sensory-region of ear and taste to cranial two-thirds of tongue; motor-to muscles of facial expression; parasympathetic-to mandibular and sublingual salivary glands.
VIII	Vestibulocochlear	Sensory	Cochlea (hearing); semicircular canals (equilibrium)
IX	Glossopharyngeal	Mixed	Sensory-to pharynx and taste to caudal third of tongue; motor -to parotid salivary glands
X	Vagus	Mixed	Sensory-to pharynx and larynx; motor -to muscles of larynx; parasympathetic-to visceral structures in the thorax and addomen
XI	Spinal accessory	Motor	Motor- to muscles of shoulder and neck
XII	Hypoglossal	Motor	Motor-to muscles of tongue

Modified from Frandson, R.D. : Anatomy and Physiology of Farm Animals. 4th Ed. Philadelphia, Lea & Febiger, 1986, p 84.

second neuron which does innervate a muscle or gland. This is in direct contradistinction to the somatic fibre which connects the spinal cord directly with an effector organ. Thus, in considering the autonomic nervous system, we speak of *preganglionic* and *postganglionic* fibres. The preganglionic fibres terminate in the ganglion consisting of cell bodies which give rise to postganglionic fibres. These later fibres innervate smooth muscles and glands.

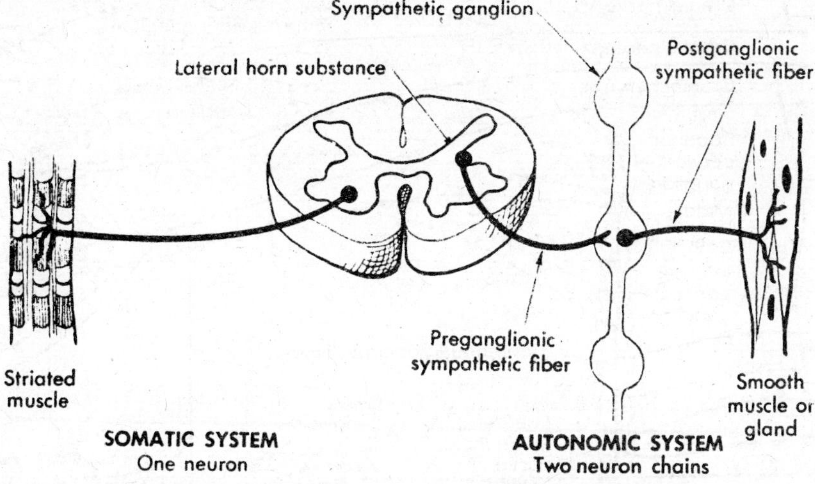

Fig. 3.40 Comparison of the somatic and autonomic nervous systems. Note that in the somatic system there is only one neuron; in the autonomic system there are always two.

The autonomic nervous system is composed of two parts: (1) *the sympathetic* and (2) *the parasympathetic* divisions. Both are parts of peripheral nervous system that innervates smooth muscle, cardiac muscle and glands, i.e., these are associated with visceral structures, while the remainder of the peripheral nervous system is associated with somatic structures.

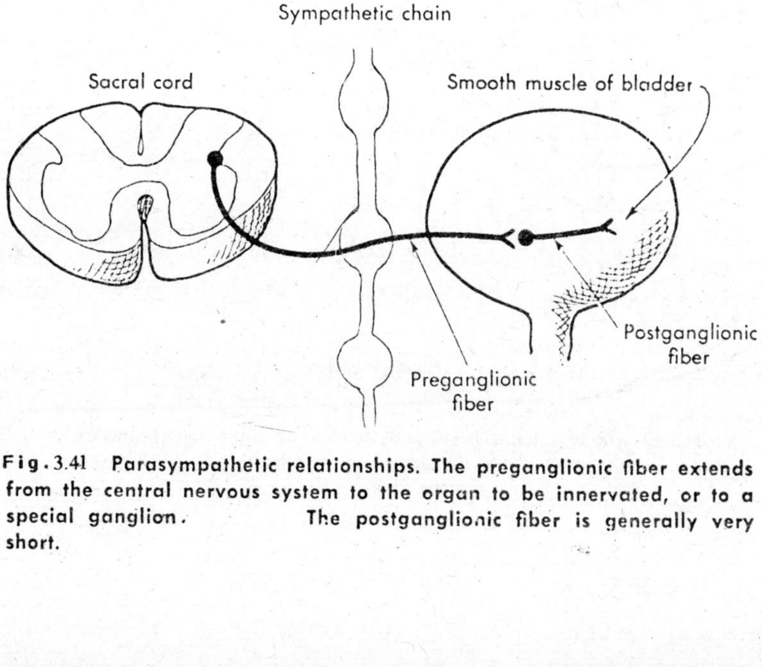

Fig. 3.41 Parasympathetic relationships. The preganglionic fiber extends from the central nervous system to the organ to be innervated, or to a special ganglion. The postganglionic fiber is generally very short.

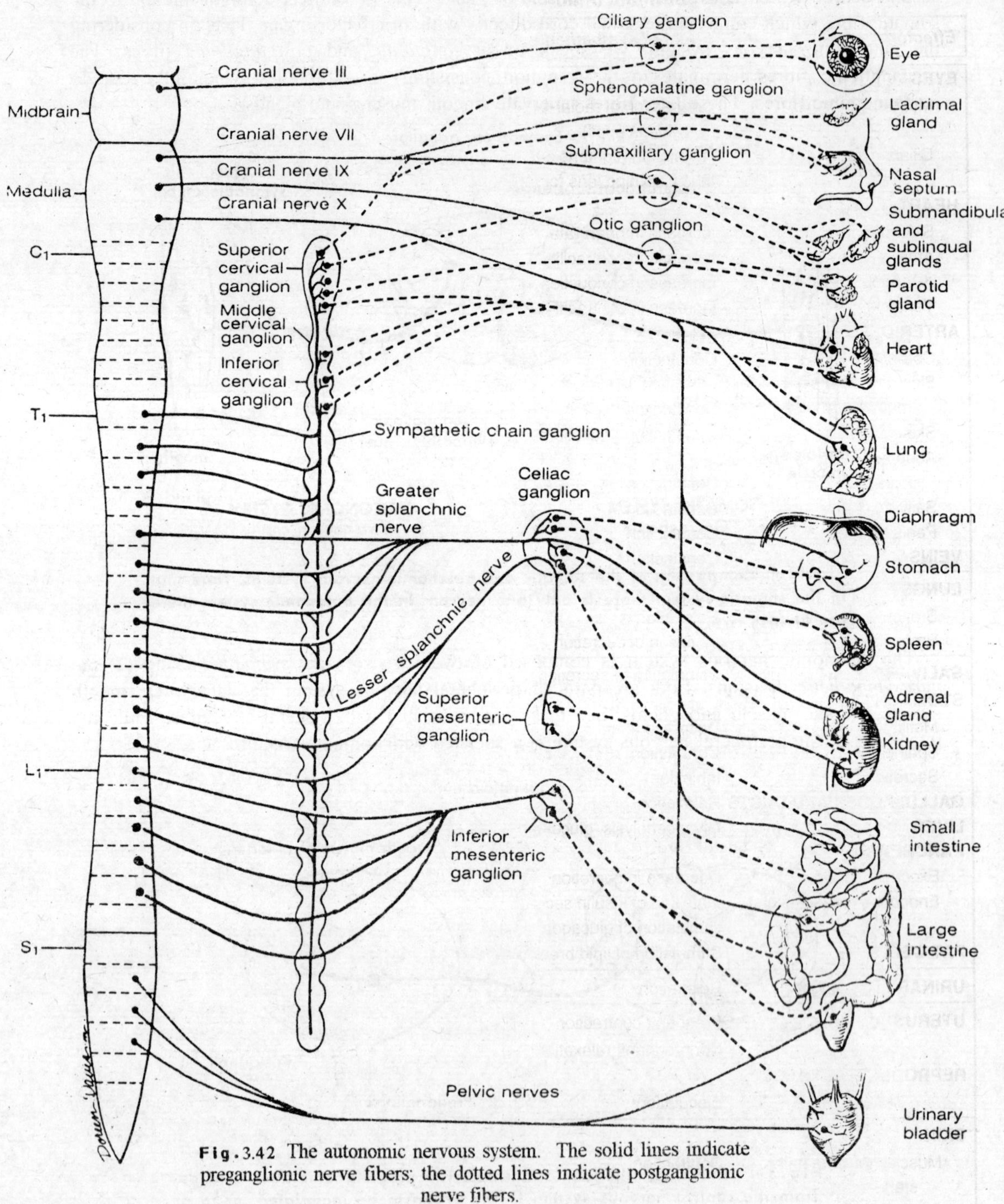

Fig. 3.42 The autonomic nervous system. The solid lines indicate preganglionic nerve fibers; the dotted lines indicate postganglionic nerve fibers.

Table 3.16

Some effects of autonomic nervous system activity

Effectors	*Effect of sympathetic nervous system*	*Effect of parasympathetic nervous system*
EYES		
Muscles of the iris	Contraction of radial muscle (widens pupil)	Contraction of sphincter muscle (makes pupil smaller)
Ciliary muscle	Relaxation (tightens suspensory ligaments thus flattening lens for far vision)	Contraction (relaxes ligament, allowing lens to become more convex for near vision)
HEART		
S-A node	Increase in heart rate	Decrease in heart rate
Atria	Increase in contracility	Decrease in contractility
A-V node	Increase in conduction velocity	Decrease in conduction velocity
Ventricles	Increase in contractility	Decrease in contractility
ARTERIOLES		
Coronary	Constriction	Dilation
Skin and mucous membrane	Constriction	——— ‡
Skeletal muscle	Constriction or dilation	———
Abdominal viscera and kidneys	Constriction	———
Salivary glands	Constriction	———
Penis or clitoris	Constriction	Dilation (causes erection)
VEINS	Constriction	———
LUNGS		
Bronchial muscle	Relaxation	Contraction
Bronchial glands	Inhibition of secretion	Stimulation of secretion
SALIVARY GLANDS	Stimulation of secretion	Stimulation of secretion
STOMACH		
Motility	Decrease	Increase
Sphincters	Contraction	Relaxation
Secretion	Inhibition	Stimulation
GALLBLADDER AND DUCTS	Relaxation	Contraction
LIVER	Glycogenolysis, gluconeogenesis	———
PANCREAS		
Exocrine glands	Decrease in secretion	Stimulation of secretion
Endocrine glands (islets)	Inhibition of insulin secretion, stimulation of glucagon secretion	Stimulation of insulin secretion
FAT CELLS	Stimulation of lipid breakdown	———
URINARY BLADDER	Relaxation	Contraction
UTERUS	Pregnant; contraction Nonpregnant; relaxation	Variable
REPRODUCTIVE TRACT (male)	Ejaculation	———
SKIN		
Muscles causing hair to stand erect	Contraction	———
Sweat glands	Stimulation of secretion	Stimulation of secretion
LACRIMAL GLANDS	———	Stimulation of secretion

‡ means that these cells are not innervated by this branch of the autonomic nervous system.

Between sympathetic and parasympathetic divisions, they differ from one another anatomically and physiologically. However, they are alike in that both contain preganglionic and postganglionic fibres. Anatomically they differ with respect to the locations of their ganglia. Most of the sympathetic ganglia lie close to the spinal cord in contrast the parasympathetic ganglia lie within the effector organ.

In both sympathetic and parasympathetic divisions, the major neurotransmitter released at the ganglionic synapse between pre- and postganglionic fibres is *acctylcholine.* In the parasympathetic divisions, the neurotransmitter between the postganglionic fibre and the effector cell is also *acctylcholine.* In the sympathetic division, the transmitter between the postganglionic fibre and the effector cell is usually *norepinephrine.*

The role of autonomic nervous system in the homeostatic control of the internal environment is detailed in Table(3.16.)

EYE

Fig. 3.43 shows a cross-sectional diagramme of the eyeball. It rests upon a pad of fat within the cavity in the skull called orbit, where it is held in position by bony walls and partly by the action of the eyelids, and partly through the agency of seven ocular muscles and the optic nerve around which they are arranged.

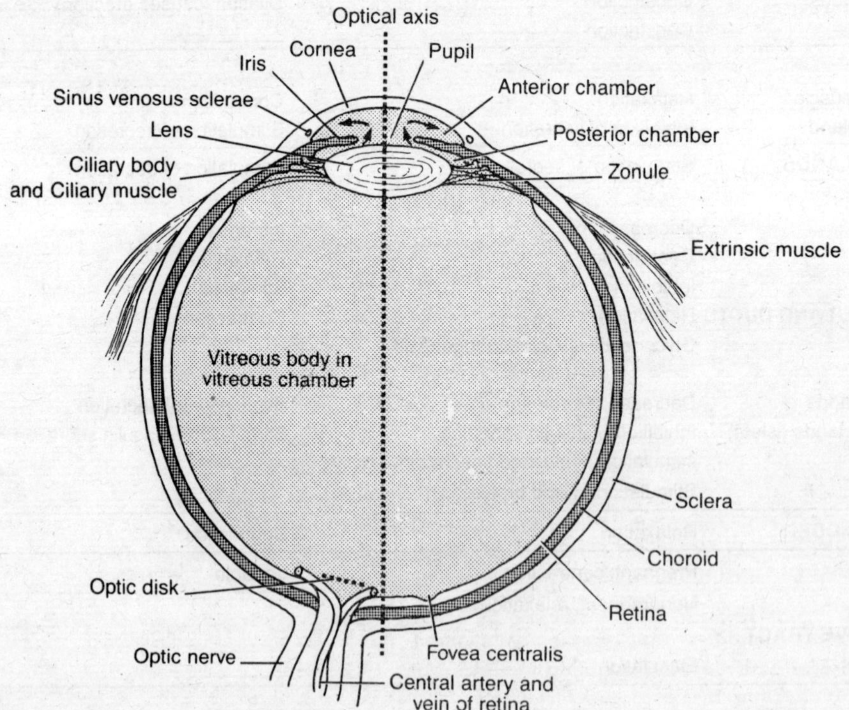

Fig. 3.43. ***Diagram of an eyeball showing its basic structure.*** From Cormack, D.C.: Cormack's Introduction to Histology. Philadelphia, J.B. Lippincott, 1984.

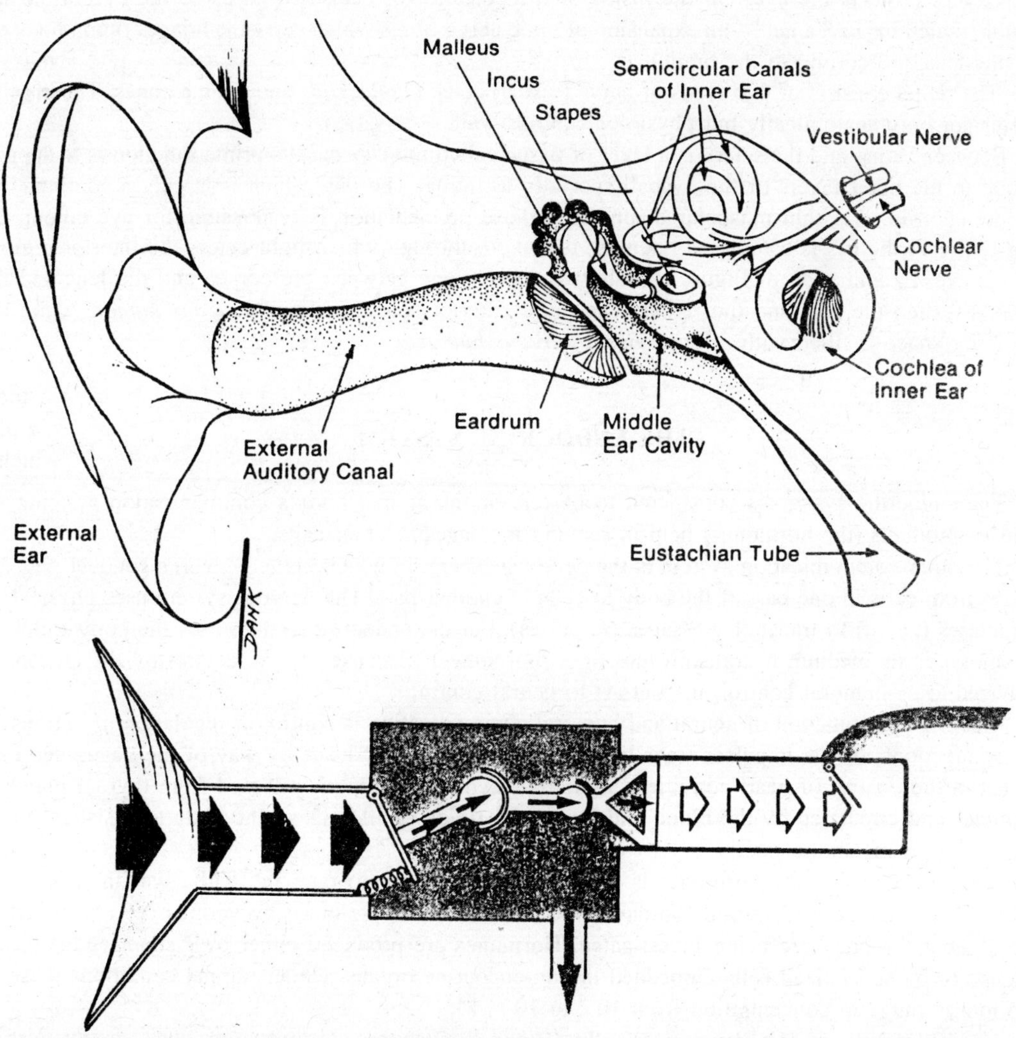

The External Ear collects, amplifies and transmits Sound Waves to the Eardrum causing it to vibrate.

Eardrum Vibrations set up a 3-Bone chain reaction in air-filled Middle Ear.

Vibrations cause Movement of Cochlear Fluid, stimulating Nerve Endings which send Sound Impulses to Hearing Center in Brain.

Ear—This drawing simplifies the complexity of the ear and explains the process of hearing. Injury or disease affecting the eardrum, three tiny bones (malleus, incus and stapes), middle ear cavity, auditory nerves or the hearing center of the brain can interfere with the reception or transmission of sound. The result is a loss of hearing ranging from slight to severe.

Fig. 3.44

The outer layer consists of dense white fibrous tissue known as *sclera*, which means hard. Sclera gives shape to the eyeball. The most anterior continuation of sclera is transparent and known as *corona*, it is also tough and resistant material and thus not only permits the passage of light but effectively protects the eye. On the inside of the posterior or back two-thirds of the eyeball is the *retina*, which means "a net"—an expansion of optic nerve fibres which carry the images (upon focused by the lens and cornia) to the brain.

The retina consists of two types of nerve (visual) cells: (1) the *rods* and (2) the cones. These cells differ not only anatomically but physiologically as well.

Between retina and the sclera is a layer of tissue called the *choroid*. Its prime function is to supply blood to the outer layers of the eyeball specially to retina. The *iris*, which is largely a continuation of the choroid, is a thin muscular diaphragm whose pigmentation is responsible for eye colour. In the centre of the iris is a rounded opening, the *pupil*, through which light enters the interior regions of the eye. Examination of Figure reveals two spaces, one between the cornea and the lens and the other between the lens and the retina. The more anterior space contains *aqueous humor*, while the posterior space is filled with a more viscid *vitreous humor*.

THE ENDOCRINE SYSTEM

The endocrine system is considered to be one of the animal body's communication systems, and its products (the hormones) help in sending messages to other cells.

The other communication system is the nervous system, in which nerve networks conduct messages from cells in one part of the body to cells in another part. The nervous system uses physical structures (nerve) to transmit messages (impulses), but the endocrine system uses the body fluids (humors) as its medium to transmit messages (hormones). Because of this, control by the later is referred to as humoral control, in contrast to neural control.

The principal function of neural and humoral communication is control or regulation of various body functions. Nerve impulses travelling from the brain to the heart by way of the vagus nerve assist in the control of heart activities. Similarly, thyroid hormone is released from thyroid gland follicles and circulated by the blood and interstitial fluids to all cells of the body to assist in the regulation of metabolic rate.

The discovery of new hormones is growing at an astounding rate. In 1970 fewer than 30 of these chemicals were identified. To-day some 200 hormones produced by various cells scattered throughout the body are being investigated. Hormones are produced either by distinct endocrine glands or by specialized cells embedded in non-endocrine organs. Under normal conditions these hormones range in concentration from 10^{-9} to 10^{-11} M.

Hormones have so long been classically defined as chemical substances produced by ductless glands that are released into the blood and carried to other parts of the body to produce regulatory effects.

This definition does not anymore stand good since some new hormonal compounds neither secreted from ductless glands nor they are released into the blood stream, viz., Prostaglandins are not produced in any one gland of the body, but are produced by most of the body cells. Furthermore, prostaglandins can be transmitted by diffusion in the interstitial fluid rather than by circulation in the blood.

Therefore, Hormones may now be defined as organic chemical messengers to perform intercellular signals, many of which are secreted by ductless glands. They reach their targets via the bloodstream or tissue fluids, eliciting changes in their specific target cells which may be the same cell that produced them or situated anywhere in the body in minute amounts.

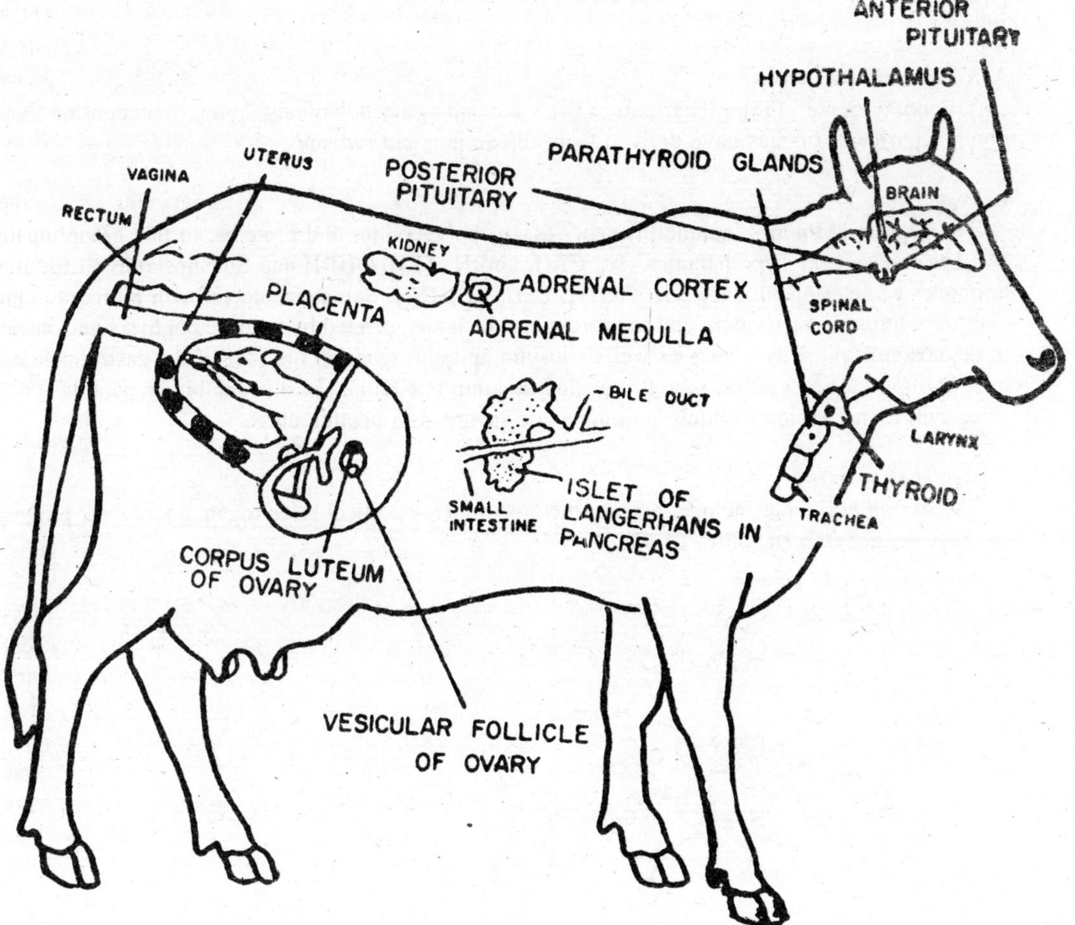

Fig. 3.45 Hormonal glands in Animal body.

Mode of Transmission

The concept of the restriction of hormone transmission to blood circulation only, must be abandoned and recognition be given to other means of transmission. Hormonal communications are classified according to the distance over which the signal acts.

1. Autocrine hormones act on the same cell that released them.
2. Paracrine hormones act only on cells close to the cell that released them. Prostaglandins and polypeptide growth factors of the hypothalamus are examples of this group.
3. Endocrine hormones act on cells distant from the site of their release. Endocrine hormones, for example, insulin and epinephrene, are synthesized and released in the bloodstream by specialized ductless endocrine glands. This is typical of most hormones.

Chemical Nature of Hormones

Hormones are biochemically categorized as (amino acid derivatives), peptides or steroids as follows.

A. *Amino Acid Derivatives*

Triiodothyronine (T_3), Thyroxin (T_4), adrenal catecholamines, viz., epinephrine and norepinephrine hormones have derived from the amino acid tyrosine.

B. *Peptides*

The peptide hormones include (a) peptides, (b) polypeptides and proteins. In this group all the five hormones of the hypothalamus viz., CRH, GnRH, TRH, GHRH and Somatostatin; all the five hormones of anterior pituitary, viz. ACTH, FSH, LH, TSH, Somatotropin (growth hormone), and two more hormones (oxytocin and vasopressin) which are secreted by neurohypophysis and stored in the posterior pituitary glands as well as insulin and glucagon; all the four of the gastrointestinal tract hormones, viz., gastrin, secretin, cholecystokinin (CCK) and gastric inhibitory peptide (GIP) along with parathyroid calcitonin hormones are included in peptide class.

C. *Steroid Hormones*

The steroid hormones include, glucocorticoids, mineralocorticoids, estrogen, androgens, progestins and the active metabolites of vitamin D.

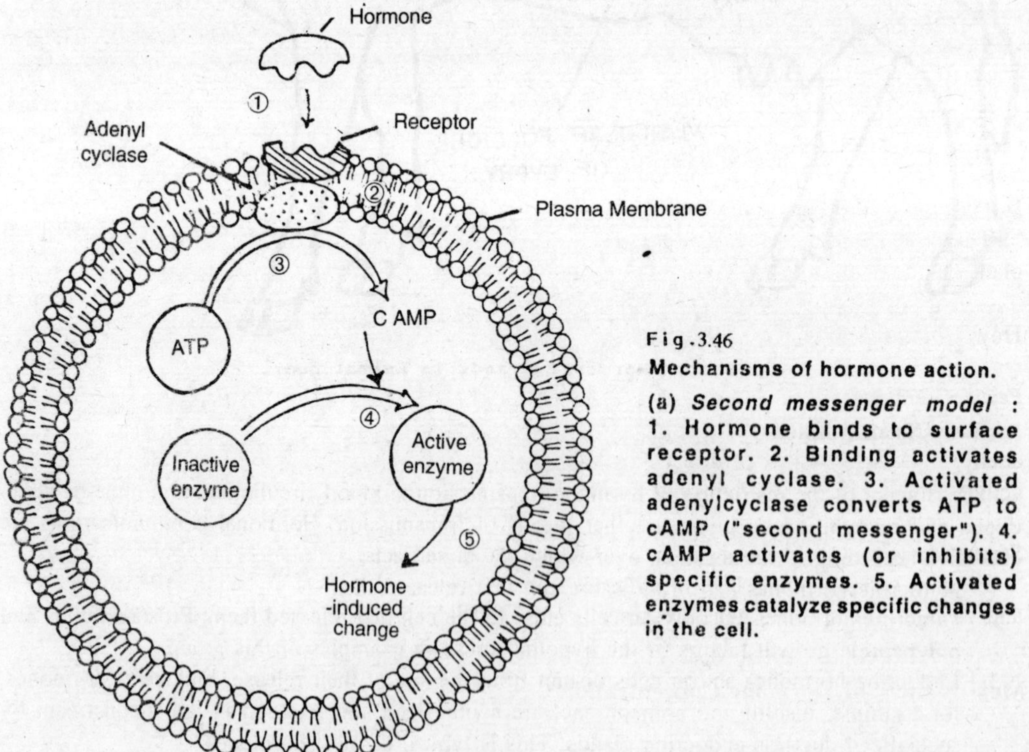

Fig.3.46
Mechanisms of hormone action.
(a) *Second messenger model* : 1. Hormone binds to surface receptor. 2. Binding activates adenyl cyclase. 3. Activated adenylcyclase converts ATP to cAMP ("second messenger"). 4. cAMP activates (or inhibits) specific enzymes. 5. Activated enzymes catalyze specific changes in the cell.

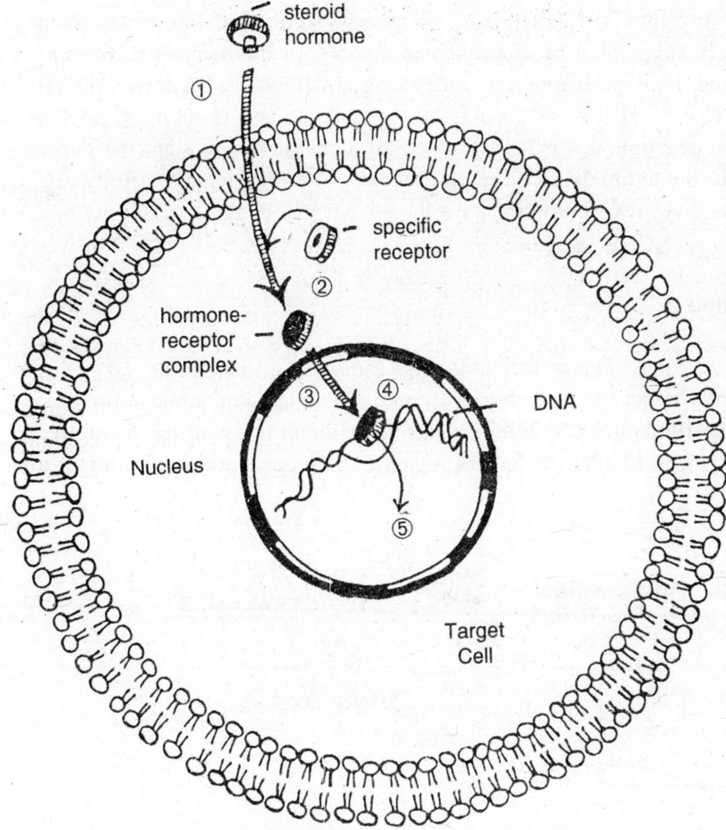

Fig. 3.47
Mechanisms of hormone action.
(b) *Steroid hormones*: 1. Hormones readily passes through plasma membrane and 2. reacts with receptor molecule. 3. The hormone-receptor complex enters the nucleus and 4. attaches to a specific site on the chromosome. 5. Attachment activates gene(s) responsible for the hormone induced change (for example, production of a hair shaft by a previously dormant hair follicle on an adolescent boy's chin).

D. *Polyunsaturated Fatty Acids*

The prostaglandins are derived from arachidonic acid, (an essential fatty acid) synthesized by plant kingdom or from excess intake of another fatty acid, linoleic acid in animal kingdom.

How Hormone acts at the Target?

Peptide Hormones

Bind to a specific receptor molecules present on the target cell's surface. Binding stimulates adenyl cyclase enzyme to produce cylic AMP (cAMP), which unleashes the cells potential by activating the enzymes responsible for the hormone induced change. (see Fig. 3.46)

Steroid Hormones

Bind to receptor molecules in cytoplasm. The resulting complex attaches to the chromosome and turns on the specific genes responsible for the response to hormone stimulation.

Measurement of Hormone Concentration

The serum concentrations of hormones are extremely small, generally between 10^{-12} and 10^{-7}M (Molar), so that they usually be measured by indirect means. Biological assays have traditionally been employed for this purpose but they are generally slow, cumbersome, and imprecise. Such assays have therefore been largely supplanted by *Radioimmunoassays.* In this technique, the unknown concentration of a hormone, H, is determined by measuring how much of a known amount of the radioactively labelled hormone, H*, binds to a fixed quantity of anti-H antibody in the presence of H. This competition reaction. is easily calibrated by constructing a standard curve indicating how much H* binds to the antibody as a function of (H). The high legand affinity and specificity that antibodies possess gives radioimmunoassays the advantages of great sensitivity and specificity.

Regulation of Hormone Secretion

Hormones exert their effects in extraordinary tiny amounts, generally in nanogram (10^{-9}g) or picogram (10^{-12}g) amounts and their targets are acutely sensitive to even slight endocrine variations. The levels of hormones and tissue fluids must be tightly controlled (reins) to avoid the disruptive effects of either deficits or excesses. A number of factors regulate the precise concentrations of a hormone are discussed below.

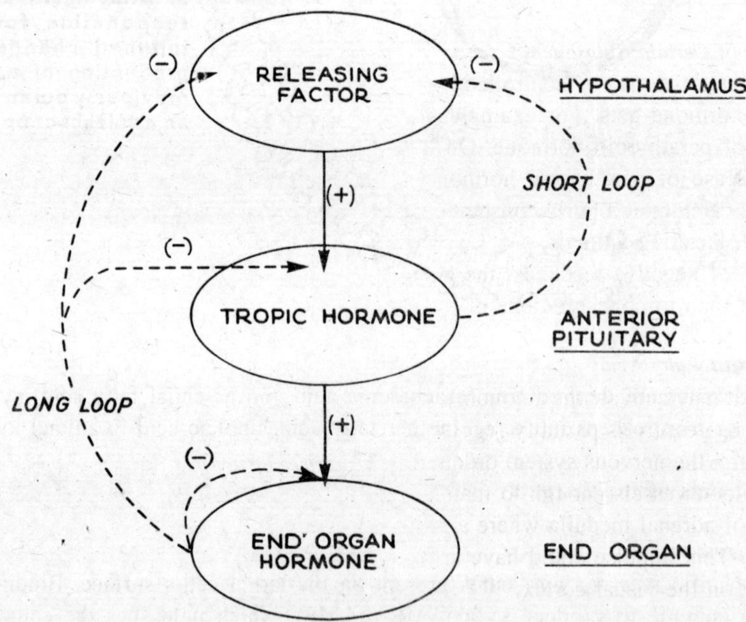

Fig. 3.48 General feedback control of endocrine systems involving the hypothalamus, anterior pituitary, and end organ.

1. *Negative Feedback Mechanism*

In many cases, the concentration of a hormone directly influences its own production. Some endocrine cells produce hormones only when the levels of those hormones in the blood drop below "normal". Deficits in the hormone spur (stimulates) the gland to secrete more, and the concentration in the blood begins to rise. Elevated concentrations have the opposite effect; they pull the reins (restrain) or hormone secretion before an excess can accumulate. For example, the production of LH by the anterior pituitary gland stimulates the testes to secrete testosterone. As more and more testosterone is produced by the testes, it enters the blood stream and is carried to the hypothalamus and the anterior pituitary gland, where it causes a decreased production of LH. Thus when testosterone secretion is low, LH production is increased.

This regulatory mechanism is called *negative feedback*. The system is similar to the way one maintains a constant driving speed in a car. When speedometer alerts the driver about excessive speed, he reduces the velocity. When he notices that the speed has gone down than that of desired one, the driver immediately exerts more pressure on his accelerator and the speed is regained.

Many glands equipped with sensor glands (specialized nervous tissue sensitive to a specific change in the environment), like the speedometer, inform them of their endocrine "speed". These glands constantly self correct to maintain stable hormone concentrations.

2. *Positive Feedback*

Some hormones enhance their own production by activating the glands that produce them. The result is just the opposite of negative feedback. With positive feedback, elevated hormone concentrations increase hormone release. Although in most situations, such self-perpetuating escalation would disrupt homeostasis, some special situation demands rapid increases in hormone concentration, for example to promote expulsion of the fetus during parturition, or during milking.

3. *Blood Levels of Certain Substances*

Hormone secretions may be controlled by the blood level of the substance (other than hormone) on which the hormone acts. For example, a high concentration of blood calcium causes a low secretion rate of parathyroid hormone. On the other hand a low concentration of blood calcium permits the release of parathyroid hormone. This interaction between calcium and parathyroid hormone keeps calcium at a fairly constant concentration in the blood stream which is an important phenomenon. in lactating animals.

In this form of negative feedback, the gland responds to the eventual effect (concentrations of calcium) rather than to concentrations of the hormone itself.

4. *Autonomic Neurons*

Sensory input may activate the autonomic nervous system either to promote or to inhibit hormone secretion. Blood pressure is partially regulated by such a mechanism. When neurons sense a drop in blood pressure, the nervous system orders the secretion of hormones that increase blood volume and constrict blood vessels enough to maintain circulatory pressure.

In the case of adrenal medulla where a peripheral nerve connection can cause increased output of epinephrine. This impulse could have arisen in the cerebral cortex after the animal recorded a frightful image on the visual cortex.

5. *Influence Genetic Make Up*

The phenotypic characteristics of the individual are only manifestations of biochemical coding which is present in the DNA of the genes. There are possible effects of genetic coding on hormone output and the effect of hormone on the protein synthesis.

HYPOTHALAMUS and PITUITARY FUNCTIONS

Since about 1950 information has been accumulating at a rapid rate to show that the hypothalamus and higher nerve centres exert marked influences over the secretion of several of the pituitary hormones. These findings are of particular importance as they provide, a partial answer to the question of how exteroceptive stimuli resulting from changes in an animal's environment are converted into changes in the nature and quantities of hormones secreted. Hypothalamus includes the optic chaisma, mammillary bodies, tuber cinereum, infundibulum and pars nervosa of the brain. However, hypothalamus as commonly used excludes the pituitary gland.

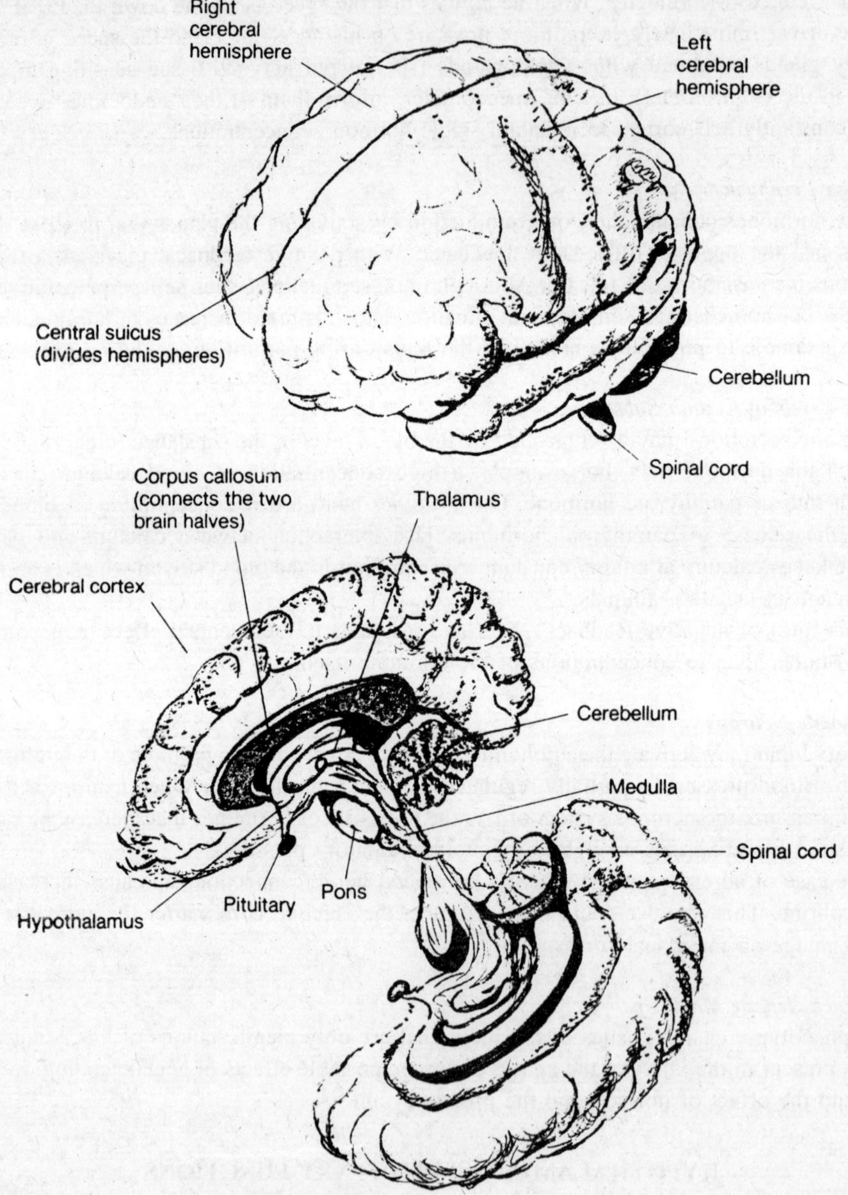

(a) The intact brain reveals mostly cerebrum
(b) Separating the two cerebral hemisphere reveals some of the brain's structural complexity.

Fig. 3.49 Two views of the brain

The anterior pituitary has frequently been called the "master endocrine gland" because the multiple hormones it secretes control the secretion of four or five hormones (depending upon animal's gender) by other endocrine glands. *However, if any "gland" deserves the title of "master", it is the hypothalamus*, since this portion of the brain, in addition to producing two hormones, viz., Oxytocin and Vasopressin, also secretes a number of other hormones which control the secretion of all the anterior pituitary hormones. The basic pattern for this overall system is (with one exception) sequences of three hormones; they begin with a hypothalamic hormone, which controls the secretion of an anterior pituitary hormones, which controls the secretion of hormone from a peripheral endocrine gland.

The last hormone in the sequence then acts on its target cells.

Hypothalamic Releasing Hormones

We have seen that the secretion of various hormones by peripheral endocrine glands is controlled by hormones from the anterior pituitary. But secretion of the anterior pituitary hormones, itself, largely regulated by still other hormones produced by the hypothalamus. Apart from this important function, the paraventricular nucleus of the hypothalamus secretes oxytocin while the supra-optic nucleus secretes vasopressin hormone, both of which flow along axons (Plate) into the posterior lobe of the pituitary gland where these are stored. Direct electrical stimulation of the hypothalamus, copulation or suckling, are among the stimuli which will induce release of these two hormones, (oxytocin and vasopressin) from posterior pituitary glands.

In contrast to the neural connections between the hypothalamus and posterior pituitary, there are no important neural connections between the hypothalamus and anterior pituitary. But there is an unusual capillary-to-capillary connections (Plate). These portal vessels offer a local route for flow of capillary blood carrying various hormones from hypothalamus to anterior pituitary.

Because most of these (five) substances stimulate release of their relevant target hormones, they are all collectively termed *hypothalamic releasing hormones*. Each of the hypothalamic releasing hormones is named according to an anterior pituitary hormone whose secretion it controls (Table); for example, the secretion of ACTH (also known as corticotropin) is stimulated by *Corticotropin releasing hormone* (CRH). However, as shown in Table , at least two of the hypothalamic hormones inhibit, rather than stimulate, release of anterior pituitary hormones. One of these inhibits secretion of growth hormone and is most commonly called *somatostatin*. The other inhibits secretion of prolactin and is termed *prolactin release inhibiting hormone* (PIH) (Fig. 3.50)

Several of the hypothalamic hormones influence the secretion of more than one anterior pituitary hormone: *Gonadotropin releasing hormone (GnRH)* stimulates the secretion of both FSH and LH; *thyrotropin releasing hormone* (TRH) stimulates the secretion not only of TSH (also known as thyrotropin), but prolactin as well (it was named TRH because its effect on thyrotropin was first discovered).

There are also cases of several hypothalamic releasing hormones which exert opposing effects, e.g., the secretion of pituitary growth hormone is controlled by two releasing hormones, viz. (1) *Somatostatin* (also known as growth hormone release inhibiting hormone) and (2) Growth hormone releasing hormone (GHRH) of hypothalamus control the response of the anterior pituitary for secreting the amount of growth hormone.

Thus it is clear that hypothalamic releasing hormones control anterior pituitary function, we must now ask. *What controls secretion* of the hypothalamic releasing hormones? Some of the neurons which secrete releasing hormones may possess spontaneous autorhythmicity, but firing of most of them requires *neuronal* and or hormonal input to them.

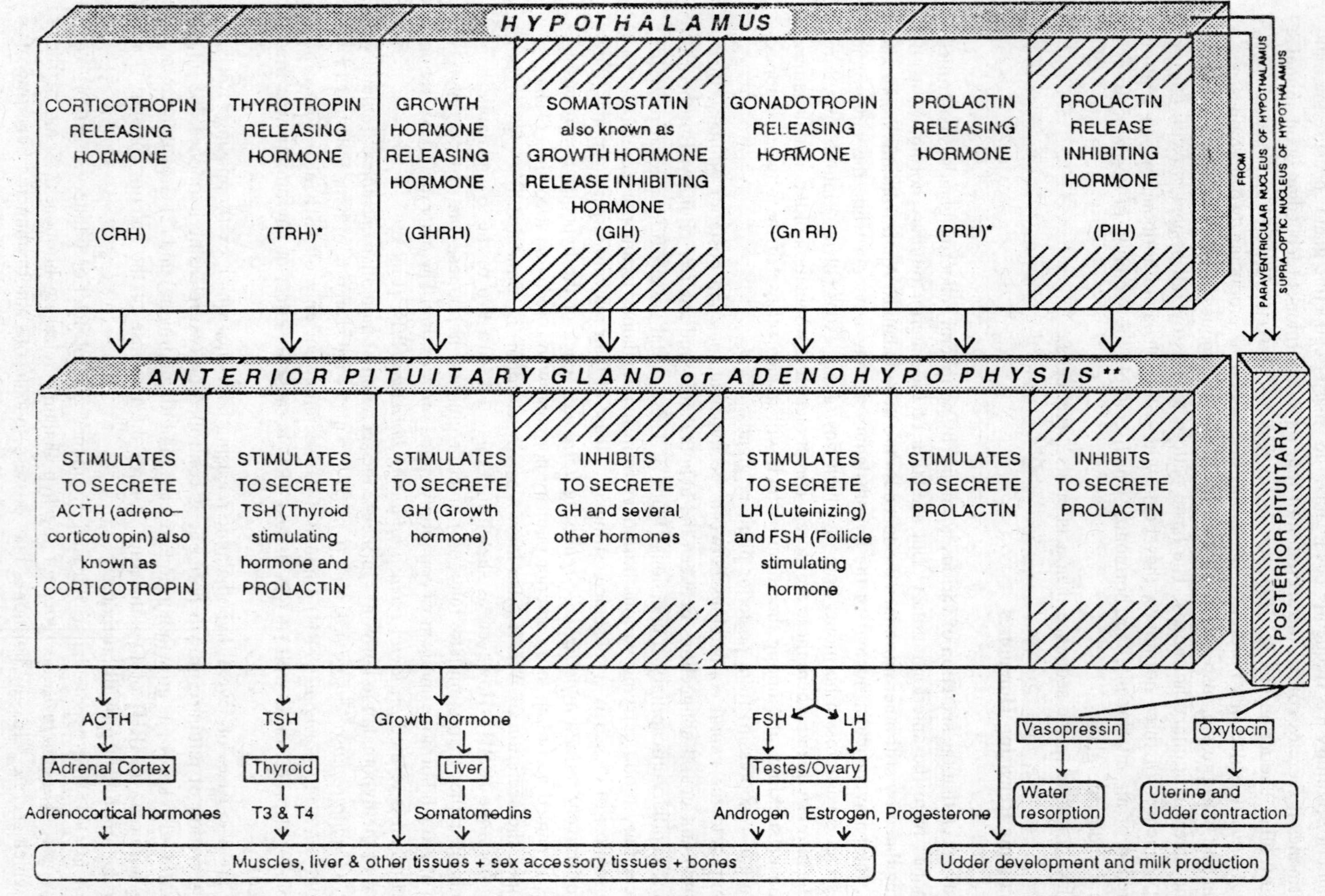

* *Note that TRH stimulates the secretion not only of TSH but of Prolactin as well; therefore, TRH is also a 'PRH'. However, it is likely that there is a second PRH, which acts only on Prolactin, and that is why PRH is listed separately here*

** *The Hypothalamus actually stimulates Anterior pituitary (AP) to produces Six hormones, viz., (1) GH, (2) TSH, (3) ACTH, (4) Prolactin, (5) FSH, and (6) LH whereas Hypothalamus also inhibits AP from producing (1) Prolactin and (2) Growth Hormone according to physiological condition.*

Fig. 3.50

Neuronal Input

The hypothalamus receives synaptic input, both stimulatory and inhibitory, from virtually all areas of the central nervous system. Figure illustrates these points for the CRH-ACTH-Cortisol system: Corticotropin releasing hormone, secreted by the hypothalamus, stimulates the anterior pituitary to secrete ACTH, which in turn stimulates the adrenal cortex to secrete the hormone cortisol. A wide variety of stresses, both physical (an injury, severe blood loss, etc.) and emotional (fright, for example) act, via neuronal pathways to the hypothalamus, to increase CRH secretion (and hence, that of ACTH and cortisol) markedly above its basal value. But even in a completely unstressed person, the secretion of cortisol varies in a highly stereotyped manner during a 24 hour period. This is because endogenous neural rhythms within the central nervous system impinge upon the hypothalamic neurons which secrete CRH.

Hormonal Feedback

A prominent feature of each of the hormonal sequences initiated by the hypothalamic releasing hormones is negative feedback exerted upon the hypothalamic—pituitary system by one or more of the very hormones in the sequence. For example, in the CRH—ACTH-Cortisol sequence (Fig.3.51) the final hormone—cortisol—acts upon the hypothalamus to reduce secretion of CRH (by causing a decrease in the frequency of action-potentials in the neurons secreting CRH). In addition, cortisol acts directly on the anterior pituitary to reduce the sensitivity of the ACTH—secreting cells to CRH. Thus by a double-barreled action, cortisol exerts a negative feedback control over its own secretion.

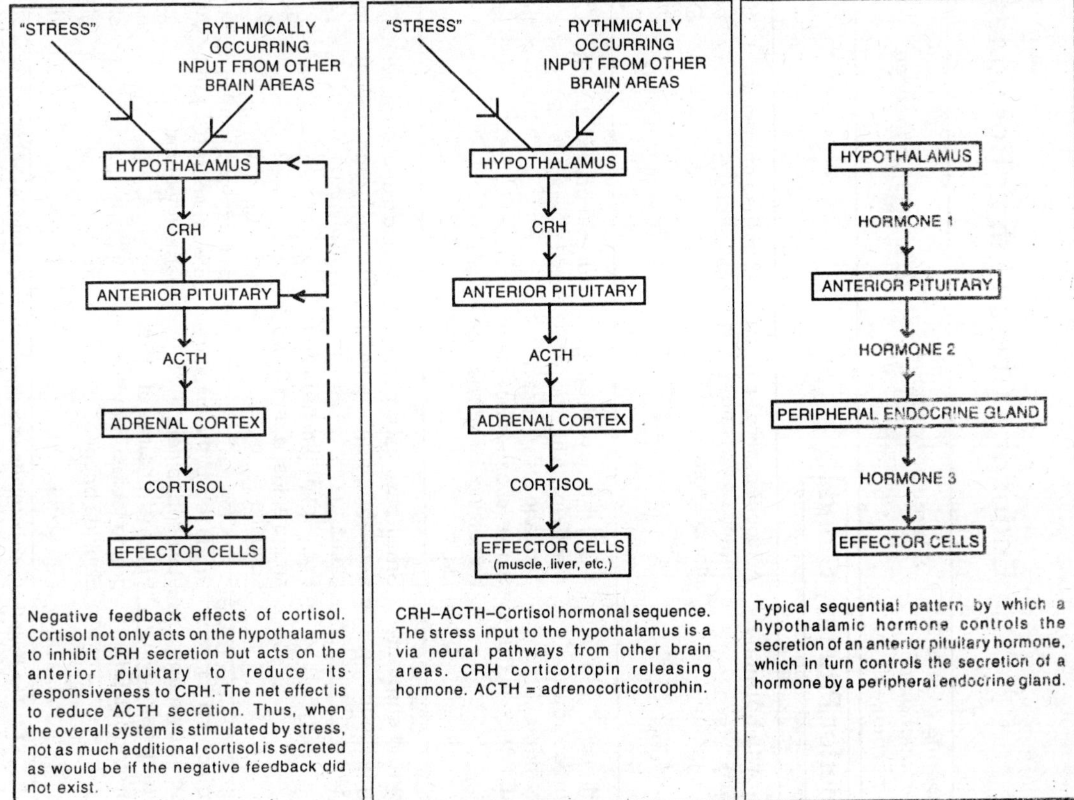

Negative feedback effects of cortisol. Cortisol not only acts on the hypothalamus to inhibit CRH secretion but acts on the anterior pituitary to reduce its responsiveness to CRH. The net effect is to reduce ACTH secretion. Thus, when the overall system is stimulated by stress, not as much additional cortisol is secreted as would be if the negative feedback did not exist.

CRH–ACTH–Cortisol hormonal sequence. The stress input to the hypothalamus is a via neural pathways from other brain areas. CRH corticotropin releasing hormone. ACTH = adrenocorticotrophin.

Typical sequential pattern by which a hypothalamic hormone controls the secretion of an anterior pituitary hormone, which in turn controls the secretion of a hormone by a peripheral endocrine gland.

Fig. 3.51

Table 3.17

Endocrine Glands - their Hormones and Characteristics

Endocrine glands & production of hormones	*Source of hormone & its Chemical nature*	*Tissue (s) influenced*	*Major physiological function (s)*	*Controlled by*
Anterior Pituitary Gland				
1. Growth hormone (GH)	Acidophilic cells, straight chain polypeptide, 191 amino acids.	All tissues of the mammalian body	Stimulates organic metabolism and thereby growth of the body. Deficiency will cause dwarfism while excess of the hormone will cause gigantism in adult.	GH release is regulated by a Releasing factor and SRIF (somatostatin) of hypothalamus.
2. Adreno-Corticotropin hormone (ACTH)	ACTH is synthesized mainly in the anterior pituitary and also in brain. Single chain polypeptide containing 39 amino acids.	Adrenal cortex (just in front of kidneys)	Causes adrenal cortex to secrete adrenal cortical hormones. When hormonal level is low there will be less adrenal cortical hormone and vice versa.	The secretion of ACTH is regulated by corticotropin releasing hormone of hypothalamus during stress.
3. Thyroid stimulating hormone (TSH)	Small basohpilic cells of anterior pituitary (AP) gland. Polypeptide chains of 209 amino acids, α and β two subunits	Thyroid gland (on either side of trachea just below larynx)	Stimulates thyroid to secrete Triiodothyronine (T_3) and Thyroxin (T_4). At high TSH level T_3 & T_4 will be produced at lower concentration and vice versa.	Secretion of TSH is controlled by hypothalamic releasing factor, TRH (thyrotropin releasing hormone) which is a neutral tripeptide.
4. Prolactin (PL) also known as Luteotropic Hormone (LTH)	Produced bythe pituitary eosinophilic cells. Peptide chains of 198 amino acids with three disulfide bridges.	Corpus luteum (CL) and mammary gland	Activates CL and causes progesterone production; stimulates mammary development. It also stimulates enlargement of crop gland and formation of "crop milk" in pegions.	Prolactin is inhibited by a hypothalamic factor—Prolactin inhibitory factor (PIF). Both estroens and the act of suckling stimulate prolactin secretion.

(Contd.)

Gonadotropin hormones **5. Follicle stimulating hormone (FSH)**	Large basophilic cells of anterior pituitary gland. (AP). Consists of two non-identical, non covalently linked subunits, the α and β chains having 236 amino acids.	Ovaries and testes	In ovaries, stimulates fllicular development, ovulation and estrogen synthesis. In testes stimulates spermatogenesis. Deficiency of the hormone will cause infertility or even sterility. Excess will damage seminiferous tubules.	Estrogens usually stimulate FSH secretion but may inhibit depending on the circumstances.
6. Luteinizing hormone (LH)	As above except that it has 215 amino acids.	Ovaries and testes.	In ovaries, stimulates oocyte maturation and follicular synthesis of estrogens and progesterones; in testes stimulates androgen synthesis.	Oestrogen stimulates but progesterone inhibits secretion of LH.

Intermediate Lobe of Pituitary Gland

Melanocyte Stimulating hormone (MSH)	Basophilic cells of the middle lobe. Three peptides (α-MSH, β-MSH, and γ - MSH) have been isolated from pituitaries of various species, α - MSH has 13 amino acids.	Skin	Increases the deposition of melanin, a brown pigment by the melanocytes of skin thus controlling cutanious pigmentation particularly in amphibians.	Hydrocortisone and cortisone inhibit the secretion of MSH. When corticosteroids are inadequate, as in "Addison's disease" MSH is secreted in excess.

Posterior Pituitary Gland

1. Oxytocin or Pitocin	Secreted by supraoptic and paraventricular nuclei of hypothalamus. Posterior pituitary (PP) only stores. Cyclic polypeptide having 9 amino acids with one disulfide bridge.	Mammary gland and uterus.	Stimulates uterine contraction during parturition (birth), secretion of milk by mammary gland and expulsion of egg in hens. Excess secretion will cause premature parturition while deficiency will delay the process.	Levels of estrogen and progesterone (inhibition)

(Contd.)

Endocrine glands & production of hormones	Source of hormone & its Chemical nature	Tissue (s) influenced	Major physiological function (s)	Controlled by
2. Vasopressin or Antidiuretic hormone (ADH)	Secreted by the neurons of supraoptic and paraventricular nuclei of hypothalamus. Posterior pituitary only stores. Cyclic polypeptide having 9 amino acids with one disulfide bridge.	Distal convulated tubule of kidney	Stimulates water resorption by kidney and increases blood pressure by contraction of blood vessels, and increases the absorption of H_2O by the Kidney.	Solute concentration of blood. A deficiency of this hormone causes the syndrome "Diabetes insipidus", characterized by large volume of urination (may be upto 30 lit / day) of low specific gravity.

Thyroid Glands

1. Thyroxin (T_4) and 2. Triiodothyronine (T_3)	Thyroid gland follicles. Both have originated from one amino acid Tyrosine. T_4 is having 4 mols. of Iodine while T_3 has got 3 mols of iodine.	All tissues of the body.	Controls basal metabolic rate; promotes metamorphosis in amphibians. Deficiency will cause Hypothyroidism: simple goiter, in young cretinism. While excess will result Hypothyroidism: exophthalmic goiter, increased metabolic rate, excitability.	Thyroid stimulating hormone (TSH) from anterior pituitary.
3. Calcitonin	"C" cells of the thyroid gland. Polypeptide having 32 amino acids	Bone and kidney	Inhibits calcium uptake from bone and kidney when it is in excess, thus regulates blood calcium levels in cooperation with another set of glands, the parathyroid glands which reverses the effect of calcitonin.	Release of calcitonin is stimulated by high levels of ionized calcium in the serum and vice versa.

Parathyroid Gland

Parathyroid	PTH is initially synthe-	Bone and kidney	PTH maintains the concentration	The action of PTH on bone

(Contd.)

hormone or Parathormone (PTH)	sized in the chief cells as Preprohormone which is then converted to Prohomone in endoplasmic reticulum. This in turn is hydrolyzed in the Golgi bodies to Parathyroid hormone. Polypeptide with 84 amino acids.		of calcium in the plasma. In bone the hormone causes rapid release of calcium and phosphorus. In kidney, PTH increases phsphate excretion along with reabsorption of calcium. Dificiency of the hormone will result Ca concentration falls with increase of P; increase excitability of nerve and muscle. While high PTH increases plasma calcium and decreases phosphorus, along with weakness, nausea and softening of bones.	and kidney are independent of any other hormones, but on the plasma concentration of calcium. (negative feedback).

Adrenal Cortex Glands

1. Glucocorticoids : i) **Corticosterone** ii) **Cortisol also known as Hydrocortisone** iii) **Cortisone** iv) **11-dehydrocorticosterone**	Zona fasciculata and zona reticularis of adrenal cortex. Steroid in structure	All tissues of the body mainly muscle and liver	(1) Enhances gluconeogenesis from protein, thus mobilizes body energy sources. (2) Anti-inflammatory action. Increase resistance to stress. (3) Chronic use causes increased secretion of HCl and pepsinogen by the stomach & trypsinogen by the pancreas; this favours gastrointestinal ulcers. (4) Favours Ca loss on prolong use resulting Osteoporosis.	In response to corticotropin releasing factor (CRF) of hypothalamus, the pituitary cell secrete ACTH leading to secretion of steroid hormone.
2. Mineralocorticoids : i) **Aldosterone** ii) **11-deoxycorticosterone** iii) **17-hydroxy-11-deoxy-crticosterone**	Zona glomerulosa cells of adrenal cortex. Aldosterone is the most important mineralocoids, being about 1000 times as effective as cortisol. All are steroid in structure.	Kidney, all tissues indirectly.	Regulates sodium retention and potassium excretion, water distribution in tissues. Also effective in promoting membrane transport in sweat glands, salivary glands and between intra & extracelluar compartments. Retention of body water expands blood volume and thus	There are 3 ways by which aldosterone increases. (1) ACTH stimulation, (2) Low plasma potassium and (3) Renin-angiotensin system. Renin a kidney enzyme acts on blood globulin, to form angiotensinogen, to form

(Contd.)

Endocrine glands & production of hormones	Source of hormone & its Chemical nature	Tissue (s) influenced	Major physiological function (s)	Controlled by
			re-establishes normal blood pressure (low blood pressure is the cause of renin secretion).	Angiotensin I which is converted by the lung to Angiotensin II. This compound is the stimulus for the secretion of aldosterone from the zona glomerulosa.

Adrenal Medulla Gland

Endocrine glands & production of hormones	Source of hormone & its Chemical nature	Tissue (s) influenced	Major physiological function (s)	Controlled by
1. Epinephrene or Adrenaline.	Formed in medulla and stored in chromaffin cells of medulla. Derivative of Tyrosine amino acid. By methylation of the side chain of nor-epinephrene, epinephrene is formed.	Heart, skeletal muscle, adipose tissue and liver.	Stimulates relaxation of some smooth muscles of the stomach, intestine, bronchioles, urinary bladder and contraction of the sphincters of stomach and bladder. Increases heart rate and blood pressure, stimulates muscle glycogenolysis and lypolysis in adipose tissue. Reduces glucose uptake by tissues.	Lower blood glucose stimulates adrenal secretion. Sympathetic preganglionic portion of autonomic nervous fibres enter the adrenal medulla controls release of the hormone. A number of other factors like fear, anger, pain, emotional states, hypoglycemia stimulate the secretion of hormone.
2. Nor-epinephrene or Nor-adrenaline	Same as above. The two hormones epinephnene and non-epinephrene of the adrenal medulla are structurally related to C group of compounds known as catechols and so these two hormones jointly known as Catecholamines	Peripheral blood vessels, smooth muscles	Exerts an overall vasoconstrictor effect without affecting cardia. Decreases peripheral circulation. Stimulates lypolysis in adipose tissue.	Catecholamines are allosteric inhibitors of their own synthesis at tyrosine hydroxylase. This when hormones are mobilized rapidly, synthesis is correspondingly reduced.

(Contd.)

Pancreas

1. Glucagon	$\propto$ Cell of the islets of Langerhans. Polypeptide consists of 29 amino acids in a straight chain.	Mainly in liver for glycogenolysis. In adipose tissue glucagon also increases break-down of lipids to fatty acids and glycerol. It also hydrolyses muscle glycogen.	Stimulates glucose release through glycogenolysis (break-down of glycogen to glucose), also stimulates lipolysis. Directly stimulates gluconeogenesis by activation of pyruvate carboxylase enzyme. Another action is stimulation of the secretion of insulin and of somatostatin.	Glucagon secretion is directly inhibited by high blood glucose level only in the presence of insulin.
2. Insulin	Insulin is formed in the β-cells as preproinsulin. On hydrolysis yields proinsulin. By loosing a portion of polypeptide it becomes insulin. It has 2 chains; a short one (A) made up of 21 amino acids and a long one (B) of 30 aminos acids. (Total 51).	Blood, muscle, adipose and several other body tissues.	1. Lowers blood sugar level. 2. Important anabolic agent in muscle, liver and fat cells as it increases synthesis of glycogen (opposite to glucagon), fatty acids and triglycerides along with protein.	Secretion is increased by glucose and calcium ions as well as by amino acids arginine and leucine. Also stimulated by somatotropin and also inhibited (to a lesser extent) by the same somatotropin. (negative feed back)
3. Somatostatin	In addition to hypothalamus the hormone has also been found in the intestine and the pancreas. In pancrea it is formed in the islets of "D" cells which is then cleaved to somatostatin.	Gastro-intestinal hormones.	It usually appears to act as on inhibitory agent to slow the output of nutrients into the circulation and to moderate the metabolic effects of insulin, glucagon and growth hormone. In this regard, somatostatin inhibits the secretion of gastrin, secretin, cholecysto kinin, pancreatic exocrine secretion, gastro-intestinal motility and the absorption of glucose by blocking entry of calcium into the hormone secreting cells.	

(Contd.)

Endocrine glands & production of hormones	*Source of hormone & its Chemical nature*	*Tissue (s) influenced*	*Major physiological function (s)*	*Controlled by*
Gonads				
A. Ovaries 1. Estrogen i) Estradiol ii) Estrone iii) Estriole	1) Ganulosa cells of ovarian follicles 2) Corpus Luteum 3) Placenta 4) Adrenal Cortex C_{18} Steroid in Structure	Reproductive organs (Primary and secondary) Mammary glands	Concerned in cyclic rhythms; produce estrous behaviour, stimulates growth and function of reproductive tract, stimulates uterine contractions, regulates gonadotropin release, develops and maintains secondary sexual characters. Develops mammary gland but inhibits milk secretion.	Luteinizing hormone (LH) and FSH from anterior pituitary.
2. Progesterone	1) Corpus luteum of ovary (goat, cow, sow) 2) Placenta (sheep, mare) 3) Adrenal cortex C_{21} Steroid in structure	1. Mammary gland 2. Uterus (nedation and maintenance of pregnancy. Hormone appears after ovulation.	Prepares uterus for implantation; stimulates endometrial secretion, maintains pregnancy, suppresses LH surges. The hormone also suppresses estrous, ovulation and stimulates mammary glands.	Mainly LH from anterior pituitary controls. If fertilization does not occur, the follicular and progestational hormones suddenly decrease. During pregnancy progesterone continues till near term.
B. Testes *Androgens* 1. Testosterone 2. 5 ∝–dihydrotestosterone	Testosterone is synthesized by the interstitial (Leydig) cells of the testes. In some tissues this is converted to 5 ∝–dihydrotestosterone which is more active. These are 19 carbon steroids. Testosterone is also found in adrenal gland.	Seminiferus tubule, interstitial cells and on all other tissues of the body which shows male characteristics	The hormone promotes the growth and function of the epididymis, vas deferems, prostate, seminal vesicles, and penis. Its metabolic effect as a protein anabolic steroid exceeds that of other naturally occuring steroids. It also contributes to the muscular and skeletal growth that accompanies puberty. Development of secondary sex characters such as male voice, the crest in the bull and boar, thick	Control is by (feedback) gonadotropin hormones. FSH stimulates sperm production by the seminiferous tubules while LH stimulates the interstitial cells (Leydig) to produce testosterone. In males LH is known as interstitial cell stimulating hormone (ICSH).

(Contd.)

			horns in the bull etc and sex drive (Libido) are due to this hormone.	

Uterus

Prostaglandin $F_2\propto$ [Hormone like compounds, (Hormonoids) occur in all cells]	Prostaglandins are produced from endocrine cells throughout the body. 20 carbon hydroxy fatty acid containing one 5 membered ring, derived from modification of arachidonic acid which is considered as one of the essential fatty acids.	$PGF_2 \propto$ controls the contractionn of smooth muscles of the uterus, bronchi and intestine acting chiefly through the agency of cGMP or Calcium ions. It is also active in CL and placenta	It affects only females except poultry. Probably the natural hormone that causes regression of CL in sheep, cattle and swine. PGF2 $\propto$ is also potent in terminating pregnancy by controling uterine muscle.	ACTH controls the release of corticosterols which in turn increases in the level of $PGF_2 \propto$.

Gastrointestinal Hormones

A. Wall of stomach 1. Gastrin	Produced by the antral portion of the gastric mucosa of the stomach. Polypeptide. Two active gastrins I and II, containing 17 and 14 amino acids respectively.	Stomach	1. Stimulates the gastric secretions of HCl and pepsinogen 2. Stimulates secretion of HCO_3 and H_2O from bile duct epithelium. 3. Stimulates secretion of pancreatic enzyme.	Gastrin release is stimulated by amino acids & partially digested protein as well as by the vagus nerve (which innervates the stomach) in response to stomach distention. Gastrin is inhibited by other gastro-intestinal hormones.
B. Wall of Duodenum 1. Cholecystokinin (CCK) (Pancreozymin)	Produced by the upper small intestine. Polypeptide with 33 amino acids.	Gall bladder, stomach, Pancreas	A. Inhibits secretion B. Stimulates: (1) gall bladder emptying, (2) pancreatic secretion of digestive enzymes, HCO_3 and H_2O by bile duct epithelium, and (3) Contraction of gall bladder and relaxation of sphinctor of oddi	CCK is released in response to the products of lipid and protein digestion, that is fatty acids, monoacyl glycerols, amino acids and peptides.

(Contd.)

Endocrine glands & production of hormones	*Source of hormone & its Chemical nature*	*Tissue (s) influenced*	*Major physiological function (s)*	*Controlled by*
2. Secretin	Produced by the upper small intestinal (duodenal and jejunal) mucosa in response to acidification by gastric HCl. Polypeptide having 27 amino acids.	Pancreas	Inhibits HCl secretion. Stimulates secretion of HCO_3 and H_2O from pancreas and bile duct epithelium. Also stimulates pepsinogen.	Presence of food in duodenum
3. Gastric inhibitory peptide (GIP)	Hormone produced by cells linning the small intestine Polypeptide having 43 amino acids.	Stomach, Pancreas	Inhibitor of gastric acid secretion, gastric mobility and gastric emptying. However, GIP's major physiological function is to stimulate pancreatic insulin release.	The release of GIP is stimulated by the presence of glucose in the gut which accounts for the observation that, after a meal, the blood insulin level increases before the blood glucose level does.

Negative feedback : Any regulatory mechanism in which the increased level of a substance inhibits further production of that substance, thereby preventing harmful accumulation.

Other Hormones or Hormone like substances

There are several substances synthesized and secreted by cells of the gastrointestinal tract and the kidney that have hormone like action, even though they do not exactly fit the classic definition of hormone.

Renin

Kidney produces a hormone like substance, *renin*, which is secreted from cells of the juxtaglomerular cells. Once secreted into blood, it activates plasma angiotensinogen to form *angiotensin*, which acts on the adrenal zona glomerulosa to cause secretion of aldosterone. The angiotensin also causes some general systemic arteriole constriction to increase arterial pressure.

REF (Renal Erythropoietic Factor)

Kidney also secretes REF, which acts on a precursor globin in the blood to form the hormone *erythropoietin*, also known as *haemopoietin* and *erythropoietic stimulating factor*. Some REF is also produced by the liver.

The REF exerts its effect on the stem cells of the bone marrow to increase the formation of more red blood cells, so that more oxygen can be carried to the tissues. It is a feedback mechanism that decreases or shuts off secretion of REF when the oxygen demands of the tissues are satisfied.

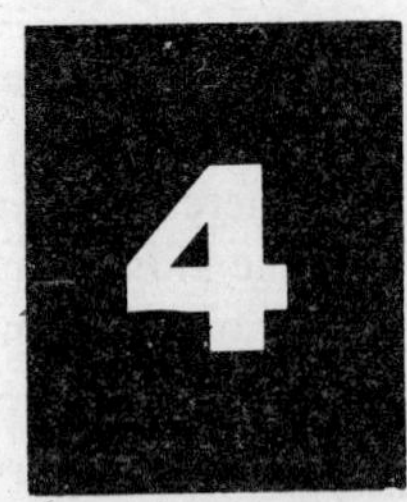

ANIMAL BLOOD

ANIMAL BLOOD

Blood may be termed as a specialised and circulating tissue composed of cells suspended in a fluid intercellular substance which circulates through a closed system of blood vessels (arteries, veins) due to pumping action of the heart. When the blood is centrifuged it separates into two distinct fractions, the upper fraction is a clear straw-coloured fluid called plasma while less than half of the tube is packed with the so-called formed elements, consisting of red blood cells, white blood cells, and platelets. When the blood is allowed to clot, a colourless fluid portion oozes out. This is serum. It differs from plasma in that the fibrinogen portion is not present in the fluid portion of the serum.

The Functions of Blood

1. Blood carries nutrients made available by the digestive tract to body tissues.
2. It carries oxygen from the lungs to the tissues.
3. It carries carbon dioxide from tissues to the lungs.
4. Waste products from various tissues are carried to the kidneys for excretion.
5. Hormones are carried from endocrine glands to other organs of the body.
6. Blood plays an important role in temperature control by transporting heat from deeper structures to the surface of the body.
7. Water balance is maintained by the blood.
8. Buffers such as sodium bicarbonate in the blood help to maintain a constant pH of tissues and body fluids.
9. The clotting ability of blood prevents excess loss of blood from injuries.
10. Blood contains important factors for defence of the body against disease

Blood Volume

This is the total amount of blood present in animal body. Blood volume can readily be calculated if the percentage of body weight normally comprised of blood is known. Average figures in percentage of body weight due to blood are: Dog–5·5–9·1 Cow–7·7, Sheep–8·0 and Horse—6·6

The volume can also be determined indirectly when a known volume of dye is injected into the blood stream and then the volume is calculated from the dilution of the dye after it is thoroughly mixed with the blood.

Components of the Blood

It has been stated that the liquid portion of the blood is the plasma. The cells or cell-like structures floating in the plasma are the formed elements.

When a sample of blood is treated to prevent clotting and permitted to stand undisturbed, the cells gradually settle to the bottom of the container, leaving a straw coloured fluid. This fluid portion of the blood, called *Plasma* and is made up of about 92% water and 8% other substances. The kidneys are responsible for maintaining constant proportions of water and other constituents of the plasma by selective filtration and resorption of water and other substances from the blood plasma. These substances include about 90% proteins and 0.9% inorganic matter; the remainder is non-protein organic matter.

The substances other than water that comprise 8% of the plasma can be subdivided on the basis of their molecular weights (MW). Those having a MW greater than 50,000 gm/mole are the proteins, which comprise 7/8 of this plasma fraction (7 gm/100 ml). Those having a MW less than 50,000 gm/mole include glucose, lipids, amino acids, vitamins, hormones, NaCl and other electrolytes, inorganic mineral salts and metabolic waste products, such as urea, uric acid and creatinine. These make up the other 1/8 fraction of the plasma. Normally, plasma comprises 50 ± 10 percent of the blood in mammals. Changes in colour of the plasma may occur under normal physiological condition : horses and cows fed on green forage typically have bright yellow plasma. After a fatty meal the plasma in most animals is milky white. However pathological changes may change the colour of the plasma. A red-coloured plasma results from increased fragility and rupture of red blood cells.

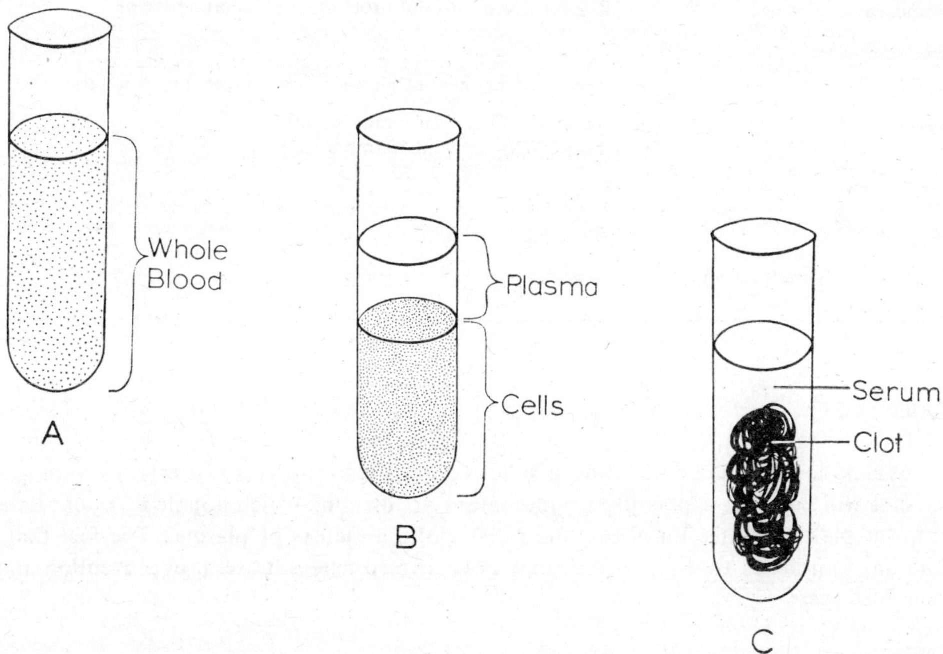

Fig 4.1 Blood. Diagram illustrating different physical states of blood. *A*, Unclotted blood, cells dispersed uniformly throughout; *B*, blood treated with anticoagulant. Cells permitted to settle, leaving clear plasma. *C*, Clotted blood. Serum separated from clot.

Table 4.1

Some important plasma constituents

Constituent/type	*Amount concentration*	*Functions/comments*
Water	90 per cent of plasma	Dissolves, suspends, ionises, electrolytes carries heat
Electrolytes	About 1 per cent of plasma (examples: Na^+, K^+, Ca^{++}, Mg^{++}, Cl^-, HCO^-_3, PO_4	They buffer, establish osmotic gradients, are responsible for excitability of cells
Proteins	6-8 per cent of plasma	General functions; give viscosity to blood, clotting, antibodies, reserve of amino acids, establish colloid osmotic pressure of plasma
Albumins	50-65 per cent of total proteins	Are responsible for most of the plasma colloidal osmotic pressure
Globulins (alpha, beta, gamma)	14.5-27 per cent of total proteins	Serve general functions: γ globulins are major source of antibodies
Fibrinogen	2.5-5 per cent of total proteins	Clotting factor
Other substances		
Glucose	About 0.1 per cent of plasma	Nutrients or wastes
Gases (O_2, CO_2)	Variable (O_2 av. 20 ml/100 ml blood) (CO_2 av. 9 ml 100 ml blood)	
Lipids	Variable	
Vitamins	Variable	
Nitrogenous materials (urea)	Variable	

Serum

When blood clots in a test tube, a solid red mass is formed. However, on standing longer, the clot will contract expressing a supernatant yellow fluid which is called *Serum*. Essentially serum is plasma minus fibrinogen and other clotting factors of plasma. The fact that serum contains antibodies that the animal may have formed makes it useful in prevention and treatment of disease.

The Formed Elements

The formed elements of the blood include red blood cells, white blood cells and blood platelets.

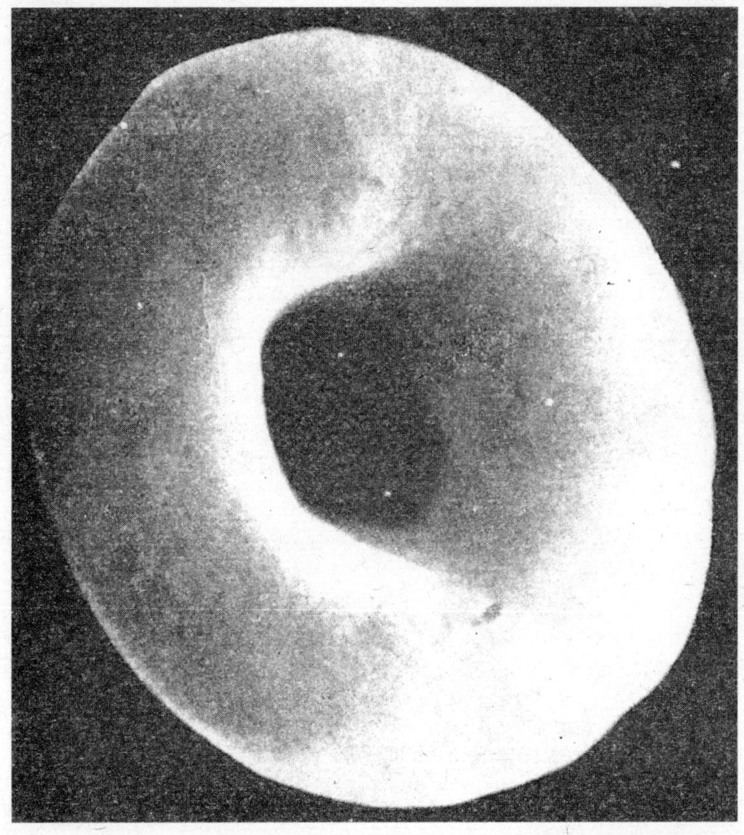

Plate 3. Electron scanning micrograph of a normal RBC x 14.000 (Chapter 4).

Red Blood Cells (RBC) or Erythrocytes

Erythrocytes constitute about 32 per cent of the total amount of the blood. Seen under the microscope they appear as biconcave discs, circular in shape, flexible and they possess no nucleus; having lost it before entering the circulation. It may be noted that the RBC of birds including chicken, ducks, turkeys etc., fish and reptiles including any of a group of cold-blooded vertebrates that crawl on their bellies, viz. snakes, lizards, crocodiles, alligators and turtles possess a nucleus, while those of camel erythrocytes are oval in outline and biconvex.

The depth and size of the concavity vary with the species. The dog RBC is a distinct biconcave disc, those in horse and cat have a shallow concavity and the pig and ruminants have RBC similar to a flattened disc.

The largest size erythrocyte is found in dog (7.0/μm) and the smallest in goat (4.1/μm). The total number of RBC not only varies for a given species, but wide variations occur with different breeds, nutritional state, physical activity and age.

Erythrocytes are formed in the red bone marrow of the proximal ends of certain long bones and also in ribs, the sternum, vertebrae and in pelvis.

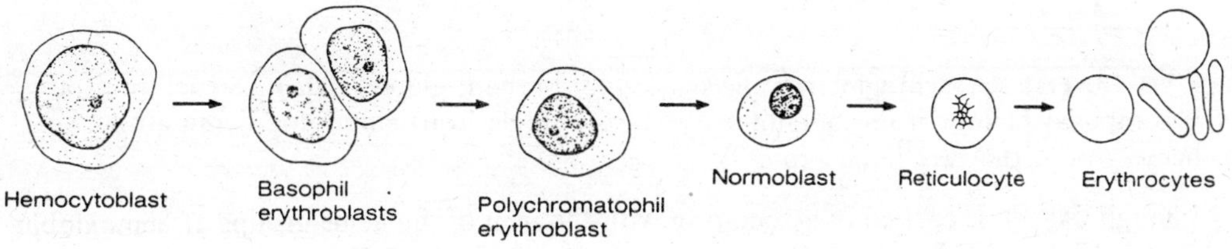

Fig 4.2. Erythrocyte formation from hemocytoblast cells in red bone marrow. The hemocytoblasts are formed from stem cells located in the bone marrow.

During formation, stem cell, inside the marrow give rise to cells called *hemocytoblasts* which in turn form cells called *basophil erythroblasts*. At this stage cells begin to synthesize a special organic compound known as *hemoglobin*. The basophil erythroblasts give rise to cells called *polychromatophil erythroblasts*. As hemoglobin synthesis continues, the nuclei of the cells shrinks, and the cells become *normoblast*. When the normoblast cytoplasm attains a hemoglobin concentration of about 34 per cent, the nuclear disappears, although the remains of some endoplasmic reticulum are still evident. These non-nucleated cells are called *reticulocytes*. Finally the reticular material itself disappears and the cells become fully formed erythrocytes.

Erythrocytes function in the transport of gases by the blood at pressures sufficient to permit rapid diffusion of oxygen from the blood to the metabolizing cells and also CO_2 from these cells to the blood. It is the hemoglobin within the erythrocyte that is responsible for this activity and is present in various domestic animals from 8 to 16 gm per 100 ml blood. Hemoglobin (Hb) consists of a protein called *globin* united with four non-protein groups called *hemes*. Each heme group contains an iron atom which is able to combine reversibly with one oxygen molecule. Thus each hemoglobin molecule can potentially associate with four oxygen molecules. When hemoglobin is combined with oxygen, it is called *Oxyhemoglobin* (HbO_2);

when it is not carrying oxygen, it is called *reduced hemoglobin.* In the body, virtually all the hemoglobin that travels to the tissues are oxygeneted, whereas about 25 per cent of the hemoglobin that return from tissues are in the reduced form. When we consider that a single RBC may contain up to *300 million* hemoglobin molecules and that there may be 5 million RBC per cubic millimeter of blood, the substantial oxygen carrying capacity of these cells becomes readily apparent.

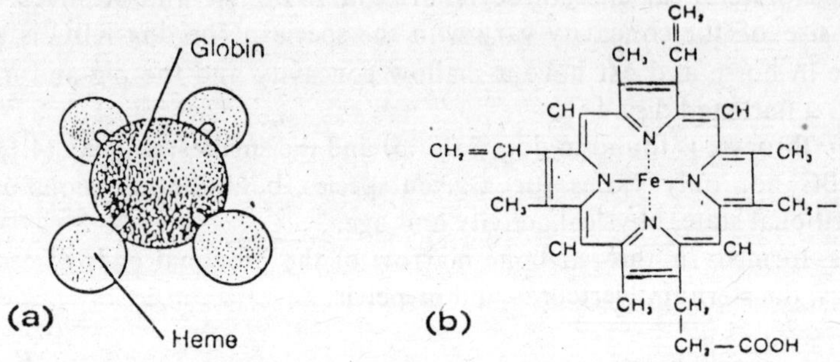

Fig. 4.3 (a) A hemoglobin molecule is composed of four iron-containing heme groups that are joined to a protein, globin. (b) Structure of a single iron-containing heme group.

Although oxygen is carried in association with the iron of the heme groups of hemoglobin, CO_2 is carried in reversible association with the protein portion of the Hb molecule. Carbon dioxide-protein complexes of the type that involve the globin are called *Carbamino compounds.*

Methemoglobin is a true oxidation product of hemoglobin which is unable to transport oxygen as the iron is in a ferric (Fe^{+++}) state rather than usual ferrous (Fe^{++}) state. The condition is produced by certain chemicals such as nitrite and chlorates. Nitrite poisoning has been reported in cattle grazing on plants grown on highly fertilized soil. In these cases, nitrates in the plants are converted to nitrites in the rumen and cause the formation of *methemoglobin* when absorbed into the blood.

Carboxyhemoglobin is a more stable compound formed when carbon monoxide (present in exhaust fumes of car, bus etc.) combines with hemoglobin. $CO + Hb \rightarrow COHb$. The Carboxy-hemoglobin is unable to carry oxygen, and the animal essentially dies of suffocation, although the blood is typically cherry red in colour.

Hemolysis is a breakdown of red cells so that the hemoglobin escapes into the plasma. It may be caused by bacterial toxins, snake venoms, blood parasites, hypotonic solution and many chemical substances. The resulting hemoglobin in the plasma gives it a reddish colour, and the condition is called *hemoglobinemia.*

Hemagluttination is a clumping of red cells of blood. Usually cells from one species will agglutinate when injected into the blood of an animal of another species or within the species when wrong types are used.

Red cells when formed normally carry out their function in the blood stream for about 120 days in man, 45–50 days in rabbit and rat, 124 days in dogs. The cells are destroyed in great numbers daily. On a calculation based on average life of RBC as 100 days it has been found that for an animal weighing 450 kg, about 35 million cells undergo degradation and synthesis every second.

Leucocytes or White Blood Cells (WBC)

These are colourless cells found along with RBC in blood plasma. They are larger (8–25

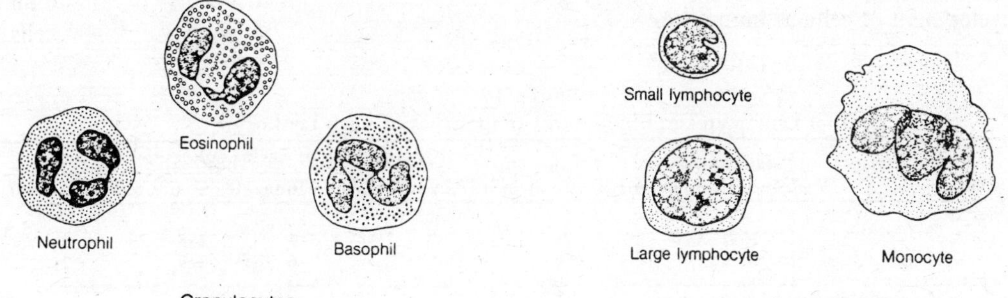

microns) and fewer than red cells, all are nucleated and contain no hemoglobin, and capable of independent movement. In addition of being present in the blood, many leucocytes are found in lymphoid tissues such as thymus, lymph nodes, spleen and lymoid areas in the linings of the gastrointestinal tract. WBC are classified as follows:

Granulocytes	*Agranulocytes*
(Contain granule within the cytoplasm, that stain with common blood stain. Nuclei appear in many shapes. Cells remain functional for 10 hours to 3 days)	(Usually show few granules in the rather sparse cytoplasm. Cells remain functional for 100–300 days).
Neutrophils Eosinophils Basophils	Monocyte Lymphocyte

The life span of the white blood cells varies considerably from only a few hours for granulocytes, to potentially months for monocytes, and years for lymphocytes.

Neutrophils. The group constitute the greatest number of all the WBCs. They reside to a great extent along the inner margins of the capillaries and small vessels. Cells are granulated, with eosin or other basic dyes these are not coloured. They can migrate from the blood vessels into the tissues and engulf bacteria (phagocytosis), are thus found in pus and are very important for defence against infection. Their number increases rapidly whenever acute infection is present.

Eosinophils. Ganulocyte type that stains with eosin is known as eosinophil. May be weakly phagocytic. Primary function seems to be the detoxification of either foreign proteins introduced into the body via the lungs or G.I. tract, or toxins produced by bacteria and parasites by secreting hydrolytic enzymes.

Basophils. Contain blue staining granules, are also rare in normal blood. Since they contain heparin (an anticoagulant), it is postulated that they release this in areas of inflammation to prevent clotting and stasis of blood and lymph.

Monocytes. The largest WBC, like neutrophils, are phagocytic. They are functional more for cases of less acute infections.

Lymphocytes. Variable in size and appears. One of the major functions is their response to antigens (foreign substances) by forming antibodies that circulate in the blood or in the development of cellular immunity.

Table 4.2
Total Leukocytes in Blood and Components of Each Leukocyte

Species	Total Leukocyte Count (Range; no./μl)	Percentage of Each Leukocyte				
		Neutrophil	Lymphocyte	Monocyte	Eosinophil	Basophil
Pig						
1 day	10,000–12,000	70	20	5–6	2–5	<1
1 week	10,000–12,000	50	40	5–6	2–5	<1
2 weeks	10,000–12,000	40	50	5–6	2–5	<1
6 weeks and older	15,000–22,000	30–35	55–60	5–6	2–5	<1
Horse	8000–11,000	50–60	30–40	5–6	2–5	<1
Cow	7000–10,000	25–30	60–65	5	2–5	<1
Sheep	7000–10,000	25–30	60–65	5	2–5	<1
Goat	8000–12,000	35–40	50–55	5	2–5	<1
Dog	9000–13,000	65–70	20–25	5	2–5	<1
Cat	10,000–15,000	55–60	30–35	5	2–5	<1
Chicken	20,000–30,000	25–30	55–60	10	3–8	1–4

From Swenson, M.J.: Physiological properties and cellular and chemical constituents of blood. *In* Dukes' Physiology of Domestic Animals. 10th Ed. Edited by M.J. Swenson. Ithaca, NY, Cornell University Press, 1984.

Table 4.3
Functions of formed elements

Element	*Function(s)*
A. Erythrocytes	Transports O_2 and CO_2 by presence of haemoglobin; buffering
B. Leucocytes	
1. Neutrophil	Phagocytosis of particles, wound healing. Granules contain peroxidase for destruction of microorganisms
2. Eosinophil	Detoxification of foreign proteins. Granules contain peroxidases, oxidases, trypsin, phosphatases. Numbers increase in auto-immune states, allergy, and in parasitic infection (Schistosomiasis trichinosis, strongyloidiases).
3. Basophil	Control viscosity of connective tissue ground substances? Granules contain heparin (liquefies ground substance) serotonin (vasoconstrictor) histamine (vasodilator)
4. Lymphocyte	Phagocytosis of particles, globulin production
5. Monocyte	Phagocytosis, globulin production.
C. Platelets (Thrombocytes)	Blood clotting

Platelets

Blood platelets, also called *thrombocytes*, are fragments of protoplasm found in the blood. Platelets function chiefly to reduce loss of blood from injured vessels. By adhering to vessel walls and to each other in the area of the injury, platelets may form a white thrombus (clot) that can occlude the vessel and prevent further loss of blood.

Blood cell formation

Unlike many other cell-types blood cells are short-lived. They survived for days or months and then are destroyed. Thus they are produced and removed continuously. For the most part, cell formation, *haemopoiesis* and cell destruction occur in the same tissues. Many of the tissues where these processes go on, also contribute to antibody production, clean the blood by filtration and remove many kinds of foreign pathogens.

In the embryo, blood cells first form in conjunction with blood vessels. Later, blood cells form in the tissues of the digestive tract, thymus, kidneys and liver. In the adult mammal, red blood cells and granulocytes are formed mainly in the bone marrow, while lymphoid cells are produced in lymphoid organs such as the spleen and lymph nodes. In phylogenetically more primitive, adult animals all cellular elements of the blood may be produced in the spleen.

Erythrocytes of adult mammals are in fact formed in the red bone marrow of the proximal ends of certain long bones and also in ribs, the sternum, vertebrae and in

Table 4.4

Tissue or Organ	*Function in Hematopoiesis*
Bone marrow	Produces erythrocytes, granulocytes, thrombocytes and hemoglobin; stores iron.
Lymph nodes and follicles	Produce lymphocytes and participate in antibody production.
Liver	Stores B_{12}, folic acid, and iron. Produces prothrombin and fibrinogen. Converts free bilirubin to bilirubin glucuronide for excretion via the bile. Retains its embryonic potential for hematopoiesis.
Spleen	Produces lymphocytes, stores erythrocytes and iron, retains embryonic potential for hematopoiesis. Destroys erythrocytes and hemoglobin through its extensive R.E. system.
Stomach	Produces HCl for release of iron from complex organic molecules. Produces intrinsic factor which functions in preparing B_{12} for absorption by the intestinal mucosa.
Reticuloendothelial system	Produces monocytes. Destroys erythrocytes and converts hemoglobin to iron, globin and free bilirubin. Stores iron.
Kidney	Presumptive organ for production of erythropoietin.
Thymus	Probable origin of antibody-producing cells for distribution to lymphocytic tissues throughout the body. Removal of the thymus in the very young leads to loss of ability to respond to antigen.

pelvis. These tissues have a rich blood supply which commonly includes large, loose, vascular channels, the sinusoids.

Avian Blood

In birds, the blood vascular system operate at a much higher pulse rate and blood pressure level. Considering that some birds live to be more than 100 years old with such an arrangement, there should be little question of its efficiency or effectiveness.

The main difference in the vascular system lies in the heart which has four chambers. The right atrium of the chicken is larger than the left but the mass of the left ventricle is nearly three times that of the right. The right A-V valve is simply a muscular flap, but the left A-V valves are membranous as in mammals. The aortic and pulmonary valves are similar to those in mammals.

The major differences in the blood of birds and mammals are that birds have nucleated erythrocytes and nucleated thrombocytes.

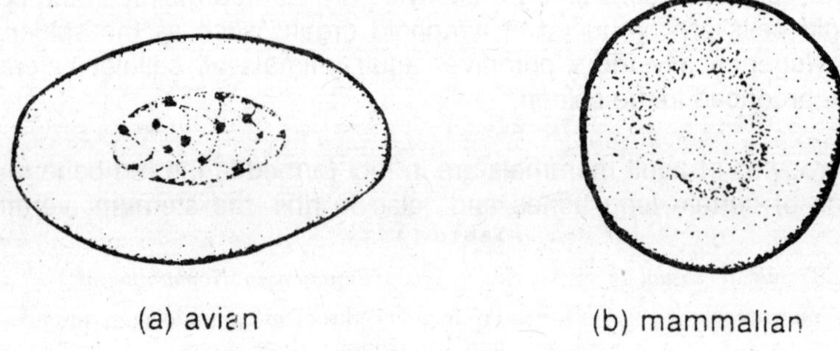

Fig.4.4. Red blood cells.

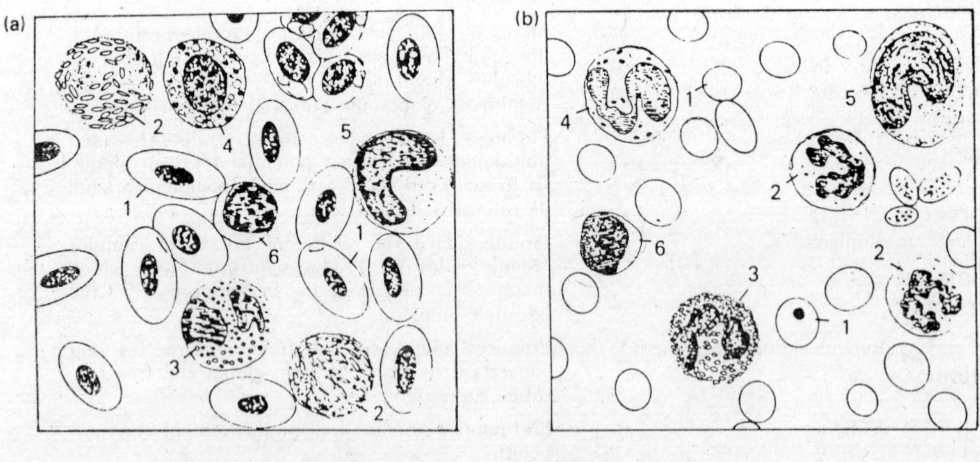

Fig 4.5 Structure of some blood cells in blood smears of (a) an avian - domestic fowl; (b) a mammal - cat

Table 4.5

WHOLE BLOOD		
Formed Elements (45%)		**Blood Plasma (55%)**
Red cells (erythrocytes)	Oxygen Carriers	Blood Serum — Fibrinogen
White cells (leukocytes)	Bacteria Fighters	Blood Serum: Electrolytes, Water; Proteins: Albumins, Globulins
Platelets	Needed in blood clotting	

The blood of a chicken makes up about 8 per cent of the body weight in chicks of 1-2 weeks of age and about 6 per cent of the weight of a mature hen. The heart of a mature small fowl such as a White Leghorn is about 350 beats per minute. Larger breeds such as Rhode Island Red have lower rates averaging about 250 beats per minute.

The haematocrit value (percentage by volume of whole blood that is composed of erythrocytes) is about 30 in young chicken and laying hen while 40 in adult males. As a rough guide, values in other domestic species are in sheep, 32; cow, 40; horse and pig 42 while in dog it is 45. The blood of the fowl clots very rapidly.

Sheep

The haematology of sheep is in general similar to that of the cow, with the exception of size and number of erythrocytes. because of the type of husbandry sheep harbor gastrointestinal parasites much more common than cattle. Modest variation due to season and nutritional state have also been observed, particularly in parasitized sheep.

Horse

For interpretation of equine haematology, it is necessary to know whether the animal is classed as "hot-blooded" or "Cold-blooded". Horses with considerable Arabian ancestry are commonly referred to as hot-blooded.

Avian Blood Components

Erythrocyte (RBC)

The red blood cells are small and oval in shape, *unlike mammals, contain a large nucleus* and average long diameter is around 13 μm, short diameter is 7 μm with a thickness of about 3.0 μm. The number of RBC varies due to age, sex, hormones, hypoxia and other factors. The number is always more in adult male averaging 3.8 million per cubic millimeter whereas in adult females the number hardly exceeds 3.0 million.

The erythrocytes are generally elliptical and quite large. The nucleus is condensed and in the centre of the cell. Hemoglobin concentration (MCHC) is lower in avian cells than in mammalian erythrocytes, probably because of the space occupied by the nucleus.

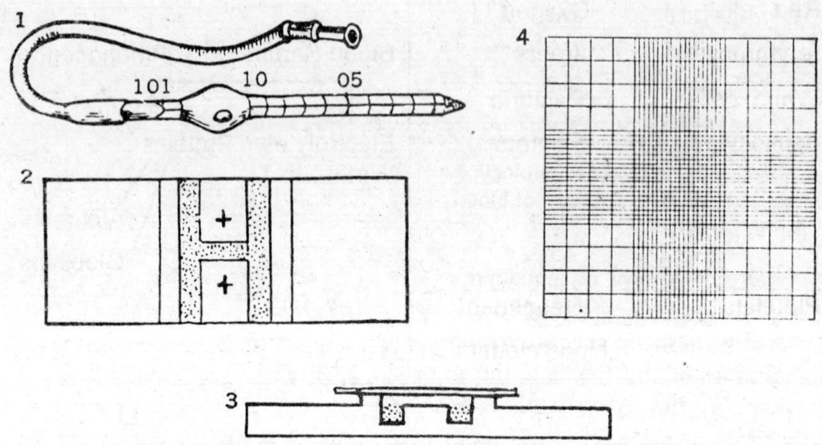

Fig 4.6 —Equipment for blood counting. Hemocytometer for counting the red blood cells. 1. Pipette for diluting blood sample; 2. glass slide, provided with two platforms on each of which ruled squares marked by +, and shown highly magnified in 4, are engraved. Each square has an area of 1/400 sq. mm.; 3, slide in cross-section with cover glass in position.

The life span of human erythrocyte is about 120 days; that of chickens averages 28-35 days. The haemoglobin content of whole blood in male averages 11.3 g per 100 ml and in female it varies between 9.0 to 10.0 g/100 ml. There is every reason to believe that avian haemoglobins contain the four iron containing heme units in mammals; but the protein moieties (globins) are different being at least of two types, one (70-80 per cent) exhibiting slow, and the other (20-30 per cent) fast electrophoretic mobilities. A mature RBC derives its energy mainly from anaerobic glycolysis and from the phospho-gluconate pathways.

Leucocytes (WBC)

The white blood cells (WBC) or leucocytes are the mobile units of the body's protecting system. They are formed partially in the bone marrow (the granulocytes) and partially in the lymph nodes (lymphocytes and monocytes), but after formation they are transported in the blood to the different parts of the body where they are to be used as rapid and potent defense against any infectious agent that might be present.

Five different types of WBC are normally found in the blood. These are (a) polymorphonuclear (granulocytes) neutrophils, polymorphonuclear eosinophils, polymorphonuclear basophils and (b) agranulocytes such as monocytes and lymphocytes. The granulocytes and the monocytes protect the body against invading organisms by ingesting them.

Total number of WBC in birds ranges from 20-30 thousand per cubic millimeter.

Table 4.6

	Total Leuko-cytes thous-ands per mm³	Lympho-cytes	Hetero-phils	Eosino-phils	Baso-phils	Mono-cytes	Thrombocytes thousands per mm³
Chicken	20.0	59.0	27.2	2.0	1.7	10.2	25.4
*Chicken	30.4	73.3	15.1	—	2.7	6.3	—
Chick	29.4	66.0	20.9	1.9	3.1	8.1	26.5
Duck	23.4	61.7	24.3	2.1	1.5	10.8	23.4

(Partly from Kolb, Lehrbuch der Physiologie der Haustiere)
**Source*: Cook, S.F. (1937). A study of blood picture of poultry and its diagnostic significance. Poultry Science, *16*, 291.

1. *Heterophils*: This type of leucocyte is sometimes designated as a polymorphonuclear—pseudo eosinophilic granulocyte, but for the sake of brevity it is usually designated "heterophil". In chickens these are generally round and have a diameter of about 10 to 15 μm. The characteristic feature of these cells is the presence of many rod or spindle-shaped acidophilic crystalline bodies in the cytoplasm. The nucleus is polymorphic with varying degrees of lobulation.

2. *Eosinophils*: Polymorphonuclear eosinophilic granulocytes are of about the same size as the heterophils. The nucleus is often bilobed and is of richer blue than that of the heterophil, giving the impression of a sharper differentiation between chromatin and parachromatin than in the nucleus of the latter.

The question has arisen as to the correctness of distinguishing between the heterophil and the eosinophil in avian blood. Some workers believe that the two cell types represent modified forms of the same group, but others think that the heterophil and eosinophil have different lineages.

3. *Basophils*: Polymorphonuclear basophilic granulocytes are of about the same size and shape as the heterophils. The nucleus is weakly basophilic in reaction and round or oval in shape; at times it may be lobulated. The cytoplasm is abundant and devoid of colour. Electron microscopy reveals that granules of basophils are variable in size and are fibrillar in nature.

4. *Monocytes*: In birds monocytes are difficult to identify or to distinguish from large lymphocyte because there are transitional forms between the two. In general, the monocytes are large cells with relatively more cytoplasm than the large lymphocytes. The cytoplasm of these cells has a blue-grey tint. The nucleus is usually irregular in outline. The nuclear pattern in monocyte is of a more delicate composition than is that in the lymphocyte.

5. *Lymphocytes*: Lymphocytes consititutes the majority of the leukocytes in the blood of the fowl. There is a wide range in the size and shape of these cells The cytoplasm is usually weakly basophilic. The nucleus is usually round and may have a small indentation.

Thrombocytes (Platelets)

Avian thrombocytes show considerable variation in size, and their shape may vary from oval to round. However, the typical one is oval, unlike mammals the cells are provided *with a round nucleus in the center* of a clear cytoplasm. A constant feature is the one or more brightly red-stained granules present at the poles of the cell when stained with Wright's stain. The total number ranges in most species between 20-30,000/cubic millimeters. Platelets are involved in blood clotting.

Thrombocytes appear to function in haemostasis in birds analogously to the platelets of mammals. Although the terms thrombocyte and platelet are synonymous in mammalian haematology, only the term thrombocyte should be used in descriptions pertaining to avian species. Birds and mammals also differ in coagulation, particularly in the intrinsic system where birds appear to lack coagulation factors XI and XII.

Table 4.7 Blood is commonly obtained from the various animals as follows :

Animal	Site	Needle size	
		Gauge	Length (inches)
Horse	Jugular vein	16–19	$1\frac{1}{2}$ to 2
Cow	Jugular vein	16–19	$1\frac{1}{2}$ to 2
Sheep and goat	Jugular vein	18–20	$1\frac{1}{2}$ to 2
Pig	Anterior vena cava	20	$1\frac{1}{2}$ to 4
Dog	Cephalic, saphenous, or jugular vein	20–22	$1\frac{1}{2}$
Cat	Cephalic or jugular vein	22–25	1
Rabbit	Cardiac puncture	18	3
Small primates	Femoral artery	22–26	$\frac{5}{8}$—1
Rat and mouse	Orbital sinus	Micro blood-collection tube	

Anticoagulants used

1. *Heparin.* Used as 1.0 per cent soln. and 0.1 ml. is sufficient for 10 ml. of blood.

2. *Sodium citrate.* It is prepared by mixing 3.8 g of sodium citrate to 100 ml. of distilled water. 0.1 ml. of this soln. is O.K. for 10 ml. of blood.

3. *Ammonium & Potassium oxalate* at 60:40 ratio can be made by taking 1.2 g of ammonium oxalate and 0.8 gms of potassium oxalate. Add 100 ml distilled water to this salt mix.

Take 0.5 cc of this soln. in a specimen tube & put it in incubator at 70°C. This is adequate for 5 ml. of blood.

4. *EDTA* (Ethylene diamine tetra acetate). It is used as 1 mg. powder for 1 ml. of blood. 1 drop of 10 per cent solution will be adequate for 5 ml. of blood.

Camel Blood

The total blood volume of an adult camel has been reported to be about 93 ml/kg body weight. The erythrocytes of camel are ovoid and non-nucleated and biconvex. There is very little change in shape and size of RBC even after an individual is put to water deprivation. The RBC are also very resistant to salt and water and do not burst or lose shape even when treated with 4.5–5.0% salt water.

Table 4.8 *Components of Camel Blood Plasma*

Components	Mean ±SD	Range
Sodium mg/lit.	147 ± 4.2	129-161
Potassium mg/lit.	5.3 ± 0.43	3.6-6.1
Calcium mg/100 ml.	9.2 ± 0.99	7-10
Inorganic phosphate mg/100 ml.	5.3 ± 0.28	3.9-6.8
Magnesium mg/100 ml.	2.5± 0.23	1.8-2.9
Copper mg%	118.3	60.172
Iron mg%	98.5 ± 19	62.133
Iron binding capacity mg%	321 ± 62	198-443
Protein g%	7.3 ± 0.51	6.3-8.7
Globuling %	3.5 ± 0.47	2.8-4.4
Urea mg%	32 ± 9	16-49
Total lipids %	195 ± 46	125-382
Uric acid mg %	0.46 ± 0.1	0.19-0.61
Cholesterol mg%	32 ± 11	21-79
Bilirubin mg%	0.32 ± 0.2	0.2-0.8
Creatinine mg%	1.9 ± 0.3	1.2-2.8
Glucose mg%	50 ± 8.2	37-67
Albumin g%	3.5	3.0-4.4
Alkaline phosphatase IU/lit		33-196
Aspartate transaminase IU/lit.		69-98
Creatinine kinase IU/lit		35.92

Table 4.9 **Normal Blood Values for Camel.**

RBC	:	Ovoid and non-nucleated
RBC size	:	Large axis, 7.7-10.1μm
	:	Short axis, 4.2-64 μm
	:	Thickness, 2.5 μm
	:	Average area, 50.6 μm2
RBC count	:	7.0 to 11 million/cmm
Haematocrit value	:	28.5% to 30%
Haemoglobin	:	11 to 15.5 g/100ml
Mean Corpuscular volume (MCV)	:	28.5μm3
Mean Corpuscular Haemoglobin Concentration (MCHC)	:	54.4%
Mean Corpuscular Haemoglobin (MCH)	:	12.0 to 15.5 pg (Picogram)
Osmotic fragility	:	Resistant to wide range of salt conc. 0.2 to 20%
Critical Haemolytic volume	:	Camel RBC can swell upto 240% original volume without rupturing.
Erythrocyte sedimentation rate	:	50-120 mm/3h
Erythrocyte survival time	:	90-120 days
Total leucocyte count	:	3-10 thousand/cmm
Neutrophil %	:	33 to 70% - 51%
Lymphocyte %	:	21 to 62% - 40%
Monocyte%	:	1 % to 7%-4%
Eosinophil %	:	0 to 4%-4%
Basophil%	:	0 to3%-0.5%
Reticutocytes %	:	0 to 0.7%-0.5%
Fibrinogen	:	200-400mg/100ml.
Platelets	:	4,03,000/μl

Source : Yagil, 1985, The Desert Camel, Karger, Basel and others.

Table 4.10

Average Blood Cell values of domestic animals

Animal	Erythrocytes Total No. millions/mm³	Erythrocytes Size (μm)	Leucocytes Total no. thousand/mm³	Neutrophil %	Lymphocytes %	Monocytes %	Eosinophils %	Basophils %
DOG	7.0	7.0	12.6	70	20	5.2	4.0	0
(range)	5.5-8.5	6.7-7.2	6.0-17.0	60-77	12-33	2.10	2-10	0
CAT	7.9	5.9	16.0	59	32	3.0	5.5	0
(range)	5.0-10.0	5.5-6.3	5.5-19.5	37-75	20-55	1-4	2-12	0
CATTLE	6.3	5.5	7.9	28	58	4.0	9.0	0.5
(range)	5.0-10.0	4.5-8.0	4.0-12.0	14-45	45-75	2-7	2-20	0.2
SHEEP	9.5	4.5	7.4	30	62	2.5	5.0	0.5
(range)	8.0-10.0	2.5-3.9	4.0-12.0	10-50	40-75	0–6	0–10	0–3
GOAT	14.0	4.1	8.9	36	56	2.5	5.0	0.5
(range)	8.0-18.0	2.5-3.9	4.5-13.0	30-48	50-70	0–4	1–8	0–1
HORSE	9.5	5.3	5.5-12.5	49	44	4.0	4.0	0.5
(range)	6.0-12.0	3.8-7.0	9.0	30-65	25-70	0.5-7.0	0–11	0–3
PIG	7.4	6.0	17.1	37	53	5.0	3.5	0.5
(range)	5.0-8.0	4.0-8.0	11.0-22.0	28-47	39-62	2-10	0.5-11	0–2
BUFFALO	7.0	–	9.0	35	54	4.0	4.0	0.5
CAMEL	8.2	7.5–6.4	20.0	38	46	5.0	9.0	0.5
FOWL	3.0	–	20.0	20–40	30–70	1.0	5–14	3.0
HUMAN	4.5–5.5	–	6–9	60-70	20–25	3–8	2–4	0.5

Source : Textbook of Veterinary Histology, Dellmann, H & Brown, E.H., Lea & Febiger, Philadelphia, 1976, except the values for human, buffalo, camel & fowl.

Table 4.11

Some Differential Characteristics in Blood Morphology of Domestic Animals

	The Erythrocytes					The Leukocytes	
Animal	Rouleaux	Central Pallor	Mean Diameter (μm)	Reticulocytes in Peripheral Blood in Health (%)	Special Features	Approximate Neutrophil: Lymphocyte Ratio	Speical Features
Dog	+	++	7.0	± 1.0	Essentially uniform in size. Crenation does not occur readily.	70:20	Basophils rare. Eosinophil granules do not fill cell; granules variable in size and stain lightly. Cytoplasm shows through and takes pale blue stain.
Cat	++	+	5.8	± 0.5	Crenation with few blunt processes. Slight anisocytosis. Eccentric blue body in 1% of cells.	60:30	Basophils rare. Eosinophil granules rod-like and stain dull grayish-orange. Majority of lymphocytes of small size. Few band neutrophils are normally present.
Cow	—	+	5.5	0	Anisocytosis is common. Giant forms may occur. Thrombocytes usually are numerous.	28:58	Eosinophil granules small, round, intensely stained, and fill cell. Azurophil granules of large size may occur in lymphocytes. Vacuoles common in monocytes.
Sheep	±	+	4.5	0	Regular in size and shape with small central pale spot. Compact groups of thrombocytes.	30:60	Neutrophil nucleus usually multilobed. Eosinophil granules well-stained, ovoid and fill cell. Frequent large azurophil granules in lymphocytes. Monocyte nucleus amoeboid.
Horse	+++	±	5.7	0	Marked rouleaux, a consistent finding. Cells uniform in size. Occasional H-J-like body. Immature RBC almost never in peripheral blood.	cold-blooded, 55:35 hot-blooded, 50:45	Eosinophil very characteristic; granules very large and fill cell. Majority of lymphocytes are small. Monocytes usually have kidney-bean nucleus.
Pig	++	±	6.0	± 1.0	Crenation with sharp points is a characteristic feature. Slight anisocytosis. Occasional polychromatophilia.	35:50	Eosinophil granules ovoid, pale pink-orange, fill cell. Band neutrophils occur in health (ave. 1%). Lymphocytes vary from small to large.

Source : Jain, Nemi C : Schalm's Veterinary Haematology, 4th edition (1986); Lea and Febiger, U.S.A.

Table 4.12
Heamatological and electrolyte values
(Mean values and ranges)

SPECIES	RBC × 10^6/mm^3	Hb g/100ml	PCV ml%	Blood vol. ml/kg	WBC × 10^3/mm^3	Sodium mEq/l	Potassium mEq/l	Inorganic phosphorus mg/100ml	Calcium mg/100ml
Monkey (M. fascicularis)	4–6	10–12	35–43	55–75	5–10	146–152	4–5	5–5.4	9.5–10
	7.3	10.5	40.5		17.0	151	4.8	6.3	10.7
Cat	5–10	8–15	24–45	45–75	5–20	147–156	4–6	4.5–8.1	5–13
	8.5	14.2	45.9		9.8	147	6.2	7.9	11.5
Rat	6–10	11–17	40–50	50–65	5–13	140–156	5.4–7.0	3–11	5–14
	3.1	10.1	34.3		19.7	155	5.3	7.0	16.8
Chicken	2–4	7–13	25–45	60–90	9–31	148–163	4.6–6.5	6.2–7.9	9–24
	6.8	17.0	53.6		12.6	147	4.5	4.2	9.9
Dog	5.5–8.5	12–18	37–59	75–100	6–18	135–180	3.5–6.7	2–9	2.9–11.7
	8.5	15.0	47.0		10.2	—	3.3–6.3	3.7–8.2	3.7–6.2
Gerbil	7–10	10–17	43–52	60–85	7–22				
	6.5	13.5	40.8		8.6	144	6.0	4.9	9.9
Rabbit	5–8	8–17	31–50	45–70	3.0–12.5	138–160	3.7–6.8	2.3–6.9	5.6–12
	5.2	14.3	43.6		11.2	123	5.0	5.3	10.2
Guinea Pig	3–7	11–17	37–50	65–90	6–17	120–149	3.8–7.9	3–7.6	5.3–12
	7.2	16.4	50.8		8.1	131	5.0	5.7	9.9
Hamster	4–10	13–19	39–59	65–80	5–11	106–146	4.0–5.9	3.4–8.2	5–12
	9.2	11.1	41.8		13.6	136	5.3	6.0	6.4
Mouse	7–13	10–14	33–50	70–80	6–17	128–186	4.9–5.9	2.3–9.2	3.2–8.5

Table 4.13 Clinical biochemistry reference values
(Mean values and ranges)

SPECIES $\bar{x}$ range	Glucose mg/100ml	B.U.N① mg/100ml	Cholesterol mg/100ml	Total Protein g/100ml	Albumin g/100ml	S.G.O.T② I.U./I	S.G.P.T.③ I.U./I	Alkaline phosph. I.U./I
Monkey (M. *fasciculars*)	60–90	18–28	100–150	7.5–8.7	2.4–3.4	34–56	21–39	15–35
Cat	117 60–145	26 20–30	105 75–150	6.0 4.5–8	2.8 2–4	18 7–29	19 9–30	12 3–21
Rat	75 50–135	14.5 5–29	27 10–54	7.6 4.7–8.2	3.7 2.7–5.1	63 46–81	24 18–30	87 57–128
Chicken	164 125–200	2.0 0.5–6	96 52–148	6 5–7	2.7 2–3.5	148 88–208	13 10–37	35 25–44
Dog	86 64–120	16.5 8–22	189 95–275	6.8 5.7–7.8	3.4 2–4	52 33–75	37 16–67	17 7–25
Gerbil	94 40–140	21 17–31	— 90–130	7.9 5–17	3.1 2.5–4.5	— —	— —	— 12–37
Rabbit	132 78–155	18.5 9–32	26 20–83	6.8 5–8	3.3 2.5–4	71 42–98	65 49–79	130 90–170
Guinea Pig	92 82–107	23.5 9–32	30 16–43	5.2 5–6.8	2.6 2.1–3.9	47 27–68	42 25–59	70 55–108
Hamster	69 33–118	22 12–26	53 10–80	7.1 4–8	3.3 2.5–4	100 38–168	24 12–36	17 3–31
Mouse	89 63–176	19.5 14–28	64 26–82	3 4–8.6	3 2.5–4.8	36 23–48	19 2–24	19 10–28

① Blood Urea Nitrogen.
② Serum Glutamic Oxaloacetic Transaminase.
③ Serum Glutamic Pyruvic Transaminase.

Table 4.14 **Normal Blood Values for Cattle**

Erythrocytic Series

	Range	Ave.
Erythrocytes ($\times 10^6/\mu l$)	5.0-10.0	7.0
Hemoglobin (g/dl)	8.0 - 15.0	11.0
PCV (%)	24.0 - 46.0	35.0
MCV (fl)	40.0 - 60.0	52.0
MCH (pg)	11.0 - 17.0	14.0
MCH (%)		
Wintrobe	26.0 - 34.0	31.0
Microhematocrit	30.0 - 36.0	32.7
Reticulocytes (%)	0	0
ESR (mm)		
1 hour	0	0
8 hours	0-3	
RBC diameter (μm)	4.0 - 8.0	5.8
Resistance to saline (%)		
Min		
Max	0.52 - 0.66	
Myeloid : erythroid ratio	0.44 - 0.52	
	0.31 - 1.85 : 1.0	0.71 : 1.0

Other Data

	Range	Ave.
Thrombocytes ($\times 10^5$)	1.0 - 8.0	5.0
Icterus index (units)	2-15	5-10
Erythrocyte life span (days)	160	
Plasma proteins (g/dl)	7.0 - 8.5	
Fibrinogen (g/dl)	0.3 - 0.7	

Leukocytic Series

	Range	Ave
Leukocytes/μl	4,000-12,000	8,000
Neutrophil (band)	0 - 120	20
Neutrophil (mature)	600 - 4,000	2,000
Lymphocyte	2,500 - 7,500	4,500
Monocyte	25 - 840	400
Eosinophil	0 - 2,400	700
Basophil	0-200	50
Percentage Distribution	0 - 2	0.5
Neutrophil (band)	15-45	28.0
Neutrophil (mature)	45-75	58.0
Lymphocyte	2 - 7	4.0
Monocyte	0-20	9.0
Eosinophil	0 - 2	0.5
Basophil		

Table 4.15 **Normal Blood Values for the Sheep**

Erythrocytic Series

	Range	Ave
Erythrocytes ($\times 10^6$ μl)	9 - 15	12.0
Hemoglobin (g/dl)	9 - 15	11.5
PCV (%)	27.0 - 45.0	35.0
MCV (fl)	28 - 40	34.0
MCH(pg)	8 - 12	10.0
MCHC (%)	31 - 34	32.5
Reticulocytes (%)	0	0
ESR (mm)	0	0
RBC diameter (μm)	3.2 - 6.0	4.5
Resistance to hypotonic		
Saline (%)		
Min.	0.58 - 0.76	
Max.	0.40 - 0.55	
Myeloid:erythroid ratio	0.77 - 1.68 : 1.0	1.1 : 1.0
	(Grunsell, 1951)	

Other Data

	Range	Ave
Thrombocytes ($\times 10^5/\mu l$)	2.5 - 7.5	4.0
Icterus index (units)	Normally < 5	
Plasma proteins (g/dl)	6.0 - 7.5	
Fibrinogen (g/dl)	0.1 - 0.5	
Erythrocyte life span (days)	140 - 150	

Leukocytic Series

	Range	Ave.
Leukocytes/ul	4,000 -12,000	8,000
Neutrophil (band)	Rare	--
Neutrophil (mature	700 - 6,000	2,400
Lymphocyte	2,000 - 9,000	5,000
Monocycle	0 - 750	200
Eosinophil	0 - 1,000	400
Basophil	0 - 300	50
Percentage Distribution		
Neutrophil (band)	Rare	--
Neutrophil (mature)	10-50	30.0
Lymphocyte	40 - 75	62.0
Monocyte	0 - 6	2.5
Eosinophil	0 - 10	5.0
Basophil	0 - 3	0.5

Table 4.16 **Normal Blood Values for the Goat**

Erythrocytic Series	Range	Ave.	*Leukocytic Series*	Range	Ave
Erythrocytes (x10⁶/μl)	8.0 - 18.0	13.0	Leukocytes/μl	4,000-13,000	9,000
Hemoglobin (g/dl)	8.0 - 12.0	10.0	Neutrophil (band)	Rare	--
PVC (%)			Neutrophil (mature)	1,200 - 7,200	3,250
Wintrobe			Lymphocyte	2,000 - 9,000	5,000
(2,250 G x 30 min)	24.0 - 48.0	35.0	Monocyte	0 - 550	250
Microhematocrit			Eosinophil	50 - 650	450
(14,000 G x 10 min)	22 - 38	28.0	Basophil	0 - 120	50
MCV (fl)					
(Wintrobe)	19.5 - 37	27	Percentage Distribution		
(Microhematocrit)	16 - 25	19.5	Neutrophil	30 - 48	36.0
MCHC (%)			Lymphocyte	50 - 70	56.0
(Wintrobe)	28 - 34	31.5	Monocyte	0 - 4	2.5
(Microhematocrit)	30 - 36	33	Eosinophil	1 - 8	5.0
MCH (pg) (Microhematocrit)	5.2 - 8.0	6.5	Basophil	0 - 1	0.5
Reticulocytes (%)	None	--			
ESR (mm)	None	--			
RBC diameter (μm)	2.5 - 3.9	3.2			
Resistance to hypotonic salaine (%)					
Min.	0.74	--			
Max.	0.44	--			
Myeloid : erythroid ratio	0.69 : 1.0				
Other Data					
Thrombocytes (x10⁵/μl)	3.0 - 6.0	4.5			
Icterus index (units)	2 - 5				
Plasma proteins (g/dl)	6.0 - 7.5				
Fibrinogen (g/dl)	0.1 - 0.4				
Eythrocyte life span (days)	125				

Table 4.17 **Normal Blood Values for the Pig**

Erythrocytic Series	Range	Ave	*Leukocytic Series*	Range	Ave.
Erythrocytes (x10⁶ μl)	5.0 - 8.0	6.5	Leukocytes/μl	11,000 - 22,000	16,000
Hemoglobin (g/dl)	10.0 - 16.0	13.0	Percentage Distribution		
PCV (%)	32.0 - 50.0	42.0	Neutrophil (band)	0 - 4	1.0
MCV (fl)	50 - 68	60	Neutrophil (mature)	28 - 47	37.0
MCH (pg)	17.0 - 21	19.0	Lymphocyte	39 - 62	53.0
MCHC (%)	30.0 - 34.0	32.0	Monocyte	2 - 10	5.0
Reticulocytes (%)	0.0 - 1.0	0.4	Eosinophil	0.5 - 11	3.5
ESR (mm in 1 hr.)	Variable		Basophil	0 - 2	0.5
RBC diameter (μm)	4.0 - 8.0	6.0			
RBC life span (days)	86 ± 11.5		*Other Data*		
Resistance to hypotonic			Thrombocytes (1 x 10⁵/μl)	5.2 ± 1.95	
Saline (%)			Icterus index (units)	< 5	
Min		0.70	Plasma proteins (g/dl)	6.0 - 8.0	
Max.		0.45	Fibrinogen (g/dl)	0.1 - 0.5	
Myeloid:erythroid ratio	1.77 ± 0.52 : 1 (Lahey et al., 1952)				

Table 4.18

Normal Blood Values for the Horse

	Hot-Blooded Breeds (based on 147 clinically normal horses)		Cold-Blooded Breeds	
	Range	Mean ± SD	Range	Ave
Erythrocytic Series				
Erythrocytes (x 10^6/µl)	6.8 - 12.9	9.0 ± 1.2	5.5 - 9.5	7.5
Hemoglobin (g/dl)	11.0 - 19.0	14.4 ± 1.7	8.0 - 14.0	11.5
PCV (%)	32.0 - 53.0	41.0 ± 4.5	24.0 - 44.0	35.0
MCV (fl)	37.0 - 58.5	45.5 ± 4.3	--	--
MCH (pg)	12.3 - 19.7	15.9 ± 1.5	--	--
MCHC (%)	31.0 - 38.6	35.2 ± 1.4	--	--
RBC diameter (µm)	5.0 - 6.0	5.5 -	--	--
Resistance to hypotonic saline (%)	0.34 - 0.56	0.45 -	--	--
Leukocytic Series				
Total Leukocytes/µl	5,400 - 14,300	9,050 ± 1,800	6,000 - 12,000	8,500
Neutrophil (band)	0 - 1,000	36 ± 104	--	--
Neutrophil (segmenter)	2,260 - 8,580	4,745 ± 1,235	--	--
Lymphocyte	1,500 - 7,700	3,500 ± 1,120	--	--
Monocyte	0 - 1,000	388 ± 288	--	--
Eosinophil	0 - 1,000	305 ± 244	--	--
Basophil	0 - 290	45 ± 62	--	--
Percentage Distribution				
Neutrophil (band)	0 - 8.0	0.35 ± 0.97	0 - 2.0	0.5
Neutrophil (segmenter)	22.0 - 72.0	52.62 ± 8.73	35 - 75.0	54.0
Lymphocyte	17.0 - 68.0	38.73 ± 8.66	15 - 50.0	35.0
Monocyte	0 - 14.0	4.32 ± 2.42	2 - 10.0	5.0
Eosinophil	0 - 10.0	3.35 ± 2.55	2 - 12.0	5.0
Basophil	0 - 4.0	0.49 ± 0.65	0 - 3.0	0.5
Other Data				
Plasma proteins (g/dl)	5.8 - 8.7	6.9 ± 0.6	--	--
Fibrinogen (g/dl)	0.1 - 0.4	0.26 ± 0.08	-	--
Icterus index (units)	7.5 - 20 (influenced by plant pigments and PCV)			
Thrombocytes (x 10^5)	1.0 - 3.5	2.25	--	--
Erythrocyte life span (days)	140 - 150			
Myeloid : erythroid ratio	0.5 - 1.5 : 1.0			

Table 4.19 **Normal Blood Values for the Chicken *(Gallus gallus domesticus)***

	Erythrocytic Series			*Leukocytic Series*	
	Range	*Ave*		*Range*	*Ave.*
Erythrocytes (x10^6 µl)	2.5 - 3.5	3.0			
Hemoglobin (g/dl)	7.0 - 13.0	9.0	Leukocytes/µl	12,000 - 30,000	12,000
PVC (%)	22.0 - 35.0	30.0	Heterophil (band)	Rare	--
MCV (fl)	90.0 - 140.0	115.0	Heterophil (mature)	3,000 - 6,000	4,500
MCH (pg)	33.0 - 47.0	41.0	Lymphocyte	7,000 - 17,500	14,000
MCHC (%)	26.0 - 35.0	29.0	Monocyte	150 - 2,000	1,500
Reticulocytes (%)	0 - 0.6	0.0	Eosinophil	0 - 1,000	400
ESR (mm)	3.0 - 12.0	7.0	Basophil	Rare	--
RBC size (um)	7.0 x 12.0				
Other Data					
Thrombocytes (x 10^3/µl)	20.0 - 40.0	30.0	Percentage Distribution		
Icterus index (units)	2 - 5	2	Heterophil (band)	Rare	--
Plasma proteins (g/dl)	4.0 - 5.5	4.5	Heterophil (matre)	15.0 - 40.0	28.0
Fibrinogen (g/dl)	0.1 - 0.4	0.2	Lymphocyte	45.0 - 70.0	60.0
Erythrocyte life span (days)	20 - 35 days		Monocyte	5.0 - 10.0	8.0
			Eosinophil	1.5 - 6.0	4.0
			Basophil	Rare	--

Source : N. C. Jain, : Veterinary Hematology, 4th Ed. (1989) ; Lea & Febiger, Philadelphia, U.S.A.

Table 4.20 **Normal Blood Values for Water Buffaloes**

Parameter	Range	Mean	Standard Deviation
RBC (X 10^{6}µl)	5.07-8.27	6.54	0.77
Hb (g/dl)	9-13.5	11.1	0.96
PCV (%)	26-34	31.0	2.0
MCV (fl)	40.6-55.2	48.2	4.60
MCHC (%)	30.5-38.5	35.2	2.34
MCH (pg)	13.5-20.5	17.10	1.85
Icterus index (units)	2-5	2	1.25
ESR (mm at 1 hr)	17-69	53	12.30
Plasma protein (g/dl)	6-9	7.8	0.70
Fibrinogen (g/dl)	0.2-0.8	0.37	0.20
Reticulocytes (%)	0	0	0
WBC (number/µl)	6,250-13,050	9,676	1,789
Bands	0-106	18	40
Neutrophils	1,285-6,893	3,257	1,262
Lymphocytes	2,554-9,637	5,065	1,595
Monocytes	63-1,349	584	301
Eosinophils	170-1,471	592	452
Basophils	0-326	131	98
WBC, percentages			
Bands	0-1	0.2	0.34
Neutrophils	13-54	32.9	8.74
Lymphocytes	26-75	52.7	12.0
Monocytes	1-11.5	5.9	2.63
Eosinophils	2-14.0	6.9	4.64
Basophils	0-3.5	1.4	1.02

Sources : Jain, Nemi. C. Schalm's Veterinary Haematology, 4th edition (1986); Lea and Febiger, U.S.A.

Table 4.21

NORMAL BLOOD VALUES FOR YAK

Erythrocyte Series	*Average Values*	*Leucocytic Series*	*Average Values*
Erythrocyte (X10^6 μι)	6.40	Total Leucocyte (10^3/μι)	6.6
Hæmoglobin (g/dl)	9.00	Neutrophil (%)	42.0
PCV (L/1)	0.36	Lymphocyte (%)	46.0
ESR (mm in 1 hr.)	0.70	Monocyte (%)	0.4
MCH (pg)	21.00	Eosinophil	10.7
MCHC (g/dl)	36.00	Basophil	0.5
MCV (fl)	58.00		

Source : Joshi, B.P., *Wild Animal Medicine*, Published by Oxford & IBH Publishing Co. Pvt. Ltd. 66, Janpath, New Delhi,

Table 4.22

Normal Values in Circulatory System

	Horse	*Cow*	*Sheep*	*Pig*	*Dog*
Sedimentation rate (mm/min)	2 to 12/10 15 to 30/20	0/30 0/60	0/30 0/60	0 to 6/30 1 to 14/60	1 to 6/30 5 to 25/60
Red blood cell count (million/cu mm)	7	7	11	7	7
Diameter of red cells (μ)	5.6	5.6	5.0	6.2	7.3
Hemoglobin (gm/100 ml)	12.5	12	11	12	13.5
Hematocrit (volume % of red cells)	42	40	32	42	45
White blood cells (thousands/cu mm)	9	9	8	15	12
Differential white count (%)					
Neutrophils	55	30	40	40	60
Eosinophils	4	5	4	2	5
Basophils	1	1	1	1	1
Monocytes	10	5	6	8	8
Lymphocytes	30	60	50	50	25
Blood pH (average and range)	7.4 (7.35 to 7.43)	7.3 (7.20 to 7.55)		7.4	7.5 (7.32 to 7.68)
Coagulation time (minutes)	11.5	6.5	2.5	3.5	2.5
Specific gravity	1.060	1.043	1.042	1.060	1.059
Heart rate/min (average and range)	32 to 44	60 to 70	70 to 80	60 to 80	70 to 120
Blood pressure (mm Hg, syst/diast)	80/50	134/88	114/68	169/108	148/100
Carotid pressure (mm Hg, average and range)	169 (159 to 194)	125 to 166	114 (90 to 140)	169 (144 to 185)	155 (120 to 176)
Blood volume (% of body weight)	9.7	7.7	8.0		7.2

*Data compiled from standard references, including Benjamin, Dukes, Payne, and Spector.

Cerebrospinal Fluid

Cerebrospinal fluid is formed by *choroid plexuses* (tufts of capillaries) in the ventricles of brain. It circulates throughout the brain and spinal cord. The fluid resembles blood plasma from which it is derived, but has less protein, glucose and K^+. It probably serves partly as a nutritive medium for the brain and spinal cord as well as cushioning these structures against shock.

Synovial Fluid

Synovial fluid is a thick, tenacious liquid found in joint cavities, tendon sheaths, and bursae. It ows its physical properties and lubricating ability due to the presence of mucopolysaccharides and possibly hyaluronic acid. Besides reducing friction in joints, synovial fluid probably helps to nourish the articular cartilages.

Fundamentals of Terminology

Medical terms generally have Greek or Latin origin. The meaning of many commonly used terms in hematology can be readily understood by learning the following word parts :

Prefix or Stem			*Prefix or Stem.*		
a	=	without	mega	=	large
aniso	=	not equal	meta	=	change
baso	=	base	micro	=	small
eosin	=	red	mono	=	one
erythro	=	red	morpho	=	form
granulo	=	granule	myelo	=	marrow
hem or hemat	=	blood	neutro	=	neutral, neither
hyper	=	excessive	normo	=	nor
hypo	=	deficient	oligo	=	scanty, few
hetero	=	denoting relationship to another	pan	=	all
karyo	=	nucleus or nut	poikilo	=	irregular
leuk	=	white	poly	=	many
lympho	=	water, relating to lymph	pro	=	before
macro	=	large	reticulo	=	net
			thrombo	=	clot

Stem or suffix			*Stem or suffix*		
blast	=	germ	osis	=	a process
chrome	=	color	penia	=	poverty
crit	=	to separate	philia	=	love
cyte	=	cell	plasia	=	to form (tissue)
meter	=	to measure	poiesis	=	making
ology	=	study of	rubri	=	red

Terminology

Anemia. A decrease in the hemoglobin value, the packed cell volume, or the erythrocyte count of more than two standard deviations below the mean normal determined by the same method on the bloods of healthy animals of the species concerned.

Basophilia and Basophilic. Terms which when applied to a cell or cells of the erythrocytic series, as observed microscopically, indicate that the cell so described shows no trace of the characteristic hemoglobin colour and the cytoplasm shows a strong affinity for basophilic dyes. With the Romanowsky strains the cytoplasm of such cell strains various intensities of opaque blue. (These terms also may be applied to cells of the neutrophilic series when, as a result of toxemia, maturation of the cytoplasm is incomplete leading to a retention of ribonucleic acid which takes a blue stain).

Chylomicron or Chylomicra. Particles of emulsified fat in the blood plasma. These particles are 0.5 to 1.0 micron in size and when present in large numbers the plasma is cloudy and after centrifugation a layer of white neutral fat may be present above the plasma. The plasma may be described as *lactescent* or *lipemic*. Examination of a drop of lipemic blood under a coverglass and by means of a microscope will reveal the chylomicra in the form of myriads of particles showing brownian movement. In the dry, unfixed blood film treated with new methylene blue stain the chylomicra appear as refractile bodies surrounding the erythrocytes.

Erythrocytosis. The presence of an increased erythrocyte count of more than two standard deviations above the mean normal determined by the same method on the blood of healthy animals and associated with an increase of total blood volume. The latter condition distinguishes true erythrocytosis from apparent erythrocytosis associated with dehydration or hemoconcentration. (Erythrocytosis has the same connotation as polycythemia).

Erythrocytic hypoplasia. Refers to hypoplasia (incomplete development) of the erythrocytic series only, and means a selective depression of erythrogenesis. (Depression anemia).

Hematocrit Value. The volume per cent erythrocytes in centrifuged blood.

Hemoglobinemia. Free hemoglobin circulating in blood plasma from red blood cell hemolysis within the vascular system.

Hypoplastic Anemia. Implies depression of all three cell types found normally in the bone marrow; namely, erythrocytic, granulocytic, and thrombocytic series. Hypoplasia is preferred to "aplasia" or "aplastic anemia" because strictly speaking, only complete absence of specific cells from the marrow should be called aplasia and this condition rarely exists in the hypoplastic anemias.

Hyperchromic. It is recommended that this term be avoided, because a significant increase in mean corpuscular hemoglobin concentration is not known to occur.

Hypochromic. An adjective describing a blood picture in which the erythrocytes have a mean corpuscular hemoglobin concentration and usually a mean corpuscular hemoglobin more than two standard deviation below the mean normal determined by the same method on the bloods of healthy animals of the species concerned.

Lipemia. Presence of lipids in visible form in blood and imparting a cloudy appearance to the plasma. Frequently of postprandial origin in the dog.

Macrocyte. An erythrocyte having a diameter exceeding by more than two standard deviations that of the mean normal determined by the same method on the bloods of healthy animals of the same species.

Macrocytic. An adjective describing a blood picture in which the erythrocytes have a mean corpuscular volume exceeding by more than two standard deviations.

Megaloblast. A cell of the rubricytic series, about the prorubricyte stage which is abnormal because of interruption of nuclear maturation. Typical of vitamin B_{12} or folic acid deficiency.

Microcytic. An adjective describing a blood picture in which the erythrocytes have a mean corpuscular volume more than two standard deviations below the mean normal determined by the same method on the bloods of healthy animals of the same species.

Normochromasia and Normochromatic. Terms which, when applied to the microscopic appearance of a cell or cells of the erythrocytic series, indicate that the cells described appear to have their full complement or hemoglobin and no residual basophilic material in the cytoplasm; in other words, that they show normal staining characteristics.

Normochromic. An adjective describing a blood picture in which the erythrocytes have a mean corpuscular hemoglobin concentration within plus or minus two standard of deviations of the mean normaly determined by the same method on the bloods of healthy animals of the same species.

Normocyte. Any erythrocyte having a diameter within plus or minus two standard deviations of the mean normally determined by the same method on the blood of healthy animals of the species is in question.

Normocytic. An adjective describing a blood picture in which the erythrocytes have a mean corpuscular volume within plus or minus two standard deviations of the mean normaly determined by the same method on the bloods of healthy animals of the same species.

Pernicious Anemia Type. (Also see megaloblast.). The qualifying adjective phrase to be applied to any cell of the erythrocytic or granulocytic series, and to the marrow and blood pictures as a whole, to indicate the presence of the morphologic changes characteristically seen in pernicious anemia and other macrocytic anemias which respond to liver extract or folic acid therapy. (Pernicious anemia does not occur in animals but this type of cell may be seen in human or in the related macrocytic anemias in animals). In the nucleated cells of the erythrocytic series the major feature of this change is a relative increase in the palestaining parachromatin with a corresponding decrease in the deep-staining basichromatin. In the cells of the granulocytic series the characteristic change is the presence of giant forms having very bizarre nuclei, and in the segmented neutrophils the occurrence of many cells with more than five lobes, hypersegmentation.

Reticulocyte. Young erythrocyte that takes up the vital stain new methylene blue. Slightly larger than the definitive red cell and also more resistant to hemolysis. They are often polychromatophilic in the stained blood film.

Table 4.23
Values of Some Constituents of Blood from Mature Domestic Animals

	Value (Range)				
Constituents	**Horse**	**Cow**	**Sheep**	**Pig**	**Dog**
Glucose (mg/dl)	60–110	40–80 80–120 (calf)	40–80 80–120 (lamb)	80–120	70–120
Nonprotein nitrogen (mg/dl)	20–40	20–40	20–38	20–45	17–38
Urea nitrogen (BUN) (mg/dl)	10–24	10–30	8–20	8–24	10–30
Uric acid (mg/dl)	0.5–1	0.1–2	0.1–2	0.1–2	0.1–1.5
Creatinine (mg/dl)	1–2	1–2	1–2	1–2.5	1–2
Amino acid nitrogen (mg/dl)	5–7	4–8	5–8	6–8	7–8
Lactic acid (mg/dl)	10–16	5–20	9–12		8–20
Cholesterol (mg/dl)	75–150	80–180	60–150	60–200	120–250
Bilirubin (mg/dl)	0–0.4	0–0.3	0–0.3	0–0.3	0.06–0.1
Direct					
Indirect	0.2–5	0.1–0.5	0–0.1	0–0.3	0.01–0.5
Total	0.2–6	0.2–1.5	0.1–0.4	0–0.6	0.10–0.6
Electrolytes (mEq/L)	132–152	132–152	139–152	135–150	141–155
Sodium					
Potassium	2.5–5.0	3.9–5.8	3.9–5.4	4.4–6.7	3.7–5.8
Calcium	4.5–6.5	4.5–6.0	4.5–6.0	4.5–6.5	4.5–6.0
Phosphorus	2–6	2–7	2–7	3–6	2–6
Magnesium	1.5–2.5	1.5–2.5	1.8–2.3	2–3	1.5–2.0
Chlorine	99–109	97–111	95–105	94–106	100–115

From Swenson, M.J.: Physiological properties and cellular and chemical constituents of blood. *In* Dukes' Physiology of Domestic Animals. 10th Ed. Edited by M.J. Swensen. Ithaca, NY, Cornell University Press, 1984.

MECHANISMS OF REPRODUCTION

MALE REPRODUCTIVE ORGANS

The two testes are the primary sex organs of the male. In mature normal animal testes perform two vital functions:

(1) They produce viable, potentially fertile spermatozoa;

(2) They produce the androgen, or male hormone, testosterone.

In all mammals except those living in the sea and birds, the testes which is the primary organ—develop in the vicinity of the kidneys, undergo an elaborate descent, ending in the scrotum. The secondary sex organs comprise the ducts leading from the testes to the exterior, the vasa efferentia, the epididymis, the vasa deferentia and the penis. The accessory sex organs comprise the prostate gland, the two seminal vesicles, and the two bulbourethral glands or Cowper's glands. The primary, secondary, and accessory sex organs are collectively termed the male reproductive tract.

The testes. The testes are suspended vertically within the scrotum, are ovoid in shape, 10–16 cm in length and 5–8 cm in width, varying with the age and size of the animal. Histologically each testis is composed of several crypts, enclosed in a serous layer called tunica vaginalis. Each crypt in turn has a number of seminiferous tubules. The wall of the seminiferous tubules consist of a basement membrane and a multilayered sperm producing epithelium having two types of cells; (a) *Germ cells*—it is here that the male germ cells, the spermatozoa, are produced; (b) *Sertoli cells*—are also called "sperm mother cells" because it is thought that the sperm heads, which become embedded in these cells, undergo a ripening process in them. The space between the seminiferous tubules occupied by interstitial cells or the *Leydig cells* which produce the male hormone. The many seminiferous tubules finally become straight and join to form the *rete testis*. Arising from the rete testis are twelve or more outgoing ducts, the *vasa efferentia*, which emerge from the testes and enter *epididymis*.

The epididymis. A tube arising at the dorsal part of the testis from the efferent duct, is considered in three parts: the caput (head), the corpus (body) and the cauda (tail). Throughout most of its length the epididymal tube is lined with secretory cells. In the caput, the tube is lined, in addition, with a ciliated, pseudostratified columnar epithelium, the flagella of which whip in the direction of efferent flow. Spermatozoa accumulate in and mature during their journey through the epididymis, which may be 33–35 metres (110–118 feet) long in the bull and longer in the boar. Epididymis has four major functions: (1) Transport—the sperm are transported from the rete testis to the efferent ducts by the fluid pressure of the testis and by the active outward beating of the cilia. It takes about 7 to 9 days for any sperm to travel from germinal epithelium to the cauda, (2) Concentration—the dilute sperm concentration originating in the testis, water is absorbed into the epithelial cells of the epididymis specially in

caput and a highly concentrated sperm is left in the tail, (3) Maturation—while migration takes place sperm cells get matured as a result of secretion from the epididymal cells, (4) Storage—

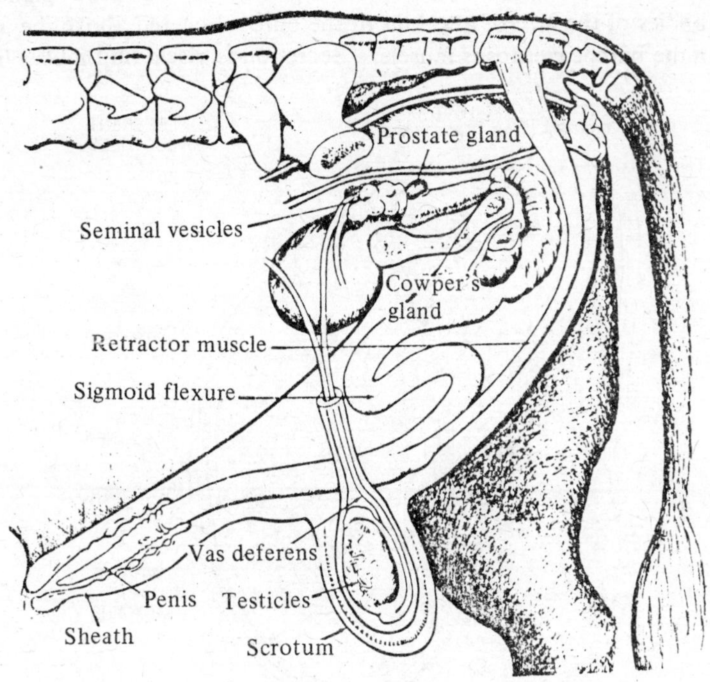

Fig. 5.1 Genitalia of the bull.

the tail of the epididymis is the sperm depot. If the epididymis in the bull is ligated, the sperm will remain alive and fertile in the epididymis upto about 60 days.

Vas deferens. The tail of the epididymis leads into the vas deferens which is a slender tube with a thick cord like wall. Like the epididymis and the testes, the vas deferens is paired and the two along with the spermatic arteries, veins, nerves and cremester muscle surrounded by tunica vaginalis (a paritonial layer) are sometimes known as the spermatic cords. Each vas deferens goes through the inguinal ring and lies very close to the vas deferens from the other testis in the pelvic cavity and finally empties into the urethra. The vas deferens is abundantly supplied with nerves and by involuntary contractions of the musculature, the vas deferens is involved in ejaculation.

The urethra. The urethra is a common passage way for the products of the testes, accessory glands and for the excretion of the urine. It extends through the pelvic area and the penis and end at the tip of the glans penis as the external urethral orifice.

The accessory organs. The accessory sex organs provide the bulk of the seminal plasma. This is rich in carbohydrate, salts of citric acid, proteins, amino acids, enzymes, water soluble vitamins and being relatively high in buffer capacity. There are three accessory organs: (1) The seminal vesicles—the two seminal vesicles are located one on either side of an ampulla.

The secretion contains high level of (upto 1%) fructose and of citric acid. (2) The prostate – is a gland consisting of two joined parts. It is surrounded by urethral muscles, and hence it often escapes notice. Prostate secretion is the source of male antagglutin and is believed to be high in mineral content. (3) The bulbo-urethral glands or Cowper's glands—are paired, round, compact bodies of the size of a walnut in the bull. Located above the urethra and are partially buried in the bulbocavernosus muscle. Secretion is viscid and mucus like.

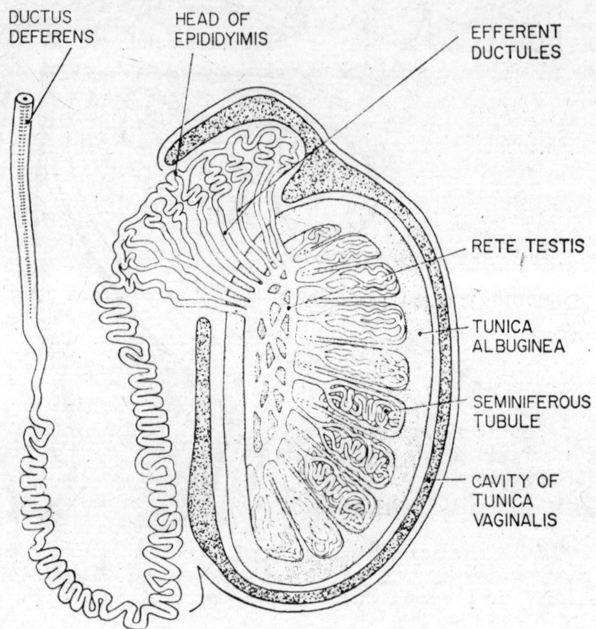

Fig. 5.2 Arrangement of tubules and ducts in the testis and epididymis.

The penis. The penis is the male organ of copulation and is composed essentially of erectile tissue. This tissue is a sponge like system of irregular blood channels which, when the male is sexually stimulated, become filled with blood under high pressure, which causes the penis to enlarge and become rigid. When not in use it forms an "S" shaped or sigmoid flexure behind the scrotal sac which is straightened out during erection. The retractor muscle which is attached on the anterior arms of the flexure helps in pulling the erected and exposed penis back into the sheath for protection against injury and infection. The tip of the penis is known as the glans and is about 3'' long. The entire penis of the bull is about 3 feet long and 1 inch in diameter.

Functions of the scrotum and the pampiniform plexus. The scrotum, with its muscles, fibrous linings, and outer skin, support the testes, protects them, and provide for the testis an environment that is 1 to 8°F cooler than the body cavity, which is a must for active spermatogenesis. The following are the mechanisms by which scrotum aids in lowering the temperature:

(1) Mere presence of the testes in the scrotum assures them of an environment cooler than the body cavity,

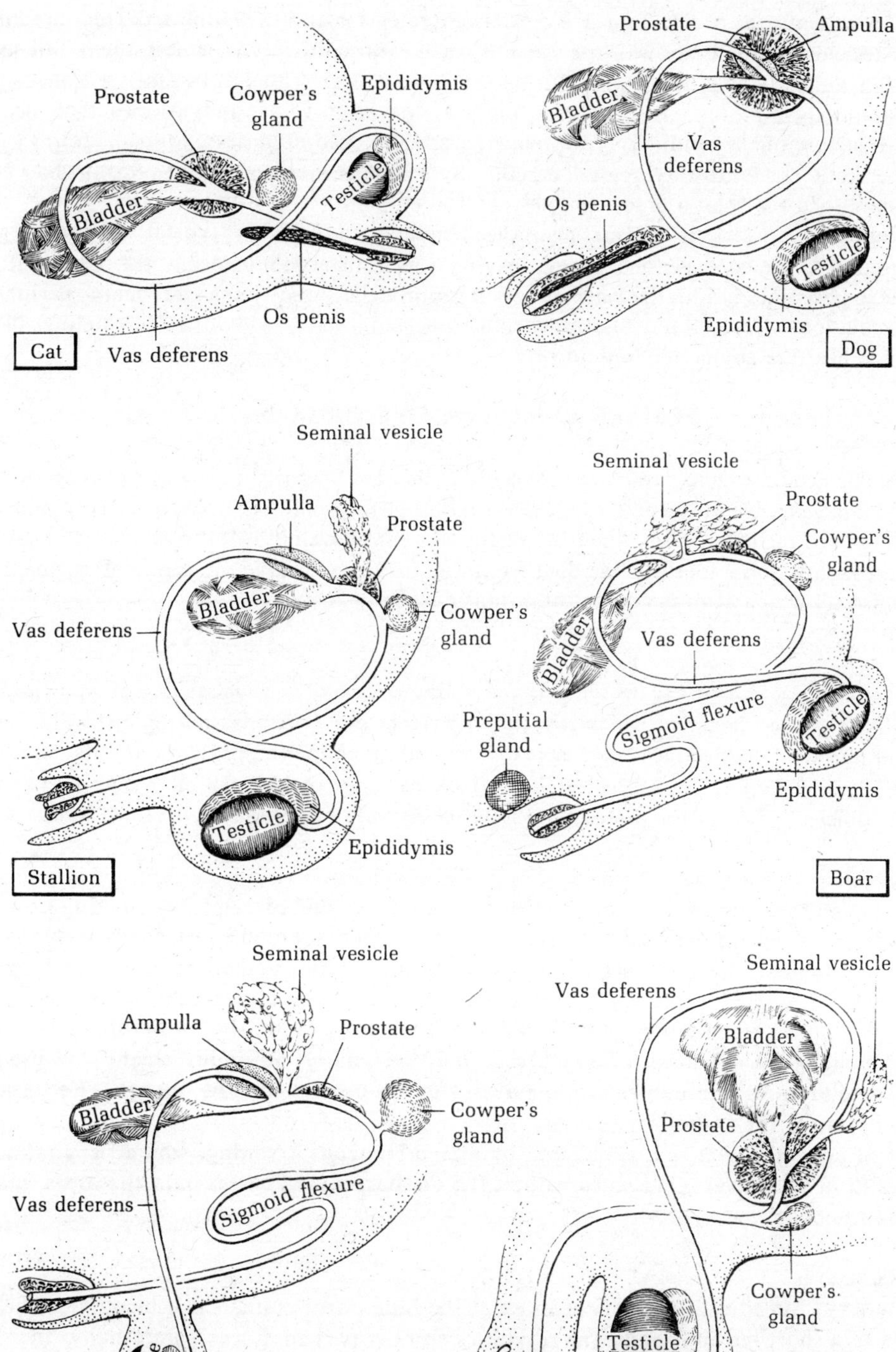

Fig. 5.3 Comparative Anatomy of the Male Reproductive Tract

(2) The two muscles of the testes i.e., external cremaster and the tunica dartos draw the testes close to the body wall for warmth when exposed to cold or lets them fall away from the body wall for cooling during exposure to warmth as in summer season.

(3) Pampiniform plexus: a wonderful looped system of veins and arteries that lies on the surface of the epididymis and which gradually becoming less looped, follows the spermatic cord into the inguinal canal. By actual measurements in rams it has been established that blood enters the plexus at a temperature of 39°C and that by the time it enters the testicle it is at or near the temperature (34.8°C) typical of that organ. Similarly, the cool venous blood leaving the testicle and entering the pampiniform plexus becomes gradually warmer as it approaches and joins the main peripheral circulation. The cellular and biochemical mechanisms by which the descending blood loses heat are completely unknown.

FEMALE REPRODUCTIVE ORGANS

The female genital organs are composed of (1) the two *ovaries*, the essential reproductive glands in which the ova are produced, (2) the *uterine* or *fallopian tubes* which convey the ova to the uterus, (3) the *uterus*—in which the fertilised ovum develops, (4) the *vagina*—a dilatable passage through which a foetus is expelled from the uterus, (5) *vulva* or terminal segment of the genital tract which also serves for the expulsion of the foetus.

Ovaries

The ovaries are a pair of organs lying in the abdominal cavity to whose dorsal wall they are connected by a broad ligament which stretches across the body wall in this region. The ovary has a dual purpose, the production of eggs or ova and an endocrine function and its sizes are ½" to 1½" in diameter, 1" in width and ½" in thickness. In each ovary there may be as many as 75,000 follicles. Except for poultry both the ovaries are functional in all farm animals.

Oviducts

The fallopian tubes, ovarian tubes or oviducts are slender and zigzag tubes running along the margin of the ligament and of 20-25 cm in length. They are not attached firmly to the ovaries but lie close to them in such a way that they seldom fail in their task of catching the egg or eggs. The oviduct has got a diameter of about 0.1 cm in case of the cow and it widens into a funnel shaped tube at the ovarian end which is called the "Infundibulum". The epithelial lining of the oviduct is often ciliated, and the ciliary motion is chiefly towards the tubes. These tubes help in conducting the ova from the ovaries to the uterus. Fertilisation generally occurs in the ampullary regions.

In case of dogs, the ovaries are enclosed by a membraneous covering which is continuous with the wall of the tubes. This ensures that the discharged ova passes into the tubes and is not lost in the body.

Uterus and Horns

The uterus of the cow like uterus of most of the other farm animals is a bicomute structure. It consists of a short medium body and a pair of spirally twisted horns. Internally the body has a very small corpus, the common cavity connecting the two horns is also known as the body of the uterus. The walls have three layers, e.g., the outer Servosa, the middle Muscularis and the inner Mucosa. The inner mucosa of the body and the horn is thrown out into a number of raised spots called caurancles which develop into cotyledons during pregnancy, and is provided with uterine glands to secrete uterine milk for early nutrition of the embryo. In the non-pregnant animals the uterus lies in the pelvic cavity which descends into the abdomen during pregnancy. This can be palpated per rectum and forms a basis of pregnancy diagnosis by rectal palpation method. It is the uterus to which the foetus becomes attached, and develops inside it until the time of birth.

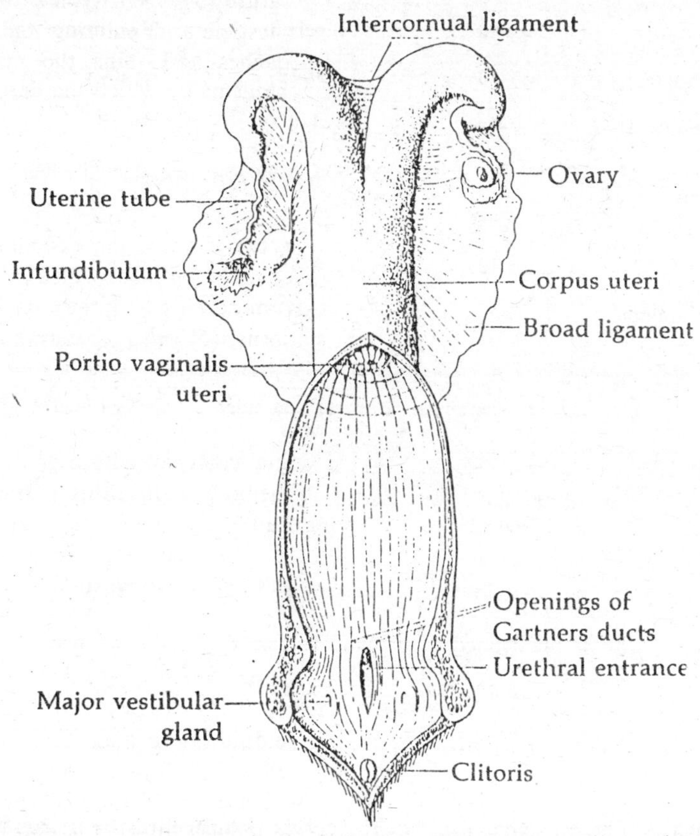

Fig.5.4 ***Reproductive tract of the cow (dorsal aspect).*** The vulva, vestibule, and vagina have been laid open and the left ovary withdrawn from the bursa. The portio vaginalis uteri is an interlocking circular fold that assists closure of the cervical lumen.

The Cervix

The cervix is also known as the neck of the womb. It is a thick walled portion of the reproductive tract and lies between the uterus and vagina. It also has the usual three layers but the muscle layers are very thick and the mucosa has longitudinal folds and transverse constrictions forming a spiral passage way through it. It is tightly closed during pregnancy and anoestrus period and relaxes only during oesttrus (heat) and parturition. It is rich in mucus secreting goblet cells which secrete the slimy antiseptic discharge generally seen as coming out of the

Table 5.1

Comparative Anatomy of the Reproductive Tract in the Adult Nonpregnant Female of Farm Mammals

Organ	Animal			
	Cow	Ewe	Sow	Mare
Oviduct				
Length (cm)	25	15–19	15–30	20–30
Uterus				
Type	Bipartite	Bipartite	Bicornuate	Bipartite
Length of horn (cm)	35–40	10–12	40–65	15–25
Length of body (cm)	2–4	1–2	5	15–20
Surface of lining of endometrium	70–120 Caruncles	88–96 Caruncles	Slight longitudinal folds	Conspicuous longitudinal folds
Cervix				
Length (cm)	8–10	4–10	10	7–8
Outside diameter (cm)	3–4	2–3	2–3	3.5–4
Cervical lumen				
Shape	2–5 Annular rings	Several annular rings	Corkscrew-like	Conspicuous folds
Os uteri				
Shape	Small and protruding	Small and protruding	Ill-defined	Clearly-defined
Anterior vagina				
Length (cm)	25–30	10–14	10–15	20–35
Hymen	Ill defined	Well developed	Ill defined	Well developed
Vestibule Length (cm)	10–12	2.5–3	6–8	10–12

The dimensions included in this table vary with age, breed, parity, and plane of nutrition.

vulva during heat. The muscular folds of the cervix project into the uterus and vagina as the uterine and vaginal so respectively. In cow it is about 4" long and 1" or more thick. The canal through the cervix is spiral.

The Vagina

It is the organ of copulation in females, extending from the cervix posteriorly up to the urogenital sinus or vestibule from which it is separated by the hymen or the hymenal constriction. It is a highly elastic organ and is responsible for the secretion of the mucus. The vagina serves as a birth canal at the time of parturition and admits the male organ in copulation. In case of the cow it is abuut 8"-10" long. The vagina is constricted at the junction with the urinogenital sinus or vestibule. The cow is peculiar in that, in addition to this posterior sphincter, it also has a constriction or anterior sphincter just at the back of the external os.

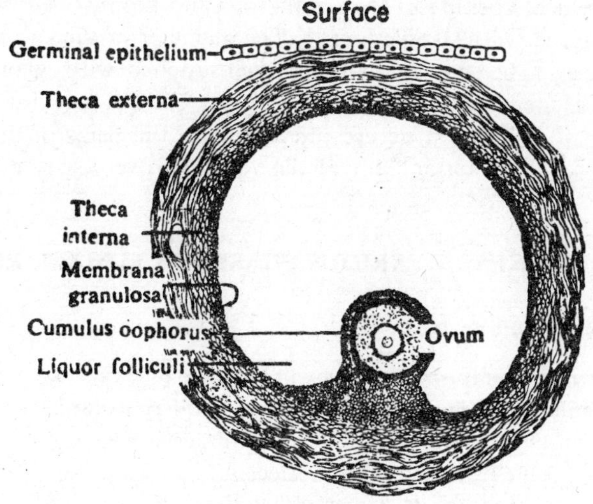

Fig. 5.5. Illustration of a graafian follicle

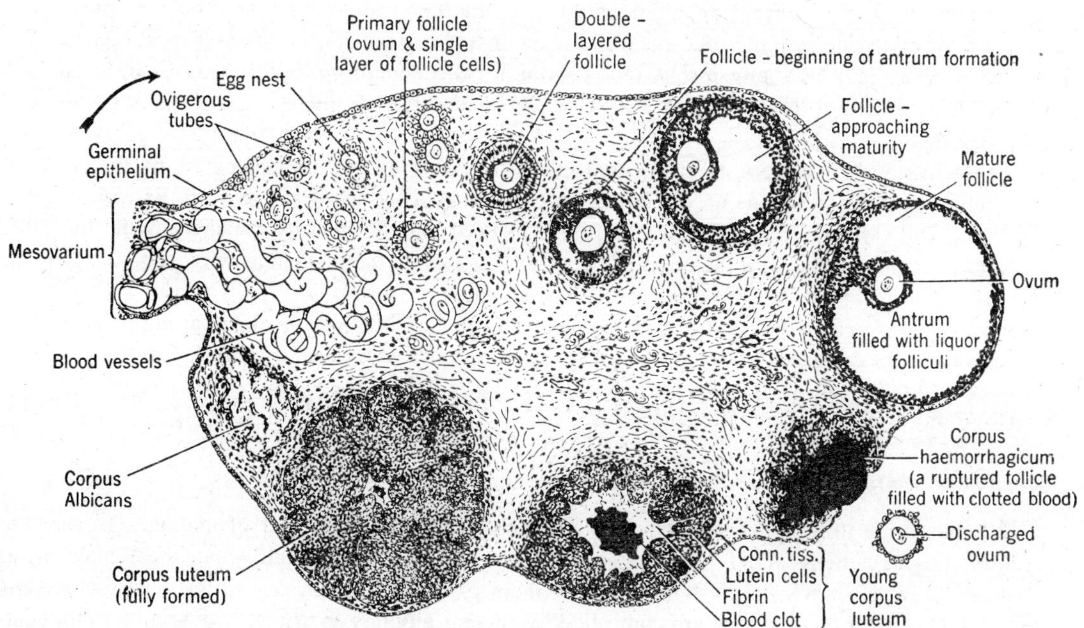

Fig. 5.6. Schematic diagram of mammalian ovary showing the sequence of events in the origin, growth, and rupture of the ovarian (Graafian) follicle and the formation and retrogression of the corpus luteum. Follow clockwise around the ovary, starting at the arrow.

The Vulva

It is the external vertical opening of the genital tract and lies just below the anus. It has two lateral vulval lips provided with tectile hairs. The diameter of the vulva is considerably larger than that of the vagina. The vulval walls are well supplied with glands which are specially active during sexual excitement.

The clitoris is a small, rod-like structure and represents the penis of the male, but unlike the penis, is solid. It lies in the posterior floor of the vulva. It is very sensory and erectile in nature.

ROLE OF HORMONES IN VARIOUS PHASES OF FEMALE REPRODUCTION

Hormones of Growth and Puberty

The body growth is mainly influenced by growth hormone (GH) also known as somatotropin (STH) secreted by the acidophilic cells of anterior pituitary gland. It has dual roles: (1) the hormone stimulates the release (mainly from the liver) of a group of growth promoting peptide hormones known collectively as Somatomedin; and (2) it exerts direct effects of its own on the protein, lipid, and carbohydrate metabolism of various organs and tissues. When the body growth is fully attained, gonadotropic hormones come into play in initiating the growth of the genitalia, GH is a protein, reduces the amount of fat stored in the body.

Among other hormones related to growth and puberty, thyroid hormone of the blood is important. This is almost entirely L-thyroxine, although there are traces of triiodothyronine. The main physiological effect of thyroxine is to increase energy production and oxygen consumption of most body tissues. A lack or deficiency in young results in a condition called *cretinism*, which induces dwarfism and idiocy. Thus a certain level of thyroxine secretion is essential for metabolic functions involved in normal growth.

Estrogens, the female hormone are produced by the ovary and to a lesser extent by the adrenals. In pregnant females estrogens are produced by the placental tissues. Estrogens are known to aid in regression and closure of the epiphyseal cartilage plate of long bones thus slowing growth. Increased estrogen secretion occurs with the onset of puberty. This fact partially explains why girls stop growing appreciably in height soon after the onset of menstruation.

Insulin also increases the uptake of amino acids and glucose into muscle and thus stimulates growth by increasing the synthesis of RNA and protein in a number of tissues, including muscle and bone.

Glucocorticoids are inhibitors of growth, one of these hormones, cortisol decreases the synthesis of DNA and protein in a number of tissues.

Hormones of Oestrous and Oestrous Cycle

Oestrous is the time when the female will receive the male in the act of mating. The oestrous cycle begins at puberty and is the interval between two oestrous periods when the female is not pregnant. During oestrous cycle there are four main phases, viz., proestrous, oestrous, metoestrous and dioestrous. All these events are controlled by several pituitary interrelated ovarian hormones.

The primordial follicles present at birth in the female are all that are present throughout the life of the animals and no more new ova are produced after birth. This contrasts with the male, in which new spermatozoa are produced throughout adult life. In females most of the follicles become atretic and never develop into mature ova. Development of most of the oocytes at birth were arrested at the primary oocyte stage in the prophase (first phase) of the first meiotic division. A hormone-independent stage of primordial follicle growth starts at puberty (defined as the beginning of reproductive life). This involves growth of the oocyte and an increase in the number of granulosa cells for several primordial follicles each day during the reproductive life of the animal.

During proestrous stage FSH as secreted by the anterior lobe of the pituitary gland stimulates the development of the Graafian follicles and is further responsible for maturation of the ovum and also controls secretion of estrogen from ovary. High levels of ovarian steroid hormones, mainly estradiol stimulates the growth and secretion by the uterus and the other genitalia resulting estrus signs.

Hormones of Ovulation

Except some species like cat, rabbit, camel where ovulation occurs following copulation, in other domestic animals it is spontaneous and usually occurs towards the end of estrus. An exception to this are cattle and buffaloes where ovulation occurs after the end of oestrous, i.e., during metoestrous.

The essential endocrine stimulus for ovulation is a sharp increase of LH. Under the stimulus of this hormone, cells in the wall of the follicle begin a change called luteinisation; during this change there is an increase in the amount of cytoplasm and a shift from the secretion of estrogen to the secretion of progesterone. At the same time, the connective tissue barrier between the follicle and the ovarian surface is gradually thinned. The role of progesterone is to stimulate collagenase activity in the follicular wall. The role of estrogen might be to give proper signal for the release of two prostaglandin compounds, viz., $PGF_{2\alpha}$ and PGE_2. The $PGF_{2\alpha}$ is involved in follicular rupture and PGE_2 in the remodelling of the follicular layers. Finally the connective tissue barrier between the follicle and the ovarian surface is gradually thinned. An increased intrafollicular pressure causes the follicle to rupture, this is ovulation.

Hormones of Corpus Luteum (CL) Formation and Maintenance

Formation of CL involves luteinization of the granulosa, by which the granulosa is converted from estrogen secretion to progesterone secretion. The process is initiated by the pre-ovulatory LH surge. The cavity of the ruptured follicle and the fibrin clot within serve as the framework on which the granulosa cells develop. Blood vessels from the theca externa invade the developing CL, so that it becomes vascularised. Maintenance of the CL is provided for by LH. Over 4 to 5 days the *corpus haemorrhagicum** is transformed into a solid yellow body, the corpus luteum. The entire process is known as luteinisation.

The CL secretes the female sex hormone, progesterone. Progesterone prepares the uterus for acceptance of a fertilised ovum or embryo. If the animal fails to conceive, the CL decreases in size, becomes pale in colour and the tissue inside become fibrous, known as *Corpus albicans*. However, if the ovum is properly fertilized and pregnancy ensues, the CL may last throughout the gestation period and functions as an endocrine gland which produces progesterone, a hormone essential for maintenance of pregnancy by blocking myometrial contractions. In the cow the level of which declines rapidly during the last 48 hours prior to parturition.

In addition the placenta also assumes the main role of progsterone production at between 150 to 200 days of gestation. Towards the termination of pregnancy direct effect of glucocorticoids or the direct effect of placental estrogen may be responsible for luteal regression, but it is most likely that regression is initiated by the action of $PGF_{2\alpha}$. The latter is released as a result of the effect of placental estrogens acting upon the fetal cotyledons.

Hormones of Parturition

The most dramatic changes in the levels of hormones during pregnancy occur shortly before parturition. The progesterone level suddenly drops. This results in the rise of estrogen level which sensitize the myometrium.

Some Theories on the Initiation of Parturition

Theory	*Possible Mechanism(s)*
Fall in progesterone concentration	Blocks myometrial contractions of the uterus during pregnancy; near term of parturition the blocking action of progesterone decreases
A rise in estrogen concentration	Overcomes the progesterone block of myometrial contractility and/or increases spontaneous myometrial contractility
Increase of uterine volume	Overcomes the effects of progesterone block of myometrial contractility
Release of oxytocin	Leads to contractions of uterus in an estrogen-sensitized myometrium
Release of prostaglandins ($PGF_{2\alpha}$)	Stimulates myometrial contractions; includes luteolysis leading to a fall in progesterone concentration (corpus luteum-dependent species)
Activation of faetal hypothalamic-pituitary-adrenal axis	Fetal corticosteroids cause a fall in progesterone, a rise in estrogen, and a release of $PGF_{2\alpha}$. These events lead to myometrial contractility

What exactly causes the changes in hormone levels and starts the uterine contractions is still uncertain. The corticosteroid levels follow the estrogen pattern, first rising then abruptly falling just before parturition. Prolactin levels essentially do the same, whereas LH levels remain relatively un-

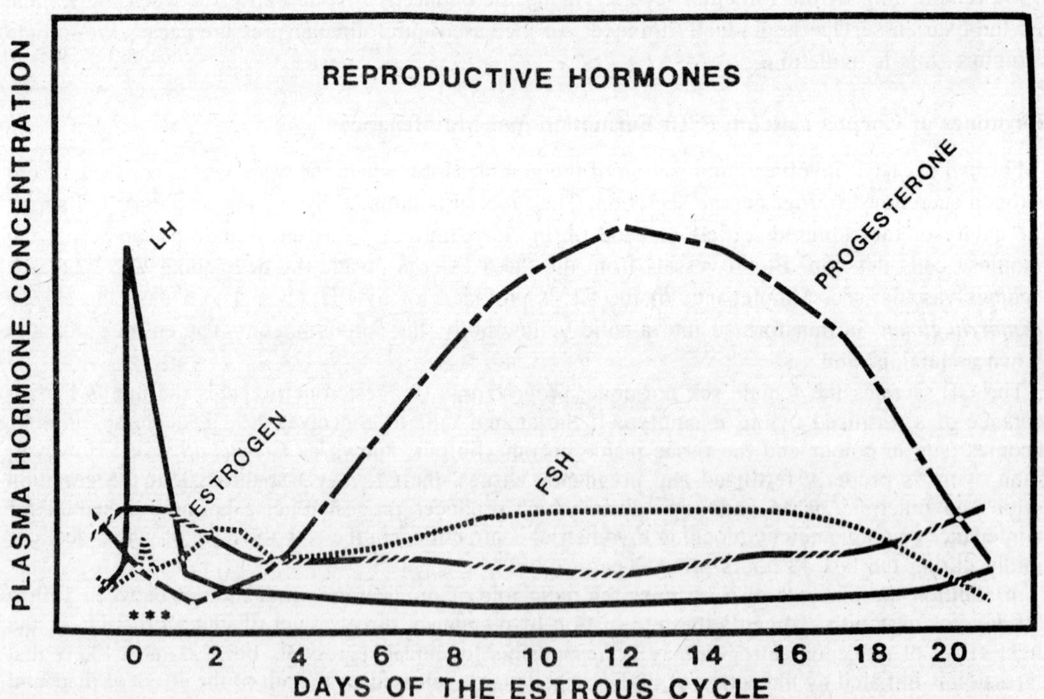

Fig. 5.7 Relative changes in reproductive hormones throughout the estrous cycle in heifers or gilts. Graph begins at estrus (***). Hormonal changes in ewes are similar except that the cycle length is about 4 days shorter.

Table 5.2

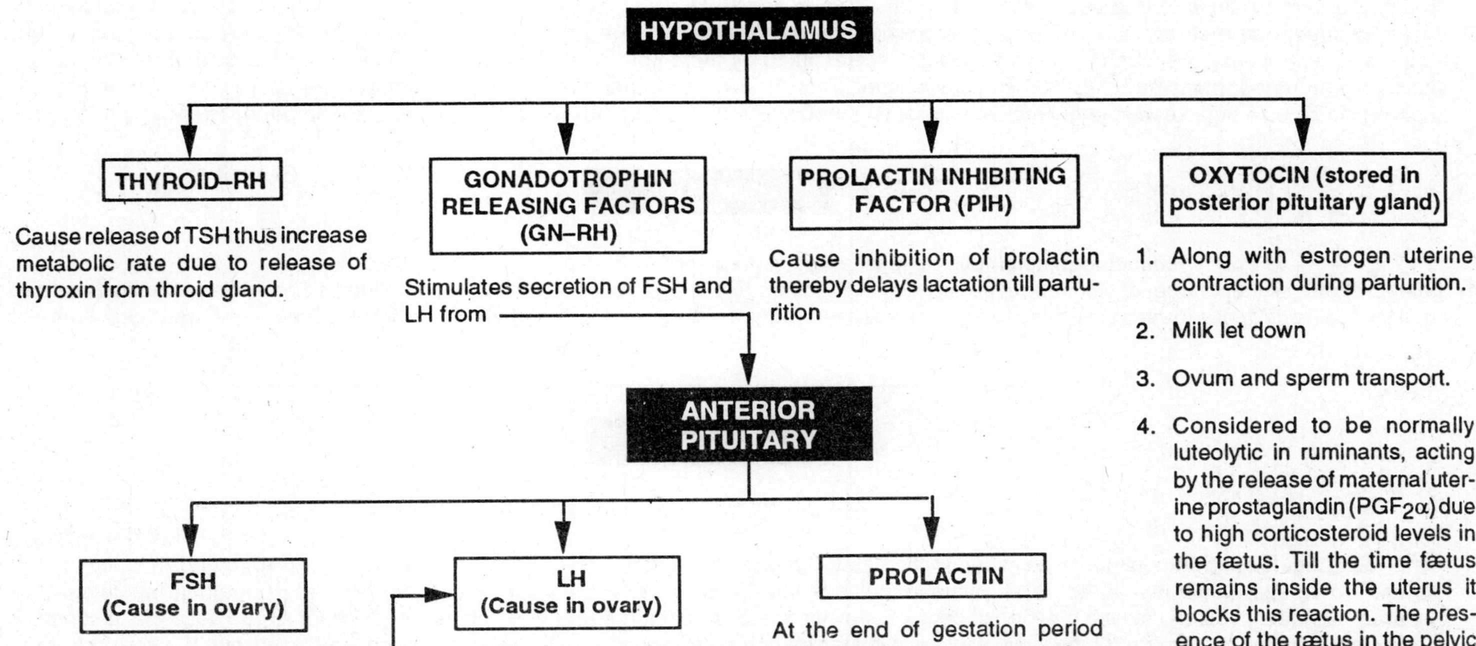
HYPOTHALAMUS
THYROID–RH
Cause release of TSH thus increase metabolic rate due to release of thyroxin from throid gland.
GONADOTROPHIN RELEASING FACTORS (GN–RH)
Stimulates secretion of FSH and LH from
PROLACTIN INHIBITING FACTOR (PIH)
Cause inhibition of prolactin thereby delays lactation till parturition
OXYTOCIN (stored in posterior pituitary gland)
1. Along with estrogen uterine contraction during parturition.
2. Milk let down
3. Ovum and sperm transport.
4. Considered to be normally luteolytic in ruminants, acting by the release of maternal uterine prostaglandin (PGF2α) due to high corticosteroid levels in the fætus. Till the time fætus remains inside the uterus it blocks this reaction. The presence of the fætus in the pelvic canal causes oxytocin to be released from the posterior pituitary. The hormone is also present in bovine CL.
ANTERIOR PITUITARY
FSH (Cause in ovary)
1. About 3 days prior to ovulation, levels of estrone and estradiol increases and cause release of surge of LH
2. Stimulation of ovarian follicle growth
3. Spermatogenesis in male testes.
LH (Cause in ovary)
1. Ovulation along with FSH
2. Stimulates androgen secretion in male
3. Development of Corpusluteum (CL)
4. Stimulates both estrogen from ovarian follicles and progesterone secretion by CL.
PROLACTIN
At the end of gestation period anterior pituitary releases prolactin due to high estrogen of placenta which promotes lactation, stimulates CL function and progesterone secretion in some species, may inhibit estrogen secretion.

(Contd.)

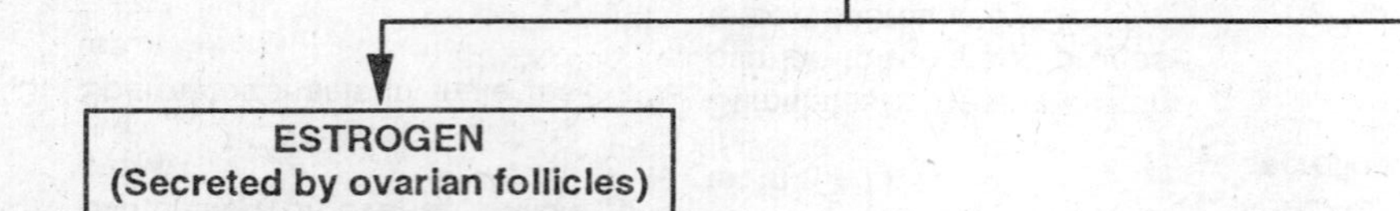

ESTROGEN
(Secreted by ovarian follicles)

Induces estrous behaviour; stimulates growth and function of reproductive tract; stimulates uterine contraction; regulates gonadotropin release; develops and maintains secondary sexual characteristics. estrogen also promotes mammary gland duct growth while proper combinations of estrogen and progesterone stimulates lobule–alveolar development, has anabolic effect, in poultry stimulates growth of oviduct and uterine secretion to calcify egg shell.

PROGESTERONE
(Secreted by CL)

Prepares uterus for implantation of fertilized ovum; stimulates endomaterial secretion for retention of the embryo in the uterus; essential for the formation of placenta and thus maintains pregnancy. Due to presence of progesterone further maturation of follicles and ovulation are inhibited; it also induces the uterine glands of the endometrium to secrete uterine milk essential for embryonic nutrition. Supresses LH surges; generally antagonises estrogenic effects (in small amounts, progesterone synergizes with estrogen to enhance to estrogenic effects on estrous behaviour. In poultry triggers LH release by hypothalamus development of oviduct.

PLACENTA

1. Secretes estrogen all through pregnancy and reaches maximum before parturition
2. Progesterone is also released from placenta in case of sheep and mare but from CL in a goat, cow and sow during pregnancy. In farm animals there is marked fall in progesterone level as parturition approaches.

UTERUS

Prostaglandin ($PGF_{2}\alpha$) secreted by maternal uterine wall is the natural luteolytic agent that terminates the luteal phase of the estrous cycle about 14 days after ovulation and allows for the initiation of a new estrous cycle in the absence of fertilization. $PGF_{2}\alpha$ is also particularly potent in terminating early pregnancy. During normal parturition an increase in the amount of ACTH being released from the adenohypophysis of the fætus. This in turn increases secretion of corticosteroid levels in the fætus causes an increase in the release of Prostaglandin $F_{2}\alpha$) from the maternal uterine wall. This may then starts myometrial contractions probably by stimulation for the release of oxytocin after the decrease of progesterone and increase of estrogen levels during initiation of parturition (except in mare).

altered. Evidence to date implicates an increase in the amount of ACTH being released from the anterior pituitary of the fetus and thereby produces enough cortisone to cause the placenta to change progesterone to estradiol. The estradiol then stimulates the uterus to produce relaxin, which softens and dilates the cervix. Corticosteroids also cause an increase in the release of a prostaglandin ($PGF_{2\alpha}$) from the maternal uterine wall. The prostaglandin may then start the myometrial contractions, after the progesterone levels have decreased.

The prostaglandin may also stimulate the release of oxytocin, secreted mainly from posterior pituitary store and additionally from ovary just before to parturition, causing uterine muscle contraction and thereby completes the parturition process.

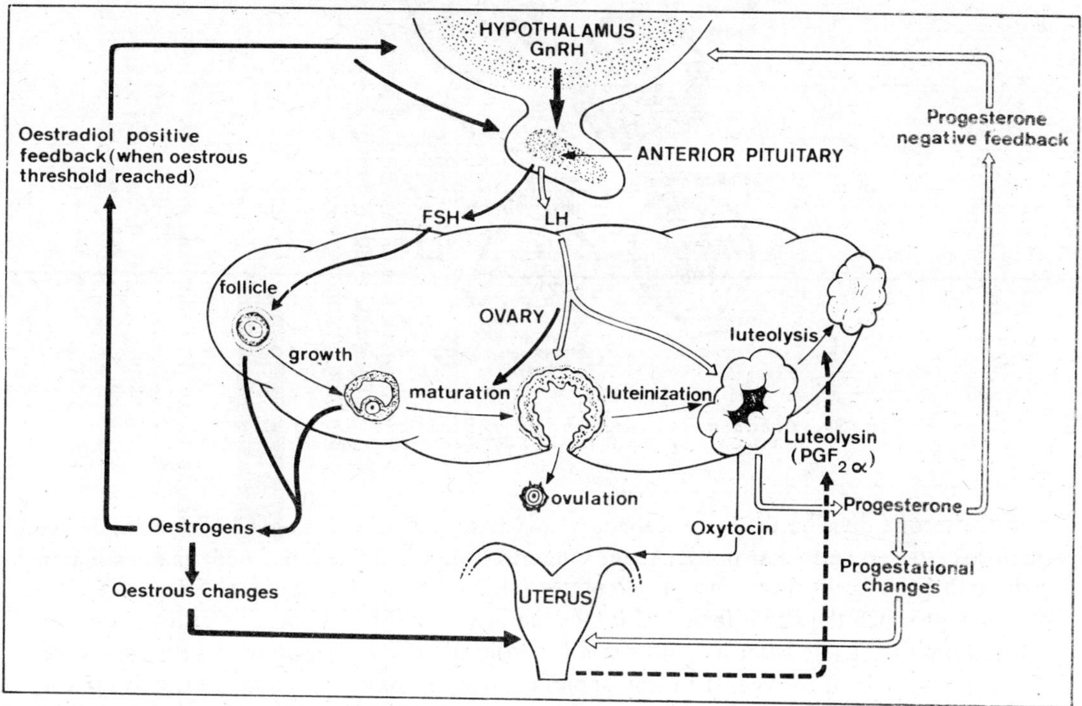

Fig. 5.8 A summary of the hormonal control of the ovarian cycle.

GAMETOGENESIS

The process by which gametes are formed is known as gametogenesis. When an individual becomes sexually mature, production of mature germ cells begins. The gonia first undergo a period of rapid growth, after which they are known as Auxocytes or Meocytes. In the male they are called spermatocyte and in the female oocytes. So we have spermatogenesis in the male and oogenesis in the female. By this process ultimately each auxocyte gives rise to 4 daughter cells.

Oogenesis

The female auxocyte or primary oocyte is very much like the primary spermatocyte. But the period of growth prior to the maturation divisions is prolonged where large amounts of yolk are formed. The nature of the maturation division is also different, for the first division, instead of giving rise to 2 secondary oocytes of equal size, produces one very large cell and one excessively minute cell called first polar body (Fig. 5.9).

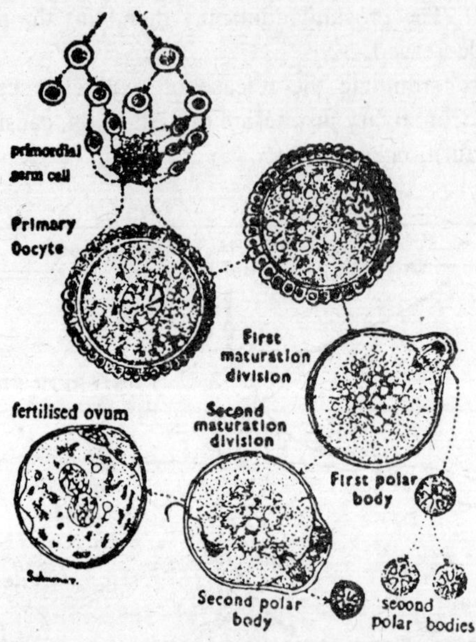

Fig. 5.9. Diagram illustrating multiplication, growth, maturation and fertilisation of mammalian egg

In the second division the large secondary oocyte again divides into 1 large cell and 1 very small cell—the second polar body. At the same time the small first polar body may or may not divide into 2 equal cells. In this way 4 cells are produced (or 3 if the small first polar body fails to develop), of which the single large cell is the mature ovum and the smaller cells are the polar bodies (Fig. 5.10). These latter are incapable of fertilisation and degenerate. As they are formed at the animal pole of the egg, the polar bodies are often of practical value in orienting the egg.

Unlike the male gametes whose maturation is completed within the testis the oocytes do not complete their maturation until after leaving the ovary, and in vertebrates at least, the second division is not completed until after the entrance of the sperm. The significance of this situation is not understood although it has been suggested that the egg shall be freshly matured at the time of the union of the pronuclei.

Spermatogenesis

Like oogenesis, spermatogenesis also passes through three equivalent stages: (1) The first is the proliferation of the primitive germ cells, (2) The second is the growth period leading to rapid enlargement or growth, (3) The third or the final stage is the maturation stage when the important nuclear changes occur.

Spermatozoa arise from the epithelial cells that leave the tubules of the testis. A study of the cross section of the normal mature mammalian testis usually reveal all stages of spermatogenesis. The cells within a tubule are of two distinct types. They are:

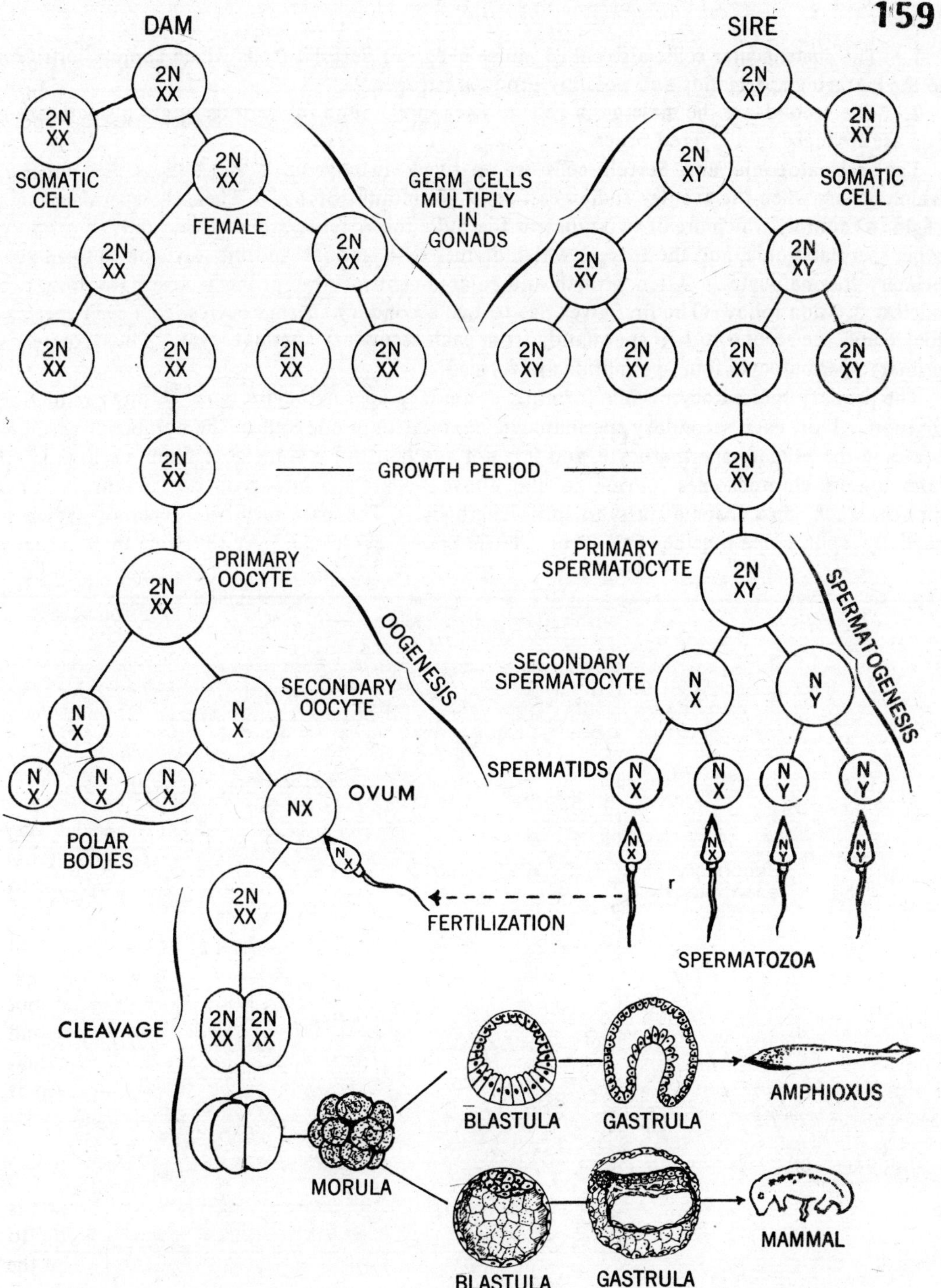

Fig. 5.10 Diagram illustrating gametogenesis (oogenesis in the dam and spermatogenesis in the sire), cleavage, and development of the embryo in amphioxus and in a mammal.

1. The sustenacular cells, also called nurse cells, or Sertoli's cells which supply nutrition to the maturing spermatids and possibly produce estrogen.

2. The second are the male germ cells. They are found in various stages of maturation and are arranged in a layered order.

The spermatogonia and Sertoli cells are relatively inactive until the bull reaches puberty, which occurs when the average Indian calf is 9-12 months of age. Then the spermatogonia begin to multiply which are of two types in the bull: the A type, which divide only to produce other spermatogonia, and the B type, which divide by a similar mitotic division to form two primary spermatocytes. After growth and enlargement of the primary spermatocytes, two nuclear division follow. The first gives rise to two secondary spermatocytes from each spermatocyte and the second to two spermatids from each secondary spermatocyte. Thus from each primary spermatocyte four spermatids are formed.

The primary spermatocyte while forming secondary spermatocytes goes through reduction division. Thus each secondary spermatocyte contains only one half of the number of chromosomes in the primary spermatocyte, and it is not any half but one member from each pair of homologous chromosomes. Prior to the above separation and reduction in chromosome number, each chromosome starts to split lengthwise. The pair members, each of which is partially split, come together and form what is known as tetrad. At this time there usually

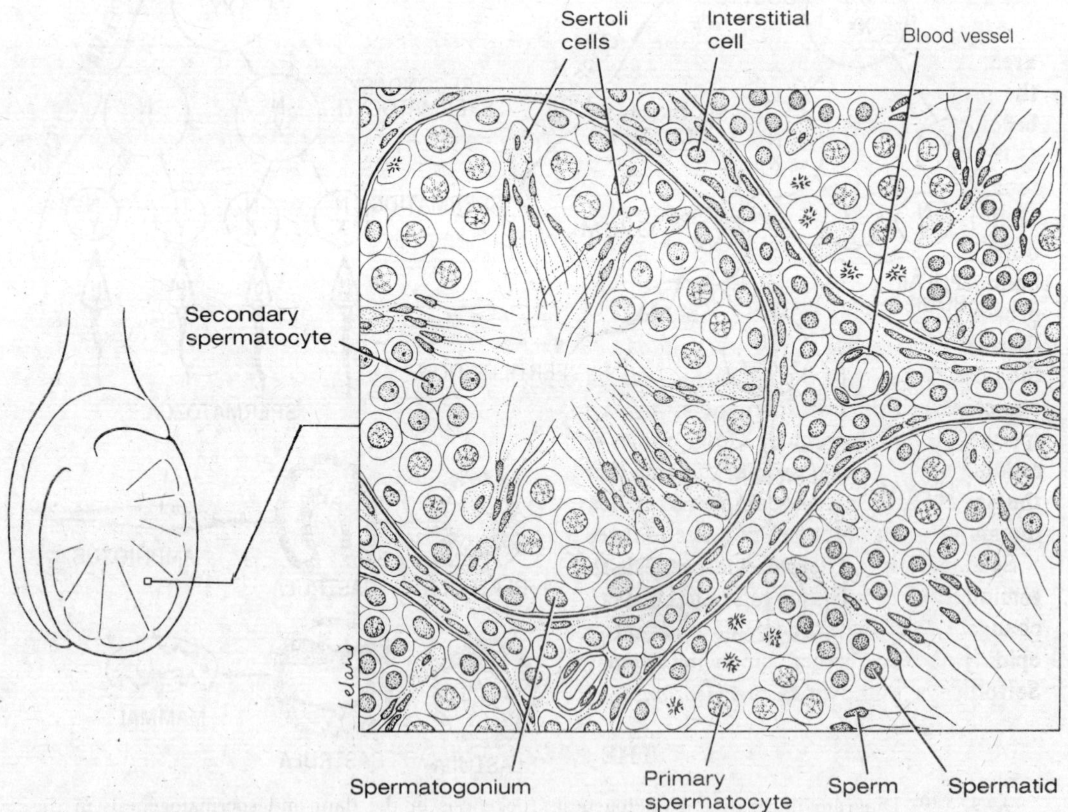

Fig. 5.11 Section of testis showing spermatogenesis within the seminiferous tubules.

occur twisting of the tetrad which allows for the exchange of chromatin material between the members of the tetrad, i.e., crossing over.

The secondary spermatocyte after its formation goes through a second meiotic division. This process involves homotypic or equational division and the separation of the earlier-formed diads. This results in the formation of spermatids, which are smaller than either the spermatogonia or primary spermatocytes and differ from them in having half the original number of chromosomes.

The newly formed spermatid then enters a series of morphological changes by which it becomes converted into an elongated element with the chromatin material packed in the head, followed by a slender middle piece and behind the middle piece is a whip like tail (Fig. 5.11).

Spermiogenesis. The term is also known as spermateliosis and is used in reference to the final maturation of the spermatids into spermatozoa. The changes involve both nucleus and cytoplasm but no divisions of the cells occur. The process begins in the seminiferous tubules and is completed in the epididymis.

The nuclear envelope of the spermatid is double and the entire nucleus is localised in the anterior area of the cell. It contains several granules of DNA of various sizes.

The Golgi complex is composed of numerous small vacuoles, congregate at the anterior nuclear pole and then flatten and form a cap over the pole. The acrosome of the spermatozoon is formed from these structures and the fluid within the vacuole.

After formation of the vacuole, the Golgi bodies migrate into the cytoplasm near the neck area, the centrioles appear. The larger of the two, the proximal centriole remains ttached to the proximate poles of the nucleus, and the other, the distal centriole, migrates posteriorly to become the end of the spermatozoon middle piece.

In the meantime mitochondria have become concentrated in the posterior area of the cell and looks like a membrane. This membrane known as the *manchetta* or *caudal tube* is the cytoplasmic area to be included in the mitochondrial sheath covering the axial filaments. The cytoplasm outside the caudal tube is later lost and the membrane of the manchetta forms the future outer boundary of the middle piece. Throughout this period the acrosome is growing from the proacrosome. Due to the development of acrosome, mitochondrial sheath, axial filament—the spermatid elongates. The tail originates from the centriole when the latter is moving towards the posterior part of the nucleus. It is initially formed of 9 fibrils arranged in circle around one central fibril and surrounded by a tubular membrane. At the neck of the fully formed spermatozoon the granular Golgi bodies remain, and after elimination of excess cytoplasm, a residual protoplasmic droplet remains there as ring centriole. The bead is not usually lost until the spermatozoon has completed at least a part of its journey through the epididymis. Thus the mature spermatozoon consists of three principal parts: the head, the neck and the tail.

Spermeation. After spermatogenesis the spermatozoa stays for about 5 to 7 days within the seminiferous tubule and gets attached to Sertoli cells for some physiological and biochemical change. The detachment of spermatozoa from the Sertoli cell takes place as they move to epididymis for further biochemical maturation. This movement of spermatozoa from the Sertoli cells is known as *spermeation*.

THE SEXUAL CYCLE

Within the breeding season, heat appears in the normal female for the most part in quite regular cycles. The cycle of heat is made up of four distinct phase which have been desig-

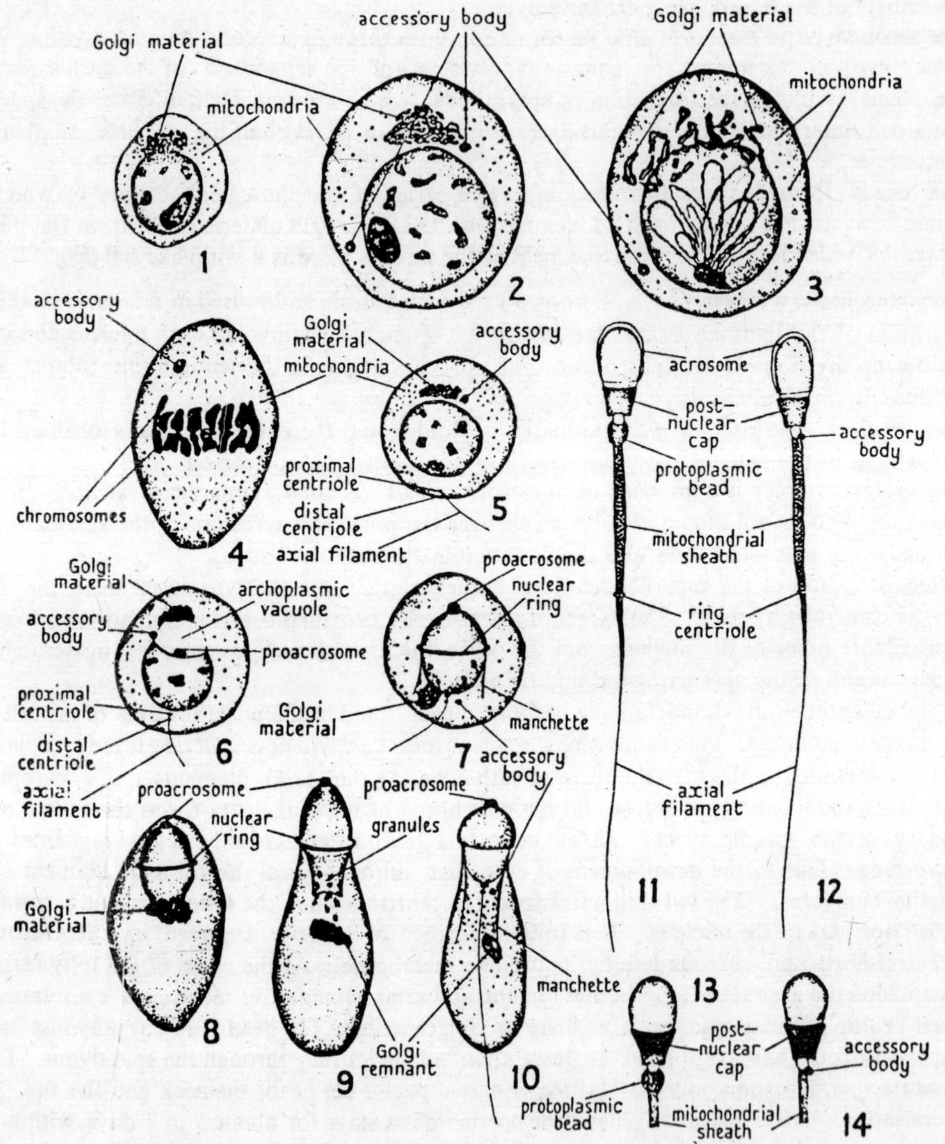

Fig. 5.12. Formation of a spermatozoon. Note the process of spermiogenesis and the responsible cellular inclusions. 1. Spermatogonium. 2. Primary spermatocyte. 3. Primary spermatocyte—early prophase. 4. Primary spermatocyte—early anaphase. 5. Young spermatid. 6–8. Spermatids. 9, 10. Late spermatids. 11. Spermatozoon. 12. Spermatozoon, showing accessory body; the protoplasmic bead is not shown. 13. Spermatozoon. 14. Spermatozoon, showing accessory body; the protoplasmic bead is not shown. (Gresson, R. A. R., and Zlotnik, I.: Quart. J. Micro. Sci. *89*:219, 1948.)

nated by Marshall as: Proestrum, Oestrum, Metoestrum and Dioestrum.

Proestrum

This marks the animals comming in heat. During this phase th^ graafian follicle within the ovary is growing, principally by the increased secretion of follicular fluid. This fluid which

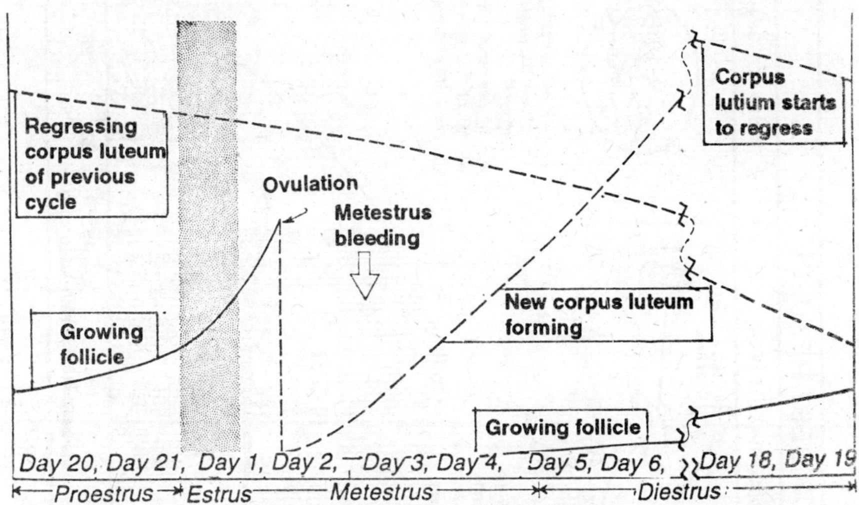

Fig. 5.13 The estrous cycle in the cow. (From Physiology of Reproduction and Artifical Insemination by G. W. Salisbury and H. L. VanDemark. Copyright by W. H. Freeman and Company, 1961.)

surrounds the ovum, contains the hormone estradiol. This is absorbed into the blood, whereupon it passes into the oviduct, or fallopian tube, and there causes a growth of the cells lining the tube, and an increase in the number of cilia which are shortly to transport the ova to the uterus. At the same time a marked increase in the vascularity of the uterine mucosa takes place in preparation for the intense wave of growth which is soon to occur. The epithelial wall of the vagina increases in thickness. The vaginal adjustment is well fitted to prevent possible damage tc the wall when coitus occurs. Vaginal smears taken at this time usually possess a few large polymorphonuclear and mononuclear leucocytes, a few nucleated epithelial cells and no confirmed cells.

Oestrum or Oestrus

This is the period of desire. The graafian follicles now "ripe", or very turgid, and the ovum is undergoing certain maturation changes. This period is brought to a close by the rupture of the follicle or ovulation. As a rule the heat period of the cow lasts 12 to 24 hours; in the ewe, 1-2 days; in the mare 4 to 5 days and in the sow 2-3 days. At this time the vulva becomes swollen and both vulva and vagina are congested with blood. Late in heat, vaginal smears possess many leucocytes, and many acid staining epithelial cells.

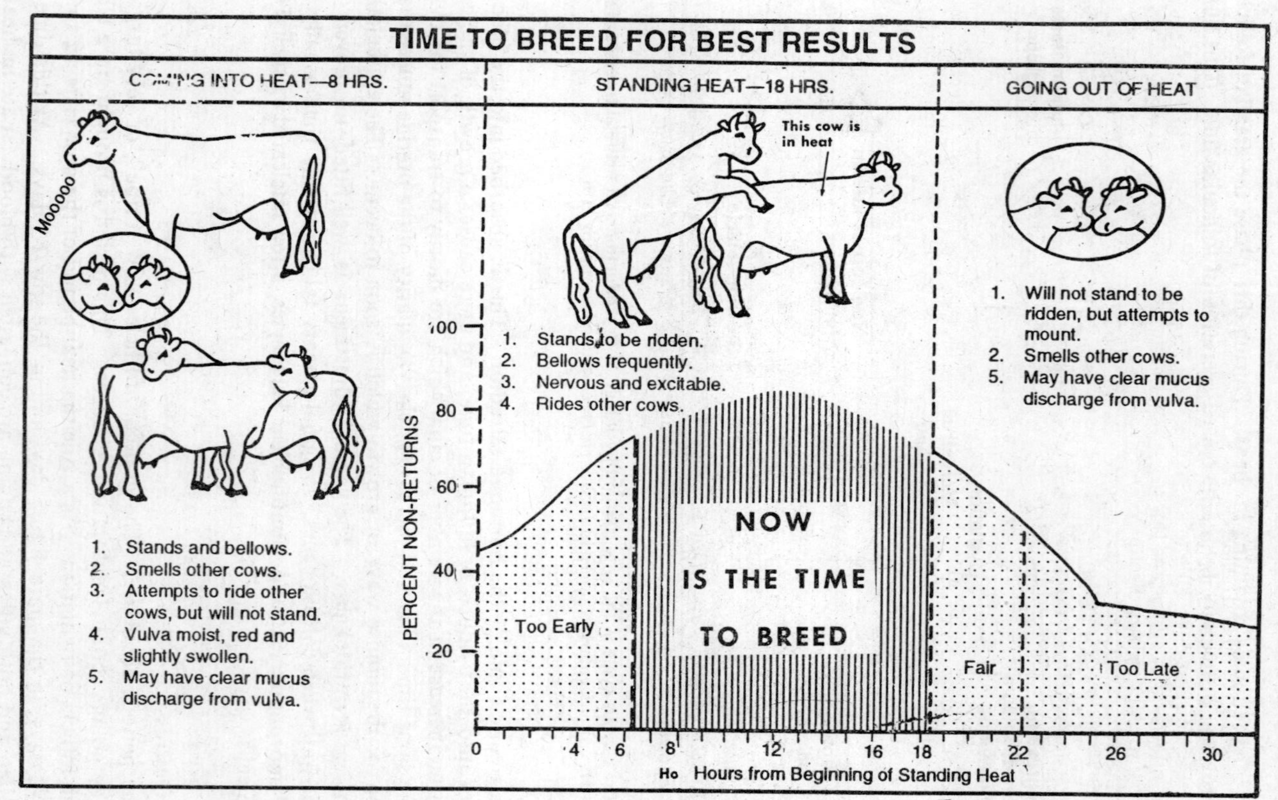

Fig.5.14 Time to breed for best results.

Table 5.3

Symptoms of Heat in Cows and Buffaloes

Symptoms at early stages of heat are not pronounced in cattle but they show activities like smelling other cows, attempting to mount on them and bellowing. They become restless and their vulva gets moist, red and slightly swollen. After a lapse of six to eight hours the heat becomes more pronounced. The cow stands still to be mounted by other cows or bulls. Due to this, this period is termed as "standing heat". This extends for 12-18 hours and shows other symptoms like bellowing, nervousness, anorexia, reduction in milk yield, moist and red vulva and clear mucus discharge.

Symptoms	***Early heat (Mounting) 0-8 hours***	***Mid-heat(Standing) 12-18 hours***	***Late heat 24 hours***
		COWS	
Social behaviour	Restless, tries to get isolated from other cows	Mixes with other cows in the herd	Normal behaviour with other cows in the herd
Excitement	Shows sign	More pronounced	Absent; calm
Appetite	Depressed	More depressed	Normal
Bellowing	Sometimes	Frequent	Very seldom
Milk yield	Falls	Further falls	Starts increasing
Licking other animals	Moderate	High	Seldom
Rise of body temperature	Slight rise	Sharp rise	Comes back to normal
Mucus discharge from vulva	Clear, watery and copious break while falling down form vulva and flows	Turbid, opaque or cloudy viscous and ropy; in reduced quantity; does not break while falling; rather hangs right from vulva down to the ground.	Seldom seen
Vulva	Wrinkles on vulva lips start disappearing; lips starts swelling	Pronounced swelling	Swelling recedes
Vaginal Mucus discharge	Clear and ropy	Pronounced	Difficult to detect
Mounting other animals	Rarely seen	Frequently observed in the first half of mid heat	Seldom seen
Standing still when other cows or bulls try to mount	Sometimes seen	Very common during the second-half of mid heat and indicate right time for insemination	Seldom seen
Urination	Frequent	More frequent	Normal
Uterine tone	Tight and turgid	Becomes more turgid	Comes down to moderate tone
		BUFFALOES	
Appetite	Normal	Depressed	Normal
Excitement	Very much	Less excited	Does not show
Bellowing	Occasional	Frequent	Absent
Swollen vulva	Slight	Moderate	Absent
Frequency of urination within 30 minutes	Occasional to two times	More frequent	Less frequent
Uterine tone	Intense(tight & turgid)	More intense (tight and turgid)	Moderate
Opening of cervix	Partial or fully open	Fully open	Almost closed
Mounting by teaser bull	Present (70% cases)	Present (90% cases)	Present (40% cases)

Source : Dairy India 1992

Metoestrum or Metestrum

This is the period when the organ returns to a normal non-congested condition. During this time the cavity of the graafian follicle from which the ovum has been expelled becomes reorganised and forms a new structure known as corpus luteum (C.L.), an endocrine gland which secretes progesterone with important functions.

1. It prevents the maturation of further graafian follicles and thus prevents the occurrence of further estrus period for a time.
2. It is essential for the implementation of the fertilised egg.
3. It nourishes the foetus during the first half of pregnancy.
4. It is intimately concerned with the development of the mammary gland.

During metestrum the vaginal wall loses most of its new growth.

Dioestrum or Diestrum

During the phase, which is usually the longest part of the cycle, the C.L. is fully grown and its effect on the uterine wall is marked. The muscles of the uterus also develop. The reactions are obviously intended to produce a copious supply of uterine "milk" for the nourishment of the embryo prior to its attachment to the uterine wall. If pregnancy supervenes, this stage is prolonged throughout the gestation, the C.L. remaining intact for the whole or most of this period. In the absence of a fertilised egg, the C.L. undergoes retrogressive changes and the cell becomes vaculated and laden with large lipid droplets. These changes are followed by a rapid resorption of the C.L.

These diestrum periods are transmitted by activities which normally occur at the end of the pregnancy, such as nest making and the secretion of milk. These periods are described as *Pseudopregnant* periods.

OVULATION

Ovulation may be defined as the discharge of the egg from the graafian follicle. In most domestic animals, ovulation is spontaneous i.e., it occurs whether or not mating has occurred. In these animals, ovulation is triggered. by a balance between circulating blood levels of hypopnyseal gonadotropins (FSH and LH). In other animals, such as the cat, rabbit and mink, ovulation is induced by copulation.

In general, ovulation occurs near the end of estrus, with a variation among different species. The time of ovulation in cow is about 12–15 hours after the end of the 18 hours estrus. In other ruminants, the ewe and the goat, the eggs are ovulated a few hours before the end of estrus, which lasts an average of 24 to 40 hours, respectively. The sow's eggs are ovulated about 36 hours after the start of the 40 to 60 hours estrus. Most mammalian eggs are ovulated when the second maturation division has reached metaphase. In the dog and probably the horse, however, the egg is ovulated as a primary oocyte and pass through its maturation in the fallopian tube.

Mechanism of Ovulation. The present day theory of the cause of ovulation is based on hormonal activity and indicates that ovulation is largely under the control of LH. The mature follicle wall consists of three layers. The outer layers separate during final pre-ovulatory changes, and the inner layer protrudes forming a papilla. Finally the inner layer gives way and the ovum with attached cells flow out. Just prior to ovulation, follicles become flaccid indicating that the follicular pressure has dropped. Current views are that at first there is release of LH from the pituitary gland brought about by neurohumoral mechanism.

It has been found that oxytocin administered to heifers at the beginning of estrus significantly hastened the time of ovulation. The result when considered together with the recent finding that oxytocin and vasopression are produced in hypothalamic nuclei, suggest but do not necessarily prove, that oxytocin may be one of the hypothalamic neurohumors involved in gonadotropin release (LH) from the anterior pituitary.

LH thus released stimulate DNA to synthesise specific messenger RNA (m-RNA). This in turn aids for the synthesis of the enzyme—*collagenases*. Collagenases in turn causes enzymatic decomposition of the collagen content of the follicular wall structure resulting in the oozing process of ovulation. In domestic animals the average fertile life of an egg varies from 12 to 24 hours after ovulation. Loss of viability is not sudden. Ageing eggs may be able to undergo apparently normal fertilisation, but may give rise to embryos that die before birth. With further ageing fertilisation may be abnormal or totally fails.

Periodically, mature eggs are discharged from the ovary. This occurs once in a year in most vertebrates but once a month in human and bovine species. The number of ova discharged at a single ovulation varies from one, as in man, bovine or the fowl to thousands in the frog, even millions in many fish. Ovulation in the cow occurs more frequently in the right ovary than in the left (20.2%), the reason of which is not known. It may be possible that anatomical location of the rumen very close to the left ovary exert sufficient perssure to diminish the blood flow in the left ovary.

FERTILISATION

The process involves penetration of the comparatively large sessile (stalkless) egg by a small motile spermatozoon, completion of the maturation process of ovum, and fusion of the nuclei to form the zygote nucleus. Spermatozoa must traverse both male and female reproductive tracts to unite with oocytes in the ampulla of the oviduct for fertilisation. In most mammals, fertilisation begins after the first polar body has been extruded, so that the sperm penetrates the ovum while the second reduction division is in progress. The process of fertilisation may be discussed under the following heads.

The Meeting of the Spermatozoon into the Egg. The arrival of spermatozoa at the site of fertilisation before the eggs suggest that sperm must be exposed for at least 4–6 hours to tubal, uterine or vaginal secretions before penetrating the cumulus oophorus and zona pellucida of the eggs in the case of cow, 1.5 hours in the sheep. This phenomenon is known as "*Capacitation*". Although the total number of sperm in an ejaculate is measured in hundreds or thousands of millions, the number travelling as far as the ampulla is relatively small i.e., not more than 1,000 in any animal. There is evidence that the meeting between spermatozoa and eggs is not entirely random in some circumstances, and that selective fertilisation can occur, eggs of one type more often involved than those of another. In other cases the phenomenon depends on chance i.e., there is an equal chance of any sperm fertilising any ovum. Previously it was thought that movement towards the egg is aided by the liberation of some chemical substances from the egg i.e., the mechanism of *chemotaxis*. It has been established that chemotaxis between eggs and spermatozoa does not operate in animal kingdom. The mass of cumulus cells might be facilitating contact by trapping sperm in the neighbourhood of the ovum.

Table 5.4
Physiologic Phenomena of Sperm and Egg Related to Fertilization

Parameters	*Oogenesis and Characteristics of Ova*	*Spermatogenesis and Characteristics of Sperm*
Mitosis in the gonad	Ceases during fetal life; no new eggs are formed after birth	Continues throughout reproductive life of the male
Meiosis in the gonad	Begins during fetal life	Begins at puberty and continues throughout reproductive life
First maturational division in gamete	First maturational division is completed in preovulatory follicle	First meiotic division results in two cells of equal size
Second maturational division	Second maturational division is completed only when egg is penetrated by sperm	Not comparable
Numberof gametes produced during reproductive life	Thousands of oogonia are found in neonate ovary	Millions of sperm are produced in each ejaculate from puberty, with reduced numbers during senility
Sex chromosome in gamete	X	X or Y
Amount of cytoplasm in gamete	As oocyte matures, the amount of its cytoplasm increases	As spermatid develops into sperm, the amount of cytoplasm decreases; acrosome and tail develop in late spermatid
Motility of gamete	Oocytes, surrounded by follicular cells, are immotile	Sperm motility develops gradually in various parts of epididymis and increases at ejaculation
Plasma membrane at fertilization	Egg acquires plasma membranes from sperm	Sperm loses its plasma membranes to egg
Survival in female reproductive tract	12 to 24 hours after ovulation	Fertilizability is maintained 24 hours after ejaculation

Source : Reproduction in Farm Animals, 4th edition, E.S.E. Hafez Lea & Febiger, Philadelphia, U.S.A.

The Entry of Sperm into Ovum. To enter the ovum the sperm has first to penetrate (1) the cumulus mass, (2) the zona pellucida, and (3) the vitelline membrane.

The sperm makes its way through the cumulus mass due to its own motility. Cumulus oophorus consists of a large number of follicle cells embedded in a jelly-like matrix composed of a hyaluronic acid-protein complex. The spermatozoon carries in the acrosome an enzyme, *hyaluronidase* capable of depolymerising the hyaluronic acid-protein matrix of the cumulus oophorus. Spermatozoa thus make an entry by dissolving a tunnel through the hyaluronic acid matrix reach upto zona pellucida—which is the next obstacle to sperm entry. The ovum is said to produce a substance *fertilizin,* which reacts with the sperm and specifically agglutinates it. Sperm cells also carries another enzyme known as "*Zona lysin*", that acts upon the substance of the zona, permitting the spermatozoon to make its way through. Thus by the action of sperm motility and enzymatic reaction sperm enters through the cumulus oophorus and zona pellucida and makes contact with the surface of the vitellus. The last stage in the penetration of ovum involves the attachment of the sperm head to the surface of

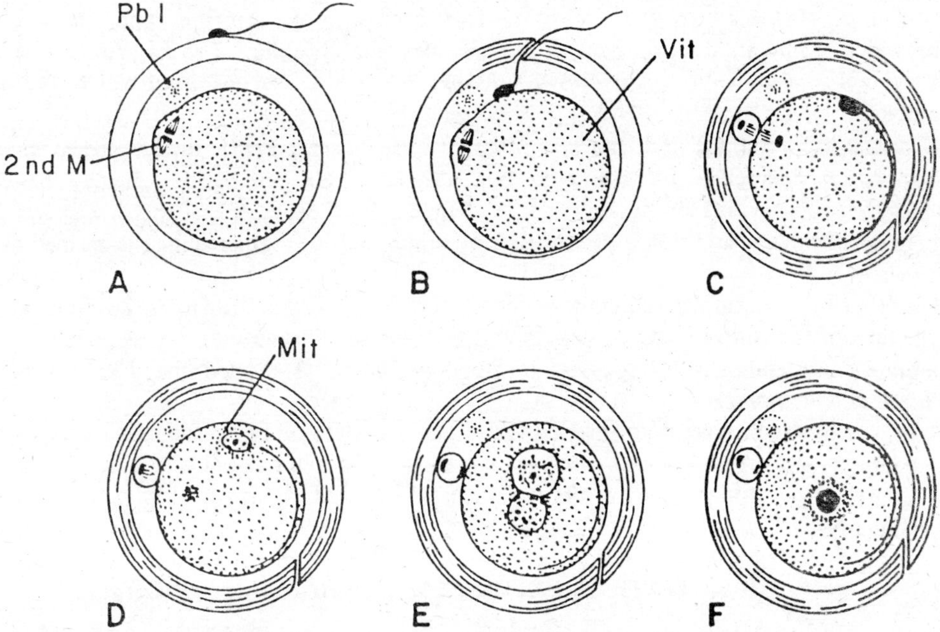

Fig. 5.15 ***Processes occurring during fertilization in swine.*** **A.** The sperm is in contact with the zona pellucida. The first polar body (*Pb1*) has been extruded; the nucleus of the ovum is undergoing its second meiotic division (*2nd M*). **B.** The sperm has penetrated the zona pellucida and is now attached to the vitellus (*Vit*). This evokes the zona reaction, which is indicated by shading as it passes around the zona pellucida. **C.** The sperm has now been taken almost entirely within the vitellus. The head is swollen. The vitellus has decreased in volume and the second polar body has been extruded. The zona has rotated relative to the vitellus. **D.** Male and female pronuclei develop. Mitochondria (*Mit*) gather around the pronuclei. **E.** The pronuclei are fully developed and contain many nucleoli. The male pronucleus is larger than that of the female. **F.** Fertilization is complete. The pronuclei have disappeared and been replaced by chromosome groups, which have united in the prophase of the first cleavage division. From Hafez, E.S.E.: Reproduction in Farm Animals. 4th Ed. Philadelphia, Lea & Febiger, 1980.

vitellus. The pause before actual entry into the vitellus lasts for about half an hour in some rodent eggs. It is this time when activation of the egg occurs. The ovum awakes from its dormancy and development begins. The sperm head with its tail then enters the vitellus.

Pronucleus Formation. The remarkable result of activation is that (cow, pig) the vitellus shrinks in volume, expelling fluid into the perivitelline space. At the same time the sperm head in the vitellus swells and acquires the consistency of a gel, losing its characteristic shape. Immediately following contact with the cytoplasmic body of the egg, fusion occurs between the plasma membranes limiting the two cells and ultimately they are enclosed within a single plasma membrane. The sperm components—nucleus, centrioles, mitochondria and tail fibres and sheath—pass into the egg cytoplasm while the sperm plasma membrane is removed.

In most species the second polar body is expelled from the ovum soon after sperm entry, and formation of the female pronucleus then begins. The two pronuclei increase progressively in volume until they are about 20 times their original size and more towards each other through the cytoplasm, so that when fully grown they are in close contact. Then, quite suddenly, they diminish in volume and finally fade out altogether, giving place to two chromosome groups. In their turn, these chromosome groups move together and form a single group which represents the prophase of the first cleavage division. The stage upto the union of the two chromosome groups is known as *syngamy*, at the conclusion of which fertilisation is complete.

Zona Reaction and Vitelline Block. Often ova are observed with several sperm clustering around the outside of the zona pellucida, but only a single one inside. It may be due to the fact that zona pellucida undergoes some change after the passage of the first sperm which renders it difficult for additional penetration by other sperms. This change is termed as *Zona reaction*.

The other mechanism against entry of more than one sperm is shown by the vitelline itself. At the time of the contact between sperm and vitelline membrane there is a reaction in the membrane, that renders it unresponsive to other sperm and is termed the *Vitelline block or the block of polpspermy*.

Extra sperm which succeed in entering the vitellus, in spite of both the zona reaction and the vitelline block, are called *supernumerary sperm*, and the ovum is said to show *polyspermy*. The disadvantage of polyspermy to the organism is thus that it leads to *triploidy*, which is a lethal condition.

IMPLANTATION, FETUS AND FETAL MEMBRANES

Implantation is the embedding of the developing embryo in the lining of the uterus. In cow implantation actually begins from 11th to 40th day *post coitum*. After fertilisation the zygote travels slowly down the oviduct; cell division occurs and this early cleavages of the fertilised egg are completed in the oviduct, the young embryo, consisting of from 8 to 16 cells (the blastocyst stage) arrives in the uterus in search of permanent attachment by about 4 days. During the first days after its arrival in the uterus, the embryo is completely dependent upon uterine secretions for its energy. The uterine glands under the influence of estrogen and progesterone hormone secrete "*uterine milk*" which is composed of protein, fat and traces of glycogen. As the blastocyst increases in size, it can no longer absorb enough nutritive material by diffusion, and thus makes it imperative that it establish a more adequate source of nutrition. About the 8th day zona pellucida begins to break up, and the cells push outward.

Layers of cells form and from these layers grow membranes that soon will nourish the developing embryo. To understand the development of these membranes, it is first necessary to have some concept of the three primary germ layers in the developing embryo. After numerous cell divisions, the embryo is a hollow sphere of cells a few layers thick. This single tissue layer is known as the *ectoderm*, and is the origin of the skin and other structures. Somewhat later, one side of this sphere is pushed in to form a double walled cup-like structure, leaving ectoderm on the outer surface; the inner surface is known as *endoderm*, Later, part of this pinches off into a tube to form the digestive tract. Proliferation of cells between the ectoderm and endoderm gives rise to a third germinal layer; the *mesoderm*. The mesoderm plays an important part in the formation of muscles.

From these three germinal layers arise not only the various tissues of the developing embryo itself, but those surrounding membranes which protect it and enable it to obtain nourishment. These membranes are collectively known as the *extra-embryonic membranes*.

The period of the embryo between 13th day to 45th day is characterised largely by the first formation of most organs and body parts. During this period the digestive tract, the lungs, the liver, and the pancreas all develop from the primitive gut. The heart and the circulatory system are started, and between 21st and 22nd day the heart begins to beat. The beginnings of the nervous system, the muscular and skeletal systems and the urogenital system are established.

From the sides of the embryo a fold grows up and over it, fusing at the top and ultimately enclosing the embryo in a double lavered sac which is known as the amnion (Fig. 5.16.). This amnion or water bag as it is commonly called, become filled with a clear watery fluid in which the embryo is suspended. Its purpose is to form a protective cushion against external shocks and pressure of the adjacent body organs and to prevent adhesions between the surface of the embryo and the surrounding membrane. At parturition, the amnion acts as a wedge to dilate the cervix at which time it usually ruptures, allowing the "waters" to escape.

As an outpouching of the hind gut of the digestive tract the *allantois* is formed. It enlarges and fills the space between the amnion and the outer membrane of the placenta, the *Chorion*.

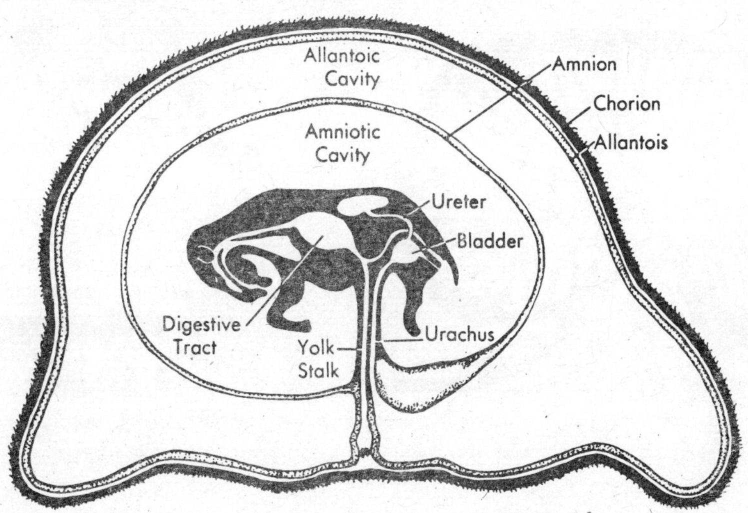

Fig. 5.16 Fetus of bovine within the placents.

The allantois functions as the urinary receptacle for the embryo and, also, collects some solid wastes. The chorion, the outer membrane, completely surrounds the embryo, amnion and allantoic cavity, is rich in blood vessels and lies in opposition to the uterine mucosa, through which, by diffusion and osmosis, an exchange of gases and nutrients occurs between the blood vessels of the fetal circulation and the blood stream of the mother. The allantois which fuses with the chorion becomes the *fetal placenta.*

The transfer of O_2, CO_2 and nutrients is affected by more or less intimate union of the chorion with the uterine mucosa of the dam to form the placenta. The mucosa, or lining, of the uterus is essentially a spongy network of blood sinuses in which the finger-like villi of the chorion bury themselves. Thus, the placenta is partly maternal and partly fetal in its origin. There is no mixing of maternal and fetal blood, however, for both nutrients and gases must

Table 5.5

Classification of types of placentation

Type of placenta	*Gross shape*	*Animals*
Epitheliochorial	Diffuse	Pig, horse, donkey
Syndesmochorial	Cotyledonary	Sheep, goat, cow,
Endotheliochorial	Zonary or discoid	Cat, dog, ferret
Hemochorial	Discoid or zonary	Primates
Hemoendothelial	Discoid or spheroidal	Rat, rabbit

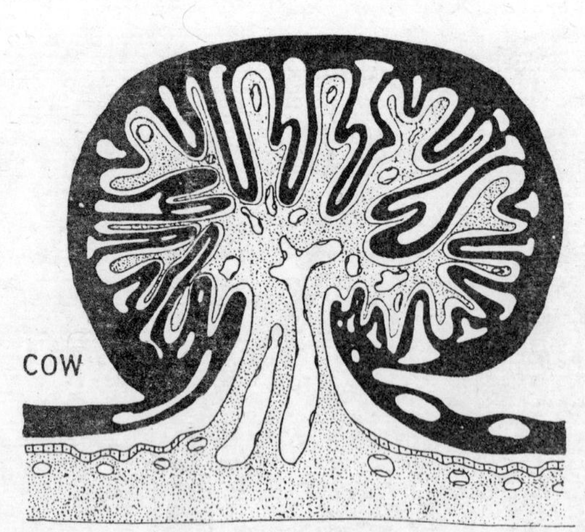

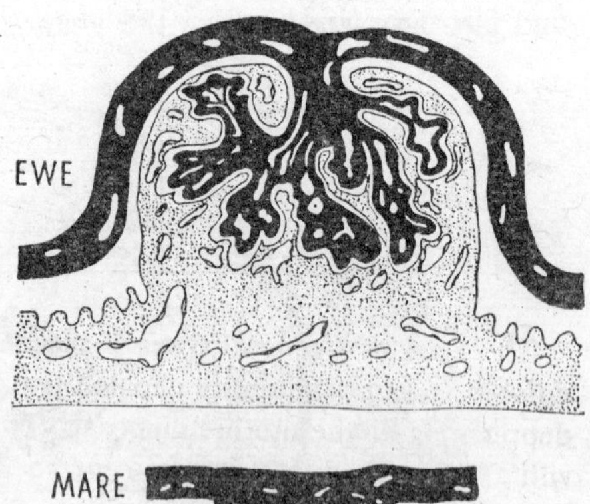

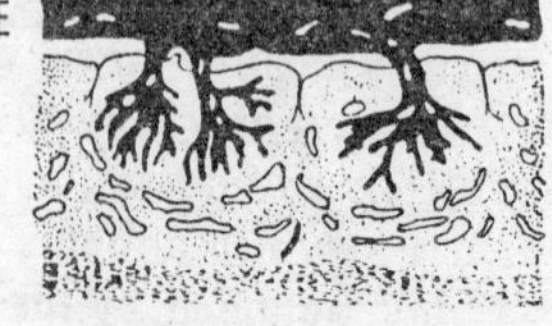

Fig. 5.17 Placental attachment of cow, ewe, and mare. Black = allanto-chorion of fetus. Stippled = maternal uterine tissue. (Hafez, *Reproduction in Farm Animals*, Lea & Febiger.)

pass through the membrane of the placenta. The food materials leave the maternal placenta and enter the fetal circulation by diffusion through the maternal and fetal placentae, after which they enter the blood vessels of the allantois which terminate in the umbilical cord. Wastes are carried back to the maternal circulation by the same system.

Table 5.6

PERIODS OF DEVELOPMENT DURING PREGNANCY

State of pregnancy		Mare	Cow	Ewe and goat	Sow	Bitch
I	Duration of period Length of fetus	14 days Ovum $\frac{1}{12}$ in	14 days Ovum $\frac{1}{12}$ in	14 days Ovum $\frac{1}{15}$ in to $\frac{1}{20}$ in	14 days Ovum $\frac{1}{15}$ in to $\frac{1}{20}$ in	10 days Ovum $\frac{1}{15}$ in to $\frac{1}{20}$ in
	Stages in development	Fertilised ovum has reached uterus from oviduct				
II	Duration Length of fetus	3 to 4 weeks $\frac{1}{2}$ in	3 to 4 weeks $\frac{1}{3}$ in	3 to 4 weeks $\frac{1}{8}$ in	3 to 4 weeks $\frac{1}{2}$ in	10 days to 3 weeks $\frac{1}{8}$ in
	Stages	Traces of fetus appear; head, body and limbs are discernible by end of this period				
III	Duration Length of fetus	5 to 8 weeks $2\frac{1}{8}$ in	5 to 8 weeks $1\frac{3}{4}$ in	5 to 7 weeks $1\frac{1}{4}$ in	4 to 6 weeks $1\frac{3}{4}$ in	3 to 4 weeks 1 in
	Stages	First indications of hoofs and claws visible as little pale elevations at ends of digits				
IV	Duration Length of fetus	9 to 13 weeks 6 in	9 to 12 weeks $5\frac{1}{2}$ in	7 to 9 weeks $3\frac{1}{2}$ in	6 to 8 weeks 3 in	5th week $2\frac{1}{2}$ in
	Stages	Stomach well defined in foal, pig, and puppy; differentiation of four stomachs in ruminants at end of this period				
V	Duration Length of fetus	14 to 22 weeks 13 in	13 to 20 weeks 12 in	10 to 13 weeks 6 in	8 to 10 weeks 5 in	6th week $3\frac{1}{2}$ in
	Stages	Large tactile hairs appear on lips, upper eye-lids, and above eye. Teats visible in female fetuses				
VI	Duration Length of fetus	23 to 24 weeks 2 ft 3 in	21 to 32 weeks 2 ft	13 to 18 weeks 1 ft 2 in	11 to 15 weeks 7 in	7 to 8 weeks 5 in
	Stages	Eye-lashes well developed. A few hairs appear on tail, head and extremities of limbs				
VII	Duration	35 to 48 weeks	33 to 40 weeks	19 to 21 weeks	15 to 17 weeks	9th week (8th in cat)
	Length	$3\frac{1}{2}$ ft	3 ft	$1\frac{1}{2}$ ft	9 to 10 in	6 to 8 in (kitten 5 in)
	Stages	Fetus attains full size. Body becomes gradually covered with hair, hoofs and claws complete, but soft				

There are two general types of placentae among farm animals. The sow and the mare have a *diffuse placenta*; the entire chorion is beset with finger-like villi which fit into corresponding depressions in the uterine mucosa. The cow and the ewe have a cotyledonary placenta; the villi are localised in a hundred or so rosettes, or cotyledons, over the surface of the chorion. These are separated by areas of smooth chorion. The villi of the cotyledons fit into pits in the spongy button-like cotyledons of the uterus. At parturition, the chorionic villi of both types are merely withdrawn, and there is no extensive destruction of the uterine tissue.

The extent to which a foetus grows in the latter stages of pregnancy is demonstrated by the actual weights obtained by the late Sir John Hammond in one of his investigations carried out on Shorthorn heifers.

Correct feeding is important throughout pregnancy, but it is even more important during the last stages, when the foetus is making very rapid growth.

Table 5.7

	Month of pregnancy								
	1	*2*	*3*	*4*	*5*	*6*	*7*	*8*	*9½*
Weight of foetus or calf (kg.) –	0.00009	0 009	0.090	0.730	1.816	2.724	10.442	16.80	34.00

PREGNANCY DIAGNOSIS IN ANIMALS

(Cows and She-buffaloes)

Pregnancy or gestation is the condition of female when a developing young is present in the uterus. The period of pregnancy, pregnant period, or gestation period, is the duration of time which elapses between service (or more correctly conception) and parturition.

The importance of detecting whether a female animal is pregnant or not is directly related to the economy of dairy management. A female may sometimes show a number of signs which are strongly suggestive for a positive case but on proper diagnosis it may not be found correct. By this way the animal might have passed quite a valuable time of her life. On the other hand if a cow is really pregnant, it can demand a change in her feeding schedule as well as the management from the very early stage. Whereas in case of failure due to infertility, sterility, etc., the causes as well as curative measures should be enquired. If it becomes impossible or uneconomical to cure an animal, culling is preferable.

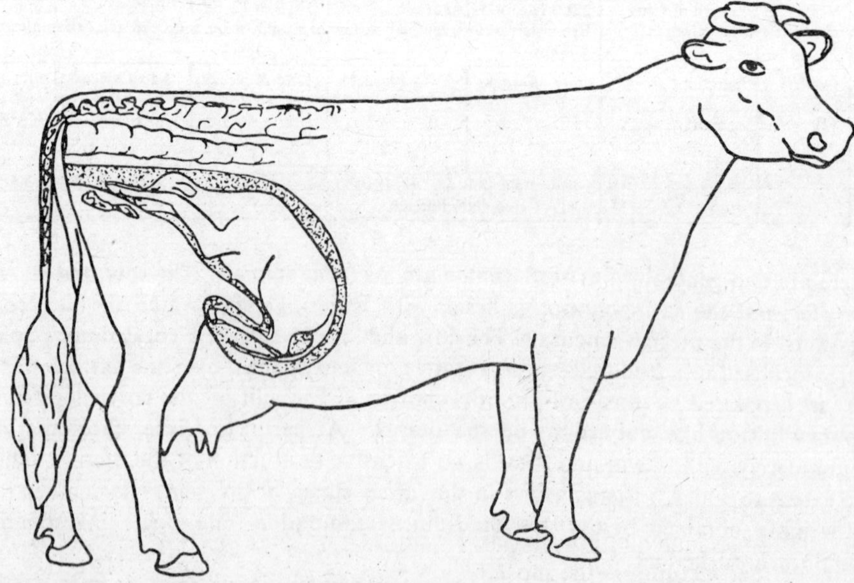

Fig. 5.18 Position of the calf in the uterus after it has been oriented for normal delivery.

An early detection of pregnancy of an animal thus becomes an indispensable job of any herd owner.

Methods of Detecting Pregnancy

The various methods by which pregnancy is detected are classified broadly into three groups which are given below:

(a) Signs of pregnancy—which are exhibited by the females and can be detected externally.

(b) Symptoms of pregnancy—which are detected per rectum and per vaginum examination.

(c) Laboratory tests—the principle of which depends upon the presence of certain hormones. It may be carried out either biologically or chemically.

Signs of Pregnancy

1. Cessation of estrus—In case of cows and she-buffaloes which have an estrus cycle of short duration with frequent recurrence cessation of the cycle after coitus is the first indication of pregnancy and generally a reliable one. Following points are to be remembered while considering the above sign:

(a) Low intensity of heat may be overlooked and thus the animals may be thought to be pregnant.
(b) Heat may be inhibited following the service due to hormonal dysfunctions.
(c) Sometimes though the animal is pregnant, signs of heat may be observed.

2. The animal concerned tends to become sluggish in temperament and more tractable.

3. The animal has a tendency to grow fat.

4. Increase in body weight of the animal at the last half of pregnancy due to the development of foetus and hypertrophy of the uterus and mammary glands.

5. Increase in the volume of the abdomen at a later stage of pregnancy.

6. Changes in the mammary gland—As parturition approaches the gland becomes firm, enlarged and glossy, teats take a waxy appearance. In dry milch cows mammary enlargement becomes prominent during the last 14 days prior to parturition.

Symptoms of Pregnancy

Per rectum examination of ovaries, uterus and uterine arteries. In bovine animals, palpation of the uterus per rectum, is the most reliable method of pregnancy diagnosis, particularly during early and mid-gestational periods. Positive conclusion is drawn by the detection of the characteristic changes which the uterus and uterine arteries undergo during pregnancy and also by the palpation of the foetus itself or its membranes. Useful supporting evidence is obtained by recognition of the presence of a fully developed corpus luteum in one ovary over a period of several months.

It is to be remembered that the person conducting the tests should have adequate knowledge of the anatomy of the animal regarding the size, position and the physiology of the uterus and ovaries both during the various stages of gestation and during the different phases of oestrus cycle.

Ovaries. In the bovine, corpus luteum of pregnancy persists in the ovary at its maximum size throughout the whole gestation period. It is firm, rounded at the top and slightly elevated from the surface of the ovary. With practice this corpus luteum of pregnancy can easily be differentiated from the graafian follicle, ovarian cyst, persistent corpus luteum, etc.

The corpus luteum may be present in either side of the pregnant horn of the uterus.

If the animal is examined some 10 days after service, again on the 22nd day and again about the 40th day and if the same ovary is found to be uniform in size with the corpus luteum, strong evidence of pregnancy is indicated. The absence of signs of heat during this period may be of supporting evidence.

The ovary can be examined up to 3 months of pregnancy after which it sinks deeper in the abdominal cavity due to increase in weight of the uterus and hypertrophy of ovarian and uterine ligaments.

Uterus. The changes which the uterus undergoes during gestation period may be arbitrarily divided into different stages.

1. *Up to Two Months*

If proper knowledge is acquired, pregnancy can be diagnosed as early as on the 30th day by examining the uterus. During this stage the foetus cannot be felt although it lies in the amniotic vesicle and the size is nearly 3/4 of an inch. In case of heifers slight enlargement of the gravid horn can be detected out, but in case of multigravida this difference is not found.

From the beginning of the 2nd month to the middle of the 2nd month, if the enlarged horn is allowed to slide between the thumb and the first two fingers, the sphere can be felt. It has a characteristic slippery feeling. After 7th week, this feeling rapidly disappears.

At the end of the 2nd month if the free part of the gravid horn is gently pinched through the rectal wall, sensation of the foetal membranes slipping between the fingers can be detected. But this is more pronounced during the 3rd and 4th month of pregnancy.

2. *During 3rd and 4th Month*

* Increase in the size of the gravid horn is more detectable, and can easily be compared with the non-gravid horn. The gravid horn is also noticeably larger than the other.

By 90 days the uterine distension can be detected with accuracy. Sometimes it is possible to detect the foetus at this stage. Tapping of the distended horn with fingers reveals like a piece of wood floating in the fluid beneath.

Early in the 4th month cotyledons can be felt. The sizes of the cotyledons are small, but

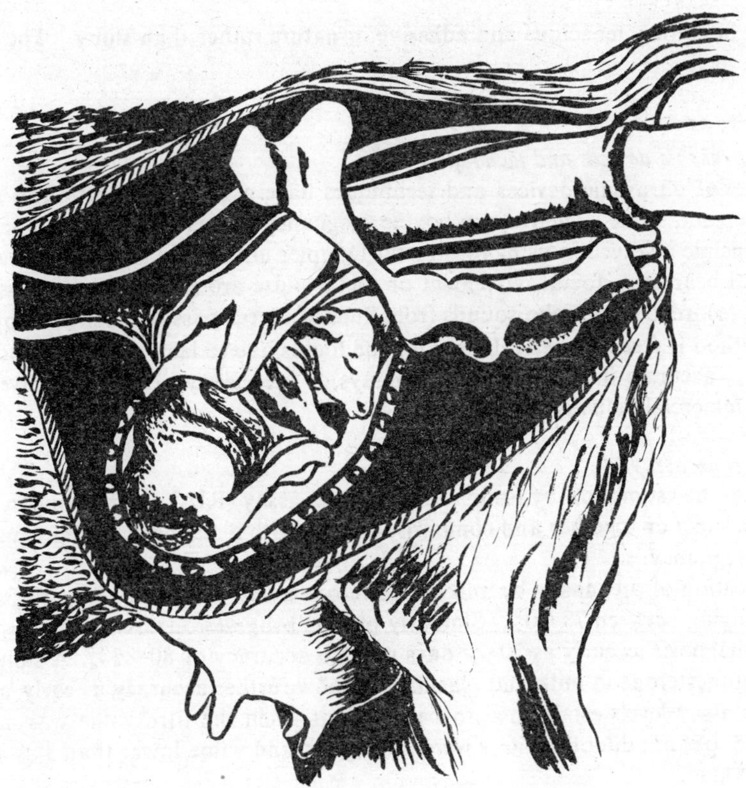

Fig. 5.19 Pregnancy diagnosis by rectal palpation method.

they grow larger as pregnancy advances. By the end of the 4th month, uterine arteries start enlarging. The middle uterine artery can be felt as a tense chord. At this time if the artery be slightly compressed between the finger and the thumb, a continuous vibrating fremitus (uterine thrill) can be detected which later changes to pulsation.

3. *From 5th Month Onwards*

From the 5th month onwards, the uterus sinks below the pelvic brim until the middle of the 6th month, but the foetus can still be felt in 50% of cases.

From the middle of the 6th month to the middle of 7th month, pregnancy can be detected from condition of the uterus, its blood vessels, the cotyledons and from the tension of the cervix.

From this period to the end of the pregnancy the presence of calf can be detected from external signs.

Differential diagnosis. In many cases pregnancy may be confused with some of the uterine abnormalities. One such case is pyometra of uterus. In case of pyometra, the uterus enlarges in both the sides, there will be no cotyledons, no double layers of the uterus, fremitus absent. Also in case of pyometra, pus will be present in vagina.

Per vaginum examination. If the vagina is examined during pregnancy by means of a speculum, the vaginal wall appears dry and wrinkled. During pregnancy the secretion of the cervical glands becomes gelatinous and tough forming a plug for sealing the canal. The seal is light brown in colour, tenacious and adhesive in nature rather than slimy. The seal develops on the 60th day.

Laboratory Tests

1. *Use of ultrasonic devices and techniques*

The use of ultrasonic devices and techniques have a wider application in small animals like the sheep and swine. Their use in bovine pregnancy testing is gathering momentum.

The principle involved in using intrarectal Doppler ultrasound is that sound waves develop due to foetal heartbeat, foetal movement or foetal pulse are reflected back at an altered frequency and recorded while echo sounds from fluid of uterus pass through an amplifier.

The method is free from any danger for the foetus due to lack of x-rays and is claimed to be over 90% accurate if tested after 35–50 days of pregnancy. Due to involvement of high cost, the commercial value is poor.

2. *Progesterone assay*

Progesterone estimation by using radio immuno assay (RIA) can be done in both milk and plasma separately or together and comparison made with a standard non-pregnant animal for detecting pregnancy.

Identification of pregnancy by milk progesterone assay can be done by 30–35 days with an accuracy ranging between 78–90%. Similarly plasma progesterone assay also provides clue for pregnancy diagnosis as early as 20–25 days with an accuracy of 80–85%. A simultaneous estimation of progesterone in milk and plasma will show further accuracy as early as 20 days.

In milk assay levels established to be pregnant when the titre value was more than 4 ng (nanogram)* per ml; doubtful titers were 3–4 ng/ml, and value lower than 3 is a definite case of negative value.

In plasma progesterone assay, levels higher than 1 ng/ml considered to be positively pregnant.

However, false results due to early embryonic death, abortions and catarrhal inflammation of genital tract also commonly observed.

3. *Pattern of vaginal smear*

Use of cervical mucus for detection of pregnancy was initiated since 1957 but still the method could not get popularity due to lack of accuracy as other endocrine factors are also responsible for producing similar fern like pattern in the vaginal mucus. Vaginal smears are first stained and fixed. Visible cells are then classified into (i) nucleated polygonal, (ii) non-nucleated polygonal, (iii) large nucleated spherical, (iv) small nucleated spherical and (v) leucocytes. The proportion of large nucleated spherical cells are criterian factors. However, a coupling of cervical mucus examination and rectal palpation showed a 90% accuracy as early as 20 days of pregnancy.

4. *Immunological techniques*

The developing embryos/foetus bears antigens which are foreign to mother and it could

---

*One nanogram = One billionth = $\frac{1}{1,000,000,000} = 10^{-9}$ gram.

One billion = A thousand millions = 1,000,000,000

One million = A thousand thousands = 1,000,000

be expected that immune rejection of the conceptus would occur. One of the reasons why the foetus is not rejected is because a depression of the maternal immune response takes place during pregnancy.

Serum from pregnant animals of several species has been shown to contain a factor, "early pregnancy factor" (EPF), which is immunosupressive. EPF can be detected as early as 6 hours after fertilization and disappears immediately when the foetus or embryo dies.

The diagnosis of the factor is estimated by Rosette inhibition test (RIT), is a time consuming but sensitive test with an accuracy of about 72%. Availability of laboratory facilities for the test although costly but under field conditions, early pregnancy diagnosis can easily be detected by the method.

5. *Faetal electrocardiography*

The graphic recording due to variation in electrical potential produced from the body surface of the heart (electro-cardiography) was adopted as a method of pregnancy diagnosis. The accuracy of the test is increased with the length of gestation and proved to be a better method for diagnosis of twin, triple or even quadruple (consisting of four) pregnancies and late foetal mortality.

6. *Barium chloride test* .

When 5-6 drops of 1% barium chloride solution is poured to 5 ml of urine, a clear white precipitate is formed in non-pregnant cows while added to the urine of pregnant cow, the increase estrogen and progesterone content of the urine prevent the formation of any precipitate. The test is 95-100% accurate. It takes less than 3 minutes and gives correct results 31–210 days after fertilization.

The test is recommended only where cows are in byres and fed special diets devoid of hormones. Remember that fresh pasture and other green forage contain significant amount of oestrogen as detected in the urine of animals on grazing.

7. *Pregnant mare serum test (PMS)*

The test is applicable with mares at present form. It is conducted by using 10 ml of blood serum collected from a mare between 50–85 days after fertilization. The serum is injected into the ear vein of a mature, non-pregnant female rabbit that has been isolated from all male rabbits for at least 30 days. A positive test showing that the mare is pregnant is indicated by dark red follicles, *corpora hemorrhagica*, in the ovaries of the rabbit 48 hours after the injection. The ovaries of the rabbit may be examined during a surgical exploratory operation, and the rabbit may then be saved for future use, or the rabbit may be butchered and the ovaries examined at that time.

8. *Scanning*

At present pregnancy can be easily diagnosed in case of sheep, cattle, horses and dogs by the use of an equipment called "*OVISCAN*".

The equipment helps to establish pregnancy within 30 days of fertilization in sheep. The flock of sheep should be scanned within 45–100 days to count the number of foetuses accurately. Although placental gonadotrophins probably are secreted by all domestic animals during pregnancy, the quantities are insufficient, except in mare to produce a reaction in the ovaries of test animals.

While considering the percentage accuracy, rectal palpation can be recorded as the best method of early pregnancy diagnosis followed by progesterone assay in cattle. Ultrasonic technique is also gathering momentum.

For sheep and goat plasma progesterone levels; laparoscopy, and the use of ultra sound (Doppler) devices are all accurate, but each requires special handling facilities, highly trained technicians, or considerable time per ewe or goat. However, the use of an external ultrasound device has consequently become popular in U.K., U.S.A. etc. for sheep and goat since it is quick and safe.

For horse rectal palpation method as early as 18 days in mare is very effective for early diagnosis. In early pregnancy, diagnosis is based on increased tone of the uterus and cervix; after 30–35 days, the uterus enlarges due to development of the chorionic vesicle. The foetus can be palpated by ballottment (pushing against the uterus with the finger) of the uterus from day 110 to term. The ultrasound method is also good particularly for detection of twin pregnancies. Biological pregnancy tests in the mare are based primarily on the detection of gonadotrophin in the serum produced by endometrial cups and effective from about day 41–100 of pregnancy. Their disadvantage is that false positives may result if abortion or embryonic death occur after the cups begin to function.

For sows ultrasonic test is highly recommended.

PARTURITION

Parturition is the expulsion of the foetus and its membranes from the uterus through the birth canal by natural forces and in such a state of development that the foetus is capable of independent life. The process is called 'foaling' in the mare, 'calving', in the cow, 'lambing' in the ewe, 'kidding' in the goat, 'farrowing' in the sow, and 'pupping' or 'whelping' in the bitch.

Parturition is an absolutely normal physiological process, being accompanied by pain, discomfort and general disturbance. This is mainly due to the difficulty that is experienced in transmitting a relatively large, bulky and living animal, through a comparatively small and rigid canal.

Prior to parturition, the pelvic ligament of the cow, specially the sacrosciatic becomes more relaxed causing a sinking of the croup (a part of the hind quarters lying immediately behind the loins) muscles. The state can also be noted by the elevation of the tail head. The vulva becomes more flaccid until it is two to six times its normal size. The udder becomes elongated and swollen. Just before parturition, the udder secretion changes from a honey-like secretion to a yellowish one, known as colostrum. Usually the cow discharges stringy types of mucus from its vagina from the seventh month of pregnancy and onwards. At a later stage the amount of mucus increases markedly and the cervical seal liquefies.

Causes of Parturition

The exact cause of parturition remains still a mystery. The different prevalent views may be summarised as follows:

1. Towards the end of pregnancy the level of estrogen usually increases and the level of progesterone decreases. The estrogen sensitises the uterus for the action of oxytocin. At the

time of parturition oxytocin is released which directly brings about strong uterine contraction and thus initiates parturition.

2. The increase in size of the foetus, along with certain unknown developments in the ovary, possibly bring about a fatty degeneration of the placental cells, with the effect that the interchange between foetus and dam ceases to be normal. Probably this condition sets up some slight amount of irritation in the uterus and the uterus is stimulated to contract in reflex and expel the foetus which is now a mere foreign body.

3. Still one more hypothesis is that due to inadequate nutrients or some other reason, the foetus releases a hornlone which enters the maternal circulation and initiates parturition.

The Forces of Expulsion

The forces by which expulsion is achieved are exerted by the plain muscle of the wall of the uterus in the first place, and secondly, by contraction of the walls of the abdomen which raises the intra-abdominal pressure. The total effect of this is called a *Labour Pain.* At first labour pain are weak, short, and infrequent. They gradually increase in strength, duration, and frequency until, at the height of the act, they cause considerable distress to the dam. From this time onwards they diminish gradually, and soon after the foetal membranes have been expelled, they cease altogether. In the early stages, all the force of the contraction is directed against the cervix of the uterus, and the pressure on the non-compressible amniotic fluid forces the membranes into the canal. This gradually dilates until a bladder like piece of chorion (the outer most of the membranes) forces its way into and through the cervix. For a time the result of the following contractions is simply to dilate this opening still wider, until finally it becomes as wide as possible, and the uterus, cervix, and vagina form one continuous passage. About this time, the chorionic bladder like swelling appears between the lips of vulva; this is popularly called the "*water bag*". The head and forelimbs soon become forced into the pelvic and the external genital passage, until the forelimbs reach the level of the vulva. The water bag soon bursts and the contained fluid is discharged. There is often a pause in the series of labour pains at this stage—a provision of nature whereby the dam gets an opportunity of resting and regaining her strength preparatory to the powerful and violent pains that are imminent. From this time onwards till the young is born, the pains attain their maximum, both as to the force and duration of the contractions. They are all exerted upon the passive foetus in an endeavour to drive it out from the abdominal cavity. The accessary contractions of the abdominal walls and the diaphragm come into play to a considerable extent, but the muscle in the uterine wall remains the chief expellant.

The head and forelimbs are gradually passed through the external genital canal to the outside where they become visible. The withers and shoulders of the young are now passing through the bony pelvic of the dam, and they correspond to the big end of the wedge whose smaller end is the forelegs and head. The wedge like shape of the young completes the dilation of the genital canal and make delivery possible.

Stages in Parturition

The act of parturition is a continuous one. For the sake of understanding, the process may be explained under the following four stages:

1. The Preliminary stage,
2. The Dilation stage,

3. The Expulsion of the foetus stage,
4. The Expulsion of the after birth stage

The preliminary stage. It continues for about some hours to even days. There is a swelling of the udder, a clear waxy fluid material oozes from the teats or may be expelled by pressure of the hand. The entire external genital organs become swollen and looks reddish. A clear, straw coloured stringy mucus is secreted, which usually soils the tail and hind quarters. The quarters droop along with the slackening of the muscles and ligament of the pelvic region, which is popularly known as '*softening of the bones*'. If the animal is not confined. it will look for a solitary place. The cow feels uneasy, bellows and becomes excited.

Dilation of the cervix stage. There is a marked increase of uneasiness followed by a mild labour pain The animal is sometimes somewhat distressed and may show signs of pain in its abdomen. It may lie and rise again several times. Labour pain becomes more acute with short intervals. The cow at this stage looks anxious, her pulse is quickened and her breathing is distressed and rapid. After about ½ to 3 hours the 'water bag', appears at the vulva. It is found empty at first, but forefeet of the young animal can be felt in it later. At this time the cervix is fully dilated.

Expulsion of the foetus stage. The phase comprises the period from the complete dilation of the os-uteri to the delivery of the foetus. The back of the cow is arched, her chest is expanded, and the muscles of her abdomen become broad and hard with each labour pain. Frequently, the rectum forcibly discharges its contents and the urinary bladder does likewise. At each contraction, the water bag protrudes further and further from the vulva till the front hoof is visible. At this stage the bag bursts and a quantity of fluid is thrown off and the animal has a short period of ease. The calf normally comes with the two front hoofs first. Close set on them is its nose. When the hoofs and the nose are at the genital of the cow, the head of the calf is at the pelvic which will have to pass through the small pelvic opening. This is the moment of the supreme effort and of the greatest point of labour pain. The heifer may cry out at this stage. At last the uterine contractions combined with the additional abdominal force on the uterus results in the driving away of the foetus through the cervix, vagina and vulva.

Expulsion of the after birth. In the cow, the attachment of placenta with the uterus is limited to the cotyledons and is very close. As a result of this, involution (shrinkage of the uterus) does not greatly affect the detachment and removal of the placental membrane from the cotyledons during the expulsion of the foetus, although loosening of the attachment occurs to some extent.

After the expulsion of the calf the uterus tends to throw out the placental membrane which is now merely a foreign body. As a result of uterine contraction the placenta separates from the cotyledons and passes into the vagina, wherefrom it is expelled.

Early discharge of the membrane is desirable, to avoid putrefaction of the placenta which may cause infection of the uterus. Expulsion within 6 to 8 hours may be regarded as normal. In case it exceeds 8 hours, manual removal is advocated.

Care of the Cow after Parturition

After parturition the exterior of the genitalia, the flanks and tail should be washed with warm clean water. The warm water used for washing may contain some crystals of potassium permanganate or *Neem* leaves boiled in water. This will give a good antiseptic wash. The cow should then be given a warm drink which should be prepared with bran and salt. The cow should be allowed to rest and some dry hay may be placed before her to take as she pleases. Some green grass may also be given. For two days the cow should not be given much concentrates. If the cow is in good condition at the time of calving the amount of feed during these two days does not matter. The amount of concentrates should then be gradually increased with the aim of reaching full dosage in three weeks.

STERILITY

To a dairy farmer, nothing is so important as the regular fertility of his farm animals. Late maturity, fewer or no calvings, long dry periods, silent breeding, frequent abortions, repeat breeding are some of the common troubles that reduce or limit reproduction in almost all classes of animals.

The troubles that cause a complete and permanent reproductive failure is known as sterility while lowered fertility is a sort of compromise between fertility and sterility and may cause reduction in reproductive efficiency from 99 per cent to 1 per cent. Of the two, lowered fertility in animals is feared more by an owner than sterility in animals simply because it is more expensive to handle.

Causes of Sterility

The most common and important cause of sterility can be grouped under several headings, as given below. However, it must not be thought that this classification is perfect or the list is exhaustive. The causes of sterility are arranged in this way merely for convenience.

1. Anatomical
2. Accidental
3. Physiological
4. Nutritional
5. Psychological
6. Pathological
7. Genetical
8. Miscellaneous
9. Faults of Management

ANATOMICAL. These include structural defects and malformations which may either be congenital or acquired. Some of these may be severe enough to cause sterility while others may affect the degree of fertility only. Some of the important ones may be summarised as under:

1. *Cryptorchidism.* It refers to the undescended condition of the testes into the scrotal sac. Such males are also known as cryptorchids or Rigs. It may be unilateral (with one undescended testes) or bilateral (with both the testes undescended). The undescended testes are exposed to a higher body temperature as a result of which the germinal epithelium is destroyed and there occurs no spermatogenesis, e.g., no sperms are formed. The condition is reported to be heritable.

2. *Scrotal Hernia.* The descent of viscera into scrotum through the inguinal canal leads to the testicular atrophy by hampering their blood supply.

3. *Importentia Coeundi.* Failure of the retractor penis muscles to relax and to allow the penis to extend from the sheath.

4. *Free-Martin* (*Neuter*). When a female calf is born as a twin to a male calf, a sterile female, known as a free-martin, results in approximately 91 per cent of the cases. The free-martin is a female in which the reproductive organs have failed to develop properly. In consequence, such an animal is not only sterile but also develops certain characteristics of the

male. The male of such a pair would breed normally. This condition is not due to a direct inheritance of the abnormal tract, but to the twinning, which is an inherited trait.

This condition is due to the fact that the choria, or membranes, which surrounded the individuals are united in such a way that the circulatory system of two are joined and the blood of one individual circulates through the body of the other. The blood of the female does not interfere in any way with the normal development of the male, but the blood of the male circulating in the female seems to inhibit her full sexual development. This is thought to be due to a hormone which is secreted by the male foetus and carried through the blood, arresting the full development of the female reproductive organs. Such females will not breed. No corrective measures are known, for attempts at hormonal correction have failed.

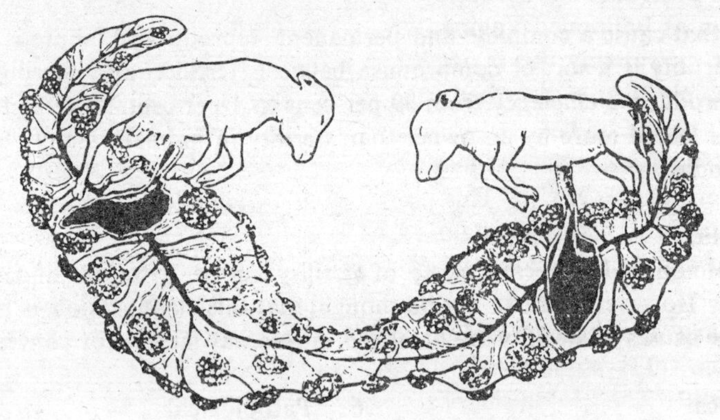

Fig. 5.20 A bovine free-martin.

Occasionally (ahout 9 per cent) a female born with a male will breed. This is due to the fact that the choria of the two animals remain distinct so that each has its own circulatory system. Then the female will breed normally.

5. *Persistent hymen* (White Heifer Disease). Hymen is a thin band of tissue between the vagina and the vestibule in virgin females and breaks with the first coitus. But sometimes this tissue gets thick and cannot be easily broken and persists barring reproduction. It may also lead to the accumulation of the oestral and other secretions of the uterus and vagina. It can be surgically operated and cured.

6. *Incomplete canalisation and fusion of the reproductive ducts.* Sometimes the reproductive ducts like vas deferens, fallopian tubes, uterine horns, etc., are not properly canalised and may remain as solid structures. At times the Mullerian ducts do not fuse or there may be the double vaginae, double cervices, etc. These conditions may act as physical barriers.

7. *Absence of parts.* This feature is quite common amongst both the sexes and may be either unilateral or bilateral. The gonads or any part of the tubal genitalia may be absent. This excludes the animal from breeding either completely or partially.

ACCIDENTAL. These include the consequences of any mechanical injury that may exclude the animal from breeding temporarily or even permanently. These are usually curable if prompt and expert treatment is resorted to.

1. *Bruising, Laceration and Inflammation of Genital Organs.* It is common in case of horses and asses which get kicked by the oestrus female if not properly secured. This may hurt the animals on testes, penis, etc. Jumping over barbed wire while running behind the females may also lead to similar injuries. Sometimes false entry of the penis during copulation leads to the bruising of the penis and rectum.

2. *Perforation of the Uterine and Vaginal Walls.* A variety of complications of this sort may arise due to abnormal parturition or service by a large and vigorous male. Under abnormal conditions the penis may be caught by the urethral orifice or enlarged Gartner's ducts and the fistulae may be formed.

3. *Prolapse of Uterus and Vagina.* This condition is generally faced during advanced pregnancy or when approaching parturition. Generally the vagina and at times also the uterus gets reversed and protrudes out through the vulva and makes parturition difficult. This condition is also known as Ballooned Vagina.

PHYSIOLOGICAL. Probably this is one of the most widespread form of sterility or reduced fertility. It is mainly due to disturbed coordination, equilibrium and imbalance among the various hormones of the body.

1. *Impaired Sexual Maturity.* It may be due to pituitary dysfunction with regard to the gonadotrophic hormones (GTH). This may lead to underdeveloped or undeveloped condition of the gonads and the accessary genitalia in both the sexes. Other hormones like thyroxin, somatotrophic, etc., which affect the general growth of the animal body may also affect sexual maturity.

2. *Lack of Gametogenesis and Libido.* Both these processes controlled by the FSH and LH components of the GTH stimulate both spermatogenesis and oogenesis in the testes and ovaries respectively. The LH on the other hand stimulates the interstitial cells of the testes in males to produce androgen which in turn induce the animal to exhibit its sex or sex drive otherwise called libido. The deficiency of any of these hormones may limit or retard reproduction in either sex.

3. *Anoestrus Condition.* The anoestrus condition of the females may be due to a variety of causes of which the main ones are noted below:

(a) *Infantile ovaries.* It may be due to genetic or nutritional causes. In these cases there will be no follicular development and the level of estrogen will be reduced so much that there hardly will be any oestrus.

(b) *Persistent corpus luteum.* The corpus luteum that remains functional beyond the normal period goes on producing progesterone which keeps the pituitary suppressed for the GTH activity. The absence of the FSH, therefore, does not stimulate the ovary to develop follicles which produce estrogens responsible for heat.

4. *Silent or Quiescent Estrous.* Frequently females go through the normal ovarian changes in the estrous cycle but do not show the signs of heat and receptivity to males. Such cows and buffaloes are also known as silent or shy breeders. This is quite common in sheep which do not exhibit any sign of their first heat after the long anestrous period. Most probably the deficiency of the progesterone due to completely regressed corpus luteum may be the reason.

5. *Short Cycles and Retarded Implantation.* This condition may be due to unhealthy or deficient C.L. This leads to the deficiency of the progesterone and frees the pituitary for GTH activity, thus stimulating the ovary for oogenesis and bringing the animal into heat even

before due interval is over. The deficiency of the progesterone may also lead to improperly prepared conditions of the uterus for implantation of the foetus leading to no conception.

6. *Cystic Ovaries or Nymphomania.* In some cases single or multi-cysts may develop on the ovary and cause short oestrus cycles or prolonged oestrum. The animal usually will not conceive if bred at these abnormal heat periods. These animals are often referred to as chronic bullers and the condition is called nymphomania. Such cysts may be removed manually or treated with certain hormones, but the cow usually will not breed until she has passed one or two normal heat periods.

NUTRITIONAL. Of all the problems concerning animals "effect of nutrition on reproduction" has received the best attention of various workers.

1. *Carbohydrates.* Experiment with low energy levels, at Pennsylvania (U.S.A.) have indicated delay in spermatogenesis, reduction in the number of spermatozoa produced and poor viability of the sperms.

2. *Fats.* As far as the fats in the diet are concerned, no planned experiments have been conducted on larger animals and ruminants. With laboratory animals it has been indicated that the unsaturated fatty acids are essential for the well-being of reproduction. Their deficiency may lead to a variety of troubles, namely, lack of libido in males, reabsorption of the foetus, abortions or dead births, etc.

3. *Proteins.* Very little work has been done on the effect of protein deficiencies on reproduction in cattle. It is difficult to imagine a practical condition of management in which protein alone could be a limiting factor. It has been suggested that spermatogenesis is more satisfactory if the animal proteins are included in the feed but critical experimentation has not supported this.

4. *Minerals.* Of the minerals that limit reproduction, phosphorus seems to be the most important. The amount of phosphorus needed by an adult cow for efficient reproduction is about 10 to 12 gm per day.

There is no evidence that calcium deficiency can be responsible for reproductive troubles in cattles, but the C : P ratio is important. This ratio should be between 1:2 and 2:1 for maximum efficiency.

Iodine deficiency has been blamed for some of the reproductive troubles namely lack of libido and poor quality semen. This is probably related to the lowered metabolism due to failure of the thyroid gland to secrete enough iodine containing hormones, the thyroxine. Its deficiency may also lead to premature, weak or dead birth.

5. *Vitamins.* Among the vitamins, vitamin A deficiency causes cornification of the mucous membranes. This is what is otherwise known as the unfavourable uterine environment. The uterus may not be in a suitable condition to transport sperm and provide effective nourishment to the embryo. Vitamin A deficiency or of carotene (precursor of vitamin A) in calves brings about the degeneration of the germinal epithelium and lack of gametogenesis in both the sexes.

The influence of vitamin C (ascorbic acid) on reproduction is not yet clear, vitamin C content in feeds is never a limiting factor, and moreover, the cow can synthesise her own vitamin C requirement, it is doubtful that ascorbic acid deficiency is an important deterrent in the dairy cow.

The effects of deficiency of vitamin E in causing reproductive failure in rats, both male and female have been established. While there have been claims as to similar failure in farm animals which have been prevented or overcome by adding a source of the vitamin to the ration, carefully controlled experiments have failed to substantiate these claims.

Vitamin D is needed during foetal growth, as well as during body growth, to ensure adequate calcium and phosphorus assimilation.

Of the other vitamins, B and K are synthesised by the ruminants in their body. There is, therefore, no evidence, that marginal deficiencies of vitamins B and K along with vitamin D (which is also pronounced in animal body specially in tropical country) affect reproduction.

PSYCHOLOGICAL. It has been recorded in a few cases when animals have become nervous and shy in nature. This may be primarily due to lack of experience in case of young animals or experience of some unnatural or painful event during first attempts at copulation. This may ultimately lead to elimination of sex behaviour and fear of reproduction.

PATHOLOGICAL

1. *Specific*

(a) Brucellosis (Bang's disease)—caused by *Brucella abortus* usually found in pregnant uterus, but can also localise in other tissues such as the udder or in the testes. The disease is responsible for 85 per cent of cattle abortions. It results in abortion between 5 and 8 months of pregnancy and can spread through contaminated feed, water, bodily discharges including milk. An estimated 25 to 30 per cent of the animals that come in contact with this disease become either temporarily or permanently sterile.

(b) Bovine venereal trichomoniasis — The disease is caused by a single celled protozoon—*Trichomonas foetus.* Under normal condition it is believed to be transmitted by infected instruments or in semen in A.I. The damage due to infection is confined to females. The organism inhabits the uterus and brings about the early destruction of the embryo usually within 3–5 weeks after conception. The animals then return in heat and may remain infected for several months. It may lead even to pyometra.

(c) Vibrio-foetus—The organism *vibrio foetus,* is a comma shaped bacterium and is responsible for occasional abortion of sheep and cattle. In this case the abortion takes place in 4 to 7 months. It is transmitted through the infected semen and can be checked by diluting it and the use of antibacterial reagents. The organism apparently interferes with the circulation of blood in the placenta thus causing abortion. Agglutination test of cervical secretions of cows has been found to be more useful for the diagnosis of vibriosis.

(d) Leptospirosis—The importance of this disease in cattle has been recognised only within the last few years. The causal organism is *Leptospira pomona* which can be transmitted to man also. It causes abortions, jaundice, mastitis, haemoglobinuria (bloody urine) and even death. Antibiotic treatment is effective in curing the disease and vaccination of animals with formalin-killed suspensions of the organism have been proved as preventive.

2. *Non-specific.* Little is known about the non-specific infection of the reproductive tract. The actual mode of infection and the causal organism of these diseases are not properly understood. The infection is probably picked up by contact and during copulation or parturition, and the causal organism may be protozoa, bacteria or virus.

1. Vaginitis—Inflammation of the vagina. It is due to some organic infection (virus like organism). It may be a vesicular or a nodular veneral disease.
2. Salpingitis—Inflammation of the fallopian tube.
3. Hydrosalpingitis—Fallopian tube becomes full of watery - fluid, and acts as spermotoxin.
4. Haematosalpingitis—Fallopian tube becomes full of blood.
5. Piosalpingitis—Fallopian tube becomes full of pus.
6. Metritis—Inflammation of the uterus.
7. Cervicitis—Inflammation of the cervix.
8. Pyometra—It is characterised by a progressive accumulation of pus in the uterus and the persistence of functioning lutein tissue in an ovary.

GENETICAL. 1. A male Drosophila without a "Y" chromosome looks normal but sterile.

2. Lethal factors and free-martin condition. A free martin if fertile to some extent is likely to give birth to a free-martin.
3. Hybrids of distant crosses are mostly sterile due to the dissimilarity of chromosome number.

Horse X Ass → Mule

Horse X Zebra → Zebroid

4. White heifer disease—This is a condition of persistent hymen. It is also said to be inherited.
5. Failure of the erection of penis—An inability to copulate due to unstraightened sigmoid flexure of the penis of the bull. This is due to failure of the retractor muscle and is a heritable feature.

MISCELLANEOUS FACTORS. Under this may be included a variety of factors e.g., age, season, temperature, light, etc. All these factors, no doubt, act by altering the endocrine balance with the animal body, either directly or indirectly.

1. *Age.* Fertility increases up to the age of about 4 years, levels off till 6 years of age and then gradually decreases afterwards in females whereas in males the peak is reached in about 2 years and then the decline sets in. These figures are for the foreign breeds which mature earlier with better feeding and care. For our own animals, the exact figures are not known.

2. *Season.* A number of conflicting views are held regarding the fertility of cattle in different seasons of the year. In general it is highest in spring, moderate in fall and low during winters and summers. Temperature seems to be the main factor responsible for it.

3. *Temperature.* This is also important in determining reproduction. High fevers, undescended testis, bandaged scrotum, and wool on scrotum also render the animals sterile either temporarily or permanently.

4. *Light.* It has been indicated that the conception rate is significantly correlated to the average length of the daylight. Ewes can be brought to heat earlier by exposing them to artificial light, while darkness induces late maturity and reduces oestrus. Longer exposures of poultry to light have beneficial effects on egg production. Now whether this is a direct effect of light or it works indirectly by inducing the birds to eat more and to produce more (for birds do not feed in dark) is not clear.

RECENT RESEARCH FINDINGS IN THE PHYSIOLOGY OF REPRODUCTION

Synchronization of Oestrus & Ovulation

Oestrous synchronization involves manipulating the reproductive processes so that females can be bred during a short, predefined interval with normal fertility. This application of technology facilitates breeding in two inportant ways: (1) it reduces and in some cases eliminates, the botheration of oestrous detection; and (2) it enables the producer to schedule the time of breeding. For example, if all the animals in a herd can be induced to exhibit oestrous at about the same time, the producer can arrange for a few days of intensive artificial insemination. Other advantages of this procedure includes: (1) it creates a more uniform group of offspring, (2) a selected male may be used for breeding purposes to a number of females, (3) the breeding and thereby parturition takes place at a particular time of the season which facilitates necessary planning in a economic way, (4) females with certain compounds can be bred without oestrus detection. Various compounds or methods used for synchronization are as follows:

1. *Prostaglandins*: Prostaglandin F_2 and its synthetic analogues induce oestrous and ovulation in cattle, horses, and sheep by terminating the functional activity of the corpus luteum. Intramuscular injection of these compounds 6 days after ovulation will induce oestorus within 2-3 days after treatment.

Table 5.8

Classes of Compounds used for Synchronization of Estrus of Farm Animals

Class of compound	Route and length of administration	Class of animal
Progestogen	Oral, intravaginal pessary, injection, subcutaneous implant; 12–21 days (approximately one estrous cycle)	Cattle, sheep, goat, swine (generally effective in acyclic as well as cycling females)
Prostaglandin F_2 or analog	Intramuscular injection, once during luteal phase of estrous cycle	Cattle, sheep, goat, horse
Progestogen with estrogen	Progestogen as above, 9–12 days; estrogen by intramuscular injection at beginning of treatment to shorten life of corpus luteum	Cattle
Progestogen and prostglandin F_2	Progestogen by intravaginal pessary, 5–7 days; prostaglandin near last day to regress corpus luteum	Cattle

[a]Primarily from Hafez, 1980 (chap. 27); Hawk, 1979 (chap. 8).

2. *Progestogen*: Progestin will also synchronize oestrus in farm mammals. These

compounds prevent maturation of follicles and the occurrence of oestrus and ovulation. After the hormone is withdrawn, females will come into oestrus and ovulate in a few days. Several progestin compounds such as medroxy-progesterone-acetate (MPA), and fluro-gestone-acetate (FGA) have been used in intravaginally where it is melted and diffused by the body temperature before absorption in body circulatory system.

3. *Teaser Rams*: When rams are suddenly introduced into the ewe flock just prior to the normal breeding season, a majority of the ewes will ovulate within a few days and have a normal fertile oestrous at their next cycle. Mating teaser rams (vasectomised) with ewes for 2 weeks before the introduction of entire rams will result in an early, compact lambing period.

Superovulation

The bull is capable of producing from several thousand to millions of sperm daily and discharges through ejaculates. A cow on the other hand normally produces one ovum (occasionally two) every 17–21 days. Now it is possible through the administration of hormones and other fertility drugs to obtain several ova (5–50) from a cow at one oestrus or even from heifer calves.

The ovaries of cows and heifers possess many thousands of potential ova at birth and produce no new ones thereafter. Since female livestock produce and utilize a limited number of ova to produce young during their lifetime, most of the original ova in the ovary do not produce young and are in effect wasted.

Superovulation consists of injecting the female with fertility drugs causing the larger follicles—each of which contain one oocyte or egg, in the ovaries—to mature and ovulate (rupture and release of the egg). Injections are administered in the middle part of the cycle (9.14 days after oestrus in cows). FSH is injected twice daily (4–5 mg per dose for 4–5 days). Additionally, on day 3 or 4 of FSH injection, prostaglandin F_2 alpha is also injected, which results in destruction of previously formed corpus luteum (C.L.) on the ovary, thereby triggering the next oestrus, commonly 2 days after administration of prostaglandin. This time she will produce and ovulate more eggs than normal. The eggs can be fertilized inside the female, or removed and fertilized *in vitro* (outside the animal body) where "matings" can be planned for each individual egg.

If the eggs are fertilized inside the female, the resulting embryos can be left to develop into twins or triplets, or they can be collected and transferred to other females called *surrogate mothers* (substitute mothers). When surrogate mothers are not readily available, the embryos can be frozen to await transfer at a later time.

Further, a single embryo can be made to produce additional offsprings. Normally a single-cell fertilized egg divides into 2 cells, which divide into 4 cells, 8 cells, and so on. At this very early stage of development, *all cells in the embryo are exactly alike genetically*. This means that splitting a four-cell embryo into 4 separate cells by microsurgery and then transferring these cells to surrogate mothers could potentially result in identical quadruplets. The technology is indeed tremendous.

In Vitro Fertilization (Test-tube Babies)

The first reported so-called test-tube human baby was born in 1978 in Great Britain. The procedure involves: (1) recovering a mature egg from the ovary; (2) placing the egg in a petri dish enriched with a culture medium similar to that of the oviducts; (3) collecting and placing viable spermatozoa in the culture medium and incubating at body temperature for 18 hours; (4) transferring the fertilized egg to a culture medium simulating (to have the external environment) the uterine condition and incubating for another 18 hours, during which cell division occurs, resulting in the formation of morula; and (5) placing the morula intravaginally into a recipient uterus, following proper hormonal preparation of the recipient female to accept the new embryo. The procedure is complicated and difficult for many reasons.

Embryo Transfer (ET) in India

In India, embryo transfer technology in cattle and buffalo was initiated in the recent past. The birth of first embryo transfer calf in cattle in India was reported in 1986, by the Andhra Pradesh Agricultural University at Tirupati. By now, many institutions have adopted ET successfully in cattle, resulting in several pregnancies and calves. The National Institute of Immunology (NIL) produced a calf through ET in January 1987. Birth of several calves is now reported under the Science and Technology (S&T) project in the National Dairy Development Board (NDDB), its regional centres and state-centres. Today, there are approximately 160 ET-born calves in cattle and 20 in buffaloes in India under the S&T project.

The NDDB started work on ET in buffaloes in 1986. So far 27 pregnancies have been achieved through surgical and non-surgical transfers. First buffalo calf through ET was born in December 1987 at the Sabarmati Ashram Gaushala, Bidaj.

In 1987, the Government of India initiated a National Science and Technology project on 'Cattle Herd Improvement for Increased Productivity using Embryo Transfer Technology' through its Department of Biotechnology. This project is under implementation through a multi-agency network on mission mode, with the National Dairy Development Board (NDDB) as the lead implementing agency, with Sabarmati Ashram Gaushala, Bidaj, as the main ET laboratory. Other four collaborating agencies are : (1) Indian Veterinary Research Institute (IVRI), Izatnagar; (2) National Dairy Research Institute (NDRI), Karnal; (3) National Institute of Immunology (NIL), New Delhi; and (4) Central Frozen Semen Production and Training Institute, Hessarghata.

The four regional ET centres are located at (1) Sree Nasik Panchwati Panjrapole, Nasik, Maharashtra; (2) Buffalo Breeding Centre, Nekarikallu, Dist. Guntur, Andhra Pradesh; (3) Animal Breeding Centre, Salon, District Rae Bareli, Uttar Pradesh and (4) Central Frozen Semen Production and Training Institute, Hessarghatta, karnataka.

The laboratory buildings, animal housing and donor and recipient herds have been established at these centres. The laboratories have been equipped with essential equipment. All the four regional centres have become operational. Each centre has been allotted certain breed and breed types for carrying out ET work. The Nasik centre has donor animals of pure Gir, HF and HF-and-Jersey cross breds. The Nekarikallu centre is exclusively working on buffaloes. The Salon centre will be producing HF and HF crossbred stock. The Hessarghatta centre is working on HF crossbred, Hallikar and Amrit Mahal breeds.

In addition, 25 ET state-centres are to be established at Erode, Trivandrum, Anand, Mehsana, Ludhiana, Jaipur, Bangalore, Goa, Kolhapur, Ujjain, Bhubaneswar, Patna, Lalkua, Prakasam, Chittor and Ernakulam Of these, the first four are fully operational. Ludhiana, Jaipur and Bangalore are equipped and would soon start functioning. The state centres will mainly transfer frozen embryos of elite parents received from the main and regional laboratories, to the recipient animals of farmers in villages.

The total project outlay is Rs. 168.46 million. The project aims at improving the production and productivity of the cows and buffaloes in the country. The thrust under the S & T project however is on the Indian buffalo, the main stay of Indian dairying. Some 0.1 per cent of our buffaloes or some 35,000 of these are in the production group of 3,500 kgs per lactation, while the country's average is only some 800 kgs. per buffalo per year or some 1,200 kgs. per buffalo per lactation. ET offers the quickest means for increasing the productivity of our buffaloes. Using embryo transfer and embryo microsurgery, we can produce, under Indian conditions 6–12 offsprings from a donor buffalo or cow in a year or 30 to 60 offsprings in her life.

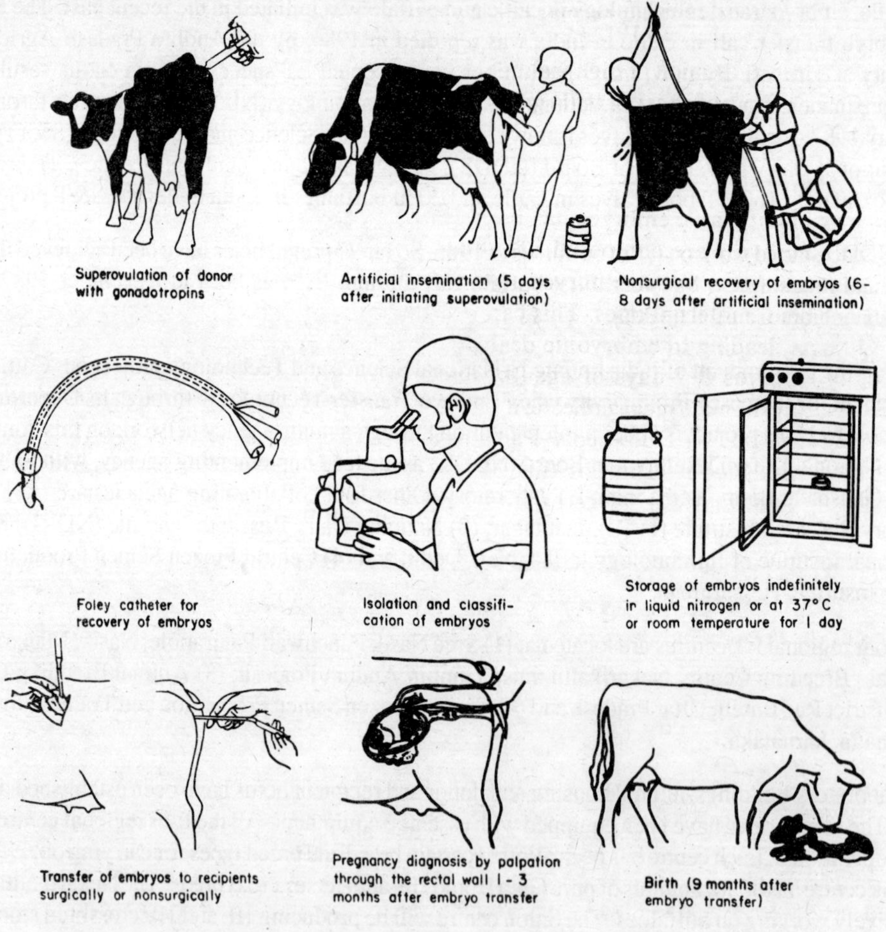
Superovulation of donor with gonadotropins
Artificial insemination (5 days after initiating superovulation)
Nonsurgical recovery of embryos (6-8 days after artificial insemination)
Foley catheter for recovery of embryos
Isolation and classification of embryos
Storage of embryos indefinitely in liquid nitrogen or at 37°C or room temperature for 1 day
Transfer of embryos to recipients surgically or nonsurgically
Pregnancy diagnosis by palpation through the rectal wall 1 - 3 months after embryo transfer
Birth (9 months after embryo transfer)

Fig.5.21 Schematic presentation of bovine embryo transfer procedures.

It is to be noted that embryo transfer cannot be considered as an independent project nor can it replace or substitute artificial insemination in animal breeding programmes. It is complementary to the existing breeding and AI programmes and has to be integrated in it to enhance the genetic gain, through existing programmes.

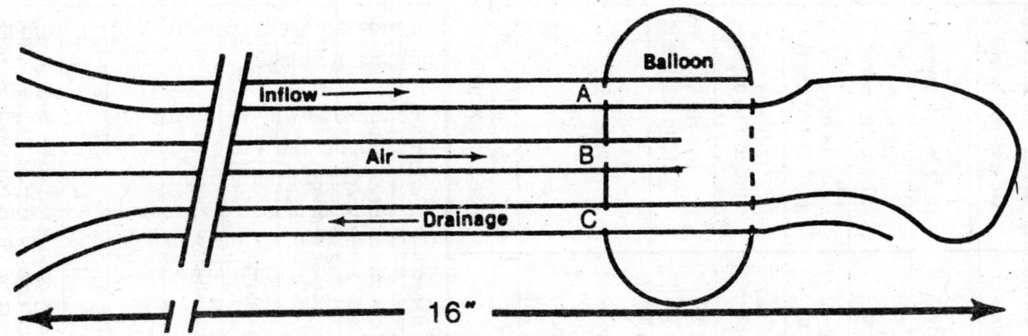

Fig.5.22 Diagrammatic depiction of a three way Foley catheter.

ET is not aimed at creation of high yielding animals for the milk producers directly. It provides only the seed stock – supply of superior bulls for the National AI network and for natural service where AI is not available.

Freezing Embryos

The freezing of viable embryos has been more difficult in comparison to freezing of bovine semen, since embryos are composed of masses of cells, rather than being a single cell as is the case with spermatozoa. When embryos are frozen and thawed, external cells are exposed to the environment before internal ones. This can result in becoming weak and lead to disaggregation of the cell mass, leading to embryonic dealth.

Recently embryos 6–7 days of age (0.2 mm in diameter) are recovered from superovulated donor cows using non-surgical collection methods. The embryos are pooled in a suitable growth medium viz., (i) Dulbecco's Phosphate—Buffered Saline (PBS), or (ii) Ham's F-10 supplemented with blood serum, or (iii) Bovine serum albumin. Other protective agents like Dimethyl sulfoxide (DMSO), glycerol, and 1,2—Propanediol are used to reduce the damage of freezing to embryos.

With this technique, embryos can be recovered, stored and transported almost anywhere in the world. However, the present technology of freezing, thawing and transferring the frozen embryos to recipients results 50% success when compared to fresh unfrozen embryos.

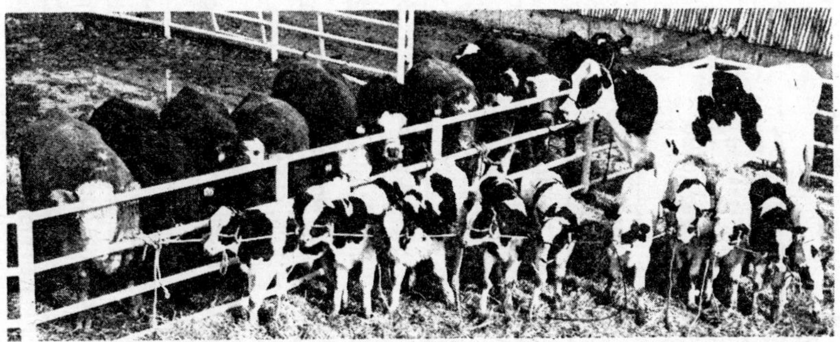

Fig.5.23 The Holstein Cow (upper right) is the genetic mother of 10 calves shown above. She was superovulated and the embryos were recovered from her uterus 7 days after conception, which were transferred to 10 recipient cows (left) for gestation to term. Colorado State University, U.S.A..

Table 5.9 AVERAGE CHARACTERISTICS OF SOME INDIAN FEMALE FARM ANIMALS REPRODUCTION BEHAVIOUR

Animal	*Onset of Puberty*	*Av. Age First Service*	*Length Estrous Cycle*	*Length Estrous*	*Gestation Period*
MARE	21 mo (16 to 24 mo)	3 to 4 yrs	21 days (19 to 21 days)	5 days ($4\frac{1}{2}$ to $7\frac{1}{2}$ days)	336 days 323 to 341 days)
COW	24 to 30 mo	25 to 30 mo	21 days (18 to 24 days)	18 hrs (12 to 28 hrs)	282 days 274 to 291 days)
EWE	9 to 14 mo (1st fall)	18 to 24 mo	$16\frac{1}{2}$ days (14 to 20 days)	30 hours (24 to 48 hrs)	148 days (140 to 160 days)
SOW	8 to 10 mo	9 to 10 mo	21 days (18 to 24 days)	2 days/Gilts : 1 day (1 to 5 days)	114 days (110 to 116 days)
BUFFALO	28 to 30 mo	30 to 35 mo	21 days	24 hrs. (6 – 47 hrs.)	316 days (310 to 320)
GOAT	8 to 10 mo	14 to 18 mo	20 days (15 to 24 days) 10% of some breeds of goat have short cycle of 6 - 10 days	40 hrs. (16 to 50 hrs.) Young have shorter duration.	150 days (145 to 155)
CAMEL	3 to 4 years	4 to 5 years	10 days (16 to 26 days)	3 to 5 days	391 days (365 to 400 days)

	Time of Ovulation	*Optimum Time for Service*	*Advisable Time to Breed after Parturition*
MARE	1 to 2 days before end of estrus	3 to 4 days before end of estrus or the second or third day of estrus	About 25 to 35 days of second estrus. About 9 days of frst estrous only if normal in every way
COW	10 to 15 hours after the end of estrus	Just after the middle of estrus to the end of estrus	60 to 90 days (85 days on an average)
EWE	12 to 24 hours before the end of estrus	18 to 24 hours after the onset of estrus	Usually the following autumn
SOW	35 to 45 hours after the onset of estrus	12 to 30 hours after the onset of estrus. 2 services at an interval of 12-14 hrs.	First estrus 3 to 9 days after weaning pigs
BUFFALO	11.40 hrs. after the end of estrus (10 to 18 hrs)	5 to 8 hrs. before the cessation of heat or 16 to 20 hrs. after the onset of heat	60 to 75 days
GOAT	25 to 35 hrs. after the onset of estrus	12 to20 hrs. after the onset of estrus.	80 to 90 days
CAMEL	Ovulation is sequel of coitus		A cow camel breeds only once in two years. She usually takes the bull about one year after calving. After parturition next oestrus or follicular wave may often delayed sometimes for as long as one year. In well fed females oestrus may occur early.

Note : Variation of reproductive behaviour in farm animals is most common due to genetic and environmental conditions.

Table 5.10 Reproduction and production parameters in Indian cattle and crossbreds

Breeds	Age at first calving (months)	Service period	Calving interval (months)	Lactation yield (kg.)	Lactation length (days)	Dry period (days)	Yield/day of calving interval (kg.)
INDIAN BREEDS							
DANGI	53.6±2.0	229.0±6.9	17.0±0.6	615.9±34.9	292.5±11.5	221.3±16.8	1.2
DEOGIR	46.9±2.1	181.0±9.0	15.4±0.4	1,423.1±60.5	313.2±08.7	157.0±08.4	3.1
DEONI	52.9±1.0	163.6±6.5	14.8±0.3	879.2±23.6	270.0±04.6	172.6±07.4	2.0
GIR	47.0±0.8	160.6±4.4	15.7±0.5	1,403.0±31.1	257.4±04.6	213.6±05.1	2.9
GAOLAO	46.2±0.4	188.3±4.8	15.6±0.3	534.5±15.2	295.2±05.2	185.2±07.6	1.3
HALLIKAR	45.1±1.5	298.3±7.5	19.7±0.9	541.9±61.1	285.1±10.1	302.0±28.5	0.9
HARYANA	58.7±0.4	166.9±0.5	19.5±0.5	1,136.7±34.0	232.5±04.3	166.9±08.0	1.9
KANGAYAM	44.1±0.4	225.0±5.9	16.7±0.3	643.6±10.5	212.0±30.0	242.0±06.9	1.3
KANKREJ	47.4±0.8	212.0±6.1	16.2±0.4	1,850.0±51.4	351.0±08.0	141.0±09.2	3.8
KHILARI	51.5±1.1	175.0±4.0	15.2±0.2	214.7±12.2	255.0±03.1	242.7±06.7	1.0
ONGOLE	39.9±0.4	229.3±5.2	17.0±0.6	613.1±60.5	217.0±08.9	366.2±23.7	1.2
RATHI	40.1±0.4	256.1±8.3	19.3±0.7	1,931.0±53.0	331.0±04.2	243.0±06.2	3.3
RED SINDHI	41.7±0.6	146.8±5.1	14.7±0.3	1,605.0±24.7	284.0±02.4	146.8±05.1	3.7
SAHIWAL	40.2±0.2	156.0±3.2	15.0±0.6	1,718.7±36.0	283.5±01.8	156.0±03.2	3.8
THARPAKAR	49.4±0.4	145.5±8.3	14.8±0.8	1,659.2±53.3	280.1±06.0	145.5±08.3	3.7
UMBLACHERY	45.6±1.1	202.0±8.9	16.1±0.5	323.9±18.5	233.7±09.1	277.9±15.8	0.7
NON–DESCRIPT	59.0±2.5	280.0±8.6	18.7±1.0	534.7±14.3	303.0±06.2	264.0±20.3	0.9
NON–DESCRIPT	54.0±2.0	295.2±9.2	19.6±0.9	492.3±11.6	268.6±04.0	300.8±26.1	0.9
CROSSBRED CATTLE (BOS INDICUS F X BOS TAURUS M)							
H X F	33.0±1.1	173.0±15.3	15.3±0.8	3,195.5±205.0	340±05.1	85.0±15.4	7.0
H X BS	29.0±0.9	134.0±12.0	14.1±0.6	2,785.5±163.2	336.0±24.5	115.0±23.2	6.6
H X J	32.9±1.2	134.0±10.7	13.5±0.4	2,868.0±215.5	308.0±04.2	98.0±05.2	7.1
G X J	24.9±1.8	101.0±10.8	12.7±0.9	2,713.0±225.5	324.0±06.2	57.0±06.3	7.1
G X F	34.9±0.5	113.3±11.6	13.2±0.3	2,254.5±097.5	288.2±06.0	105.9±16.3	5.7
RS X F	29.2±0.6	090.0±10.8	12.2±0.4	2,326.2±094.3	283.8±08.3	84.1±18.2	6.3
RS X RD	28.3±1.2	071.0±10.3	11.7±0.3	2,213.8±115.5	267.0±09.4	85.0±17.0	6.2
RS X J	29.0±0.9	109.6±09.9	13.6±0.5	1,501.7±082.3	305.8±07.2	98.4±12.8	3.7
R X J	31.3±1.2	104.0±11.2	12.6±0.5	2,801.6±096.4	321.0±08.4	60.0±11.9	7.4
T X F	33.6±0.6	119.8±12.4	13.2±0.4	2,600.0±049.5	311.1±17.8	96.2±17.7	6.6
S X F	33.6±0.8	133.6±11.5	13.7±0.4	2,356.8±020.0	294.6±05.1	121.8±12.4	5.7
S X J	32.6±0.6	120.0±15.4	13.3±0.6	2,659.7±029.0	314.0±16.8	92.0±06.3	6.7
J X BS	34.5±5.1	147.2±77.3	14.4±2.9	2,188.0±607.0	292.0±12.9	141.3±18.8	5.0
L X J	31.0±3.5	218.2±17.9	17.7±0.8	1,151.0±045.0	328.6±04.0	109.3±23.2	3.7

H–Hariana, S–Sahiwal, RS–Red Sindhi, G–Gir, T–Tharparkar, L–Non descript, R–Rathi, F–Friesian, BS–Brown Swiss, RD–Red Dane, J–Jersey.
Source : Animal Genetic Resources in India, NDRI, 1981, pp 28, 30.

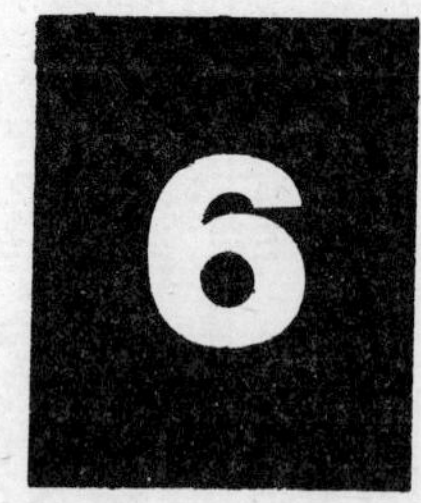

MECHANISMS OF HEREDITY

STRUCTURE OF THE CELLS

Discovery of living cells would have been difficult, if not impossible, before the compound microscope was invented by Zacharias Jansen of Holland in 1590. Robert Hooke of England applied the term 'Cell' to the cavities he saw in sections of cork. Ten years later, Marcello Malpighi published *Anatomy of plants*, the first systemic study of cell structure.

In 1839 Theodor Schwann an animal anatomist, formulated the cell theory which set forth the concept that "the elementary parts of all tissues are formed of cells though very diversified in manner."

In Animal Biology, the term cells refer more specially to the individual units of living structures. Most cells range in diameter from about 10 to 100 micra with cells that are multiplying, ranging about 20-30 micra in diameter. Sizes of cells vary considerably from one type of cell to another. With the exception of yolks of bird's egg (which are considered to be single cell), the distance from the interior of the cell to some portion of the cell membrane (surface of the cell) is seldom over 50 micra.

Diverse kinds of cells serve the specialised functions of the various tissues. The smallest body cells are found in the blood stream, while the largest (longest) are the nerve cells. Shape and size may depend on the function of the cells served. For example, muscle cells must be long if they are to shorten; nerve cells must be long to reach from the brain or spinal cord to organs in outlying areas, red blood cells have a flattened shape to permit rapid passage of gases (O_2, CO_2) through their membranes. Certain features are, however, common to all cells. All possess a cell membrane, a nucleus and cytoplasm containing number of cellular organelles and soluble proteins essential to the biochemical and physiologic functions of that cell. These common points have given rise to the concept to the typical cell. The typical cell, like the so-called average man, is an image arrived at by extrapolation, which does not actually exist in animal body. It is a convenient means of demonstrating a cell structure in general. In multicellular organisms the cells are differentiated to carry out specific functions, such as secretion, absorption, maintaining structure and conveying impulses.

Plasma Membrane

The entire cell is surrounded by a plasma membrane which is between 75 and 100 Å in width. The membrane is made up of a double layer of lipid molecules oriented parallel to each other and a layer of protein is absorbed on both surfaces of the membrane. The bi-layer

---

μ = micron or 1/1000 mm (millimetre); about 1/25,00 inch
mμ = millimicron or 1/1000 micron; about 1/25,000,000 inch.
Å = angstrom or 1/10 mm.

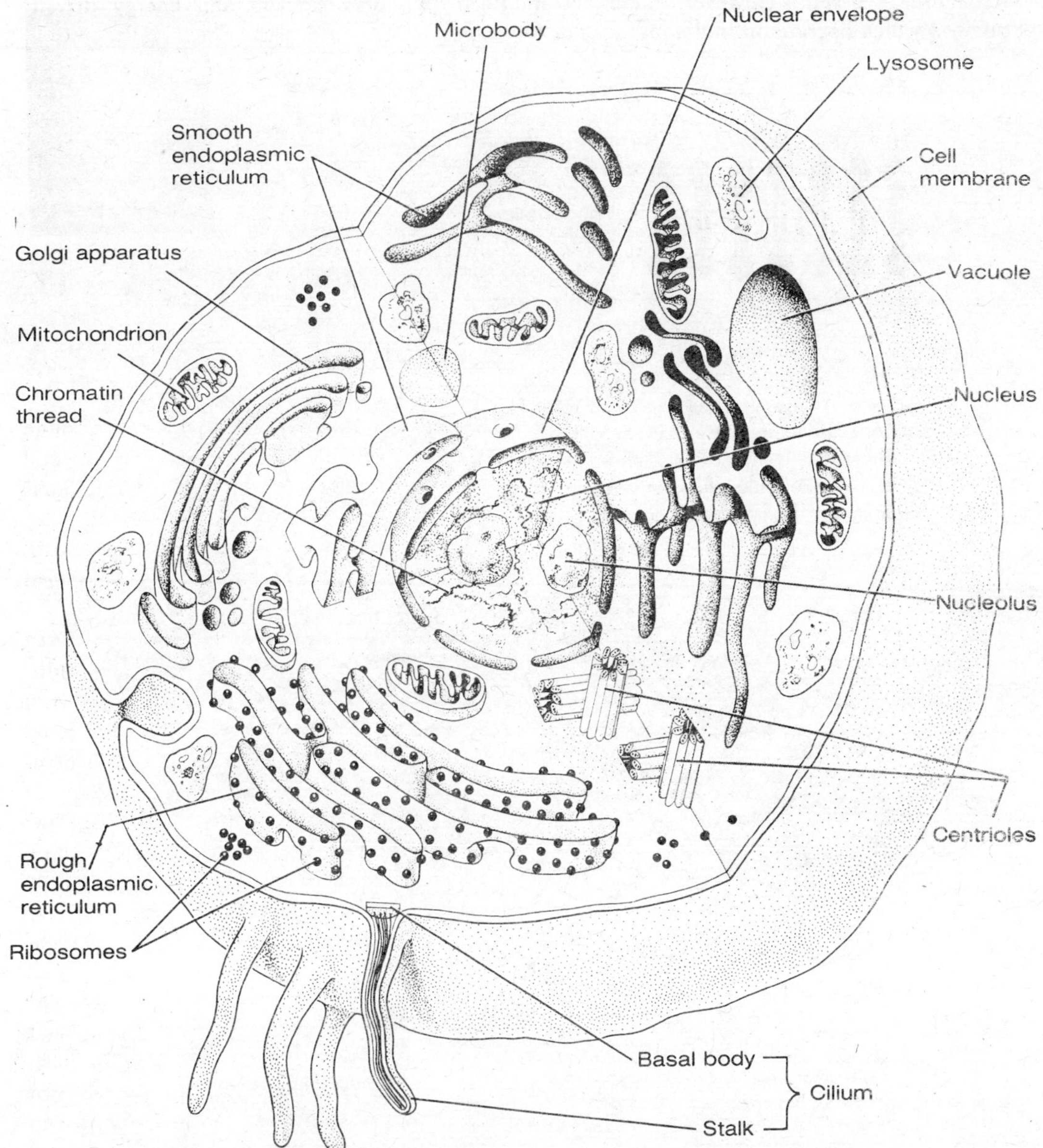

Fig. 6.1 Diagram of a typical cell based on what is seen in electron micrographs.

of lipids has non-polar carbon chains at the centre of the membrane with the polar ends pointing outwards. This entire membrane is referred to as a unit membrane. The plasma membrane also has a number of pores, leading to the interior, which are lined with protein molecules. The endoplasmic reticulum and the Golgi apparatus of the cytoplasm are continuous with the pores of the plasma membrane. The cell membrane itself produces an almost impermeable barrier between the aqueous portion of the cytoplasm and the aqueous solution surrounding the cell. However, these are modified by pores carriers and energy driven "pumps" which operate on individual ions or molecules.

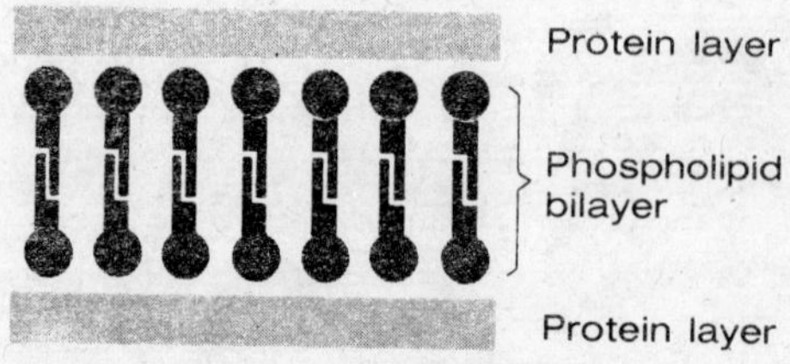

Fig 6.2 A theory of cell membrane structure that was widely accepted for many years maintained that the cell membrane is composed of a phospholipid layer two molecules thick, covered at each surface by a layer of protein.

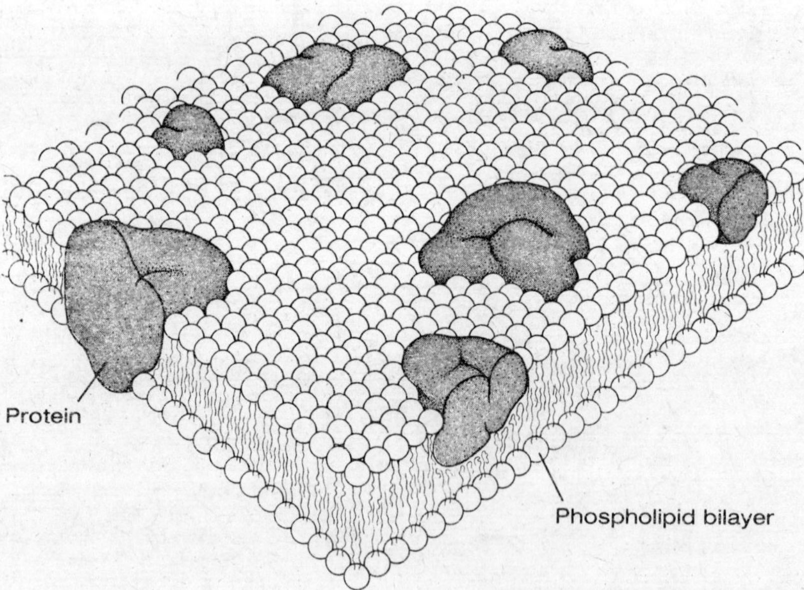

Fig 6.3 A current theory of cell membrane structure proposes that the cell membrane consists of a "sea" of phospholipid two molecules thick in which "islands" of proteins are distributed.

Functions of Cellular Organelles

Cell Organelle	*Functions*
Cell or plasma membrane	Differentially permeable memberane through which extra-cellular substances may be selectively sampled and cell products may be liberated.
Cell wall (plants only)	Thick cellulose wall surrounding the cell membrane giving strength and rigidity to the cell.
Nucleus :	Regulates growth and reproduction of the cell.
Chromosomes	Bearers of hereditary instructions; regulation of cellular processes (seen clearly only during nuclear division).
Nucleolus	Synthesizes ribosomal RNA; disappears during cellular replication.
Nucleoplasm (nuclear sap)	Contains materials for building DNA and messenger molecules which act as intermediates between nucleus and cytoplasm.
Nuclear membrane	Provides selective continuity between nuclear and cytoplasmic materials.
Cytoplasm :	Contains machinery for carrying out the instructions sent from the nucleus.
Endoplasmic reticulum	Greatly expanded surface area for biochemical reactions which normally occur at or across membrane surfaces.
Ribosomes	Sites of protein synthesis (shown as black dots lining the endoplasmic reticulum in Fig. 6.1).
Centrioles	Form poles for the divisional process; capable of replication; usually not seen in plant cells.
Mitochondria	Energy production (Kreb's cycle, electron transport chain, beta oxidation of fatty acids, etc.)
Plastids (plants only)	Structures for storage of starch, pigments, and other cellular products. Photosynthesis occurs in chloroplasts.
Golgi body or apparatus	Production of cellular secretions; sometimes called dictyosomes in plants.
Lysosome (animals only)	Production of intracellular digestive enzymes which aid in disposal of bacteria and other foreign bodies; may cause cell destruction if ruptured.
Vacuoles	Storage depots for excess water, waste products, soluble pigments, etc.
Hyaloplasm	Contains enzymes for glycolysis and structural materials such as sugars, amino acids, water, vitamins, nucleotides, etc. (nutrient soup or cell sap).

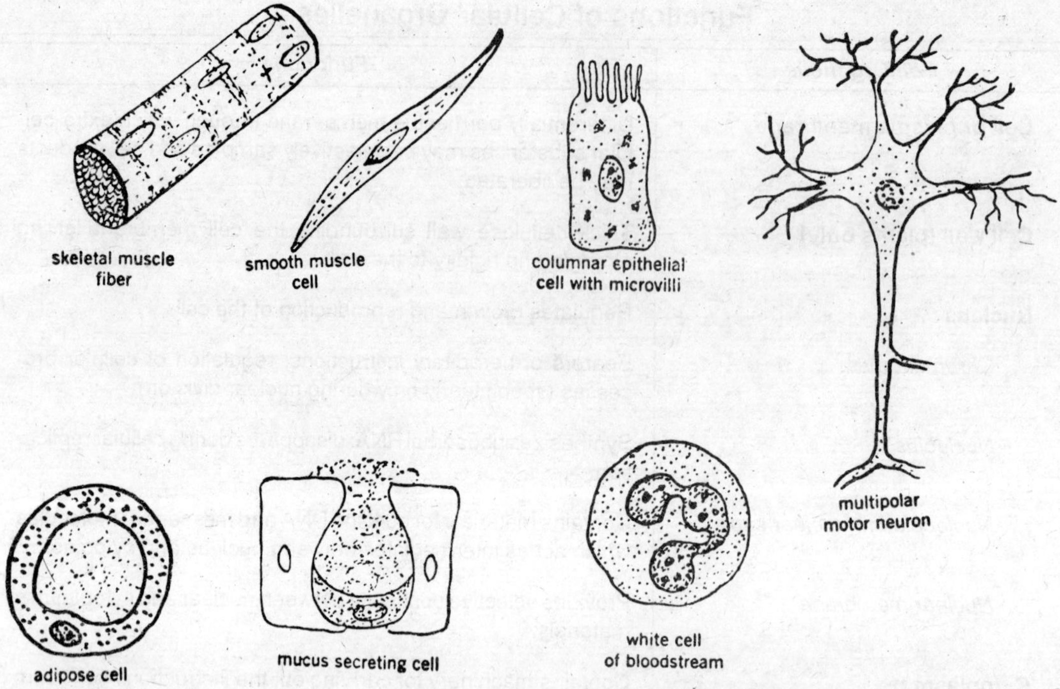

Fig.6.4. Types of common animal cells.

Nucleus

The nucleus is a roughly spherical body in the cell with a diameter between 5-7 micra. In most tissues, one nucleus is found in each cell. The nucleus is surrounded by a double membrane, the outer membrane being continuous with the endoplasmic reticulum. The nucleus is connected with the cytoplasm by a system of pores in the double layered membrane. It has been estimated that the nuclear membrane has pores ranging in diameter from 400 to 800Å and that these pores cover approximately 10 per cent of its surface area. These pores are large enough to permit the passage of protein molecules.

The nucleus contains the genetic material, which is made up of chromatin material. This is primarily deoxyribonucleic acid (DNA) that is complexed with a basic protein, a histone. The combination of these two form nucleo-histones. The DNA molecule, which has a molecular weight in the millions, contains a combination of four bases, a pentose sugar-deoxyribose, and a phosphate group. The four bases are composed of two purines, adenine and guanine; and two pyrimidines, cytosine and thymine. Each base is attached to the one carbon position of deoxyribose. The pentose sugars are joined in a strand by a phosphodiester bond between the 3 and 5 carbon of the adjacent pentose sugars. The genetic information is coded by the sequence based on the polynucleotide. The DNA is composed of two strands that curl around each other to form a double helix. The strands are joined together by hydrogen bonding between the pairs of bases. Adenine is always bonded to thymine and guanine is always bonded to cytosine. Prior to mitosis the chromatin material congregates, into the chromosomes the number being specific species.

The DNA is responsible for the activity of the cytoplasm and accomplishes this by the

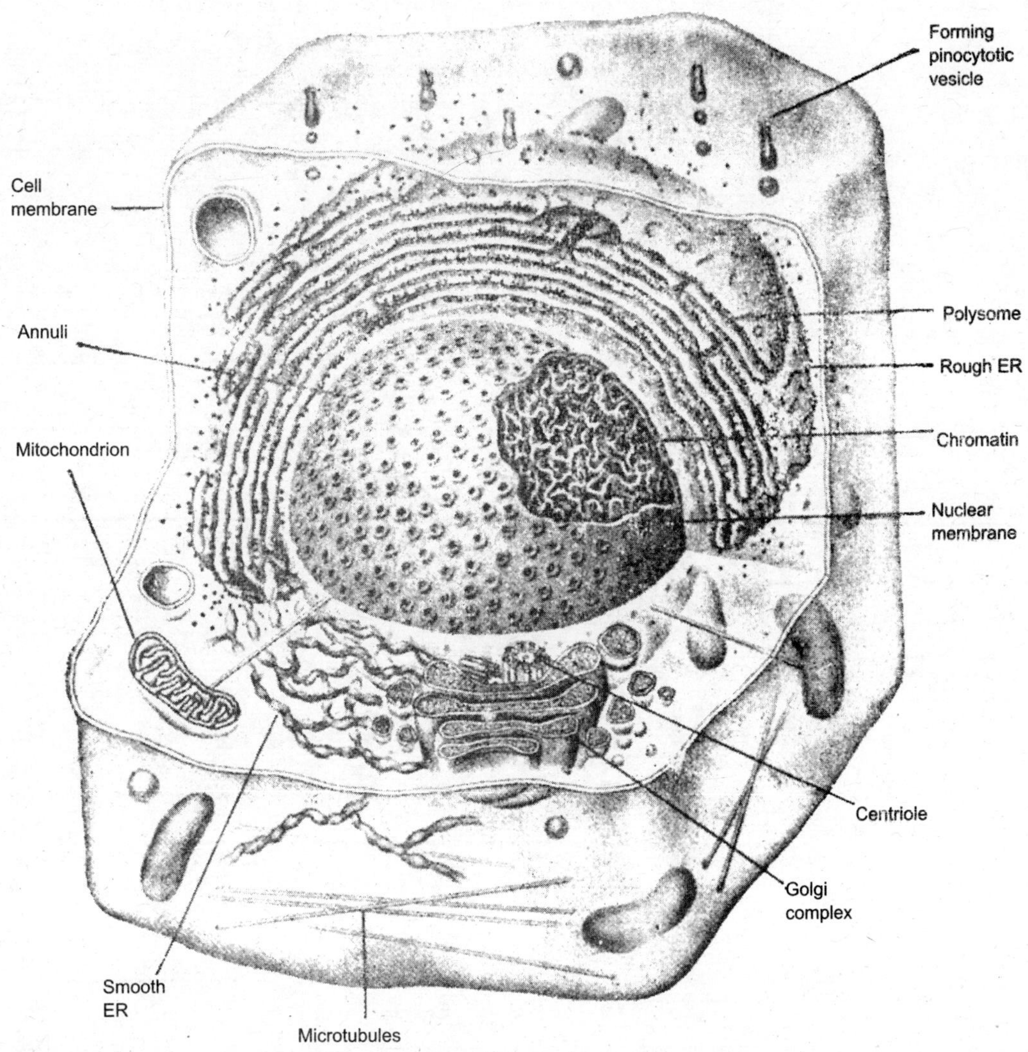

Plate 4. Animal cell showing internal features (Chapter 6).

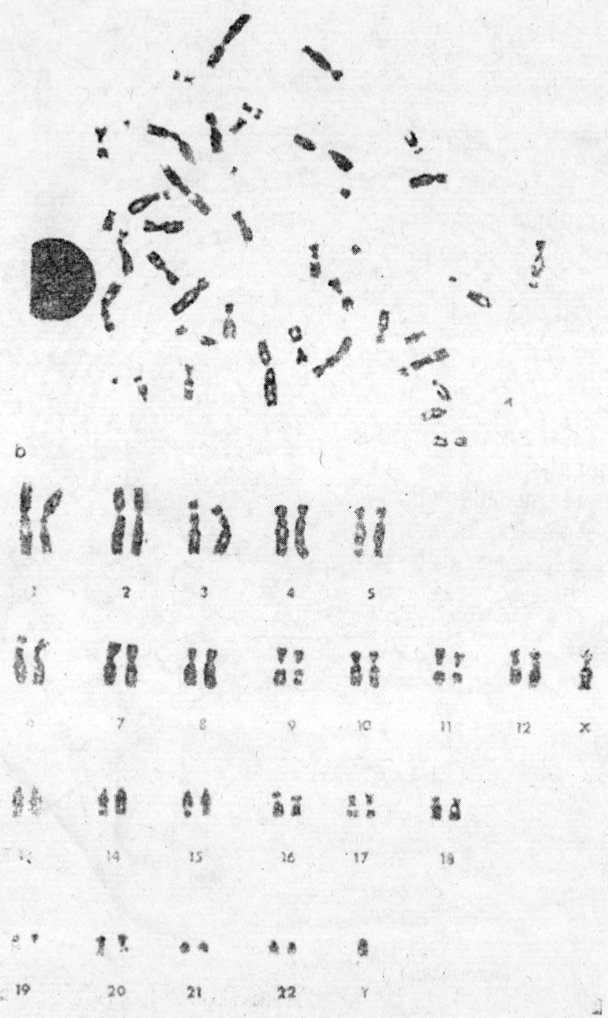

Plate 5. Human chromosomes (male cell from a culture of peripheral blood) (Chapter 7).

synthesis of ribonucleic acid (RNA). RNA is comparable to DNA, except the pyrimidine, uracil replaces the thymine of DNA and the pentose ribose replaces deoxyribose. Moreover, RNA is a single strand unit.

Three types of RNA are present in the cell. Messenger RNA (m-RNA) carries the coded information from the DNA to the ribosomes on the endoplasmic reticulum and these serve as a template for the synthesis of proteins and enzymes from amino acids. This is controlled by the particular base sequence in the m-RNA. A triplet of bases on m-RNA serves as the code for the placement of amino acid, i.e., a triplet of adenine-adenine is the code for lysine (an amino acid). The sequence of basis in m-RNA is determined by a portion of the DNA strand in which the base of the m-RNA being synthesised lies opposite the bases of DNA similar to the arrangement in the double stranded DNA. The exception being that uracil lines up opposite adenine. The second RNA is the ribosomal RNA, which becomes part of the ribosomes lining the endoplasmic reticulum. The third RNA is the transfer RNA or soluble RNA (s-RNA) recognises specific amino acids in the cytoplasm, activates them, and carries them to specific site on the m-RNA. The recognition of the amino acid and the site on the m-RNA is determined by a specific triple of bases on each s-RNA. There is at least one specific s-RNA for each amino acid. The triplet of bases on the s-RNA pairs with the triplet on the m-RNA, and in this way the m-RNA determines the sequence of amino acids in a protein.

It is generally believed that the amount of DNA per cell is constant for species. DNA can be demonstrated in the nucleus by the Feulgen strain and other basic stains. The nucleus contains one or more nucleoli, which shows dense granular textures. The nucleoli do not have a membrane separating them from the nucleus but are intermeshed with the chromosomal DNA. These nucleoli appear to be primary sites for protein and ribosomal RNA synthesis.

The nucleus contains 8 to 20 per cent of the RNA in the cell. The nucleus is capable of performing all of the metabolic reactions of the cytoplasm but at a much lower level of activity. The principal function of the nucleus is to serve as the site for the regulation and transmission at hereditary characteristics.

Endoplasmic Reticulum

The endoplasmic reticulum (ER) is series of membrane-bounded tubules, vesicles and cisternae that extend from the nuclear membrane outward to the plasma membrane. They pack the basal portion of the cell as well as the sides of the nucleus. Most of the tubules are rough surfaced and have dense particles attached on the outer surface of the membrane. The dense particles are ribosomes and take up basophilic dyes because of their high RNA content. Ribosomes that are not attached to the endoplasmic reticulum are found throughout the cytoplasm. The ribosomes are the major site of protein formation within the cell. The protein molecules to be exported from the cell are transferred to the interior of the membrane and apparently travel to the Golgi apparatus before being excreted. Prior to the advent of electromicroscopy it was thought that the cytoplasm was a homogeneous mass of material. It now appears as if the entire cytoplasm consists of a series of membranes and much of the secretion process and functional work of the cell is done by the passage of micromolecules through membranes. This is particularly true of the large amount of ER, which divides the cytoplasm into compartments.

The ribosomes not attached to the ER are probably sites where proteins are synthesised for use in the cell. Vacuoles as part of the ER or Golgi apparatus are located throughout the cell may be reservoirs for essential secretory materials or waste products of the cells. The ER allows the cell to maintain efficient contact with its environment.

Ribosomes from animals consist of approximately equal amounts of RNA and protein. The ribosome is composed of two sub units and has an approximate size of 230 Å.

Golgi Apparatus

The Golgi apparatus is a series of smooth lined membrane tubules and cavities that are continuations of the lipoprotein membranes of the ER. The Golgi apparatus appears to play no direct part in protein synthesis but is involved in exporting protein synthesised by the ribosomes. It is the first area in the cell in which electron micrographs can identify protein particles. It has been suggested that the Golgi may function as a condensation membrane to concentrate smaller proteins into larger drops or granules that can be observed with the electron microscope. It may also function by removing water from the maturing secretions. It has been shown that the zymogen granules of the pancreatic cells take on an identifiable form in the Golgi apparatus by a progressive concentration of secretory products, which then move to centrally located condensing vacuoles. From here they move away from the Golgi zone and accumulate in the apical region of the cell and wait to be released into the lumen after the intake of food. The membrane of the Golgi vacuole becomes the limiting membrane of the zymogen granule. The zymogen granule is released into the lumen without a rupture of the cell membrane. The Golgi apparatus plays a role in the export of steroids and protein in the rat liver, since lipoprotein molecules are apparently exported through the Golgi apparatus.

Mitochondria

Located throughout the cytoplasm are fried rice shaped objects measuring about 15,000 Å in length and 5,000 Å in diameter. These mitochondria have a two layered wrapping with the inner membrane projecting into the interior by a number of sacs or protrusions called cristae. The cristae are transverse to the long axis of the cell. The surface of both the outer and inner membranes and cristae are sprinkled with small particles that carry out the chemical activities of mitochondria. The inner membranes contain the enzymes of the citric acid cycle metabolites.

The mitochondria are considered the power house of the cell in that they supply over 90 per cent of the energy requirements. The mitochondria, regardless of the cell species or type, have the same basic structure and apparent function. Their size and the shape vary with the isolation procedure and whether the cells are viewed and the shape vary with the isolation procedure and whether the cells are viewed *in situ*. It has been calculated that mitochondria make up for 18 per cent of the total volume and 22 per cent of the total cytoplasmic volume of the rat liver cell.

The mitochondria supply energy to the cell by the oxidation of substrates and the conversion of released energy in the form of bond energy of ATP. This involves three steps: (i) carrying out oxidation reaction that supply electrons, (ii) transferring the electrons along a chain of intermediates that synthesise ATP and (iii) catalysing synthetic reactions that are powered by ATP. These processes appear to be located on both the inner and the outer membranes of the cells. Mitochondria can actively accumulate certain ions from the surrounding cytoplasm to a process that appears to be related to the respiratory chain phosphorylation.

It has been questioned for a period of time whether the mitochondria are self-reproducing or whether they arise from other organelles. Recent evidence indicated that mitochondria contain DNA that can be used as template to synthesise messenger RNA or protein formation. It also appears that mitochondria arise from *de novo* synthesis within the cell. Mitochondria also oxidise and actively synthesise fatty acids.

Lysosomes

Another particle scattered throughout the cell is the lysosome. Lysosomes are slightly smaller than mitochondria and contain most of the active degradative or hydrolytic enzymes of the cell. The lysosomes have a dense matrix with vacuoles or droplets in them. They have a very dense

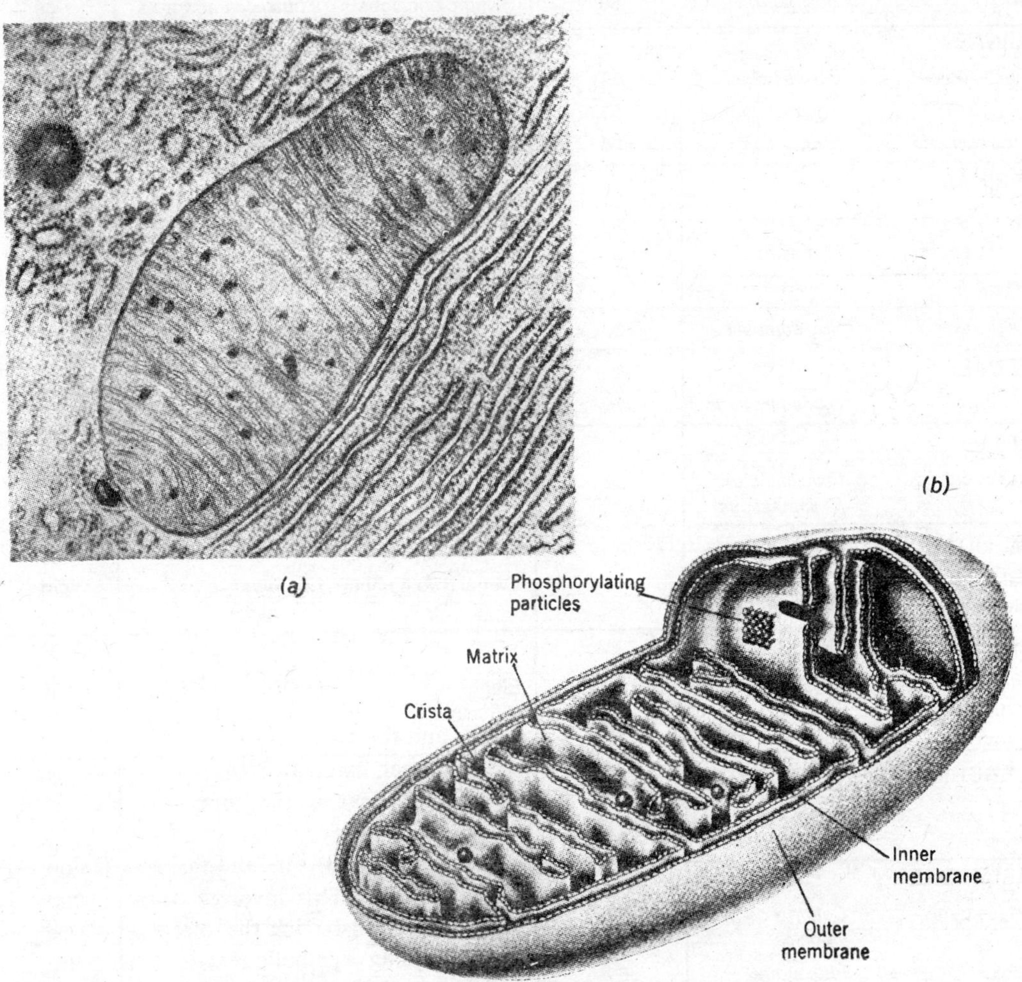

Fig.6.5. A mitochondrion. (a) Electron micrograph (x53,000) of a mitochondrion. (b) Perspective showing the interior of a motochondrion.

Table 6.1 Chromosome numbers (2N) of Common domestic Animals

Family and Common Name	Scientific name	Chromosome Numbers (2N)	Common name	Scientific name	Chromosome Numbers (2N)
BOVIDAE					
Domestic cattle (Zebu) with hump	*Bos Indicus*	60	Yak	Bos grunniens	60
Domestic cattle (Europian) Humpless	*Bos taurus*	60	Nil gai	*Boselaphus tragocamelus*	46
Europian bison	*Bison bonasus*	60	Cattalo	--	60
American bison	*Bison bison*	60	Water or River buffaloes	*Bubalis bubalis*	50
Gaur	*Bos gaurus*	58	Swamp buffaloes	*Bubalis carabanesis*	48
EQUINAE					
Domestic horse	*Equus caballus*	64	African Zebra	*Equus burchelli*	44
Ass (Donkey)	*Equus asinus*	62	Mule	--	63
Tibetan wild ass	*Equus kiang*	56	Zebroid	--	55
CAPRINAE					
Domestic goat	*Capra hircus*	60	Barbary sheep	*Ammotragus lorvia*	58
Domestic sheep	*Ovis aries*	54			
SUIDAE					
Domestic swine	*Sus domesticus*	60			
CANIDAE					
Dog	*Canis familiaris*	78			
FELIDAE					
Domestic cat	*Felis catus or F. domesticus*	38			
CAMELIDAE					
Camel (single hump)	*Camelus dromedarius*	74	Camel (two humps)	*Camelus bactrianus*	74
ELEPHANTIDAE					
Elephant (Indian)	*Elephas maximus* or *Elephas indicus*	56	Elephant (African)	*Loxodonta africana*	56
MELEAGRIDIDAE					
Turkey	*Meleagris gallopavo*	80			
PHASIANIDAE					
Japanese quail	*Coturnix coturnix japonica*	78	Fowl	*Gallus domesticus*	78
Pheasant	*Phasianus colchicus*	80	Pea fowl	*Pavo cristatus*	80
ANATIDAE					
Goose	*Anser anser*	80	Duck	*Anas platyrhynchos*	80
Muscovy duck	*Cairina moschata*	80			

peripheral rim with a less dense core. The lysosomal membrane usually remains intact, but it is extremely sensitive to rupture under a variety of physiological conditions. Its rupture causes the release of the enzymes, which can cause a breakdown of the cell. The lysosomes may also be engaged in intracellular digestive processes in which material is taken into the cell, broken down after the release of the hydrolytic enzymes, and the breakdown products excreted. Lysosomes may also function as scavangers for removing unneeded or foreign material from the cell. The particular function of the lysosomes in a cell may vary with the type of cell.

In higher organisms the gametes have only half as many chromosomes as the somatic cells. Only one member of a chromosome pair enters into each gamete by the process of reduction division or meiosis. In cattle, for example, the somatic or zygotic number is 60 and the gametic number is 30; in horse the number is 64 and 32, respectively. The somatic, zygotic or diploid number (characteristics of body cells of the species) is $2n$; the gametic or haploid number is designated by n. The set of chromosomes in a nucleus is referred to as the chromosome complement.

CELL DIVISION

A cell never appears spontaneously but always originates from some pre-existing living cell by division. In higher organisms the cell divisions are of two types: (1) mitosis and (2) meiosis. Mitosis is the usual division of somatic cells and in this two daughter nuclei are formed whose chromosome number is the same as that of the original parent nucleus. Meiosis is a reductional division and the daughter nuclei produced by this division have half as many chromosomes as in the parent nucleus. Meiosis takes place in the gonads and precedes gametogenesis.

Mitosis

For purposes of study, the mitotic cell division is divided into six stages: (a) interphase, (b) prophase, (c) prometaphase, (d) metaphase, (e) anaphase and (f) telophase. These stages are readily discernible by some landmarks but the whole process of cell division is continuous and one stage passes imperceptibly into the next. The process of cell division may be broadly divided into karyokinesis or nuclear division and cytokinesis or cytoplasmic division. Karyokinesis precedes cytokinesis.

(*a*) *Interphase*. Interphase or resting stage is characterised by the large nucleus, with intact nuclear membrane, prominent nucleolus or nucleoli and the chromosomes in the form of reticulate mass. The term resting stage in the chromosomes is a form of misnomer because the nucleus in this phase is metabolically most active. During this stage each chromosome builds up a copy of itself out of the materials in the protoplasm and thereby duplicates itself. Each chromosome has two chromatids at the end of this stage.

(*b*) *Prophase*. At this stage, chromosomes become visible in the nucleus. They gradually become shortened and thickened due to dehydration and despiralisation. The centrosome divides into two parts, each containing a centriole. The daughter centrosome move to the two opposite ends of the nuclear membrane and act as poles. The nucleoli gradually decrease in volume.

(*c*) *Prometaphase*. During this stage the nuclear membrane dissolves and the spindle mechanism is formed. The spindle mechanism consists of astral rays originating from the centrosomes, the gelatinous spindle and the traction fibres connecting the centromeres of various

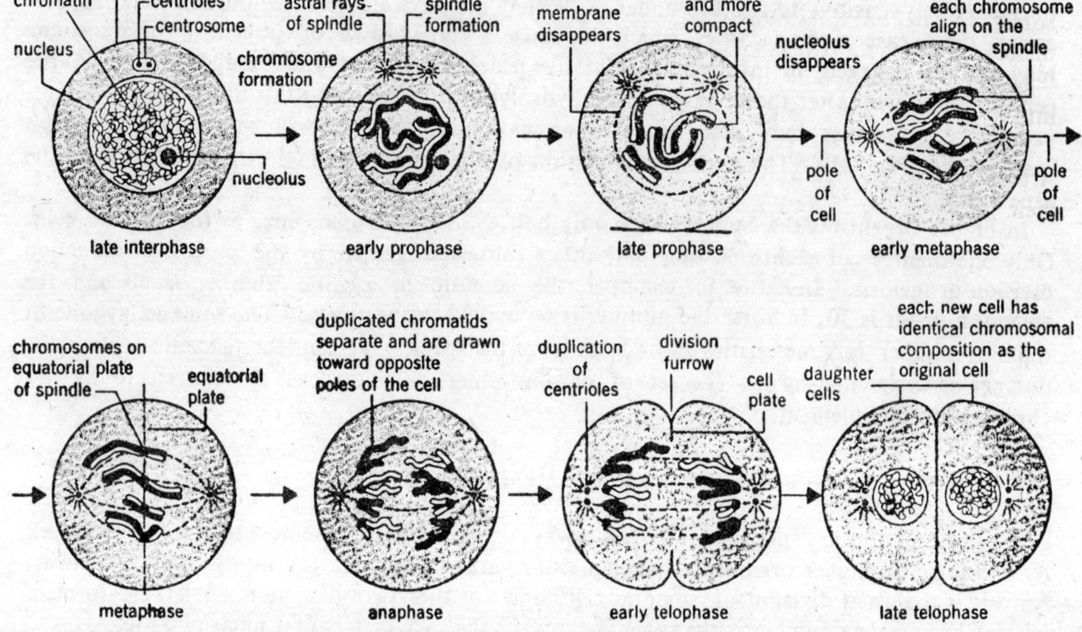

Fig. 6.6 Diagram of mitosis in the somatic cell of an animal.

chromosomes to either centrosome. The nucleolus disappears at this stage.

(*d*) *Metaphase.* At metaphase the chromosomes, which are now very short and thick, orient themselves in the equatorial region of the spindle. Each chromosome has two chromatids which are to be separated but are held together by a functionally single centromere.

(*e*) *Anaphase.* The centromere of each chromosome divides into two at anaphase, and the two sister chromatids are converted into two independent chromosomes which move to opposite poles. Certain chemicals, e.g., colchicine, prevent anaphase movement by poisoning the spindle and thereby double the chromosome number.

(*f*) *Telophase.* The spindle disappears and two daughter nuclei are reconstituted from the two groups of anaphase chromosomes moving to the poles. The chromosomes uncoil in the telophase nucleus. The nucleus membrane and the nucleolus reappear.

Cytokinesis takes place after the nuclear cell division. A cleavage furrow appears as an indentation of the outer membrane at the position of the equatorial plate. This indentation gradually moves inward and divides the cytoplasm into two halves.

Significance of mitosis. It mitosis, each chromosome is longitudinally duplicated and the two halves are distributed into two daughter nuclei. Due to this process each daughter nucleus gets qualitatively and quantitatively the same genetic constitution as the original nucleus. These help to maintain the constancy of species.

Meiosis

In animal the doubling of gametic (haploid) chromosome number which results from fertilisation is compensated for by a having of the resulting zygotic (diploid) chromosome number at some other stage of the life cycle. Such reduction is brought about by a single chromosomal replication followed by two successive nuclear divisions. The process is known as meiosis or reduction division and occurs during the gametogenesis of animals.

Meiosis is divided into division I and division II. In division I, the prophase is subdivided into five consecutive stages: leptonema, zygonema, pachynema, diplonema and diakinesis.

Leptonema. During this stage the chromosomes are highly stretched and bead like structures, chromomeres are often visible. The chromosomes may remain attached with one of their ends by a portion of nuclear membrane, forming the so-called bouquet configuration.

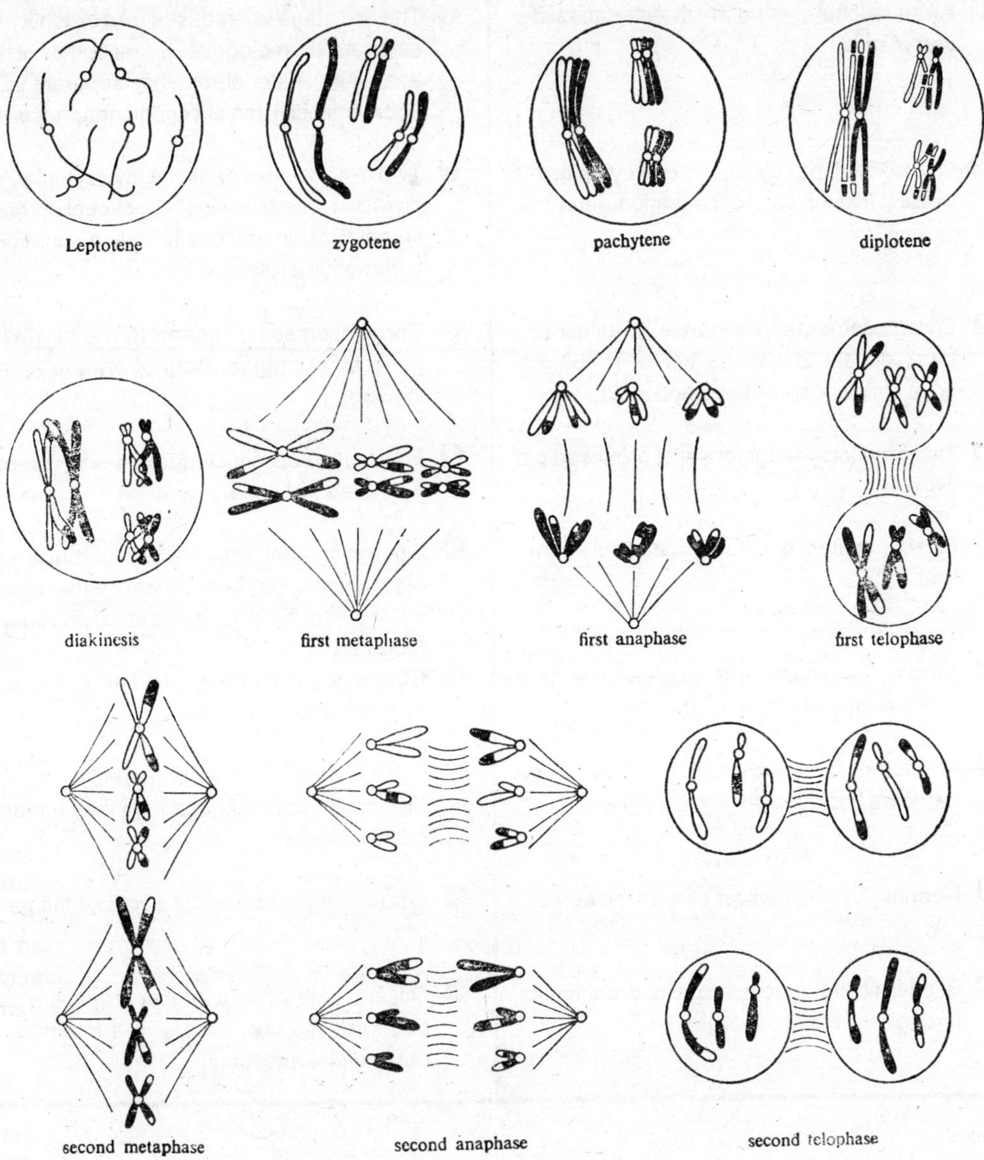

Fig. 6.7 Stages in heterotypic division of meiosis.

Table 6.2

Differential Characteristics between MITOSIS and MEIOSIS

Mitosis	*Meiosis*
❶ An equational division which separates sister chromatids.	❶ The first stage is a reductional division which separates homologous chromosomes at first anaphase; sister chromatids separate in an equational division at second anaphase.
❷ One division per cycle, i.e. one cytoplasmic division (cytokinesis) per equational chromosomal division.	❷ Two divisions per cycle, i.e. two cytoplasmic divisions, one following reductional chromosomal division and one following equational chromosomal division.
❸ Chromosomes fail to synapse; no chiasmata form, genetic exchange between homologous chromosomes does not occur.	❸ Chromosomes synapse and form chiasmata; genetic exchange occurs between homologues.
❹ Two products (daughter cells) produced per cycle.	❹ Four cellular products (gametes or spores) produced per cycle.
❺ Genetic content of mitotic products are identical.	❺ Genetic content of meiotic products different; centromeres may be replicas of either maternal or paternal centromeres in varying combinations.
❻ Chromosome number of daughter cells is the same as that of mother cell.	❻ Chromosome number of meiotic products is half that of the mother cell.
❼ Mitotic products are usually capable of undergoing additional mitotic divisions.	❼ Meiotic products cannot undergo another meiotic division although they may undergo mitotic division.
❽ Normally occurs in most all somatic cells.	❽ Occurs only in specialized cells of the germ line.
❾ Begins at the zygote stage and continues through the life of the organism.	❾ Occurs only after a higher organism has begun to mature; occurs in the zygote of many algae and fungi.

Zygonema. The chromosomes in somatic cells usually occur in pairs. Two chromosomes, one from the paternal and another from the maternal parent form a pair and they are homologous with each other. During zygotene phase, pairing or synapsis of homologous chromosomes takes place. The pairing starts at one or more points and progresses in a 'zipperlike' fashion till completion. When pairing is completed, the apparent number of chromosomes become half of that of the original cell but each visible body within the nucleus is a bivalent rather than a single chromosome.

Pachynema. This is the stable stage of pairing. The bivalents become thicker in appearance. The nucleolus is prominent of this stage and remains attached to a particular chromosome. At later stages of pachynema each chromosome of a bivalent divides longitudinally into two chromatids. Exchanges between homologous but not sister chromatids may take place by the end of this stage. This phenomenon is called crossing over and it leads to genetic recombination.

Diplonema. During this stage the homologous chromosomes (which have divided into chromatids) of a bivalent start separating. The separation is not complete because the chromatids are held together at certain points, marked as chiasmata. The longer chromosomes have more chiasmata. At each point of contact only two chromatids, one from each homologue, are found to cross over. The chiasmata move towards the end of the bivalent and this process is called terminalisation. The positions of chiasmata at this stage do not indicate the exact places of cross over because the chiasmata shift from their place of origin.

Diakinesis. The bivalents become shorter and thicker during this stage. Apart from these two characteristics of the bivalents, diakinesis is often indistinguishable from diplonema. During diakinesis the terminalisation is completed, the nucleolus often disappears and the bivalents lie well spaced out in the nucleolus often adjacent to the nuclear membrane.

Metaphase I. The nuclear membrane disappears and the bivalents are arranged at the equator. The spindle mechanism originates as in mitosis. Each bivalent has two undivided centromeres which are on the longitudinal axis of the spindle whereas in mitotic metaphase each chromosome has one undivided centromere lying on the equatorial plate.

Anaphase I. The two homologous chromosomes constituting a bivalent separate and move to the two opposite poles. Hence the separation is reductional. Due to this separation a number of chromosomes move towards each pole, while the original somatic number was $2n$.

Telophase I. The separated chromosomes reconstitute two daughter nuclei. Each daughter nucleus has only n number of chromosomes. Very often Telophase I and next interphase are not observed in rapidly dividing gonads and the daughter nuclei start the Division II.

Division II. This division is equational like usual mitotic division. The centromere of each chromosome divides into two and the two sister chromatids separate. Finally four haploid nuclei are produced.

Meiosis makes possible of (a) the interchange of material between homologous chromosomes and (b) the distribution of one member of each chromosome pair to each gamete.

Common Genetical Key Terms

Allele One of the two or more alternative forms of a gene. Alleles are those genes which may appear at the same locus in homologus chromosome.

Autosomes The chromosomes present in the same number in both sexes of any species.

Chromatid The parts of the chromosome after it has split down its length in cell division.

Chromatin Collection of DNA-protein fibers which during prophase, condense to form the chromosomes.

Chromomere is a densely staining granule visible as an apparent component of the chromosome during early meiosis

Chromonema The coiled core of a chromatid, thought to contain the genes.

Chromosome Dark-staining rod like or rounded bodies visible under the microscope in the nucleus of the cell during metaphase stage of cell division. These are compact bundle of deoxyribonucleic acid molecules, portion of which represents gene. Chromosomes occur in pairs in body cells, and the number is constant for a species. Chromosomes are made of protein and nucleic acids.

Crossing over Exchange of parts by homologous chromosomes during synapsis of meiosis prior to the formation of sex cells or gametes. Thus the homologous chromosomes exchange genes.

Deletion Loss of a portion of a chromosome following breakage of DNA.

Dihybrid cross A cross involving two pairs of alleles, each of which regulates different characteristics.

Diploid Containing a double set of chromosomes. This is the normal chromosome complement for all somatic cells of most animals. Often written 2n.

Dominant Condition where one allele masks the effect of other (recessive) allele for the same trait. A gene is said to be dominant when its characteristic effect is expressed in the heterozygote as well as the homozygote i.e., Aa and AA genotypes are indistinguishable.

Epistasis Modification of normal gene expression in which a particular gene at one locus masks the expression of at least one other gene at a different chromosmal location.

F_1 First generation progeny from crossing inbred lines.

F_2 Second generation progeny produced by randomly mating F_1 progeny.

Filial The Latin word meaning "progeny". Used in genetics to represent the generation or progeny resulting from intermating succeeding generations originating from the cross of two inbred lines. Filial is generally denoted by F with the subscript 1 to denote the generation after crossing.

Gene A portion of a DNA molecule (occupy a specific locus on the chromosome) through which inheritable characteristics are transmitted to succeeding generations in all living organisms. They provide information for the synthesis of various enzymes and each and every type of proteinous compounds of the body. Genes are basic units of inheritance. There are at least two alleles for a gene, one of which may be dominant over the expression of the recessive allele.

Genetics The branch of biology concerned with the physical basis of the transmission of inherited characters, i.e. about the heredity and variation of organisms.

Genetic recombination The reshuffling of gene combinations caused by breakage of DNA and its reunion at a different chromosomal point.

Genotype An individual's genetic make up (composition).

Heredity The passage of genetic traits to offspring which consequently are similar or identical to the parent(s).

Hereditary The transmission of qualities from parent to offspring by processes which occur first in the nuclei of germ cells. The words genetic and hereditary are often used interchangeably.

Heretability The strength of inheritance of the trait. Denoted by h^2. A technical term used to describe what fraction of the differences in a trait is due to differences in genetic value rather than environmental factors.

Heterosis The increased level of performance as compared to the average of the parental types is known as hetirosis or hybrid vigour.

Heterozygous A term applied to organisms that posses two different alleles for a trait. Often, one allele (A) is dominant, masking the presence of the other (a), the recessive.

Homologous Members of a chromosome pair, which have a similar shape and the same sequence of genes along their length.

Homologous chromosome From the Greek **homo**, meaning "like", and "logus" meaning "proportion". Homologus refers to chromosomes that are structurally alike. Two chromosomes, one inherited from the sire and the other from the dam, which pair and synapse at meiosis, have the same morphology, and contain genes governing the same characteristics.

Homozygote An individual possessing like genes for a pair of allelomorphs, e.g., AA or aa. Having only one type of allele for a given trait.

Homozygous A term applied to an organism that has two identical alles for a particular trait.

Hybrid A heterozygote, or progeny of genetically unlike parents.

Incomplete dominance A phenomenon in which heterozygous individuals are phenotypically distinguishable from either homozygous type.

Inheritance The act of receiving something previously in another's possession as if by legacy.

Karyotype The chromosomes of a plant or animal as they appear at the metaphase of a somatic division.

Law of independent assortment Alleles on non-homologous chromosomes segregate independently of one another.

Law of segregation During gamete formation, pairs of alleles separate so that each sperm or egg cell has one gene for a trait.

Linkage The tendency of genes of the same chromosome to stay together rather than to assort independently. Genes that reside on the same chromosome constitute a **linkage group**.

Linkage mapping A technique used to construct genetic maps that show relative positions and distances of the genes on a chromosome.

Locus Point occupied by a gene on a chromosome i.e., relative position of a gene on a chromosome.

Monohybrid A monohybrid is an individual which is heterozygous for one pair of allelic genes.

Monohybrid cross A cross involving one pair of alleles, each of which controls an alternative form of the same characteristic.

Multiple allele Three or more possible alleles at the same locus on one pair of homologus chromosomes for a given trait, such as ABO blood groups in humans.

Mutagens Chemical or physical agents that induce genetic change.

Mutation Random heritable changes in DNA that introduce new alleles into the gene pool. Gene mutation occur within a gene (as opposed to chromosomal mutations). Substituting one nucleotide for another results in a **point mutations.**

Phenotype An individual's observable characteristics resulting from the expression of its genotype and its surrounding environment.

Pleiotropy Where a single mutant gene produces two or more phenotypic effects.

Polygenic inheritance An inheritance pattern in which a phenotype is determined by two or more genes at different loci. In humans, examples include height and pigmentation.

Polyploid An organism or cell containing a reduptication of a chromosome number, e.g. triploid, tetraploid etc., having three, four etc., times of the normal haploid or gametic number.

Recessive An allele whose expression is masked by the dominant allele for the same trait.

Recombination The rejoining of DNA pieces with those of a different strand or with the same strand at a point different from where the break occured.

Regulatory genes Genes whose sole function is to control the expression of structural gene.

Sex chromosome The one chromosmal pair that is not identical in the karyotypes of males and females of the same animal species.

Sex influenced dominance An inheritable trait that is expressed as a dominant in one gender and as a recessive in the other, as a result of sex hormone differences, e.g. baldness in humans.

Sex limited gene expression An inheritable trait that is expressed in only one sex, as a result of sex hormone differences, e.g., beards in men.

Sex limited traits Traits controlled by genes located on the X-chromosome.

Species Taxonomic subdivision of a genus. Each species has recognizable features that distinguish it from every other species. Members of one species generally will not interbreed with members of other species.

Synapsis The pairing of homologous chromosomes during prophase of meiosis I.

Variation The structural or functional difference between closely related individuals within a species.

X-chromosome The sex chromosome present in two doses in cells of a female, and in one dose in the cells of a male.

Y-chromosome The sex chromosome found in the cells of a male. When Y-carrying sperm unite with an egg, all of which carry a single X-chromosome, a male is produced.

Zygote A fertilized egg before first cleavage. The diploid cell that results from the union of a sperm and egg.

HEREDITY

The most striking attribute to living organisms is their ability to transmit hereditary characteristics from cell to cell and generation to generation. The existence of heredity must have been noticed by early man as he witnessed the passing of traits such as hair and eye colour from parents to their children. Man, however, did not begin to understand the physical basis of heredity until about the middle of the nineteenth century. Three levels of study have been integrated to give us our present knowledge of genetic mechanism:

1. The phenotypic level—genetic mechanisms have been implied from patterns of transmission of phenotypes from parent to progeny.
2. The cellular level—genetic mechanisms have been inferred from knowledge of the process of cell division.
3. The molecular level—the chemical reactions by which certain genes produce their effects have been elucidated.

Phenotypic Inheritance—The Laws of Mendel. Gregor Johann Mendel (1822-1884), an Austrian monk, has been called the "father of genetics" because he was the first to uncover and record the laws of inheritance. Mendel experimented with crosses among inbred lines of garden peas (*Pisum sativum*) during the years 1856-1864. The results, which Mendel published in 1866, set forth the rules of inheritance. However, the process of mitosis, meiosis and fertilisation had not yet been worked out and Mendel's experiments were forgotten until 1900 when three botanists, Correns (Germany), DeVries (Holland), and Tschermak (Austria) independently rediscovered his paper.

Mendel's methods of experimentation are classic in their adherence to scientific principles. He first carefully tested his inbred lines for purity, then studied one character at a time by crossing inbred lines. After learning the pattern of inheritance for several traits, Mendel studied two traits together. Replication was another feature of Mendel's experiments as he raised large numbers of plants in each generation. Large numbers were necessary because, although the progeny phenotypes, ultimately occurred in constant proportions, the results from small samples were (and are) quite variable because of the chance processes of gamete formation and fertilisation.

Laws of Segregation. Mendel had tall type (mature plant height 2 to 2.5 metres) and dwarf type of peas (mature plant height 0.25 to 0.5 metres) in his collection. He self-fertilised each of these types and found that both types bred true for six generations. He crossed tall with dwarf and observed that the hybrid progeny (F_1) were all tall. Upon self-fertilisation the F_1 tall plants produced an F_2 which contained 787 tall and 277 dwarf plants, i.e., the ratio tall: dwarf was in the proportion of 3:1. He self-fertilised the F_2 tall plants and found that one-third of them produced tall individuals while two-third produced tall and dwarf individuals in 3:1 ratio. The F_2 dwarf plants bred true.

The dwarf character was masked in the F_1 plants by the contrasting tall character. The concept of *dominance* and *recessiveness* was formulated from these observations. The masked characteristic (dwarf) is *recessive* and the masking characteristic is (tall) *dominant*. The dominant character is symbolised by capital letters (T) for tall and the recessive by the same letter but a small one (t) for dwarf. Hence the F_1 can be symbolised by Tt. Mendel assumed that a pair of hereditary units controlled the inheritance of a particular character and symbolised them with some letters of the alphabet. The dominant character is symbolised by capital

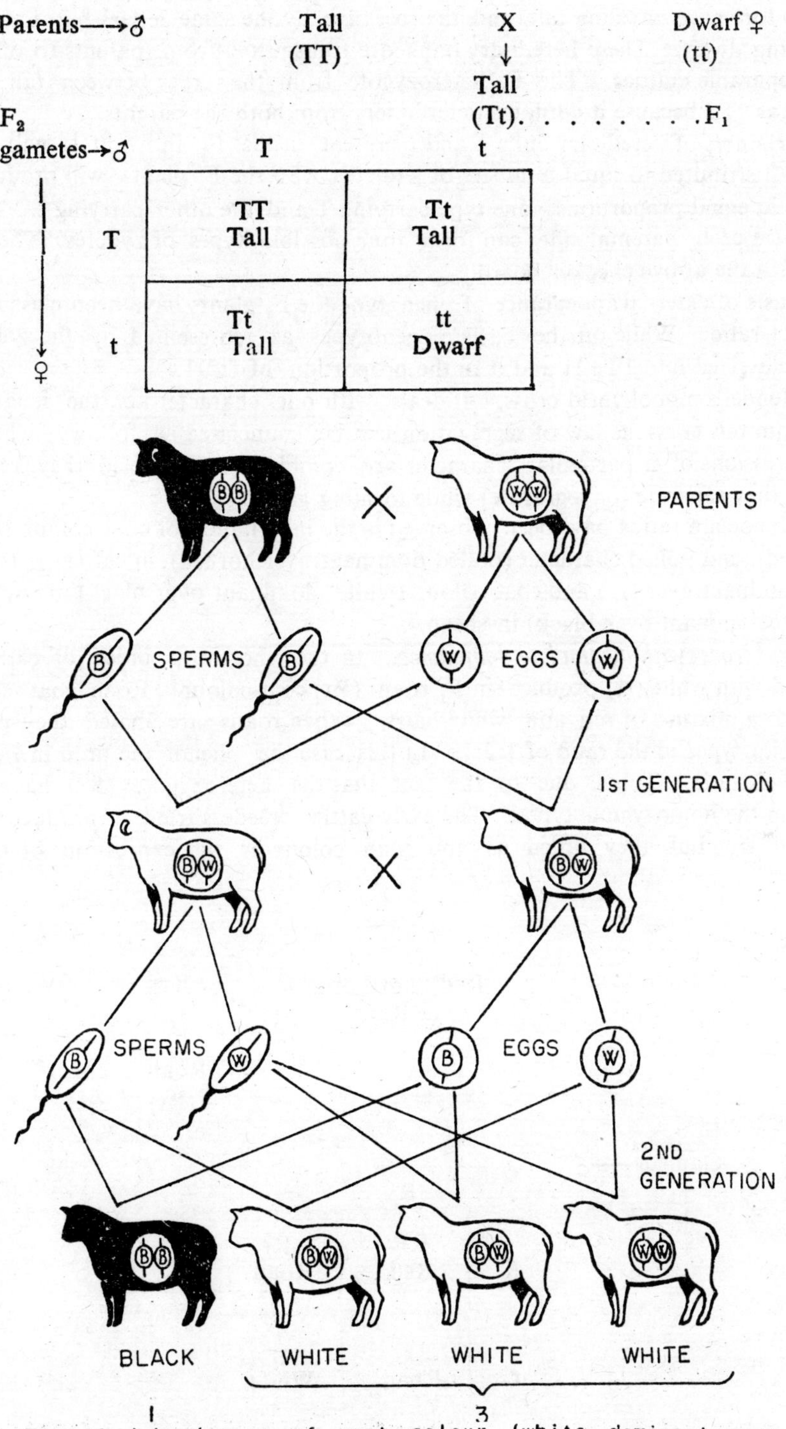

Fig. 6.8. Inheritance of coat colour (white dominant over black)

letters (TT) for pure breeding tall and the recessive by the same letters but small one (tt) for pure breeding dwarf. These hereditary units are transmitted from parents to offspring in the form of separable entities. The F_1 heterozygote from the cross between tall and dwarf is symbolised as 'Tt' because it contains determiners from both the parents.

The determiners of hereditary units T and t present in the F_1 individuals will separate out and will be distributed to equal numbers of gametes. So the F_1 plants will produce two types of gametes in equal proportions—one type carrying T and the other carrying t. Two types of gametes form each parental side can form four possible types of zygotes. These results are represented in the above checker board.

On the basis of external appearance of phenotype the F_2 plants have been classified into tall: dwarf in 3:1 ratio. While on the basis of genotypes as represented by the symbols, the F_2 plants are classified into TT, Tt and tt in the proportion of 1:2:1.

This is Mendel's monohybrid cross. It deals with one character i.e., the height of mature plants. From this cross the law of segregation can be enunciated as follows—when two contrasting expressions of a particular character are combined in a hybrid they remain unblemished and they separate (or segregate) while forming gametes.

Simple Mendelian ratios have been observed in the inheritance of coat colour (black dominant over red), and polled character (polled dominant over horned) in cattle: of the nature of ear (erect dominant over lap) and coat colour (white dominant over black) in swine; of fleece colour (white dominant over black) in sheep.

Monohybrid cross with incomplete dominance. In the shorthorn breed of cattle red (RR) when crossed with white (rr) produce in F_1 roan (Rr) coat colour. Roan coat colour is produced due to a mixture of red and white hairs. When roans are mated they produce red, roan and white types in the ratio of 1:2:1. In this case the phenotypic ratio in F_2 is the same as the genotypic ratio. This is due to the fact that the heterozygote (Rr) has a phenotype different from the homozygous types. The early cattle breeders tried to produce roans which would breed true but they failed as the roan colour is the expression of heterozygous condition.

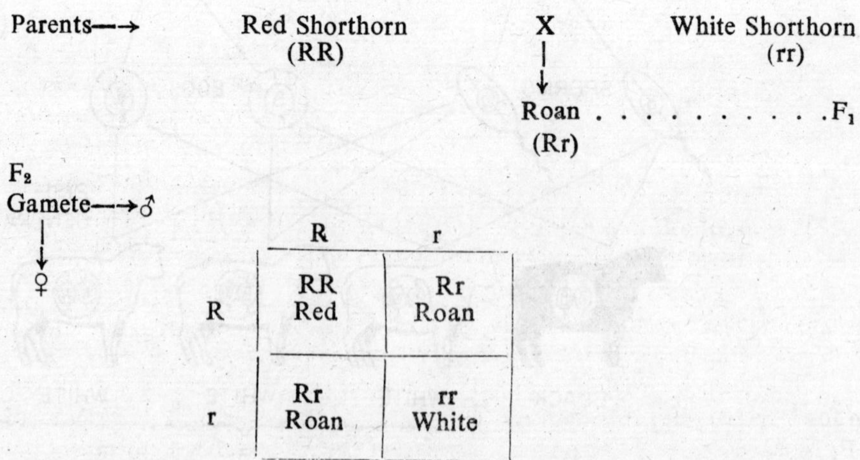

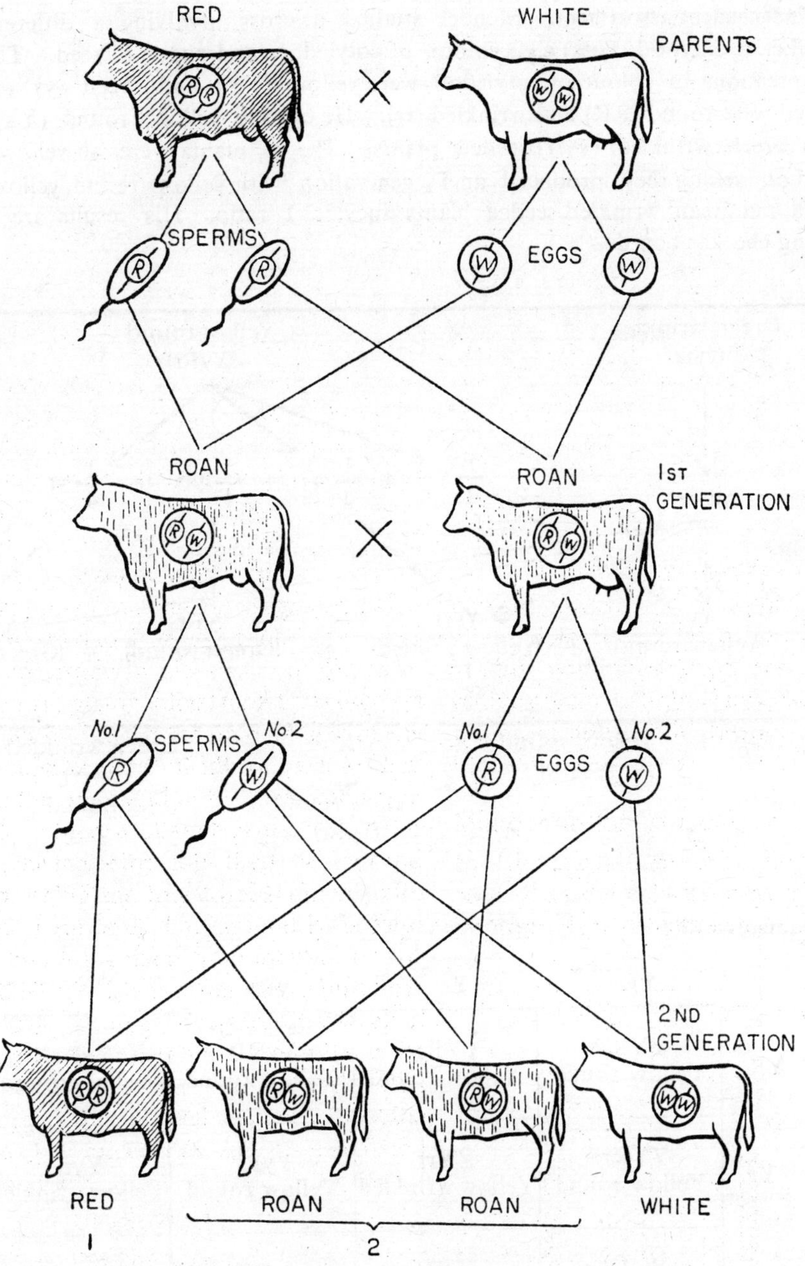

Fig. 6.9 Inheritance of incomplete dominance.

In fowl this type of inheritance is found in the cross of black and white feather types where the F_1 is of blue Andalusian type. In plants, the example of a pink hybrid from a cross between red and white flowered four-O'clocks is classical.

Laws of independent assortment. Mendel studied a cross involving a difference of two characters (i.e., a dihybrid cross) e.g., colour of cotyledon and shape of seed. The two contrasting expressions in colour of cotyledon were yellow (YY) and green (yy) and those in shape of seed were round (RR) and wrinkled (rr). He crossed yellow, round (YYRR) seeded plants with green, wrinkled (yyrr) seeded plants. The F_1 plants were all yellow and round seeded and on selfing they produced an F_2 generation with yellow round, yellow wrinkled, green round and green wrinkled seeded plants in 9:3:3:1 ratio. His results are depicted in the following checker board.

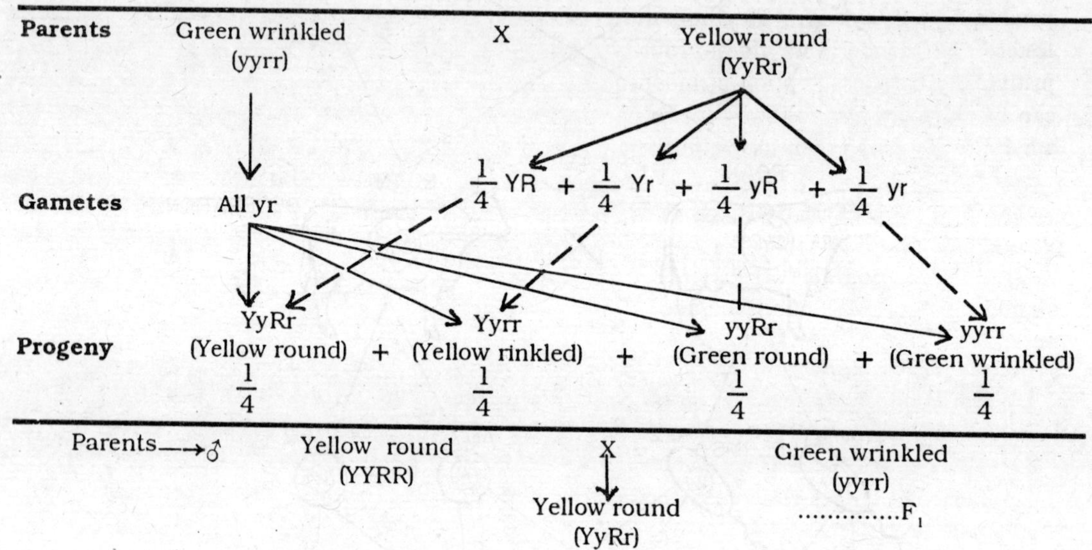

F_1
Gametes → ♂
↓
♀

	YR	Yr	yR	yr
YR	YYRR Yellow round	YYRr Yellow round	YyRR Yellow round	YyRr Yellow round
Yr	YYRr Yellow round	YYrr Yellow wrinkled	YyRr Yellow round	Yyrr Yellow wrinkled
yR	YyRR Yellow round	YyRr Yellow round	yyRR Green round	yyRr Green round
yr	YyRr Yellow round	Yyrr Yellow wrinkled	yyRr Green round	yyrr Green wrinkled

Mendel explained these results with the assumption that the two characters, i.e., colour of cotyledon and shape of seed, segregated independently of each other. The F_1 (Yy) will produce two types of gametes Y and y with regard to colour of cotyledons; and R and r types with regard to shape of seeds. When two characters are considered at a time, the gametes produced by F_1 will be of the four possible types YR, Yr, yR, and yr. Mendel tested this assumption with a test-cross, involving the F_1 and the double recessive parents, i.e., green wrinkled.

The double recessive parent produces only one type of gamete carrying two recessive heredity units and hence they will not interfere with the expression of the genotypes of gametes produced by F_1 hybrid. The four different phenotypes observed in equal proportions in the testcross of Mendel were due to four types of gametes produced by F_1 plants. This testcross justifies the basic assumption of independent assortment. The law of independent assortment can be enunciated as follows—if two pairs of unrelated contrasting characters are combined in a hybrid they group themselves independently of each other during gamete formation.

CYTOLOGICAL BASIS OF MENDELIAN INHERITANCE

Cytologists uncovered the secrets of metosis, meiosis, and fertilisation between the time Mendel's paper was published and its rediscovery in 1900. Mendel's main contributions were:

1. To demonstrate that hereditary factors are discrete entities which are constant from generation to generation.
2. To demonstrate that hereditary factors occur in pairs in each individual.
3. To demonstrate that each hereditary pair of each progeny contains one factor from each parent.

Rediscovery of Mendel's paper caused great excitement among cytologists because the Mendelian factors paralleled, in phenotypic response, many of their observations about chromosome behaviour during cell division. Sutton and Boveri (1902-1904) summarised the cytological basis for Mendel's laws in the following ways:

1. Fertilisation in plants and animals is effected by the union of egg and sperm. These two gametes form the physical link between the parents and offspring. The hereditary factors must be transmitted through these gametes.
2. Only the nucleus of the sperm takes part in fertilisation, thus the nucleus must contain the male hereditary factors. It may be concluded that the nucleus is the vesicle for all hereditary factors.
3. The chromosomes are the only elements which divide exactly and are distributed equally to the daughter nuclei during cell division. Hence the chromosomes must carry the hereditary factors.
4. The chromosomes occur in pairs of somatic cells. In each pair one chromosome is paternal in origin and the other is maternal. The hereditary factors also occur in pairs as demonstrated by Mendel.
5. The members of a chromosome pair segregate during meiosis and, as a result, each

gamete receives only one member of each homologous pair. The Mendelian factors behave similarly.

During meiosis members of each chromosome pair segregate independently of other chromosome pairs. Mendelian factors for different traits also segregate independently during gamete formation.

Much additional work has shown that chromosomes are the carriers of the hereditary factors. Morgan and his school fully elucidated the particulate nature of the hereditary factors (now known as genes) and their association with chromosomes. The number of genes far exceeds the number of chromosomes, thus many are located on the same chromosome. The chromosome pairs have been identified, named, and the genes which occur in each region (locus) of specific chromosomes have been determined for some animal species.

Chemical basis of heredity. Mendelian geneticists and cytologists demonstrated that genes are discrete bodies carried on the chromosomes. Biochemists discovered that chromosomes were strands of DNA surrounded by histones, and that DNA was the genetically active portion, but the method by which DNA produced the genetic properties was not known until the Watson-Crick model of DNA was proposed (1953) and tested.

Previous knowledge about the genetic mechanism required that the DNA structure explain the following four properties of genes.

1. The gene must carry genetic information from cell to cell and generation to generation.
2. It must duplicate itself with great precision.
3. It must mutate, even though rarely, and copy the mutated gene with great precision.
4. There must exist some mechanism for translating the genetic information into action in the developing individual.

The Watson-Crick model represented the DNA molecule as two strands coiled around each other to form a double helix. (Refer to the preceding chapter on the structure of the cell for a more complete description). This structure has been supported by many experiments, and is most useful in explaining how DNA possesses the above properties.

DNA carries genetic information. The property of information storage clearly lies in the order of the purine and pyrimidine bases in the DNA molecule. There are only four types of bases in a DNA molecule, but each gene is thought to contain 1000 to 1,500 pairs, thus there are at least 4^{1000} different ways in which these bases could be ordered into sequences. The capacity for storage of information on genes is enormous, but this is necessary if these genes are to direct the growth and development of a zygote into a man, rose, or a buffalo.

Storage of genetic informatian is analogous to a book written in language which contains only four letters and three letter words. Each letter is a specific base (adenine, guanine, thymine or cytosine) and each sequence of three letters specifies formation of a specific amino acid.

Duplication of DNA. The property of exact duplication is the result of the complementary strands of the double helix. The structure of the DNA molecule is such that each base will pair with only one other base (i.e., adenine with thymine and guanine with cytosine). Thus, if the sequence of bases on one strand is known the sequence on the other strand can be obtained by lining up the complementary base for each base of the known strand. DNA duplicates by separation of the two strands of the helix. This separation breaks the hydrogen bonds which hold the bases together and allows each base to attract and bound a complementary base from the surrounding cell contents. Once the paired strands begin to separate they continue to spread apart something like a zipper. The DNA molecule is duplicated at completion of the spreading apart and attraction of new complementary bases.

The molecular basis of mutation The third property of the gene is mutation; a sudden change in the structure of the gene which is passed on to copies of the chromosome. From the structure of the DNA molecule it is obvious that any change in one or more of the bases would create a new arrangement which would be duplicated.

Mutation could involve substitution of one base pair for another, the insertion of one or more extra base pairs between existing base pairs, the deletion of one or more base pairs, or more complex arrangements. Many mechanisms are known to cause mutation:

1. Some chemicals change the structure of bases. Nitrous acid changes cytosine to uracil which bonds with adenine. This could cause adenine to replace cytosine.
2. Base analogues are substances which are structurally similar to the regular bases and sometimes substitute for them, but are not so specific in pairing and sometimes pair with a different base changing the sequence of the complementary strand.
3. Ultraviolet light causes thymine molecules to join tightly together causing stress on the molecule and leading to errors in duplication.
4. X-rays and other ionising radiation break the DNA strand allowing extra bases to be inserted before rejoining.
5. Proflavine and other chemicals are known to cause small insertions and deletions.

The structure of the DNA molecule has cleared much of the mystery which surrounded the magic of mutations. In summary we may say that a mutation is a change in the sequence of bases in a DNA molecule which causes coding for formation of a protein different from that produced by the original gene. The phenotypic result of this change depends on the new protein which is produced or the lack of the protein produced by the original gene.

Translating genetic information into action. The fourth property, a mechanism for translating genetic information into tissues, pigments, and secretions was long a puzzle to geneticists. The information encoded in DNA was found to contain the sequence of amino acids in specific proteins. It was then discovered that RNA molecules copied the base sequence of DNA, moved to the ribosomes, and provided the template on which protein molecules were formed. It is only logical that proteins are the active agents in causing development activity since certain proteins (enzymes and hormones) have long been known as the catalysts which govern the types and rates of chemical reactions in the body. Thus, in general, we can say that the phenotypic response is determined by the sequences of bases in DNA which code for formation of specific proteins which catalyse reactions among the chemicals in the cell which are present because of environmental conditions and previous chemical reactions.

Many aspects of the process of translation are not fully understood. One of these is the mechanism for turning genes on and off, for it appears that many genes are inactive much of the time. Also, it is obvious that the genes which function in a muscle cell are different than those which catalyse the secretion of milk even though the full compliment of genes is present in every cell of the body. It may turn out that the switching on and off genes is also under genetic control.

Examples of gene function. Gene action can be determined only if it affects some trait in the individual. Most of the knowledge of gene action has come through studies of genetic defects resulting from mutation. These studies have shown that the function of genes is chemical in nature.

One of the first known causes of the genetic control of a specific chemical reaction was found in the rare metabolic disease in man called alcaptonuria. This disease is characterised by the hardening and blackening of the cartilage of the bones and the blackening of the urine when exposed to the air. The black urine is due to an accumulation of homogentistic acid. In the normal person, the enzyme that is present is responsible for the change of homogentistic acid to aceto acetic acid, which is clear in the urine. The person with alcaptonuria lacks this enzyme, so homogentistic acid accumulates in abnormal amounts in the urine.

Another group of genetic defects in human appears to involve the production of abnormal forms or the failure to produce a certain protein. A gammaglobinemia seems to fit into this group, and has been described only recently. This term refers to the failure of production of gammaglobulin in the body and its lack in the blood. A new born baby receives supply of gammaglobulin from its mother before birth, but this supply gradually decreases to near zero at four months of age. Normally the baby's own gammaglobulin production begins at about three weeks of age and reaches a high level by five to eight months. The lack of gammaglobulins results in increased susceptibility to bacterial infections because of the lack of resistance from antibodies in the blood.

Another example of genes in man that appears to function in the control of a production of a particular protein is that revealed by the gene defect causing sickle-cell anaemia. In the individual having this disease, the red blood cells have the shape of a sickle instead of the normal round shape. This disease is confined largely to populations in areas where malaria is prevalent. In normal humans, only haemoglobin A is found in the red blood cells. The sickle-cell gene apparently results in the production of an abnormal form of haemoglobin called haemoglobin S, which provides some protection against malaria. Individuals homozygous for the sickle-cell gene are very anaemic, however.

Evidence is also accumulating that hormone production by the pituitary gland, or the action of these hormones may be under genetic control. If true, this would fit in very well with the theory that mutations result in the production of defective proteins. Hormones from the anterior pituitary are protein in nature.

Dwarfism in mice has been shown to be a genetic effect resulting in a lack of growth hormone secreted by the anterior pituitary gland which stimulates body growth.

Further study of such inherited defects should be quite helpful in determining how genes function in growth and reproduction in all species including farm animals, and could lead to improved methods of more efficient and economical livestock production.

When genes express themselves. Many people are of the opinion that traits determined by genes are always present or visible at birth. This is not true, because the time at which genes express themselves is variable. In sheep an inherited condition has been found in which the lambs are born with short tails. The genes for this trait express themselves early in the embryonic life when the bones were being formed. Genes for eye colour in humans usually begin to show their effects a few weeks after birth, and not at birth. A form of muscular dystrophy in humans is not expressed until the age of seven to fifteen years. Hereditary baldness affects most individuals only after maturity, at 25 to 30 years of age. The gene for Huntington's Chorea, a nervous disorder in human, may not affect the individuals until he is past 50 years of age.

MULTIPLE ALLELES

In simple genetic experiments one form or condition of a character is contrasted with another form or condition of the same character, as two eye colours, two wing shapes, two colour patterns. The genes which are responsible for these two conditions are said to be allelic with one another. They are located on the same position in homologous chromosomes and in the reduction division they regularly go to different cells. Each gamete receives only one. These two genes are known as allelomorphs or alleles. Allelic genes always segregate in monohybrid ratio. Monohybrid segregation is the standard test of allelism.

A gene can have more than two alternative forms. These different forms of the same gene are called multiple alleles. The members of a multiple allele series will show monohybrid segregation crossing with each other. Multiple alleles arise due to mutation.

The Albino series of coat colour in rabbit. In rabbit, albinos with white coat and pink eyes are recessive to wild type with grey coat colour. Albinos are also recessive to Himalayan type with white coat but black nose, ears and feet. In these two cases the F_2 generation shows typical 3:1 segregation. This indicates that genes at a single locus govern coat colour, which has five alternative expressions—Albinos, Himalayan, Wild, Chinchilla and Light grey. Chinchilla is recessive to wild but incompletely dominant over Himalayan and albino. Light grey type is produced in F_1 of the crosses of segregation ratio is 1:2:1. In this series of coat colour the Albino is recessive to all other expressions while Wild type is dominant. The genotypes of the different expressions can be represented as follows:

Wild type	CC Cc^{ch}, Cc^{h}, Cc^{a}
Chinchilla	$c^{ch}c^{ch}$
Light grey	$c^{ch}c^{ah}$, $c^{ah}c^{a}$
Himalayan	$c^{h}c^{h}$ $c^{h}c^{a}$
Albino	$c^{a}c^{a}$

Multiple alleles exist in many other cases. There are 12 different alleles in the white eyes series of Drosophila. The genes or blood groups and Rh factor in man have multiple alleles. The cellular antigens in cattle have a long series of multiples, numbering about 300. In plants, self-sterility is controlled usually by a long series of multiple alleles.

MODIFIED DIHYBRID RATIO DUE TO INTERACTION OF GENES

The classical Mendelian dihybrid ratio is 9 : 3 : 3 : 1. However, there are cases where this dihybrid ratio is modified phenotypically in various ways. It has been found that in these cases the fundamental laws of transmission of heredity remain the same. These apparent exceptions are due to the fact that the two pairs of genes influence in the expression of the same character and the modification is due to the interaction between these two pairs. The only deviation in this case is that more than one pair of factors are responsible for each single character while Mendel supposed that each pair of factors is responsible for one character.

The type of comb in poultry is a classical example of two genes influencing the same character, the birds with 'rose comb' in Wyandotte, 'pea-comb' in Brahamas and 'single comb' in Leghorn can breed true. Crosses between rose-combed and single combed varieties showed that rose is dominant over single and in F_2 a segregation of 3 : 1 appeared. The same result is obtained in crossing between pea-combed and single-combed varieties and it has also been found that pea is dominant over rose. However, in crossing between rose-combed, and pea-combed varieties the F_1 birds become walnut-combed, a new variety and in F_2 generation walnut, rose, pea and single-combed birds appear in the proportion of 9:3:3:1 respectively.

The above ratio shows that two pairs of factors are acting together in the expression of the comb. This can be explained as follows:

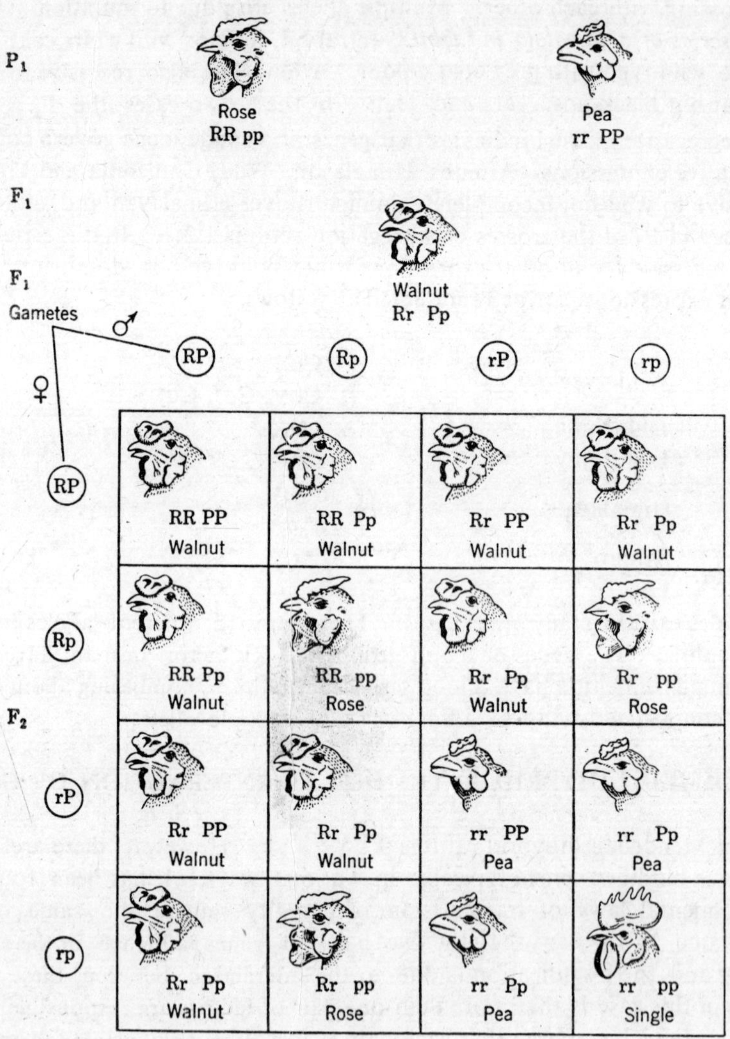

Fig. 6.10 Diagram showing interaction of factors for comb form in fowls. The cross of a pure rose-comb bird with a pure pea-comb one gives all walnut-combed offspring. The 16 possible combinations of the F_1 gametes, with their genotypes and the phenotypes resulting from factor interaction, are shown in the F_2 checkerboard. (*From Sinnott and Dunn.*)

In the F_2 generation the walnut variety is due to the presence of at least one dominant factor from both the pairs, while the single variety is due to the presence of both pairs of recessive factors. The walnut-comb depends on the presence of two dominant genes (R) and (P). One of these genes alone (R) produces the rose comb, the other alone (P) produces the pea-comb. The combination of the recessive alleles (r) and (p) produces the single type of comb, (rrpp).

The 9: 7 ratio due to double recessive epistasis. In the flower Daisy, when a yellow centred type of one locality is crossed with a purple centred type, all are centred in F_1 and in F_2 purple and yellow centred are in the ratio of 3: 1. It is apparent that yellow is recessive to purple. Another yellow centred type of different locality when crossed with the purple centred one, the results obtained are the same as in the previous experiment. As both the yellow types and the purple types breed true, all of them are homozygous.

But when these two yellow varieties from different localities are crossed together in F_1 all purple, and in F_2 the ratio between purple and yellow is 9 : 7 respectively. If both the yellow centred varieties are due to the same pair of factors, all would have been yellow in F_1. So two yellow varieties are genetically different, and yellow 1 and yellow 2 are due to different recessive factors.

The F_2 ratio 9 : 7 shows that two pairs of factors are concerned for the expression of the same character in Daisy. The pink centred variety is due to double dominant factors, one coming from each yellow variety. So each yellow has one pair of recessive and one pair of dominant factors.

It can be explained on a checker board as given below.

This modification is due to double recessive epistasis in which (p) is epistatic over (R) and (r) thus combinations like (ppRR) or (pp Rr) are all of yellow variety due to the masking effect of (p). Similarly in the case for combinations like (PP rr) or (pp rr) is yellow because

PPrr Yellow$_1$ X ppRR Yellow$_2$

↓

Pp Rr Pink. . . . . F_1

P_2

Gametes→♂
↓
♀

	PR	Pr	pR	pr
RR	PP RR Pink	PP Rr Pink	Pp RR Pink	Pp Rr Pink
Pr	PP Rr Pink	PP rr Yellow	Pp Rr Pink	Pp rr Yellow
pR	Pp RR pink	Pp Rr Pink	pp RR Yellow	pp Rr Yellow
pr	Pp Rr Pink	Pp rr Yellow	pp Rr Yellow	pprr Yellow

of the absence of any colour factor. The origin of pink centred flowers can be explained also by the complementary action of the two dominant genes P and R.

The 15: 1 ratio due to double dominant epistasis. In the poultry some breeds have a feathered shank while in some others the shank is unfeathered. All the types breed true. The F_1 individuals are with feathered shank in a cross between feathered shank and unfeathered shank types. This indicates that feathered shank is dominant over unfeathered. In F_2 generation feathered and unfeathered shank are found in the ratio of 15 : 1. This shows that it is

FF SS Feathered X ff ss Unfeathered

↓

Ff Ss . . . . F_2
Feathered

F_2
Gametes→♂
↓
♀

	FS	Fs	fS	fs
FS	FF SS Feathered	FF Ss Feathered	Ff SS Feathered	Ff ss Feathered
Fs	FF Ss Feathered	FF ss Feathered	Ff Ss Feathered	Ff ss Feathered
fS	Ff SS Feathered	Ff Ss Feathered	ff SS Feathered	ff Ss Feathered
fs	Ff Ss Feathered	Ff ss Feathered	ff Ss Feathered	ff ss Unfeathered

a case of modified dihybrid ratio in which two pairs of factors are responsible for the expression of the character of the shank.

So if (F) and (S) be the two pairs of factor then homozygous feathered shank bird will be of (FF SS) combination and the homozygous unfeathered shank will have (ff ss) combination. This can be explained on a checker board as given below.

It is a case of double dominant epistasis, feathered shank is expressed due to the presence of at least one dominant factor of these two pairs of alleles, while unfeathered condition is possible only when both pairs of alleles are in recessive combination.

This 15: 1 ratio in F_2 can be explained also by duplicate factor hypothesis, which assumes that two pairs of genes are controlling a single trait and the presence of one dominant gene can produce the dominant phenotype.

The 13: 3 ratio due to inhibiting factor or dominant and recessive epistasis. The white plumage of White Leghorn fowls is found to be completely dominant over the coloured plumage different coloured varieties, and a cross between white leghorn and any other coloured birds results in all white birds in F_1 generation. However, the white plumage of some other varieties, e.g., white silky, white wyandottes, etc., are found to be recessive to coloured plumage, and due to a gene distinct from that which produces the white of leghorm.

It has been inferred that white Leghorn contains a potential gene of colour but its expression is inhibited due to the presence of another pair of factors, called inhibiting factor. Denoting this inhibitor by (I) and the colour gene by (C), the homozygous White Leghorn is (IICC) and the white silky is (ii cc). The presence of the least one (I) will mask the expression of the colour gene. It can be explained on a checker board as given below.

In F_2 generation the white and coloured types appear in 13: 3 ratio. Here the combinations (II CC), (CII Cc), (Ii CC), or (Ii CC) are white due to the presence of inhibiting action of (I) over colour gene (C), while combination (II cc), (Ii cc) and (ii cc) are white due to the absence of any colour gene.

II CC X ii cc

White Leghorn ↓ White silky

Ii Cc. . . . . F_1

White

F_2

Gametes→♂

↓

♀

	IC	Ic	iC	ic
IC	II CC White	II cc White	Ii CC White	Ii Cc White
Ic	II Cc White	II cc White	Ii Cc White	Ii cc White
iC	Ii CC White	Ii Cc White	ii CC Coloured	ii Cc Coloured
ic	Ii Cc White	Ii cc White	ii Cc Coloured	ii cc White

Other modified dihybrid ratio where two pairs of factors acting on the expression of same character are also found such as:

(a) 9 : 3 : 4 ratio due to recessive epistasis.
(b) 12 : 3 : 1 ratio due to dominant epistasis.

Pleiotrophy

When a gene is studied carefully it is usually found to produce several effects. Many examples could be cited but perhaps the most extreme is the gene, "polymorph", in Drosophila which has been demonstrated to affect eye colour, growth rate, fertility, wing size, body hair, viability, wing vein arrangement and several other characters. A gene which produces several superficially unrelated effects is said to be pleiotrophic.

The chemical nature of the gene and its guidance of development through production of proteins, enzymes, and hormones provides some insight into the phenomenon of pleiotrophy. Although the chemical reaction catalysed by a specific enzyme or hormone usually produces a specific chemical product, this chemical can enter into many other reactions. The appearance of the same chemical in many biochemical pathways which produce different end products would suggest that pleiotrophy is the rule rather than the exception.

Polygenes

The converse of pleiotrophy, many genes affecting one character, is **called polygenic Inheritance.** Polygenes are the basis of the inheritance of quantitative traits, and genes at many different loci have been shown to effect some traits. As an example, some 20 specific gene loci have been demonstrated to affect the pigment of the eye in Drosophila, and many more than 20 loci have been shown to influence the colour of the maize plant.

QUALITATIVE AND QUANTITATIVE TRAITS

Traits are often grouped into those which exhibit qualitative differences and those which show quantitative differences. Qualitative traits are those which exhibit discontinuous variation; i.e., those in which variations fall into a few clearly defined classes. The variations in quantitative traits, on the other hand, are continuous in that there are small gradations in expression from one extreme to the other.

Almost all of the traits whose inheritance is well-known are in the qualitative class. The discontinuous nature of the variation in qualitative traits makes it possible, through breeding tests, to determine the genotypes of individuals in each phenotypic class because:

1. Most of the variation in qualitative traits can be attributed to one or a few major genes.
2. These traits are little affected by environmental modifications.

However, most traits of economic importance in farm livestock vary continuously. Major genes have not been found for such quantitative traits as body weight, egg production, milk yield, or growth rate, much evidence exists to show that these traits are inherited. Some of these evidences are as follows:

(i) These traits respond to selection.
(ii) Relatives resemble each other more closely than unrelated individuals for these traits.
(iii) Breeds perform quite differently, even when raised together and given the same care.

Quantitative traits usually are characterised by:

1. Polygenic inheritance (i.e., genes at many loci).
2. Large environmental effects.

Although environmental effects can cause a discontinuous array of genotypes to appear as continuous phenotypes, the inheritance of quantitative traits is usually polygenic. Major genes have not been detected for most quantitative traits despite intensive study. This supports the hypothesis that none of the genes contributing to the overall genetic merit has sufficiently large effect to be detected, thus suggesting that a large number of loci are involved. The nature of weight, milk yield, etc., would suggest that many factors affecting the overall health, vigour, and metabolic process would also influence these traits.

Models for quantitative inheritance. All types of gene action probably are present among the genes affecting quantitative traits. Dominance and epistasis are almost certain to occur. Some evidence from inbreeding studies indicates that heterozygosity may be beneficial for some quantitative traits. The effects of gene are also greatly modified by the environment.

Additive model. The simplest model for quantitative inheritance is to assume that there are two alleles at each locus and the presence of each favourable allele (capital letters) adds one unit more to the genetic value than the alternative allele. The colour of the wheat kernel provides an example of this model as the genotypes below illustrate.

Genotypes	*Phenotypes*
AABB	very dark red
AABb, AaBB	dark red
AaBb, AAbb, aaBB	medium red
Aabb, aaBb	light red
aabb	white

Thus, for each A or B gene which was substituted for an a or b gene the degree of redness increased one shade. If very dark red wheat were crossed with white wheat the F_1 would all be medium red and the F_2 would exhibit the full range of variation in the following proportion: (1/16, 4/16, 6/16, 4/16, 1/16).

If we consider the same model with three contributing loci we get the following distribution of F_2 genotypes:

Genotype	*Frequency*
6 favourable genes	1/64
5 favourable genes	6/64
4 favourable genes	15/64
3 favourable genes	20/64
2 favourable genes	15/64
1 favourable genes	6/64
0 favourable genes	1/64

Several things may be noticed from this model:

1. The average of the parent, F_1 and F_2 generations are identical. In fact, the average of the progeny from any mating is expected to be the same as the average of the parents.

2. As more loci are added the expected frequency of the extreme types in the F_2 becomes smaller and smaller.

3. The distribution of genetic values tends to become more like a continuous distribution as more loci are added to the model.

4. The genetic values toward a normal distribution as loci are added.

Although this model is a gross over simplification, it gives some insight into the results one might expect for quantitative traits. The rarity of the extreme genotypes in the F_2 provides a test for the number of loci involved. Appearance of the extreme types in the F_2 indicates control by a few major genes, whereas the failure to find these types indicates that many loci must be involved. Also, if the F_1 and F_2 generations average the same as the parental average, there is some support for concluding that the controlling genes are not dominant.

Dominance model. A slightly more complex model is one where two dominant genes affect the trait in the following manner:

Genotypes	*Size (arbitrary units)*
Aabb, AAbb	3
AABB, AaBB, AABb, AaBb, aabb	2
aaBb, aaBB	1

We see that the presence of AA or Aa increases the size by one unit relative to aa and that BB or Bb decrease the size by one unit relative to bb; i.e., A and B are dominant to a and b, respectively. If we make matings among these genotypes we get:

Parents	*Expected progeny*	*Parental average*	*Progeny average*
Aabb × Aabb	$\frac{1}{4}$AAbb + $\frac{1}{2}$Aabb + $\frac{1}{4}$aabb	3	2.75
Aabb × aabb	$\frac{1}{2}$Aabb + $\frac{1}{2}$aabb	2.5	2.5
aaBb × aaBb	$\frac{1}{4}$aaBB + $\frac{1}{2}$aaBb + $\frac{1}{4}$aabb	1.0	1.25
AaBb × AaBb	all nine genotypes	2.0	2.0
	⋮		

Many of these matings produce progeny which average the same as the average of the parents, but some do not. Upon closer examination we see that:

1. Tall parents to produce progeny which average shorter than their parents.
2. The progeny of short parents tend to average taller than their parents.
3. Intermediate sized parents tend to produce progeny with more variation in size than parents of either extreme.
4. If random mating occurs for several generations, the distribution of progeny genotypes will be the same as the distribution of parent genotypes.

This general tendency for progeny of extreme parents to be less extreme than their parents is called regression. It can be shown that regression also occurs if there is epistasis or environmental effects. The results of regression can be illustrated as follows (crow):

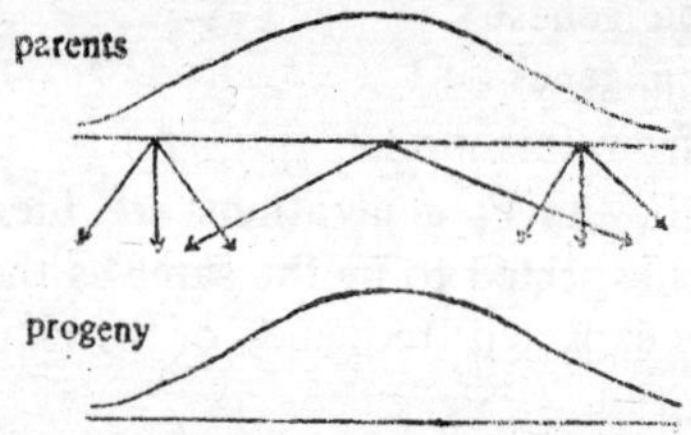

Fig.6.11 Result of Regression

If we generalise the above model to include many loci and the effect of dominance, epistasis and environmental effects, we can draw several conclusions. In each generation large parents produce progeny some of which are larger than themselves but most of which are smaller. Conversely, small parents produce progeny some of which are smaller than themselves, but most of which are large. However, intermediate size parents produce progeny more extreme than themselves in both directions with the end result that the distribution of progeny is very similar to that of the parents. Also, the parents of most large progeny are themselves large and the parents of most small progeny are smaller than average.

LINKAGE

The phenomenon by which the parental types appear in greater frequency than is expected in F_2 is known as linkage. This is due to the location of genes on the same chromosome. In such cases Mendel's law of Independent Assortment does not hold good.

Bateson and Punnet (1906) first reported an exception to Mendel's Law of independent assortment in *Lathyrus odoratus,* the sweet pea. On crossing a homozygous type with purple flower and long pollen with another homozygous type with red flower and round pollen the following results were obtained:

Purple long (PL/PL) × Red round (pl/pl)

PL/pl........F_1
Purple long

The F_2 results were as follows:

Segregates	*Observed frequency*	*Ratio*	*Expected frequency*	*Ratio*
Purple long	4,831	11	3,910.5	9
Purple round	390	1	1,303.5	3
Red long	393	1	1,303.5	3
Red round	1,338	3	434.5	1
	6,952		6,952.0	

Here it is observed that parental combinations, viz., purple long and red round are in great excess while the recombination or new combination, viz., purple round and red long are less than expected. So, it is clear that these two characters of flower colour and pollen shape did not assort in all the possible combinations in an independent fashion. Purple and long from one grand parent and red and round from the other, tend to hold together, so that more of these combinations are obtained than the expected ratio in the F_2 whereas the new combinations are observed in lesser quantity. Since the parental characters tend to stay together, this feature of heredity is called linkage.

Bateson and Punnet pointed out that when the dominants entered from the same parents they tend to remain together and did not assort themselves freely so that recombinations were fewer, while in the second cross when the dominants entered from different parents they tend to keep apart. The former was termed as coupling and the latter as repulsion. No satisfactory explanation of coupling and repulsion was developed until Morgan in 1910 found similar situation in Drosophila. Morgan said that coupling and repulsion are but two aspects of a single phenomenon called linkage. He showed that this tendency of linked genes to remain in their original combination was due to their presence in the same chromosome. Furthermore, he advanced the basic idea that the degree of strength of linkage depends upon the distance between the linked genes on the chromosomes. This proved to be a very fruitful idea, for it soon developed into the theory of the linear arrangement of genes in the chromosomes, and has led to the construction of genetic or linkage maps of chromosomes.

An example of linkage in poultry. Screbrousky in 1928 reported a case of linkage of comb shape and leg length in chickens. Rose comb (R) is dominant to single comb (r), and the creeper (C) is dominant to normal leg length (c). Creeper chickens have short legs that cause them to take very short steps, so that they appear to creep when they walk. Individuals homozygous for the creeper gene die early in life, and thus this gene is a semilethal gene.

When the testcross was made between a male heterozygous for both rose comb and creeper legs and female homozygous for the single comb and normal legs, the progeny produced were as follows:

Rose comb creeper	×	Single comb normal
RC/rc	↓	rc/rc
	Offspring	
22 RC/rc	Rose comb, creepers	
1 Rc/rc	Rose comb, normal	
33 rc/rc	Single comb, normal	
4 rC/rc	Single comb, creepers	

Thus the genes for rose comb and creeper legs were carried on one member of a chromosome pair, and the genes for single comb and normal legs on the other member. Some crossing-over occurred, however, as shown by the appearance of some rose comb normal and some single comb creepers in the progeny. The amount of crossing-over was about 8 per cent.

Genes located further apart on the same chromosome cross-over more often than those that are close together. In fact, the further apart they are the more difficult it becomes to distinguish crossing-over from the independent assortment of characters; thus some linkages remain undetected. For this reason, there may be more instances of linkage in the traits of farm animals than we have been able to discover.

The degree of crossing-over has been used to determine approximately the loci of certain genes in some species. Maps of chromosomes have been made showing approximate location. Mapping have progressed quite rapidly for the fruit fly (Drosophila) and to a lesser extent for mice and human. Very little chromosome mapping has been done for the various species of farm animals.

Linkage may be classified in two ways:

(1) According to the type of chromosome.

(a) *Autosomal*—When the genes in question are linked on autosomes (i.e., chromosomes other than the sex determining ones) e.g., deafness and defective teeth growth in man.

(b) *Heterosomal or Sex Linkage*—When the genes are located in sex chromosomes, e.g., colour blindness and hemophilia in man.

(2) According to the distance between the linked genes.

Calculation of linkage. The degree or intensity with which two genes are linked together is called the linkage value, which can be calculated from F_2 frequency and is always expressed in terms of percentage. Out of several methods, the simplest and commonest one is given below:

Shaw reported in linseed the following linkage:

Petal deep lilac	Petal lilac
Stigma deep purple	Stigma white

F_1 – Lilac petal, white stigma.

F_2 the observations were as follows:

1.	Lilac petal white stigma	... ...	357 (a)
2.	Lilac petal deep purple stigma	... ...	37 (b)
3.	Deep lilac petal white stigma	... ...	33 (c)
4.	Deep lilac petal deep purple stigma	... ...	94 (d)

Using this example the linkage value is illustrated below by taking one important and simple method.

Additive Methods (*Emerson's*).

$$P^2 = \frac{E-M}{n}$$ where : P=Linkage value
n=Total population (a to d)
E=Sum of End classes (a+d)
M=Sum of Middle classes (b+c)

I—P=Cross-over value expressed as percentage.

$$P^2 = \frac{(357+94)-(33+37)}{521} = \frac{381}{521}$$

P^2 =0.73: P=0.854; I -P=0.146 or 14.6%

Cross-over value=14.6%: Linkage value=85.4%

Shaw obtained some new combinations in the above cross although not as many as expected according to the law of independent assortment. He expected 195 and got only 70. Morgan ascribed the origin of recombination types to interchange of parts between homologous chromosomes, which he called "Crossing over". Crossing over is the exchange of corresponding segments between chromatids of homologous chromosomes, by breakage and reunion during late pachynema. The phenomenon is inferred, genetically, from the recombination of linked

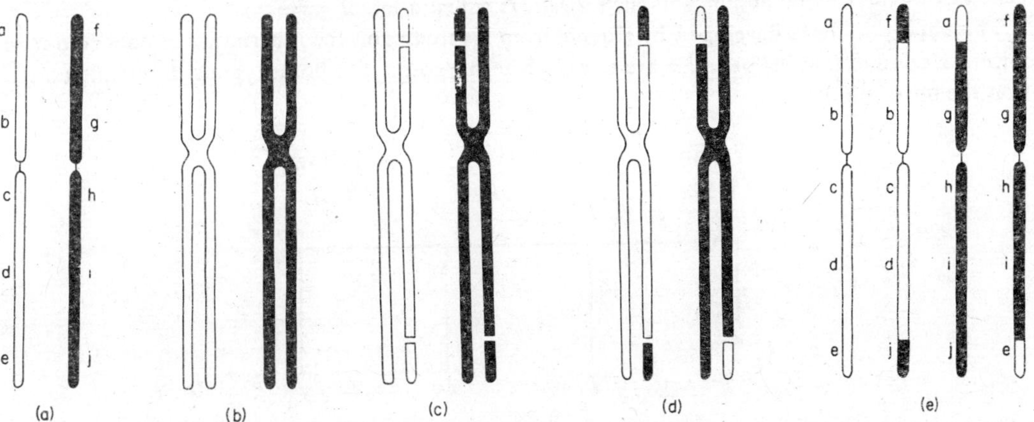

Fig.6.12 Crossing over. (a) Pairing of homologous chromosomes; a-f, b-g, c-h, d-i, e-j are pairs of allelic genes. (b) Each chromosome replicates and is now composed of two chromatids. (c) Breakage occurs in some of the chromatids. (d) Crossing occurs as a result of incorrect joining. (e) Four new chromosomes; in each, crossing over has resulted in the recombination of the genetic material.

factors in the progeny of the heterozygotes, and cytologically from the formation of chiasmata between homologous chromosomes.

Chromosome behaviour during crossing over at meiosis. During meiosis the homologous (maternal and paternal) chromosomes come together and form pairs (which is known as synapsis) during the zygotene stage. This pairing is evidently brought about by mutual attraction of the homologues. During the transition between the pachytene and the diplotene stages, each of the paired chromosomes divides into two chromatids so that the bivalent is now in four strand condition. Then the paired homologues exchange bits of chromatids (i.e., crossing over) and after that the separation of chromatids begins due to repulsion. However, the separation is not complete and homologues are found to be held together at one or more points. Such points of contact on either side of the centromere are known as chiasmata. The chiasmata are cytological indications of crossing over. A long chromosome forms a larger number of chiasmata than a short one. Due to crossing over, maternal and paternal chromosomes are not transmitted unchanged because they carry genes that were originally located in different members of the homologues.

Due to linkage the genes tend to remain in original parental combinations, but crossing over often breaks the linkage and produces recombination types.

Crossing over value. The frequency of crossing over between two genes.

Effective crossing over. That which is detectable in breeding experiments.

Somatic crossing over. Crossing over at mitosis as opposed to meiosis.

Unequal crossing over. Crossing over that produces one chromatid containing a gene twice and another lacking that gene.

LETHAL FACTOR

It has been observed that certain factors when present in a particular combination in an organism causes its death. It is due to the fact that the very combination of that gene blocks certain vital developmental or metabolic process of the organism concerned. This action of the gene is known as lethal action and such a gene is called a lethal gene.

This conception was developed by Cuenot from his studies on the inheritance of coat colour in mice. He found that yellow mice are always heterozygous. On homozygous dominant condition the mice will die.

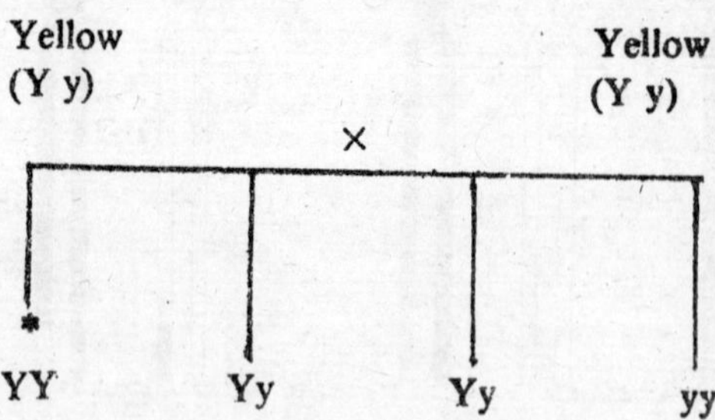

*YY combination is fatal because it prevents the pigment formation of red blood corpuscles of the animals and hence only the heterozygous type Yy will survive as yellow mice, yy is not yellow. Some of these genes have such drastic effect that they cause the death of the young during pregnancy or at the time of birth. Such genes are referred to as lethal (deadly) genes.

Still other genes do not cause death, but definitely reduce vigour. These will be referred to as detrimental genes.

A lethal gene may have its effect any time from the formation of the gamete until birth or shortly afterward. In a strain of horses, a sex linked recessive lethal has been reported that kills approximately one-half of the male offsprings of carrier female, so there are approximately twice as many females as males at birth. It is possible that such genetic defect may also be present in other species of farm animals. Frequently when a cow is mated and apparently conceives, she does not show signs of oestrus at a later date. Possibly conception takes place, but the zygote or embryo dies because of lethal gene effects; it is reabsorbed, and the female resumes the normal oestrus cycle. There is good evidence that lethal genes may cause losses in swine during pregnancy, because inbreeding increases embryonic death losses whereas cross breeding decreases them. This suggests that genes with non-additive effects are involved.

Semilethal genes are responsible for some death losses in farm animals. Dwarfism in Herefords, resulting from the mating of Comprest with Comprest is such an example. The dwarfs are born alive, as a general rule, but almost invariably they die before they are one year of age.

Most detrimental and lethal genes are either recessive or partially dominant and must be present in the homozygous state to have their full effect.

Detrimental recessive genes are generally present at low frequencies in a population.

Typical Illustration of Lethals in Cattle

Achondroplasia 1. Affected calves have short vertebral columns, inguinal hernia, rounded and bulging forehead, cleft palates and very short legs. The homozygous dominants are bulldog, the heterozygous are Dexters. About one fourth of the bulldog calves are aborted after their death in the sixth to eighth month of pregnancy following accumulation of amniotic fluid in the dam. The mode of inheritance is dominant, requiring to genes to have the lethal effect.

Achondroplasia 2. This condition has been described in the Telemark cattle of Norway and is similar to bulldog calf. Affected calves are carried to full term but die within a few days after birth due to respiration obstruction. The mode of inheritance appears to be recessive.

Achondroplasia 3. Described in Jersey breed, the defect is quite variable in the expression and is usually, but not always, lethal. Both the axial and appendicular skeleton may be affected. The head is deformed, being short and the legs are slightly reduced in length. In extreme cases, the calves are stillborn or die soon after birth. A recessive gene seems to be involved.

Agnatha. This lethal condition has been reported in Angus and Jersey cattle. The lower aw is several inches shorter than the upper, and it has been observed only in male calves, so it may be a sex linked recessive.

Cerebral hernia. Described in Holstein-Friesian calves. The affected calves have an opening in the skull because of a failure of ossification of the frontal bones. The brain tissue protrudes and is easily seen. Affected calves are stillborn or die soon after birth, probably due to a recessive.

Bulldog head (*Prognathism*). Observed in the grade Jersey herd. The skull is broad, the eye-sockets large, the nasal bones short and broad, and the forehead broader than normal. The condition is associated with impaired vision in partial or full daylight. Recessive factors are responsible.

Prolonged gestation. Gestation is prolonged to 310 to 315 days, with calves weighing from 50 to 60 kg at birth. Calves are thought to be homozygous for a lethal recessive gene.

Umbilical hernia. The hernia appears at the age of 8 to 20 days and persists until the calves are 7 months of age. At that time the hernial sac seems to contract, permitting the hernial ring to close. Appears to be limited to males and is dominant.

White heifer disease. The hymen is constricted, the anterior vagina and cervix are missing and the uterine body is rudimentary. Sex limited recessive genes seem to be involved

SEX CHROMOSOME AND SEX LINKAGE

Discovery of Sex Chromosomes

Each species of plant and animal has a characteristic number of chromosomes. In the human, the number is 23 pairs, in cattle 30 pairs, in wheat 21 pairs, sheep 27 pairs and goat 30 pairs.

McClung and Wilson during the first decade of the present century identified a pair of chromosomes out of the total chromosomes present in each nucleus of a certain female bug as sex chromosomes, since they carry the principle determiners for sex as well as for certain other characteristics. The two chromosomes identified in females are known as X chromosomes. Wilson found that in case of male bugs only one such X chromosomes is present. Hence the male bug always contains an odd diploid chromosome, one less than the female. Thus the females regularly have 7 pairs and males have 6 pairs and one odd, i.e., 13 chromosomes.

Thus the chromosomes themselves are divided into two categories, the autosomes (chromosomes having no relation with sex) and the heterosomes (sex chromosomes)

In mammals in general (including man) the females have two 'X' chromosomes, and the male has one 'X' and one 'Y' and both sexes are alike in their autosomes. The 'Y' chromosome is usually different from 'X' in size.

In some other animals a reverse situation exists. They are the moths, some flies, birds including poultry and some fishes. In them, it is the male that has two similar sex chromosomes, the female has two unlike ones. To indicate this reverse heterosomic relation between the sexes, some geneticists have designated the heterosomes of these groups as Z and W. The male has the constitution ZZ, the female ZW. Sometimes the W chromosome is missing and the female has a single Z.

The sex chromosomes (X and Y) often are of unequal size, shape and/or staining qualities. They, however, pair during meiosis indicating that the two chromosomes contain at least some homologous segments. Genes on the homologous segments are said to be *incompletely or partially sex linked* and may recombine by crossing over as do the gene loci on homologous autosomes with the difference that they do not segregate independently of sex as autosomal genes do. In man these include the gene for total colour blindness; that for *Xeroderma*

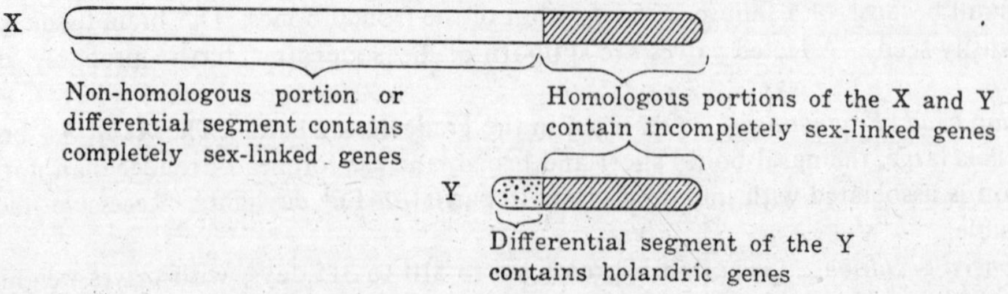

Fig. 6.13 Diagram of X and Y chromosomes showing homologous and non-homologous regions.

pigmentosum (a skin disease characterized by pigment patches and cancerous growths on the body). A few genes are also known to reside in the non-homologous portion of the Y-chromosome in man. In such cases the trait would always be transmitted from father to son. Such completely Y-linked genes are called *holandric genes* and the inheritance of such gene is called *holandric inheritance*. Examples of such inheritance are *hairy pinna* and *webbed toes*. Both the traits are transmitted from father to son.

Genes in the heterosomes. From these relations of the heterosomes it is clear that, the genes situated on them, will be inherited in a special fashion. In the mammals and in most iusects, females will have two genes of each kind found in X chromosomes, and will transmit one of such genes in every egg, but males will have only one gene of such kind.

These peculiarities in transmission have made it possible to discover genes located in the heterosomes. Many genes for various ordinary characters have located in the heterosomes. Many genes for various ordinary characters have been proved to exist in 'X' chromosomes, only a few in the Y chromosomes. The same peculiarities exist in Z and W chromosomes: many genes are known for the Z chromosome, few for W.

The type of sex determination in which the female has two 'X' chromosomes and the male has one 'X' and one 'Y' chromosome is very widespread being found in many insects, some invertebrates, some fishes, and mammals including man and in many dioecious plants. In

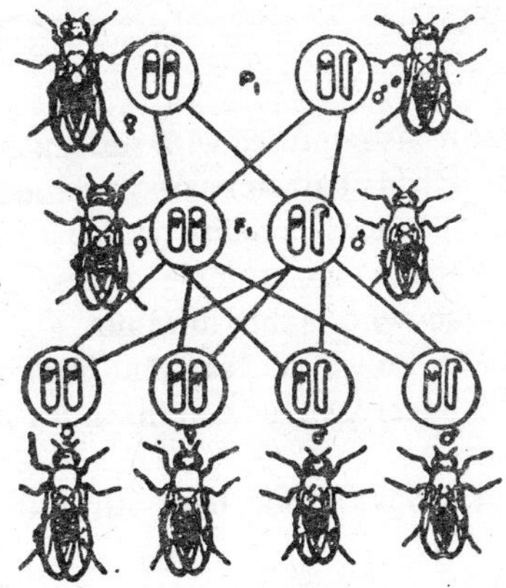

Fig.6.14 Sex-linked inheritance in Drosophia. The cross of red-eyed female by white-eyed male. The course of the sex chromosomes carrying the sex-linked gene W-w is traced from the parents to the F_2. Females at right.

man for example, somatic cells have 46 chromosomes. Each egg carries 22 autosomes and an 'X'. In the male two kinds of spermatozoa are formed, half of which carry an 'X' and the other half a 'Y' chromosome. The sex of the offspring are determined at fertilisation by the kind of spermatozoa that happens to fertilise the eggs: the 'X' bearing sperms produce girls and the 'Y' bearing ones boys.

In all the above cases, the male is the heterozygous or heterogametic sex because of two kinds of sperm and the female is homozygous or homogametic because all eggs are sexually alike.

But in some animals the relations are reversed, the female is heterogametic. Animals of this type are thus called ZW and ZZ types. In domestic fowl for example the female forms eggs of two sorts, half with Z chromosome, which when fertilised by any sperm develop into ZZ males, and half with 'W' chromosome which on fertilisation with 'Z' types of sperm will produce ZW females.

Sex Linkage

Approximately 20 known genes in man are inherited through the X chromosome. The commonest sex linked human trait is red-green colour blindness. The trait occurs in about 8% of men and only 0.5% of women.

E.B. Wilson in 1911 pointed out that all the facts about the heredity of colour blindness could be explained by the assumption that the recessive gene responsible for this condition is contained in the 'X' chromosomes.

It is easy to analyse why colour blindness is found more often among males in man. A father transmits his 'X' chromosomes to all his daughters but not to his sons. A mother passes one of her two X's to each of her children. Therefore, all the sons of a colour blind mother are colour blind regardless of what kind of colour vision her husband may have; but if the husband has normal vision all the daughters have normal vision. These daughters are, however, carriers of the gene for colour blindness. They contain the recessive gene covered up by its dominant allele. Such girls married to men with normal colour vision, will produce all normal girls but among the boys about ½ will be normal and others colour blind. A colour blind daughter can be produced only if a colour blind man happens to marry a carrier or a homozygous colour blind woman.

Sex Influence Heredity

Sometimes sex influenced heredity is confused with sex linked heredity. But it will be cleared if we think about the fact that sex linked characters are governed by the genes which are present in the sex chromosomes and sex influenced heredity as due to the genes in the autosomes.

The baldness in man may be taken as an example of sex influenced heredity. A man who is BB or Bb becomes bald and one who is bb does not. A woman with BB becomes bald, but one with Bb or bb is normal. So we can say that homozygous condition is the same in both the male and female, but the heterozygous condition Bb behaves differently in males and females.

The development of this sort of behaviour has been attributed to different types of hormones present in the male and female.

Sex Reversal

Sometimes female chickens (ZW) which have produced enough of eggs have been known to undergo not only a reversal of secondary sexual characteristics such as development of spurs, cock-feathering, and crowing, but also the development of testes and even the production of sperm cells. This may be due to some diseases responsible for destroying the ovarian tissue, and in the absence of the female sex hormones the rudimentary testicular tissue present in the center of the ovary proliferates. In solving problems of such kind, it should be remembered that the functional male derived through sex reversal will still remain genetically female (ZW).

Example

The gene for pattern baldness in humans exhibits dominance in men, but acts recessively in women.

Table 6.3

Genotypes	Phenotypes	
	Men	Women
$b'b'$	bald	bald
$b'b$	bald	non-bald
bb	non-bald	non-bald

MUTATIONS

The phenomenon causing sudden discrete and heritable change in the genotype of an organism is called mutation.

The change if it is in germinal cells is transferable from one generation to the other. The effect is mostly unfavourable to the individual concerned but sometimes it may be favourable also.

Types of Mutation

Gene mutation. Genes arise only from genes, and heredity is due, in the last analysis, to accurate gene replication. The process of gene reproduction or replication is exact but occasionally it goes wrong; a copy of gene differs from its original and the modified gene goes on reproducing its changed structure. This is gene mutation, or point mutation. In this case usually one character is affected at one time.

Chromosomal mutation: In an organism the chromosome complement usually divides or reproduces itself accurately: but from time to time it may be altered by duplication-inversion in some chromosomes or change in the number of chromosomes. Such an individual with change in chromosome structure or number is called a mutant. The type of mutation effects large number of characters. Change in fertility is an indicator of chromosomal mutation.

Stage at which Mutations Occur

Mutation may occur at any stage in the development of an organism. It may occur during the formation of gametes when the progeny concerned will show the change. If on the other hand mutation occurs in the first mitotic division of the zygote then the individual concerned will show partly mutated and partly non-mutated tissues. Mutation may also occur at a later stage when the organism has attained maturation and if number of cells affected are large *the chimeric* tissues may arise. This mutation may be (1) Gametic, (2) Zygotic, or (3) Somatic in origin.

Probable Agencies Inducing Mutation

Mutations can be autogenous or exogenous. The most common external causes including mutation, are natural radiations, to a less extent nutritional conditions and ageing. The agents that are used in artificial induction of mutations are (1) different types of radiation—X-rays, r-rays, ultra-violet rays, infra-red rays etc., (2) temperature shocks, (3) mutagenic chemicals like cumarin, colchicine, ausculin, 8 hydroxyquinoline, mustard compounds and many other chemicals.

Results of Mutations

A great many of the mutants are lethal, the offsprings never reach maturity. Whereas in others they are not lethal in action as for example, the white eye mutant in Drosophila. In white eye mutants, other characters are also affected and the mutants become less robust, sluggish and short lived.

The best known mutant among farm animals is polledness, or hornlessness. Another mutation, now extinct, occurred many years ago in the Ancon breed of sheep, resulting in low backed, long bodied, short crooked legged animals.

Regarding mutations in domestic animals, Babock and Clausen state that:

Any system of herd improvement founded on the search for and utilisation of mutants is doomed from the beginning to failure for mutants of a beneficial character appear so rarely as to have almost no practical significance.

General Characteristics of Mutation

1. Gene mutations are sudden variations resulting from chemical, structural or positional changes of genes. If they occur in the germ cells, they become a part of the hereditary material, if they occur in the soma or body, they may affect only one cell or whole groups of cells, but these somatic mutations do not become part of hereditary material.
2. Mutation generally occurs in one gene at a time.
3. Mutation rates differ in different genes, it varies from very low frequency in some genes to relatively high frequency in others and the rates may be inherent or may be influenced by the environment.
4. Mutations are more likely to occur in some parts of the chromosomes than in others.
5. Mutation from a normal type to a new allele is called direct mutation, and from mutant allele back to the normal type is called reverse mutation.
6. Mutations have different types of effects, from almost no visible changes up to lethal effect.
7. Mutations are usually recessive and generally harmful or lethal.
8. Mutations may occur at any time, probably most frequently at maturation division.
9. Mutations that are dominant show up at once.
10. Mutations that are sex linked recessives show up at once in males.
11. Spontaneous mutations occur in appreciable frequency.
12. Mutations can be induced by radiation, temperature changes, chemical agents, and are proportional to the dosage, within viable limits, of the treatment given.
13. Mutations can be detected by breeding experiments.

VARIATION

Every individual, even of the same species, varies from other in some of its characteristics. This variation may broadly be classified into two types:

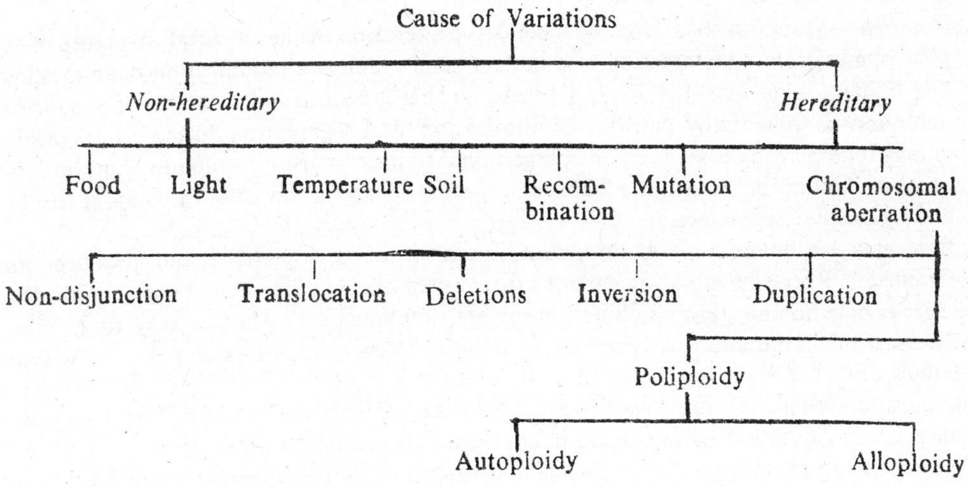

1. Hereditary variation is genic in origin and may be transmitted from one generation to the other.

2. Non-hereditary variation—which is not of genetic origin but due to the effects of environmental factors, e.g., feeding, light, etc.

Variation due to Non-Hereditary Causes

Environmental factors play a great role in bringing about variation among individuals. It can be found that different animals of the same species and of the same age but provided with different levels of nutrition, grow differently. One which is provided with a higher level of nutrition grows faster than another provided with a higher level of inferior type. Same is the case with the growth of plants in soil. A plant growing in soil, which provides its optimum requirements, grows better than the other which is growing in a deficient soil.

Similarly grasses under shade become pale due to want of sunlight.

Temperature also affect the morphological as well as physiological expression of plants and animals, cows of temperate zone when brought to tropical countries do not thrive well.

From the above examples, it may be concluded that environmental factors play a great role in bringing about variation, both in animals and in plants. Environmental factors, however, do not change the genic make up of an individual, but they determine the extent to which the inherited characters may be expressed. So by changing the environmental conditions, it is possible to change the expression of the inherited characters to different degrees. But these changes cannot be transmitted to the offspring.

Mechanisms causing genetic variation. Hereditary variations are defined as the variations in the composite genotypes individual animals. These variations originate from changes in the hereditary material which are transmitted to resultant progeny. The mechanisms by which these genetic changes originate are as follows:

1. *Recombination.* Variation may occur through recombination, i.e., new combinations of existing genes, which occur through gamete formation, crossing over and fertilisation. The first appearance of many characters is due to recombination of already existing factors, rather than mutation. Modified dihybrid ratios, as discussed previously, are examples of recombination and appearance of new varieties.

2. *Mutation.* Mutation has been defined as the alteration in the chemical structure of a gene. That is, mutation is the creation of a mutant gene which is a modification of an existing gene. The mutant gene acts like any other gene in that it codes for formation of a specific amino acid and is potentially capable of duplication and segregation during cell division. Mutation may take place in a somatic or in a germinal tissue. Variations due to mutation in somatic tissues cannot be transmitted through sexual reproduction, but in plants it can be transmitted by asexual reproduction.

Mutation may be dominant. A dominant mutation of a somatic tissue produces an immediate effect. Recessive mutation cannot express their effects immediately unless both the recessive genes of a homozygous combination mutate simultaneously which is very rare.

Recessive sex-linked mutation will produce an immediate effect in males of XO or XY type and in female ZO or ZW type.

Dominant mutation in germinal tissue will produce an immediate effect in the next generation, while recessive mutation will show up in later generations due to inbreeding.

The rate of mutation is very low. Though it varies for different genes, many have been found to have mutations of approximately 1 in 100,000 gametes. In spite of this low rate, many of the variations in organisms trace their origin to alterations of single genes.

3. *Chromosome aberrations.* Abnormal behaviour of chormosomes also plays a major role in altering the basic genetic arrangements. Some of these changes are hereditary.

(*A*) *Non-Disjunction*

Sometimes one (or more) homologous pairs of chromosomes fail to separate during gamete formation. This results in formation of some gametes which lack an entire chromosome and an equal number of gametes have an extra chromosome. Zygotes formed by uniting a normal gamete with one lacking a chromosome are usually not viable, probably because of lethal recessives on the unpaired chromosome. Zygotes formed by uniting a normal gamete with a gamete containing an extra chromosome are often viable, but develop into abnormal individuals. Progeny resulting from non-disjunction of chromosomes have sometimes been found to be fertile and to transmit their abnormal chromosome arrangement, but the rarity of these arrangements, except for the sex chromosomes, indicate that they are basically unstable and either are eliminated by selection or revert somehow to a diploid state.

(*B*) *Abnormalities Resulting from Chromosome Breakage*

(i) *Deletion.* A deletion is the loss of a segment of a chromosome containing one or more genes. Deletions result when a broken segment fails to rejoin the segment containing the centromere. Deletions may contain many or few genes and they may occur on any segment of the chromosome. Deletions result in loss of the genes and cause death, abnormalities, or no change, depending on the function of the genes lost.

One mechanism of creating a deletion is illustrated in Fig. 54. In this example the chromosome shown in A can form a loop as in E. If two breaks occur at the point where the ends of the loop cross, the segment containing A may rejoin with the segment containing D omitting the loop and gene C.

(ii) *Inversion.* An inversion occurs when a segment of a chromosome breaks off and rejoins the opposite ends from the original arrangement, resulting in the inverse order for genes on this segment. This arrangement could also result from looping if the ends of the loop rejoin with the opposite straight segment as shown in G and H of Fig. 6.15. Inversions change the

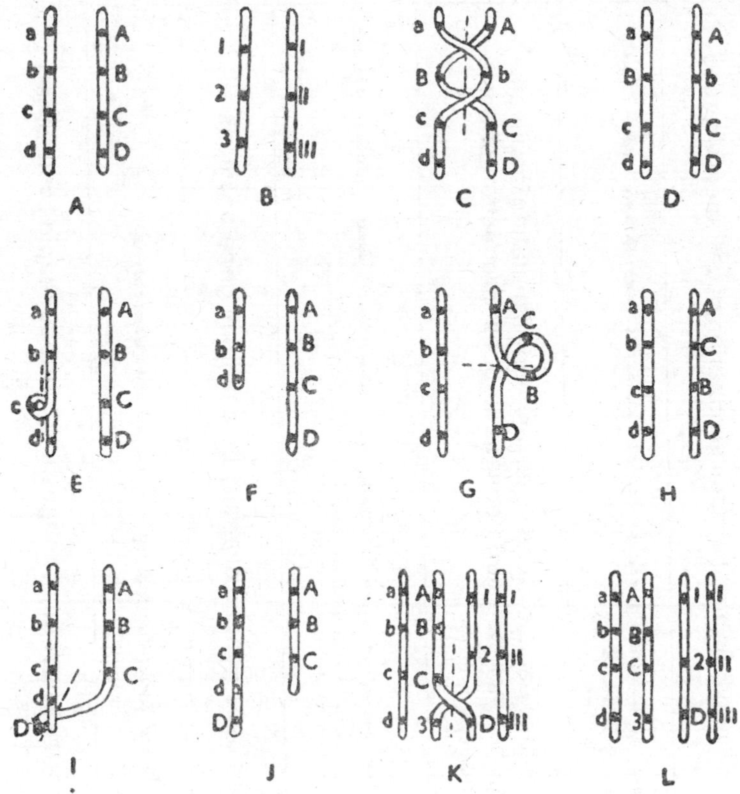

Fig. 6.15 Diagram to show crossing over and various chromosomal aberrations.

gene orders but do not result in loss of genes. However, they prevent crossing over in some animals.

(iii) *Duplication.* If a part of one chromosome breaks and the broken part gets attached to the homologous pair, a condition is obtained where certain genes are present in a double dose in one chromosome while the same genes are deficient in the other chromosome of the pair. This condition is known as duplication.

If one member of the chromosome pair shown in A comes to lie across the other as shown in I and a break occurs in the plane of the dotted line, the chromosome on the left in J will have a duplication and contain both gene d and gene D, whereas the chromosome on the right will have a deficiency in the section containing gene D.

(iv) *Translocation.* When a piece of chromosome becomes broken off and attached to another chromosome, usually of another pair, the phenomenon is called translocation. This causes a change in the relation of linkage group. A new sex linkage is formed when translocation occurs in sex chromosome.

Translocation may be simple, when one chromosome of a pair breaks and gets attached to another chromosome of a different pair. Reciprocal translocation is the exchange of parts between non-homologous chromosomes.

Table 6.4

Type of Alteration	Example of How Change May Occur	Some Possible Effects • Favorable • *Harmful*
DELETION	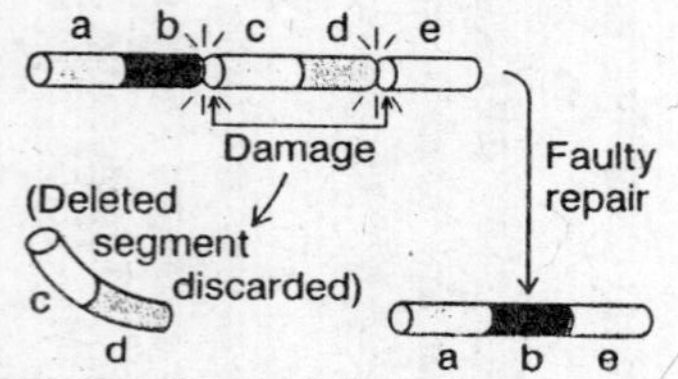a b c d e Damage (Deleted segment discarded) c d Faulty repair a b e	Rarely favourable : perhaps elimination of detrimental genes *Loss of critical genes is lethal: disrupts chromosome separation during meiosis*
DUPLICATION	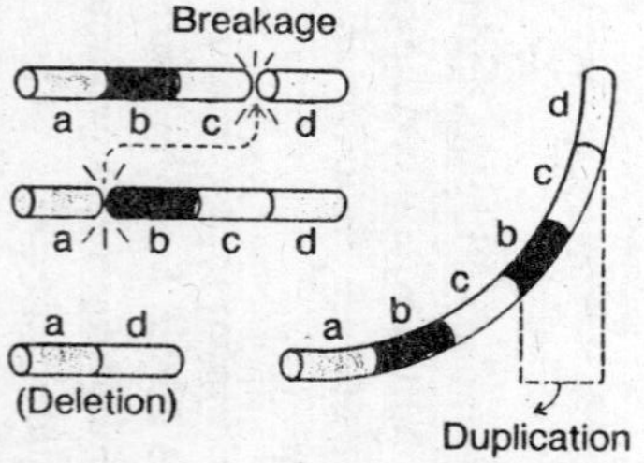Breakage a b c d a b c d a d (Deletion) a b c b c d Duplication	Provides backup genes to cover needs if mutation inactivates a gene; increase gene dosage to boost production of some products *May interfere with chromosome separation; may disrupt gene function if duplication occurs within a gene*
INVERSION	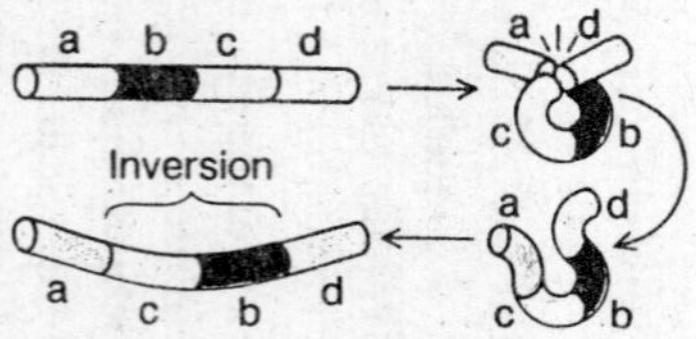a b c d Inversion a c b d a d c b a d c b	Increases genetic diversity by changing gene positions *Reduced fertility; loss of control of gene expression*
TRANSLOCATION	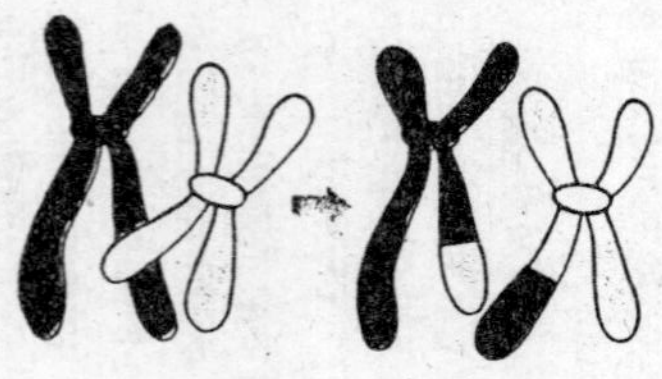	Enormous genetic changes may generate rapid evolutionary advances *May activate genes that cause cancer; reduce fertility; may result in gain or loss of whole chromosome*

In Fig. 6.15 one member of the chromosome pair shown in A may come to lie across one member of the chromosome pair shown in B, as seen in K. If a break occurs in the plane of the dotted line, sections of non-homologous chromosomes are changed, or translocated, as shown in L.

Translocation has been found to be important in the formation of new species by providing a format or chromosome structure sufficiently different that matings of individuals with the new structure and those with old do not produce viable progeny.

4. *Polyploidy.* It means occasional increase in the number of chromosomes adding or subtracting a part or the whole set of haploid complement. It is more frequently observed in plants than in animals and has played a major role in the evolutionary process.

7

ANIMAL BREEDING

Even the best feeding and management cannot coax performance beyond the genetic limit of an inferior animal. Improving the genetic merit of livestock populations is important at all levels of management, but it appears to be particularly important that, in periods of improving management and nutrition, animals be bred which have the genetic capability to better utilise additional feed and better management. A sound breeding programmc is a necessary part of the total animal production system whether the husbandman breeds his own replacements or purchases them from another breeder.

The productive capacity and physical appearance of animal populations can be changed greatly by selective breeding. Examples of these changes are numerous in the history of agriculture. Breeds of cattle which produce tremendous volumes of milk have evolved from foundation stock which produced barely enough milk to support one calf. Mink growers can breed mink which produce pelts in any of a wide variety of colours. Poultry breeders have developed some lines of chicken in which hens lay an egg nearly every day of their adult lives, and other lines which do not lay many eggs but do gain weight rapidly with efficient conversion of feed into meat. These changes in the form and function of animals have largely been achieved not by the creation of new genes but by locating the existing genes, increasing their frequency, and recombining genes in progeny so that many favourable genes are present in the same animal.

Selection—The Tool of the Breeder

Man improves his livestock by limiting the reproduction of inferior animals and by choosing superior animals for mating to produce the progeny which constitute the next generation. Through selection of breeding stock, the breeder is manipulating the frequencies of genes by deciding which genes in the population will have an opportunity to be present in a gamete which develops into a viable progeny. Genes must be manipulated in sets (not individually). However, since the entire gene compliment of the individual animal is segregated and transmitted according to laws of gamete formation and recombination, the random nature of segregation and recombination makes selection a slow and complex process except in a few relatively simple situations.

Although selection is slow, it is a very powerful tool for change. The most elegant proof of the effectiveness of selection is the variety of animal and plant life which has evolved on earth through natural selection. New genetic material is created by rare accidental mutations but selection is the process by which favourable genetic material is multiplied and distributed throughout the population so that it is not lost with the death of the animal in which the mutation occurs. In a relatively short span of time few mutations occur, but many mutant genes are present at low frequencies. Selection within a man's lifetime will produce changes mostly by increasing the frequencies of genes already present in the population.

Natural Selection

Natural selection is defined to be that selection which occurs without the planning of man. In the wild state, natural selection operates because more progeny are left by animals whose geno-types better enable them to procure food, escape predators, resist disease, attract mates, or otherwise survive and produce. Even in the "artificial" environments provided by man, there is some natural selection because certain genotypes reduce fertility or prevent conception and others produce susceptibility to disease or impair the length of life.

VARIATION

Selection is possible only when differences exist between members of the population. Variation among animals in size, colour, speed, stamina, growth rate, disease resistance, milk production and numerous other traits have often been recorded. This is indeed fortunate because genetic variation is the raw material from which the breeder creates superior stock. Without variation in the genetic make up of his herd, the breeder could not hope to produce progeny better than their parents, yet this same variation which is necessary for progress is also responsible for mediocre progeny.

Sources of Variation

Variation arises from two sources:

1. Genotypes—the particular combination of genes which directs the development of the animal.
2. Environment—the conditions of nutrition, climate, competing animals, stress, exposure to disease organisms, and other non-genetic conditions which influence the animal expression of a trait.

Genetic variation is transmitted to future generations, but that due to environmental differences is not transmitted. The relative importance of these two sources of variation determines, to a large extent, the speed and ultimate chance of achieving a desired goal through selection. The breeder tries to select the animals with the best genotypes, but often environmental effects cover up the true genotypic values.

Environmental variation. Environmental variation is often large and many of the environmental influences which cause variation are not well defined. The overall result of environmental variation is the masking of genetic differences, and the primary problem of most breeders is the elimination of (or allowance for) environmental influences so that true genetic differences may be identified. Identical twins are ideal for studying environmental variation because their genetic make-up is identical, as demonstrated by their identical sex, colour, blood antigens and other traits which directly reflect the genotype without environmental modification. When raised under different nutritional levels, these twins show dramatic differences in growth rate, milk production, and reproductive performance. Even when grown together in the same pen, indentical twins often show large differences for traits such as milk production which are greatly affected by random environmental effects.

Although different environments allow different degrees of expression for the same genotype, the environment does not directly alter the hereditary make-up of the animal. Removing the horns of cattle for many generations has not prevented the development of horns on progeny of horned parents. Docking the tails of sheep and horses, clipping of hair, and notching of ears are further proof of the non-transmittance of environmentally acquired characteristics. Stunted and underdeveloped animals from a good genetic background have often produced superior progeny.

Genetic variation. The genotype is the collection of genes which comprises the hereditary material of each cell of the animal. In a population of animals, a wide variety of genotypes are present. This variation in genotypes is the result of differences anong the paired genes at the same locus from one animal to the next. The existence of heterozygous animals at a particular locus is proof of at least two alleles in the population at that locus. When two heterozygotes (Aa) are mated, they produce three progeny genotypes, heterozygotes (Aa) and two different homozygotes (AA and aa), providing a demonstration of genetic variation.

The exact number of gene loci in any of the species of farm livestock is not known, but a conservative estimate would run into the thousands, and this is very likely to be far too low. Some of these loci undoubtedly contain only one allele which is absolutely essential to the life of the organism, but breeding studies have revealed that populations contain more than one allele at most loci. Aso, multiple alleles contribute to genetic variation. More than 300 alleles have been identified at one locus of cattle, and multiple alleles have been recorded at many other loci.

Differences among genotypes constitute the genetic variation present in a species at any one time. However, the transmission of genetic variation from one generation to the next is of considerable importance to the breeder because his goal is the reduction of the most favourable genotypes. Genes, not genotypes, are transmitted to progeny because only one gene from the pair at each locus of the parent goes to each gamete. Thus, a parent which is homozygous at a particular locus can produce a progeny homozygous at this locus only if the other parent contributes the same allele. Causes of genetic variation during transmission of genes can be attributed to several sources:

1. Recombination of genes
2. Gene interactions
3. Mutations
4. Chromosome aberrations
5. Chromosome number changes

Variation from recombination of genes. Recombination of genes is the primary source of genetic variation, and its potential is immense. First, consider a single pair of chromosomes. During gamete formation one chromosome will go to each gamete, thus two gametes are formed from each primary germ cell and these gametes are different if only a single locus is heterozygous on this chromosome pair. Crossing over frequently occurs during meiosis so that, when several loci are heterozygous, many additional types of gametes are actually formed from segregation of the chromosome pair in different primary germ cells of the same animal.

To give a specific example consider five loci for two parents with the following genotypes:

sire: Aa bb CC DD Ee
dam: Aa Bb CC Dd Ee

In the progeny there could be three genotypes (AA, Aa, aa) at the A locus, two genotypes (Bb, bb) at the B locus, one genotype at the C locus, two genotypes (DD, Dd) at the D locus, and three genotypes (EE, Ee, ee) at the E locus.

Thus, $3 \times 2 \times 1 \times 2 \times 3 = 36$

genotypes are possible from this specific mating, although all would not occur with equal frequency if some loci located on the same chromosome. Progeny from this mating could range from AABbCCDDEE to aabbCCDdee although these extremes are not likely to occur at high frequencies. These progeny would all have identical pedigrees, but only at the C locus would the same pedigree guarantee identical genotypes.

Table 7.1

Kinds of gamates and progeny genotypes from various Species heterozygous at one locus on each chromosome

Species	*Number of chromosome pairs*	*Possible gamete types from one animal*		*Possible progeny genotypes from mating heterozygotes*	
Ascaris	1	2^1	2	3^1	3
Ascaris megalocephala	2	2^2	4	3^2	9
Fruit fly (D. melanogaster)	4	2^4	16	3^4	81
Corn (zea mays)	10	2^{10}	1,024	3^{10}	59,049
Swine	19	2^{19}	524,288	3^{19}	1,162,261,476
Mouse	20	2^{20}	1,048,576	3^{20}	3,486,784,401
Man	23	2^{23}	8,388,608	3^{23}	94,143,178,827
Sheep	27	2^{27}	134,217,728	3^{27}	7,625,597,544,036
Catle, Goat	30	2^{30}	1,073,741,824	3^{30}	205,891,132,094,649
Horse	32	2^{32}	4,294,967,296	3^{32}	1,853,020,188,851,841
	n	2^n		3^n	

The random process of fertilisation assures that each gamete has equal chance to form a zygote. Thus, if we consider the simplest case of mating two heterozygous animals with no crossing over, there are four possible ways to pair one chromosome from the sire with one from the dam. Two of these combinations produce identical heterozygotes if the two parents are heterozygous for the same alleles at the same locus, leaving three different genotypes as the absolute minimum from recombination of heterozygotes.

Chromosome pairs have been shown to segregate independently. Thus, if a single locus on each of n chromosome pairs is heterozygous, there are 2^n possible gametes from each individual and at least 3^n progeny genotypes could be formed by mating animals with heterozygous genes on each chromosome pair. The number of possible gametes and progeny genotypes for the above situation for various species is shown in Table 7.1.

The enormous numbers in Table 7.1 must be considered the minimum numbers of possible gene combinations. We do not know how many genes are present on each chromosome, but if each contains as few as 100, a cow would possess 6,000 genes. If each of these 3,000 pairs were heterozygous a single cow could produce 2^{3000} different types of gametes and there would be at least 3^{3000} different genotypes possible by independent assortment and crossing over. These numbers exceed the number of cattle on earth, thus genetic variation from recombination is indeed tremendous.

Variation from Gene Interactions

Genes are said to interact when a gene gives a different response in the presence of some other gene than in its absence. Interactions cause genetic variation because the same gene may produce a different response in one progeny than in another by the same parents. The importance of gene interactions is in dispute. Attempts to partition genetic variance have found only a small part of the genetic variation in quantitative traits to be due to gene interactions. However, dominance and epistasis have been demonstrated to contribute substantial variation in many traits governed by one or a few loci.

Selection for variations due to gene interactions is selection for added genetic values of certain gene combinations above and beyond the average effects of the same genes in random combinations. To be successful this selection requires that certain combinations of genes be transmitted from parent to progeny, and breeding programmes to be capitalised on transmission of genotypes require inbreeding and/or progeny testing and are much more complex than simple selection which capitalises on the direct effects of each gene.

Gene interactions are of two types:

1. Dominance—one gene masks the effect of another at the same locus.
2. Epistasis—a gene at one locus influences the effect of gene at another locus.

Dominance. An example of dominance is the gene in cattle which causes the growth of horns when present in the hh combination, but is recessive to the allelic gene H so that heterozygotes (Hh) do not develop horns. Selection for polled (hornless) cattle is less effective than selection for horns because one-fourth of the progeny of polled heterozygous parents (Hh) would develop horns whereas all horned animals breed true.

Epistasis. The gene c, found in many species, provides an example of epistasis. Animals homozygous for this gene (cc) are albinos because the gene blocks the formation of pigments in the hair and skin. This gene is epistatic to a number of genes at different loci which determine the colour and patterns of pigment when the (cc) homozygote is not prevented from giving expression in the albino genotype. Some albino individuals may possess residual genotypes for a very desirable colour, but these can only be identified by progeny testing since the albino genes have blocked the expression of the remainder of the genotype for colour.

Consequences of gene interactions. The overall result of gene interactions is the production of genotypes which are not readily transmitted to progeny. For quantitative traits this produces confusion and reduced efficiency of selection which is similar to environmental variation because it causes selection of parents which do not transmit their superiority to their offspring.

Genetic variation from other sources. Mutations, chromosomal aberrations, and irregularities in chromosome numbers are the ultimate sources of all genetic variation, yet they happen so rarely as to constitute such a small part of the total genetic variance that it is hardly measurable. Some mutations, such as the dominant gene for hornlessness in horned breeds of cattle and certain colour mutants of mink, have been quickly recognised and used, but most viable mutations are either recessive or produce relatively small effects which are never recognised. Variations in chromosome number have been dramatically used in some varieties of plants, but are usually lethal in animals probably because of the high proportion of lethal genes and the low reproductive rates of most animal species.

Implications of Variation

Environmental Variation

Variation due to non-genetic effect are not transmitted to offspring. These variations have long been sources of frustration to breeders. Two types of environmental variation are involved:

1. Non-random
2. Random

Non-random environmental variations are those which are constant from one animal to the next in the same group. Examples of non-random environmental variations are those which result from climate, level of feeding, husbandry practices, or other influences which affect all animals in the same group. The presence of these differences is often known, but their influence usually is not. For example, in dairy cattle it is known that feeding level greatly influences milk production. The breeder often needs to know whether the cows in a certain well fed herd are genetically superior to those in another herd which are fed poorly. To rephrase the question, the purchaser wants to know from which herd he should purchase cows to get those which will perform best in his herd. He knows that the higher average yield in the well fed herd is partly due to feeding level, but he does not know how well cows from the poorly fed herd would have performed had they been in the well fed herd. The problem of known non-genetic effects is not limited to between herd comparisons, as records in the same herd but by cows calving in different seasons, years or at different ages are also difficult to evaluate because of non-random environmental effects.

Random environmental effects are those which influence individual records of animals but are not constant for all individuals being compared. Examples are lameness, minor infections, social dominance, and chance accidents. In general, random environmental influences are those which might produce differences between identical twins raised together in the same pen. These random non-genetic influences cause a large share of the total variation for many quantitative traits and often their causes are not recorded or even known. If these influences are truly random they have two important properties:

1. A good genotype is equally likely to be associated with a good or bad set of random environmental influences. This means that, on the average, the best phenotypes will have the best genotypes.
2. If several records are averaged, the favourable environment of some records cancels the unfavourable environment of others. This means that random environmental effects becomes less important as more records are included in each average. If the number of records in each average becomes large enough the difference between averages will include only genetic and non-random environmental differences.

Errors in choosing the best genotypes result when the candidates for selection are affected by different environments. If all environmental effects are random, these mistakes reduce the efficiency of selection, but the selected group is genetically superior to those rejected. However, if one group receives a consistently better environment than another, the selected animals will always be from the group with the better environment unless:

1. Adjustment is made for the effect of the environment.
2. The genetic difference between animals is greater than the difference in environmental effects.

Environmental iufluences can be reduced in several ways:

1. Make the environment as uniform as possible for all candidates for selection. This will reduce errors, but many environmental effects cannot be controlled.
2. Adjust for known environmental influences. Adjustment for influences such as season or age can sometimes be based on their effect on previous records on animals of similar genetic merit.
3. Obtain additional records on each animal since random environmental effects are usually not repeated.
4. Choose the best individuals within similar environments. For example, choose one or a few of the best individuals from each herd rather than all individuals from the "best" herd.
5. Try to discover the environmental conditions which influenced each record.

Implication of Genetic Variation in Breeding Programme

Recombination of genes during transmission from one generation to the next introduces the elements of chance into breeding programmes. The chance recombinations of genes produce characteristic distributions of progeny when large numbers of progeny are obtained from the same parents, but the results of individual matings can be predicted with certainty in only a few simple cases. Recombination of genes for quantitative traits produces some progeny which are far superior to their parents and others which are distinctly inferior, but the majority of progeny are not greatly different from the average of their parents for quantitative traits.

If dominance, epistasis, or random environmental influences have affected the phenotype, the progeny will tend to average nearer to the group average than their parents. This is very important because it means that only a portion of the superiority of outstanding individuals will be transmitted to the progeny. Outstanding individuals should be used for parents, however, because their progeny will average better than the progeny of any other parents.

Relationship of Reproductive Rate to Selection Intensity

The amount of selection which can be practised is limited. In selecting foundation or replacement breeding stock from outside the herd there are many candidates from which to choose but accuracy of selection is very low due to the diverse non-genetic influences which affect their performance. Within the herd the amount of selection which can be practised is limited by:

1. The reproductive rate
2. The success in raising replacements

The reproductive rate is usually the factor which limits the intensity of selection. For example, an average cow gives birth to about 5 calves (2.5 heifer calves) during her lifetime. To maintain a constant population size each cow must, on the average, leave one female progeny. This means that two heifers from every five born must be saved to be replacements for the breeding herd. This is very low compared with poultry where each hen may produce 100 to 300 eggs. If all her eggs are fertilised and incubated a hen may produce upwards of 40 female progeny from which one must be selected to replace her mother. If the productive rate is high, we can get many progeny from a few highly selected parents, whereas low reproductive rates prevent intense selection because almost all progeny must be used for breeding.

The reproductive rate places a limit beyond which selection intensity cannot increase. However, selection intensity is further restricted by failure to raise all progeny through either death or sale of progeny before they reach sexual maturity.

Females of the species of farm livestock generally have low reproduction rates. Cattle, buffalo and horses usually produce one offspring per year, sheep and goats usually have 1, 2 or 3 progeny each year, and swine often produce 10 progeny twice in a year. These rates are low relative to poultry which produce 100 or more progeny per year and many plants which produce several hundred seeds.

Males, however, generally have much higher reproductive rates than females for species of farm livestock. One male can usually service at least 20-30 females and, by use of artificial insemination, several thousand progeny may be obtained from a single sire in a year. Selection of superior sires is particularly important because each sire leaves many progeny relative to the few progeny of each female.

CHOOSING TRAITS FOR SELECTION

Many factors enter into the choice of traits to be selected for. The following are among the most important:

1. The goal of the selection programme
2. The heritability of the traits
3. The economic value of improvement in each trait
4. The range in variation of expression of each trait
5. Correlation among the traits
6. The cost of the selection programme

A. Selection Goals

Often the goal of the selection programme makes the choice of traits quite obvious. The breeder of the race horses must select for speed if he is to be successful and his choices of traits are limited to alternative ways to measure speed. Similarly, the breeder of dairy cattle may set out to breed cows with superior milk production and not be concerned with any other characteristics of his cows, thus his choice of traits is specified by his selection goals.

The more usual case, however, is for the selection goals to be less definite, such as "to breed a more profitable animal". Consider the case of dairy cattle where primary income is derived from the sale of milk. Obviously increased milk production must receive primary emphasis in a selection programme. However, some cows require far more feed per litre of milk produced than others. Some cows do not breed regularly, are susceptible to mastitis, are difficult to milk, have poor conformation, produce undesirable meat, or are otherwise unprofitable. How much emphasis should be given to improve these traits? The answer to this question is difficult, but it must be answered before proceeding with a selection programme. A definite goal is a prerequisite for a successful selection programme.

B. Heritability

Heritability (h^2) is defined to be the fraction of the superiority of parents which is, on the average, transmitted to their offspring. For example, suppose a breeder takes an unselected group of mature cattle with average weight of 44.5 kg and divides them into two groups, averaging 48.5 kg and a light group averaging 40 kg. Suppose he then keeps the groups in separate pastures so that the heavy bulls mate only with large cows and small bulls mate only with light weight cows. After mating he intermixes the groups so that their progeny will have the same environment, but he identifies the calves from each group of parents. When the progeny reach maturity he weighs them and finds that progeny from parents in the heavy groups average 47.5 kg whereas progeny from light-weight parents average 42.2 kg. The difference between the parent groups was 8.8 kg whereas the difference between their progeny groups was 5.3 k. thus heritability is 5.3/8.8=6.0 since one-half of the superiority of the heavy parents was transmitted to their progeny. The non-transmittable part of the parent superiority is due to environmental effects and gene interactions.

Recent estimates of heritability for some traits of farm livestock are:

Table 7.2

Heritability Estimates

1. Dairy Cattle

Trait	*Estimate*	*Trait*	*Estimate*
Lactation		Udder cleft	.14
Fat percentage	.55 – .70	Conformation	
Fat yield	.20 - .40	Body capacity	.27
Lactose percentage	.35	Back	.23
Lactose yield	.36	Dairy character	.19
Milk yield (305 day)	.20 - .30	Feet	.11
Protein - lactose - mineral percentage	.50	Fore udder	.21
Protein-lactose-minerals	.20 - .30	Final score	.31
Protein percentage	.50 - .60	Front end	.12
Solids-not-fat percentage	.50 - .60	General appearance	.29
Solids yield (total)	.20 - .30	Head	.10
Milking/udder traits		Hind legs	.15
Average milking rate	.30 - .40	Mammary system	.22
Height of fore udder	.08	Rear udder	.21
Machine-on time	.22	Rump	.25
Milking time	.02 - .30	Stature	.51
Milking yield at 2 min	.35 - .45	Teat placement	.31
Peak flow rate	.35 - .45	Udder support	.21
Percentage milk front quarters	.25 - .35	Mastitis	
Rear udder height	.09	Cell count (log)	.14 .38
Teat diameter	.38	Clinical frequency	0.0 - .38

1. Dairy Cattle (Contd.)

Trait	Estimate	Trait	Estimate
Nature of pathogens	.18	Feed intake (Lactation)	.26
Fertility		Feed intake (31 - 60 days)	.24
Abortion	.05	Feed intake (121 - 150 days)	.22
Calving interval	0.0 - .10	Feed intake (181 - 210 days)	.14
Cystic ovaries	.05	Growth/body size	
Days open	0.0 - .09	Average daily gain	.3 - .5
Gestation length	.50	Birth weight	.40
Nonreturn rate	0.0 - .03	Chest depth	.38
Retained placenta	.16	Chest girth	.36
Services/conception	0.0 - .09	Chest width	.31
Stillbirths	.01 - .08	Feed conversion	.40
Twinning	.11	Heart girth	.40 - .60
Feed efficiency		Mature size	.30 - .50
Feed efficiency (lactation)	.56	Rump length	.37
Feed efficiency (31-60 days)	.44	Width at hips	.38
Feed efficiency (121-150 days)	.44	Wither height	.50 - .70
Feed efficiency (181-210 days)	.34		

2. Poultry

Trait	Estimate	Trait	Estimate
Body weight		Intermediate survivor production	.19
2 wk (embryo)	.18	Long term survivor production	.22
2 wk (male)	.01 - .05	Hen-housed production	
2 wk (female)	.31	Short term	.33
4 wk (male)	.43	Long term	.15
4 wk (female)	.31	Rate of production	
6 wk (male)	.30	Short term	.11
6 wk (female)	.38	Long term	.15
8 wk (male)	.38	Egg mass	.25
8 wk (female)	.39	Sexual maturity	.39
10 wk (male)	.54	Sexual maturity	.39
10 wk (female)	.51	Broodiness	.16
12 wk (female)	.58	Pauses	.10
24 wk (pullets - light)	.57	Persistency	.20
24 wk (pullets - heavy)	.53	Oviposition interval	.59
Mature (hens-light)	.52	Early egg weight	.45
Mature (hens-heavy)	.49	Early egg weight	.57
Weight gain		Mature egg weight	.46
Up to 10 wk (female)	.35	Yolk weight	.43
4-10 wk (male)	.44	Yolk size	.39
Feed consumption		Albumen weight	.38
Up to 10 wk (male)	.73	Blood spots	.13
Up to 10 wk (female)	.87	Specific gravity	.35
Feed efficiency		Egg shape	.35
Up to 10 wk (male)	.14	Shell color	.35
Up to 10 wk (female)	.29	Haugh units	.42
Egg production		Miscellaneous traits	
Shor term, survivor production	.22	Fertility	.02

2. Poultry (Contd.)

Trait	Estimate	Trait	Estimate
Hatchability (percentage)	.09	Breast angle (female)	.40
Hatchability (probit)	.19	Body depth	.19
Hatching time	.49	Keel length	.47
Growing mortality	.02	Shank length	.13
Annual mortality	.08	Shank diameter	.61
Breast width	.17	Dressing percent	.41
Breast angle (male)	.39		

3. Swine

Trait	Estimate
Reproduction	
Birth weight	.09
Number farrowed	.05 - .15
Number weaned	.05 - .15
Weaning weight (pig)	.10 - .20
Age at puberty	.30 - .40
Gestation length	.41
Services per connection	0.0 - .10
Carcass	
Dressing percentage	.25 - .35
Length	.40 - .60
Lion eye area	.40 - .60
Backfat thickness	.40 - .60
Belly thickness	.40 - .60
Percentage lean cuts	.40 - .50
Percentage of shoulder	.47
Carcass score	.46
Performance	
Average daily gain	.25 - .40
Feed/unit gain	.30 - .40
Pig weight (140 - 180 days)	.20 - .30
Pig weight (98 days)	.15
Conformation	
Body length	.45 - .60
Leg length	.65
Number of ribs	.74
Number of nipples	.20 - .40
Type	.38

4. Sheep

Trait	Estimate
Reproduction	
Fecundity	.10 - .30
Semen quality	.05 - .15
Number nipples	.22
Wool characters	
Grease fleece weight	.30 - .60
Clean fleece weight	.30 - .60
Percentage clean yield	.10 - .60
Staple length–weaning	.40 - .50
Staple length – yearling	.40 - .60
Fiber diameter	.20 - .50
Wrinkle score	.20 - .80
Growth	
Birth weight	.10 - .30
Weaning weight	.10 - .30
Yearling weight	.30 - .40
Mature weight	.40 - .60
Rate of gain	.30 - .40
Gain/unit feed	.20 - .40
Visual scores	
Weaning	.10 - .30
Yearling	.10 - .20
Face cover	.40-.60
Carcass	
Weight	.30 - .50
Conformation	.20 - .30
Fatness	.15 - .30
Loin eye area	.20 - .30
Lean yield weight	.30 - .50
Percentage lean	0.0 - .1
Carcass (constant weight)	
Weight/day of age	.30 - .50
Fatness	.40 - .60
Quality grade	.30 - .50
Loin eye area	.30 - .50
Lean yield weight	.25 - .40
Percentage lean	.25 - .40

Source : Handbook of Animal Sc. (1991), Edited by Putman, Academic Press, Inc.

Heritability measures the ability of the trait to respond to selection. Traits with high heritability show a much stronger response to selection than do those with low heritability. In general, reproductive traits usually have low heritability (0.00 to .10), yield (milk, eggs, wool) characters have moderate heritability (.15 to .35), and anatomical measurements usually have moderate to high (.40 to .60) heritability.

Traits with extremely low heritability (such as fertility) are poor risks in a selection programme since most variations are non-transmissible and response to selection will be slow if it occurs at all.

C. Economic Value

The relative economic value of alternative traits is an important consideration in a selection programme. Traits with high economic value often have low heritability, thus, both factors must be considered jointly if we are to make a good choice of traits. Perhaps the best way to compare economic values is to compute the expected response of each trait to specific intensity of selection, then to compare the economic values of the expected responses.

Many traits can be quickly eliminated, however, because they have little or no economic value.

D. Variability of the Trait

Selection operates on the variability in expression of the trait by choosing parents which are above average. Obviously if all animals are quite. uniform for a trait there will be little selection response because any selected group of parents will not be much better than those not selected. Some traits are much more variable than others, thus the innate variation of the traits should be carefully considered in choosing traits for selection.

Variation can be increased by improving exotic types, and sometimes this can result in new combinations of genes which are superior to either parent type.

E. Correlated Traits

Sometimes traits tend to be inherited together. These correlations may arise in several ways.

1. The traits may be of different measures of some underlying trait. For example weight and height are both measures of body size, thus taller animals are usually also heavier and these two traits are said to be correlated.

2. Pleiotrophy. If the same genes produce responses in several traits these traits will be correlated.

3. Linkage. Genes on the same chromosome tend to segregate together causing correlations. In the long run, however, crossing over produces an equilibrium between coupling and repulsion phases, thus correlation due to linkage are transitory.

Correlated responses are common. Selection for increased milk yield produces a correlated decrease in the per cent of fat in the milk of dairy cows. Selection for an increased rate of gain produces a correlated increase in feed efficiency in swine. Thus, both direct and correlated responses result from selection, and some correlated responses are positive while others are negative.

Correlated responses may be used advantageously in a selection programme. For example, feed efficiency is expensive to measure because it requires both weight gain and feed intake on each individual whereas weight gain requires neither feed weight nor individual feeding. The high correlation between rate of gain and feed efficiency causes almost as much correlated improvement in feed efficiency from selection for rate of gain as would be obtained by direct selection for feed efficiency.

Conversely, some correlated responses show slow progress. Egg size and number of eggs produced are negatively correlated, thus selection for more eggs results in smaller eggs whereas selection for larger eggs results in fewer eggs being laid. The breeder would often like to get both larger eggs and more eggs. The optimum combination for selection depends on the market situation and the price differences between large and small eggs. Selection for both more and larger eggs is effective, but is much slower than if they were not negatively correlated.

In summary, definite goals are essential for a successful selection programme. The success in achieving these goals depends on the existence of genetic differences, the degree to which phenotype differences are heritable, and the correlated responses in other traits. In comparing selection programmes the breeder must evaluate the value of the expected response and the cost of the programme relative to the costs and responses of alternative selection programmes.

HOW MANY TRAITS SHOULD BE CONSIDERED IN SELECTION?

Selection intensity is so restricted by the low reproductive rates of farm animals that it is critical that selection intensity be concentrated on a few important traits. Simultaneous selection for several traits reduces the selection intensity for any single trait. It has been shown that if n traits are equally important and independent then the intensity of selection will be $\frac{1}{\sqrt{n}}$, as intense for each trait as if selection were for only one trait. Thus:

Table 7.3

n traits	*Relative intensity*
1	1.00
2	.71
3	.58
4	.50
16	.25
n	$\frac{1}{\sqrt{n}}$

We see that selection for two traits produces response in two traits, but only .71 as much response in each trait as if selection has been for that trait only. From this relationship we can conclude that:

1. Selection for unimportant traits is harmful because it reduces progress in important traits.
2. Primary emphasis should be placed on one or few traits which are economically important and have the capacity to respond.
3. Selection for unimportant traits should take the form of culling only extremely undesirable individuals so that the intensity of selection for important traits will be little affected.

Of course, many traits are correlated (not independent), but this alters the above conclusions only by increasing the emphasis given to traits positively related to economically important trait and decreasing the emphasis on negatively related traits.

The foregoing is not intended to argue that selection should be exclusively for one trait, but that selection should not be wasted on traits which are not heritable or which have low economic value.

DEGREES OF RELATIONSHIP

The relationship between two animals can be defined as the fraction of genes obtained from common ancestors. Two animals may belong to the same breed but their relationship may be zero if they have no common near ancestors. Two animals with identical genotypes have a relationship of 100. They are alike in 100 per cent of genes, e.g., identical twins. The degree of relationship, therefore, ranges from 0 to 100.

Relationship may be of two kinds, direct and collateral. You are directly related to your father, for you are his offspring. That is you and your father have more genes in common (50%) than do unrelated members of the human population. Similarly one half of your genes are indentical with those of your mother. You and your cousins are collateral relatives, because you both have some ancestors in common. Your cousin probably has some identical genes that came to each of you from your common grand parents C and D.

$$\text{You}\begin{cases} A \begin{cases} C \\ D \text{ (Grand parent)} \end{cases} \\ B \end{cases} \qquad \text{Cousin}\begin{cases} Y \text{ (Uncle)} \begin{cases} C \\ D \text{ (Grandparent)} \end{cases} \\ Z \end{cases}$$

The key to measurement of relationship is number of generations between the animals being studied and their common ancestors. The formula for relationship between individuals, say X and Y, is therefore.

$$R_{xy}=\Sigma[(\tfrac{1}{2})^{n+n'}]$$

Σ=Summation of. The contribution of all common ancestors is summed.

$\frac{1}{2}$=the halving sampling process of inheritance in each generation.

n=number of generations between X and the common ancestor or the number of times the halving process has undergone between X and the common ancestor.

n′=number of generations between Y and the common ancestor.

Example:

Relationship between you and your father

$$=(\tfrac{1}{2})^{1+0} \qquad =1/2=50\%$$

There is one generation between you and your father and the genetic meterial has been halved once in getting from your father to you. There is no generation between your father and himself and n′ is therefore 0.

Relationship between son and grandfather (where son = X and grandfather=C) is as below:

$$X\begin{cases} A\begin{cases} D \\ C \end{cases} \\ B \end{cases}$$

Rxc=(1/2) 2+0 =1/4=25%

There being two generations between X and C, n is equal to 2. There is no generation between C and itself, hence n′ is 0. Full brother and sister are 50% related:

$$\text{Brother } X\begin{cases} A \\ B \end{cases} \qquad \text{Sister } Y\begin{cases} A \\ B \end{cases}$$

Rxy is to be determined. First find the number of common ancestors. In this case there are two common ancestors A and B. Then find the relationship through each of them. Then sum the relationships.

Relationship through A = Rxy = $(1/2)^{1+1}$ = 1/4 or 25%

Relationship through B = Rxy = $(1/2)^{1+1}$ = 1/4 or 25%

Sum of relationship = 50%

Therefore Rxy = 50%

A simplified form of expressing the pedigree and measurement relationship where there are two or more common ancestors is as follows:

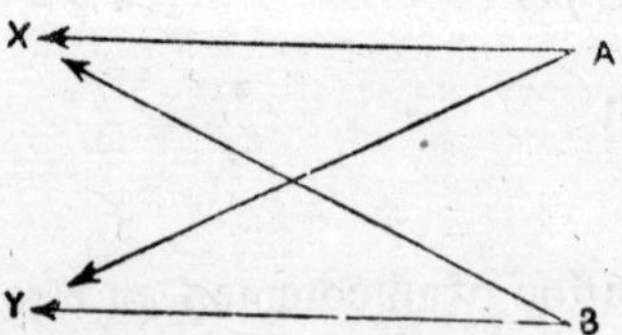

Pedigree of full brother and sister.

In this each arrow indicates one generation. By counting the number of arrows from the common ancestors to each of the individuals it is easy to find out n and n′. The results may be tabulated as follows:

Relationship between X and Y

Common Ancestors (C.A.)	n	n′	Contribution
A	1	1	$(1/2)^2$: .25
B	1	1	$(1/2)^2$: .25
		Sum of relationship=	.50

First cousins are related 12.5 per cent.

$$X\begin{cases}A\begin{cases}C\\D\end{cases}\\B\end{cases}\qquad Y\begin{cases}Z\begin{cases}C\\D\end{cases}\\S\end{cases}$$

Relationship between X and Y

C.A.	n	n′		Contribution
C	2	2	$(1/2)^4$	6.25%
D	2	2	$(1/2)^4$	6.25%
				RXY=12.50%

The figure 12.5 per cent means that X and Y probably have 1/8 or 12.5 per cent more identical genes than unrelated animals of their species and breed.

Half first cousins are related 6.25 per cent.

$$X\begin{cases}A\begin{cases}C\\B\end{cases}\\B\end{cases}\qquad Y\begin{cases}E\begin{cases}C\\H\end{cases}\\F\end{cases}$$

C.A.	n	n′	Contribution
C	2	$2(1/2)^4$	6.25%

Double first cousins are 25 per cent relation.

A { C { M, N ; D { O, P   B { F { M, N ; E { P

Applying the relationship formula, we have the relationship through M = $(1/2)^4$ and the same from N, O and P, so that the summation for all four is 4X $(1/2)^4$ = 25%.

Simultaneous direct and collateral relationship.

D { E { B, C ; F { B, H   E { B, C

In this pedigree D and E are related both directly and collaterally. E is the ancestor (sire) of D (direct). B is an ancestor of D through F and E collaterally.

C.A.	n	n'	Contribution
E	1	0	$(1/2)^1$: 50 %
B	2	1	$(1/2)^3$: 12.5%
		RDE = Sum	: 62.5%

Coefficient of Inbreeding

When animals which are related, in other words those having genes in common, are mated more homozygosity results in the offspring in relation to average animals of the same breed in the foundation stock. Inbreeding, therefore, increases homozygosity and decreases the heterozygosity in individuals.

The average percentage increase in homozygosity or decrease in heterozygosity in an inbred animal in relation to an average animal of the same breed of the foundation stock is known as the 'coefficient of inbreeding". It is obtained by multiplying the relationship among parents, i.e., Rxy by 1/2; since the new generation produced is once further removed from the common ancestors and a further halving of the genetic material occurs. The formula for the coefficient of inbreeding of individual (Fx) is

$$Fx = [\Sigma (\tfrac{1}{2})^{n+n'1}]$$

n = number of generations or halving from the sire to the common ancestor.

n' = number of generations from the dam to the common ancestor.

Σ = summation of.

Examples:

Full brother or sister mating:

$$X \begin{cases} A \begin{cases} C \\ D \end{cases} \\ B \begin{cases} C \\ D \end{cases} \end{cases}$$

C.A.	n	n′	Contribution
C	1	1	$(1/2)^{1+1+1} = 12.5\%$
D	1	1	$(1/2)^{1+1+1} = 12.5\%$
			$F_x = 25.0\%$

Parent and offspring mating is the same as full brother and sister mating:

$$X \begin{cases} A \\ B \begin{cases} A \\ C \end{cases} \end{cases}$$

$$Fx = (1/2)^{0+1+1} = (1/2)^2 = 25\%$$

Half brother and sister mating:

$$X \begin{cases} B \begin{cases} D \\ E \end{cases} \\ C \begin{cases} D \\ F \end{cases} \end{cases}$$

D is the only common ancestor to the parents of X; Hence

$$Fx = (1/2)^{0+1+1} = (\tfrac{1}{2})^2 \; 12.5\%$$

What does this figure 12.5% mean ? The animal X is 12.5 per cent less heterozygous than an average animal in the herd which is unrelated. Suppose the animals D, E and F are 50 per cent homozygous (i.e., 50 per cent heterozygous). The animal X is 12.5 per cent less heterozygous or 50 per cent of 12.5 = 6.25 less heterozygous than 50 per cent. In other words, the animal X will be only 43.75 per cent heterozygous.

SYSTEMS OF BREEDING

The aim of the breeders, as stated in the beginning of the chapter, is to evolve outstanding and improved types of animals which can render better service to man. Selection and system of breeding constitute the only tools available to the breeder for improvement of animals, since new genes cannot be created, though they can recombine into more desirable groupings.

Systems of breeding have been broadly divided as under:

1. Inbreeding: Breeding of the related animals.
2. Outbreeding: Breeding of the unrelated animals.

Inbreeding

This means the mating of related individuals. Each animal has two parents, four grandparents, eight great grandparents biologically and so on, having 1,024 ancestors in the 10th generation and 10,48,576 ancestors in the 20th generation. Relationship, therefore, becomes a vague term and must be specified. So in order to be more specific we should say that inbreeding involves the mating of related individuals within 4-6 generations. It has also been defined as the mating of the more closely related individuals than the average of the population.

Inbreeding can again be divided into following groups

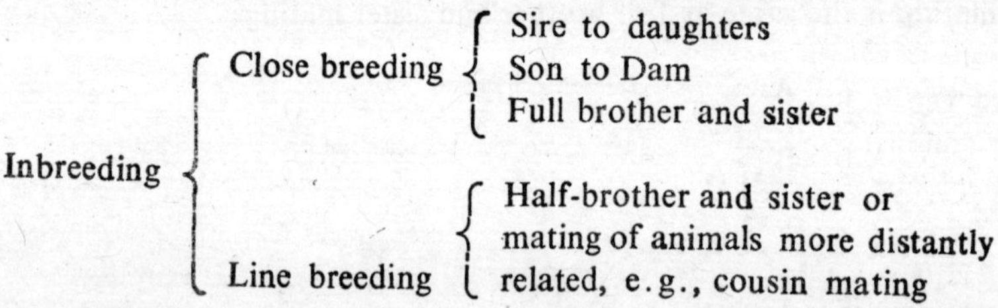

Close Breeding

This means the mating of full sister to full brother or sire to his daughter or dam to her son. These types of matings should be used only when both parents are outstanding individuals, and then only at increased risk of bringing undesirable recessive genes into homozygous form in the progeny.

Advantages of Close Breeding

1. Undesirable recessive genes may be discovered and eliminated by further testing in this line.
2. The progeny are more uniform than outbred progeny.

Disadvantages

1. The undesirable characteristics are intensified in the progeny if unfavourable gene segregation occurs.
2. It has been observed that the progeny becomes more susceptible to diseases.
3. Breeding problems and reproductive failure usually increase.
4. It is difficult to find out the stage of breeding at which it should be discontinued in order to avoid the bad effects of the system.

Line breeding

This means the mating of animals of wider degrees of relationship than those selected for close breeding. It promotes uniformity in the character. Homozygosity is not reached so quickly as in close breeding. Neither desirable nor harmful characters are developed so quickly.

It is a slowed method for the fixation of hereditary outstanding bull or cow and the progeny is mentioned as being line bred to certain ancestors.

Advantages of Line Breeding

1. Increased uniformity.
2. The dangers involved in close breeding can be reduced.

Disadvantages of Line Breeding

1. The chief danger in line breeding is that the breeder will select the animal for pedigree giving no consideration to real individual merit. This may in some cases result in a few generations which receive no benefits from selection.

Consequences of Inbreeding in General

The effects of both close breeding and line breeding are similar. The only difference is in the degree of their intensity. They are more intense in close breeding and less so in line breeding. These may be described as follows:

1. It increases homozygosity (like alleles) and decreases heterozygosity (dissimilar genes) and hence favours the development of genetic uniformity amongst the animals.
2. It is the best method of getting true strains from unknown stocks as it sorts out the characters in the homozygous condition and thus help in the selection of the desirable and culling of the undesirable individuals. Strains which breed true are not obtained in animals, however, and in plants are obtained only when close inbreeding is accompanied by intense selection.
3. The outward effects of inbreeding may include the following.

(*i*) *Effect on growth rate.* With the exception of a few laboratory animals some moderate decrease in growth rate and mature weight have been noted. The studies on rats on the other hand have shown that they withstand inbreeding (up to 100 generations over 40 years) without any apparent bad effect on growth rate. The reproductive rate of rats is very high, however, relative to farm stock.

(*ii*) *Effect on reproductive performance.* In almost all the cases a reduction in the reproductive efficiency has been noted. It may delay testicular development and puberty, reduce gametogenesis or increase the embryonic death rate.

(*iii*) *Effect on vigour.* It has been noted that the death rates among the inbred groups of animals are higher than those in outbred ones. They are also adversely affected by environmental conditions. They have higher percentages of *Runs* (animals which are undesirable due to variety of reasons).

(*iv*) *Effect on production.* Productive traits usually show moderate decrease with increased inbreeding.

(*v*) *Appearance of lethals and abnormalities.* Hereditary abnormalities or lethal factors are likely to appear more often in the inbred animals than in the outbred ones.

Of the two components of inbreeding, i.e., close breeding and line breeding, it is safer to go in for the latter one. A few recommendations have also been made with regard to them.

It is recommended for the seedstock breeds in the following situations:

1. Better than average herds.

2. If the owner is well informed regarding both its possibilities and pitfalls.
3. Herds with two or more sires to keep the inbreeding level under control and not allowing it to rise to dangerous levels.
4. For some experimental purposes.

It is further recommended that the herds of the following types should never be subjected to inbreeding:

1. The grade or commercial herds.
2. Poor herds below average.
3. Herds with one sire and where the owner has got no knowledge about genetics.

Inbreeding is useful if we want to evolve a more uniform line in any animal species. A line is often desirable for scientific purpose when animals or plants from a number of lines can be mated to get a breed with many desirable qualities. However, that is the job of a scientist or precisely of a geneticist. A fine line of animals may not be commercially profitable at all. A farmer is, therefore, advised not to conduct this experiment in breeding unless he knows genetics.

Out-breeding

Out-breeding is the breeding of unrelated animals and this involves the following types of breeding:

1. Out-crossing
2. Cross breeding ⟶ { 1. Criss-crossing; 2. Triple crossing; 3. Back crossing }
3. Species Hybridization
4. Grading-up

Out-Crossing

It consists in the practice of mating of unrelated pure bred animals within the same breed. The animals mated have no common ancestors on either side of their pedigree upto 4–6 generations and the offspring of such a mating is known as the out-cross.

Advantages

1. This method is highly effective for characters that are largely under the control of genes with additive effects, e.g., milk production, growth rate in beef cattle, etc.
2. It is an effective system for genetic improvement if carefully combined with selection.
3. It is the best method for most herds.

Cross breeding

It is the mating of animals of different breeds. It is generally used where the crossed progeny is directly marketed and are not needed for breeding and further multiplications. It has become quite common in pigs and in the production of hybrid chickens. With beef cattle also it is practised to a certain extent. Cross breeding for milk production has been tried with varying degrees of success. It is generally used for the production of new breeds.

Methods of Cross breeding

1. *Criss-crossing.* When the two breeds are crossed alternatively, the method is known as criss-crossing. This method is proposed for utilising heterosis in both dams and progeny.

Breed A females are crossed with breed B sires. The cross-bred females are mated back to sires of breed A and so on. In this system the cross breeds soon come to have about 2/3 of their inheritance from the breed of their immediate sire with 1/3 from the breed being used.

A } A 50
B } B 50
A } A 75, B 25
B } A 37.5, B 62.5
A } A 68.5, B 31.5

2. *Triple crossing.* In this system three breeds are crossed in a rotational manner. It is also known as rotational crossing.

Three breeds are used in this system. The females of crosses are used on a sire of pure breeds in rotation. The crossbreds will soon come to have 4/7 of inheritance of the breed of the immediate sire, 2/7 from the breed of maternal grand-size and 1/7 of the hereditary material of the other pure breed.

A } A 50
B } B 50
C } A 25, B 25, C 50
A } A 63, B 12, C 25
B } A 31, B 57, C 12
C } A 15, B 28, C 57
A } A 58, B 14, C 28
B } A 28, B 58, C 14

3. *Back crossing.* Back crossing is mating of a crossbred animal back to one of the pure parent races which were used to produce it. It is commonly used in genetic studies, but not widely used by breeders. When one of the parents possesses all or most of the received traits, the back cross permits a surer analysis of the genetic situation than F_2 does.

A heterozygous individual of the F_1 when crossed with a member of the homozygous recessive parent race, the offsprings group themselves into a phenotypic ratio of 1 : 1; if on the other hand, the individual of the parent race were to be homozygous dominant all the offsprings will be phenotypically alike.

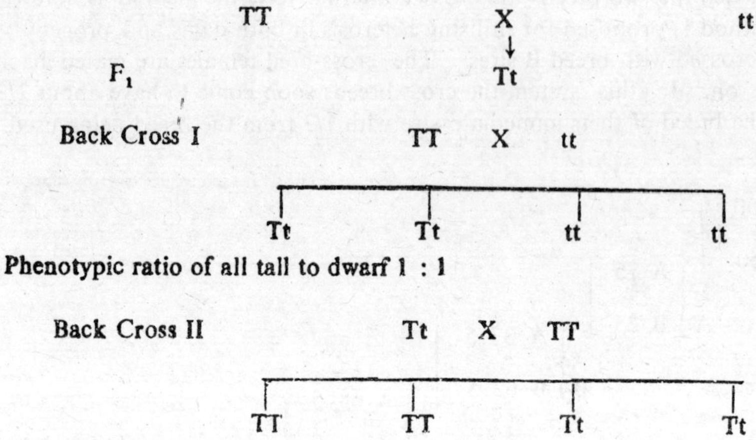

Phenotypic ratio of all tall to dwarf 1 : 1

Back Cross II Tt X TT

TT TT Tt Tt

All being tall, there is no ratio of tall to dwarf.

Advantages of Cross breeding

1. It is valuable as a means of introducing desirable characters into a breed in which they have not existed formerly.

2. It serves a good purpose in evolving a new breed owing to the fact that it disturbs the balance and brings about recombination in the germ plasm to cause variations. Selection can then fix the favourable variations in the population.

3. It is an extremely handy tool to study the behaviour of characteristics in hereditary transmission.

4. The cross-bred animals usually exhibit an accelerated growth and vigour or heterosis, which means the blending of desirable dominant genes from two breeds in the first generation. Such animals are more thrifty than either of the parents; they grow rapidly, produce more milk, wool, eggs, etc., than would be expected from their pedigree. The productive traits usually show the greatest improvement from cross breeding.

Disadvantages of Cross breeding

1. The breeding merit of crossbred animals may be slightly reduced because of the heterozygous nature of their genetic composition, and the fact that all animals transmit only a sample half of their own genetic meterials to their offspring. This may otherwise be explained that crossing has a tendency to break up established characters and destroy combinations of characters which have long existed in the strains and which, under the system of pure breeding, have long existed in the strains and behaved in a manner like unit characters in transmission.

2. Cross breeding requires maintenance of two or more pure breeds in order to produce the crossbreds which undoubtedly involved a considerable investment as rapid progress need not be expected in any line of breeding unless sufficient numbers can be kept to allow for rigid selection.

Chromosome Numbers and Reproductive Ability in Equine, Bovine and Caprine Hybrids

Species and Chromosome Number (2N) Sire	X	Dam	*Hybrids Chromosome Number (2N)*	*Reproductive Ability*
Ass (donkey), 62 *(E. Asinus)*		Domestic horse, 64 *(E. caballus)*	63 (Mule)	Sterile
Domestic horse, 64 *(E. caballus)*		Ass. (DonkeY), 62 *(E. asinus)*	63 (Hinny)	Males are sterile, females are fertile, only in very exceptional cases
Grevy zebra, 46 *(E. Grevyi)*		Domestic horse, 64 *(E. caballus)*	55 (Zebroid)	Sterile
African zebra, 44 *(E. burchelli)*		Ass (Donkey), 62 (E. asinus)	53 (Zebronkey)	Sterile
Ass (Donkey), 62 *(E. asinus)*		(Mountain zebra, 34 (?) *(E. zebra)*	48	Sterile
American bison, 60 *(Bison bison)*		Zebu, 60 *(Bos indicus)*	60	Females are fertile
American bison, 60 *(Bison bison)*		Domestic cattle, 60 *(Bos taurus)*	60 (Cattalo)	Male F, are sterile
Domestic cattle, 60 *(Bos taurus)*		American bison, 60 *(Bison bison)*	60 (Cattalo)	Male F, are sterile
Domestic goat, 60 *(Capra hircus)*		Barbary sheep, 58 *(Ammotragus lorvia)*	59 (?)	Full-term fetuses, but no live hybrid
Domestic goat, 60 *(Capra hircus)*		Domestic sheep, 54 *(Ovis aries)*	57	Embryos are resorbed or aborted at six weeks pregnancy

Heterosis or Hybrid Vigour

Heterosis or Hybrid vigour is a phenomenon in which the crosses of unrelated individuals often result in progeny with increased vigour much above their parents. The progeny may be from the crossing of strains, breeds, varieties, or species. One of the explanations for this increased vigour is that genes favourable to reproduction are usually dominant over their opposites. As a species or breed develops, it becomes homozygous for some dominant genes, but some undesirable genes are also present at high frequencies. When one breed is crossed with the other, one parent supplies a favourable dominant gene to offset the recessive one supplied by the other and vice versa.

(1)

The dominance theory of heterosis. Hybrid vigor is presumed to result from the action and interaction of dominant growth or fitness factor.

Example :

Assume that four loci are contributing to a quantitative trait. Each recessive genotype contributes one unit to the phenotype and each dominant genotype contributes two units to the phenotype. A cross between two inbred lines could produce a more highly productive (heterotic) F_1 than either parental line.

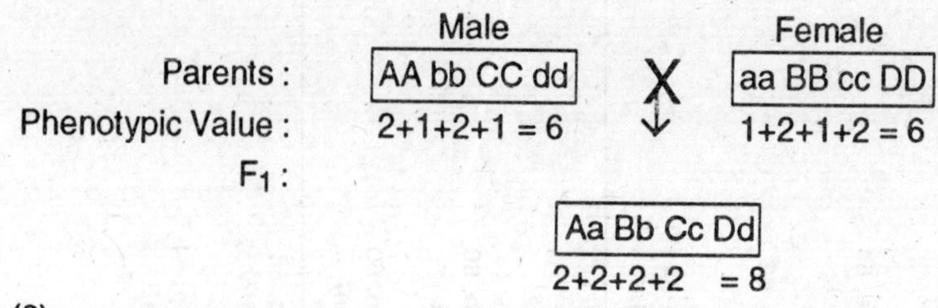

(2)

The overdominance theory of heterosis. heterozygoisty per se is assumed to produce hybrid vigor.

Example :

Assume that four loci are contributing to a quantitative trait, recessive genotypes contribute 1 units, to the phenotype, heterozygous genotypes contribute 2 units, and homozygous dominant genotypes contribute $1^1/_2$ units.

	Male		Female
Parents :	aa bb CC DD	X	AA BB cc dd
Phenotypic Value:	$1 + 1 + 1^1/_2 + 1^1/_2 = 5$		$1^1/_2 + 1^1/_2 + 1 + 1 = 5$
F_1:			

Aa Bb Cc Dd

2+2+2+2 = 8

The offspring, therefore, has a larger number of loci with dominant genotypes than does either parent and is likely to be more vigorous.

Another explanation for hybrid vigour is overdominance, where the heterozygous condition (Aa) is superior to either homozygous condition (aa or AA).

Heterosis is employed to produce commercial stocks with high individual merit. The successful exploitation of heterosis depends upon how superior the crosses are over the pure bred, and the cost of replacement of pure bred stock. For these reasons it is more commonly practised in poultry, swine, and sheep among whom fertility is high and the cost of replacement of pure bred stock is likely to be low. There is no advantage to cross breeding, however, if one parent line of breed is better than the crossbred progeny.

Grading Up

Grading is the practice of breeding sires of a given breed to non-descript females and their offspring for generation after generation.

Explanation of Grading

It is evident from the above definition that grading up is the successive use of purebred bulls of a certain breed of non-purebred herds. The continued use of good purebred sires for only a few generations are all that are required to bring the herd to the point at which it has all the appearance, actions, and practical value of pure breeds. The following Table shows the rapidity with which purebred sires will change the genetic composition of the non-descript one.

	Offspring	
	Per cent replaced	Per cent non-descript
1st Generation	50	50
2nd ,,	75	25
3rd ,,	87.5	12.5
4th ,,	93.75	6.25
5th ,,	96.87	3.13
6th ,,	98.44	1.56
7th ,,	99.22	0.78

From the above Table, we can see that the offsprings come closer to a 100 per cent improved breed, as we go on grading. Grading is a process by which a few purebred sires can rather quickly transform a non-descriptive population into a group of pure breeds. The grading process does not create anything new but it may transfer the good qualities of an improved breed.

For a grading up programme it is advisable to use a breed that has thrived well under local conditions. Otherwise graded animals may not adapt themselves to the local environment.

Advantages of Grading

1. Purebreds can be obtained just after a few generations (after 7th to 8th generations).
2. The start can be made with a little money in comparison to the purchase of an entire herd of purebreds.
3. It helps to prove the potentialities of the sire and adds to its market value.

4. It is a good start for new breeders who can slowly change over to pure breed systems.

Limitations of Grading

1. Pure breeds are not always better than grade or country animals for the use to be made of them.

2. Pure breed stocks which give good results in one set of environmental conditions do not always give favourable results in some different environmental set-up. The pure breed dairy cattle from temperate zones often degenerate when used in tropical areas. Moreover, their offspring fails to show vigour and constitution for high reprodution. To make grading successful, the pure breed must have the ability to perform under the environmental set-up where their offspring is going to perform.

SELECTION METHODS

There is only one way to select and that is to "keep the best and cull the poorest". The various selection methods are techniques for identifying or estimating the genetic values of individual candidates for selection. The procedure discussed here apply to selection for quantitative traits.

A. Performance Testing

A performance test is a measure of the phenotypic value of the individual candidate for selection. Since the phenotypic value is determined by both genetic and environmental influences the performance test is an estimate, not a measure of the genetic value. The accuracy of this estimate depends on the heritability of the trait, i.e., on the degree to which the genetic value is modified by the environmental influences. If heritability is 1.00 or if environmental effects are completely removed (usually impossible) the performance test is an exact measure of the genetic value. If non-random environmental effects are removed the phenotype is an unbiased estimate of the genetic value because the random environmental effects are equally likely to be positive or negative.

Advantages of Performance Test

a. High accuracy. Among simple procedures the performance test is the most accurate. Among more complex procedures performance records must usually be included to obtain near maximum accuracy.
b. Environmental influences can be minimised by testing candidates for selection in the same pen or in similar environmental conditions.
c. The measure is direct, not on a relative basis.
d. All candidates for selection can be tested in contrast to progeny testing where only a few parents can be tested, i.e., it allows a high selection differential.
e. Generation intervals are usually short.
f. Testing can usually be done on the farm under normal management conditions.

Disadvantages of Performance Test

a. Accuracy becomes low when heritability is low.
b. Phenotypes are not available for one sex in sex-limited traits such as milk yield or egg production.

c. Traits which are not expressed until maturity may become expensive or difficult to manage by performance tests since most selection decisions must be made before maturity.

Performance tests should be the backbone of most selection programmes. Although much publicity has been given to other selection methods, it remains a fact that most of the progress in livestock improvement to date has been due to selection on the individual's own phenotype (i.e., performance test).

B. Pedigree Selection

Pedigree selection is useful when inadequate information is available about the individual, such as when selection decisions must be made before the individual expressess the trait (carcass merit or mature weight) and when dealing with sex-limited traits (milk yield or maternal ability). If a performance record is available on the individual the addition of pedigree information usually adds little to the accuracy of estimation of the breeding value of the individual.

Pedigree selection is based on the fact that relatives possess many of the same genes, thus an estimate of the breeding value of one animal provides some information about the breeding value of his relatives. In fact, the accuracy of pedigree selection from single relatives is equal to the accuracy of the performance test on the relative multiplied by the fraction of genes this relative has in common (i.e., relationship) with the candidate for selection. Essentially a pedigree evaluation is only an extension of performance testing since each individual is performance tested and performance records are used to evaluate related animals.

In general, estimation of the breeding value of an individual for quantitative traits has low accuray when based on the records of ancestors. This low accuracy is due to both incomplete heritability and to segregation of genes for traits with polygenic inheritance. In addition, ancestor records were usually made several years ago under environmental conditions quite different from those now existing. The value of the pedigree was greatly exaggerated by breeders of the past, although it is very useful when used properly.

Since each progeny obtains one half of its genes from the sire and the other half from the dam, the sire and dam sides of the pedigree should be accorded equal weight. This holds true if there is equal information, but if many more close relatives on one side of the pedigree have records this side should receive more emphasis. This is particularly true if the sire has a large number of progeny with records.

If we evaluate the genetic variation, we find that 25 per cent of the variation among breeding values of full-sibs is "determined" by each parent and the remaining 50 per cent is attributable to the segregation of the genes of the parents during gamete formation. The contribution of each parent to the phenotypic variation, however, is $.25\ h^2$ because the genetic values are modified by the environment (h^2 denotes heritability). If we carry this partitioning back additional generations we find that the fraction of phenotypic variance accounted for by each grandparent is $.0625\ h^2$, by each great-grandparent is $.0156\ h^2$, etc., each generation decreasing to 1/4 of the preceding generation. From this rapid reduction in "accountable" genetic variation as we go furthes back in the pedigree, we see that, although all of the progeny genes are descended from the distant ancestors, the segregation of genes during each generation of gamete formation has so mixed up the genes that most genetic variation is due to recombination, and that the descendants closely resemble only very close relatives.

When unequal information is available on the various candidates for selection, it becomes difficult to know how much emphasis is to give to each kind of record. For example, we wish to choose one herd replacement from two candidates; candidate A has been performance tested sire. The best available method is to compute the index:

$$I=b_1(X_1-\overline{X})+b_2(X_2-\overline{X})+\ldots+b_i(X_i-\overline{X})$$

where b_1 is a weight for the first type of record, b_2 is a weight for the second type of record, etc. X_1 is a phenotypic record on the first type of relative, X_2 is a phenotypic record on the second type of record, and $\overline{X}$ is the population (or herd) phenotypic average. By this method the animals with the highest indexes should be selected since they have the best chance to be genetically "best". The weights (b_i) depend on:

1. Heritability
2. The relatives which have records available.

When one record on the relative is available the weight for this record is:

$$b=Rh^2$$

where h^2 is heritability and R is the relationship between the relative that made the record and the candidate of selection. Thus if candidate A has a record (X_A) on his dam and candidate B has a record (X_B) on his granddam their respective indexes would be:

$$I_A=.5h^2(X_A-\overline{X})$$

$$I_B=.25h^2(X_B-\overline{X})$$

Candidate A would be chosen if I_A is greater that I_B and candidate B would be chosen if I_B is greater than I_A. Note that the weights are directly proportional to the relationships, thus giving much more emphasis to close relatives. Also, performance tests fit directly into this index since the relationship of an individual with itself is 1.0.

When there are several sources of information about the same candidate, the weights to combine information are more difficult to compute because some information is "duplicated". For example, if we have a record on the dam and a record on the maternal granddam, we must reduce the weights somewhat because the maternal granddam transmits her genes only through the dam. If heritability were 1.0 the weight for the granddam would be zero, but if heritability is less than 1.0 the granddam does contribute some information about the genetic value of the candidate in addition to that from the dam's phenotype. In general, however, the weights for ancestors are considerably reduced if a closer relative also has a record available. The weights for some frequent combinations of records are listed in Table 7.4. To illustrate the use of Table 28, suppose we wish to choose the prospective herd sire which will best improve weaning weight from two candidates (A and B) in the same herd. The pedigrees for the two candidates are:

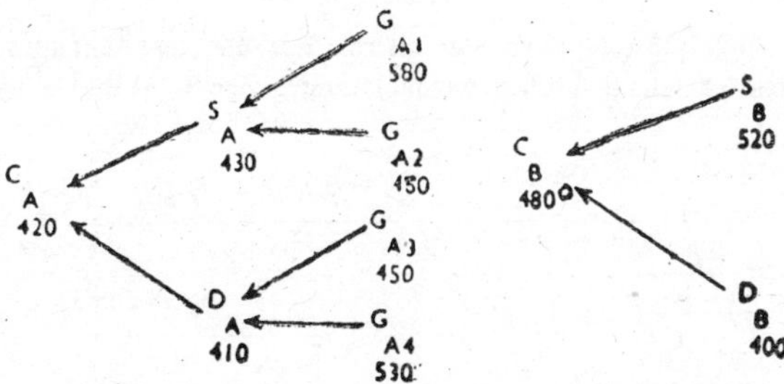

The herd average weaning weight (H) for this herd has remained constant at 400 pounds for several years. The heritability of weaning weight is about .35, thus the index equations would be:

$$I_A = b_C (C_A - H) + b_S (S_A - H) + b_D (D_A - H) + b_1 (G_{A2} - H)$$
$$+ b_2 (G_{A2} - H) + b_3 (G_{A3} - H) + b_4 (G_{A1} - H)$$
$$= .26\,(420-400) + .10\,(30) + .10\,(10) + .04\,(180) + .04\,(60) + .04\,(50) + .04\,(130)$$
$$= 26.0$$

$$I_B = b_C (C_B - H) + b_S (S_B - H)\ b_D (D_B - H)$$
$$= .27\,(480-400) + .11\,(520-400) + .11\,(400-400)$$
$$= 34.8$$

Thus, candidate B would be chosen on the basis of fewer records because his own record and his sire's record are high whereas the high records behind candidate A were made by more distant relatives. If the records were made in different herds it would be necessary to substitute the appropriate contemporary herd average for H for each record.

Several principles will be clear from examination of Table 7.4.

a. The emphasis given to relatives falls off rapidly as the relationship becomes less.
b. Distant relatives are much more important when records on close relatives are not available.
c. Distant relatives add little information when close relatives have records.
d. Selection accuracy increases as heritability increases.
e. Information on relatives is more important when heritability is low.
f. Adding information on additional relatives always increases accuracy, provided they are weighted properly.

Advantages of Pedigree Selection

a. It provides information when performance tests are not available for the candidates.
b. It provides information to supplement performance test information.
c. It allows selection to be completed at a young age. Pedigree records may be used to select animals for performance or progeny testing in a multi-stage selection scheme.
d. It allows selection of both sexes for sex limited traits; i.e., bulls can be selected on the milk records of their female relatives.

Table 7.4

Weighting factors for single phenotypic records on relatives for constructions of selection indexes to compare candidates for selection when unequal information is available on the candidates

Individuals with records	*Selection Index Weights*							
	Candidate	*Parents*		*Grand parents*				*Accuracy**
	b_C	b_D	b_S	b_1	b_2	b_3	b_4	
Heritability = .20								
C	.20							.45
C+P	.19	.08						.48
C+S+D	.18	.08	.08					.51
C+S+D+4GP	.177	.076	.076	0.33	0.33	.033	.033	.53
P		.10						.22
S+D		.10	.10					.32
S+D+4GP		.09	.09	.04	.04	.04	.04	.36
GP				.05				.11
4GP				.05	.05	.05	.05	.22
Heritability = 30								
C	.30							.55
C+P	.28	.11						.58
C+S+D	.27	.11	.11					.61
C+S+D+4GP	.26	.10	.10	.04	.04	.04	.04	.63
P		.15						.27
S+D		.15	.15					.39
S+D+4GP		.13	.13	.06	.06	.06	.06	.44
GP				.075				.14
4GP				.075	.075	.075	.075	.27
Heritability = .50								
C	.50							.71
C+P	.47	.13						.73
C+S+D	.43	.14	.14					.76
C+S+D+4GP	.42	.125	.125	.04	.04	.04	.04	.77
P		.25						.35
S+D		.25	.25					.50
S+D+4GP		.21	.21	.07	.07	.07	.07	.53
GP				.125				.18
4GP				.125	.125	.125	.125	.35

Symbols

b_i is the index weight of a single record on relative i for relative i
C is the candidate for selection
S is the sire of C
D is the dam of C
P is a sire, dam, progeny, or full-sib of C
GP is a grandparent or half-sib of C
4GP are the 4 grandparents of C
the grandparents are denoted 1, 2, 3, and 4

*Accuracy is measured as the multiple correlation between the index and the true breeding value for the animals indexed from this information.

Disadvantages of Pedigree Selection

a. Accuracy, relative to alternative selection procedures, is usually low.

b. Too much emphasis on relatives, especially remote relatives, greatly reduces genetic progresss.

c. Progeny of favoured parents are often environmentally favoured.

d. Relatives often make records under quite different environments, thus introducing non-random bases into the selection system.

C. Progeny Testing

Progeny testing is a special form of pedigree evaluation where the parents are chosen on the basis of phenotype performance of their progeny. Of course, this is a two stage selection system because some preliminary selection determines which animals first produce progeny followed by further culling of those which produce poor progeny.

The great appeal of progeny testing is due to the high accuracy which can be obtained when many progeny are obtained. However, a record on one progeny provides equivalent information to that from a record on one parent or a full-sib. It takes 2 to 3 progeny to provide accuracy equivalent to one record on each parent and as heritability increases from zero to .90, it takes from 4 to 31 progeny to provide selection accuracy equivalent to one performance test record on the candidate for selection. However, the selection accuracy increases as more progeny are obtained until perfect accuracy is reached with a large enough number of progeny as shown in Table 7.5. The selection index weights and accuracy are computed from the following equations:

$$I=b(X-H)$$

$$\text{Selection index weight}=b=\frac{2nh^2}{4+(n-1)h^2}$$

$$\text{Accuracy of index}=\sqrt{\frac{nh^2}{4+(n-1)h^2}}$$

=correlation between index value and true genetic merit of the candidate

where, n progeny each have one performance test record

X is the average for the n progeny records

H is the average of contemporary herdmates of progeny

h^2 is heritability

These values are tabulated in Table 7.5

Selection indexes computed as described in this section are directly comparable to those described for performance testing and pedigree evaluation. The weights of 2.0 may seem strange but they result because the average value of progeny is the same as the average of their parents. This means that each parent transmits one-half of its superiority to the progeny, thus twice the progeny superiority equal's this parent's superiority if the other parent is of average value.

Table 7.5

Weights and accuracy of selection index for progeny test of one record on each of a progeny

	Selection index weights					*Accuracy*				
	Heritability					*Heritability*				
Progeny	.1	.2	.3	.5	.75	.1	.2	.3	.5	.75
1	.05	.10	.15	.25	.38	.16	.22	.27	.35	.44
2	.10	.19	.28	.44	.63	.22	.31	.37	.47	.56
3	.14	.27	.39	.60	.82	.26	.37	.44	.55	.64
4	.19	.35	.49	.73	.96	.31	.42	.49	.61	.69
6	.27	.48	.65	.92	1.16	.37	.49	.57	.68	.76
10	.41	.69	.90	1.18	1.40	.45	.69	.67	.77	.84
20	.68	1.03	1.24	1.48	1.64	.58	.72	.79	.86	.91
50	1.12	1.45	1.60	1.75	1.84	.75	.85	.89	.94	.96
100	1.44	1.68	1.78	1.87	1.92	.95	.92	.94	.97	.98
1,000	1.92	1.96	1.98	1.99	1.99	.98	.99	.99	1.00	1.00
10,000	1.99	2.00	2.00	2.00	2.00	1.00	1.00	1.00	1.00	1.00

To be successful, progeny testing requires a high reproductive rate because :

a. If heritability is high, pedigree and performance testing each produce faster genetic progress.

b. If heritability is low:

   1. Many progeny are needed to obtain an accurate progeny test.
   2. After completing progeny tests large numbers of progeny must be produced from superior parents to offset the progeny of inferior parents obtained during the progeny testing stage.

Advantage of Progeny Testing

a. High accuracy when many progeny are obtained.

Disadvantages of Progeny Testing

a. Long generation interval.

b. Requires high reproductive rate.

c. Few candidates can be tested, thus low selection intensity. To be successful many more parents must be tested than will eventually be used heavily.

3. *Requirement for Successes in a Trogeny Test Programme*
   a. Mates of the tested candidates must be of equal merit.
   b. The average environment of all progeny groups must be the same. This is best done by:
      1. One progeny of each sire per herd.
      2. Progeny from the candidates randomly distributed among pens or herds. Definitely do not put all progeny of a parent in the same pen or herd or in adjacent stalls in the stable.
   c. High reductive rate.
   d. Several to many tested candidates for each one selected for heavy use.

Alternative Methods of Progeny Testing

The selection index method of progeny testing is presented because:

1. It is more accurate.
2. The values are directly comparable with indexes from performance and pedigree records.

Alternative forms of progeny tests have been widely used and will be discussed with a reference to the selection index procedure.

1. *The progeny (or daughter) average.* In this method the candidate whose progeny have the highest average is selected. This assumes that:

   a. All parents have an equal number of progeny.
   b. Equivalent environments were provided for all progeny groups.
   c. The mates of each candidate for selection are equal.

When these conditions are met the progeny average is equally as good as the selection index for comparison of progeny tested candidates, but does not allow a progeny tested candidate to be compared with a performance tested candidate. The selection index procedure becomes distinctly superior when some candidates have many more progeny than other candidates.

2. *The daughter-dam comparison.* In this method the sire whose progeny excel their dams by the largest amount are selected. This assumes equal merit of mates of the sires and equal environmental conditions for all records of dams and daughters. Two factors usually make this procedure very ineffective:

   a. Environmental changes—the dams usually make their records at a different time than their daughters, thus large non-random environmental effects usually remain in the daughter dam difference.
   b. The importance of the dam is overemphasised relative to including her in a selection index. Also, when one candidate has many more daughter-dam pairs than another, the procedure is very inefficient. Accurate comparisons of daughter-dam proofs with performance and pedigree records are difficult.

3. *The equal parent index.* This is an extension of the daughter-dam comparison to correct the merit of mates by adding twice the daughter-dam difference to the dam average. This usually provides slight improvement since the major drawbacks of the daughter-dam procedure remain.

4. *The contemporary comparison.* This is more a principle than a selection method. A

contemporary comparison is a comparison of two individuals of the same age which are raised together in the same pen or the same environment. In this situation, differences in performance are due to genetic differences and random environmental influence, thus providing the most accurate possible comparison of genetic values. The selection index uses the principle when all records are expressed as deviations from the contemporary herd or environmental average. Comparisons within a contemporary group are very accurate, but usually we want to combine information on animals from one contemporary group with information on animals in a different contemporary group. When heritability is high it is better to compare performance records directly, but when heritability is low (less than .50) differences between group means are mostly determined by environmental effects and it is usually preferable to express all records as deviations from the contemporary group means. For example, from the data given below if we wish to compare the milk production of the following cows

Table 7.6

Cow	*Cow production*	*Contemporary herd average*	*Contemporary comparison*
A	7,000 lb	6,500 lb	+ 1000
B	6,000 lb	6,500 lb	− 500
C	12,500 lb	11,000 lb	+ 1500
D	9,000 lb	11,000 lb	− 2000

by contemporary comparison the cows would rank C, A, B, D, but on actual records, they would rank C, D, A, B. Obviously the better ranking procedure for herd comparisons depends on how much of the difference between herd averages is due to genetic differences and how much of this difference due to feeding and management. Many studies have shown that most differences between herd averages are environmental if heritability is low.

D. Show Ring Selection

Selection on the basis of show ring performance has had considerable vogue in the past. Essentially this selection has been directed toward bringing the conformation of the animals to some ideal conformation. This improvement has been based on two goals:

1. Improvement of conformation.
2. Correlated response.

Improvement of conformation has economic value because a part of the sale price is determined by the conformation of the individual. The ideal type was chosen so that, in the opinion of the judges, the animal possessing this conformation was most likely to be a profitable producer. In other words, the judges were attempting to stress traits of conformation which are correlated with productive ability.

With the advent of record keeping it was found that direct selection for performance traits resulted in much faster progress than selection via correlated conformation traits. Also, when subjected to intensive study, many of the correlations between performance and show ring traits were found to be of non-genetic origin. If the correlations are of genetic origin, direct selection for performance should improve conformation as well as the reverse situation. The show ring has been a good forum for discussion of what constitutes ideal type and good management and has produced dramatic changes in the conformation of some species. This has resulted primarily from education of the breeders, however, for most animals which are presented in the ring are good and the selection differential among these animals is usually so small as to produce little change.

Advantages

1. It enables breeders to exchange ideas and experiences.
2. It allows comparisons among superior animals both within and between breeds.
3. It allows new breeders to make contact with established breeders.

Disadvantages

1. Emphasis is usually placed on traits of little economic importance.
2. Clever fitting and showmanship can mask defects of various kinds.
3. Differences between exhibited animals are usually small.
4. Conformation and production traits usually have low genetic correlations.

Summary

Performance tests should be the basis of selection programme. Pedigree records, when weighted appropriately, improve the accuracy of selection and are useful for preliminary selection of candidates to be performance of the progeny tested. Progeny tests are useful when the population size is large, the reproductive rate is high and heritability is low.

Choosing Breeding Animals

The future of the herds depends upon the animals saved for breeding. It is often said that the sire is half of the herd because each sire contributes half of his genes to many progeny whereas each cow in the herd transmits half of her genes to only a few progeny. Thus, the following considerations are especially important in selecting herd sires:

A. Choose healthy individuals free from serious genetic defects.

B. Check the reproductive organs. Be sure the testicles are descended. Have your veterinary check semen quality. Buy pregnant females and sires which have been successfully mated if possible. Infertile breeding animals leave few progeny.

C. Choose mature animals if good ones are available.

   1. Top progeny tested parents are the best bet if available.
   2. Parents of demonstrated top performance are next best.
   3. Progeny of outstanding proven parents are next.
   4. Offsprings with poor parents but above average grandparents and other relatives are usually no good prospects.

D. Choose unproven young animals from good parents in preference to below herd average candidates, since those below herd average have been proven to be poor risks as breeding animals.

E. Good proven sires are often available by artificial insemination.

FERTILITY AND BREEDING EFFICIENCY

In animal husbandry there is no more important economic problem than fertility of the animals. The profit that is obtainable through meat, milk, eggs, wool, etc., is dependent on the reproductive efficiency of the farm stock. Unfortunately fertility does not respond well to selection, thus improvement must come from feeding and management (especially health).

Fertility is the ability of an animal to produce large number of living young. This is a relative term; consequently 'high' and 'low fertility' are terms used to describe differences between number of young per litter or differences in the frequencies of pregnancies. This applies to both males and females.

Prolificacy is used to denote whether many or few offsprings result from a given mating or from a certain individual during its lifetime. It is more or less restricted in its application to the female or groups such as breed, strain or herds.

Fecundity is the potential capacity of the female to produce functional ova, regardless of what happens to them after they are produced. For instance, a hen may have high fecundity but her eggs may have low fertility or hatchability. That is, she may lay many eggs, but only a few of those start development if incubated or perhaps only a few of those which start to develop will go far enough to hatch.

The inability to produce any offspring at all is sterility. Either sex may be sterile. It may be temporary for a short period or permanent. It is an absolute term meaning that individual is incapable for the time at least, of producing any young at all. The sterile female is often called a *barren*.

Breeding efficiency measures the reproducing ability of an adult animal. Any true dairyman would be interested to know the breeding efficiency of his herd because of efficient herd management. These findings will definitely bring an impetus among the new dairyman. It is practically impossible to get a herd with a reproductive efficiency of 100 per cent, and so it should be used only as a goal. There are many methods by which breeding efficiency can be measured; some of these are as follows:

1. *The number of services per conception.* The number of services an average cow would require for conception is one of the methods for measuring breeding efficiency of that cow. Workers at Nebraska station in U.S.A. found that under their conditions the number of services required per conception for fertile cows ranged from an average of 1.63 to 1.80 for various groups, but the figure came to 2 services per cow when total services to cows were included. The general rule permits less than 2 services per conception for satisfactory breeding record.

2. *The percentage of non-returns.* This method of measuring breeding efficiency of bulls is very common to most of the Artificial Breeding Associations of U.S.A. A non-return is an animal that has been bred and for which there is no request for another breeding. The method is not exact, since all non-return animals may not necessarily become pregnant. An acceptable record is 70 per cent non-returns upto 60 days after breeding, or 60 per cent non-returns upto 90 days after breeding.

3. *Length of the calving interval.* Finding the breeding efficiency of any cow by this method would be more ideal if the cow calved every 12 months. A fertile herd takes less than 13 months between calving.

4. *Pregnancy period.* This method is more precise in nature. A cow during her productive life must remain pregnant only for 9 months in every year. In such cases, the cow is rated as having 100 per cent breeding efficiency.

Gilmore and others have developed a formula for finding out the reproductive efficiency of dairy animals which is as follows:

$$\text{R.E.} = 12\times \frac{\text{Number of calves born}}{\text{Age of cow (months)} - \text{age at first breeding}} \times 100 \text{ (months)} + 3$$

Factors Affecting Breeding Efficiency

Number of Ova

The first limitation on fertility is the number of functional ova released during each cycle of ovulation. In unipara as the cow, mare, etc., usually a single ovum is released, in sheep one or two and occasionally three, whereas in swine several ova even up to 25 are released in a single ovulation period.

Percentage of Fertilisation

The second limitation on fertility is fertilisation of ova. Failure to be fertilised may result from several causes. The spermatozoa may be few or low in vitality. The service may be either too early or too late, so that the sperms and the eggs do not meet at the right moment, to result in fertilisation. The spermatozoa retain their ability to fertilise for only a few hours after they are released in the female genital tract. If service occurs too early, sperms are dead by the time ova are liberated. In late service the ova must have descended considerably down in the fallopian tube and gets impenetrable by the sperms due to the mucoid coating. In dairy cattle the period of ovulation seems to be 14 hours after the end of heat. Occasionally a given mating produces no results although both the individuals later prove fertile in other matings.

Embryonic Death

From the time of fertilisation till birth, embryonic mortality may occur due to a variety of reasons. Hormone deficiency or imbalance may cause failure of implantation of fertilised ova which die subsequently. Death may occur as a result of lethal genes for which the embryos are homozygous. Other causes may be accidents in development, overcrowding in the uterus, insufficient nutrition, or infections in the uterus. The percentage of those which die between birth and maturity varies greatly with different kinds of animals. This may be due to genetic causes, or bad nutrition or management.

Age of First Pregnancy

Breeding efficiency can be lowered seriously by increasing the age of first breeding. Females bred at a lower age are apt to appear stunted during the first lactation, but their mature size is affected little by their having bred early.

Frequency of Pregnancy

The breeding efficiency can be greatly enhanced by lowering the interval between successive pregnancies. The wise general policy is to breed for the first time at an early age and to rebreed at almost the earliest opportunity after each pregnancy. In this way the lifetime efficiency is increased. Cows can be rebred in 9 to 12 weeks after parturition. Swine breeding programme can be adjusted to raise two litters per year.

Longevity

The length of life of the parent is an important part of breeding efficiency, because the return over feed-cost is greater in increased length of life. Also it affects the possibility of improving the breed. The longer the life of the parents, the smaller the percentage of cows needed for replacement every year.

Twins

Twins as a rule are preferred in animals if they can grow up easily to maturity. Twins, however, are rare in cattle and horses ranging from 0.03 to 1.5 per cent of all births.. In sheep, it is relatively more and variations occur according to breeds. Single lambs are usually larger and grow more rapidly whereas twins give more lamb-meat per ewe. Identical twins, which are a subject of popular interest, are of little practical importance to the breeder.

Twinning

Two kinds of twin calves may be born, 1) identical or monozygotic and 2) non-identical or dizygotic or fraternal twins.

Identical

Twins of this kind originate from the same fertilized egg. After this egg undergoes its first division, the two cells formed separate instead of remaining joined together. Each of the new cells divides in the normal way until a fully developed embryo is formed. Thus the nuclei in the normal body cells of both the calves are identical with the nucleus of the fertilized egg from which they grew. These twins share a common amnion.

Non-identical

Twins of this kind are formed from two separate fertilized eggs. Occasionally two eggs are released from the ovaries simultaneously; each egg is fertilized by one sperm. Each fertilized egg develops into an embryo. Thus the nuclei in the body cells of one calf are completely different from the nuclei in the body cells of the second calf.

Cloning

Cloning in simple terms is production of multiple and identical copies. Cloning of plants is an easy practice but successful cloning of an animal from a body cell, a feat thought as impossible has become possible by the team of scientists led by reproductive biologist Ian Wilmut at the Roslin Institute, U.K. They had produced a full fledged lamb from a cell taken from the udder of an ewe. The udder cells taken from a six year old Finn Dorset ewe were first cultured in calf-serum less culture medium and then fused with enucleated unfertilised eggs taken from a Scottish Black Face ewe - a diff. breed. Twenty-nine embryos which grew out of this experiment were cultured till 32 - cell stage and then placed in the wombs of Black Face ewes and from these one full - fledged lamb-Dolly was born five months later. The team of scientists has found this quite easy in case of sheep cells but it is not sure whether it is possible in other animals. The possibilities that their success raises are many. For one sheep and cattle of exotic variety can be cloned from body cells. Cells can be genetically modified using recombinant DNA technology and then used to grow sheep or cattle.

Measures to Promote Breeding Efficiency

Most of the individual variations in fertility in a breed are probably matters of management. Keeping the animals free from disease as far as possible, and in a reasonably good nutritive condition, timely observance of heat and mating of the females are some of the ways to get high fertility. Flushing or special feeding a few weeks before the breeding season has been found to reduce the number of services per conception and also increase the number of offsprings per conception in sheep.

Artificial insemination has not only cut down the cost of maintenance of males in cattle, but has increased the intensity of selection of sires and dissemination of efficient sires' semen.

Variations within and between breeds in reproductive efficiency tells that this is a genetic phenomenon. Selection for traits like age of maturity has been found to give success and this may be so for other traits as litter size or fertility as a whole. The important practical step is to keep reasonably complete and up-to-date records of each individual's production and reproduction with emphasis on selection, which will be the guidance for future breeding programmes.

Some of the management suggestions which will tend to improve breeding efficiency are listed below:

1. Do not breed cows following parturitions until all vaginal discharge has ended and at least 60 days have elapsed.
2. Keep an accurate record of dates of parturition, heat periods, services, etc.
3. Breed cows near the end of heat period.
4. Have a competent veterinarian make an examination in cases of failure to come into heat, irregular periods, abortion and retained placenta, and follow his recommendations as to correction of the problem.
5. Have proper sanitation, isolation and care when disease is found in the herd.
6. Have regular pregnancy examinations by a competent veterinarian.
7. Be sure to feed well balanced ration.
8. Maintain regularity in your dairy and handle your stock with full affection.

ARTIFICIAL INSEMINATION

Artificial insemination is the introduction of male reproductive cells into the female reproductive tract by an artificial means. It is commonly abbreviated as AI when associated with domestic animals. In humans, artificial insemination is abbreviated as AIH when the husband's semen is used and AID when the semen is that of a donor.

The foremost value of AI in farm animals lies in its use as a tool for the rapid improvement of quality of genes in future generations by maximum possible use of best series on a mass basis.

Thus artificial insemination is primarily an economical measure in that fewer bulls are required and maximum use can be made of the best sires.

History and Development of AI

An old Arabian document dated 700 of the Hegira (1300 A.D.), records that an Arab chief of Darfur, introduced a wad of wool into the vagina of a mare (a female horse) recently bred to an excellent stallion belonged to an enemy chieftain. After 24 hours he then hurried home and introduced the cotton into the vagina of his own mare. The mare then came in foal.

In 1777, Lazzaro Spallanzani, priest of Modena and a professor of physiology at the University of Pavia, began a series of successful experiments using AI on reptiles. In 1780, he used AI successfully to inseminate a Spanish bitch.

In 1899, Elias I. Ivanoff, a Russian researcher, began a series of studies using AI and was successful in pioneering the method in birds, horses, cattle and sheep. Mass breeding of cows through AI was first accomplished in Russia, where 19,800 cows (an average of 100 cows per bull) were bred in 1931. The Russians were thus the first to appreciate the potential of AI; they were also giving training to many technicians and by 1938 many thousands of cattle and horses and millions of sheep were being successfully bred. Cooperative Cattle AI associations were established in Denmark in 1936 and in the U.S.A. in 1938 and in Britain in 1942. Since the Second World War the practice of AI in dairy cattle has grown tremendously in all milk producing countries of the world, in Denmark, Japan and Israel over 90% of cattle are artificially bred, in the U.S.A. over half the dairy cattle population are artificially inseminated.

Artificial insemination was first attempted in India in 1939 by Dr. Sampath Kumar at the Palace Dairy Farm, Mysore, and some healthy calves were obtained. Comprehensive studies on problems of artificial insemination with special reference to Indian conditions began in 1942 at the Indian Veterinary Research Institute (I.V.R.I.), Izatnagar, under a scheme sponsored by the Indian Council of Agricultural Research (I.C.A.R.). It was soon found that the technique could successfully be used under Indian conditions but that its successful application depended largely on organisation. The field work started at Izatnagar showed that there were a number of problems to be solved, and in 1945–47 the Government of India opened four regional centres at Calcutta, Bangalore,

Patna, and Montgomery (now in West Pakistan), to study these problems and to prepare for the development of artificial breeding on an all-India basis. The work carried out at these centres demonstrated the feasibility of this method of breeding in India, under both urban and rural conditions, in spite of many difficulties. The Montogomery centre was closed on August 15, 1947, on the partition of the country and the Bangalore centre closed in 1951. The State Governments of West Bengal and Bihar took over the centres at Calcutta and Patna respectively by the end of 1950 and the Government of Mysore had by then started artificial insemination work in Bangalore city.

During the First Five-Year Plan (April, 1951 to March, 1956), a master project, the Key Village Scheme, was launched, which provides for the all-round improvement of cattle and buffaloes in the country. To bring about rapid genetic improvement in the stock, artificial insemination was accepted as a major activity of the scheme. Under this Scheme 600 key villages and 150 artificial insemination centers were established during the period 1952 to 1956. One centre was attached to a group of four key villages. Each key village had 500 cows and/or she-buffaloes, so that one artificial insemination centre was responsible for 2000 animals.

Under the Second Five-Year Plan (April, 1956 to March, 1961) the scope of work has been further extended and by 1957, 400 artificial insemination centres were operating. Besides the artificial insemination centres in the Key Village Scheme almost all the states had additional artificial insemination units working in areas outside the Key Village units. Some private agencies or co-operative organisations dealing with livestock have also adopted artificial insemination for breeding work.

A semen bank has been established at the National Dairy Research Institute at Bangalore with a view to supplying semen from Jersey bulls for cross-breeding work and also from bulls of superior Indian dairy breeds for selective breeding or upgrading work. Semen from this bank is being flown to different parts of the country.

The use of AI in other species has generally lagged behind its use in cattle largely because of the problem of the satisfactory storage of semen. In the United Kingdom, France and Germany 5% or less of the total number of matings of sows and gilts are by AI, in Holland it is 20% and in some Scandinavian countries it is over 30%.

According to present status AI is currently used in dairy and beef, cattle, goats, buffalo, sheep, swine, horses, turkeys, bees, dogs, red fox, fish, mink, humans and many other species in many countries of the world.

The first buffalo calf through AI was born in 1943 at the Allahabad Agricultural Institute in U.P. India.

Advantages of AI over Natural Breeding

1. The main advantage of A.I. is that it increases the usefulness of superior sire to an extraordinary degree. It makes available sires of inheritance for milk and butter fat production to all dairymen within a limited area. Previously only a few could get the advantage of good bulls.
2. The services of superior sires are greatly extended. By natural services, a bull can be bred to 50 to 60 cows per year; on the contrary New York Artificial Breeders Co-operative have sired 10,000 in one year by one bull. It would have taken about 200 years to accomplish this by natural service of that bull.
3. The breeder does not need to maintain a herd sire and thus can avoid the botherations accompanied with the management of a bull. It helps to regulate the breeding programme

and the space between successive calvings without unnecessarily prolonging the dry period.

4. The dairyman does not have the problem of searching and purchasing a new herd sire every two years to avoid in-breeding.
5. The technique of A.I. can be made use of in cross breeding for hybrid vigour by quickly transporting the semen by air to different continents.
6. The intensity of the spread of genital diseases are lessened if A.I. is conducted under complete sanitary conditions by the specially trained persons.
7. Overcomes the difficulty of size and weight.
8. Increases rate of conception.
9. Outstanding animals located apart can be mated.
10. Helps in better record keeping.
11. Old heavy and injured sires can be used with advantages.

Limitations of A.I.

1. Requires well trained operations and special equipments.
2. Requires more time than the natural services.
3. Necessitates the knowledge of structure and function of reproduction, on the part of the operator.
4. Improper cleaning of the instruments and insanitary conditions may lead to lower fertility.
5. Market for the bulls is reduced while that for the superior germ plasm is increased.
6. Selection of the sire should be very rigid in all respect.

Problems Under Indian Conditions

1. The sentimental views of people do not relish castration of scrub bulls which are very essential.
2. The lack of understanding of A.I.; some say that it produces weaker calves, etc.
3. It hampers the prospects of the breeders in the disposal of their bull calves.
4. Severe climatic conditions are detrimental for preservation and transportation of semen.

THE TWO COMPONENTS OF SEMEN

Spermatozoa

Whole semen as ejaculated, generally appears as viscous, creamy, slightly yellowish or greyish fluid and consists of spermatozoa or sperm suspended in the fluid medium, called seminal plasma. Its composition depends, in the first place, on the proportion of sperm and plasma and is further determined by the size, storage capacity and secretory output of several different organs which comprise the male reproductive tract. The volume of the ejaculate and concentration of spermatozoa or the sperm density in ejaculated semen, vary widely from one species to another.

In the majority of species, including man, mature spermatozoa have a filiform structure owing to the presence of a flagellate appendage, although non-flagellar forms of sperm cells are not uncommon in certain lower animals, e.g., among crustacea nematodes. The peculiar filiform structure determines, to a considerable extent, the remarkable permeability of the sperm cell, which is perhaps best illustrated by the so called 'leakage' phenomenon, i.e., the remarkable case with which even large molecules such as cytochrome or hyaluronidase can detach themselves from the sperm structure and pass with the extracellular environment. The high degree of permeability explains the cellular speed with which exchange reactions can take place between the spermatozoa and the surrounding medium, whether this be the seminal plasma or an artificial pabulum.

In a typical flagellar spermatozoon it is usually possible to distinguish three regions, viz., sperm head, middle piece and tail; but even among closely related species, one encounters an extraordinary diversity of form, size and structure. Moreover, on examination of the semen from single individual, one often finds in addition to the normally shaped spermatozoa, a variety of degenerated, abnormal or miniature forms which represent every conceivable deviation from the normal structure, from tapering and double cells with a double head or tail to giant (Fig. 8.6) and monster cells containing several nuclei and several tails in a mass of cytoplasm.

Although a high degree of sperm abnormality is undoubtedly associated with sub-fertility, normal semen is seldom completely uniform and human semen, for example, is reckoned to contain as a rule, at least 20 per cent of abnormal forms. In the bull and in stallion the percentage

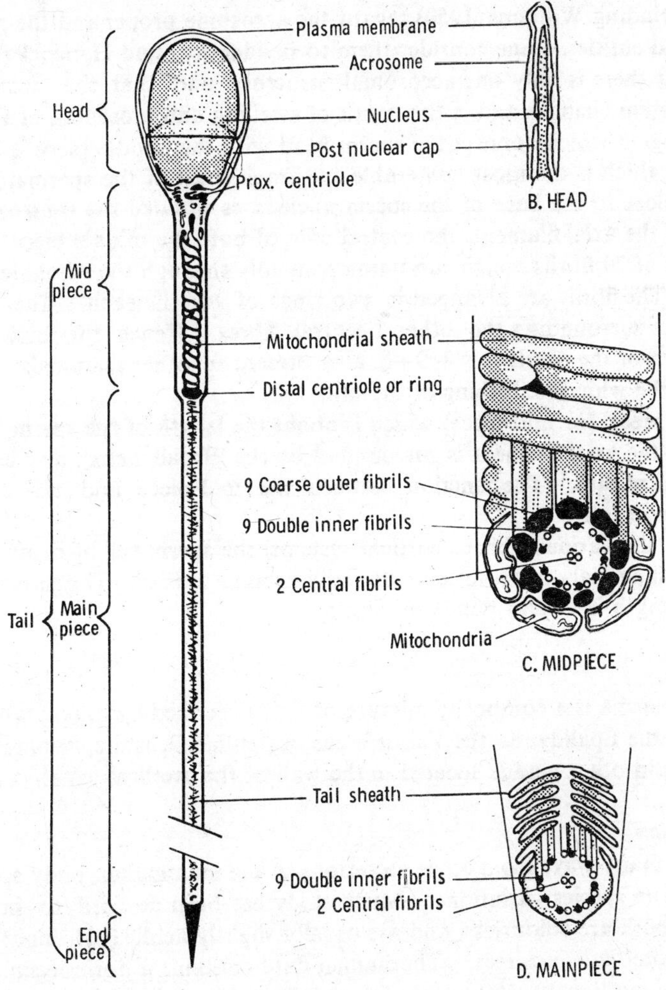

Fig. 8.1. A normal bull spermatozoon.

of abnormal forms in semen is similarly high; in the ram, on the other hand, it appears to be much less.

The shape of the head in normal spermatozoon varies greatly. It is ovoid in the bull, ram, boar and rabbit; it resembles an elongated cylinder in the fowl and has the form of a hook in the mouse and rat.

In the bull the spermatozoon is about 68 ± 3μ in length. Of this length the tail makes up about 50μ, the head about 8 — 10μ, the neck 1μ and the midpiece 8 — 10μ.

The main part of the head is occupied by the nucleus, filled by closely packed chromatin which consists largely of desoxyribonucleoprotein. (Fig. 8.1).

The anterior part of the nucleus is covered by a cap-like structure known as the *Acrosome.* Several investigations have revealed that in spermatozoa, yet another cap, a loose protoplasmic structure named *Galea capitis* which envelopes the apical part of the sperm head and can break away spontaneously to form the so-called spermatic veil or floatin cap. However, whereas most authors including Williams (1950) regard the acrosome proper and the galea capitis as two distinct structural entities, some consider them to be identical and Hancock (1952) for instance is convinced that there is only one acrosomal structure and that the detachable cap arises through postmortem changes and is the result of swelling and loosening of the acrosome itself.

The narrow region which connect the sperm head with the middle piece is known as the Neck (or Neck-piece) which is the most vulnerable and fragile part of the spermatozoon.

In the neck, close to the base of the sperm nucleus, is situated the centrosome which marks the beginning of the axial filament, the central core of both the middle piece and tail. The axial filament consists of 20 fibrils which run uninterruptedly through the whole length of the middle piece and tail. The fibrils are arranged in two rings of 9 fibrils each. The nine members of the inner ring are surrounding the other 2 central fibres. Hence for bull spermatozoa, the numerical pattern of the fibrils is 9 + 9+2, also present in other mammals. These fibrils are responsible for the whip-like lashing of the tail.

In the middle piece (or mid-piece) which is about the length of the sperm head, though only one-tenth wide, the axial filament is surrounded by the 'Broad helix', also called 'Spiral Body' or mitochondrial sheath. The junction between the mid-piece and tail is marked by the presence of a ring centriole.

In addition to the various fibrous cortical systems, the sperm cell of many species including man and higher mammals, is protected externally around the tail. The terminal tailpiece which is about 3μ in length is a solid bundle of fibrils.

Seminal plasma

The seminal plasma is a composite mixture of fluids secreted by organs which in the higher species comprise the Epididymis, the Vas deferens, Ampullae, Prostate, Seminal Vesicles, Cowpers glands and contain other glands located in the wall of the urethral canal.

Prostatic Secretion

This differs in many ways from other secretions of the mammalian body and its composition shows considerable species variations. Much study has been devoted to human and bovine prostatic fluids; both are colourless, and are usually slightly acidic (pH about 6.5). It contains several strong proteolytic enzymes. The human fluid contains a fibrinolysin so powerful that 2 ml of the same can liquefy 100 ml of clotted human blood in 18 hours at 37°C.

The prostatic secretion represents the main source of citric acid and acid phosphate for whole human semen. In men the prostatic secretion also provides the main source of calcium.

Among the chemical peculiarities, the prostatic secretion is rather high in content of zinc.

Table 8.1

Semen volume and sperm density and number in ten animal species

Species	Semen volume (ml)	Range	Sperm concentration ($\times 10^6/ml$) = million/ml	Range	Total sperm ejaculate ($\times 10^6$)
Man	3.5	2.0-6.0	100	50-150	3,500
Bull	8	0.5-12.0	1,200	300-2,000	9,600
Buffalc	2.5	0.5-4.5	600	200-800	1,500
Ram	1.0	0.7-2.0	3,000	2,000-5,000	3,000
Goat	1.0	0.2-2.5	3,000	1,000-5,000	3,000
Boar	215	125-500	250	25-1,000	53,750
Stallion	125	30-320	120	30-800	15,000
Jack	50	10-115	400	95-600	20,000
Dog	10	1-25	125	10-540	1,250
Rabit	0.5	0.2- 2.0	300	100-700	150

SOURCE: *The Artificial Insemination of Farm Animals*, edited by Enos J. Perry, 4th edition, Oxford & IBH Publishing Co., 1969.

Seminal Vesicle Secretion

In several species including the rat, guinea-pig and bull, boar, stallion, etc., the seminal vesicles alone contribute more fluid than the rest of the accessory glands together.

Compared with the prostatic fluid the seminal vesicle secretion is usually less acidic and is sometimes distinctly alkaline. It has a higher dry weight, and contains more potassium bicarbonate, acid soluble phosphate and protein.

In certain animals, e.g., the dog and the cat, the seminal vesicles are altogether absent.

The normal seminal vesicle secretion is usually slightly yellowish but occasionally, specially in man and bull, it can be deeply pigmented. The yellow pigmentation is probably of composite origin but much of it is due to flavins.

The reducing power of the vesicular secretion is one of its most characteristic chemical properties.

It is also important to note that the seminal vesicles are the main sources of fructose in higher mammals. The identification of the seminal sugar as fructose by Mann (1945) opened the way for detailed studies of the fructose generating capacity of the accessory tissues.

COLLECTION OF SEMEN

Collection from the Bull

The primary objective in semen collection is to obtain maximum output of high-quality spermatozoa per ejaculate. Factors known to influence semen output are: 1. Age of the bull (maximum output occurs between 5 and 8 years of age). 2. Season of the year (winter months are best for total sperm production). 3. Frequency of ejaculation (increased frequency of ejaculation results in more total sperm being obtained, but with fewer sperm per collection). 4. Pre-ejaculation sexual preparation (This consists essentially of exciting the bull by allowing him to see, approach, sniff at the teaser and by 'false mounting' in which ejaculation is prevented). 5. Correct techniques of semen collection methods (proper conditioning of Artificial vagina or Electrical stimulatory equipment). 6. Several studies indicate that oxytocin and certain other hormones of the anterior pituitary influence sperm output. Prolactin, growth hormone and testosterone increases immediately after ejaculation. 7. Recent research at Colorado State University in U.S.A. also showed that scrotal circumference (SC) or testicular size is correlated positively with fertility ($r = 0.58$). Since the correlation of SC with actual testicular weight is $r = 0.95$, this means that SC is a reliable predictor of the amount of sperm-producing tissue within the testes. Therefore, the larger the testes, the greater the sperm production potential.

Several methods of obtaining bull semen for AI have been developed, the most common of which are: 1) Artificial vagina (AV) and 2) Electro-ejaculation methods.

Before discussing the details of AV and Electro-ejaculation, the pre-requisites required for semen collection by either of these methods are discussed below:

Selection of Breeding Bulls

Bulls should be so selected whose pedigree is known and particularly should have born of a high yielding dam (mother).

Preparation of Young Bull

Quality bull calves should be procured at 6–12 months of age. At 9 months of age a nose ring made of copper is fixed. They may be stationed at centrally located bull farms and reared under best of environment, feeding and management. At 12 months of age the bulls will be screened for freedom from vibriosis, trichomoniasis, brucellosis and other chronic diseases like Johne's and tuberculosis.

The bull calves so selected must be finally screened Karyologically to detect any chromosomal abnormality. It has been reported that screening for chromosomal abnormality alone improves fertility by 15%. The technology is now available at Tamil Nadu Veterinary and Animal Sciences University, Madras.

At 18 months of age the bulls should be trained for semen collection. At 24 months of age the semen will be collected and evaluated, before final selection. Once selected, bulls should be on balanced ration comprising sufficient greens. Maintenance ration is enough since semen production does not require any extra ration.

Time for Collection

Semen collections should be made during early morning hours before feeding when bulls are alert and fresh. Another advantage is that if the semen is collected during early hours, fresh lots can be used on the very day which may raise the fertility rate to a certain extent.

The Collection Yard

The semen collection yard should be located nearer to the laboratory. If the place is windy, protective walls should be erected. The ground should be covered with rough concrete flooring which should remain dustless during collection. If the collection is made on earthen flooring, water may be sprinkled to avoid dust in the air. It is also desirable to have some sort of cover on top of the yard to prevent direct sun shine or rain.

The teaser animal is tied up inside a service crate which will restrict the movement and at the same time, it provides safety to the teaser, bull and personnel. The wooden crate should be so constructed that, it should not prevent the fore limbs of the bull from embracing of the teaser and thus hinder normal thrust. The dummy should never be taller than the bull to be collected. The angle between the back of the teaser and that of the bull should not exceed 45° during ejaculation.

Cleanliness of Bull

The bull from which semen is to be collected should be clean and free from dirt, to avoid contamination of semen. Grooming with a brush or wiping the underline with a damp towel a few minutes prior to collection could be done. If the underline is extremely dirty, washing may be necessary and in that case it should be done long before the collection so that the animal is dry at the time of collection. *Wet underline is more conducive to the transmission of microbes than a dry one.* The long hairs at the sheath of the penis should be cut to 4–7 cm. Too short hairs do not protect the opening of sheath and also aid in developing a tendency to masturbate.

Selection of Teaser Cow

As far as possible the teaser cow should be of the same breed, size and colour of the bull. It should also be physically strong and docile so that she is able to bear the weight of the bull and does not show irritable temperament when she has to stand in the service crate for long time for collection of semen from a number of bulls. It is better to select a cow which has gone through 2–3 calvings. The teaser cow should neither be in oestrus nor be pregnant. It is better to tie her tail with a rope on one side.

Pre-ejaculation Sexual Preparation

Sexual preparation of bulls may be defined as prolonging the period of stimulation beyond that adequate for mounting and ejaculation. It has been noted that motile sperm output per ejaculation in bulls can be increased as much as two fold when two or three false mounts (and active restraint) are given as rapidly as possible (preferably by 10 minutes) before ejaculation.

Stimuli other than false mounting may also be used to increase sperm output in bulls. These stimuli include moving the stimulus animal, exchanging stimulus animals, changing locations of preparations, changing the personnel handling the bulls, and combination of these. Additionally undefined stimuli from a teaser animal near a bull cause the bull to ejaculate more sperm. The undefined stimuli are not visual since blinded bulls also respond to sexual preparation with increased sperm output. Part of the stimuli must involve olfactory (sense of smell) mechanisms since bulls mount estrous cows twice as fast as non-estrous cows and yield larger volumes of semen and greater sperm numbers.

Tying of Aprons to the Bull

There are some advantages in tying of aprons behind the elbows which will hang so much so that it does not touch ground while the bull is in standing position. The apron cloth should be of coated rexin on one side facing penis of the bull.

The size of the apron is about 65 × 62 cm with semicircular cut at one end. For keeping the apron straight and without any folding it should have two metallic rings on each corner fixed up and rubber strap going round the heart girth of a bull. The advantages of using bull apron are as follows:

1. It prevents cross infection from bull to bull, which otherwise may take place through contact of penis to the rump of the teaser.
2. It prevents losses of semen ejaculates which might happen in certain bulls by tactile stimulation (due to rubbing the penis against the skin of the rump of teaser) and thereby throwing semen outside before penis is directed in AV.
3. The apron prevents the direct contact with the skin of teaser and thereby more hygienic ejaculates can be obtained.

Artificial Vagina (AV) for Bull

The first AV for bulls was designed in 1930 by Russian scientists. Several modifications of the early model have been devised by English, Americans and Danish scientists. The Danish model is now most commonly used in U.S.A., India and many other countries. There are different kinds of AV for different kinds of animals conditions of which are almost aiming to that of natural vagina.

The AV is simple in construction and stimulates natural copulation. It consists of: (a) A strong outer rubber cylinder having an inner diameter of 6 cm with a length between 30 cm for young bulls and 40 cm for adult bulls. The cylinder has rims on either side. A valve is fixed at about 5 cm from one end to admit water and air in the preparation of AV. The outer edges of the cylinder are upturned and refilled so as to have the firm grip by the inner sleeve. (b) A thin inner latex or of PVC liner of a diameter between 7.0 to 8 cm with a length of 50 to 55 cm, which is turned back over each rim of the outer cylinder and tightly held by thick rubber bands. (c) A latex rubber cone between 20 to 25 cm in length is mounted on the cylinder to the end where water and air inlet valves are closer. (d) A graduated glass collection tube of 10 ml capacity is fixed to the conical end of rubber cone. (e) An insulation bag covering the glass tube and rubber cone is fixed on the rubber cylinder with strap for protecting semen in tube from cold and direct sun rays.

Preparation of AV

The AV for a particular bull should be chosen depending upon the length of its penis. For

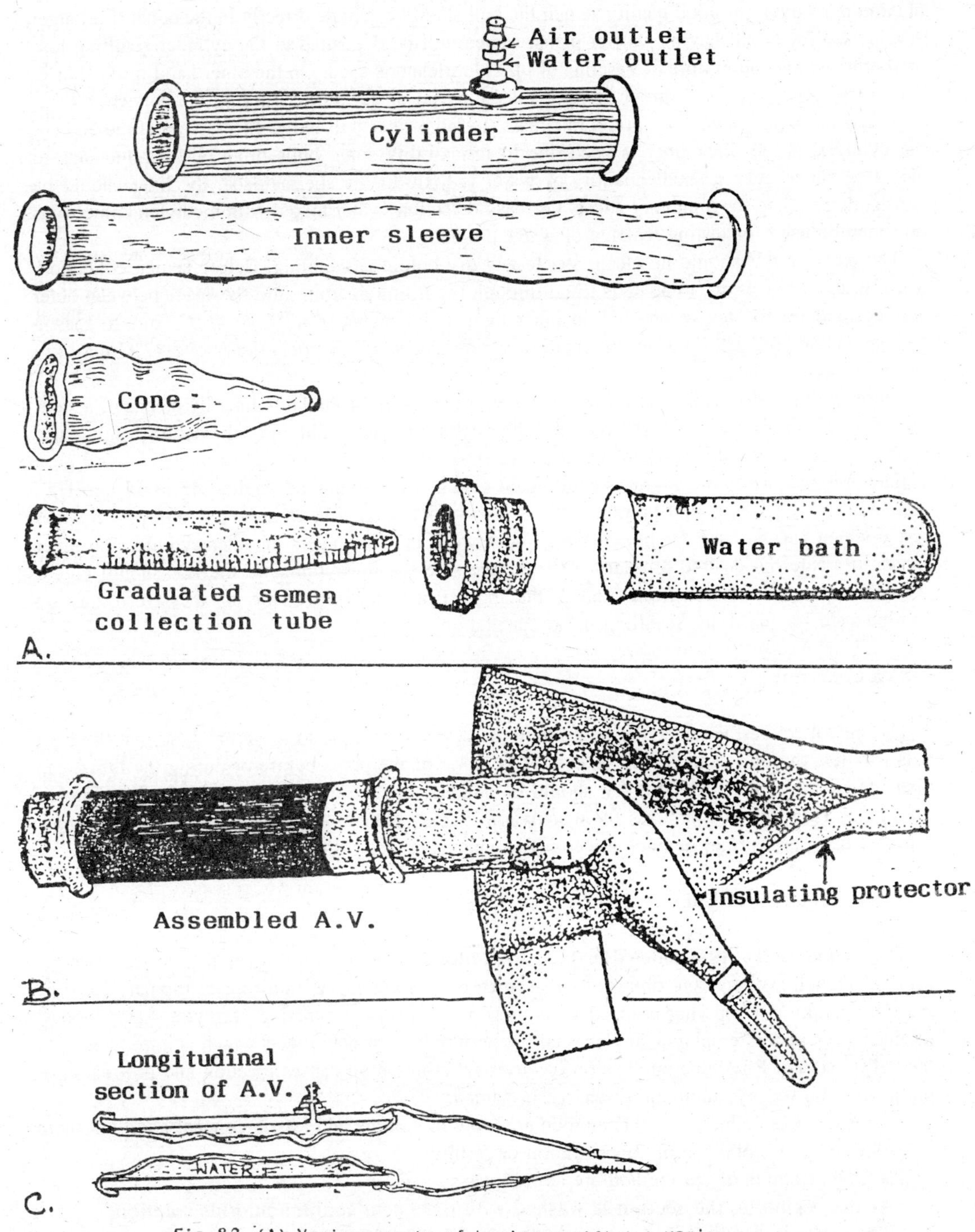

Fig. 8.2 (A) Various parts of bovine artificial vagina (A.V.) (B) Assembled A.V. (C) Longitudinal section of an A.V.

maximum recovery of good quality semen the bull should ejaculate directly in the cone. If a longer AV is used for a bull having shorter penis, semen will be deposited in the cylinder resulting loss of sperm and also admixture of vaseline or other lubricant as used. On the other hand if too shorter AV is used, the penis will throw off the collection vial or get hurt by hitting the collection tube.

The liner should have appropriate thickness, too thin liner will bulge excessively at the ends of the cylinder, if too thick liner is used due to inflexibility some bulls might show reluctance to ejaculate. Since even a small quantity of water is toxic to the spermatozoa, the liner should be constantly checked for minute crevices. For easy detection, water mixed with methylene blue solution may be used for testing leakage of water droplets.

The parts of AV should be clean, sterile and dry before assembling. Before semen collection, warm water between 45° to 50°C is filled through the filling aperture into the space between outer cylinder and inner latex to provide an inner temperature between 42°C to 46°C. Due to season and individual liking the inside temperature varies. An inside temperature above 47°C may kill sperm in the ejaculate.

Sterile soft paraffin is now smeared over the inner surface of the latex liner by means of a stout glass rod. The warm water apart from providing natural warm condition of the natural vagina also facilitates the even distribution of the paraffin.

The pressure inside the vagina should again match with the natural vagina (45 to 55 mm Hg). Younger bull requires higher pressure. AV is always provided with an air screw along with water screw which can be used for blowing the air between the two layers of outer cylinder and inner sleves to create the desired pressure. At right pressure the inner lining of the AV should give a star like appearance if seen from front. If the amount of water or pressure is excessive it may act as hindrance for the thrust resulting in no ejaculation.

Semen Collection

During collection the collector should hold the AV at 45° angle to the ground, so that the long axis parallels the line of the penis. Excessive bending of the penis before or during the thrust can distract and injure the bull. The AV should be handled in such a way that the penis just touches the lining. This stimulus, arouses the ejaculation. Semen collections can take place twice a week (one ejaculate each time) or once a week (two ejaculates per collection).

Electro-ejaculation in Bulls

The technique was first adopted in 1922 by Battelli for collection of semen from guinea pigs. In 1948 French investigators obtained bull semen by introducing a multiringed, bipolar electrode into the rectum and applying upto 30 volts (700 miliamperes, alternating currents). Later models of electro-ejaculators employ a single rectal probe with bipolar electrodes, which is introduced into the bull's rectum. Rhythmic application of electrical stimulation causes erection and protrusion of the penis followed by automatic discharge of semen.

Semen samples collected by this method are more in volume and less in concentration but there is no difference in total sperm concentration or fertility.

The salient points of the method are as follows:

1. At the beginning the rectum is washed with 6 per cent sodium chloride solution.
2. The probe is then inserted up to about 12 inches and held in a position of rectal floor.
3. Alternate current increasing in voltage gradually from zero to 5 volts and returning

again to zero within every 5 to 10 seconds is initially passed.

4. The subsequent stimulations made progressively higher so that at about fifth stimulus a maximum of 10-15 volts is reached. Erection and ejaculation occur at 10 to 15 volts when 0.5 to 1 ampere current is flowed. The source of electric current is AC/220-250 volts/single phase/50 cycles.

The home consumption of electrical current in India is between 200-250 volts, 50 cycles. The voltage is reduced by a step down transformer between 10-15 volts and low voltage current when passed through the rheostat, the changes in voltage can further be made as desired by the operator. This is done by varying the resistance without opening the circuit.

Advantages

1. Semen can be collected from males that are too young or old or unable to mount due to weak or injured legs.
2. No female or dummy is required for collection.
3. Less chance of contamination.

Disadvantages

1. The methods are highly technical and need considerable skill and practice.
2. The semen generally gets contaminated with urine.
3. Some males resist too much to this method and refuse collection.
4. Sciatic nerves are temporarily affected during the operation but is relatively minor if the electrodes are kept over the ampullar region.

Collection of Semen from Buffalo Bull

By AV Method

Semen from buffalo bulls are easily collected in a short AV measuring 20 to 30 cm. in length. Other aspects of collection is to be followed as in the cow bull. Buffalo bulls are most susceptible to temperature variations.

Collection of semen from Sheep and Goat

Artificial vagina and electrical stimulation methods are the only methods employed for collection of semen from rams and bucks.

It has already been discussed that the AV method is preferred since it is quick and simple, is not stressful to the male, and results in collection of better quality semen. Semen can be collected several times per day by artificial vagina. Electrical stimulation may be used when semen is required from a male which can not be trained for collection by AV. It has the disadvantages that it causes considerable discomfort to the animal, frequent collections can not be made, and semen may be contaminated with urine during collection. Semen collected by this method is generally of larger volume but lower sperm concentration than that collected by AV. Electrical stimulation is however, useful for testing large numbers of males for fertility, including teaser rams or buck prepared by surgical intervention.

Collection by AV

The AV as used for rams and bucks is similar to that used for bulls. It consists of an outer casings (20 cm × 5.5 cm of ram, 15 cm × 5.5 cm for buck) made from heavy rubber and an inner liner made of rubber or synthetic material. The shorter AV corresponds to the length of the buck's penis. The liner should extend at least 5–8 cm. beyond the ends of the outer casing so that it may be folded back and secured at the ends with rubber bands to form a water tight jacket.

Before use the liner is rinsed with 70% alcohol in distilled water and allowed to dry. Next the jacket is half-filled with water at 48–50°C.

One end of the inner liner is then lightly lubricated with vaseline to a depth of not more than 3 cm using a sterile glass rod. At the other end a sterile calibrated semen collecting glass is inserted to a depth of 1.5–2.0 cm. While holding the glass in position the vagina is inflated by blowing air through the air outlet. The temperature of AV just before semen collection should be 42–45°C and can be checked by insertion of a clean thermometer. In order to prevent cold shock to the spermatozoa, the semen collecting glasses should be warmed to 30–37°C. Before collection the prepuce of the male should be wiped, cleaned to prevent semen contamination.

The teaser female should not have long wool or hair, or be soiled at the rear end. The operator takes a kneeling position at the right side of the teaser and holds the AV in the right hand along its flank and with the open end facing towards the male and downwards at an angle of 45°.

When the male enters the pen he may engage in courtship behaviour, but the operator should be prepared for the ram or buck suddenly mounting the teaser female. When the male mounts, the erect penis is directed into the open end of the AI. The left hand is used to gently grasp the sheath and deflect the penis into the open end of the AV. A vigorous upward and forward thrust signifies that ejaculation has occurred. The male should be allowed to withdraw his penis before an attempt is made to remove the vagina. The semen collecting glass can then be removed, labelled, covered and placed in a waterbath at 30°C.

The frequency at which semen may be collected depends on the age, condition and temperament of the animal. Rams may mount and ejaculate 20–25 times or more a day. At such frequency the volume and concentration of semen (and consequently the number of spermatozoa per ejaculate) decreases with successive ejaculates. However, a regime of 3–5 collections daily for 4–5 day periods separated by 2–3 day rest periods should not cause a marked reduction in semen quality or quantity.

For goat bucks 2–3 collections daily on alternate days can be regarded as a normal regime. Intervals of 0.5–1.0 hour between successive daily collections are advisable to obtain ejaculates of good volume and concentration.

Collection by Electrical Stimulation

There are different types of electrical stimulators. Those in current use have a bipolar rectal electrode like the one of Ruakura Ram Probe. This is a self-contained stimulator operated by batteries giving a 10 or 15 volt output. When the rectum of the male is dry the 15 volt output is recommended.

For collection, the male should be restrained in a lateral position on a suitable table or clean floor. Long wool or hair should be clipped from around the sheath, and the prepuce should be wiped with cotton wool. The rectal probe is moistened or lubricated with vaseline and inserted into the rectum to a depth of 15–20 cm, taking care to avoid injury. The penis should be extended by straightening the sigmoid flexture so that the glans penis can be grasped with a clean hand and the penis withdrawn from the prepuce. A piece of gauze is then secured behind the glans penis and the glans and the urethral process are inserted into a clean, sterile test tube. It is best to hold the penis and test tube with one hand so that other hand is free to massage the penis in a forward direction between electrical stimuli.

The rectal probe is pressed towards the floor of the pelvis by an assistant and a short stimuli (3–8 seconds) are applied at 15–20 second intervals. After several stimuli accessory gland secretions will flow, followed by semen. When a large amount of clear fluid is obtained initially this should be discarded to avoid diluting the semen. There is considerable variation between males in the amount of stimulation required to produce a satisfactory ejaculate. However, apart from the discomfort and muscular contractions occurring during treatment there are no permanent ill effects.

Collection of Semen from Boar

Pressure is especially important for collecting semen from the boar. The boar ejaculates when the curled tip of the penis is firmly engaged in the sow's cervix or in AV specially made to suit male boar or the operators gloved hand and pressure is exerted on the coiled distal end of the penis throughout ejaculation.

The ejaculate from the boar consists of the following four fractions:

1. *Pre-sperm fraction*—Very thin like water, having no colour. The quantity is about 10 ml and is sperm free. The deflection of this secretion is over at the height of excitement. Its importance is in rinsing the urethral tract which usually has a high bacterial count. This fraction is always preferred to discard.

2. *Sperm-rich fraction*—The volume of second fraction is about 40–80 ml, is dense and milky and contains about 80% of spermatozoa.

3. *Low-sperm fraction*—The third fraction consists of 150 to 200 ml of thin fluid with low-sperm concentration. This fluid originates from the secretions of seminal vesicles and prostate gland which is known as seminal plasma.

4. *Post-sperm fraction*—The fourth fraction is gelatinous and secreted by bulbourethral glands. It tends to seal cervix of the sow during mating, preventing loss of semen.

Semen Collection by AV in Boar

Mating is a prolonged process in boar, varying from 3-25 minutes, and waves of high and low sperm concentrations exist in the flow. The tip of the penis locks into the entrance of the uterus, cervix and ejaculation occurs directly into the uterus. For boar, the Norwegian type of artificial vagina is more common, the length of which is about 18 cm while the diameter is like that of bull. (Fig. 8.5).

It contains two inner tubes, one for air and the other for water. When the boar mounts the dummy, the collector guides the penis into the AV through the Y-shaped hole in foam rubber piece. The collector then tries to catch and hold the penis through the vagina with his right hand (Fig. 8.3). Ejaculation is produced by digital pressure on the spiral portion of the glans penis.

Latest design of a very simple AV for boar consists of only one simple smooth rubber liner (Fig. 8.4) where by applying continuous pressure by hand near distal end of penis, semen is collected.

Some 200 cc of semen is produced, but of this about 50 cc consists of a gelatinous material sperm, and this is strained off before insemination or storage.

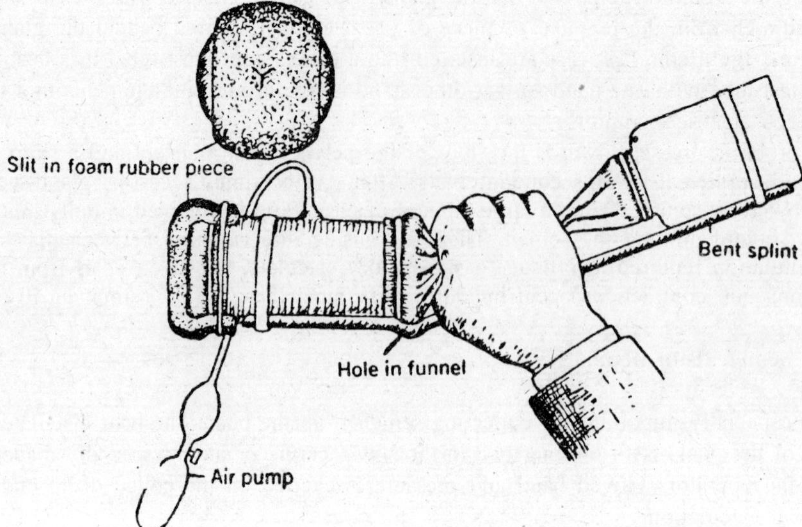

Fig.8.3. Method of grasping the penis of the boar prior to ejaculation by A.V. method.

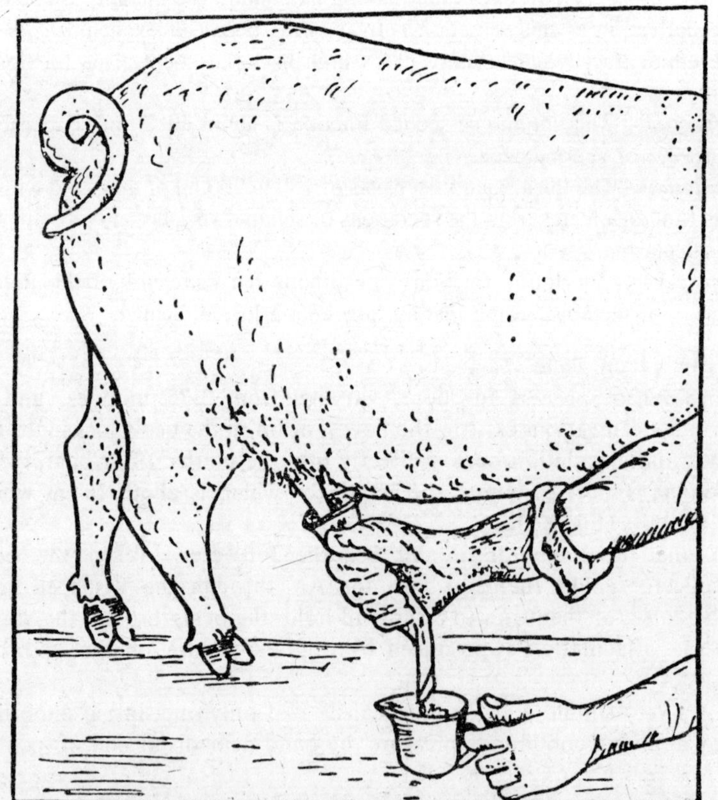

Fig.8.4. Semen collection from boar by use of a smooth rubber liner and continuous pressure exerted by hand near the distal end of penis.

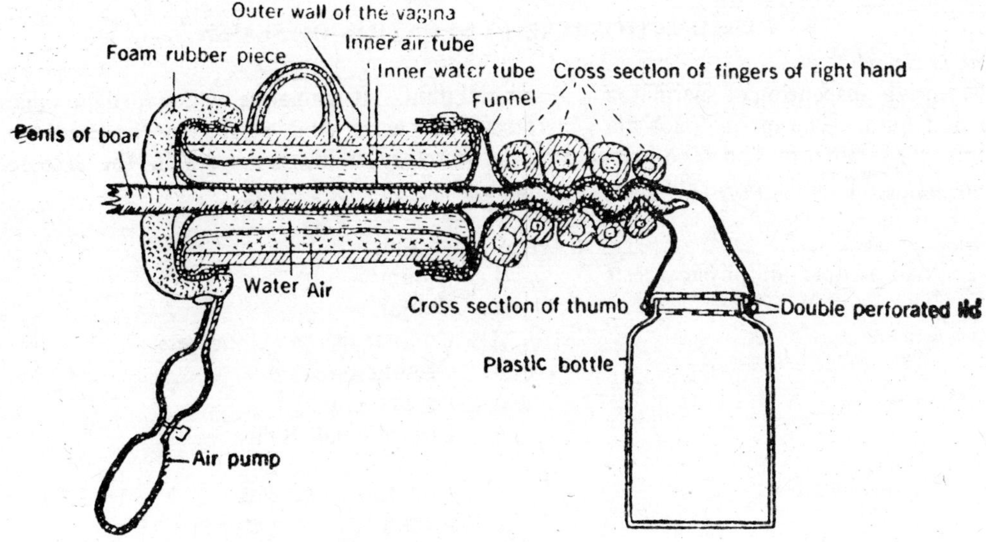

Fig.8.5. Semen collection from boar by A.V.

Collection of Semen from Stallion

Methods in current use employ either AV or latex condom. The Cambridge or Russian model and the Missouri or American model are considered suitable. The AV technique is similar to that employed for the bull. It is essential in practice that the mare shall be in full oestrus. The AV is, of course, larger than that used for bulls and in the case of larger stallions it requires to be held by two operators at the time of collection. As the stallion mounts the mare, the operator nearer the stallion guides the penis into the AV with his left hand which he then transfers to the under surface of the penis in order to detect the peristaltic ejaculatory waves. With his right hand he helps the other operator to hold the AV at a slightly inclined angle until organism is detected; then the collecting end is lowered so that the semen flows into the attached collecting vessel.

The Missouri and Mississippi models are most popular in USA. Mississippi model is made of one piece of rubber tubing 91.5 to 122 cm long and 18 to 20 cm in flat diameter. Water temperature is between 41–45°C inside the artificial vagina.

Many of the semen collectors prefer to collect stallion semen by placing a condom over the penis just prior to intromission. Ejaculation occurs into the condom which is stripped from the penis as the stallion dismounts.

Prior to ejaculation, the penis should be washed with warm soapy water and rinsed with clean water to remove smegma and other debris on the surface of the penis.

Unlike with bovine or ovine spermatozoa, the poor viability of equine spermatozoa is partly due to poor initial sugar content of semen and its early exhaustion during metabolism.

The first fraction of the ejaculate is of watery consistency and is devoid of spermatozoa. In next phase the ejaculate comes from the testes and possess high concentration of spermatozoa and thereby milky white in appearance. During the third and final phase a glairy, viscous material resembling white of an egg is expelled. This is the secretion obtained from seminal vesicles and Cowper's glands.

EXAMINATION AND EVALUATION OF SEMEN

What is Serren?

Semen is a suspension of spermatozoa in seminal fluid. It is opaque, white to light cream-coloured fluid. The spermatozoa are generated in the testes and stored in the epididymis whereas the seminal plasma is contributed by the secretory fluids produced in the accessory organs like epididymis, prostrate gland, seminal vesicle, cowper's gland.

EXAMINATION OF SEMEN

A. Macroscopic and physical tests
1. Volume
2. Colour
3. Consistency and cloudiness
4. Osmotic pressure
5. Specific gravity
6. Electro conductivity

B. Microscopic tests
1. Counting of sperms
2. Motility of spermatozoa
3. Live and dead count
4. Morphological abnormalities

C. Chemical tests
1. Fructolysis
2. Respiration co-efficient
3. Methylene blue reduction
4. Hydrogenion concentration
5. Catalase test

D: Bacteriological tests

A. Macroscopic and Physical Tests

1. *Volume.* The volume is measured directly with the help of the graduated, pipette or cylinder. The average per ejaculate from Bull—5 to 8 c.c., Stallion—100 c.c., Boar—200 c.c. Cock—0.6 c.c.

2. *Colour.* Colour is not necessarily a criterion of good quality but gives a check during collection. Pathological indication in colour: yellow—pus and urine; pinkish or reddish-admixture of fresh blood; deep red and brownish colour probably indicates degenerative blood tissue; greenish—purulent degeneration.

3. *Consistency and cloudiness.* Gives an indication of colour and consistency:

Thick Creamy	...	Excellent
Thin Creamy	...	Very good
Thick Milky	...	Good
Thin Milky	...	Fair
Watery	...	Extremely poor

4. *Osmotic pressure.* Determinations of the osmotic pressure in terms of freezing point depression (in Centigrade).

Bull	...	0.54–0.73
Ram	...	0.55–0.70
Stallion	...	0.58–0.62

Whereas the specific gravity of the sperm cell is due to the highly condensed nuclear and protoplasmic protein constituents, the specific gravity of the seminal plasma is the direct outcome of the actual osmotic pressure exerted by electrolytes and is thus related to the depression of the freezing point. It would seem that generally more reliance should be placed on the results obtained with seminal plasma than with whole semen.

5. *Specific gravity.* The average specific gravity of whole semen is 1.028 in man, 1.011 in dog and 1.035 in bull, with fluctuations due in first place to the variable ratio between sperm and seminal plasma. The latter is so much lighter than the spermatozoa (1.240–1.334) in bull that in practice the specific gravity of semen is often found to be directly proportional to sperm concentration. In bull semen, low specific gravity is usually associated with low sperm concentration and poor quality whereas high values accompany good density and good quality.

6. *Electro conductivity.* It has been claimed that the spermatozoa possesses at the head and tail small but directly opposite electrical charges. However, all that can be claimed with certainty is that an electric charge is associated with the sperm cell but that its magnitude depends largely on the concentration of the various positively and negatively charged ions in the surrounding medium. The following values for electro-conductivity in semen at 25°C expressed in reciprocal ohms $\times 10^{-4}$ were given by Bernstein and Shergin (1936) Bull 89.5—116.3, Ram 48.5 to 80.5, Stallion—111.3 to 129.5.

B. Microscopic Tests

1. *Counting of sperms* (by Heamacytometer). The counting chamber contains in the centre 16 big squares divided into 256 small squares. The size of the small square is 1/400 sq mm and the height of the cover glass above it is 1/10 mm. Therefore, the space in each small square is 1/4000 cu mm.

Semen dilution to be made with 0.9% NaCl containing 0.01% mercuric chloride to suppress the motility of the sperm,

0.1 cc. of semen to 9.9 cc of Normal Solution—1: 100...A
1.0 cc from A to 9.0 cc of Normal Solution—1000
0.2 cc from A to 9.8 cc of Normal Solution—1: 5000
0.1 cc from A to 9.9 cc of Normal Solution—1: 10,000

It is better to add a colouring fluid, e.g., Rose Bengal Eosin etc., to give colour to the sperms for better visibility under a microscope.

$$\text{No. of sperms in 1 cc of semen} = \frac{\text{No. of sperms counted} \times 4000 \times \text{dilution factor} \times 100}{\text{No. of squares counted}}$$

Counting of sperms can also be made by the help of (a) Visual estimation of concentration—by Blom's comparator, (b) Estimation by comparison with Opacity tubes, (c) Estimation by Absorptiometer.

2. *Motility of spermatozoa.* A drop of sample is taken just after collection and after properly mixing on a clean dry hollow ground slide kept at body temperature. It is then examined under the low power and rated on the basis of the swirling currents.

Interpretation:

0 = No motility.

+ = Less than 20 per cent of the sperms showing progressive motion.

++ = 20–40 per cent showing progressive movement but no wave.

+++ = 44–60 per cent showing progressive movement with slow wave.

++++ = 60–80 per cent showing progressive movement with wave more intense.

+++++ = 80–100 per cent showing progressive movement with rapid waves.

As a rule +++ or more are recommended for A.I. purposes.

The movement of sperms may be:

(1) Progressive or rapid
(2) Rotatory
(3) Oscillatory

3. *Live and dead count.* One drop of semen is mixed with 2 drops of 50 per cent Eosin solution in distilled water, one drop of 10 per cent Nigrosin added and mixed. A film is then made from the mixture. Living spermatozoa appear unstained and dead stained pink against a brownish purple background. Care should be taken to ensure that the semen and stain are at the same temperature as otherwise artefacts may be produced.

4. *Morphological abnormalities.* The sperms may be abnormal (Fig. 8.6) with regard to their:

Head—Micro-head; mega head; altered shape including narrow pear-shaped head; double head; detached galea capitis; abnormal staining reactions.

Neck—Rupture or absence of attachment to the head; fixation misplaced to one side; presence of protoplasmic droplet.

Middle Piece—Enlarged, narrowed, adherent protoplasmic droplet coiled at anterior end.

Tail—Coiled at anterior end, split, broken at junction with mid piece, looping.

It is the general view that in normal bull semen the percentage of abnormal forms should not exceed 15 to 20 per cent. The presence of more than 2 to 3 per cent of spermatozoa with proximal protoplasmic droplets is also considered abnormal.

The number of abnormal sperms are influenced by a variety of reasons, e g., (1) Season of the year—very high in the rains during May and June, with young bulls it is high in summer but in old ones it is so in winters. (2) Previous coitus or collection—when the sexual rest between the ejaculations is long there will be an abnormal number. (3) Method of collection—among different methods of semen collection, it is minimum with AV and maximum with sponge method.

C. Chemical Tests

1. *Fructolysis.* Following the discovery by Mann that the main anaerobic source of energy in bull and ram semen is fructose, a test of these animals on their fructolytic ability has been devised. Normally, active cells metabolise fructose when incubated anaerobically at 37°C. Fructose is not utilised by either azoospermic (devoid of sperm) or necrospermic (immotile) semen. The rate of fructolysis may thus be used to distinguish normal from subnormal activity.

The anaerobic incubation of freshly ejaculated semen is accompanied by a gradual decline in

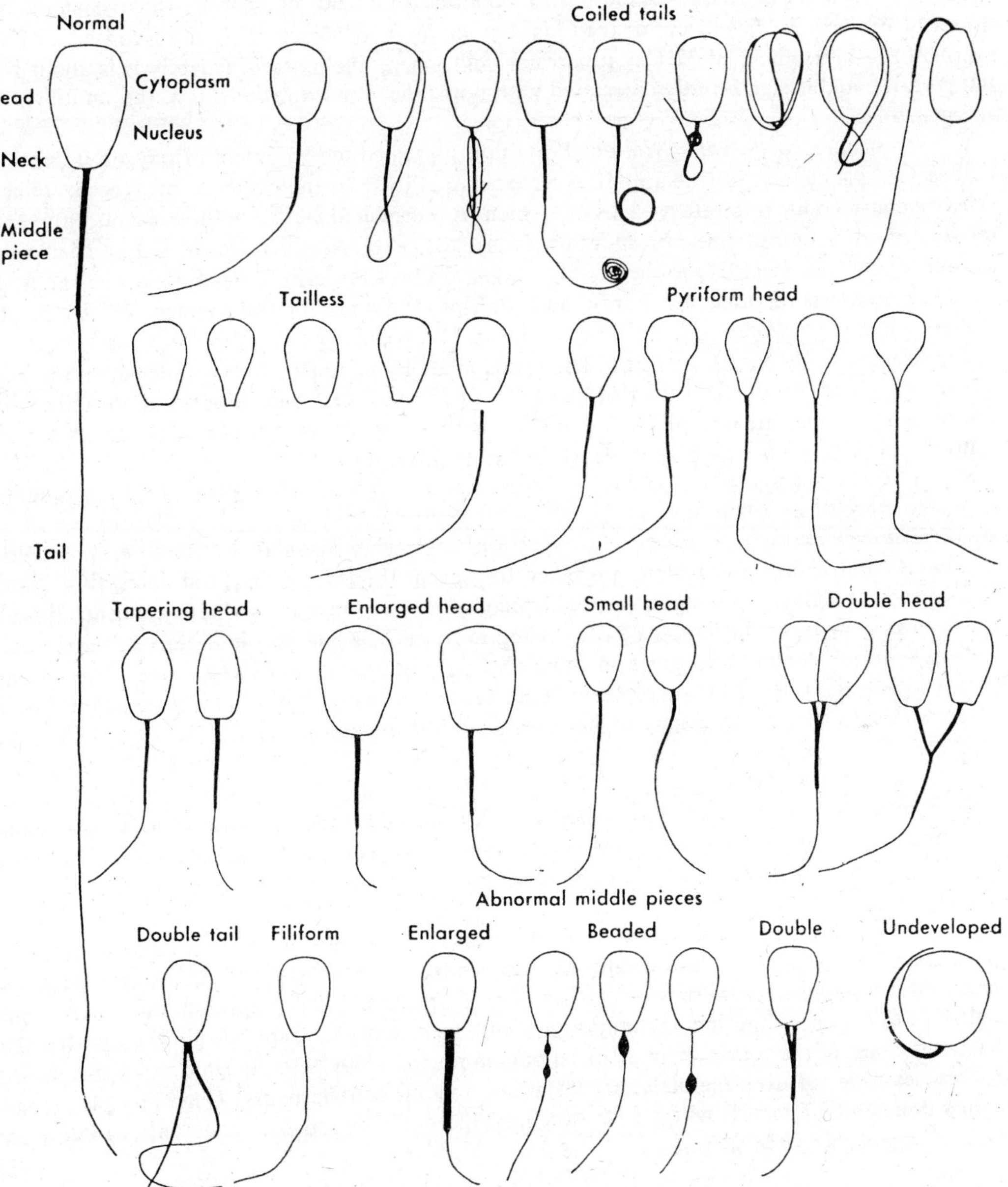

Fig.8.6. Diagramatic representation of Sperm abnormalities.

the content of fructose with a simultaneous accumulation of lactic acid. In the presence of suitable buffers, the process of fructose utilisation (fructolysis) in semen with good sperms motility proceeds almost linearly until practically all the sugar is used up. On this basis a photometric method has been worked out for the measurement of sperm fructolysis and the 'Index of Fructolysis' has been defined as the amount of fructose (in mg.) utilised by 10^{-9} spermatozoa in one hour at 37°C. In normal bull semen, the index of fructolysis is about 1–2 but it varies, and is significantly correlated with both the concentration and the motility of spermatozoa.

2. *Respiration coefficient.* Walton (1938) first suggested measurement of oxygen uptake in bull semen as a method for the appraisal of semen quality. In the presence of oxygen, semen shows a considerable respiratory activity which is correlated both with concentration and motility of spermatozoa. Sperm respiration is usually expressed in terms of ZO_2, a coefficient introduced by Redenz (1933) to denote μlO_2 taken up by 10^8 sperm cells during one hour at 37°C. ZO_2 values reported by Lardy and Philips (1943) are for Bull semen, 21; Ram, 22; Rabbit, 11; and Cock, 7.

3. *Methylene blue reduction test.* The test is made by mixing 0.2 cc of semen with 0.5 cc of egg yolk citrate dilutor and then adding to this 0.1 cc of methylene blue solution (50 mg in 100 cc of sodium citrate dilutor). The mixture is then placed in a water bath at 38°C. A control blue with methylene blue is also kept for comparison.

A good quality semen should reduce the colour in 3.5 to 6 minutes, while the poor quality may take more time to reduce.

4. *Hydrogen ion concentration.* The reaction of freshly ejaculated semen may become alkaline at first, unless precautions are taken to prevent the loss of CO_2; but later this change is followed, at least in those specimens which contain fructose and a high concentration of spermatozoa, by a rapid decrease of pH, owing to fructolysis and accumulation of lactic acid. Excessive initial alkalinity of semen in some species, notably in bulls and rams, often accompanies low fertility, the alkaline reaction being associated with absence or low concentration of sperm and with a correspondingly higher proportion of seminal plasma.

D. Bacteriological Tests

Gunslaus, Salisbury and Willet (1941) observed that the collection of semen under anything less than ideal aseptic conditions may result in enormous contamination of the semen by microorganisms. Even under the most ideal conditions, certain types of bacteria are always found in the semen of the bull.

A report by the U.S.D.A. (1942) indicates that Diptheroids were predominant types of organisms. Staphylococci were found to occur next in frequency. *Pseudomonas araginosa* and coliform organism were present occasionally. Ognianov (1947) reported that *E. coli* was injurious to semen by causing agglutination of bull spermatozoa. Caporale (1941) reported that bacterial count of the semen from artificial vagina ranged from 100 to 960,000 organisms per ml.

Samples collected from the males are tested for various contaminants. Generally plate count is first done and afterwards where necessary the differential counts are made only to know the type of organisms in the sample.

DILUTION OF SEMEN

The main objectives of extending (increasing in volume) semen are: (1) to increase the volume of the ejaculate obtained from quality adult males so that a large number of females may be mated from a single dose of his ejaculate. In natural mating, one ejaculate is used to inseminate one female, whereas by extension of the same volume of semen, several hundred (500–1,000) females can effectively be made pregnant. (2) Moreover, ejaculated sperm do not survive for long period and thus to preserve fertilizing capacity of the spermatozoa for a long period various agents are added. The agents that comprise good extending media have the following functions:

1. Provide nutrients as a source of energy
2. Provide lipoproteins and/or lecithin to protect sperm cells against low-temperature shock
3. Provide a buffer to prevent harmful shifts in pH as lactic acid is formed
4. Maintain the proper osmotic pressure and electrolyte balance
5. Inhibit bacterial growth
6. Provide a source of reducing substances to protect the sulfhydryl containing cellular enzymes
7. Provide a buffer for a proper balance of mineral elements essential to the life of sperm cells
8. Increase the volume of the pure semen so that it can be used for multiple inseminations.

Functions of Common Extender Ingredients

Glucose: Provides energy

Egg yolk and milk: Protect against cold shock of the sperm cells as they are cooled from body temperature to 5°C and by providing lecethin, proteins, lipoproteins and similar compounds found in egg yolk or milk. These substances also contain nutrients utilised by sperm.

Buffers: A variety of buffers are used for maintaining a neutral pH and an osmotic pressure of approximately 300 milliosmoles, which is equivalent to that of semen, blood plasma and milk. A satisfactory extender for one animal or one set of condition may not be acceptable for others. This has resulted in a number of diluents for various species.

Antibiotics: Penicillin, streptomycin, polymycin B or other combinations of antibiotics that cover a broad bacterial spectrum are used to enhance the keeping quality of semen. Procain penicillin is toxic to spermatozoa. Antibiotics will not completely eliminate *Corynebacterium pyogenes, Brucella, Trichomonas fetus, Mycobacterium, Rickettsiae* and *Fungi*. Addition of glycerol further reduces the efficacy of antibiotics. Hence addition of antibiotics is not an extra precaution and cannot be taken as an effective tool to permit use of semen from infected bulls or unhygienic semen processings.

Glycerol: Most widely used cryoprotective agent for bull spermatozoa particularly for frozen semen. The exact mechanism and the loci of activity is not clearly understood. The possible modes of action proposed are:

1. Modifies size and shape of ice crystals formed.
2. Binds water and decreases freezing point of solution and less ice is formed.
3. Prevents denaturation of proteins and rupture of plasma membrane.
4. Reduces the soluble concentrations.

Fructose: Provides glycolysable substrate for the sperm, prevent sperm agglutination, maintain required osmotic tension and electrolyte balance and gives added cryoprotection during deep freezing.

Composition of Extenders

For many years the emphasis in AI programmes was on the use of liquid extended semen generally preserved at 5°C for 2 to 4 days for the purpose of increasing usefulness of superior sires. An average bull in commercial AI service is currently being used to make pregnant to couple thousand cows annually in contrast with only 50–60 cows normally bred to bull under natural mating conditions annually.

A number of media have been developed that provide adequate nutritional components, (pH 6.5 to 6.7), buffering capacity, and protection against bacterial contaminants and temperature shock. The semen and extender are initially mixed together at the same temperature.

While preparing diluents either for liquid/chilled semen or for frozen the following basic principles should be borne in mind.

1. Accurate weighing of various recommended ingredients of the dilutor to provide exact osmotic tension, pH and electrolyte levels.
2. Exclusion of toxic materials and simultanious inclusion of protective components.
3. Rigid control on pathogenic contamination.
4. Decide dilution rate so as to provide optimum number of viable spermatozoa per dose at the time of insemination.
5. Maintain absolute sanitation of the room, technician, all metal and glass equipments and use quality reagents.

Dilutors for Bull

Based on the various composition of dilutors used for bull semen they may be classified as below. *Whatever may be the diluents, always add diluent to semen, never the reverse, as this may cause shock to the spermatozoa and reduce their motility.*

A. Milk or skim milk based
B. Egg-yolk based
C. Coconut milk based
D. Other commercial diluents.

A. Milk Based Dilutors

In recent years boiled whole-milk, skim milk, reconstituted milk powder and milk whey diluents have been employed in commercial A.I. These diluents are economical, easy to prepare and provide good protection for spermatozoa. The foremost objection to whole milk as dilutor is that the fat globules make microscopic examination difficult. Use of skim milk or even homozenised milk or milk of goats, which is "naturally" homozenised can partially solve the problem. Fresh milk has got *lactenin*, an antibacterial substance present in milk albumin also exerts effect on spermatozoa which if heated to about 92–95°C for 10 minutes will reduce sperm killing activity to a great extent.

Greater success has been claimed with milk diluents from Pakistan. In India the diluent designed by Girish Mohan (1974) using low fat cow milk heated up to 93°C for 20 minutes in a water bath followed by overnight cooling in a refrigerator and removing fat particles by filtering through cotton plug gave improved results comparable with egg yolk citrate dilutors.

Studies at Texas A & M University indicate that evaporated milk can be used with glycerol as dilutor in freezing stallion semen.

B. Egg-yolk Dilutors

In 1934, Milovanov observed the beneficial effects of adding egg yolk to extending fluids.

Today, egg-yolk citrate is one of the commonly used semen extenders. Only the yolk portion is used because egg white contains a substance (lysozyme) toxic to spermatozoa.

The eggs used to provide the yolk should not be more than 4 to 5 days old. The shell of the egg should be thoroughly washed with warm water, sterilised by wiping with a piece of cotton wool moistened with alcohol, and dried. After cracking the egg and separating the white, the yolk is placed on a filter paper in such a way as not to rupture its membrane. All white can be removed from the yolk by gently rolling the yolk on the filter paper. The yolk is then run into a sterile beaker by folding and squeezing the filter paper. The membrane of the yolk should remain on the filter paper and be discarded.

Before adding it to the diluent, the egg yolk should be mixed in beaker with the aid of a sterile glass rod, specially when it has been obtained from more than one egg. The egg-yolk-tris-fructose-citrate diluent should be freshly prepared on each day of before use.

1. ***Sodium Citrate Dilutor***

Salisbury *et al.* (1948) formulated the dilutor having 2.9% sodium citrate dihydrate solution with equal volume of egg yolk. The extender is very popular for use in bull semen. The medium maintains semen fit for insemination for 72–96 hours at 4 to 7°C. Moreover it gives clearer view of the microscopic examination and proved to be more efficient due to incorporation of antibiotics.

Original egg-yolk citrate dilutor has first been modified by Salisbury by adding glucose solution and later on by number of other scientists by incorporating glycine and other ingredients. Such modifications which also includes reduced proportion of egg-yolk from 50% to 20% resulted into better keeping quality of semen, economy and efficiency even at higher dilution rate.

2. ***Modified Salisbury's Diluent (EYGC)***

The dilutor is now known as egg-yolk-glucose-sodium citrate diluent. The method of preparation is as follows:

i) Dissolve 2.9 g of crystalline sodium citrate dihydrate ($Na_2C_6H_5O_72H_2O$) in 100 ml of glass distilled water ... 50 parts

ii) Dissolve 5 g of Analar grade glucose in 100 ml glass distilled water ... 30 parts

iii) Egg-yolk ... 20 parts

iv) Add 1000 I.U. of crystalline penicillin and 1000 micrograms of dihydrostreptomycin per ml just prior to addition of semen to dilutor

To prepare the egg-yolk for the egg-yolk buffer extender, fresh yolk of the hen's egg is always preferred. At first fresh egg should be washed in water and wiped with 70% alcohol. After allowing the egg to dry, the shell is broken with a sterile knife into two equal halves with one half holding the yolk, the excess albumin being collected in a beaker. Transfer of the yolk between the two halves of the shell will allow most of the albumin to be separated off and the yolk is then carefully transferred to a beaker containing distilled sterile water at a temperature of about 50°C. The traces of albumen adhering to the yolk will coagulate; the water is poured out and the egg-yolk transferred to a clean filter paper. Rolling back and forth on this paper dries the surrounding membrane, which is then ruptured. The yolk is then allowed to flow into a measuring cylinder, remaining the membrane on the filter paper.

The egg-yolk citrate buffer is usually prepared fresh each day before use.

3. *Cornell University Extender (CUE)*

In U.S.A. Cornell University workers, Foote* and Bratton (1960) formulated a diluent termed Cornell University Extender (CUE) which permitted longer storage at 5°C is narrated below:

(a)	Sodium citrate dihydrate(g)	...	14.5
	Sodium bicarbonate(g)	...	2.1
	Potassium chloride(g)	...	0.4
	Glucose(g)	...	3.0
	Sulphanilamide(g)	...	3.0
	Glycene(g)	...	9.37
	Citric acid(g)	...	0.87
	Distilled water (final volume) (ml)	...	1000.00

(b) Add 20% (by volume) egg-yolk and 80% of buffer solution (a) along with penicillin and Dihydrostreptomycin @ 100 I.U. and 1000 microgram per ml of final dilutor.

The dilutor although proved a better type of dilutor but since it has many components and each requires careful weighing and adding and therefore found to be less popular for routine use.

4. ***Illini Variable Temperature Diluent (IVT)***

Van Demark and Sharma (1957) developed the first successful technique for preserving diluted semen at room temperature and termed it the "Illini Variable Temperature" (IVT) technique and, the medium, IVT-medium. The diluent is made up of:

(a)	Sodium citrate dihydrate	...	20 g
	Sodium bicarbonate	...	2.1 g
	Potassium chloride	...	0.4 g
	Glucose	...	3.0 g
	Sulphanilamide	...	3.0 g
	Distilled water added to make the volume	...	1000.00 c.c.

(b) The above buffer mixture is gassed with CO_2 until the pH reaches to 6.3

(c) Add 1000 microgram of streptomycin and 1000 I.U. penicillin per ml. along with 10% egg-yolk.

The semen diluted in this diluent is stored in 1 ml ampoules in dark at room temperature. As high as 75% conception rate was reported from 111 inseminations carried out with semen stored at room temperature for 7 days.

The IVT diluent has received wide attention in different parts of the world. The results are not consistent. Ulaganathan (1970) observed that the sperm survivability in the IVT diluent improved by the addition of ascorbic acid. Further investigations are necessary.

5. ***Tris Buffer Diluent***

It is used as common extender for frozen semen.

(a)	Tris hydroxy methyl amino methane	...	3.97 g

* Prof. R.H. Foote was the minor advisor of the author while he was persuing his Ph.D. studies at Cornell University during 1966–70.

	Citric acid	... 1.73 g
	Fructose	... 1.27 g
	Distilled water	... 99.13 ml
	(pH adjusted to 6.8 with citric acid or NaOH)	
(b)	Tris buffer, as in (a)	... 74 ml
	Egg-yolk	... 20 ml
	Glycerol	... 6 ml

(c) To a diluent add penicillin at a dose of 1000 I.U. and streptomycin at 1000 microgram per ml.

C. Coconut Milk Based Dilutors

The use of coconut milk (water) extender (CME) for the preservation of active sperms for 7 to 10 days at room temperature was first worked out by Norman *et al.* (1960, 1962). It is made up of sterilized coconut water and a 4.3% sodium citrate solution plus 100 mg per cent calcium carbonate, 80 mg per cent penicillin and 90 mg per cent streptomycin. The pH is adjusted to 7.4 with 10% solution of NaOH. The same workers in 1962 observed that CME to which 5 per cent egg-yolk was added maintained motility better than EYC and skim-milk extenders.

Exposure to light produces photo-oxidation which results into poor motility and depression of metabolic rate. Tomar and Sharma (1974) modified the CME by selecting the following components:

2% sodium citrate dihydrate solution	... 50 ml
Coconut water	... 25 ml
Egg-yolk	... 12.5 ml
Egg-albumin	... 12.5 ml

Limited availability of superior quality coconut water all round the year and all over the regions in India restricts its popularity.

D. Other Commercial Diluents:

Fruit and vegetable juices have been used in some countries for extending bovine semen, with apparently acceptable results. Such juices as tomato broth and carrot juice, which are abundant and economical, have been used.

In New Zealand an ambient temperature dilutor, known as *Caprogen* has been found very effective in maintaining maximum fertility for a 24 hour period. The dilutor includes caproix acid in an IVT-CUE type of extender followed by gassing with nitrogen.

Recently at N.D.R.1. Karnal in Haryana, a diluent named as 'Citrate Acid Whey' (CAW) at pH 6.8 found to be the best diluent for preservation of buffalo semen. When CAW was compared with EYC, the former could preserve the sperms for 5 days at refrigerated temperature (5°C) with 60% motility as against 2 days in the case of the later diluent.

The CAW is now available in a packet containing cow skim milk powder and citric acid together. The entire contents of the packet is dispersed in 100 ml distilled water. The curdled material is filtered after 10 minutes through cotton plug and the pH is adjusted to 6.8 using 10% NaOH. The preparation is now ready for diluting semen. CAW packet can be preserv-

Table 8.2

Comprehensive morphology of the spermatozoa of buffaloes and cattle

Spermatozoa measurement	Buffaloes Mean (μ)	Buffaloes SD (μ)	Cattle Mean (μ)	Cattle SD (μ)
Head length	7.436	0.442	9.126	1.326
Head breadth (anterior)	4.264	0.520	4.732	0.494
Head breadth (posterior)	3.172	0.442	2.730	0.520
Ratio head breadth (anterior) to head breadth (posterior)	1.340	0.330	1.790	0.320
Neck	0.442	0.208	0.650	0.338
Length of middle piece	11.648	0.936	12.558	0.624
Breadth of middle piece	1.092	0.286	1.006	0.286
Length of tail	42.882	3.042	46.280	6.084

SOURCE: Mahmoud, I.N. (1952) Some characteristics of the semen of Egyptian buffaloes, *Bull. Fac. Agric. Fouad I Univ. (Cairo)*., No, 15, 16 pp. Abstracted: *Anim. Breed. Abstr*., 21, 260 (1953).

Table 8.3

Differences in the mean values of various characteristics of cattle and buffalo semen as observed in 117 cases

Semen characteristics	Cattle	Buffalo	Significance
Sperm density/mlx 10^1	1,389.6	1,234.9	*
Live sperm/ml × 10^6	1,036.5	891.7	*
O_2 uptake μl in saline/hour	112.2	81.2	**
O_2 uptake μl in phosphate/hour	85.8	64.6	**
O_2 uptake μl in Kreb's/hour	116.6	70.0	**
Fructolysis/10^9 sperm/hour	1.79	1.54	*
Fructolysis/10^9 live sperm/hour	2.45	2.15	*

*Significant at 5 per cent level.
**Significant at 1 per cent level.

SOURCE: Sinha, R.C., Sengupta, B.P. and Roy, A. (1966), Climatic environment and reproductive behaviour of buffaloes, IV. Comparative study of oxygen uptake and aerobic fructolysis by Murrah (*B. bubalis*) and Haraina (*B. indicus*) spermatozoa during different seasons, *Ind. J. Dairy Sci*., 19, 18-24.

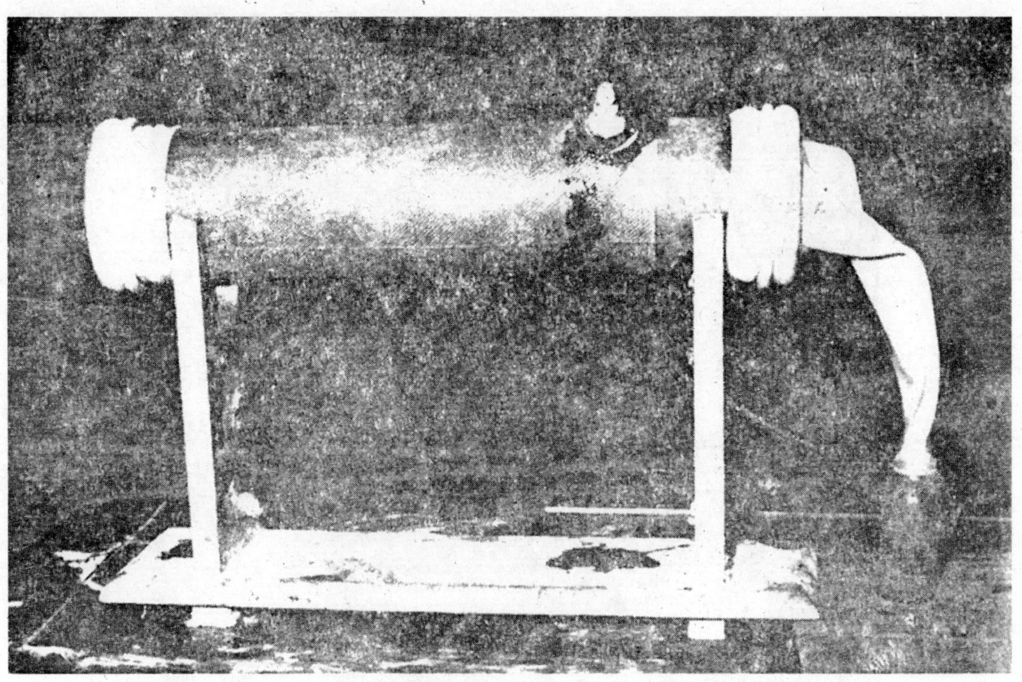

Plate 6. Assembled Artificial Vagina (Chapter 8).

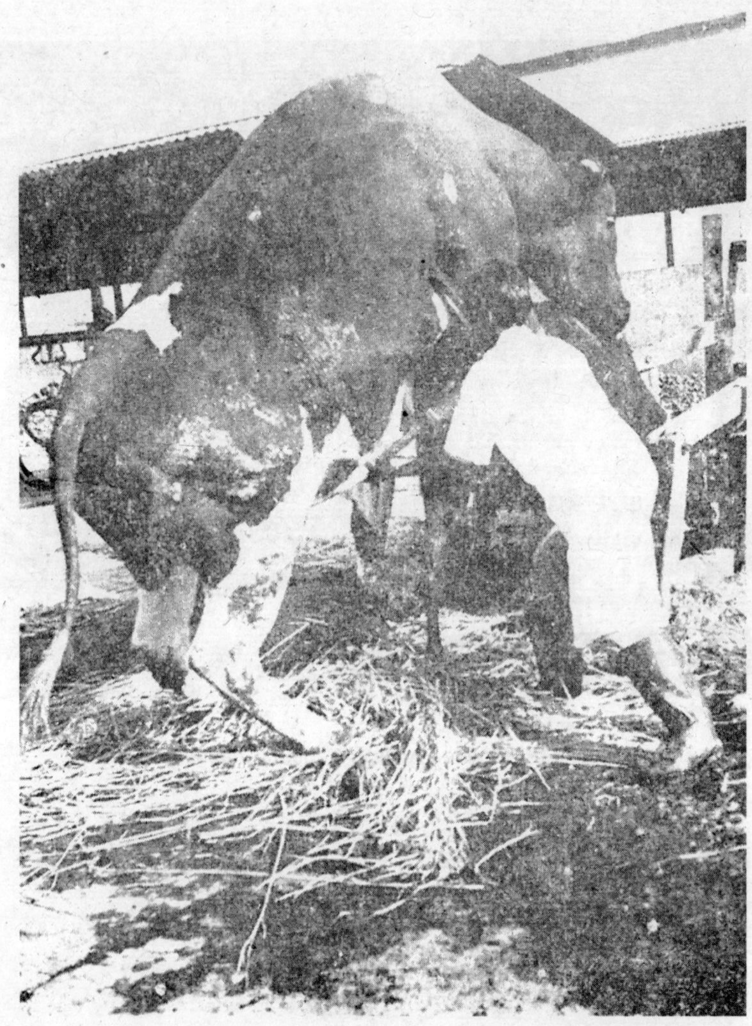

Plate 7. Collection of semen from the bull by the help of Artificial Vagina (Chapter 8).

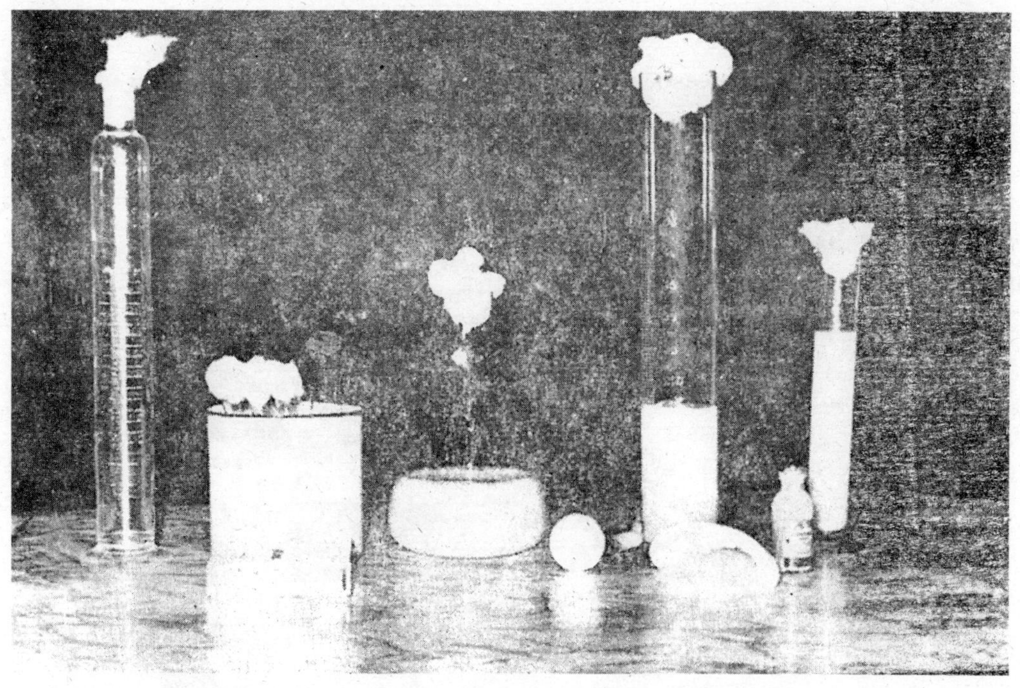

Plate 8. Preparation of Egg yolk buffer Extenter, (Chapter 8).

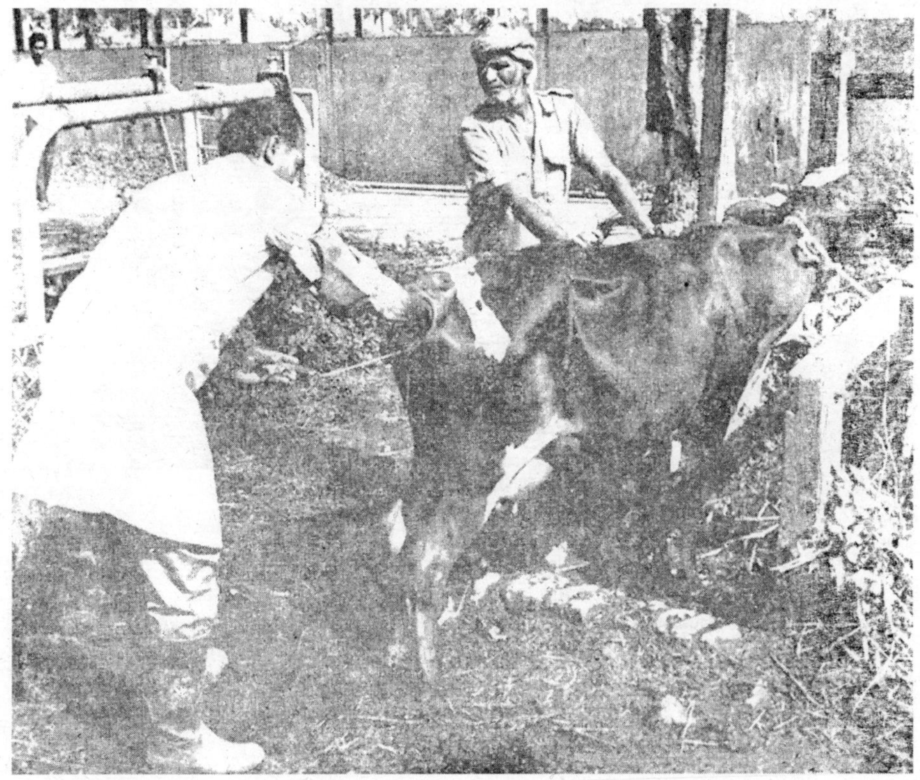

Plate 9. Artificially insemination of a cow (Chapter 8).

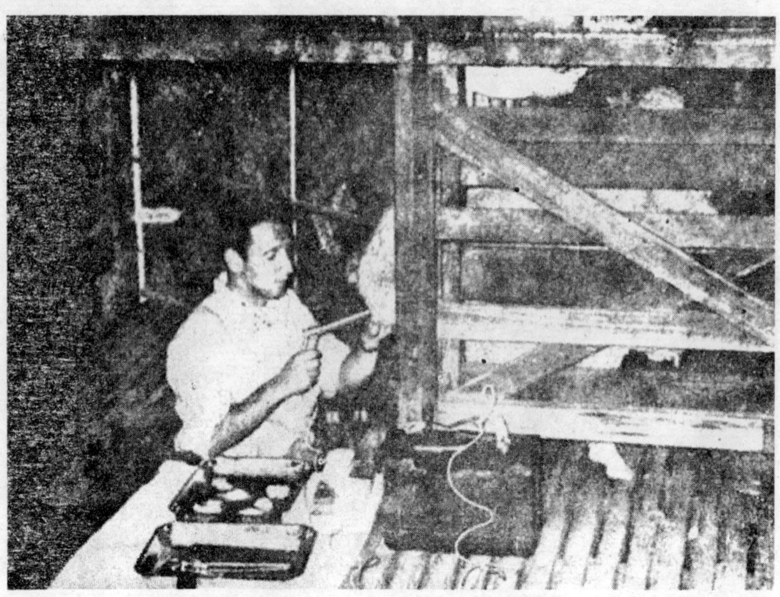

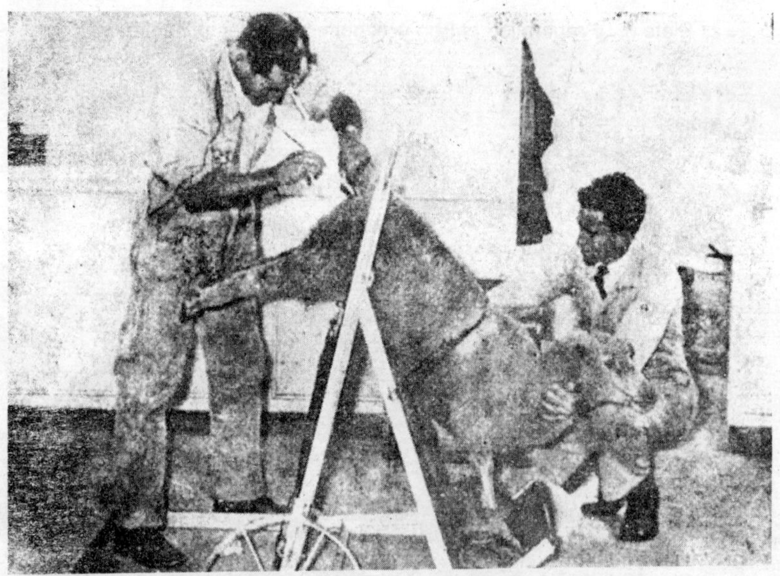

Plate 10. Two methods of artificial insemination for ewes.
Above : Rail-crate, as developed at New South Wales.
Below : Pit insemination in practice. Only one man is involve in catching and handling ewes (Chapter 8).

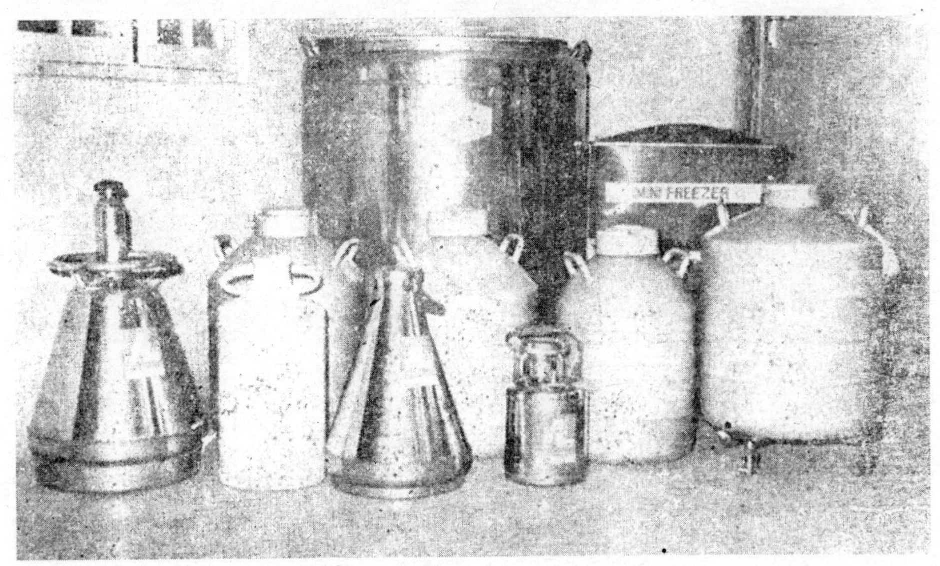

Plate 11. Oxygenic Containers (Chapter 8).

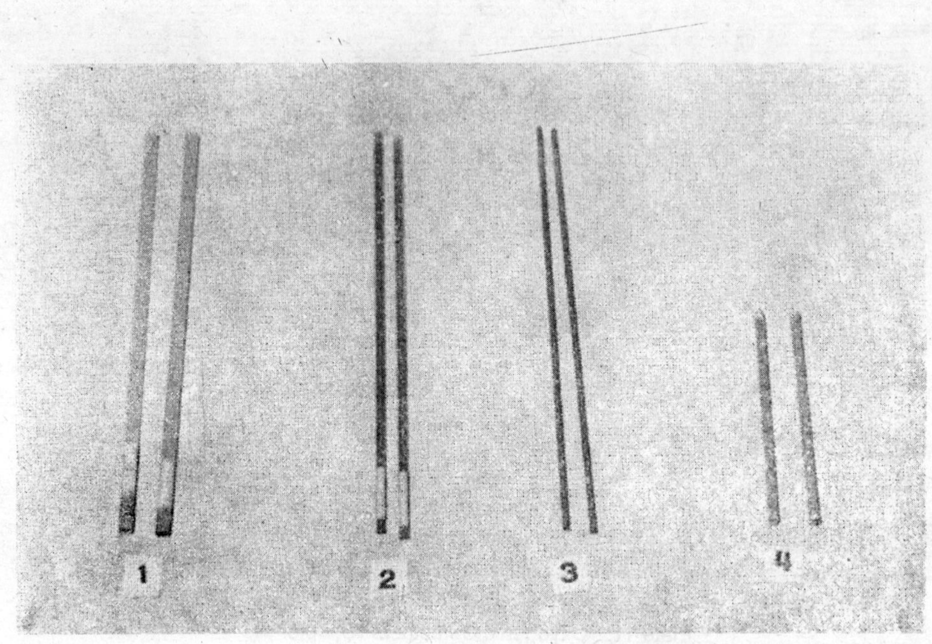

Plate 12. French Maxi, Medium, Mini and German Straws (Chapter 8).

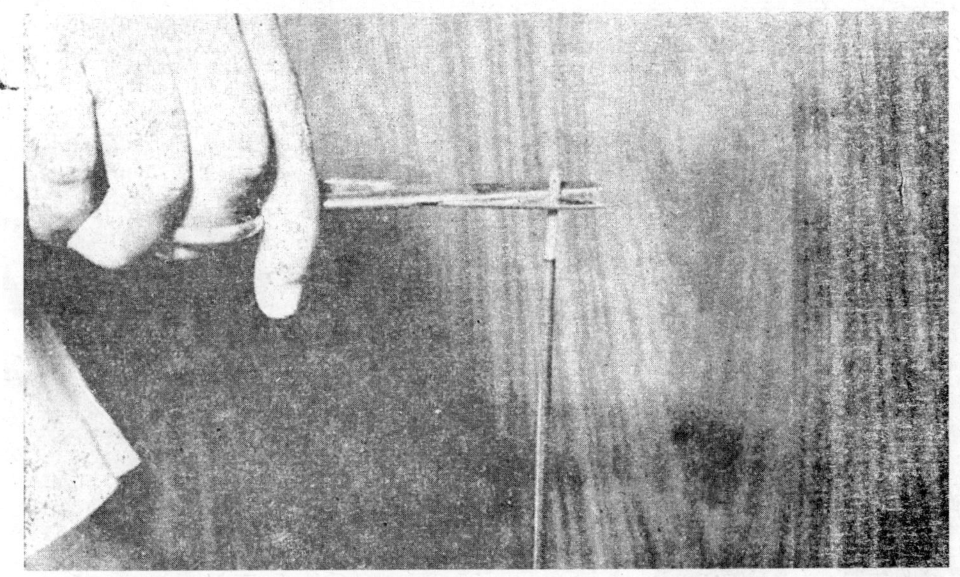

Plate 13. Cutting of straws at 90^0 Angle (Chapter 8).

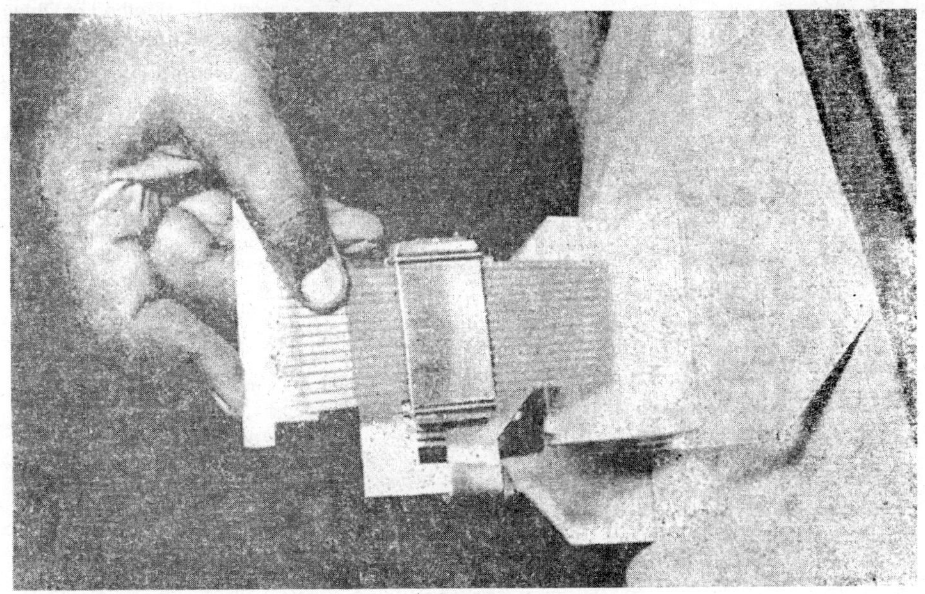

Plate 14. Filling of Semen (Chapter 8).

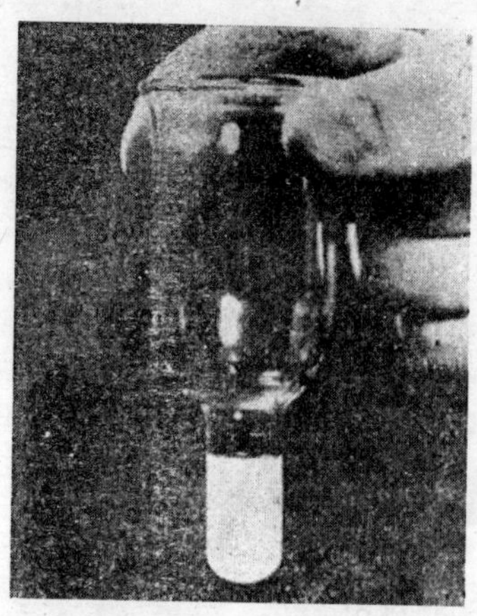

Plate 15. Assessment of semen volume in a Calibrated Collecting glass (Chapter 8).

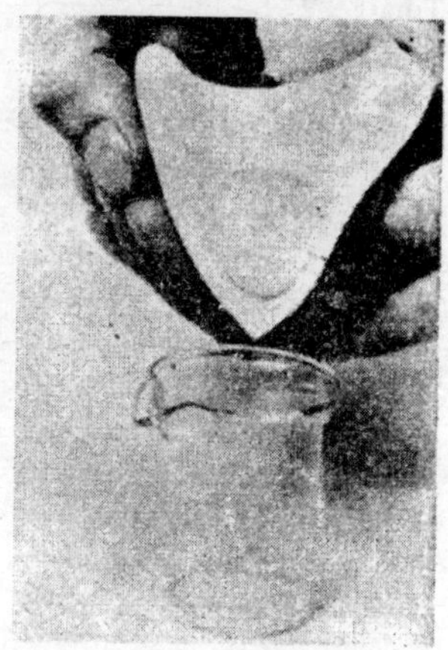

Plate 16. Method of Obtaining Egg yolk for semen diluents (Chapter 8).

Table 8.4

Composition of buffalo and zebu semen

Constituent	*(mg/100 ml semen or seminal plasma)* Buffalo	Zebu	*Statistical significance*
Total reducing substances	700 ± 52	769 ± 42	—
Fructose	355 ± 17	611 ± 39	**
Calcium	40 ± 2	75 ± 5	**
Chloride	373 ± 55	249 ± 26	*
Inorganic phosphatase	6.4 ± 0.6	5.9 ± 0.5	—
	(6.3 ± 0.4)	(5.6 ± 0.4)	
Acid-soluble phosphatase	72 ± 3.9	29 ± 3.9	**
	(64 ± 2.2)	(27 ± 2.9)	**
Total phosphorus	103 ± 8.9	47 ± 2.5	**
	(95 ± 7.2)	(42 ± 4.9)	**
Acid phosphatase activity	308 ± 44	145 ± 11	**
(Bondansky unit)	(307 ± 41)	(167 ± 11)	**
Alkaline phosphatase activity	(252 ± 37)	(134 ± 14)	*
(Bondansky unit)	(266 ± 42)	(152 ± 18)	*

Figures in parentheses indicate values in seminal plasma.
*Significant at 5 per cent level.
**Significant at 1 per cent level.
SOURCE: Roy, A., M.D. Pandey, and J.S. Rawat, Composition of Bovine Semen, *Indian J. Dairy Sci.*, 13 : 122 (1960).

ed for about eight months but once CAW is perpared, it can not be stored more than a day in a refrigerator as it loses its potency due to microbial fermentation of wheep.

Similarly another successful buffalo dilutor has been developed in Pakistan where they suggested use of homogenised milk as diluent for buffalo semen.

Dilutors for Sheep and Goat

The dilutents commonly used for dilution of ram semen are (i) tris, or (ii) citrate as buffers, glycose or fructose as the energy source and egg yolk to protect the sperm cell membrane against cold stock.

These diluents are also used for goat semen, but with a reduced egg yolk content to avoid a reaction which occurs due to the egg yolk coagulating enzyme present in the seminal plasma of goat bucks and it is higher when semen is collected by electroejaculation. The problem can be overcome by one of the following methods: (i) using a low concentration of egg yolk in the diluent, (ii) using a medium containing no egg yolk (for example milk), or (iii) removal of seminal plasma, and thereby the enzyme, by centrifugation.

Composition of two most common recommended diluents are given below:

1. Egg yolk-tris-fructose Diluent

		Ram	Goat buck
Tris(hydroxymethyl) aminomethane(g)	...	3.634	3.634
Fructose(g)	...	0.50	0.50
Citric acid/monohydrate (g)	...	1.99	1.99
Egg yolk (ml)	...	14.00	2.5*
Glass distilled water	...	100 ml	100 ml

2. Egg-yolk-glucose-citrate Diluent

		Ram	Goat buck
Sodium citrate ($2H_2O$) (g)	...	3.634	3.634
Glucose (g)	...	0.80	0.80
Egg yolk (ml)	...	20.00	2.50*
Glass distilled H_2O	...	100.00	100.00

To a diluent add penicillin at a dose of 1000 I.U. and streptomycin at 1000 microgram per ml.

** When using the above to diluents for buck semen, the coagulation reaction will not occur if the concentration of egg yolk does not exceed 2.0% after dilution. This should be considered during calculating the dilution rate of the semen. With the above egg yolk concentration there will be no harmful effect provided the buck semen is not diluted more than 1 + 3 (semen + diluent); if a greater dilution rate is required, the amount of egg yolk should be reduced accordingly.*

When preparing the above diluents, first the chemicals should be weighed and dissolved in a 100 ml capacity measuring cylinder by adding 75–80 ml of glass distilled water (ram) or 90–95 ml (buck). After addition of egg yolk and making up the final volume (100 ml) with distilled water, the diluent is mixed by rocking the measuring cylinder several times backwards and forwards to obtain an even distribution of the egg yolk.

Dilutors for Boar Semen

The following dilutors are commonly used for extending boar semen.

A.

Sodium citrate	20 gm
Sodium bicarbonate	2 gm
Potassium chloride	0.4 gm
Glucose-D	3.0 gm
Sulphanilamide	1.0 gm
Penicillin	1.0 million I. U.
Streptomycin	1.0 gm
Glass distilled H_2O	1000 ml

pH value 8.0 to 8.2 at 35°C.

B.

Glucose-D	120.0 gm
Ethylenediamino acetate	7.4 gm
NaOH(Basic soln. 4%)	16.0 gm
Sodium citrate 35.5%	20.0 ml
Penicillin	100,0001 I. U.
Streptomycin	0.5 gm
Glass distilled H_2O	2000 ml

C.		D.	
Glucose-D	40.0 gm	Glucose-D	120.0 gm
Sodium bicarbonate	1.0 gm	EDT-A	7.4 gm
Sodium citrate	3.8 gm	Sodium bicarbonate	2.4 gm
Cheloplex Helaton	2.6 gm	Sodium citrate	7.5 gm
Egg yolk	100.0 ml	Penicillin	100,000 I.U.
Combiotic	2.5 ml	Streptomycin	1.0 gm
Glass distilled H_2O	1000 ml	Glass distilled H_2O	2000 ml

The above dilutors can preserve boar semen for 3 to 6 days at a temperature of +10°C to +15°C

Dilutor for Stallion

It is very much in practice to use undiluted stallion semen for insemination of mares when the number of mares to a stallion is very limited. When large number of mares are assigned to one stallion, the semen has to be diluted and extended for use either for a single or repeated inseminations.

On account of the sensitivity of the stallion sperm it is recommended that dilutor at body temperature should be added to semen by slow rotating movements as soon as collection is obtained. Before this operation the viscous fraction is separated from the sperm bearing fraction.

Diluted semen is held in waterbath at 20 to 27°C and is used for inseminations within a few hours of the extension. When egg yolk dilutor is used the cooling process can be very rapid. The entire diluted semen is then placed in a refrigerator or into a thermoflask containing ice water at a temperature of 5 to 10°C.

The composition of a most effective dilutor is as follows:

Glucose	...	30 gm
Lactose	...	20 gm
Sodium potassium tartarate	...	10 gm
Glass distilled H_2O	...	1000 ml
Fresh egg yolk	...	200 gm
Para-amino benzoic acid	...	6 gm

The egg-yolk is freed of albumin membrane and chalazae. The dilution rate varied from 1 : 3 to 1 : 5. Fairly good results are obtained even after 48 hours storage and long transport.

Method of Dilution

Dilution of semen should be done soon after collection and routine examination. Both the semen and the diluent are placed in a waterbath at 30°C and must be at the same temperature at the time of dilution. The diluent should therefore be placed in the waterbath before collection of semen. Addition of cold diluent to semen may result in cold shock to the spermatozoa with consequent reduction of fertility. For dilution, a calibrated glass pipetter, or an inseminating pipette attached to a 1.0 ml syringe can be used .The pipette used should be thoroughly washed and sterilised and dried before hand. The dilution is done sucking an appropriate volume of diluent into the pipette (depending on the rate of dilution) and adding it slowly to the semen held in the collecting glass or other container. *Always add diluent to semen*, never the reverse, as this may cause shock to the spermatozoa and reduce their motility. After addition of the diluent, the semen and the diluent should be gently mixed. The diluted sample can then be examined under the microscope for motility and abnormality in sperm body.

INSEMINATION TECHNIQUES

Insemination in Cow

For inseminating cows or buffaloes there are two common techniques viz. 1) Speculum and 2) Rectovaginal methods.

Speculum Method

A sterilised speculum is lubricated preferably with liquid paraffin. The operator on dilating the vulvar lips introduces the speculum into the vaginal passage and on dilation locates the cervix by means of the head light torch. Insemination pipette containing 0.8 to 1.2 ml of diluted semen is then introduced through the vaginal passage and inserted half way into the cervix where semen is syringed.

The method although seems to be easier for less trained operators, but may prove dangerous if the vaginal speculum is not made 100% sterilized after each insemination. Moreover, the speculums are required in different sizes to suit cows of various sizes. The introduction of stainless steel speculum is found to be difficult owing to round opening of the tip measuring about 5 cm in diameter.

Recto-vaginal Technique

The method is relatively simpler, easy to operate and is widely used in practice all over the world. Due to non-requirement of speculum, there are less chances of spreading disease through ineffective sterilization of speculum. Moreover, by this technique it is possible to carry out intra uterine inseminations which is not possible by the speculum method.

A cow usually remains in heat for 12–24 hours and should be inseminated between 4–6 hours before the end of oestrous. Cows first seen in oestrous in the morning may be inseminated in the afternoon of the day; those first observed in oestrous in the afternoon should be inseminated in the next morning.

For the purpose of insemination, the cow at proper time should be well restrained and the tail is secured on one side of the service crate. The operator with protective clothing, viz., smock (a loose, shirtlike, outer garment worn to protect the clothes), rubber gloves and gumboots should first lubricate his left rubber gloved hand with soft soap and water and then passes it into the rectum to take out any dung at this region. By right hand the exterior of the vulva is cleaned with cotton wool swab soaked in normal saline and then with his left hand fingers should dilate the vulvar lips for inserting the insemination pipette, (a 2 ml plastic or glass syringe attached with rubber connection to a 40.0 cm glass pipette having an outside diameter of 6 mm and an inside diameter of 1 mm) well into the vagina in the upward and forward direction. The lubricated hand should then be passed into the rectum and back raked if necessary taking care that the balooning is not caused by outside air rushing into the rectum.

The operator should then try to locate and grasp the cervix properly through the rectal folds and the inseminating pipette—already in vagina—is then further directed close to the os(mouth of

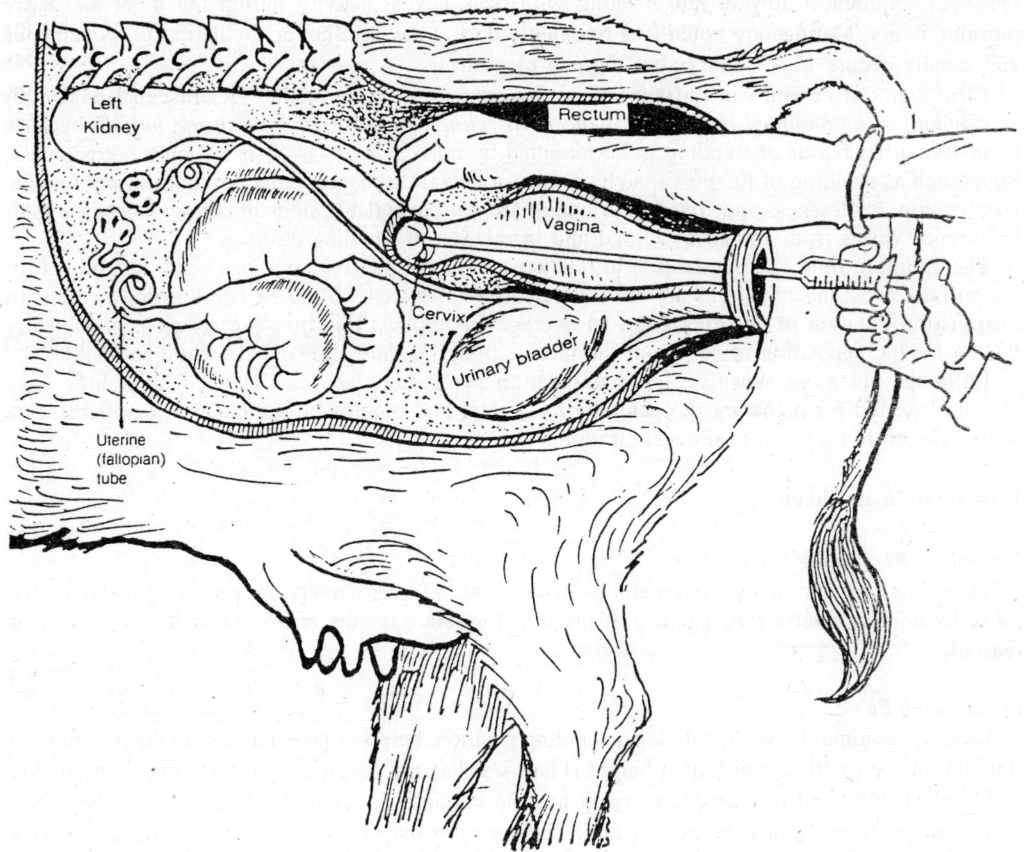

Fig.8.7. Recto-vaginal method of Insemination.

the cervix) when it should be carefully inserted the cervix proper and semen is deposited either *deep in the cervix or at beginning of the body of the uterus.* Too deep deposition in the uterine horns or deposition inside the beginning of cervix or in vagina should be avoided for better performances. When insemination is performed deep in the cervix, spermatozoa are likely to live longer in the cervix than in the uterus. Moreover, cervical semen deposition is preferred to uterine deposition, since conception rates are equal but there is less uterine injury, infection, and chance of spreading disease. Furthermore, is less likely to be interrupted in cows showing signs of oestrus during pregnancy when semen is deposited in the cervix rather than in the uterus. Semen deposition in the uterine horn is undesirable, because the non-ovulating uterine horn might be selected. (Pregnancies occur more frequently in the right uterine horn of cows). Deposition of semen in the vagina results in dilution, contamination, and lowered conception rate. Of course, when a bull inseminates a cow naturally, approximately 5 to 10 billion spermatozoa are deposited in the vagina. However, when semen is deposited artificially into the cervix, considerably fewer sperms are required to achieve conception.

Insemination in Buffalo

The oestrous cycle is about 21 days and 'standing' oestrous is usually less than 24 hours.

Oestrous commences toward late evening with peak sexual activity during the night and early morning hours. Matings are noted less frequently during daylight hours. Ovulation is spontaneous and usually occurs 15–18 hours after the end of oestrous.

Clear signs of oestrous in buffalo are not as pronounced as in cattle. Heterosexual behaviour or *standing to be mounted by a male is the most reliable sign of oestrous in the buffalo* because homosexual behaviour or standing to be mounted by other females is observed only occasionally. Signs such as swelling of the vulva, a clear mucoid vulval discharge, reduction in milk production, vocalization, restlessness and frequent urination are not dependable signs of oestrous because their occurrence varies from animal to animal and in relation to standing oestrous.

The optimum time of insemination in relation to oestrus and ovulation has been determined for the buffalo. Most inseminations are usually performed between 12 and 14 hours from the onset of oestrous(the duration of oestrous is on an average 32 hrs). At this time the cervix is sufficiently dilated for the deposition of semen in the uterine body by the rectovaginal technique of AI.

Buffaloes are more sensitive for manipulation per rectum and easily bleed on a little hard pressure exerted for palpating the genitalia in general and ovaries in particular. All possible care should therefore be taken to prevent straining.

Insemination in Sheep

Methods of Restraining Ewes

There are two commonly used methods of restraining ewes, namely the use of an inseminating pit or by holding over a rail. The use of inseminating crate is now obsolete due to many obvious reasons.

Inseminating Pit

Ewes are commonly inseminated in a standing position, held against a fence with the inseminator standing in a pit with eye at vulval height (Plate). It has the advantage that one man can quickly and easily handle and restrain the ewes. It has the possible disadvantage that ewes are held in a horizontal position so that the semen after insemination may have a back flow from the cervix area.

Rail

In many of the developed countries ewes are commonly inseminated by holding over a rail in the yards. It has the obvious advantages of simplicity, absence of specialized equipment, and the fact that ewes are held head down, so facilitating deposition and retention of semen in the cervix. If large numbers are to be inseminated the method is rather clumsy and tiring, two men being required to lift the ewes over the rail from one side.

A modification developed in Australia. It incorporates the rail principle in a simple crate. The inseminator assists in the loading operation, so eliminating one catcher, and the use of a lever to elevate the animal's rump reduces the physical labour. It is a highly satisfactory method of restraint which involves the inseminator in somewhat more labour than does the pit technique, but has the advantage of sloping the ewes.

Insemination Procedure in Sheep

Indian sheep are seasonally polyestrous, having three main mating seasons, viz. March to April or summer, June to July or autumn and September to October, post-monsoon. The fertility is high during autumn in plain areas and in summer in hilly areas.

Table 8.5

Comparative Oestrous and Oestrous Cycle in Sheep and Goat

Oestrous cycle lengths (days)			Length of Oestrous (hrs)	Time of Ovulation
Species	*Mean*	*Range*		
Sheep	16.7	(14–19)	24 – 36	Near end of oestrous
Goat	20.6	(18–22)	26 – 42	Shortly after end of oestrous

In contrast to goat, in sheep relatively quiet heat (oestrous) is the rule. Oestrous in the ewe is extremely difficult to detect if there is no ram in the flock. But, with a ram in the immediate environment, it is usual for the ewe in oestrous to associate closely with it for most of a 24 hour period. Ewes frequently initiate the first sexual contact by seeking out the ram and thereafter following the ram while heat persists. Sometimes the ewe will rub herself against the ram. Further behavioural evidence of oestrous sometimes appears as tail shaking but this only occurs at mating. Different grades of intensity occur in the sex drive of ewes, although the general mating pattern is similar in all. Many ewes in oestrous actively seek out the male and, when a choice of ram is possible, it is the most active ram which is generally chosen. Although the normal period is recognised as being just over 24 hour, oestrous can last for upto 3 days in some ewes. Mutual riding among ewes, one of which is in oestrous, has not been reported.

When the ewe is presented for insemination, the lips of the vulva should be cleaned by wiping them towards the anus with cotton wool soaked in normal saline. A sterilized speculum lubricated with white vaseline is slipped into the vagina with a rotary motion and the cervix is located and imprisoned in the opening of the speculum. The semen is drawn into the insemination pipette along and inserted greatly into the opening of the cervix for depositing about 0.1 ml semen. Because of the peculiar structure of the cervix in ewe it is not possible to deposit semen in uterus. It may be placed (i) in the opening of the cervix, (ii) on the cervix as it projects into the anterior end of the vagina.

It is recommended that at least 50 million motile sperms should be inseminated for liquid semen while for frozen semen the number should increase up to 200 million motile sperms. With progestogen treatment of ewes to induce oestrous at a synchronised time, sperm number requirements may be as great as 1500 million cells. Double inseminations 12 hours apart increase fertility.

It is to be noted that optimum time of insemination is mid oestrus i.e., 12 to 18 hours after the onset of heat.

The volume of insemination is very important, for example, insemination of more than 0.2 ml of semen into the cervix of the ewe or doe is of no advantage as much of the semen would flow back into the vagina. Recommended inseminate volumes for sheep and goat are the following:

For vaginal insemination	0.30–0.50 ml
For cervical insemination	0.05–0.20 ml
For intrauterine insemination	0.05–0.10 ml

These volumes should contain at least the recommended minimum number of motile spermatozoa. For sheep and goat many more spermatozoa are needed than for insemination of cows. This is due to the differences in anatomical structure of the cervices of ewes, does and cows. Whereas the cervix of the cow in oestrous is open and allows deep cervical or intrauterine insemination that of the sheep is impenetrable by an inseminating pipette, and in goats only a proportional cervices are penetrable. As a general rule, less spermatozoa are required for uterine than for cervical insemination and less for cervical than for vaginal insemination. The *minimum safe limit* for the number of *motile* spermatozoa per inseminate is given in Table 8.6

Table 8.6

	Type of Semen		
	Fresh	*Liquid-stored*	*Frozen-thawed*
Vaginal insemination	300	not effective	not effective
Cervical insemination	100	150	180
Intrauterine insemination . . . . via cervix (goat only)	60	60	65

Insemination in Goat

The length of oestrous cycle in goat varies between 18 to 22 days which lasts for 24 to 36 hours. Ovulation occurs 12 to 36 hours after the start of oestrous. Mating or insemination should be arranged accordingly which may be specific to individual goat. Ovulation is more frequent on the right ovary.

Oestrous in does is characterised by the following symptoms.

1) Continuous bleating (to make sound)
2) Wagging of the tail rhythmically from side to side
3) Redness and swelling of the vulva
4) Mucus discharge from the vulva
5) Mounting of other goats and allowing mounting by others
6) Lack of interest in feeding
7) Drop in milk production in some lactating does

Table 8.7

Semen characteristics of Jamunapari bucks

Colour	:	Creamy to slight yellow
Consistency	:	Thick, opaque
Volume	:	0.815 ml
Motility	:	5%
pH	:	6.5
Concentration	:	1.5 million per ml
Average % of live sperms	:	90.7
Average % of abnormal sperms	:	5

During insemination the doe in oestrous is held and speculum lubricated with liquid paraffin is inserted and cervix is located by the inseminator. The pipette containing 0.1 ml to 0,2 ml semen is then inserted through the speculum with the help of right hand and semen is blown on the mouth of cervix by slightly pressing the rubber bulb or by means of a syringe. The pipette should not be penetrated deeply. Freshly diluted semen with a minimum number of 20–50 million sperms per 0.1 ml is required for obtaining the optimum conception rate.

Insemination in Pig

Young females exhibit oestrous for the first time at about 6 months of age but because of the small litters resulting from matings during the first few heats, they are not generally served until they are about 8 months old.

Oestrous itself lasts for 2 to $2\frac{1}{2}$ days and recurs every 19–23 (average 21) days throughout the year. Gilts, however, tend to remain on heat for only about one day. Environmental light and temperature changes seem to have little influence on this basic pattern.

The observable signs of oestrous are not very precise. The vulva gradually reddens, enlarges 2–3 days before oestrous and shows its maximum development just prior to the $2\frac{1}{2}$ day period during which the sow will stand to the boar.

The sow is best inseminated without being restrained to avoid possible loss of spermatozoa. With some rubbing and pressure on the back, the sow in full oestrous usually stands calmly during insemination. The insemination tube cannot easily be guided into the cervix as the portion of the vagina tapers directly into the cervix have longitudinal folds. For this reason it is not possible to pass the cathetor into the uterus, but with the inflated cuff most of the 50 ml volume of raw or extended semen will be forced into the uterus. High sperm numbers in large volume are required in sows for maximal fertility for unknown reasons.

Insemination in Mare

In India, early spring is considered the best breeding season for horses. There is less mortality in spring foals as compared to winter foals due to warm weather.

Fertility rises during estrous to a peak two days before the end of estrous, then falls off abruptly. Mares with heat periods of 1 to 3 days should be bred on the first day. Mares with longer heat periods should be bred on the second and fifth day of heat. Repeat 2 days later if still on heat.

Early in the breeding season, some mares show intense sexual desire during long heat periods but do not ovulate. These mares probably will not conceive until their heat periods become shorter and more regular. Other mares may have only "silent heat" periods in which ovulation occurs but no sexual desire is evident. Many of these mares will conceive if the heat period is identified by rectal palpation and appearance of the vulva, vagina and cervix.

As stated above best time to breed a mare is near ovulation time (1–2 days before the end of oestrous). The mare should be restrained backed against baled straw to protect the inseminator.

The area around the vulva should be cleaned by rubbing the area with cloth soaked in mild antiseptic before the insemination to minimize contamination. The left arm in a polythene sleeve, lightly lubricated, is inserted into the vagina and the index finger easily negotiates the dilated and straight cervical canal.

The sterile plastic insemination cathetor, to which the syringe containing the semen is attached, and held in the right hand, is introduced and pushed gently along the left arm and alongside the finger into the cervix. The semen is then gently injected from the syringe into the uterus. It has been estimated that for optimum fertility between 1 and 2 billion living sperms should enter the uterus and the volume of semen should be 10–50 ml according to the size of the mare. In this way, without dilution of semen, 4 mares could be inseminated on the same day from one ejaculate.

Table 8.8

Insemination requirements and related phenomena in mammals

Item	*Cattle*	*Sheep*	*Horse*	*Swine*
1. Frequency of semen collection (per week)	3-5	7-25	7-10*	3-5
2. Characteristics of average ejaculate+ Volume (ml)	5-8	1	125	215
3. Sperm concentration (million/ml)	1200	3000	122	270
4. Total sperm/ejac. (million)	9600	3000	15,000	58,000
5. Motile sperm (%)	70	75	70	60
6. Morphological normal sperm (%)	80	90	70	60
7. Recommended diluent	Yolk-citrate +modification	Yolk-glucose citrate	Glucose-gelatin	Yolk-glucose bicarbonate
8. Storage temperature for liquid semen (°C)	5	5	15	15-5
9. Rate of dilution ‡ (1 ml of semen diluted to ml)	105	9	2	4
10. Storage of liquid semen (days)	4	1 or 2	1	1
11. Optimum time to inseminate	middle or end of estrus	toward end of estrus	third day of estrus	first and/or 2nd day of estrus
12. Dose of insemination (vol. ml) (motile sperm no. million)	1 1	0.2 50-60	20-40 1500	50 2000
13. Deposition of semen	Cervical	Cervical	Uterine	Cervical
14. No. of possible females bred/ejaculate	800	40	7	17
15. No. of possible females bred per week	3200	600	60	80
16. Conception on 1st insemination (% pregnant)	65	70	65	70

*One or two days rest should be provided each week.
+Normal and healthy mature males with nearly ideal collection technique.
‡Adjusted to conc. of sperm—practical rate listed.
(From Trimberger, G. W., in *Reproduction in Farms Animals*, Hafez, E.S.E. (Ed.), **Philadelphia, Lea & Febiger, 1962**).

However, using semen fresh, or stored upto two hours on normal mares, it has been found that an inseminating dose of 100 million sperms is satisfactory.

The minimal number of frozen sperm required for high conception rates has not been established.

DEEP FREEZING OF SEMEN

In India Artificial Insemination (AI) utilizing liquid (chilled) semen from exotic dairy breeds has been playing vital role for nearly four decades. The advent of "Frozen semen technology" has by this time become remarkable by any measure in turning this century to the gateway of white revolution.

As early as 1938 a German scientist, Jahnel found that by deep freezing testicular tissue of rabbits, sperms could survive freezing to –192°C. During 1949 Polge, Smith and Parkes accidentally added 15–20% glycerol to a fowl sperm solution and observed very good motility after freezing to –79°C. Thus the remarkable property of glycerol in maintaining life of deep frozen sperms were established. Later on it was observed that the resistance against deep freezing is quite different in different species. It is known that bull semen cannot withstand a sudden drop in temperature so called temperature shock. For that reason Smith and Polge (1950) cooled the glycerol treated bull semen slowly to –79°C and got a much better survival of the semen than that by rapid cooling. The first insemination with deep frozen semen were performed by Steward (1951) in cooperation with Polge and Rowson. Out of 5 inseminated cows one became pregnant.

Subsequent developments have been the introduction of new freezing techniques, improved semen dilutors and additives.

Principle of Deep Freezing

The general principle of deep freezing of semen is to dilute the semen with an extender containing glycerol. After equilibration the suspension is frozen according to special rules and thereafer stored in liquid nitrogen (–196°C) as the cooling medium.

As intra and extra cellular water of media crystalised as ice, the salts get concentrated in the residual fluid which becomes progressively more hypertonic. Thus the sperm cells become subject to severe osmotic stress and in particular to increase concentration of electrolytes when the water is freezing out. Glycerol has the ability to attach itself a considerable quantity of water, which is then not available to form ice but can still act as a solvent. The use of glycerol therefore enables freezing to be carried out slowly enough to avoid thermal shock without exposing the sperm cells to lethal concentrations of electrolytes.

Merits and Limitations of Frozen Semen

Merits

1. Frozen semen permits maximum utilization of semen from a given sire. No semen need to be discarded because of age, as with liquid semen.
2. Long term preservation removes barrier on time and distance in AI International semen transport has come into existence today.
3. Can be undertaken for:
   a) Selective breeding
   b) Grading
   c) Cross breeding
   d) Progeny testing of bulls

4. Transportation costs of semen are minimised compared to liquid semen usage, as large consignments can be delivered at infrequent intervals and full utilization can be made at each bull's semen producing capacity.
5. Minimises requirement of breeding bulls to be maintained at breeding farm.
6. Provides round the clock breeding facility even at the villages.
7. Frozen can safely be used in an outbreak of disease (foot and mouth) without dislocation in semen transport.
8. Complies with highest hygienic standards in artificial breeding.
9. Comparative studies on cost factor between liquid and frozen semen has been done at National Dairy Research Institute, Bangalore. It has been observed that the average cost of A.I. with liquid semen came to Rs. 60.85 as compared to frozen semen which is Rs. 18.63. Further the cost involved per calf born was Rs. 235.47 and Rs. 53.13 respectively in using liquid and frozen semen.
10. Frozen semen is extremely valuable in carrying on the influence of superior sires even after 50–100 years of their death.

Limitations of using Frozen Semen

1. About 30 per cent of bull's semen does not withstand the rigors of freezing.
2. The cost involved initially is high.
3. Frozen semen limits number of sires used, if our selection methods are not perfect. This may lead to wider damage among future progenies.
4. Requires sound technical experts for handling the frozen semen.

Dilutors for Deep Freezing

The idea that the sperm cell will remain in living condition without expenditure of any significant metabolic energy for an indefinite period inspired the scientists to preserve living cell in the frozen state. Further it was the spectacular discovery of Polge in 1949, which showed that the death of spermatozoa on freezing could be avoided by suspending the cells in a medium containing glycerol. Thus a practical answer to freezing technique was evolved.

At least 50 per cent of the bull sperm from an unselected population remains inactive or dead during freezing and thawing due to (1) internal ice-crystal formation which affects the structure of the spermatozoa, (2) the increase in solute concentration as water is withdrawn from the suspension medium, (3) by interaction of these two physical factors, an ideal extender should qualify for giving cryoprotection during freezing. For bovine spermatozoa the basic components for an ideal extender are:

Buffers

Out of varieties of inorganic and organic buffers which have been tried for deep freezing of bovine semen, an organic buffer known as 'Tris' (Hydroxymethyl amino methane) first used by Graham (1972) at pH 7.0 which has been found to be most popular even to-day. The buffer can be successfully used for bull, buffalo, ram, dog, poultry and even for human. It (i) prolongs life of sperm at room temperature, (ii) penetrates cells (iii) acts as intracellular buffer, (iv) less toxic during freezing and (v) provides better clarity under microscope.

Fructose

Addition of fructose provides (i) glycolysable substrate for the sperm, (ii) prevents sperm agglutination, (iii) maintains required osmotic tension and electrolyte balance, (iv) aids extra cryoprotection during deep freezing.

Glycerol

The possible ways by which it functions are: (i) modifies size and shape of ice crystals of the media, (ii) binds water and decreases freezing point of solution resulting reduction of ice crystals, (iii) acts through salt buffering mechanism, (iv) reduces solute concentration, (v) prevents denaturation of proteins and thereby protects plasma membrane.

Egg Yolk

(1) When mammalian sperms are cooled to 5°C they are subjected to 'cold shock' which causes leakage of intracellular enzymes, minerals, lipoproteins, ATP from inside the cell. Lecithin, proteins, lipoproteins and other similar compounds present in yolk provides an effective means of guard against cold shock. (2) In addition to this, the valuable nutrients of egg yolk are very slowly utilised by sperms. (3) Egg yolk also protects the enzymes having disulphide bridges (SH group) as well as of antiagglutinic factor presents in seminal plasma.

Antibiotics

Semen under normal condition generally gets contaminated with both pathogenic and non-pathogenic micro-organisms. Organisms which are contagious and can infect cow through pathogens are: *Brucella abortus, Vibrio fetus, Trichomonas fetus, Leptospira pomona, Mycobacterium tuberculosis, M. paratuberculosis* (Johnes disease) and viral agents that cause infectious bovine rhinotracheitis (I.B.R.), Foot and Mouth disease.

Table 8.9

Semen Extenders for Artificial Insemination with Frozen Semen

Ingredients	Bull	Bull	Boar	Ram	Buck (Goat)	Stallion
Tris (hydroxymethyl) Aminomethane (g)	24.20	—	2.00	36.34	24.20	—
Tes [N-Tris (Hydroxymethyl)] Methyl-2-Aminoethanesulfonic Acid (g)	—	—	12.00	—	—	—
Glucose (g)	10.00	—	32.00	5.00	10.00	50.00
Citric acid monohydrate (g)	13.40	—	—	—	13.40	—
Lactose (g)	—	—	—	—	—	3.00
Raffinose(g)	—	—	—	—	—	3.00
Orvus ES paste (g)	—	—	5.00	—	—	—
Penicillin (units/ml)	1000	1000	—	—	1000	1000
Streptomycin (g/ml)	1000	1000	—	—	1000	1000
Polymyxin B (units/ml)	500	500	—	—	—	—
Cow milk (ml)	—	930	—	—	—	—
Egg yolk (ml)	200	—	200	150	100	50
Glycerol (ml)	70	70	10	50	80	50
Distilled water to final volume (ml)	1000	—	1000	1000	1000	1000

Source : Primarily from Hafez, 1980 (chap.26); Pursel and Johnson, 1975; Salamon 1976; Sexton, 1980.

Refrigeration greatly suppresses the multiplication of organisms, but does not necessarily stop it. Organisms which survive freezing temperature of –196°C are *Pseudomonas aeruginosa, Trichomonas fetus, Leptospira pomona*, Foot and Mouth virus and infectious Pustular Vulvovaginitis virus.

Penicillin and Streptomycin are the two antibiotics widely used since 1950 and are still in use. They are found to be relatively harmless to sperm cells and particularly in combination, inhibit broad spectrum microorganisms. 500 to 1000 I.U. of crystallin penicillin-G and 500 to 1000 micrograms of dihydro-streptomycin per ml of extended semen is enough for routine use. *Procain penicillin is toxic to the spermatozoa.*

Antibiotics will not completely eliminate Corynebacterium pyogenes, Brucella, Trichomonas fetus, Mycobacterium, Pseudomonas and they will have no effect on viruses, Rickettsie and on Fungi.

Hence addition of antibiotics is not a 100% safety from pathogenic contamination of semen. Semen from healthy bulls managed under full hygienic environment and handled by an experienced hand is always preferred.

Methodology for Freezing Semen

1. *Preparation of Diluent*

Diluent is always prepared fresh, generally an hour before collection of semen so that the medium gets stabilised. As has been mentioned earlier, Tris yolk glycerol dilutor is the choice of preference for frozen semen. It is prepared by mixing :

Fresh egg yolk	1 part	or	20 cc
Tris buffer*	4 parts	or	80 cc
Glycerol (vol/vol)	7%	or	7 cc

**Composition of Tris buffer*

Tris (Hydroxy methyl amino methaneh)	30.481g
Citric acid	17.000g
Fructose	12.500g
Glass distilled water ...	850 ml
Penicillin	10 bcs
Streptomycin	1 g

The diluent is kept ready in water bath at 30°C for further dilution. As far as possible eggs should be fresh (not more than 7 days old) and stored in refrigerator. Eggs should never be water washed since egg is covered by a thin protective membrane which disappears on washing and thereby allows microbes to enter into egg through the micro-pores on the shell.

2. *Collection of Semen*

The bull center should have a schedule to prescribe days for collection from each bull. The usual practice is to collect semen from a healthy bull once a week and twice from young bulls all of which should be sound, having good libido and sexual behaviour.

Semen collections should be made during early morning hours before feeding is done. The teaser cow should be well cleaned before she is brought to the service crate. It is better to tie her tail with a rope on one side so that swinging of the tail does not cause any obstruction in proper mounting. The dummy should not be taller than the bull to be collected.

The artificial vagina prewarmed with hot water and refilled to bring the inner temperature of 40°C to 46°C when ready for use. Half to two third capacity of the A.V. should be filled with warm water. The inflation of air should be done in such a way that the opening of the A.V. should close, resulting in building out of the inner lining to form a cushion. Insulation bag may be fixed on the graduated glass tube to avoid temperature shock.

During collection, A.V. should be held at 45° angle to the ground, so that the long axis parallels the line of the penis. Excessive bending of the penis before or during the thrust can distract and injure the bull. The A.V. should be handled in such a way that the penis just touches the lining. The condition inside AV should equal to that of inside the natural vagina and this condition stimulates the ejaculation. The vagina must never be pressed on the penis. Generally 15 minutes of teasing and 1 or 2 false mounts will suffice.

3. *Evaluation of Semen*

Immediately after collection semen is evaluated for volume, colour, consistency and presence of foreign matter. One drop of semen is placed on glass slide and is evaluated under phase contrast microscope for initial forward motility. Samples showing more than +3 are taken for further processing. From this, 0.1 ml of semen is taken for estimating concentration of spermatozoa either by photoelectric colorimeter method or by haemocytometer counts. Till the final dilution rate is decided, semen is pre-diluted to a known low volume of extender and stored in water bath. The individual motility of the sperm is assessed with the diluted semen using phase contrast microscope. Sample showing more than 60 per cent of motility is taken for further processing.

4. *Dilution of Semen*

The basic idea of dilution of semen is (1) to preserve fertilising capacity of the spermatozoa for a long period and (2) to increase services to a number of females.

The dilution rate is decided based on the motility rate, sperm concentration and capacity of straw used. In general a minimum of 30 million motile sperms in each dose is recommended. As soon as the final volume of diluted semen has been determined the remainder of the diluent is added and the flask containing diluted semen is gradually cooled to +5°C in a refrigerator over a period of 45 to 60 minutes.

5. *Equilibration of Semen*

Before storing the diluted semen at frozen state (–196°C), the practice is to preserve it at much higher temperature (+5°C) for about 6 hours. This pre-freeze storage of diluted semen is known as '*Equilibration*' of diluted semen. This is so done for the glycerol to bring about its beneficial action on the spermatozoa. Glycerol permeates sperms and gives better resistance to withstand freezing stress.

During this equilibration period, filling of straws with diluted semen is carried out inside a cold handling cabinet maintained at +5°C. Equilibration period of 6 hours is generally practised. At the end of equilibration period, the pre-freeze motility is again recorded. Samples showing more than 60 per cent motility are taken for "Test freezing". This is done by filling processed diluted semen in 2 to 3 straws for each sample which are initially kept either in big semen containers or in mini-freezer firstly in liquid nitrogen vapour having a temperature between –120 to –130°C and then plunged in liquid nitrogen. The entire treatment will take about 10–15 minutes. After this the revival rate is determined and satisfactory samples are taken up for filling and further processings.

6. *Different Packaging System of Frozen Semen*

Packaging frozen semen in various single dose containers for storage and delivery systems started in U.S.A since 1954 where use of glass ampoules was first developed. Japanese scientists developed a technique for freezing semen in pellets. French, Danish and German were responsible for introduction of straw technique. Other packing techniques such as pipettes, bulk sausages, gelatin capsule etc. have been reported for frozen semen without any acceptance due to high cost and lower fertility.

(i) The Ampoule Method

This method was mainly used in U.S.A. Semen is placed in glass ampoules, sealed, frozen and preserved in liquid nitrogen. For insemination the ampoule is thawed in warm water, ampoule is cut, semen drawn into glass catheter and used as liquid semen.

Merits

(1) Since the semen is sealed inside ampoule, contamination during storage is avoided.
(2) Identification of sample is possible as the bull no. etc. can be marked on the ampoule.

Demerits

(1) As the semen is frozen in a larger volume the freezability and fertility are less.
(2) It occupies more storage space in frozen semen containers.
(3) About 8–10 per cent semen is lost while handling semen at the time of thawing and insemination.
(4) Use of glass catheters for Artificial Insemination has several drawbacks as experienced with liquid semen. Hence this method is not popular.

(ii) The Pellet Method

Freezing is done by depositing 0.1 to 0.2 ml of semen on the depressions created on the dry ice (solid CO_2). The semen gets frozen and after 10 minutes the pellets (like tablets) are collected in a goblet and stored in liquid nitrogen at –196°C. At insemination a pellet is dissolved in 0.9 ml of warm diluent and used just like liquid semen.

Merits:

(1) Economical method
(2) Occupies less storage space.

Demerits:

1. Identification is difficult.
2. As the semen is stored uncovered they may get contaminated with organisms if present in liquid nitrogen or other pellets.
3. When the pellets are handled by forceps they break and get attached to forceps and results in loss of sperms.
4. The freezability is moderate.
5. Cumbersome procedure involving the necessity of seperate thawing solution, glass rod for Artificial Insemination etc. Thus the potential for spread of disease is high and the pregnancy from wrong bull is not uncommon with this technique.

(iii) The Straw Technique

Plastic straws were introduced in Denmark in 1940 for packing liquid semen. The first technique for freezing of semen in straws using liquid nitrogen vapour was developed by Adler in 1960. These techniques were later modified and refined by Cassou in 1965 and most of the procedures currently employed with 'French straw' made of polyvinyl chloride was introduced. In the year 1972 a plastic straw called *'mini tube'* or *German straws* or *'Lanshut system'* was developed in West Germany. A straw known as 'U.S.' or *Continental straws* made of polypropylene was developed in United States.

Straw technique has got several advantages over pellet or ampoule methods and hence it is popular all over the world.

Merits:

1. Semen is processed in thin film, with its greater surface area to volume ratio, there is rapid heat exchange and better revival rate.
2. Reduced volume of semen is better tolerated by uterus.
3. The diameter of A.I. catheter is small and hence passing cervix in heifers and cows in late heat is easy.
4. Complete delivery of semen into the uterus is possible.
5. Identification of sample by colour of straw, printing, colour of PVA sealing powder or coloured plastic beads is possible.
6. Use of steel gun is safer compared to glass catheter.
7. Use of disposable plastic sheath for each A.I. excludes spread of disease during Artificial Insemination.
8. This occupies less storage space compared to ampoules.
9. With full automation for filling and sealing, it meets hygienic standards in semen processing.

The dimensions of French and German Straws are given below:

Table 8.10

	Length	Diameter	Volume
French Medium	135 m.m.	2.8 m.m.	0.5 ml
French Mini	135 m.m.	2.0 m.m.	0.25 ml
German	65 m.m.	2.8 m.m.	0.25 ml

7. ***Printing of Straws***

Before the diluted semen is filled into straws, the straws have to be lebelled by printing the breed, name or no. of bull, date of collection, etc. by using an automatic straw printing machine. The printing must become dry before the straws are taken up for filling.

8. ***Filling of Straws***

Filling of straws can be done manually as well as by automatic machine. Manual method is cheaper and easy, as such the method is described hereunder.

It requires vacuum pump, filling comb, rubber tube, straw clips and polyvinyl alcohol (PVA) powder. The straws (15 medium or 20 mini) are clipped together by using straw clips. The clipped straws are cooled to +5°C in the cold handling cabinet. The straws in the clamps are fitted on the filling comb, which in turn is fixed to vacuum pump through the rubber tube. Semen is taken in the bath of the bubbler and filling is done by operating vacuum pump. Due to negative pressure semen is drawn into the straws.

Appearance of two distinct bands in the factory seal indicates complete filling of straws. An uniform air space is created in all the filled straws by pushing the open ends of the straws on to the teeth of the bubbler. The bubbler and the bath are discarded after use is required in order to allow for expansion of the semen during freezing.

In its absence the sealing will be pushed out by the frozen semen. Further this air space also prevents contact of scissors with semen at the time of cutting of straw before insemination, thus preventing possible contamination.

9. *Sealing of Straws*

The sealing powder, PVA is available in 10 different colours. The French straws are also available in 16 different colours. The combination of both assures 160 positive identifications. The powder is spread on a clean glass dish to provide a thickness of 4–5 mm. The open ends of filled straws are dipped into the powder and when the powder penetrates 4–5 mm into the straw a satisfactory seal is made. This is known as 'laboratory seal' which will appear as a single band. Immediately after sealing, the straws are placed in water bath at +5°C for the equilibration period to be completed. At the same time this allows the sealing to become firmer and the excess powder on the ends falls to the bottom of water bath. The entire operation of filling and sealing has to be done at +5°C within the cold handling cabinet. At end the tubes are rolled and dried carefully with pre-cooled towels since ice will form on damp straws and this will reduce freezability and storage space.

10. *Freezing the Straws in Liquid Nitrogen Vapour*

Liquid Nitrogen vapour can be obtained from wide mouthed stainless steel container (LR 320, LR 250) where the straws are also finally stored. For the sake of economy and easy to work, the equilibrated straws after withdrawing from water bath at +5°C (which were placed in a freezing rack) are now placed in a mini freezer by holding in a horizontal position inside the straw racks at 4 to 5 cm above the level of liquid nitrogen, thereby exposing to the vapours of liquid nitrogen. The temperature of semen reaches –130°C to –150°C by about 10–15 minutes. The main advantage of horizontal freezing is the efficiency and simplicity of the method. The racks hold the straws at a constant level and the straws are frozen at even rate all along the length of the straw.

11. *Storage of Frozen Semen*

Frozen semen may be stored at:

(i) –79°C by using solid CO_2 (dry ice) and alcohol.
(ii) –190°C by using liquid air
(iii) –196°C by using liquid nitrogen
(iv) –296°C by using liquid helium

Storage of frozen semen in liquid nitrogen is the most convenient and accepted method all over the world. Soon after the temperature of straws reaches about –140°C in Mini Freezer, the straws are collected by pre-cooled forceps and finally transferred into pre-cooled goblets (a wide mouthed polythene tube like container without handles to hold the straws filled-in with semen). Goblets available in different capacities and sizes, e.g., bigger goblets hold 360 medium straws, small goblets 100 straws and even smaller holds out 25 straws. These goblets are then immersed in liquid nitrogen and kept in already identified canisters, stainless steel container (with long handle) to hold goblets deep inside liquid nitrogen of highly insulated double wall stainless steel wide mouthed semen containers (LR 320, LR 250).

12. *Thawing of Frozen Semen (Melting)*

Thawing means to melt or become liquid. Thawing of frozen semen should be done immediately before use and as quick as possible to prevent recrystallisation of the water into bigger crystals. After thawing, frozen spermatozoa do not survive long as unfrozen semen and also do not withstand re-freezing. Therefore, one must be certain that the semen is going to be used soon once it has been thawed.

The time and temperature to be allowed for thawing depends upon size of the packaging used. A universally adopted system does not exist. The most widely practised temperature of 37–40°C for 30 seconds is suitable to get optimum survival of spermatozoa. Following steps should be taken while thawing the semen:

1. The straw should be removed with the forceps from the liquid nitrogen.
2. The straw should be shaken vigorously once or twice to remove liquid nitrogen from the cotton plug.
3. Immediately after this procedure straw should be placed in warm water (37–40°C) for only 30 seconds.
4. Dry the straw with a tissue paper; also wipe the scissor.
5. Warm the chamber of the insemination gun by rubbing vigorously.
6. Hold the straw vertically with the cotton plug or ball downwards.
7. Cut the straw at right angles to remove the powder plug or sealed plug through the air space.
8. Withdraw the piston of the syringe.
9. Place the straw in the warmed up chamber of syringe.
10. Take the sheath from the container and fix the sheath over the straw to ensure the firm union between the straw and sheath.

13. *Procedure for Loading the A.I. Gun*

1. Identify the canister from which the desired semen is to be taken. Ascertain the colour of the straw by reading of identification tag.
2. Remove the lid from the container, lift the proper canister upto the level of the frost line. Never lift the canister above the neck level.
3. With a pair of tweezers grasp an individual straw and remove it, at the same time lower the canister immediately back into the container.
4. With the wrist movement give one or two jerks to the straw to expel liquid nitrogen trapped at end of factory seal.
5. Dip the straw into a clean waterbath at 37–40°C for 30 seconds. During this period the entire straw must be *completely* submerged in water bath.
6. Remove the straw from bath, dry the straw with a clean tissue paper or cotton. Inspect the straw carefully and discard straw with cracks or defective seals. Semen must never come in contact with water.
7. Place the straw in the chamber of insemination gun. To obtain a perfect fit with medium straw, it is essential that the laboratory seal is removed by cutting *at right angle* through middle of the air space. The air space could be brought to the top by gentle tapping of straw.

Make sure that the clipped end of straw has a straight *clean* cut with no jagged edges. Straws cut at other angles or cut too short will result in back flow and wastage of semen at the time of insemination.

8. Fit a sheath over the straw and the chamber of the insemination gun and obtain a perfect fit between the extremity of the straw and the cone of the sheath. Move the sheath about 1" up and check whether the straw follows the sheath, if it is not correctly fixed it will not move upwards with the sheath. Fix the sheath by locking the plastic "o" ring at the flange of the gun with a rotating motion. Do not touch the sheath in the tip or middle portion, handle only the base portion.
   Sheaths are sterilized and packed in 50 or 40 numbers in a plastic packet. The base of the sheath packet should be cut open by means of a small cut made at an angle. The sheath packet should be kept inside a sheath container made of aluminium and closed with rubber stopper on either side. After removing each sheath, the container should be tightly closed to keep it free from dust and contamination.
9. Extrude a tiny drop of semen to remove air bubble, to move the factory seal and to ensure good fitting of the sheath.
10. *The post-thaw survival of spermatozoa is poor*. For maximum reproductive efficiency, thawed semen should be used *immediately*. So, do not thaw more than one straw simultaneously.

Table 8.11

Artificial Insemination of Domestic Animals with Frozen Semen

	Cattle	Sheep	Goats	Swine	Horses	Turkeys
Volume of inseminate (ml)	0.2—1	0.05—0.2	0.02—0.2	50	20—50	0.025—0.05
Number of motile sperm per inseminate (10^6)	30	120—150	100—150	5000	1500	100
Time of insemination	8—16 hr after onset of estrus	10—24 h after onset of estrus	12—30 h after onset of estrus	12—30 h after onset of estrus	Every 2 days during estrus	Weekly
Site of semen deposition	Uterus-Cervix	Cervix	Cervix or uterus	Uterus	Uterus	Vagina

Source : *Handbook of Animal Sc.* (1991), Putman, P.A. (ed)., Academic Press, Inc.

Equipment Required for an A1 programme

To simplify the list, all items of equipment are categorised under headings appropriate to their specialised area of use. However, items of equipment which are used in more than one area are not necessarily duplicated in each section. It is therefore important to refer to the whole list for checking equipment. The numbers of items suggested only serve as a guide and should be modified according to individual requirements.

A. Collection of Semen

1. AV outer casings (30 × 6 cm for young bulls, 40 × 6 cm for adult bulls, 20–30 × 6 cm buffalo, 20 × 5.5 cm for ram and 15 × 5.5 cm for buck) at least 6 for each species.
2. AV liners and cones to suit above outer casings at least 12 for each species.

3. Rubber or synthetic bands for attaching AV liners to the outer casings.
4. Water heater or stove for heating water.
5. Funnel for filling AV with water.
6. Vaseline or medical jelly and glass or plastic rod.
7. 70% alcohol and wash bottle.
8. Semen collecting graduated tube (cow, buff) or collecting glasses for sheep and goat at least 12.
9. Incubator for pre-warming collecting glassware.
10. Dust proof glass cabinet.
11. Apron, gumboot.

B. Examination of Semen

1. Microscope with controlled light source and spare bulb.
2. Warm stage for microscope.
3. Pre-cleaned microscope slides and cover slips.
4. Waterbath with thermostatically-controlled heater. Two waterbaths with test tube racks and thermostatically controlled heater. One to be kept at 37°C for thawing semen, the other at 30°C where the semen and diluents are originally placed to maintain uniform temperature of both before mixing and used for holding the thawed semen until insemination.
5. Racks for holding collecting glasses in waterbath.
6. Haemocytometer(s), complete with cover slip, mixing pipette (red bead) and tube, 3% saline.
7. Colorimeter, complete with extra clean colorimeter tubes, the recommended filter, calibration chart, 0.9% saline and calibrated pipettes (corning) measuring 1, 2, 5 and 10 ml capacity.
8. Stain for spermatozoa (eosin-nigrosin).

C. Dilution of Semen

1. Ingredients for synthetic diluents, including glycerol for freezing semen technique.
2. Balance for weighing ingredients for diluents.
3. Stoppered measuring cylinders of appropriate capacity (25, 50 & 100 ml) 6 for each capacity.
4. Filter paper, circular, 9–11 cm diameter.
5. Glass distilled water plant.
6. Graduated glass pipettes, 2 and 5 ml (12 of each).
7. Clean glass test tubes (2, 5, 10 and 30 cc capacity) (corning).
8. Glass conical flasks (100, 250, 500, 1000 and 3000 cc) (Corning).

D. Liquid Semen Storage, Freezing and for Thawing of Semen

1. Refrigerator, cold cabinet or cold room (set at either 5°C or 15°C).
2. Wide-mouthed thermo flask (5)
3. Appropriate diluent
4. Corning type glass beakers 250 ml (6)

(a) *For liquid semen storage:*

5. Vials (5–8 ml) with stoppers, source of ice cubes or small plastic bottles containing frozen water, or semen straws and PVA (Polyvinyl alcohol) powder available in many colours.

(b) *For frozen storage (Depending on method used)* :

6. Vials or glass tubes (16 mm × 125 mm)
7. Stainless steel forceps, 25–30 cm.

8. Asbestos globes.
9. Semen straws, 65 mm and 135 having diameter of 2–2.8 mm.
10. Racks (for freezing the straws) suspended in polystyrene container.
11. Liquid nitrogen containers for supply of liquid nitrogen, 20, 30, 40 and 60 litres capacity.
12. Plastic goblets for holding straws in the canisters in the liquid nitrogen container.
13. Straw printing machine.
14. Straw filling and sealing machine.
15. Straw clip.
16. Filling comb.
17. Freezing ramps and racks.
18. Air-conditioner for the laboratory.
19. Canisters.
20. Frozen semen containers of different capacities (20, 30 and 40 litres).

E. Liquid Nitrogen Production (LN_2)

1. Liquid nitrogen plant with spares are available at

(i) Bharat Heavy Plate & Vessel Ltd.
Visakhapatnam 530 012
ANDHRA PRADESH

(ii) India Oxygen Ltd.
Oxygen House
P-34, Taratala Road
CALCUTTA 700 088

(iii) Industrial Cryogenic & Chem. Plants Ltd.
Ganesh Chandra Avenue
Post Box 342
CALCUTTA 700 001

(iv) Philips
Gloeilampen
Holland
The NETHERLANDS

2. Voltage stabilizer for plant and chiller.
3. Generator.
4. Hydrogen gas cylinder.
5. Defrosting unit LN_2 plant.
6. Liquid nitrogen storage tanks 200, 400 or 800 litres mounted on wheels.
7. Pressure pump and transfer device.

F. Equipment for Field Insemination Centre

1. Frozen semen container
2. Dip stick to measure LN_2
3. Insemination gun
4. Sheaths and Sheath containers
5. Thermos flask
6. Water heater (stove)
7. Scissor and Gloves
8. Cotton, Towels, Large plastic tray, Soap.

Factors affecting the Survival of Spermatozoa

Semen which may be of good quality when collected may subsequently deteriorate. Semen of all species are sensitive to environmental and other changes and extreme care should be taken to avoid damage when handling semen. The factors which can affect survival of spermatozoa are the following:

1. Temperature

The temperature of semen in most of the domestic animals except for on ejaculation is about that of the body (37.5°C). Exposure of semen to temperatures above this increases the metabolic rate, exhausts the energy reserves and decreases the life-span of spermatozoa. Temperatures above 45°C will kill spermatozoa.

Reduction of temperature will reduce the metabolism of spermatozoa, but a sudden drop in temperature, particularly to below 10°C, will cause irreversible loss of their viability. Motility is not regained on rewarming and fertilising ability of the spermatozoa is lost. This is called *cold shock* and can occur through careless over-exposure to cold air or by use of a cold collecting glass or microscope slide. Care must also be taken when semen is diluted to ensure that the diluent is at the same temperature as the semen.

Slow cooling of spermatozoa to 2–5°C is not fatal. The reduction in metabolism at this temperature helps to prolong the viability of the spermatozoa. On rewarming, motility is restored and the spermatozoa may still be fertile.

2. Sunlight

Direct sunlight is detrimental to semen. Short exposure to sunlight may reduce the viability of spermatozoa and 30–40 minutes exposure will kill them. Consequently, it is best to avoid exposure of semen to direct sunlight at all times, and all collection and handling procedures should be carried out indoors and away from sunny windows. It is also wise to avoid prolonged exposure to strong fluorescent lights or ultra-violet radiation.

3. Contact with Metal

Contact with metal of any kind is harmful to spermatozoa. For this reason only glass utensils or equipment made of inert synthetic materials should be used for collection, dilution and storage of semen, and for insemination.

4. Contact with Water

Water reduces the osmotic pressure of the seminal plasma and may thereby kill the spermatozoa. Thus, water is a powerful spermicidal agent and semen should never be allowed to come into contact with it. All equipment should be thoroughly dried before use, including the artificial vagina and collecting glasses. Caution must be exercised when maintaining semen in a waterbath so that water is not accidentally splashed into the semen.

5. Impurities and Bacteria

Bacteria, dust, hairs, urine and other such contaminants that may get into semen will reduce the viability or kill the spermatozoa. Contamination of semen occurs most frequently during collection and can best be avoided by thoroughly cleaning the prepuce of the male beforehand. After collection, the semen should be protected from airborne contaminants by keeping it covered with aluminium foil or a watch glass. Special attention should be paid to protection of semen from flies and other insects. Aerosol fly-sprays or antiseptic sprays should not be used as these too are very harmful to spermatozoa and can persist in the atmosphere for some time after use. Proliferation of microbes in the semen can be controlled by addition of antibiotics to the diluent.

6. Disinfectants

Disinfectants and antiseptics are harmful to spermatozoa and their use should be avoided. For sterilisation of equipment, 70% alcohol in water is suitable, but all equipment should be thoroughly dried before use. For glassware, dry heat sterilisation can be used.

7. Long Exposure to Air

Oxygen in the air increases the metabolic activity of spermatozoa and lactic acid accumulates in the semen. Lactic acid may reduce the pH of the semen below the optimum of 7.0, and the viability of the spermatozoa will be reduced accordingly. Semen should therefore be used for insemination, or storage, as soon as possible after collection.

8. Buffering Capacity of Diluent

The media used for dilution of semen should have the capacity to maintain the optimum pH in diluted semen. Shifts in pH either above 7.0 (alkaline) or below 7.0 (acid) reduce the viability of spermatozoa. The recommended semen diluents contain buffers, that is, substances able to maintain the medium surrounding the spermatozoa at optimum pH.

9. Osmotic Pressure of Diluent

The components (solutes) dissolved in the medium surrounding the spermatozoa may exert a pressure on the cell membrane. This is known as osmotic pressure, and it increases with the concentration of solutes in the medium. Media in which the concentration of solute is equivalent to that within the cell membrane are said to be isotonic. Media with lower solute concentration are hypotonic, and those with higher concentration are hypertonic. Both hypotonic and hypertonic media are harmful to spermatozoa; there is only a narrow range of tonicity over which a diluent can be altered without affecting viability of spermatozoa. Spermatozoa remain motile longest when suspended in isotonic diluent.

Characteristics of Semen of different Species

The composition of semen varies markedly between species. The volume of semen and the concentration of spermatozoa in semen are generally compatible with the reproductive anatomy and mating habits of the particular species. The characteristics of semen of different species are given in Table.

In sheep, goats and cattle ejaculation is spontaneous and lasts only seconds. During copulation semen is deposited into the anterior vagina. This type of semen deposition is known as *vaginal deposition*, and the semen of these species is relatively low in volume and high in concentration; higher volumes would be wasted since the semen could not be contained within the vagina of the female. In pigs and horses semen is deposited by the male into the uterus of the female; large volumes of semen are deposited and ejaculation is protracted. This type of semen deposition is known as *uterine deposition*.

The volume and concentration of semen varies not only between but also within species. Apart from individual variation, factors such as age, climatic conditions, nutrition, and frequency of ejaculation will affect the quantity and quality of semen.

Table 8.12

Average Characteristics of Semen from Farm Animals

	Cattle	Sheep	Swine	Horses	Rabbits	Dogs	Chickens	Goats	Buffalo	Turkeys	Cats
Volume (ml)	6	1	225	60	0.6	5	0.5	0.8	4	0.3	0.05
Sperm concentration (10^9/ml)	1.2	3.0	0.2	0.15	0.5	0.3	3.5	2.4	1.0	7.0	1.5
Total sperm (10^9)	7	3	45	9	0.03	1.5	1.8	2.0	4	3.5	0.1
Motile sperm (%)	70	75	60	70	80	85	85	80	60	60	75
Morphologically normal sperm (%)	80	90	60	70	80	80	90	90	80	85	90
Ejaculates /week	4	20	3	3	6	3	3	20	3	3	—
Living cells/ insemination (10^6)	10	120	1200	100	25	100	60	60	10	125	5
Range of pH	6.4–7.8	5.9–7.3	7.3–7.9	7.2–7.8	6.6–7.5	6.7–6.8	6.3–7.8	6.2–7.0	6.4–6.8	6.5–7.0	—

Factors Influencing Fertility during Artificial Insemination

In an AI programme, if the animals are healthy, in good condition, and free of abnormalities of the reproductive tract, still there are a number of factors which may influence the results. These are listed below:

1. Number of Spermatozoa

The number of normal, viable spermatozoa inseminated below a minimum limit affects fertility. The number required varies according to the storage state (fresh, liquid-stored or frozen-thawed) and the site of insemination.

2. Method and Technique of Insemination

Fertility varies with the method of insemination. Intra-uterine insemination (by laparoscopy in sheep or via the cervix in goats) is more successful than cervical or vaginal insemination, particularly for frozen semen. For vaginal insemination only fresh semen should be used and females should not be 'synchronised' with pharmacological agents. Increasing the depth of cervical insemination improves fertility.

3. Time of Insemination

Insemination too early or too late in relation to ovulation is detrimental to fertility. The time of insemination is more critical when liquid-stored or frozen-thawed rather than fresh semen is used since stored spermatozoa have a shorter viable period in the female reproductive tract. Females with a short oestrous may have reduced fertility.

4. Type of Oestrous (Natural or Controlled)

Fertility of sheep after cervical insemination is often lower when oestrous has been synchronised by pharmacological agents, though this problem can be overcome by use of exogenous gonadotrophins or intra-uterine insemination. In goats there is little influence of synchronisation on fertility. The type and level of treatment with pharmacological agents can affect fertility.

5. Age of Females

Fertility is generally lower in young or primiparous animals than in mature animals.

6. Season of Treatment

Fertility is usually lower when animals are inseminated outside the normal breeding season.

7. Stress Factors

Careless or rough handling of females at insemination or in the period of establishment of pregnancy affects fertility.

8. Embryonic and Foetal Mortality

Environmental and nutritional stress, or disease, during pregnancy may result in embryonic or foetal mortality. Placental insufficiency or, in cattle, buffalo and goats particularly, failure of the corpus luteum of pregnancy, may result in abortion.

Table 8.13

Major Causes of Reproductive Losses after Insemination[a]

Type of Loss	Cattle[b]	Sheep	Swine	Chickens	Turkeys[b]
Improperly timed insemination (%)	10	—	—	—	—
Ovulation failure (%)	2	1	1	—[c]	—[c]
Lost or ruptured ova (%)	5	5	1	10	10
Fertilization failure (%)	13	12	5	5	10
Embryonic death (%)	18	17	28	10	20
Stillbirths and neonatal deaths (%)	6	10	10	—	—

a Hafez, E.S.E., ed. (1980) *Reproduction in Farm Animals*, 4th edn. Lea and Febiger, Philadelphia, U.S.A.

b Hawk, H.W., ed. (1979) *Beltsville Symposia in Agri. Research* 3; *Animal Reproduction.* Allanheld, Osmun, Montclair, New Jersey, U.S.A

c Failure to lay an egg daily could be considered to be ovulation failure in poultry.

9. Hygiene

Careless handling or contamination of equipment may result in a reduction in viability of spermatozoa or spread diseases of the reproductive tract.

It is important to note that, when disappointing results are obtained, the AI technology itself is unlikely to be at fault. The fault will almost certainly be found in (i) improper application of that technology, (ii) improper management, or (iii) environment factors.

MAMMARY GLAND AND LACTATION

Mammals appeared on earth about 150 million years ago and are believed to have evolved from an advanced type of reptiles. One of the most important characteristics common to all mammals is their ability to secrete milk. The mammary gland of the cow is probably the most advanced form from an evolutionary point of view. But examples of very primitive type of mammary gland also exist in nature. The pigeons produce a white slimy substance in their crop called pigeon "milk" which they regurgitate into the mouth of their young. The duckbill platypus possesses mammary glands similar to that of the cow morphologically but has no nipples. The milk exudes from 100 to 150 separate gland tubes that open at the base of the "mammary hairs" which the youngsters lap to obtain the milk.

Anatomy and Architecture of Mammary Gland

The mammary glands (mammae) are modified sudoriferous (sweat) glands and is located outside the abdominal cavity.

Mammary Glands of Cows and Buffaloes

The *mammary glands* or *udder of the cow* is covered with fine hair except teat which is totally hairless. A desirable udder should be capacious, possess a relatively level floor, and be strongly attached, extending well forward with a rear attachment high and wide. The texture of the udder should be soft, pliable and elastic; well collapsed after milking. The teats should be uniform, of convenient length and size, cylindrical in shape, well spaced and free from obstructions.

Exterior of the udder. The udder is a skin gland and is located entirely outside the abdominal cavity. Its only connection with the abdominal cavity is through the inguinal canal, a potential tube about four inches long, through which blood and lymph vessels and nerve fibres leave the abdominal cavity to enter the udder.

The right and left halves of the udder are indicated by the intermammary groove (Fig. 9.3). The fore and rear quarters may be smoothly joined or may be demarcated by varying degrees of grooving.

The rear quarters are usually larger than the front quarters and contain 1/4 to 1/2 more secretory tissue and thus the two front quarters normally produce about 40 per cent of the total milk yield and the two hind quarters about 60 per cent.

The gross internal structure is shown in Fig. 9.6.

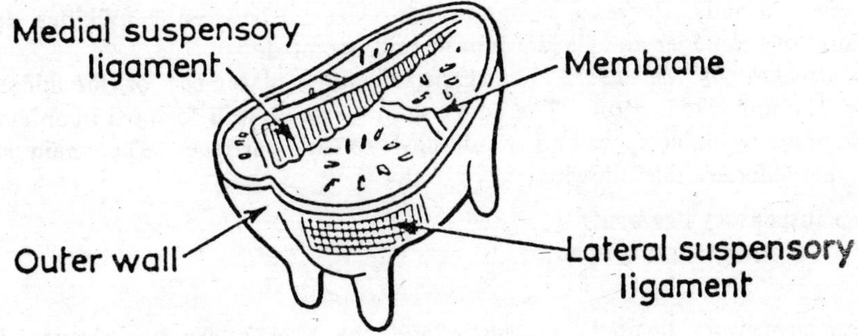

Fig. 9.1. Cross section of udder, showing the four separate quarters.

Mammary (External Pudic) Artery
Supramammary Lymph Node
Mammary (External Pudic) Vein
Mammary Lymph Vessels
Subcutaneous Abdominal (Milk) Vein
Parenchyma (Glandular Tissue)
Front Quarter
Hind Quarter
Gland Cistern
Teat Cistern
Rosette of Furstenberg
Streak Canal

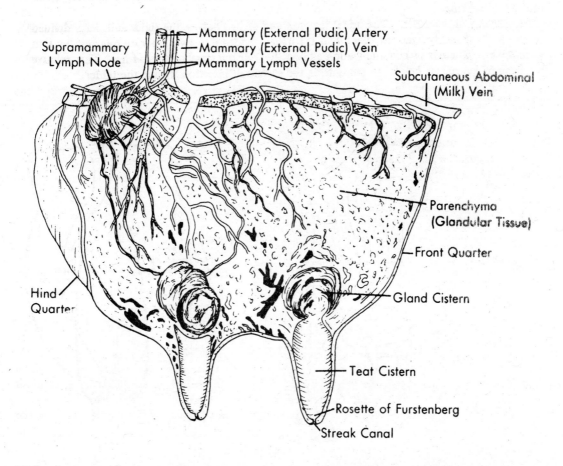

Fig. 9.2 Sagittal (dividing the full udder into right and left halves) section of udder of a cow.

The udder usually increase about 1/3 in size between milkings, depending upon the quality of the udder and the amount of milk secreted.

Suspensory structures of the udder. The shape, size and placement of the udder is very important for best milk production. The udder should extend weill forward in order to make maximum use of the available space and should have an easy carriage. The main structures that support the udder are the following.

1. Median suspensory ligament
2. Two lateral suspensory ligaments
3. Skin

The median suspensory ligament is elastic and the laterals are non-elastic. For this reason, filling of the udder causes the teats to protrude outward. In this way a maximum amount of milk can be accommodated with a minimum lowering of the udder. The median suspensory ligament is primarily responsible for the udder "breaking down". The skin covering the gland has little supporting action, but it protects the udder and minimises swaying when the cow is walking.

Morphology of the udder. The udder is composed of two halves, the right and left, divided by median suspensory ligament. Each half is further divided into two separate quarters by thin membranes. There is no communication among the four quarters of the udder. This relative isolation of quarters is helpful in minimising the spread of infection within the udder.

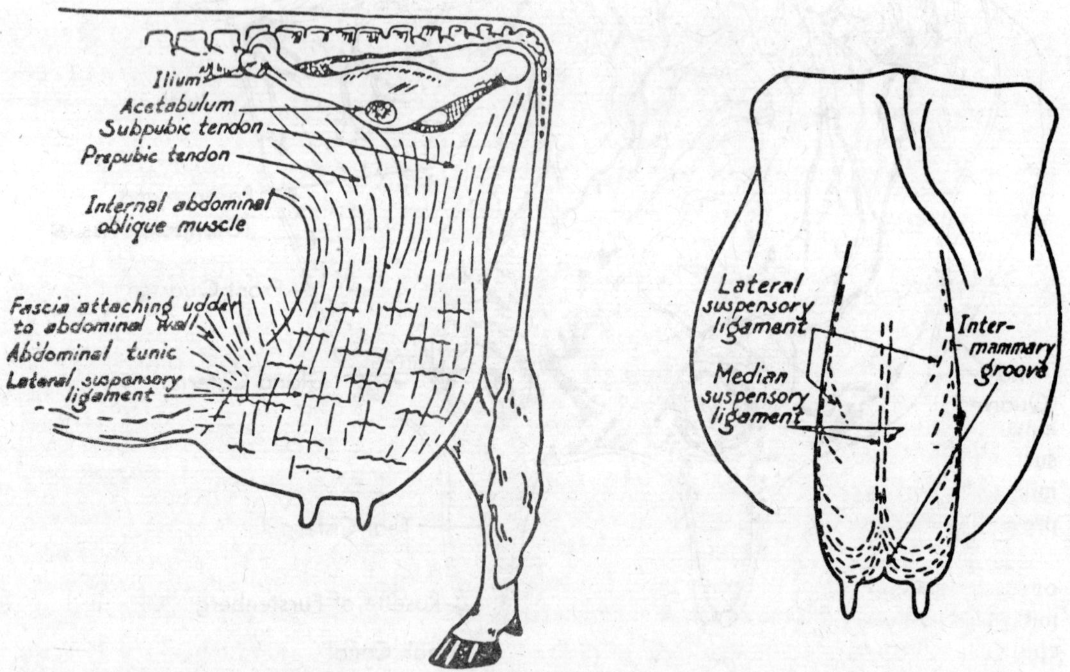

Fig. 9.3. Suspensory apparatus of the udder.

Each quarter is composed of secretory tissue and some supporting connective tissue. The secretory tissue consists of numerous *alveoli* or tiny chambers (Fig. 9.6) lined with many secretory cells. Each alveolus is supplied with tiny capillaries which lie outside the secretory cells (Fig. 9.4). Small muscle fibres, called myoepithelial cells also surround each alveolus which cause contraction of the alveoli and produce "let-down" of milk.

Each alveolus is drained by a small duct called "terminal duct". A cluster of alveoli and their ducts resembling a bunch of grapes, constitute a lobule (Fig. 9.6). A group of lobules are surrounded by a septum of connective tissue and form a lobe. The terminal ducts unite to form *intralobular* ducts. These ducts unite successively to form larger ducts called *interlobular*, *intralobar* and *interlobar* ducts. The interlobar ducts join to form galactophores that empty into the *gland cistern* or *milk cistern*, a sinus at the tip of the udder. The gland cistern is continuous immediately below with the *teat cistern*. The teat cistern is joined with the *streak canal*,

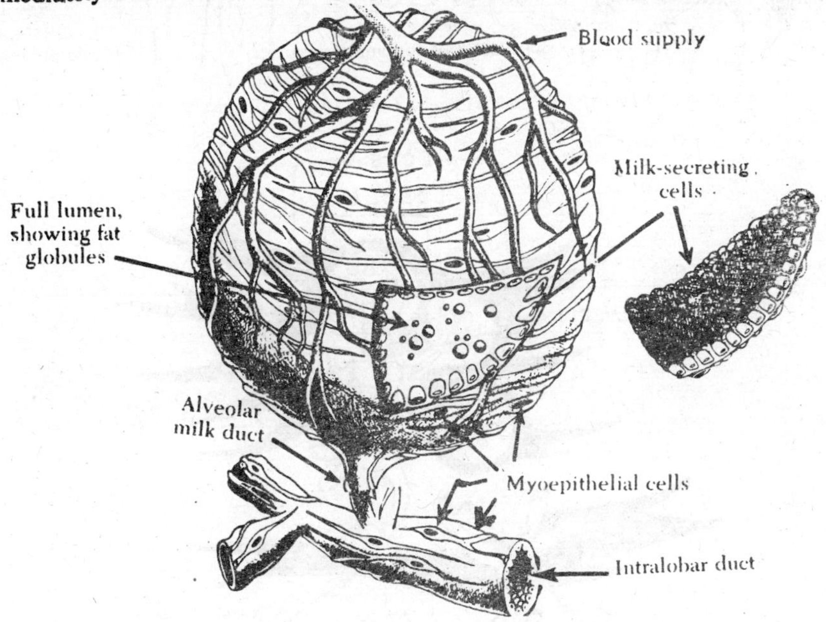

Fig. 9.4 The blood vessels and myoepithelial cells surrounding an alveolus.

a narrow tube ¼ to ½ inch long, that opens at the lower end of the teat. The streak canal is surrounded by a true muscular *sphincter* which remains constricted and prevents leakage of milk until milking commences. The streak canal and its sphincter are also responsible for preventing entrance of bacterial and other contaminants into the teat.

Milk collecting system. Milk from the lumen of the alveoli is passed via many thousands of small ducts into eight to twelve main milk ducts. These lead into the gland cistern, and the milk leaves the teat via the streak canal or papillary duct. Each cell of the udder including of epithelial cells of alveoli are in intimate contact with blood, lymph and nerve supply.

Blood which supplies milk constituents to the udder, comes from the heart via two large arteries each about 10 mm in cross section. Then, after passing round the alveoli in the udder, the blood enters the venous system and returns to the heart via two routes. One route is inter-

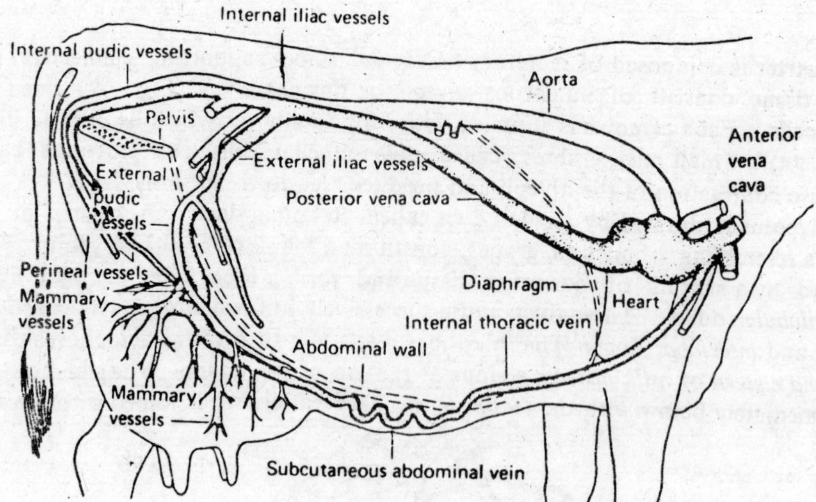

Fig.9.5. Circulation of the bovine udder.

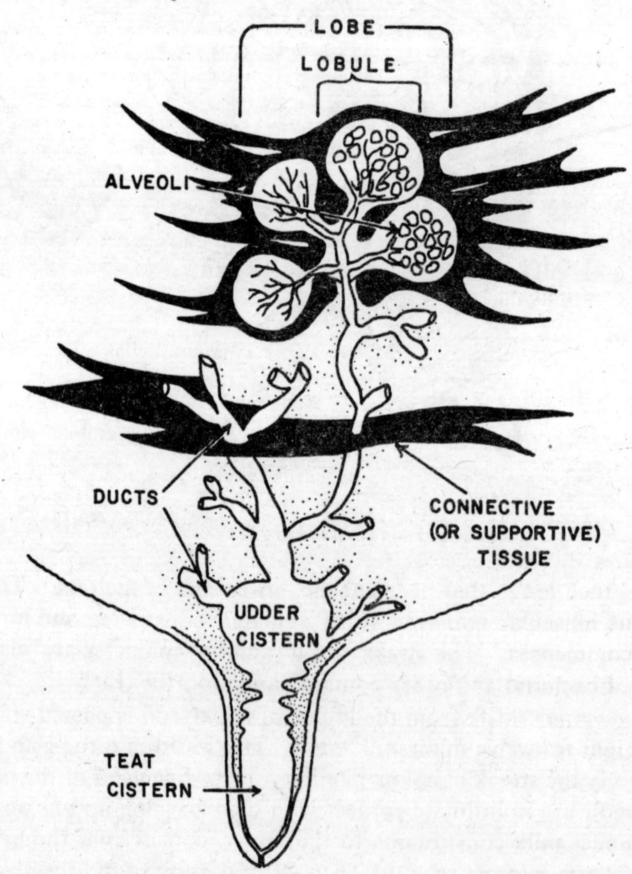

Fig.9.6 Connection of the duct with the lobule-alveolar system.

nal, whereas the other is partly external via a vein which passes along the abdominal wall just under the skin and enters the body at a depression termed the *milk well.* This abdominal vein is known as *milk vein,* and its size is often taken as an indication of the cow's potential for milk production; but it is extremely doubtful whether this has any significance.

Mammary Glands of Dogs and Swine

The bitch usually has five pairs of teats (or mammary glands). The cranial two pair are known as cranial thoracic and caudal thoracic, the middle two pair are cranial abdominal and caudal abdominal, and the caudal pair are known as inguinal. The bitch has 8–20 ducts per teat.

The normal number of teats in the domestic hog is 7 pairs or 14 teats, with the first pair just behind the junction of the sternum and ribs and the last pair in the inguinal region. The number of teats may range from 4 pairs to 9 pairs and supernumery teats are sometimes found between normal teats. The animal has 2–3 ducts per teat. Each teat cistern is continuous with a gland cistern. No hair is present on the teat but is present at its base and on the gland.

Mammary Glands of Sheep and Goat

The udders of the sheep and the goat differ from that of cow in that in both the species there are only two teats. Each half of the udder has only one teat, one streak canal, one teat cistern, and one gland cistern. The teat is sparsely covered with fine hair.

Mammary Glands of Horse

Mammary glands of the horse consist of two teats, one teat on each side attached to one half of the udder. Each teat has two streak canals and two teat cisterns, each of which is continuous with a separate gland cistern and its system of ducts and alveoli. The udder and teats of the mare are covered with the fine hair, as well as with numerous sebaceous (oil) glands and sudoriferous (sweat) glands. An woman has 15–24 ducts per teat while in mare there are 2–4 ducts per teat.

The Circulatory system

The blood supply to the udder is profuse particularly during lactation. For production of one ml of milk 400 to 500 ml of blood must pass through the udder. That is why the udder must possess an extensive vascular system. Arterial blood enters the base of each half of the udder through and *external pudic artery,* also called mammary artery. The artery passes downward through the inguinal canal in a more or less tortuous manner, and divides into several branches that supply the front and hind quarters on the same side. Another small artery that may be single or paired is the *perineal artery* which passes downward from the vulva just deep to the skin on the median line. This artery usually supplies a small amount of blood to the caudal part of both halves of the udder.

There are three primary routes for venous blood to return to the heart for oxygenation. The first route is through the *subcutaneous abdominal vein* (milk vein). The second route is the *external pudic vein.* (parallels the external pudic artery). The third possible route is the *perineal vein* through the pelvic arch.

Many have attempted to use the size and prominence of the milk veins (superficial veining) as an index of milking ability, which could not be established upon scientific experimentation.

Lymphatic system

The lymphatic system comprises numerous lymph vessels and nodes (glands) that carry *lymph* from mammary tissue to the heart via the venous blood system. In the cow the flow is upward and toward the rear of each half of the udder, where it passes through *supramammary lymph glands.*

Lymph in the mammary gland is similar in composition to blood plasma except lymph has half as much protein as blood plasma. The vessels are more permeable than the walls of the capillaries. This allows the larger particles, such as proteins and lipids, to move more easily into the lymph vessels. The vessels are difficult to identify, because they have a small amount of connective tissue in their wall and moreover the lymph in them has a very clear colour.

Lymph glands act as filters that remove or destroy foreign substances (bacteria) that may have gained entrance into the tissues. The action is performed actually by white blood cells which are produced by lymph glands. Thus lymph glands (nodes) and vessels are especially important in controlling inflammation at parturition and in removing sloughed or injured tissue. Swelling in the udder at the time of parturition results from the accumulation of large quantities of lymph and is called *edema,* which inhibits milk ejection. Thus lymphatic system by removing extra lymph from the udder has proved to be a built-in safeguard of nature for the udder health.

Nervous system

The mammary glands are supplied with *afferent sensory fibers* as well as *sympathetic efferent fibres.* Parasympathetic fibers are not present in the mammary gland.

Sensory and sympathetic nerves reach the udder by way of the inguinal nerves (from 1, 2, 3, lumber nerves). *The* perineal nerves arise from the second, third and fourth sacral nerves and enter the udder at its posterior caudal portion along with the perineal arteries and veins.

The primary functions of the sympathetic nerve, are to control blood supply to the udder and innervation of smooth muscles surrounding the milk collecting ducts and the sphinctor muscles within the teat. Stimulation of sympathetic nervous system causes a vasoconstriction of the blood vessels and this has an inhibiting effect on milk secretion.

The sensory nerves carry the sensory stimuli from the udder to the central nervous system, an important step in milk let-down.

UDDER GROWTH

Embryonic and Fetal Development. The mammary gland originates from the *ectoderm.* The first anlage or discernible sign of the mammary gland is the mammary band which consists of a single layer of cells on the ventral surface of the embryo just back of the umbilicus. The mammary band differentiates into two narrow bands of cells called the mammary line. At intervals on the mammary line further proliferation results in the formation of mammary buds, the number of which determines the number of glands that will develop. A downgrowth of the mammary bud into the mesenchyme (embryonic connective tissue) results in the formation of primary sprouts, the number of which determines the number of ducts in the mature teat. Canalisation of the primary sprout occurs resulting in the formation of a lumen. The primary sprout is the antecedent of the streak canal, teat cistern and gland cistern. Secondary sprouts grow out at angles from the primary sprout, canalise and later divide into tertiary sprouts. These secondary and tertiary sprouts are the forerunners of the duct system of the udder. At birth, only primary and secondary sprouts are present: tertiary sprouts appear later

From Birth to Puberty. In the Holstein cow, between birth and two months of age there is little growth of the udder. But between two months and the time of puberty (7-8 months),

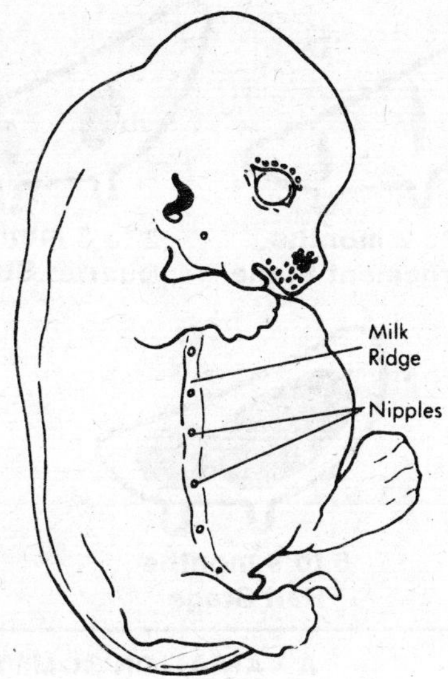

Fig. 9.7. Drawing (x515) of 20 m.m. pig embryo showing milk ridge (milk line).

line).

the mammary gland grows 3½ times faster than the body weight and reaches the peak pubertal development at 10 to 12 months of age. The mammary gland does not grow much after this period until the animal becomes pregnant. These time ranges may differ slightly for Indian breeds of cows but the fact that a very rapid phase of mammary growth starts quite early in life—well in advance of the age of puberty—and plateaus only after a few estrous cycles should be true.

During the Estrous Cycle. After the attainment of puberty, the animal undergoes recurrent estrous cycle. The mammary gland undergoes cyclic changes during the course of the estrous cycle, the duct system growing during the estrogenic phase and regressing during the progestational phase. Cumulative growth of the mammary gland occurs for the first 4 to 5 cycles; thereafter, there is not much net gain with each recurrent estrous cycle.

During Pregnancy. The largest portion of the mammary growth occurs during pregnancy. During the first three months of pregnancy only the duct system proliferates From the third month on there is rapid growth of the secretory tissue (lobule-alveolar system) which continues even after the calf is born. Secretion of colostrum begins a short time before the birth of the calf and results in a great enlargement of the udder at this time.

During Lactation. No direct studies in the cow are available but based on studies in the laboratory animals, it seems that considerable growth of the secretory tissue in the mammary gland takes place during the early part of lactation.

Hormonal Requirements for Mammary Growth. In general, estrogens promote duct growth while proper combinations of estrogen and *progesterone* stimulate lobule-alveolar development. In the cow and goat estrogen alone can stimulate considerable lobule-alveolar growth but

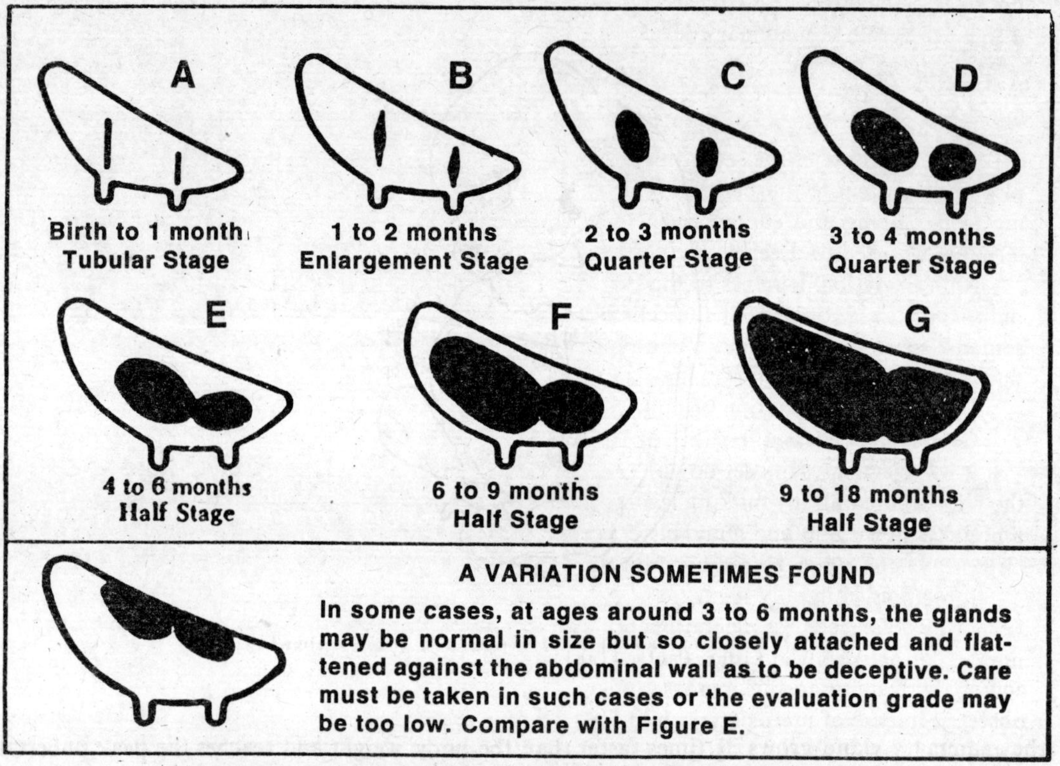

A
Birth to 1 month
Tubular Stage

B
1 to 2 months
Enlargement Stage

C
2 to 3 months
Quarter Stage

D
3 to 4 months
Quarter Stage

E
4 to 6 months
Half Stage

F
6 to 9 months
Half Stage

G
9 to 18 months
Half Stage

A VARIATION SOMETIMES FOUND

In some cases, at ages around 3 to 6 months, the glands may be normal in size but so closely attached and flattened against the abdominal wall as to be deceptive. Care must be taken in such cases or the evaluation grade may be too low. Compare with Figure E.

Drawings showing mammary gland development in heifer calves of different ages, from right side of udders.

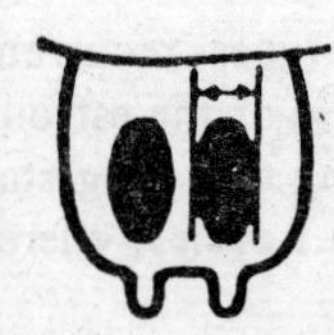

View from the rear. Widths are measured from side to side at the widest point and are averages of the right and left glands.

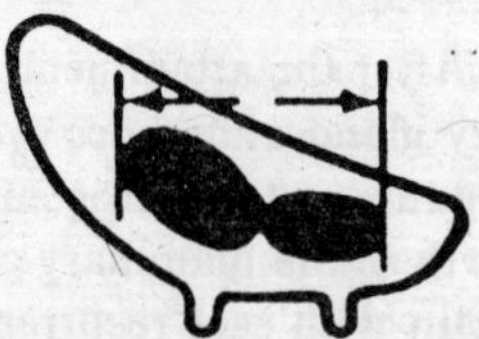

View from side Lengths are measured from the extreme front to the extreme rear of the glands, and are averages of the right and left halves.

How mammary gland measurements are made.

Fig.9.8. Mammary gland measurement in heifer calves.

alveoli developed are occasionally abnormal. For growth comparable to terminal stages of pregnancy, prolactin and growth hormone are also required. Prolactin alone possesses the ability to produce considerable lobule-alveolar growth. It seems that under normal conditions, the major hormones directly involved in the development of the mammary gland to a functional state are prolactin, estrogen and progesterone. Hormones from the adrenal and thyroid gland affect mammary development but only indirectly. The placenta elaborates several hormones including the estrogens, progesterones and a prolacta-like hormone and thus plays a significant role in mammary development during the later part of pregnancy.

Lactation

Lactation implies the secreting and giving of milk (removal) by the mammary glands. It is also used to denote the period of milk production which in case of cow is 305 days commencing from calving and ending when the cow ceases to be milked at least twice a day. The terminology used to describe the various aspects of lactation is as follows:

Milk Secretion. It refers to the synthesis of milk by the epithelial cells and the passage of milk from the cytoplasm of the cells into the alveolar lumen. The rate of secretion of milk remains constant for the first 12 hours after the previous milking and declines slowly thereafter due to back pressure of the synthesized milk to the epithelial cells.

Lactogenesis. Initiation of milk secretion.

Galactopoiesis. Maintenance of lactation.

Milk Ejection (Milk let-down). As the secretion of milk is a continuous process, most of the milk secured at any milking is already present in the udder when the milking starts. A small amount is in the teat and gland cisterns, but most of it is in the alveoli and ducts to the gland cisterns, where it may be removed by either hand milking or by machine milking.

Involution. Literally it means shrinking of an organ to its normal size after enlargement i.e., of alveolar cells. As lactation progresses, there is a tendency for a gradual decrease in number of active alveoli and also in efficiency of activity thereby there is a loss of secretory activity with simultaneous increase of connective tissue stroma. The same phenomenon is also observed in case of uterus after child birth.

Hormonal Regulation of Lactation

Initiation of Lactation (Lactogenesis)

By the end of pregnancy. the cow's udder is fully developed for nursing. The absence of lactation during pregnancy is believed to be caused by suppressive effects of progesterone and estrogens on the milk secretary process of the epithelial cells. However, immediately after parturition, the sudden loss of estrogen and progesterone secretion by the placenta removes any inhibitory effects of these two hormones and allows marked production of prolactin, also called *lactogen*, *luteotropin*, *galactin*, and *mammotropin* by the adenohypophysis. There are enzymes within the epithelial cells that are essential to the activation of the cells to convert blood constituents into milk. Prolactin functions to stimulate increased enzyme activity which in turn stimulates milk secretion otherwise mammary gland will fail to secrete milk. The sudden onset of milk secretion requires in addition to prolactin an adequate background secretion of both growth hormone and the adrenocorticosteroids.

Maintenance of Lactation (Galactopoiesis)

Crude extracts of bovine pituitary glands were found to be essential for maintenance of lactation as it is for the initiation of milk secretion. Along with prolactin which is a must for continued production, STH (growth hormone), ACTH (adrenocorticotropic hormone), TSH (thyroid stimulating hormone), and oxytocin from pituitary glands are also essential. Among other hormones from non-pituitary origin, parathyroid, placental lactogen and insulin are also significantly concerned with maintenance of lactation.

TSH of pituitary stimulates thyroid gland to secrete thyroxin which regulates the vital metabolic processes of the body and influences the general well-being of animals. It increases the appetite, heart rate, flow of blood to the udder and rate of milk secretion. Thyroxin secretion rates show seasonal trends, with increase in winter and decline in summer. This partially explains why milk secretion slows in hot weather.

Growth hormone (Somatotropin) is secreted by pituitary gland. This hormone appears to influence substances from which milk is made, e.g., by increasing the availability of blood amino acids, fats, and sugars for use by the mammary gland cell in milk synthesis.

Parathyroid hormone regulates blood level of Calcium and Phosphorus. Recent studies indicate that Vitamin D (D_2 or D_3) will maintain normal lactation in parathyroidectomized animals. It has further been noted that feeding high levels of Vitamin D (20 million IU for 3 to 7 days prepartum) will significantly reduce the incidence of parturient paresis (milk fever) in cows.

Adrenals particularly of cortisone in large daily doses (10-20 mg) inhibits milk secretion in rats, whereas lower doses (1.5-1.0 mg) increase it, and a low dose (0.25) has no effect. Thus it may be concluded that adrenal corticoids are essential for milk secretion, but excess amount inhibit lactation.

Oxytocin is secreted from the posterior pituitary gland and is a must for the ejection (milk let-down) of milk.

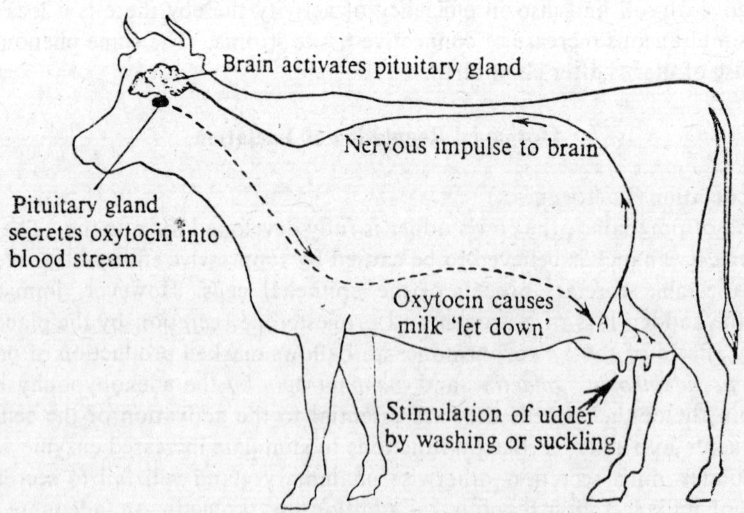

Fig. 9.9. Milk 'let down'.

Placental lactogen has got the properties of both growth hormone and prolactin but is identical with neither. In cattle, the bovine placental lactogen (bPL) has been identified. Since the source of bPL is lost when the placenta is expelled, its effect must occur prior to peak milk secretion in the subsequent lactation.

Insulin promotes mammary cell growth and cell division during gestation and lactation but alone is incapable of inducing synthesis of milk proteins by the daughter cells.

MILK SECRETION RATE

It has already been stated that milk is secreted by the alveolar cells of the udder. The daily milk yield of mammals is thus dependent upon the number of secretory tissue in the mammary gland and the rate of secretion per unit of tissue. The secretion rate is controlled

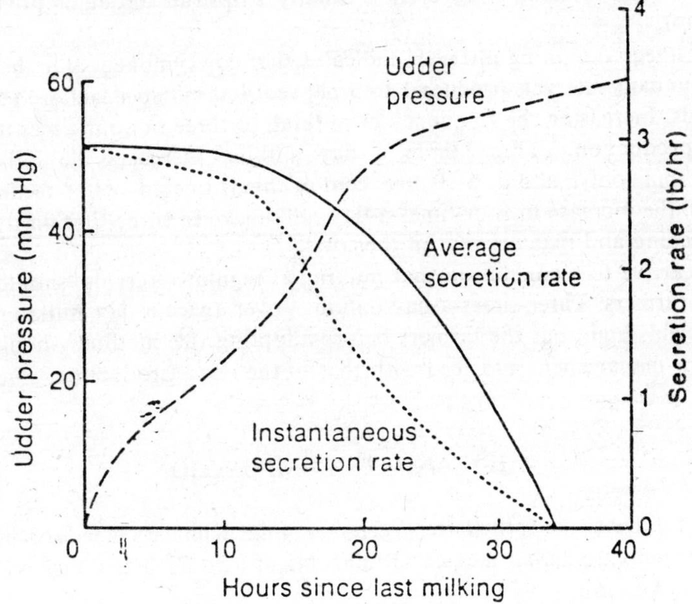

Fig.9.10 Relationship of udder pressure to secretion rates of dairy cows.

in part by the pressure in the alveolar lumina due to the accumulation of milk. Measurement of pressure in the teat cisterns at various intervals after milking indicates that three distinct phases occur in milk pressure curve. Within one hour after milking, a marked increase in pressure to approximately 8 mm Hg occurs in the teat cistern (Fig 9.10.). This hydrostatic pressure is caused by the residual milk moving from the alveoli and smaller ducts into the cisterns. This is followed by a slower increase in pressure due to the accumulation of milk in the secretory tissue and its further oozing into the teat and gland cisterns. This is followed by an accelerated rate of pressure increase and constitutes the third phase of the pressure curve.

Residual Milk

The residual milk is the amount of milk left in the udder after a normal milking. It can be obtained only after the injection of oxytocin and remilking the animal. The amount of residual milk is proportional to the amount of milk present in the udder at the beginning of the milking. On an average it has been observed that it is about 13.9 and 17.8 per cent for a cow milking only once a day and for a cow when milking intervals were 10 and 14 hours respectively. Older cows have higher percentages of residual milk than first-calf heifers, and cows with high percentages of residual milk have a lower persistency of lactation. The percentage residual milk is also higher in low producers than high producers.

Udder Pressure and Secretion Rate

The pressure required to stop the secretion process has not been definitely determined and it probably varies from cow to cow. In general after the pressure reaches a certain point, the rate of milk secretion decreases. Secretion totally stops at about 35 hours after the last milking (Fig.9.10).

The effect of unequal milking intervals indicates that cows milked at either 9 and 15 hours or 8 and 16 hour daily intervals produce 1 to 3 per cent less milk per lactation than cows milked at equal intervals. Increasing the frequency of milking to three or four times daily increases the level of milk production. Three times a day milking increases the milk production by 15-25 per cent, but only about 5-10 per cent of this is due to better feeding and management. Most of the increase in four-times-a-day milking over three-times-a-day milking is due to the better feeding and management of the cows.

We may thus arrive to a conclusion that milking at regular intervals should always be the aim of all dairy farmers. Three-times-a-day milking over twice-a-day milking (at equal intervals) although yields high, but the farmers before adopting the method should first compare the cost for extra management and feed with that of the extra production due to thrice-a-day milking.

MILK AND ITS COMPOSITION

Milk may be defined as the entire lacteal secretion of the mammary glands of mammals obtained by the process of milking during the period following at least 72 hours after calving or until the milk is free from colostrum.

Milk is a white opaque fluid with some exceptions where it is tinge yellowish particularly in some breeds. Because of its content of almost all essential nutrients (except iron which is very low 0.2 mg per 100 g of milk), milk is being used throughout the world for feeding infants and as a supplement to the diets of children and adults. In milk fat along with some fat soluble vitamins (Vitamin A, D, E and K) are present as an *emulsion* (colloidal dispersion of one liquid in another immiscible or partially miscible liquid), protein along with some mineral matters in colloidal suspensions, lactose together with some water soluble minerals and vitamins are in true solutions.

For commercial purposes it is usual to divide the milk constituents into 1) Fat and 2) non-fatty solids also known as Solids Not Fat (SNF). Water serves as the medium in which two sets of constituents are carried.

Chemical composition determines the ultimate nutritive value of the milk for the consumer and also has a direct effect on the output of various dairy products to be manufactured. For example a batch of 50,000 lit. of milk will produce approximately 52 kg less milk powder, if the SNF content of milk is reduced by only 0.1 per cent.

Now that the importance of milk composition is appreciated, milk producers are paid not only on the basis of total quantity but also on the basis of either fat or SNF content.

The main constituents of milk are indicated diagrammatically as below:

Virtually all the major constituents are synthesized in the udder from various precursors which are absorbed selectively from the blood. The cows diet is the ultimate source of most of the materials used in milk synthesis, and alterations in the amount and type of food affect both milk yield and composition. The products of digestion which are absorbed from the rumen and small intestine into the blood-stream are controlled not only by the ration of the cow but also by the types of micro-organism which become established in the rumen. The relationship between diet and the constituents in milk is therefore complex.

Water is the main constituent of milk and is secreted in association with water soluble constituents of which the most important quantitatively are lactose, sodium, potassium and chlorine. The yield of milk is closely related to the amount of lactose (a dissacharide composed of one molecule of glucose and one molecule of galactose) synthesized within the epithelial cells of the alveoli. Water must be available to maintain the ratio of lactose synthesized for normal milk production. Milk fat is a mixture of triacylglycerol containing mostly of saturated and partly of unsaturated fatty acids, and is derived from the fatty acids of the blood triacylglycerides or synthesized from acetate and beta-hydroxybutyrate of the blood plasma. Like lactose synthesis where glucose of *blood* is utilized by the alveolar cells to produce galactose for ultimate production of lactose, the protein of milk, which is mainly in the form of casein, is derived primarily from the amino acids of the *blood.* The ash in milk contains the major elements Ca, P, Mg, K, Na, Cl, Fe, Mn and I_2. Finally there are considerable amounts of vitamins A and B in milk, with smaller quantities of vitamins C, D, E and K which are not synthesized in the udder, but are absorbed from the blood like all mineral elements.

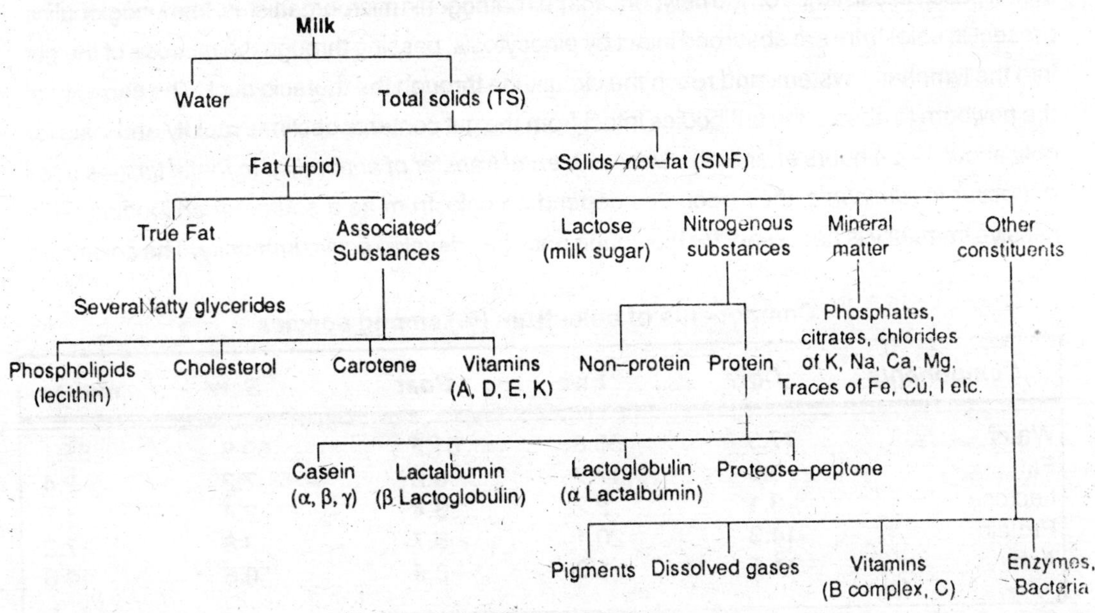

Fig.9.11 Milk constituents.

The first secretion of the mammary gland following parturition is known as *Colostrum* which is designed by Nature to give young a good start in life.

Standards for different classes of milk as per Prevention of Food Adulteration Act is given below:

Table 9.1

Constituents	Cow	Buffalo	Goat & Sheep	Standardised[E]	Recombined Toned	Double Toned	Skim
Milk Fat	3.5[A]	5.0[B]	3.0[C]	4.5	3.0	1.5	0.5[D]
S N F	8.5	9.0	9.0	8.5	8.5	9.0	8.7

A Chandigarh, Haryana, Punjab, 4.0%, Orissa 3.0%

B Assam, Bihar, Chandigarh, Delhi, Gujarat, Haryana, Maharastra, Punjab, Uttar Pradesh 6.0%

C Chandigarh, Haryana, Kerala, M.P., Maharastra, Punjab, Uttar Pradesh 3.5%

D Maximum

E Phosphatase test negative Pesticides/insecticides tolerance mg/kg fat in milk

Chlordane, Fenitrothin	-	0.05
Aldrin, Heptochlar	-	0.15
Lindane	-	0.20
DDT	-	1.25

It greatly differs from milk produced later during lactation. The major difference, and probably the most important one, between normal milk and colostrum is that the latter contains a large proportion of albumin, globulins and minerals. Colostrum is richer than normal milk in most nutrients (including vitamins), apart from lactose and fat. However, its major effect is to confer passive resistance on the newborn against pathogenic microorganisms. Immunoglobulins present in colostrum are absorbed intact by pinocytosis, passing through the mucosa of the gut into the lymphatic system, and reach the circulation through the thoracic duct. The capacity of the newborn to absorb the antibodies intact from the gut contents declines rapidly and lasts for only about 12-24 hours after birth. *Since placental transfer of antibodies to foetal tissues does not occur in ruminants,* their neonates depend on colostrum as a source of antibodies. This passive immunity is necessary for the young until they develop active immunity. The colostrum

Table 9.2

Components of colostrum (%) among species

Components	*Cow*	*Ewe*	*Goat*	*Sow*	*Mouse*
Water	77.5	58.8	81.2	69.8	85.1
Fat	3.6	17.7	8.2	7.2	2.4
Lactose	3.1	2.2	3.4	2.4	4.7
Protein	14.3	20.1	5.7	18.8	7.2
Ash	1.5	1.0	0.9	0.6	0.6

Source : Long, C. (ed), 1961; Biochemist's Handbook, London, E. & F. N. Spon, Ltd.

of ruminants contains a trypsin inhibitor which protects the immunoglobulins from digestion. The globulin fraction in colostrum declines quite rapidly with successive milkings. Within three or four days after parturition milk loses its colostral properties and becomes normal.

Table 9.3

Composition of colostrum (first 24 hours after calving) and of milk

Component	*Colostrum*	*Milk*
Total Solids (%)	22.5	12.5
Fat (%)	3.5	4.0
Protein (%)	14.3	3.3
Casein (%)	5.2	2.6
Albumin (%)	1.5	0.5
B-Lactoglobulin (%)	0.8	0.3
a-Lactalbumin (%)	0.27	0.13
Serum albumin (%)	0.13	0.04
Immunoglobulin (%)	5.5-6.8	0.09
Lactose	3.0	4.6
Ash	1.8	0.8
Calcium (%)	0.26	0.13
Phosphorus (%)	0.24	0.10
Magnesium (%)	0.04	0.01
Sodium (%)	0.07	0.06
Potassium (%)	0.14	0.16
Chloride (%)	0.12	0.10
Iron (mg per 100 g)	0.20	0.05
Copper (mg per 100 g)	0.06	0.02
Vitamin		
Carotenoids (ug/g fat)	35	7
Vitamin A (µg/g fat)	45	8
Vitamin D (ng/g fat)	30	15
Vitamin E (µg/g fat)	125	20
Thiamine (µg per 100 g)	60	40
Riboflavin (µg per 100 g)	500	150
Niacin (µg per 100 g)	100	80

Source : Roy, J H. B. (1980) The Calf. 4th edition, London: Butterworths & Walker, D.M. - (1979). Digestive Physiology and nutrition of ruminants vol.2, 2nd edition (D.C. Church, editor) page 258 - 280

Table 9.4

Comparative physical characteristics of colostrum and milk

	Characteristic	Colostrum	Milk
1.	Taste	Slightly bitter	Sweet
2.	Odour	Abnormal	Normal
3.	Acidity	0.2 to 0.4	0.12 to 0.14
4.	Freezing point (°C)	(–) 0.606	(–) 0.52 - 0.56
5.	Chloride %	0.148 to 0.156	0.14
6.	Specific gravity	1.05 to 1.08	1.029 to 1.032
7.	Refractive index at 20°C	More than milk	1.344 to 1.348
8.	Electrical conductivity	More than milk	0.005 mho
9.	Viscosity at 20°C	More than milk	1.5 to 2.0 centipoise

Table 9.5

Comparative Average Composition Of Blood Plasma and Milk of the cow
(After Maynard et al.)

Blood Plasma	(Percentage)	Milk	(Percentage)
Water	91.000	Water	87.00
Glucose	0.050	Lactose	4.90
Serum albumin	3.200	Lactalbumin	0.52
Serum globulin	4.400	Globulin	0.05
Amino acids	0.003	Casein	2.90
Neutral fat	0.060	Neutral fat	3.70
Phospholipids	0.240	Phospholipids	0.04
Cholesterol ester	0.170	Cholesterol ester	trace
Calcium	0.009	Calcium	0.12
Phosphorus	0.011	Phosphorus	0.10
Sodium	0.340	Sodium	0.05
Potassium	0.030	Potassium	0.15
Chlorine	0.350	Chlorine	0.11
Citric acid	trace	Citric acid	0.20

Milk Biosynthesis

Milk synthesis takes place inside the epithelial cells lining the alveoli.

Some milk components viz. vitamins, minerals and some proteins are not synthesized in the epithelial cells but rather are filtered from the blood through the epithelial cells and forms components of milk. Others, such as lactose, fat and most of the milk proteins are synthesized inside the epithelial cells from various blood precursors. All filtered components and the precursors pass into the alveolar cells through the plasma

Table 9.6

Composition of milk from different species

Species	Fat %	Protein %	Lactose %	Ash %	Total Solids %
Antelope	1.3	6.9	4.0	1.30	25.2
Ass (donkey)	1.2	1.7	6.9	0.45	10.2
Bear, polar	31.0	10.2	0.5	1.20	42.9
Bison	1.7	4.8	5.7	0.96	13.2
Buffalo, Indian	7.4	3.8	4.9	0.78	16.8
Buffalo, Philippine	10.4	5.9	4.3	0.80	21.5
Camel	4.9	3.7	5.1	0.70	14.4
Cat	10.9	11.1	3.4	—	—
Cow					
Red Sindhi	4.9	3.4	4.9	0.70	13.7
Gir	4.7	3.3	4.9	0.66	13.3
Tharparkar	4.5	3.4	4.8	0.68	13.2
Sahiwal	4.5	3.3	5.0	0.66	13.3
Ayrshire	4.1	3.6	4.7	0.70	13.1
Brown Swiss	4.0	3.6	5.0	0.70	13.3
Guernsey	5.0	3.8	4.9	0.70	14.4
Holstein	3.5	3.1	4.9	0.70	12.2
Jersey	5.5	3.9	4.9	0.70	15.0
Zebu	4.9	3.9	5.1	0.80	14.7
Deer	19.7	10.4	2.6	1.40	34.1
Dog	9.3	9.5	3.7	1.20	20.7
Dolphin	14.1	10.4	5.9	—	—
Elephant	15.1	4.9	3.4	0.76	26.9
Goat	3.5	3.1	4.6	0.79	12.0
Guinea Pig	3.9	8 1	3.0	0.82	15.8
Horse	1.6	2.7	6.1	0.51	11.0
Human	4.5	1.1	6.8	0.20	12.6
Kangaroo	2.1	6.2	trace	1.20	9.5
Mink	8.0	7.0	6.9	0.70	22.6
Monkey	3.9	2.1	5.9	2.60	14.5
Opossum	6.1	9.2	3.2	1.60	24.5
Pig	8.2	5.8	4.8	0.63	19.9
Rabbit	12.2	10.4	1.8	2.00	26.4
Rat	14.8	11.3	2.9	1.50	31.7
Reindeer	22.5	10.3	2.5	1.40	36.7
Seal, grey	53.2	11.2	2.6	0.70	67.7
Sheep	5.3	5.5	4.6	0.90	16.3
Whale	34.8	13.6	1.8	1.60	51.2

Source: Schmidt, G.H. 1971. *Biology of Lactaion*, W.H. Freeman and Company, San Francisco, U.S.A.

membrane which exert considerable selectivity concerning which blood substances are to be allowed to pass inside the cells. Some blood components pass with ease while others are excluded; thus the plasma membrane is often called a *selective semipermeable membrane.* During the first few days of lactation and during udder infections the secretary cells and the membranes are less functional, so that the composition of colostrum and mastitic milk more closely resembles that of blood serum.

Milk secretion is a continuous process in lactating cows. It reaches its maximum rate just after milking and its lowest rate just prior to milking. *It is assumed that 400-500 ml of blood must pass through these cells for producing one ml of milk.*

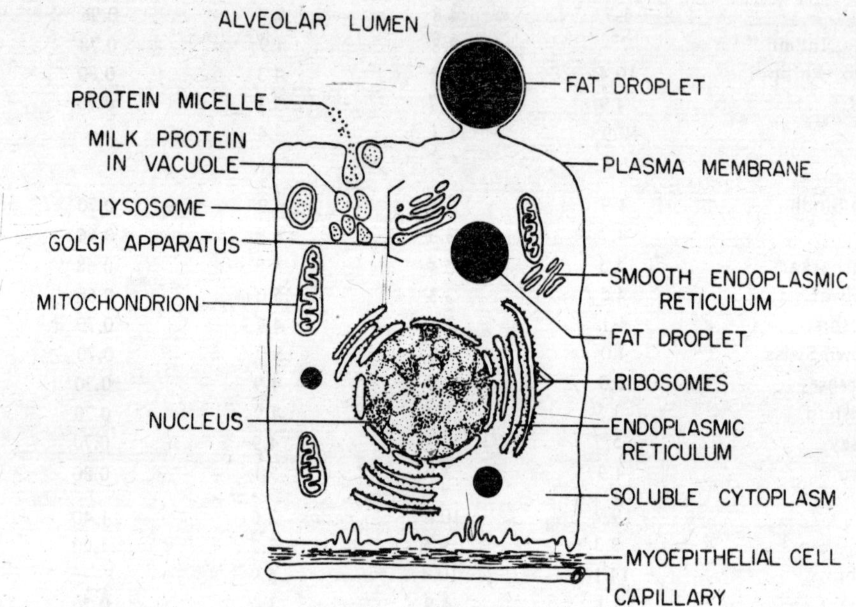

Fig. 9.12 Diagrammatic sketch of a lactating epitheleal cell. (From: Foley, R. D., Bath, D. L., Dickenson, F. N. and Tucker, H. A., Dairy Cattle: Principles, Practices, Problems, Profits, Lea and Febiger, 1972).

Techniques for Determining Milk Precursors

1. **Arteriovenous Differences (AV).** By collecting arterial and venous blood samples from vessels entering and coming out of mammary glands, it is possible to assay constituents of arterial blood supplying milk precursors to the mammary glands merely by comparison of the difference in quality and quantity.

2. **Perfusion of Excised Glands.** The entire udder being a skin gland, can easily be removed from the rest of the body parts of a cow. Thus when such an udder is surgically removed and suspended in a normal position in the laboratory, blood is pumped (perfusion) through the gland by an artificial heart and purified by an artificial lung, it is possible to detect the qualitative and quantitative differences of blood components for the formation of milk.

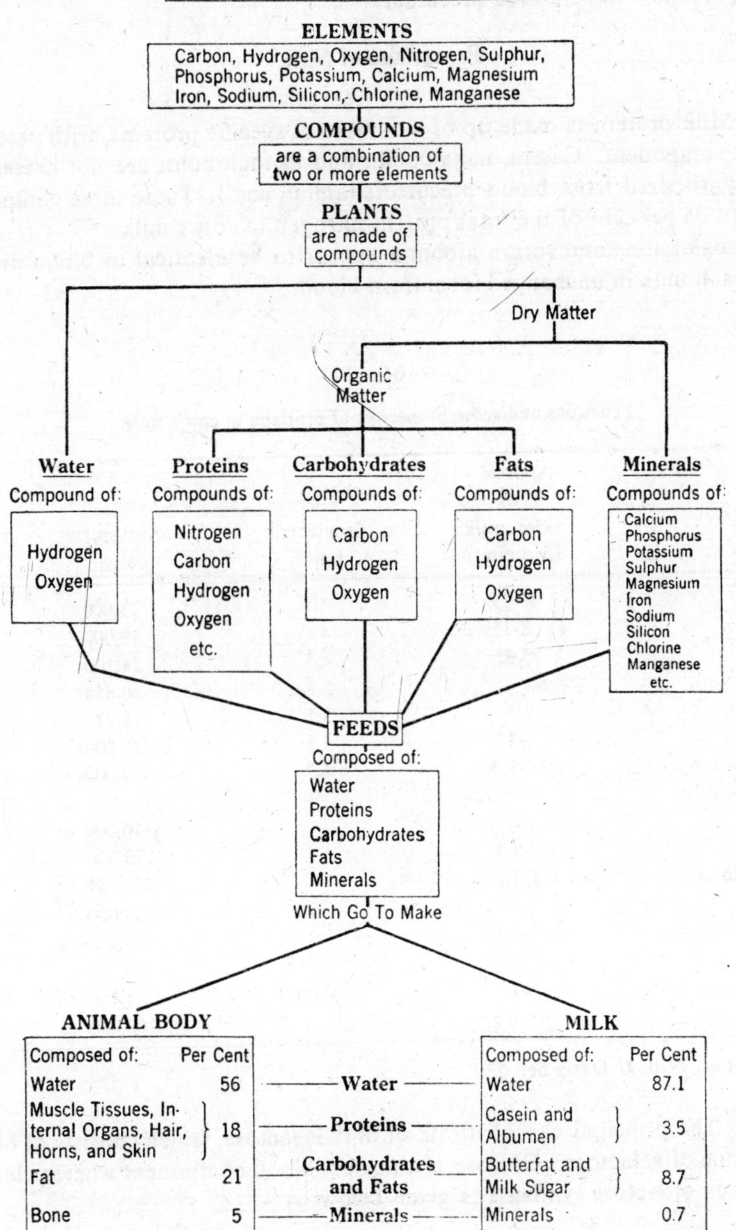

Fig 9.13

Chart showing interrelation of common component elements of plant and animal life that go to make up feed and finally milk.

3. **Radioactive Isotopes.** A substance believed to be a milk precursor is lebelled with a radioactive isotope and injected into an experimental animal. If the compound appears in milk, it may be assumed to be a milk precursor.

Precursors of Milk

1. **Protein.** Milk protein is made up of a number of specific proteins, with casein being the most important component. Casein, lactalbumin and lactoglobulin are not present in blood, they must be synthesized from blood precursors (amino acid). These three components comprise about 90 to 95 per cent of the total protein nitrogen in cow's milk.

The immunoglobulins and serum albumin appear to be identical in blood and milk and are thus diffuses in milk in unchanged form from blood.

Table 9.7

Fractions and some properties of protiens in cow's milk

Protein (contemporary nomenclature)	Approx % of skim milk protein	Isoelectric point	Molecular weight	Number of variants identified
a_s-Casein	45-55	4.1	23,000	6
K-Casein	8-15	4.1	19,000	2
β-Casein	25-35	4.5	24,100	7
γ-Casein	3-7	5.8-6.0	30,650	4
α-Lactalbumin	2-5	5.1	14,437	2
β-Lactoglobulin	7-12	5.3	36,000	6
Blood serum albumin	0.7-1.3	4.7	69,000	
IgG immunoglobulin				
IgG1	1-2		150,000 to	
IgG2	0.2-0.5		170,000	
IgM immunoglobulin	0.1-0.2		900,000 to 1,000,000	
IgA immunoglobulin	0.05-0.10		300,000 to 500,000	
Proteose-peptone fraction	2-6	3.3-3.7	4,100 to 200,000	

Source: Rose et al. 1970. J. Dariy Sei. 53:1.

2. **Lactose.** The principal carbohydrate of milk is lactose, which consists of one molecule of glucose and one of galactose. Glucose is a normal blood component whereas lactose is not. Proposed pathway of lactose synthesis is given below:

$$\text{Glucose} + \text{ATP} \xrightarrow{\textit{Hexokinase}} \text{Glu } 6 - \text{P} + \text{ADP}$$

$$\text{Glucose } 6 - \text{P} \xrightarrow{\textit{Phosphoglucomutase}} \text{Glu } 1 - \text{P}$$

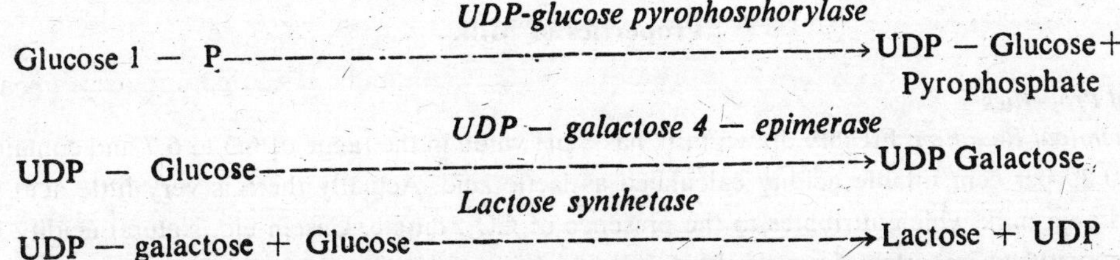

3. **Fat.** Milk fats are synthesized from acetate, beta-hydroxy-butyrate, glucose and free fatty acids. Most of the lipids in milk are in the form of triacylglycerides. Non-ruminant mammary glands utilize glucose for both energy and as the source of carbon for lipogenesis, whereas ruminants depend more on acetate (a salt of acetic acid) for fatty acid synthesis. The acetate in the ruminants along with other volatile fatty acids, are the products of polysaccharide metabolism in the rumen. This explains why cows on high grain and low forage rations often secrete milk having a low fat content. However, fatty acids having more than 16 carbon atoms such as oleic, stearic and higher fatty acids originate primarily from blood glycerides. Glucose is important in the synthesis of the glycerol moiety of the fat molecule.

Table 9.8

Percentage of fatty acids in triglycerides of milk fat

Fatty acid	Carbon length	Human	Pig	Goat	Cow
		% moles in triglycerides			
Saturated					
Butyric	4	—	↑	7	10
Caproic	6	—		5	3
Caprylic	8	—	2	4	1
Capric	10	2		13	2
Lauric	12	8	↓	7	3
Myristic	14	9	2	12	9
Palmitic	16	23	29	24	21
Stearic	18	9	6	5	11
Unsaturated					
Oleic	18:1	34	35	17	31
Linoleic	18:2	7	14	3	5
Other	—	8	12	3	4

Source: Hilditch and Willams. 1964. The Chemical Composition of Natural Fats, 4th Ed. New York: John Wiley

4. **Minerals.** Minerals of milk are derived from the blood and reach milk through simple filteration.

5. **Vitamins.** All sorts of vitamins enter through alveolar cell membranes through filtration.

6. **Water.** Water forms about 87 per cent by weight of milk. It is filtered from blood. Milk and blood are isotonic. Both have 6.6 atmospheres (atm) to Osmotic pressure. This means that there is no osmotic pressure developed on either side of the semipermeable membranes of the milk secreting cells.

Properties of Milk

Chemical Properties

1. *Chemical Reaction*: Freshly drawn milk has a pH value in the range of 6.5 to 6.7 and contains 0.14 to 0.20 per cent titrable acidity calculated as lactic acid. Actually there is very little acid in freshly drawn milk which attributes to the presence of CO_2, citrate, Casein etc. Natural acidity in milk is considered important from the heat stability point of view.

2. *Buffering action of milk*: Fresh milk acts as a complex buffer because of the presence of CO_2, proteins, phosphates, citrates and a number of other minor constituents. This property of milk is considered important from the curdling and also from heat stability points of view.

Physical Properties

1. *Taste and odour*: The normal taste of slightly sweetness and mild aromatic flavour and aroma come from milk sugar (lactose) and milk fat. At the time when milk is produced under uncleaned surroundings or from animals at their late lactations, the taste and aroma is adversely affected. Feeding of certain weeds or fodder, onions, garlics etc. and infection of udder will produce abnormal flavour and taste in milk.

2. *Colour*: Generally, looks white due to the reflection of light caused by fat globules along with other colloidally dispersed substances.

The intensity of golden yellow colour increases, due to the presence of a pigment, carotene. This again gets entry into the blood through green forages and golden yellow grains. In case of buffalo the most abundant beta-carotene gets fully converted into colourless vitamin A, hence buffalo milk looks absolutely white. After removing milk fat, the skim milk shows greenish tint which is due to the presence of riboflavin or lactochrome.

3. *Specific gravity*: Milk is heavier than water. The specific gravity of cow milk varies from 1.018 to 1.038. It varies with the temperature, being lower at higher temperature and vice versa. The specific gravity of individual constituents in milk is approximately as follows. Water 1.0; Fat 0.93; Protein 1.346; Lactose 1.666; Minerals (salts) 4.12.

4. *Boiling point:* Water boils at 100°C under normal atmospheric temperature and pressure. The presence of dissolved milk constituents enhance the boiling point from 100.2°C to 101°C with an average of 100.5°C in both cow and buffalo milk.

5. *Freezing point:* This is the temperature at which the liquid phase may freeze or crystallize and the solid phase may melt or liquify. Pure distilled water freezes at 0°C under normal atmospheric pressure, milk freezes at temperature slightly lower than that of water due to soluble constituents which raise the boiling point, viz., lactose, soluble salts, etc. Freezing point of milk of cow or buffalo ranges from –0.535°C to –0.55°C with an average of –0.545°C. The addition of 1% water of milk will raise the freezing point by 0.006°C.

6. *Surface tension*: Is a phenomenon attributed to the attractive forces or cohesion between the molecules of the liquid exposed to surface areas. These forces of attraction converge to the centre of molecules from all directions.

The surface tension of milk at 20°C is 54.5 dynes per cm. It decreases as the temperature is raised or fat per cent is increased.

7. *Viscosity*: The viscosity of a substance refers to its resistance to flow caused by intra-molecular attraction. At normal temperature the viscosity of milk varies from 1.5 to 2 centipoises (m Pa.s.) The viscosity of milk is always higher than viscosity of water due to the presence of dissolved solids in milk.

Factors affecting Milk Composition

The variation in composition and daily yield of milk is a regular phenomenon in any milking animals. Broadly, the factors which are responsible for such variations can be divided into (1) Physiological, which will be governed by the genetical make up and (2) Environmental, such as age, number of previous lactations, pregnancy, nutrition status, etc. The dairyman has hardly got any control over the physiological factors but he has some control over the environmental factors. A thorough understanding of the factors those change the environment of the dairy cattle can be used to take advantage of some of the changes in milk composition and yield that occur during a normal lactation.

Variations in the composition of milk may result from one or more of a number of causes described below:

1. *Breed*

The composition of milk varies with a number of non-nutritional factors, one of the most marked being the effect of breed. The within-breed variation in milk composition is also very common. The fat and crude protein content of the milk are related inversely to the lactation yield. Lactose values tend to be slightly higher in the milk from breeds with high fat content and thus the SNF contents (protein + lactose + ash) are also higher. Because of this fairly close relationship between fat and SNF contents, the selection of cows producing a higher fat content should also ensure a high SNF content.

There are some exceptions noted among strains and individual animals, where some individuals have high fat and low SNF and vice versa. Recorded differences are only partly genetic in origin as they reflect also environmental differences including diet, climate and other management practices.

Animals belonging to all Indian milch breeds produce more milk with compositional variations.

2. *Changes occurring during a Normal Lactation*

Lactation period of an animal is the period from the time animal gives birth to a young one till she goes dry. Throughout this period which generally considered for about 305 days, there is a variation of both in composition and total yield.

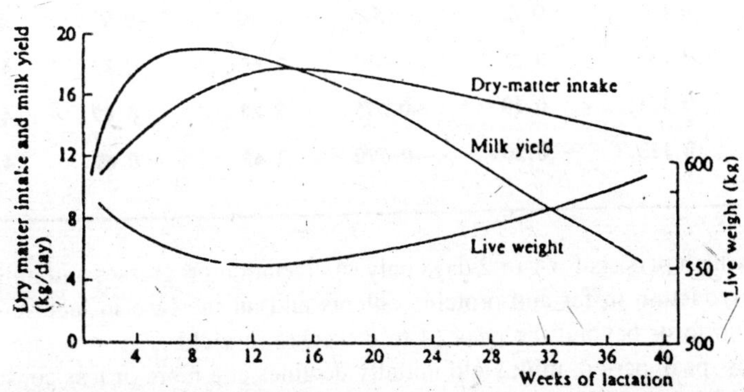

Fig. 9.14 Aschematic representation of the lactational curves of milk yield, live weight and voluntary feed intake of cows.

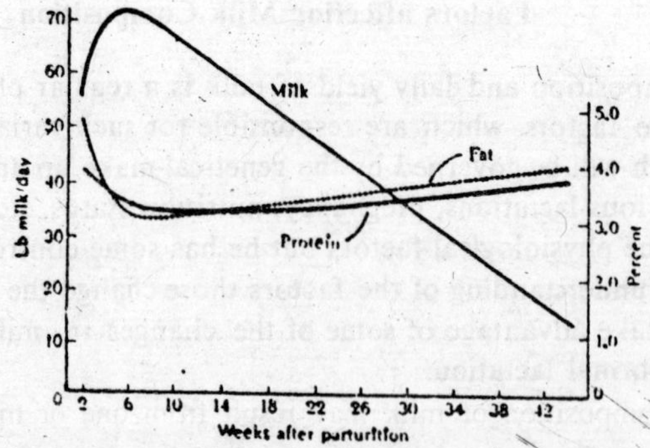

Fig. 9.15 **Lactation curves of milk fat and protein percentages of Holstein Cows.**

Immediately after the young one is born, the cow produces secretion which is quite different from the normal milk and is known as *Colostrum*, lasts for 3 to 5 days after parturition (Table 9.9) It has a high content of fat and protein, and a low content of lactose, the contents of all protein fractions are high but there is an exceptionally high proportion of globulins, mainly *immunoglobulins*, which persists for 1 or 2 days only. As lactation progresses and milk yield increases, there is a rapid reduction in fat and protein contents and an increase in lactose content, changes which continue up to or beyond the peak (4 to 8 weeks) in yield.

Table 9.9

Changes in the composition of colostrum

Days after calving	*Specific gravity*	*Chloride (%)*	*Acidity (% "lactic acid")*	*Freezing point (°C)*	*Casein (%)*	*Albumin and globulin (%)*	*Lactose (%)*	*Fat*	*Clot on boiling*
0	1.067	0.153	0.41	—0.605	5.08	11.34	2.19	5.1	+
1	1.034	0.156	0.24	—0.575	2.76	1.48	3.98	3.4	+
2	1.032	0.149	0.22	—0.580	2.63	0.99	3.97	2.8	+
3	1.033	0.137	0.23	—0.575	2.70	0.97	4.37	3.1	0
4	1.033	0.135	0.21	—0.555	2.68	0.82	4.72	2.8	0
5	1.032	0.131	0.19	—0.575	2.68	0.87	4.76	3.75	0
7	—	0.113	0.20	—0.570	2.42	0.69	4.96	3.45	0

During the post-peak period, milk yield initially declines at a more or less constant rate of about 2–2.5% per week and there is definitely a slight reversal of the previous changes in milk composition (Fig. 9.16) This becomes more marked as the milk yield decline is accelerated towards the end of lactation.

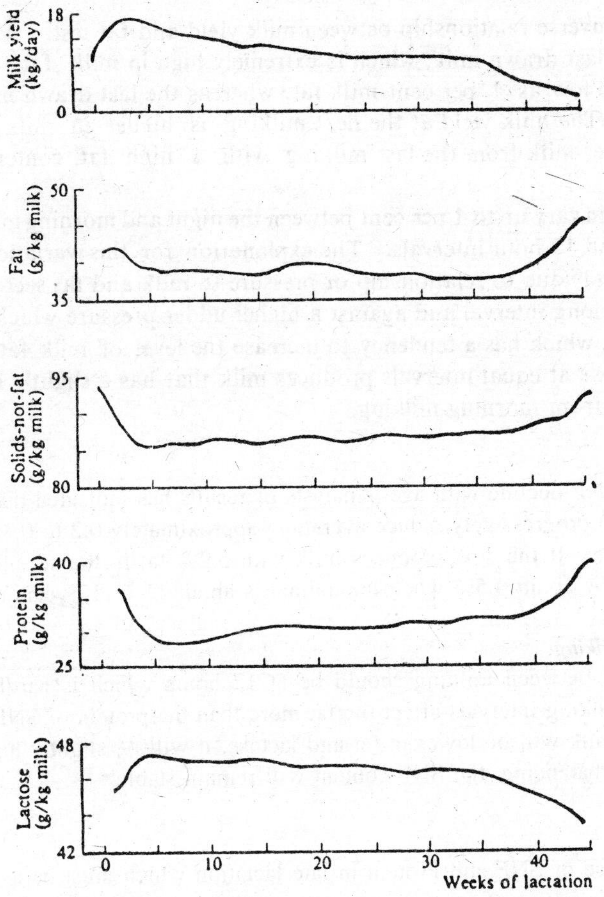

Fig.9.16 Lactational changes in milk yield and composition in dairy cows.

The size of fat globules is bigger during the first few months and it remains fairly constant during the fifth, sixth and seventh months of lactation and again become smaller during the last month of lactation period.

The fatty acid composition of milk fat also changes throughout lactation. The fat of colostrum removed at first milking has a lower proportion of short-chain fatty acids, especially butyric acid and a higher proportion of palmitic acid than the fat of milk removed at subsequent milkings throughout the 1st week of lactation. The relative proportions of short chain fatty acids, except butyric acid, increase throughout the first 8–10 weeks of lactation, that of palmitic acid is fairly constant and the proportion of stearic and octadecanoic acids tends to decrease. Subsequent changes associated with stage of lactation are small.

3. *Day-to-day Variations*

Percentage composition of milk as well as milk yield vary considerably from day-to-day. In general daily variation of milk yield are caused by excitement, estrus, incomplete milking, other irregularities previous to milking, disease, under feeding and related factors. Depression in milk yield that last for several days are usually accompanied by higher fat tests as because

there is a general inverse relationship between milk yield and fat test. An incomplete milking fails to obtain the last drawn milk, which is extremely high in milk fat. First-drawn milk, or foremilk may be as low as 1 per cent milk fat, whereas the last drawn milk may be as high as 8–15 per cent. The milk yield at the next milking is higher in milk fat content since it contains the leftover milk from the last milking with a high fat content from the present milking.

Fat test may again vary up to 1 per cent between the night and morning milkings when the cows are milked at 14 and 10 hour intervals. The explanation for this variation will involve probably two factors: (1) due to relationship of pressure to milk and fat secretion, in which milk produced during a long interval and against a higher udder pressure which has a lower fat test, (ii) due to exercise, which has a tendency to increase the level of milk fat. Consequently the evening milk of cows at equal intervals produces milk that has a slightly higher fat test than does that obtained from morning milking.

4. *Age of Cow*

Protein, fat and SNF decline with age. Analysis of results has indicated that in case of fat and SNF (mainly lactose) progressively reduce averaging approximately 0.2 to 0.4% respectively over the first five lactations. If the cow produces milk with 5.2% fat in the second or third lactation, the fat content may be about 4.5% when the animal is about 11 or 12 years of age.

5. *Interval between Milking*

The ideal interval between milking should be at 12 hours which is hardly followed by any dairymen. Uneven milking intervals affect the fat more than the protein or SNF percentages. With a long interval, the milk will be lower in fat and lactose, it will be slightly higher in protein and as a result of counterbalancing, the SNF content will remain stable.

6. *Pregnancy*

There is an increase of SNF and Protein in late lactation which must be associated with pregnancy, since open (nonpregnant) cows do not show increases in these components with advancing lactation. Pregnancy has no apparent effect on the fat content of milk.

7. *Excitement*

This may result in incomplete milk removal and thus a lower fat test. The SNF content remains unchanged.

8. *Environment Temperature*

Temperatures above 70°F (21°C) and below 30°F(–1.1°C) cause an increase in the fat content of milk, whereas protein and SNF quantities decline at higher temperatures and increase at lower temperatures.

9. *Exercise*

Slight exercise apparently increases the fat content from 0.2 to 0.3% without reducing the quantity of milk secreted. Moderate to heavy exercise in high producing cows, however, will result in reduced milk secretion and a corresponding increase in fat test. Exercise causes no apparent change in the SNF content of milk.

10. *Disease*

Very little is known about the influence of certain diseases on protein and SNF. An increase in body temperature frequently will be accompanied by an increase in fat % and a decrease in milk yield and SNF content. Udder infections, such as mastitis, cause a decrease in milk fat, SNF, protein, lactose and a notable increase in the mineral and chloride contents of milk. Mastitic milk frequently has a salty taste, which is attributed to a high concentration of chlorides. Scientists at Texas in U.S.A. and others have noted that mastitic milk contains more chloride, sodium, copper, iron, zinc and magnesium, but less calcium, phosphorus molybdenum, and potassium than normal milk.

Ketosis reduces milk yield and also markedly increases the fat content of the milk. The effect of other diseases on milk composition is not so clear.

11. *Feeds and Feeding*

(a) *Changes in milk fat content.* One of the most marked changes in milk composition due to diet is the effect on fat content.

Milk fat is highest when the fermentation in the rumen favours the production of acetic acid, and thus diets which depress this acid will depress the content of milk fat. These are as follows:

1. High concentrate rations
2. Low roughage rations
3. Grass from lush (tender and full of juice) pasture
4. Finely ground hay
5. Heat treated feeds
6. Feeds in pelleted form
7. Fish oils will depress the fat content of milk from 1 to 0.5% for as long as they are fed.

It has been noted that the above rations decrease milk fat by decreasing the acetic acid production on one hand and on the other hand by increasing propionic acid content.

Research findings suggest that the fat depression in milk can partially be rectified by feeding the following materials:

1. Sodium or Potassium bicarbonate
2. Calcium hydroxide
3. Magnesium carbonate
4. Magnesium oxide
5. Sodium bentonite
6. Partially delactosed whey

Some of the above compounds increase the rumen pH and others decrease propionate production and increase rumen acetic acid production. The drawback in using these substances is that most of them are unpalatable and decrease appetite.

The following types of rations will help to increase milk fat percentage:

1. Feeding of rations having at least 17% fibre.
2. Use of a screen that is more than 1/8 inch in diameter if ground forage is used.
3. Feeding of unground forage at a minimum rate of 1.5 kg hay per 100 kg of body weight per day.
4. Vegetable oils have been shown to cause a temporary increase in milk fat.

(b) Changes in Milk Flavour

Several weeds such as wild onions, and garlic when fed to milch animals results into objectionable flavour in milk.

(c) Changes in Proteins and SNF Content Changes in protein and SNF contents of milk is less pronounced by environmental factors, while the mineral and lactose contents are not at all variable under normal farm conditions. Underfeeding of dairy cows results in a 0.2 per cent reduction in protein and SNF percentages and a depression in milk yield. Increasing the plane of nutrition to 25 per cent above normal standards results in an increase in SNF and protein percentages to the same extent. High level of nutrition results in an elevated propionic acid production in the rumen.

(d) Changes in mineral and vitamin content. Among minerals, the major elements (calcium, phosphorus, potassium, chlorine and sodium) cannot be changed by altering the levels of these elements in the ration of a cow. Trace minerals with the exception of iron and copper can be increased by increasing the levels of those minerals in the ration upto a certain extent. For iodine which is transferred in maximum amount, it is only 3–5 per cent of the amount present in the ration appears in milk.

Among vitamins, some of the fat soluble vitamins, A, D and E can be increased in milk through dietary process. Marked seasonal variation occur in the vitamin A content is increased when the cow is exposed to enough of green forages specially during rainy season. The carotene present in all green forages are converted into vitamin A. Vitamin D content of milk can similarly be increased by providing sun-cured roughages or by exposing the cows to direct sunlight.

(e) Changes in specific gravity of milk. When the dairy cow goes off feed there is a decrease in the volume of milk produced, accompanied by increase in the fat, mineral, protein and total solids with a simultaneous reduction in lactose and specific gravity of milk.

12. *Dry period and body condition*

The length of the dry period and the body condition at calving are related. Cows must be in good body condition at calving and must have had a dry period to attain maximum production. The dry period is important for replenishing body supplies if the cow is in poor body condition at calving and also to regenerate milk secretory tissue.

13. *Season of the year*

Milk production is usually less during the summer because of the higher environmental temperatures and the prevalence of green-forage scarcity. Thus the season of calving has got a marked effect on the total production. Cows freshening shortly before winter months produce more total yield than those calving at other times of the year. The increase is probably due to more favourable temperature and more digestible feeds available during the winter.

14. *Calving interval*

The interval between calvings is another important management problem the farmer must deal with. The decision should be made on the basis of individual factors such as feed consumption, labour cost and reproductive efficiency, etc. It has been shown that it is most profitable for cows to calve at twelve month intervals. This requires to breed the cows within 2 to 3 months after freshening. More milk can be obtained in a single lactation with longer calving intervals but total production over two or more years is greatest with the yearly calving interval.

Factors affecting Milk Yield (Quantity)

1. *Species*

The milk yield varies from species to species. Buffalo yield more than average Indian pure breed milch animals. Sheep and goat are nowhere in comparison to buffalo or pure dairy type cattle.

2. *Breeds*

Among major factors, breed is one of the most important constituents. Animals belonging to milch breeds produce more milk, e.g. Sindhi (1135 litres/lactation) as compared to dual purpose breed, e.g. Haryana (1100 litres/lactation).

3. *Individuality of Animals*

The strain and the individuality of cows within a breed also are different in producing total yield. Larger cows normally secrete more milk. Cows normally will not secrete more milk daily than the equivalent of 8–10 per cent of their body weight, whereas goats may secrete enough milk daily to equal 20 or more per cent of their body weight.

4. *Stage and Persistency of Lactation*

There is considerable variation in the persistency of milk secretion following peak production within 2 months after lactation. Some cows are very persistent and their rate of milk secretion declines slowly (6–8 per cent of their previous month). The production of other cows may decline very rapidly (8–12 per cent), so that they show poor persistency.

5. *Frequency of Milking*

As milk accumulates in the lumen of the alveoli and fills the storage areas of the udder, pressure develops inside those areas. This tends gradually to inhibit further milk secretion. The more frequent removal of milk permits maximum intensity of the milk manufacturing process. Therefore, frequent evacuation of the udder is essential for maximum milk production. It has been shown that milking cows three-times-a-day increases milk production 10–25 per cent over two-times daily milking. Milking four-times-a-day instead of three results in another 5–15 per cent increase in production. Of course, this will involve some more expenditure.

6. *Pregnancy*

During the first 5 months of pregnancy, the decline in milk yield in pregnant cows is similar to the equivalent lactation period in non pregnant cows. However, following the fifth month of pregnancy, cows begin to decline more rapidly in milk yield.

The average gestation period of dairy cows is 283 days. The aim is to have each cow mated about 85 days after calving. If mated earlier than 85 days, the total yield for the lactation is reduced as in this case after about 20th week of pregnancy milk yield will start falling more rapidly.

7. *Age*

It is believed that there is a slight additional growth of secreting cells of dairy cattle during each pregnancy until cows reach about 7 years of age. This is manifested by the increase in yearly milk.

8. *Estrus*

The activity of a cow when in heat generally reduces milk secretion, however, this is temporary. To minimise milk loss during estrus, cows should be confined.

9. *Dry period*

Cows are normally bred 70 to 90 days (average of 85 days) after parturition. It is expected that they will lactate about 305 days and then be given a 60 day dry period before the next calving.

The dry period is important for replenishing body supplies including regeneration of secretory tissue. Allowing dairy cows a dry period has been shown to result in significantly higher production during the succeeding lactation.

10. *Gestation*

A significant reduction of milk yield occurs towards the end of pregnancy. Although the exact reason is not yet known but according to one hypothesis it has been suggested that level of nutrient required for foetal development are highest; however, this appears to be only 1 to 2 per cent of the daily requirement of the cow. Another convincing explanation is that of a change in hormone production, in which large amounts of estrogen and progesterone are released into blood stream, which are detrimental to high milk yield. During fourth to fifth months of gestation there is an increase of SNF.

11. *Temperature and Humidity*

Severe weather conditions drastically affect milk production. Temperatures between 40–75°F have no effect on the milk production. In this range (Comfort Zone), no body processes are directly involved in maintaining body temperature. At a very high temperature feed consumption is greatly reduced, there is an increase in water intake, an increase in body temperature and respiration resulting decrease in milk yield with lowered milk fat, SNF and total solids.

High relative humidity accentuates the problem of high temperatures.

12. *Changes Occurring during a Normal Lactation*

13. *Feed*

The speed of synthesis and diffusion of various milk constituents is dependent on the concentration of milk precursors in blood, which reflects the quality and quantity of the food supply. Nature provides for maintenance, growth, and reproductive needs before energy is made available for lactation. Inadequate feed nutrients probably limit the secretion of milk more than any other single factor in a dairy cow. Although good nutrition alone cannot guarantee high milk production, poor nutrition can prevent attainment, of a cow's full potential just as surely as poor management, low genetic potential on an unfavourable environment. The maintenance of lactation (galactopoiesis) is closely related to an adequate feed intake by the lactating animal.

14. *Stress*

Recently, more attention has been focused on the role of stress in the secretion of milk. As animals are selected to secrete higher levels of milk, any sort of stress will play an increasingly important role in lactation.

15. *Effect of Milker*

The amount of milk drawn from a cow is definitely influenced by the change of milker. Due to change of milker, the slight variation in milking process, upsets the cow and thereby affects milk yield.

16. *Disease*

Any one of many diseases may significantly reduce the amount of milk secreted. Disease may affect heart rate, and therefore, the rate of blood circulation through the mammary gland, which influences milk secretion is also affected.

Milking of cow and its care

Milking is an act of removing milk from the udder. The method involves experience and skill. It is important that the cow be milked at a very fast rate at regular times to make each milking a pleasant experience. Cows like to be milked—if it is done properly. Milking programme is made up of the following coordinated steps.

1. *Time of milking.* Milking should be done twice or thrice a day, but at regular intervals. The intervals should be as equal as possible in case of twice a day milking. Abrupt changes in the time of milking affects the total yield.

2. *Milking order.* Cows that have mastitis or a history of chronic mastitis are a source of infection to non infected cows. Hence, it is well to milk "clean" cows first. A desirable milking order in a herd is:

(a) First, calf heifers that have been free of mastitis.
(b) Older cows that have been free of mastitis.
(c) Cows that have been a previous history of mastitis, but which no longer show symptoms.
(d) Cows with quarters producing abnormal milk.

3. *Preparing the cow and milker.* The milker and the animal have a mutual liking for each other. The animal should not be excited or beaten before milking; otherwise she may hold up the milk. The "let down of milk" in case of buffaloes is rather time consuming and the milker should not lose his patience.

At the onset of milking the udder and teats should be washed with any antiseptic lotion or boiled *neem* leaves and then dry it with clean cloth. The milker should wear clean dress, cover their hairs with caps or towels and must trim their nails regularly. Milkers having filthy habits like spitting, blowing nose and even talking while milking should be cautioned.

4. *Use clean utensils.* Sanitary milking pails with dome-shaped top should be used instead of open buckets. After each milking the milking pails should first be washed with warm water, scrubbed and rinsed well with clean cold water. Afterwards they are stacked in racks upside down until next milking.

5. *Keep cows free from flies etc.* While milking, all efforts to be made if necessary by taking the help of an assistant, to keep the milking cows undisturbed by flies, unnecessary noise or

by any other acts which will draw sudden attention of the cows. In all such cases the influence of oxytocin resulting let-down will be counter-balanced by the secretion of another hormone, adrenaline, which will stop further let down of milk. Cows remaining at comfortable state will yield more milk than a roughly handled and excited cow.

6. *Milk "let-down" or ejection.* As has already been discussed, just after the last milking of the cow, the alveoli, ducts, gland and teat cisterns all are gradually filled with milk. Milk in the cisterns and larger ducts may be removed easily but milk in all smaller ducts and alveoli does not flow out easily. The cow and other mammals need a stimulation of central nervous system which are in continuous as nerve endings in the teats. These are sensitive to touch, pressure or warmth. Suckling by calf or massaging the udder by milker acts as stimuli and thereby, (1) impulses are conducted along the nerves to the posterior pituitary at the base of the cow's brain; (2) the posterior pituitary stores and releases the hormone oxytocin into the blood stream; (3) the blood transports oxytocin back to the udder; and (4) the oxytocin causes the smooth muscle-like cells surrounding each alveolus to contract, thereby forcing the milk out of them into the large ducts and cisterns of the udder.

The stimulation of the udder lasts for a limited time only (less than one minute) since oxytocin is destroyed in the bloodstream very fast. Hence, once the "let-down" has occurred, it is important that the milk be removed within approximately 5–7 minutes to obtain the greatest amount. This is so because a second stimulation can not be obtained soon after the first.

Complete milking has to be done otherwise the residual milk may act as a breeding place for organisms responsible for mastitis.

7. *Feeding during milking.* To keep the animal busy at the time of milking, it is a good practice to feed a portion of the concentrate mixture at milking time. While the animals remain busy in eating, the milk can be easily drawn.

8. *Milking procedure.* Hand milking and machine milking are the two methods of which in India the hand milking is the most common practice among individual farmers while machine milking is practiced in organised government and military dairy farms.

(a) *Hand milking*

Cows are milked from left side. After let-down of milk, the milker starts milking teats either cross wise or fore quarters together and then hind quarters together or teats appearing

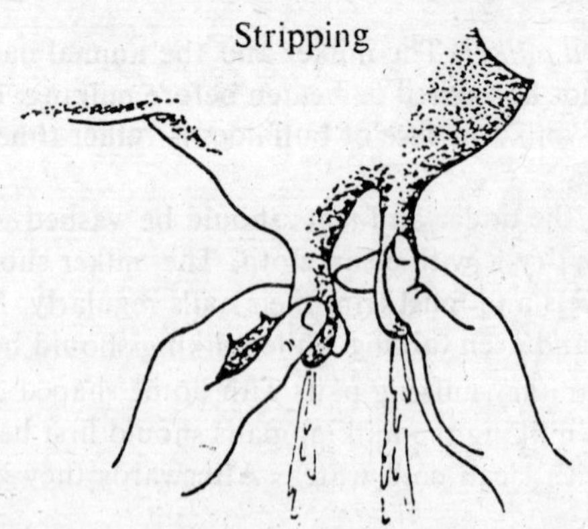

Fig. 9.17 Hand milking by Stripping method.

most distended milked first. The first few streams of fore milk from each teat should be let on to a strip cup. This removes any dirt from the teat canal and gives the operator a chance to detect mastitis.

Milking is done either by *"stripping"* or by *"full-hand"* method. Stripping is done by firmly holding the teat between the thumb and the fore-finger and drawing it down the length of the teat and at the same time pressing it to cause the milk to flow down in a stream. Fisting or full-hand milking is done by grasping the teat with all the five fingers and pressing it against the palm. The teat is compressed and relaxed alternately in quick successions, thus the

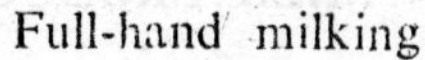

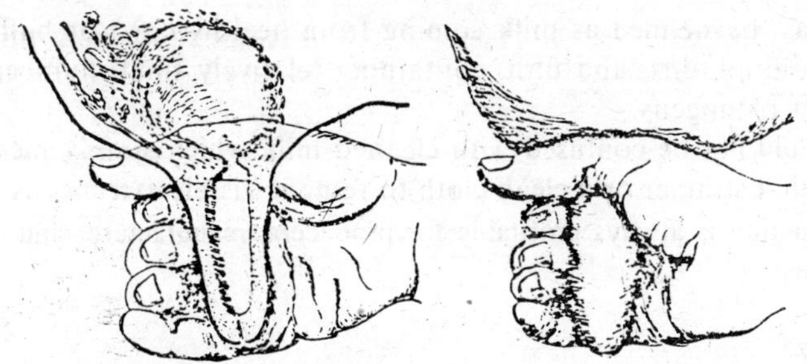

Fig. 9.18 Hand milking by Full hand method. Fingers loose, milk flows into the teat sinus.

method removes milk much quicker than stripping as there is no loss of time in changing the position of the hand. Further full-hand method is superior to strippings as it stimulates the natural suckling process by calf and moreover the method exerts an equal pressure on the large teats of cows and buffaloes.

Many milkers during milking tend to bend their thumb against the teat. The method is known as *"knuckling"* which should always be avoided to prevent injuries of the teat tissues. Thus milking should always be done with full hand unless the teats are too small or towards the completion of milking. The first few strips of milk from each quarter should not be mixed with the rest of the milk as the former contains highest number of bacteria.

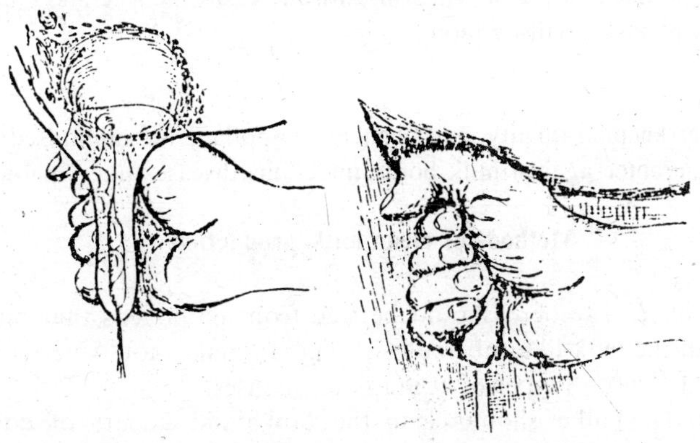

Fig. 9.19 Hand milking by Full-hand method. Fingers progressively compress teat and force the milk out.

(b) *Machine milking*

Modern milking machines are capable of milking cows quickly and efficiently, without injuring the udder, if they are properly installed, maintained in excellent operating conditions, and used properly. The milking machine performs two basic functions.

1. It opens the streak canal through the use of a partial vacuum, allowing the milk to flow out of the teat cistern through a line to a receiving container.

2. It massages the teat, which prevents congestion of blood and lymph in the teat.

CLEAN MILK PRODUCTION

Clean milk may be defined as milk coming from healthy cows or buffaloes, possessing good flavour, devoid of dirt and filth, containing relatively small number of bacteria and essentially free from pathogens.

Clean milk should not be confused with cleaned milk which simply means milk that has been passed through a strainer or a clean cloth to remove visible extraneous material.

Clean milk production is always profitable for producers, manufacturer and consumers due to the following reasons:

A. *Producer's interest.*

1. It renders protection against diseases like septic sore throat, which is essentially of human nature but can become established in cow's udder. Similarly mastitic milk can easily contaminate other healthy animals. Diseases like Typhoid fever, Dysentery etc. are transmitted to the milk by direct contamination through human contact. As such producers must always be careful about maintaining of hygienic conditions in their farm.

2. Unless due attention regarding cleanliness is perfectly observed, the milk is likely to get contaminated by other microbes through body dust of the animal or through water or through other agencies, consequently the life of unprocessed raw milk will definitely be shortened. The producer will find it very difficult to dispose his products at time consuming distant places.

B. *Manufacturer's interest*

A good raw material is always essential for finished product. It enables the manufacturer to produce high quality products, a factor which in turn increases the sale and consumption of milk products. The margin of profit will be more.

C. *Consumer's interest*

1. It provides better keeping quality, and chances of spoilage are minimised.
2. It gives them guarantee against milk borne infectious diseases like typhoid, diarrhoea etc.

Methods of clean milk production

1. *Health of the herd.* The herd should be free from pathogens that might be spread to human beings through the milk like tuberculosis. The animals should periodically be checked in every year particularly for all types of contagious diseases.

2. *Clean animals.* The milker should clean the flanks and udders of cows just prior to milkings to prevent dirt from getting into the milk.

3. *Clean surroundings.* The place at which the animal is tied at milking time, if found to be dusty, sprinkle water.

4. *Control flies.* Fly control measures are important to dairymen since they can carry typhoid, dysentery and other contagious diseases.

5. *The milkers cleanliness.* They themselves should be free from communicable diseases and must be of clean habits as will be noted from their clean clothes, trimmed nails, do not spit around or talk while milking.

6. *Clean utensils.* All types of milking utensils should be as clean and free from pathogens as possible. Best way to achieve this is to rinse the utensils immediately after use. Following washing with ordinary water, the utensils should be washed with warm water containing a suitable detergent. Soap should not be used as it leaves a greasy film.

7. *The type of milk pan.* Sanitary milking pails with dome-shaped top should be used instead of open buckets or vessels during milking.

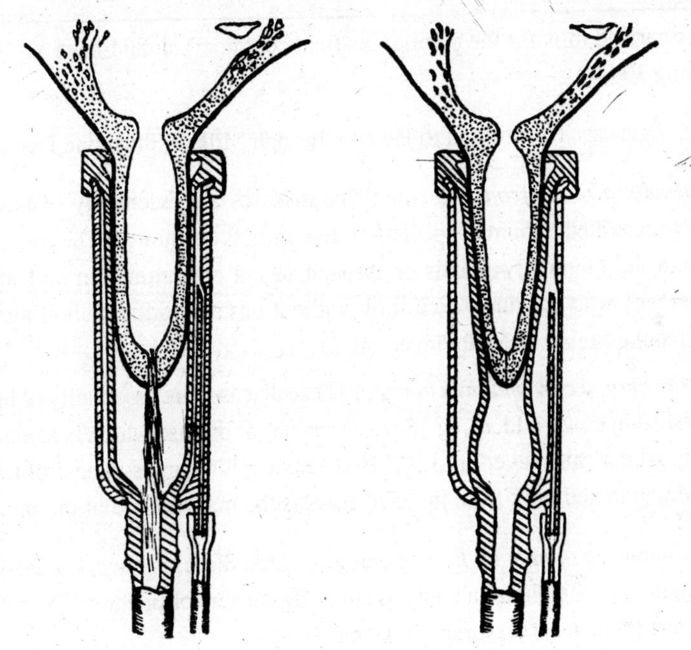

Fig. 9.20 *Machine Milking.*

8. *Straining.* Straining is done to remove sediment and other foreign materials. It should not be used as a cover for unclean milk. If cloth is used, it should be washed and dried daily otherwise dirty cloth will spoil the quality of milk further rather than to improve it.

9. *Feeding.* Feeding of the animals should be made an hour before milking. At the time of milking for the purpose of keeping milking cows busy, provide only concentrates which will be less dusty.

10. *Cool and store milk properly.* After milking, milk should preferably be cooled by keeping milking pails in cold water in winter. In summer ice cubes may be added to water if cost permits.

Bacteriological Standard of Raw Milk

Table 9.10

Bacteriological standard of raw milk as followed in India

Standard Plate Count/ml (or g) (SPC)					Grade
Not exceeding	2,00,000				Very good
Between	2,00,000	and	1,000,000-		Good
Between	1,000,000	and	5,000,000		Fair
Over	5,000,000				Poor

Note : The pasteurized milk (at the plant, in its final container) should have a SPC/ml (or g) not exceeding 30,000

Diseases Transmitted to Human through Milk (Milk-brone Diseases)

1. *Infection of milk directly from the cow* : The diseases are essentially of bovine origin that may secondarily be transmitted to human specially if raw milk is consumed. The causative organisms enter the milk through the mammary glands or through faecal contamination and thus cause a diseased condition in persons who consume such milk without pasteurization or boiling. Examples : Bovine tuberculosis; Undulant fever or Malta fever etc.

2. *Infection from man to cow and then to milk* : These diseases are essentially of human nature, but can become established in cow's udders, eg., Septic sore throat disease which is actually an acute tonsilitis begins suddenly with a chill, fever upto 105°F, severe swelling and soreness of the throat with painful swallowing. Contaminated milk from infected cows is the main source of the infection.

3. *Direct contamination of milk by human beings* : These diseases may be transmitted to the milk by direct contamination through human contact, either by carriers or patients. Examples : Typhoid fever, Paratyphoid fever; Dysentery; Gastroenteritis, etc.

4. *Indirect contamination of milk by human beings* : These are human diseases, the pathogenic organisms which enter the milk through contaminated bottles or other utensils, water supply, insects and dusts. Examples : Typhoid or Paratyphoid fever ; Dysentery or Diarrhoea ; etc.

Milk Production & Availability in India

After stagnating between 1950 and 1970 at around 17–21 million tonnes, India's annual milk production registered an impressive growth in the decade of the seventies to cross the 30-million-tonne-mark in 1980 and the 50 million-tonne-mark in 1989. The per capita milk availability has been increasing despite the growth in population by over 50 per cent – from 548 million to 844 million in this period, as shown.

Per Capita Availability
(grams/day)

2000	220
1994–95	193
1990–91	193
1984–85	148
1980–81	128
1950–51	132

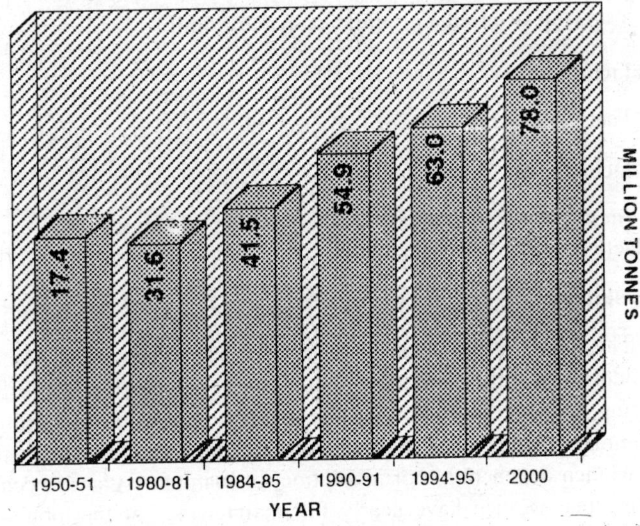

Common Terms Related to Mammary Gland and Lactation

Galactopoiesis

Maintenance of lactation after initiation for a certain period. The term is also known as *Lactopoiesis*. In general a cow after calving reaches her peak yield in about 6 to 8 weeks after parturition, remains at that level for a short period and then declines at the rate of about 10% per month. Various factors are responsible for the maintenance of this lactation pattern. The graphic curve plotted on the basis of the pattern may bend drastically downwards resulting lower yield. Group of hormones, e.g., prolactin, STH, ACTH, TSH and oxytocin exert their effect in maintaining the normal lactation curve on the basis of their ratio of concentration among themselves in blood. The hormones necessary for maintenance of lactation have been shown to be essentially the same as those concerned with its initiation in many species. However, some anterior pituitary hormones other than prolactin and ACTH have been found to cause a marked increase in the milk production of lactating cows. Somatotrophin (STH) injections as well as thyrotrophin (TSH) injections cause marked increases in milk production in lactating cows. On the other hand, injection of prolactin has very little effect on increasing the milk production of lactating cows, while large doses of ACTH or adrenal corticoids inhibit lactation in ruminants. The results of the effects of ACTH on lactation in laboratory animals are somewhat conflicting, both positive and negative responses having been reported. In general, excess ACTH in the circulation may inhibit lactation.

In most species of animals, however, maintenance of milk secretion is also dependent upon the milking or suckling stimulus and the removal of milk from the mammary glands. If the animal is not milked or milk is incompletely removed from the mammary gland, the lactation period is greatly reduced. An inadequate feed supply and the status of health condition are the vital factors causing variation in the production pattern and thereby affect maintenance of lactation.

Galactophore

A milk duct

Galactophorus

Carrying or producing milk; conveying milk

Galactopoietic

That which stimulates or increases the secretion of milk (lactogenic).

Galactosidase

An enzyme which catalyses the splitting of lactose into a molecule of glucose and a molecule of galactose.

Involution

The return of an organ to its normal size or condition after enlargement, as of the uterus after childbirth or of the mammary gland tissues commencing from advanced lactation and completes during drying off process. Following the complete cessation of lactation, there is a rapid shrinkage of the mammary glands due to disappearance of the alveoli (disquamation). The process is called involution. In women degeneration or involution, of mammary glands occur rapidly after menopause. It is interesting that women have nearly full maintenance of the lobule-alveolar system during non-lactating state, whereas the cow has intermediate maintenance and the rat minimal maintenance of the lobule alveolar system during the dry period.

Lactate

To secrete or to produce milk.

Lactation

It begins just slightly before the parturition or immediately after parturition. Lactation can be defined as the secretion of milk by the glandular secretory tissue of milk animals and their collection in the various duct system terminating in the "let-down" when subjected to specific stimuli. Thus lactation is a general term that includes lactogenesis, galactopoiesis and milk ejection in dairy animals, that is referring to the entire milk production parameters.

Artificial induction of lactation may be brought about by means of hormones. In U.K. barren anoestrous ewes have been rendered good foster-mother to lambs by a single dose of 40 mg stilboestrol diproprionate in oil.

Lactation Period

Lactation period of an animal is now accepted for first 305 days in milking stage commencing from the time animal gives birth to a young one till she goes dry naturally or by conditions created by the owner after twice a day milking.

Lactation Stage

Each lactation period may be divided as early stage (first 100 days), mid stage (101 to 200 days) and late stage (201 to 305 days). Stage of lactation affects the composition of milk quantitatively as well as qualitatively along with feed requirement.

Lactation Number

A cow in her life time may calve as high as fifteen to sixteen times depending on breed character (genetical) and on health condition. Usually the number averages between 8 to 10 times resulting equal number of lactations.

Lacteal

Pertaining to milk. Also used for the special lymphatic capillaries of the small intestine that take up chyle.

Lactogenesis

A process by which mammary alveolar cells acquire the ability to secrete milk. The first stage includes increases in mammary enzymatic activity and differentiation of cellular organelles that coincides with limited secretion of milk before parturition. The second stage is associated with copious secretion of all milk components shortly before parturition in most species, continuing for several days after parturition.

Lactogenic

Stimulating the secretion of milk

Mamogenesis

Growth and development of mammary gland

Milk

The whole lacteal secretion obtained by the complete milking of one or more healthy lactating females.

Milking

The extraction of milk from cows udder by hand or by milking machine.

Milk Ejection

It is the thrown out of the synthesized milk from the alveoli and ducts portion of the gland by the squeezing action of the hormone oxytocin.

Milk let-down

During milking, milk secretion inside the alveolus again commences thus the alveoli ducts, gland and teat cisterns get filled up with milk. This does not flow easily unless extra pressure is given to each and every alveoli including the cistern and larger ducts. Stimulation of the teats or udder results in a neuroendocrine reflex secretion of oxytocin from the posterior pituitary gland which on reaching the myoepithelial cells (covering each and every alveoli) causes them to contract and thereby removal of milk from the mammary gland is made possible.

The phenomenon associated with contraction of the myoepithelial cells is generally referred to as milk let-down. This effect ends in 10 to 15 minutes because of dissipation of oxytocin. Until milk let-down, the pressure within the mammary gland is relatively low (0–8 mm Hg.), but it increases to 30–50 mm Hg. at the beginning of myoepithelial cell contraction.

ANIMAL NUTRITION

COMPOSITION AND CLASSIFICATION OF FEED STUFFS

Livestock feeds are generally classified according to the amount of a specific nutrient they furnish in the ration. They are divided into two general classes—*roughages* and *concentrates.* Roughages are bulky feeds containing relatively large amount of less digestible material, i.e., crude fibre more than 18 per cent and low (about 60 per cent) in T.D.N. on air dry basis. Concentrates are feeds which contain relatively smaller amount (less than 18 per cent) of fibre and have a comparatively high digestibility and as a result higher nutritive value having more than 60 per cent T.D.N.

The number of substances used as feeding stuff to different species of livestock may exceed over 2,000 items. All that is being attempted in this section is to indicate the outlines of classification of the conventional feeds into broad categories and to give typical examples of different groups under this classification.

ROUGHAGES

Roughages are subdivided into two major groups—succulent and dry, based upon the moisture content. Succulent feeds usually contain moisture from 60-90 per cent, whereas dry roughages contain only 10-15 per cent moisture. For the sake of convenience, succulent feeds are again classified into various types such as pasture, cultivated fodder crops, tree leaves, silage and root crops. Dry roughages have been further classified as hay and straw based on the nutritive values and methods of preparation.

Succulent Feeds

1. PASTURE. Of the succulent feeds, pasture is the most convenient and economic for maintaining larger livestock. Young rapidly growing grasses are rich in protein and highly palatable.

2. CULTIVATED FODDER CROPS. In the absence of sufficient grazing ground of good quality for maintaining cattle, sheep, goat on pasture all the year round, the importance of growing fodder crops to provide feed economically for production of milk for draught animals, need no special emphasis. For the sake of convenience, these are classified into two groups—leguminous and non-leguminous. Among leguminous fodders, cowpea (*Vigna catjung*), cluster bean (*Gaur-cyamopsis psoraloides*), are the most common *kharif* leguminous crops. They contain from 2-3 per cent D.C.P. and about 10 per cent T.D.N. on fresh basis and yield about 100 quintal of forage per acre. Berseem (*Trifolium alexandrium*) and lucerne (*Medicago*

Table 10.1

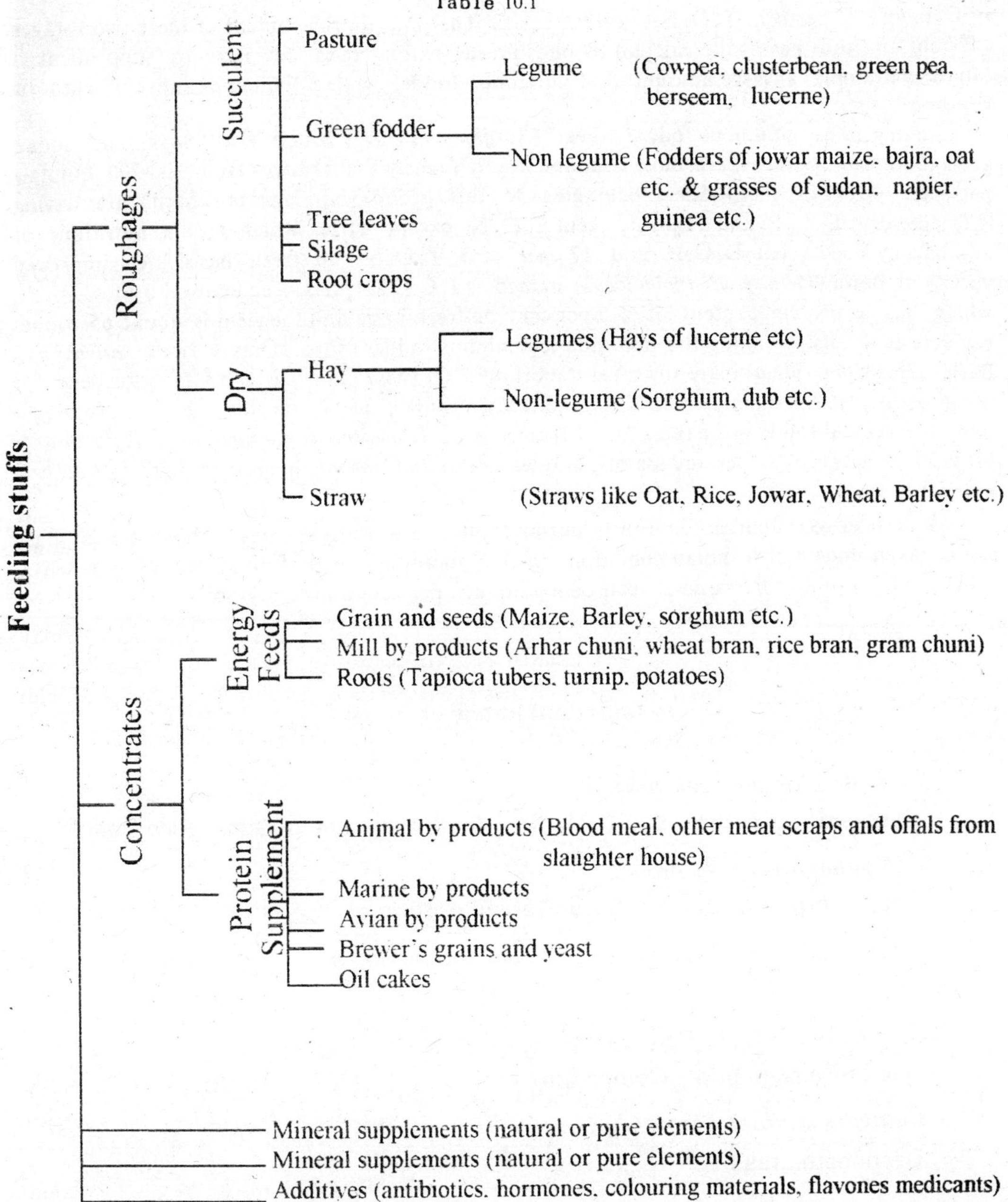

sativa) are two other common leguminous fodder in India. The former is an annual crop, grown during the rabi season; the latter is a perennial one having maximum growth in winter and spring but is retarded during the monsoon. Both these crops can yield over 300 quintals per acre in 5-6 cuttings. The disadvantage is that, both the fodders are liable to produce "bloat" if given in large quantities and thus it is advisable that they should always be given along with some dry fodder. Lucerne and berseem contain on an average 2.5 to 3 per cent

D.C.P. and 12 per cent T.D.N. on fresh basis. The phosphorus content of these two forages are poor and thus have wide calcium to phosphorus ratio. It is advisable to supplement a ration containing a large amount of leguminous fodder with a limited quantity of wheat or rice bran.

Among non-leguminous fodder Jowar (*Sorghum vulgare*), Maize (*Zea mays*) and sudan grass (*Sorghum sudanens*) are most common *kharif fodder*. Yield ranges from 100-200 quintals per acre. Most of the fodders belonging to this group (non-legume kharif) are having 0.5-1 per cent D.C.P. and 11-15 per cent T.D.N. except maize, which is the nutritious of all, having 1 per cent D.C.P. and 17 per cent T.D.N. on fresh basis. An improved variety of Bajra (*Pennisetum typihoideus*) named as I.C. 2291, has been evolved by I.C.A.R., which has a protein content of 2.5 per cent on fresh basis and the yield is about 65 tonnes per acre in 4 cuts. Among the *Rabi* non-leguminous fodder crops, Oats (*Avena sativa*) and Barley (*Hordeum vulgare*) are the most important. Of these two, oat is by far excellent for milch cattle. It has 2 per cent D.C.P. and 17 per cent T.D.N. on fresh basis. Non-leguminous perennial fodder crops consists of Napier grass (*Pennisetum purpureum*), Hybrid Napier grass (cross between Napier and Bajra), Guinea grass (*Panicum maximum*), Para grass (*Bracharia mutica*).

All these grasses flourish vigorously during summer and rainy seasons. About 4-6 cuttings can be taken under north Indian conditions so that an annual yield of 30-40 tonnes per acre is the yield. Two to three animals can be maintained per acre on these grasses.

Table 10.2

Important forage crops

I. Cultivated fodder - Legumes

Berseem Lucerne Senji Metha Shaftal Cowpea Guar Rice Bean

II. Cultivated fodder - Cereals

Oats Sorghum Bajra Maize Teosinte Barley

III. Cultivated fodder - Other than cereals and legumes

Brassica

IV. Cultivated fodder - Perennial grasses

Napier-Bajra hybrid Guinea grass

V. Cultivated fodder - Annual grasses

Deenanath grass

VI. Perennial Range Grasses

Setaria Anjan grass Dhaman grass Marval grass

3. TREE LEAVES. The utilization of tree leaves for feeding to livestock is not common. They are, however, used for feeding sheep and goats, and are sometimes fed to cattle during periods of fodder crisis. In the early stages of their growth, leaves contain fairly high amounts of crude protein and a comparatively low percentage of crude fibre. As maturity progresses, there is a gradual decrease in protein content with a concomitant increase in crude fibre. The tree leaves and shrubs are generally rich in calcium but poor in phosphorus.

Investigations conducted at I.V.R.I. have shown that leafy fodder from the following species of trees and shrubs are suitable for use as maintenance ration for livestock: Jharberi (*Zizyphus numlaria*); Katchnar (*Bauhinia variegata*); Pipal (*Ficus religiosa*); Babul (*Acacin arabica*) Bel (*Aegle marmelos*).

4. ROOT CROPS. Root crops like turnips, swedes, mangolds, fodder beet, carrot are used extensively in U.K. and other European countries for feeding during winter, when other succulent fodders are not available. The main characteristics of root crops are their high moisture content (75–92 per cent) and relatively low crude fibre content (5–11 per cent of the dry matter). An important root crop in southern India is tapioca (*Manihot utilissma*) which is grown extensively in Kerala. The yield per acre varies from 5–6 tons. The tuber is used industrially as a source of starch.

5. SILAGE. The most economical method of raising livestock is to feed them on grasses and legumes directly from the fields. Seasonal influences, however, limit the supply of these feeds at a uniform rate throughout the year. They are, therefore, conserved as hay or silage for use at the time of crisis.

Dry Roughages

1. HAY. A method of conserving green crops is that of hay making. The aim in hay making is to reduce the moisture content of the green crop upto 15–20 per cent to inhibit the action of plant and microbial enzymes. Thus a green crop in a mature state is preserved for a long time. According to the type of forages which are dried, hays are categorised as leguminous, or non-leguminous. Among the leguminous plants, the most suitable is lucerne (known as alfalfa in U.S.A.). Properly prepared lucerne hay contains 14–15 per cent of D.C.P. and 50 per cent T.D.N. Berseem and cowpea are more difficult to be converted into hay. The former has got a hollow stem, while the latter has very thick stem both of which make drying a difficult process. Non-legume hays made from grasses are not as good feeds as legume hays. These are less palatable and contain less protein, mineral matters and vitamins than legume hays.

2. STRAWS. Of all feeding-stuffs, straws are perhaps the poorest in protein and have the largest percentage of crude fibre. They are comparatively poor in phosphorus, in available calcium and also in trace elements, but are rich in silica. Their D.C.P. content is practically nil while that of T.D.N. is about 40%. In western countries straws are never fed to livestock but are usually used as bedding. In India usually 1–2 kg of a concentrate mixture is added to a basal regime of straw to form a maintenance ration. In addition, a mineral mixture rich in calcium and phosphorus at the rate of 20–25 gm daily/head is recommended. If legumes are available, 10–20 kg such feeding stuffs can be used in place of concentrate mixture for maintaining cattle kept on a basal regime of straw. In general straws of leguminous fodder like cowpea, pea, groundnut, mung, gram, etc., have higher mutritive value varying from 2 to 3 per cent D.C.P. and 30–40 per cent T.D.N.

Straw consists of the stems and leaves of plants after removal of the ripe seeds by threshing and are produced from most cereal crops and from some legumes.

Straw either from rice or wheat shall continue to be as one of the staple feeds for cattle and buffaloes throughout the rice and wheat producing areas of Asia because of 1) scarcity in the availability of good quality fodders and 2) straws are potential source of energy for ruminants having 70% carbohydrate on dry matter basis. However, in its present form the rumen microflora are able to utilize not more than 40 to 45% digestible energy due to the presence of high lignin and silica content. The protein digestibility of rice straw is almost zero while for wheat straw it may be around 2%.

The ester linkages between lignin of straw (6% on dry matter basis) and the cell wall polysaccharides (cellulose and hemi-cellulose) renders the carbohydrates to become more resistant to rumen microbial enzyme. Silica (13% on dry matter basis present in straw) also behaves just like lignin. The influence of the presence of these two components is additive on the digestibility of fodders.

Palatability of straw as such does not exceed 2.5% causing voluntary intake upto the extent of satisfying energy for maintenance requirement when fed as a sole feed along with small quantities of protein supplements.

The oxalic acid content of rice straw averages 1.6%, out of which 1.35% is in soluble form and 0.25% in insoluble form.

The total content of oxalic acid in straw is affected by (1) nitrogen fertilizers which can increase oxalate content along with increase in calcium and magnesium found more in leaves than in stem. (2) Stage of plants also affects its total quantity, more during early growth and minimum at maturity.

Rumen microbes can degrade oxalates to some extent but its rate of degradation is less with mature plants. Its excretion is mostly through faeces as an inert calcium oxalate. Metabolic effects of oxalic acid may be summarised as below:

1. It forms a complex with calcium and renders it unavailable for absorption and thus most of calcium is excreted through faeces as an inert calcium oxalate. (Loss of feed calcium!)
2. Urine excretion increases after its absorption in excess and can lead into metabolic alkalosis because of the formation of CO_3 and HCO_3 with corresponding intake of more water.
3. Persistent oxalic acid action of chronic type may result in kidney damage leading to uremia.
4. The high yielding cows or buffaloes may be more prone to a disease '*milk fever*' caused by a condition of fall in the level of blood calcium (hypocalcaemia).
5. Kidney or bladder calculi may be formed along with increase in blood clotting time due to calcium deficiency.
6. In acute toxicity, vagus nerves may be affected leading to stoppage of ruminal motility and even may cause suppression of microbial activity in rumen thereby lowering cellulose digestion.

Straw feeding has also been blamed for development of *Degnala* disease, particularly with rice straw.

The disease is characterized by development of oedema, necrosis and gangrene of the extremities besides tail and ear lobes. Factors like housing of animals, feeding practices and fertilizers have no bearing on the occurrence of the disease.

Inadequate post-harvest drying of rice straw (*parali*) before stacking, stacking at low lying places or near the water/irrigation channels are found to be associated with the occurrence of the disease. The straw, incriminated with the causation of disease outbreaks is in most of the cases found to be mouldy and moist. As such involvement of mycotoxins contaminated rice straw in causation of this disease has been implicated of which Fusarium species (*F. equiseti*) were consistently isolated from all the rice straw samples associated with disease outbreaks.

To overcome the above limitations the following treatments of straws might be of great help to enhance the nutritive value of straws:

(a) *Soaking of Straws*

Paddy straw when soaked for few hours before feeding (one kg straw in one litre of water) is believed to have beneficial effect through removal of oxalates, silica, dust and pebbles. At the same time the straw becomes soft. However, soaking straw results in the reduction of dry matter to the extent of 17 per cent.

(b) *Alkali Treatment of Straws*

It has been observed that addition of 3.3 per cent of NaOH to straws improves the palatability and digestibility. Solutions containing 1.25% NaOH in water @ one litre solution to one kilogram of straw, removes significant amount of lignin and also reduces oxalates thus normal calcium absorption is retained to a great extent.

(c) *Ammonia Treatment*

An alternative approach is to use anhydrous ammonia or solutions of ammonia in water (ammonium hydroxide). The use of NH_3 has the added advantage that it increases the crude protein content of the straw, it acts as a fungicide and it avoids the problems arising from alkali residues found with sodium hydroxide. Any excess ammonia quickly volatilizes when the treated material is exposed to air. However, the method involves expenditure.

(d) *Urea Treatment*

A cheaper, and safer form of ammonia is urea. Urea decomposes to ammonia when acted upon by the enzyme urease.

$$\underset{\text{(Urea)}}{NH_2 - CO - NH_2} + H_2O \xrightarrow[\text{urease}]{} \underset{\text{(Ammonia)}}{2NH_3} + CO_2$$

For every 100 kg of straw a solution of 40 kg water and 4 kg urea is sprayed uniformly and the entire stock is then covered by polythene sheet or by gunny bags or by leaves of banana for about 3–4 weeks. The treated straw will then be ready for serving adult cattle and buffaloes with more palatability, digestibility and above all the enhanced nitrogen content of straw will then be used for protein synthesis by rumen microbes.

(e) *By Making Silage*

The quality of straw can also be improved by making silage along with other succulent fodders such as, barseem, water hyacinth, poultry litter, potato haulum (stalks or stems of cultivated cereals, bean, potato, peals etc.).

Finally, urea pre-treatment only upgrades rice straw to a maintenance feed and supplementation with specific nutrients is required for production.

CONCENTRATES

A concentrate is usually described as a feed or feed mixture which supplies primary nutrients (protein, carbohydrate and fat) at higher level but contains less than 18 percent crude fiber with low moisture. In general concentrates are feeds that are high in nitrogen-free-extract and TDN and low in crude fiber (CF).

On the basis of the crude protein (CP) content of air dry concentrates, these are classified as either *Energy rich Concentrates* when CP content is less than 18 percent or *Protein rich Concentrates* when the CP value exceeds 18 percent.

Energy rich Concentrates

These are described under the following categories : (A) Grains and Seeds, (B) Mill by-products, (C) Molasses and (D) Roots.

A. Grains and Seeds

Grains are seeds from cereal plants – members of the grass family, *Gramineae*. Cereal grains are essentially carbohydrates, the main component of the dry matter being starch which is concentrated in the endosperm. All cereal crops are annuals (*Khariff*).

The crude protein content of grains and seeds varies between 8-12% which again is deficient in lysine and methionine. The oil which is mostly present in the embryo is highest in oats

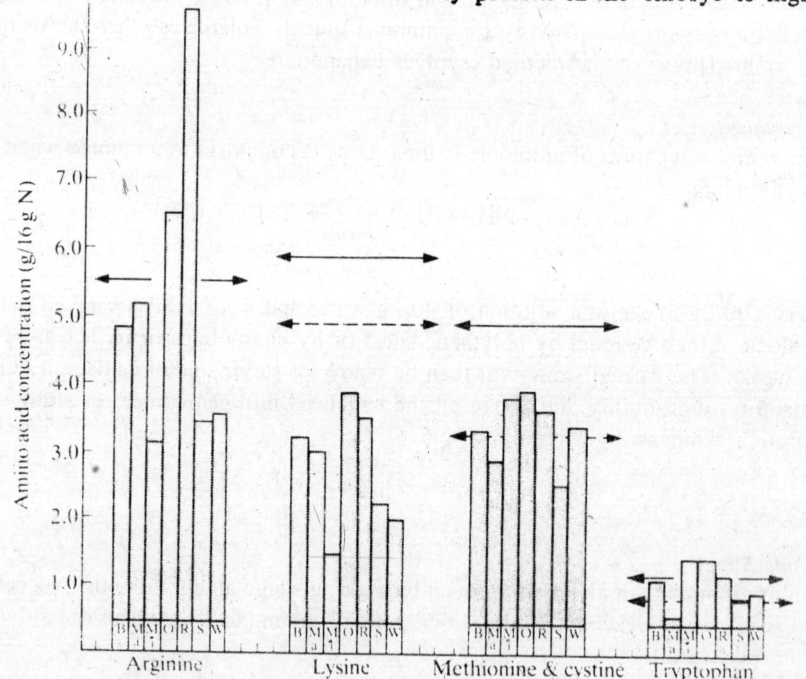

Fig. 110.1. Limiting essential amino acids of some cereal grain proteins (g/16 g N). Straight lines indicate requirements for chicks, dotted lines for growing pigs. B = Barley Ma = Maize Mi = Millet O = Oats R = Rice S = Sorghum W = Wheat

(4-6%) and lowest in wheat (1-2%). Cereal oils are unsaturated, the main fatty acids being linoleic and oleic, and because of this, cereals tend to become rancid quickly, and also produces soft body fat in non-ruminants. The crude fiber content of the hàrvested grain is highest in oats and rice which contain a husk or hull formed from the inner and outer paleae

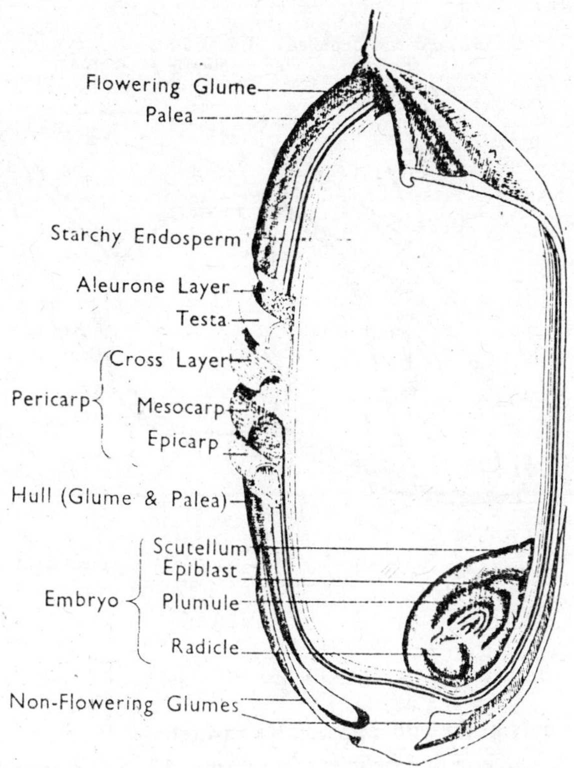

Fig. 10.2. Longitudinal section of Rice grain.

(the inner and upper bract enclosing the grain) and is lowest in the nacked grains, wheat and maize. All cereals are deficient in vitamin D and in calcium (less than 0.15%) but an moderately rich in phosphorus (0.3 – 0.5%) and vitamin E.

Some problems are inharent in the use of grains ; among them (i) grains are most costly on a weight basis, (ii) must be processed before they can be fed (iii) extremely deficient in calcium and certain vitamins, (iv) in ruminants, high concentrate rations may cause digestive disturbances, such as acidosis and parakeratosis of the rumen.

Maize or Corn (*Zea maize*)

1. Most popular and palatable grain for all kinds of livestock. Cattle and sheep are often fed ground ear corn (grain + cobs).
2. Contains about 65% starch, 85-90% TDN, about 10% proteins, deficient in tryptophan and lysine. Two types of protein are present, of which *Zein* occurs in the endosperm. The other protein *maize gluteln* occurring in lesser amount in both endosperm and germ is a

better source of tryptophan and lysine. A new variety *Opaque* - 2 has been evolved having high lysine content. The other variety, *Floury* - 2, has both increased methionine and lysine.

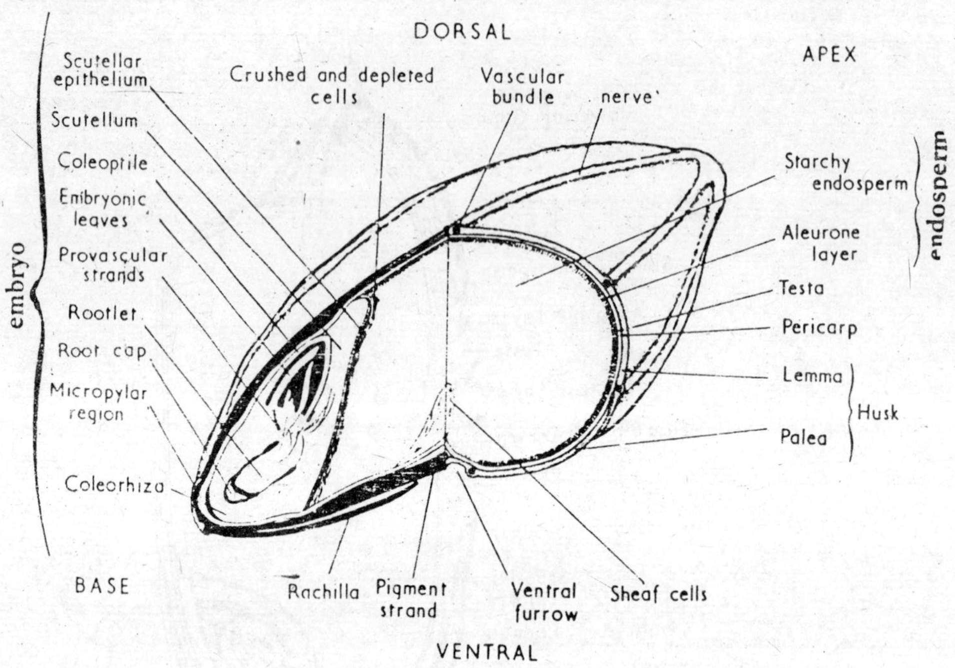

Fig. 103. Longitudinal section of Barley grain.

3. Yellow maize is only grain with appreciable carotene.
4. Extremely low in calcium and deficient in vitamin B_{12} but fair in phosphorus content.

Barley (*Hordeum vulgare*)

1. A palatable but fibrous (7% CF) feed used along with or in place of oats in rations for horses, young growing stock and breeding animals including pigs.
2. Barley should always have the awns removed before they are offered to poultry or swine.
3. The grain may be used to replace up to one-half of the maize in rations for fattening animals without materially affecting their performance.
4. Barley is usually steam rolled (flaked), crimped or coarsely ground before feeding.
5. The crude protein varies from 8-12%.

Oats (*Avena sativa*)

1. Oats are higher than maize in CF (10-18% *vs* 2%) and accordingly lower in TDN (71% *vs* 87%).
2. Are usually rolled, crimped or ground for feeding.
3. Oats can be used for all farm animals. For pigs and poultry, ground oats have a considerably higher feeding value than whole oats. Hulled oats are more palatable but

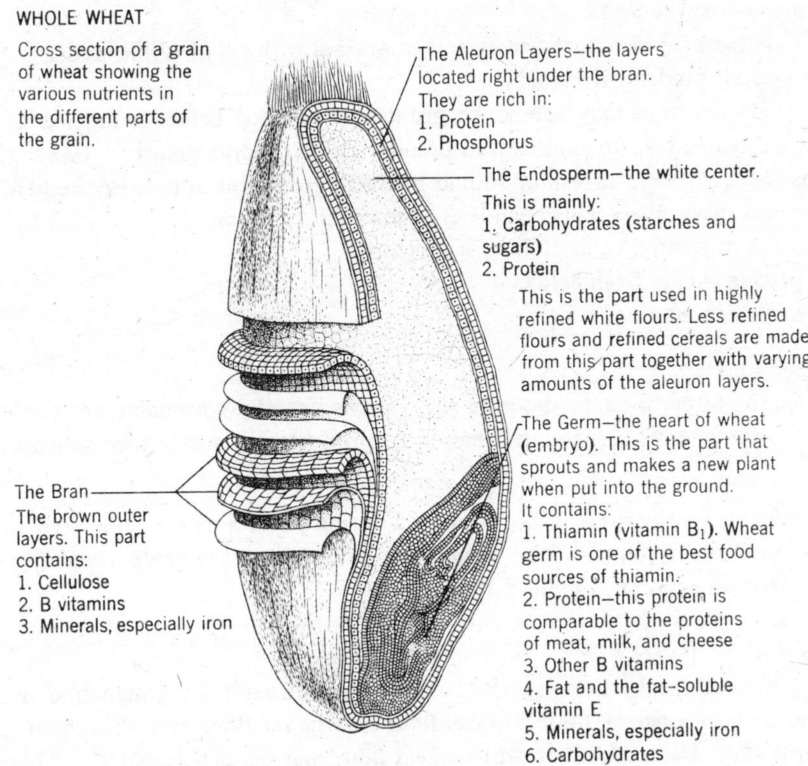

WHOLE WHEAT
Cross section of a grain of wheat showing the various nutrients in the different parts of the grain.
The Aleuron Layers—the layers located right under the bran. They are rich in:
1. Protein
2. Phosphorus
The Endosperm—the white center. This is mainly:
1. Carbohydrates (starches and sugars)
2. Protein
This is the part used in highly refined white flours. Less refined flours and refined cereals are made from this part together with varying amounts of the aleuron layers.
The Germ—the heart of wheat (embryo). This is the part that sprouts and makes a new plant when put into the ground.
It contains:
1. Thiamin (vitamin B1). Wheat germ is one of the best food sources of thiamin.
2. Protein—this protein is comparable to the proteins of meat, milk, and cheese
3. Other B vitamins
4. Fat and the fat-soluble vitamin E
5. Minerals, especially iron
6. Carbohydrates
The Bran
The brown outer layers. This part contains:
1. Cellulose
2. B vitamins
3. Minerals, especially iron

Fig. 10.4 The whole wheat kernel, its structure, composition, and nutritive value.

for cattle and older pigs it is usually not economical to hull the grain before feeding. The high fiber content limits the use of oats in pig and poultry and usually not more than 25% oats is included in rations for growing pigs, while ground oats of good quality are used upto 30% in rations for growing chickens and upto 50% in ration for layers.

Sorghums (*Sorghum vulgare*)

There are many varieties of sorghum but the composition of their grain does not differ enough to affect the feeding qualities to any great extent. All varieties are tall annual maize-like grasses grow up to more than 2 m high.

1. Most sorghum varieties are similar to shelled corn (maize grain) in chemical composition except that most grain sorghum is slightly higher in protein but low in oil than maize.
2. The grains are ground before feeding to all classes of livestock except for sheep which unlike other kinds of livestock will masticate the grains more thoroughly. Whole grains can also be fed to pigs and poultry but cracked or ground grain gives better feed efficiency.
3. When sorghum grain is replacing yellow maize, it should be supplemented with 3% dried green feed to compensate carotene of maize grain.

Bajra (*Pennesetum typhoides*)

This is a milet, annual in nature, warm-season grasses with small edible seeds.

1. Relished by all kinds of livestock.
2. As the seeds are hard they should be ground or crushed before being fed to cattle and hogs, while whole seeds or unthreshed bundles can be fed to poultry. Bajra grain which still has the hulls after threshing should be finely ground as otherwise the hard hulls will splinter into sharp fibers which can lead to internal irritation.
3. It resembles in feeding value to that of sorghum.
4. Crude protein ranges from 8-12%.
5. It is also rich in tannins.

B. Mill by-products

Quite often, the terms used to describe the various cereal by-products are confusing. Let us first discuss these terms along with some of the products commonly used as livestock feed.

1. *Bran*

Outer coarse coat (pericarp) of grain separated during processing e.g., rice bran, wheat bran, maize bran. Laxative in action. Rice bran must have 14% crude protein and less than 14% crude fiber. Protein content is about 8-18%.

2. *Flour*

Soft, finely ground meal of the grains. Consists primarily of gluten and starch from endosperm e.g., corn (maize) flour ; wheat flour ; sorghum flour etc. Sorghum grain flour must have less than 1% crude fiber while wheat flour may contain 1.5% CF. Flour contains about 16% protein.

3. *Germ*

It is the embryo of any seed. Wheat germ meal must contain at least 25% crude protein & 7% crude fat.

4. *Gluten*

When flour is washed to remove the starch, a tough, viscid, nitrogenous substance remains—this is known as gluten e.g., corn gluten, sorghum gluten. Gluten feed is generally not fed to non-ruminants due to bulkiness, poor quality protein and unpalatability. Protein content varies from 25-45% with CF from 4-8 percent.

5. *Grain screenings*

Small inperfect grains, weed seeds and other foreign material of value as a feed that is separated through the cleaning of grain with a screen. All cereal and legume grains are processed in this way and the by-products obtained therefrom. Protein percentage varies from 10-15% with 7-25% crude fiber. Quality varies according to percentage of weed seeds and other foreign material Should be finely ground in order to kill noxious weed seeds.

6. *Groats*

Grain from which the hulls have been removed, e.g., oats ; rice etc. Improved feeding value over whole grain is achieved. Protein percentage varies from 8-16% while fiber is between 1-3 percent.

7. *Hulls*

Outer covering of grain. Generally not utilised as livestock feed.

8. *Malt sprouts*

The radicle of the embryo of the grain removed from sprouted and steamed whole grain e.g., barley, wheat, rye malt sprouts.

These are obtained as by-products of liquor processing. Barley sprouts used as livestock feed must contain 24% crude protein.

9. *Meal*

Feed ingredient of which the particle size is larger than flour, e.g., corn and oat meal contains protein between 9-18% and of C.F. between 3-10%. Oat meal must contain less than 4% fiber.

10. *Middlings*

A by-product of flour milling industry comprising several grades of granular particles consisting of varying proportions of bran, endosperm and germ, each of which contains different percentages of crude fiber.

The product is having protein percentage of 15-20% and that of CF is between 4-8 percent. Deficient in calcium, carotene and vitamin D.

11. *Polishings*

By-product of rice, consisting of a fine residue that accumulates during polishing of rice kernals after initial removal of hulls and bran. It contains about 10-15% protein, 12% fat, and CF between 3-4%. It is an excellent source of energy and vitamin B complex. Due to high fat content rancidity can pose problems.

It is an excellent feed ingredient for cattle, buffaloes, sheep, swine and poultry.

12. *Red dog*

By-product of milling spring wheat consists primarily of the aleurone with small amounts of flour and fine bran particles. Protein is about 17-20% with CF 2-4 percent.

13. *Shorts*

A by-product of flour milling consisting of a mixture of small particles of bran and germ, the aleurone layer and coarse fiber. It has protein percentage between 17-20% while that of CF is between 6-7 percent.

C. Molasses

There are various types but all are concentrated water solutions of sugars, hemicelluloses, and minerals obtained usually as by-products of various manufacturing operations of the juices or extracts of selected plant materials.

(a) Cane or blackstrap molasses

This is the by-product of sugar industry from which a maximum of sugar has been extracted. About 25-50 kg of molasses results from production of 100 kg refined sugar. Cane molasses contains 3% protein, 10% ash comprising excellent source of minerals except phosphorous. It is also rich in niacin and pantothenic acid.

(b) Beet molasses

This product is obtained as a by-product of the manufacture of beet sugar. In making sugar from sugar beets, the beets are shredded into cossettes and the juice is extracted. In this process two valuable by-products are obtained, one is sugar beet and the other is beet pulp. Protein values are higher than cane molasses (6-10% *vs* 3%).

(c) Citrus molasses

When oranges or grape fruits are processed for juice or section, there remains 45-60 percent of their weight in the form of peel, rag and seeds as wastes. The liquid obtained from pressing these wastes contains between 10-15 percent soluble solids of which 50-70 percent is sugar. This material, which may amount for more than half of the total weight of the waste, can be concentrated into citrus molasses, which is normally a thick viscous liquid, dark brown to almost black in colour and has a bitter taste ! This bitter taste does not affect its usefulness in cattle feeding.

The molasses has got higher moisture content, 27-30%. On the other hand, protein content is about 14%.

(d) Wood molasses

By giving high pressure at high temperature in presence of dilute acid, wood is converted to molasses. After removal of the digester, the sugar solution is cooled to 138°C and neutralised with lime. The resulting sugar solution contains 5-6% simple sugars and is concentrated to syrup used for feeding. 1 ton of wood will yield about 0.5 tons of sugar.

In the manufacture of paper, fibre boards, pure cellulose from wood, there results an extract which contains soluble carbohydrates and minerals of the wood material which may also be processed into molasses for livestock feeding.

The molasses has a bitter taste but highly acceptable to cattle, particularly used for beef cattle.

Use of Molasses in Livestock Feeding

A. The different types of molasses are similar in feeding value and are available in both liquid and dehydrated forms.

B. Molasses is usually used in rations for cattle, buffaloes, sheep and horses

1. As a source of energy
2. As an appetisor
3. To reduce the dustiness of a ration
4. As a binder for pelleting
5. To stimulate rumen microbial activity
6. To supply unidentified factors
7. To provide a carrier for NPN and vitamins in liquid supplements
8. In the case of cane molasses, to provide trace minerals
9. In ruminant rations, molasses is restricted to the level of 10-15% of the ration. Excessive amounts of molasses (greater than 15%) will cause the feed to become messy as well as create digestive disturbance along with disrupted rumen microbial activity.
10. Poultry are rather sensitive to molasses as excess levels cause diarrhoea. Levels are restricted to from 2-5%.

Molasses Brix

The term is used in referring to the amount of sugar content of molasses.

Brix is determined by measuring the specific gravity of molasses, the value is then applied to a conversion table from which the level of sucrose (or degrees Brix) can be determined. As sugar content increases, degrees Brix likewise increases.

Since molasses also contains lipids, protein, inorganic salts, waxes, gums and other material, the Brix classification can often be misleading, because each of these components has an influence on the specific gravity of the solution. However, Brix value reflect the relative level of sugar present and so has over the years been used as a convenient basis for expressing molasses quality. Both cane and beet molasses have got generally 79.5 degree Brix.

D. Roots and Tubers

A root crop consists of the fleshy subterranean (underground) parts of a harvested plant, grown primarily for its sugar content and is normally not given to animals as such e.g., turnips, sugar beet, carrots, swedes, mangolds.

Tubers are short, thickend, fleshy stems usually formed underground such as e.g., potatoes, cassava, sweet potatoes etc. Tubers differ from the root crops in containing either starch or fructan instead of sucrose as the main storage carbohydrate. They have higher dry matter and lower crude fiber contents and consequently are more suitable than roots for feeding to pigs and poultry.

Root and tuber crops have traditionally been used more extensively as livestock feed in Europe. Due to large amounts of moisture (80 – 90%) in these feeds when fresh, only limited amounts are fed to high producing animals which requires considerable amount of dry matter. The crude protein content is low and consists to a large extent of non-protein nitrogen. It is also poor in calcium and phosphorus content.

In India, the only tuber which is used in large scale as livestock feed is cassava tuber.

Cassava (*Manihot utilissma*) is a tropical shrubby perennial plant upto 4 m high with finger-like leaves. Cultivated for its edible roots. Cassava tubers are mainly used for the production of tapioca starch for human consumption although the tubers are often used as feed for cattle, pigs and poultry. Cassava root meal can be included upto 10% in rations for growing chicks and upto 20% in rations for layers with good results. For unknown reasons cassava meal seems to cause health problems when included in turkey rations. If the ration is supplemented with 0.15% methionine, the meal can constitute upto 50% of the poultry ration in substitution of maize. Cassava is usually limited to 20-30% of the pig ration.

The various other products obtained from cassava are discussed along with unconventional livestock feeds in India in this book.

Toxicity : Cassava roots must be processed very carefully by boiling or grating and squeezing, or grinding to a powder and then pressing as they contain two cyanogenetic glucosides (1) *Linamarin* and (2) *Lotaustralin*, which are acted upon enzymes readily liberate hydrocyanic acid (HCN). The peeled tubers contain much less HCN than unpeeled as most of the HCN is contained in the skin.

Varieties can be divided in two groups (1) Bitter varieties containing 0.02 – 0.03% HCN. Needs processing before used as feed ; (2) Sweet varieties, containing less than 0.01% HCN and can be used raw for feeding.

Protein Rich Concentrates

Ingredients that contain more than 18 percent of their total weight in crude (total) protein are generally classified as protein feeds. Protein is one of the critical nutrients, particularly for young, rapidly growing animals and high producing adults, although it may be secondary to energy or other nutrients at times. In addition, protein supplements usually are more expensive than energy feeds, so optimal use is a must in any practical feeding system. The primary functions of protein feeds are to supply (1) those amino acids not provided in adequate amounts by the cereal portion of non-ruminant rations, or (2) nitrogen precursors of microbial protein in the case of ruminants.

Protein supplements may be further categorical according to source of origin as (1) plant proteins, (2) animal proteins (avian, mammalian and marine), (3) non-protein nitrogen, and (4) single-cell proteins.

A. PLANT PROTEINS

Oilseed Meals

A number of oil bearing seeds are grown for vegetable oils for human food, and for paints and other industrial purposes. In processing these seeds, protein rich products of great value as livestock feeds are obtained. The by-products left after extraction of oil from oil seeds are used for feeding of all kinds of livestock. According to the method of processing use, cakes are classified into (i) *ghani*, (ii) expeller and (iii) solvent extracted. Of these, ghani-pressed cakes contain the maximum amount of ether extract while solvent extracted cakes contain trace of oil. Conversely the protein content is highest in solvent extracted cakes and lowest in the ghani cakes.

The seeds from which oil is to be removed is cracked and crushed to produce flakes (a small thin mass) of about 0.25 mm thick, which are cooked at temperature upto 104°C for 15-20 minutes. The temperature is then raised to about 110°115°C until the moisture content is reduced to about 3 percent. The material is then passed through a perforated horizontal cylinder in which revolves a screw of variable pitch. The residue is a by-product of oil extraction and usually has an oil content between 2.5 and 4.0 percent. The cylindrical presses used for extraction are called expellers and the method is referred to expeller process.

Oilseeds having oil content less than 35% is suitable for solvent extraction. If oilseeds having higher oil content is to be so treated, it first undergoes expeller syetem to lower the oil content to a suitable level. The first stage in solvent extraction is to crack the seeds and then crushed to produce flakes. After this the solvent like hexane is allowed to percolate through the flakes. The oil content of the cakes by this process is usually below 1% and it still contains some solvent, which is removed by heating.

Oilseed cakes (meals) are in general very good sources of protein, about 95% of the nitrogen is present as true protein. It usually has a digestibility of 75% to 95%. Certainly they are of

Table 103

Average composition and nutritive value of common Indian feeding stuffs
(on dry matter basis)

A. Green Fodders :

Name	Botanical name	CP	CF	NFE	EE	DCP	TDN	Total ash	CA	P
Anjan	*Cenchrus ciliaris* Linn.	10.00	35.30	42.60	1.12	5.49	56.0	10.98	—	—
Bajra	*Pennisetum typhoides* (Burm. f.) Stapf & C.E. Hubb.	6.90	31.80	48.90	1.52	4.31	59.24	10.88	—	—
Bermuda grass	*Cynodon dactylon* Pers.	6.76	24.15	55.99	0·62	3.68	43.04	12.48	0.35	0.26
Berseem	*Trifolium alexandrinum* Linn.	15.45	26.06	35.88	2.36	12.51	59.18	20.25	1.66	0.33
Cowpea	*Vigna unguiculata* (L.) Walp	28.12	26.66	33.05	3.00	20.26	62.19	9.17	1.43	0.30
Dal grass	*Hymenachne amplexicaulis* C. Muell (syn. *H. amplexicaulis* Ness.)	9.38	22.10	54.32	2.30	5.81	57.24	12.20	0.13	0.21
Dhus	*Erianthus longisetosus* Anderss. ex-Benth.	7.50	32.20	48.80	3.40	3.03	56.25	9.19	0.21	0.01
Ghiabati	*Ipomoea pes-tigridis*	11.41	23.75	50.39	2.20	7.45	60.90	12.25	1.17	0.39
Clusterbean (*guar*)	*Cyamopsis tetragonoloba* (L.) Taub.	18.13	31.91	37.65	1.87	6.13	48.83	10.44	2.49	0.39
Guinea grass	*Panicum maximum* Jacq.	7.88	38.38	37.01	1.19	5.83	65.09	15.54	0.51	0.39
Sorghum (prime)	*Sorghum bicolor* (L.) Moench	7.75	32.30	49.61	1.73	3.44	54.03	8.55	—	—
Joya-jha	*Ischaemum rugosum* Salisb.	6.63	33.72	47.84	2.18	4.42	56.61	9.63	0.49	0.27
Karrah	*Carthamus tinctorius* L.	15.6	23.6	48.3	1.9	9.19	58.14	11.2	1.30	0.34
Kharika	*Microstegium ciliatum* A. Camus	6.04	37.50	44.95	1.80	2.66	49.85	9.71	0.32	0.12
Lucerne	*Medicago sativa* L.	19.90	29.61	34.68	1.81	15.92	57.79	14.10	2.00	0.32
Maize	*Zea mays* L.	6.74	35.95	47.07	2.09	4.14	67.77	8.15	0.52	0.28
Morara	*Melilotus indica* All.	16.02	35.15	37.99	1.94	13.30	64.01	8.90	0.75	0.22
Napier	*Pennisetum purpureum* Schum.	6.16	28.07	47.47	2.26	3.85	55.39	16.04	0.33	0.35
Natal grass	*Rhynchelytrum repens* (Willd.) C. E. Hubb. [syn. *Tricholaena rosea* Nees.]	5.61	41.61	43.39	1.40	2.42	53.12	7.99	0.34	0.11
Oat	*Avena sativa* L.	9.90	26.60	50.50	2.22	7.10	69.70	10.88	—	—
Para grass	*Brachiaria mutica* Stapf	11.98	28.22	45.70	1.01	7.91	59.54	15.16	0.32	0.35
Rhodes grass	*Chloris gayana* Kunth	9.36	36.16	42.14	1.16	5.13	58.43	11.08	0.30	0.10
Senji	*Melilotus indica* All.	15.46	31.62	41.95	3.32	12.61	64.04	9.50	1.35	0.18
Spear grass	*Heteropogon contortus* (L.) Beauv. ex Roem. & Schult.	6.97	34.52	47.94	1.35	0.84	44.77	9.22	—	—
Star grass	*Cynodon plectostachyum* Pilger	5.44	37.60	45.24	0.90	2.39	46.42	10.82	0.37	0.11
Sudan grass	*Sorghum sudanense* (Piper) Stapf	8.80	29.90	42.90	1.60	4.30	48.5	8.00	0.25	0.17
Sugarcane	*Saccharum officinarum* L.	5.47	37.18	49.78	1.48	0.00	46.30	6.09	0.41	0.20
Sunflower	*Helianthus annuus* L.	11.04	23.98	45.26	3.44	8.55	52.50	15.38	—	—
Ulu	*Imperata cylindrica* Beauv.	5.52	32.40	51.00	3.21	2.59	43.66	8.18	0.29	0.19
Urochloa	*Urochloa pullulans* Stapf	5.81	33.29	46.27	1.42	2.81	50.87	13.21	0.51	0.31
Velvet bean	*Mucuna cochinchinensis* Cheval	15.14	19.27	48.53	2.13	10.66	63.38	14.93	—	—
Venezuela	*Melinis minutiflora* Beauv.	4.38	37.78	47.99	1.02	1.61	55.79	8.83	0.54	0.31

(Contd.)

B. Subsidiary Fodders : ——

Name	Botanical name	CP	CF	NFE	EE	DCP	TDN	Total ash	CA	P
Bahera	*Terminalia bellirica* Roxb.	8.63	18.59	60.06	4.71	0.86	54.45	8.01	2.08	0.27
Bang	*Quercus incana* Roxb.	10.20	31.34	48.38	4.84	5.76	43.75	5.24	0.99	0.15
Bankli	*Anogeissus latifolia* Wall. ex Bedd.	7.45	24.15	55.36	3.55	0.57	47.78	9.49	3.03	0.34
Bamboo leaves	*Dendrocalamus strictus* Nees.	14.19	27.64	44.46	1.73	9.34	48.91	11.98	1.12	0.26
Banyan	*Ficus benghalensis* L	9.63	26.84	51.59	2.64	1.99	44.53	9.30	1.81	0.18
Bel	*Aegle marmelos* (L.)Corr. ex Roxb.	15.13	16.45	52.83	1.54	10.76	56.65	14.05	4.24	0.30
Ber	*Ziziphus mauritiana* Lam.	8.59	30.13	48.83	1.74	3.09	30.65	10.72	2.19	0.33
Chamror	*Ehretia laevis* Roxb.	13.50	17.98	51.17	6.00	8.45	54.78	11.35	1.48	0.27
Dhaura	*Lagerstroemia parviflora* Roxb.	7.77	17.30	58.18	5.70	0.86	59.14	11.05	2.59	0.25
Gauj	*Millettia extensa* Benth. ex Baker	22.68	32.50	30.93	4.57	15.51	44.34	9.32	1.91	0.29
Gular	*Ficus glomerata* Roxb.	11.16	12.27	59.00	2.43	6.69	53.82	15.14	2.66	0.31
Haldu	*Adina cordifolia* Benth. & Hook. f.	9.50	14.00	64.08	4.80	2.66	50.90	7.62	1.77	0.37
Jaman	*Syzygium cumini* (L.) Skeels	7.76	15.94	68.44	2.24	0.05	47.13	5.62	1.35	0.20
Jhahrberi	*Ziziphus nummularia* (Burm.f.) Wight & Arn.	11.63	33.82	46.76	1.59	5.45	57.10	6.20	1.90	0.31
Jhingan	*Lannea coromandelica* (Houtt.) Merr.	11.44	16.12	59.05	4.20	4.87	55.15	9.19	1.75	0.28
Kachnar	*Bauhinia variegata* L.	15.80	31.80	41.20	1.95	9.16	55.54	9.25	2.69	0.26
Khair	*Acacia catechu* Willd.	13.03	22.55	50.96	4.55	2.90	46.33	8.91	2.73	0.14
Kumbi	*Careya arborea* Roxb.	10.37	25.92	48.56	7.68	0.15	46.27	7.47	1.59	0.26
Kusum	*Schleichera oleosa* (Lour.) Oken	10.37	32.34	49.21	1.93	3.40	48.23	6.15	1.73	0.31
Lasora	*Cordia dichotoma* Forst. f.	12.81	24.55	39.56	2.42	5.14	26.93	20.66	4.24	0.30
Mahua	*Madhuca indica* J. F. Gmel.	9.81	20.31	59.36	3.80	0.00	37.06	6.72	1.61	0.13
Marorphali	*Helicteres isora* L.	13.25	19.80	53.02	3.04	9.68	58.32	10.89	2.24	0.30
Mulberry leaf-stock	*Morus australis* Poir.	11.4	2.72	34.02	39.42	7.84	48.35	9.32	1.56	0.26
Neem	*Azadirachta indica* A. Juss.	16.12	20.69	52.06	3.40	8.38	53.55	7.73	1.39	0.24
Pakar	*Ficus lucescens* Blume	10.20	21.80	52.50	2.60	2.80	45.60	12.90	2.49	0.20
Phaldu	*Mytragyna parviflora*	7.73	19.57	60.65	3.27	1.47	50.00	8.79	2.25	0.25
Phaniant	*Quercus glauca* Thunb.	9.62	29.04	49.60	4.14	4.61	39.77	7.60	1.34	0.10
Pipal	*Ficus religiosa* L.	9.66	26.96	45.82	2.66	5.47	39.22	14.90	4.10	0.22
Pula	*Kydia calycina* Roxb.	12.47	23.71	46.10	3.31	7.88	45.18	14.41	3.06	0.35
Ratendu	*Saurauia napaulensis*	12.25	18.40	51.65	4.23	1.19	34.01	13.47	2.74	0.24
Rohini	*Mallotus philippensis* Muell-Arg.	13.37	29.65	44.64	3.65	7.86	42.10	8.69	1.31	0.22
	Other fodders									
Bajra kadbi	*Pennisetum typhoides* (Burm. f.) Stapf & C. E. Hubb.	3.10	40.44	48.54	1.15	0.93	53.45	6.77	0.39	0.36
Gram straw	*Cicer arietinum* L.	6.01	44.45	35.70	0.53	2.41	37.08	13.31	—	—
Sorghum *kadbi*	*Sorghum bicolor* (L.) Moench	3.80	30.46	55.42	1.73	1.17	56.42	8.59	0.52	0.20
Kodra straw	*Paspalum scrobiculatum* L.	3.06	34.39	48.27	1.37	0.00	52.63	12.91	—	—
Ragi straw	*Eleusine coracana* Gaertn.	3.67	35.93	51.38	0.92	0.23	55.63	8.10	0.79	0.07
Rice straw	*Oryza sativa* L.	2.40	36.49	43.74	0.87	0.00	41.62	16.49	0.29	0.11
Wheat straw	*Triticum aestivum* L.	3.26	38.91	45.24	1.16	0.00	48.24	11.83	0.30	0.07
Subabool	*Leucaena latisiliqua* (Linn.) Gillis	15.40	16.80	44.39	3.36	—	—	20.05	—	—
Wooly finger	*Paspalum dilatum* Poir.	7.8	33.8	41.8	1.20	—	—	10.2	0.26	0.22

(Contd.)

C. Concentrate Feeds :

Name	Botanical name	CP	CF	NFE	EE	DCP	TDN	Total ash	CA	P
Arhar (pigeonpea)	*Cajanus cajan* (L.) Millsp.	20.50	—	70.20	1.90	14.35	74.05	7.40	—	—
Babul pod	*Acacia jacquemontii* Benth.	10.95	13.76	58.03	0.97	5.73	62.35	5.69	1.21	0.06
Bagomolasses		2.64	13.60	67.02	0.41	0.00	47.0	16.63	0.89	0.06
Barley	*Hordeum vulgare* L.	10.1	6.80	77.40	2.91	7.27	74.60	2.79	—	—
Bizada-cake (water-melon seed-cake)		23.55	39.03	27.55	4.83	20.4	52.7	5.05	0.19	0.43
Blackgram	*Vigna mungo* (L.) Hepper	25.89	5.33	63.76	0.74	13.47	63.35	4.29	0.14	0.33
Cane-molasses		0.9	—	93.1	—	—	60.0	6.0	0.74	0.08
Clusterbean	*Cyamopsis tetragonoloba* (L.) Taub.	39.30	—	49.30	4.70	32.14	78.82	6.70	—	—
Clusterbean-meal		42.5	8.5	53.0	5.5	42.52	83.49	5.0	1.0	0.76
Coconut-cake		23.44	12.91	42.28	13.00	21.10	90.10	8.37	0.40	0.74
Cottonseed		18.02	26.74	30.98	20.66	12,49	88.77	4.66	0.24	0.65
Cottonseed-cake (undecorticated)		22.84	24.11	37.40	9.15	19.38	79.56	6.50	—	—
Fish-meal		71.40	1.85	4.67	1.56	59.98	64.1	20.52	—	—
Gram	*Cicer arietinum* L.	18.06	9.83	63.66	4.93	11.96	81.33	3.50	0.26	0.41
Gram husk		5.75	48.40	38.95	0.91	0.00	61.33	5.99	—	—
Greengram *chuni*	*Vigna radiata* (L.) Wilczek.	18.8	16.0	54.70	2.50	10.0	56.2	8.0	—	—
Groundnut-cake (decorticated)		51.75	7.39	26.94	8.22	46.58	78.92	5.70	0.20	0.56
Guga-cake	*Guizotia abyssinica* Cass.	32.74	17.64	31.45	4.42	32.74	49.4	3.75	0.56	1.13
Horsegram	*Dolichos biflorus* Linn.	25.0	6.0	63.0	1.00	18.0	70.0	5.00	—	—
Jaman seed	*Syzygium cumini* (L.) Skeels	8.50	16.90	51.70	1.18	5.82	45.53	21.72	0.29	0.08
Kendu	*Diospyros tomentosa* Roxb.	7.12	25.28	56.01	2.20	0.00	34.09	9.39	1.79	0.16
Kidney bean *chuni*	*Phaseolus vulgaris* L.	20.5	10.9	57.8	7.8	16.3	66.9	7.10	0.52	0.34
Lentil	*Lens culinaris* Medic.	24.80	—	69.80	0.80	19.56	80.34	4.60	—	—
Linseed	*Linum usitatissimum* L.	19.22	6.78	32.64	36.11	15.57	117.55	7.77	0.26	0.62
Linseed-cake		30.51	9.48	43.24	6.57	25.93	70.70	10.20	0.37	0.96
Maize	*Zea mays* L.	10.60	2.20	82.10	3.30	5.86	76.00	1.85	—	—
Maize-cake		23.67	9.88	48.03	14.97	19.88	81.39	3.45	0.23	0.52
Maize germ-oilcake		23.6	8.04	51.84	15.70	19.82	85.14	0.82	—	—
Maize-gluten		24.92	1.76	65.13	3.36	23.92	68.51	4.83	—	—
Maize grit		25.62	6.59	50.28	1.86	20.63	66.96	15.75	—	—
Maize husk		8.12	15.67	72.50	1.52	4.54	75.30	2.19	0.31	0.09
Mahua-cake	*Madhuca indica* J. F. Gmel.	19.38	—	62.2	12.0	7.95	60.03	6.40	0.20	0.53
Mahua flower		5.97	8.73	78.82	0.33	2.1	68.6	6.25	—	—
Mango seed kernel	*Mangifera indica* L.	8.50	2.81	74.49	8.85	6.1	70.0	5.35	0.13	0.13
Mesta-cake	*Hibiscus cannabinus* L.	24.93	22.63	38.31	4.25	18.13	45.67	9.88	0.60	0.69
Moth	*Vigna aconitifolia* (Jacq.) Marechal.	26.60	—	65.20	1.60	20.62	80.20	6.60	—	—
Moth chuni		20.5	10.9	53.80	7.80	16.1	69.7	7.0	—	—
Nigerseed oil-cake	*Guizotia abyssinica* Cass.	36.57	12.47	26.77	3.30	18.93	58.67	20.89	—	—
Nahor seed	*Mesua ferrea* L.	18.57	14.4	58.53	12.57	—	—	0.74	0.43	0.21
Panevar seed	*Cassia tora* L.	21.12	—	64.5	7.73	16.64	59.4	5.56	0.87	0.72

(Contd.)

Name	Botanical name	CP	CF	NFE	EE	DCP	TDN	Total ash	CA	P
Pineapple bran		4.31	16.48	72.58	1.99	1.0	47.0	4.64	0.44	0.19
Oat	*Avena sativa* L.	10.07	12.71	65.88	6.55	7.86	78.48	4.79	0.1	0.141
Ragi-grain	*Eleusine coracana* Gaertn.	6.9	0.87	80.83	4.42	3.87	75.30	6.99	0.40	0.14
Raintree pods	*Samanea saman* Merr.	15.91	11.8	67.02	1.51	8.9	63.5	3.75	0.31	0.15
Rape-cake	*Brassica campestris* L.	36.37	7.70	33.19	13.41	30.92	86.77	9.33	—	—
Rawan	*Vigna unguiculata* (L.) Walp.	26.40	—	64.30	0.90	20.28	68.24	7.90	—	—
Rice bran	*Oryza sativa* L.	12.20	14.59	39.85	12.98	6.76	64.40	22.08	—	—
Sain	*Terminalia alata* Heyne ex Roth.	8.91	21.82	54.10	4.88	0.00	34.94	10.29	3.19	0.26
Sainjna	*Moringa oleifera* Lam.	15.62	17.89	48.71	4.35	11.09	61.49	13.43	3.20	0.29
Sal	*Shorea robusta* Gaertn. f.	10.06	27.43	55.41	3.22	1.14	42.60	3.88	0.71	0.12
Sandan	*Ougeinia oojeinensis* (Roxb.) Hochr.	11.61	26.50	47.57	4.32	3.72	45.57	10.00	2.39	0.30
Sarson seed	*Brassica campestris* L.	21.58	6.25	22.50	43.65	20.58	111.80	6.02	0.49	0.71
Salseed-meal	*Shorea robusta* Gaertn. f.	9.22	0.95	83.35	2.35	—	41.0	3.63	0.12	0.9
Sheesham	*Dalbergia sissoo* Roxb.	10.20	24.37	46.19	4.03	9.07	52.44	9.21	2.25	0.22
Silk cotton seed-meal		11.7	8.60	8.0	63.72	9.7	55.7	7.95	0.53	0.10
Siris	*Albizia lebbek* Benth.	16.81	31.52	36.16	3.97	11.59	49.30	11.54	2.56	0.15
Soybean seed	*Glycine max* Merr.	41.60	6.00	28.80	17.40	37.44	87.80	6.20	0.41	0.77
Spent lemon grass		6.60	34.33	51.39	1.43	0.64	49.76	6.25	0.29	0.07
Spent tapioca pulp	*Manihot esculenta* Crantz.	2.11	0.21	81.60	12.5	—	71.12	3.58	0.35	0.03
Sugarbeet pulp		12.01	25.98	48.01	0.91	3.46	59.11	13.09	3.60	0.19
Sunnhemp seed	*Crotalaria juncea* L.	35.0	10.0	46.00	3.7	30.8	71.37	5.30	0.26	0.71
Tamarind seed	*Tamarindus indica* L.	15.40	—	77.43	3.89	5.34	60.14	3.28	0.31	0.23
Tapioca	*Manihot esculenta* Crantz.	2.92	10.90	76.27	0.44	1.46	83.28	9.47	0.58	0.12
Til-cake	*Sesamum indicum* L.	46.30	4.92	27.85	9.91	42.60	86.92	11.02	—	—
Tobacco seedcake		29.95	22.33	24.66	10.37	26.33	69.37	12.69	—	—
Tomato waste		22.0	20.1	20.6	30.5	14.3	41.0	6.8	0.40	0.47
Toria-cake	*Brassica campestris* L. var. *toria* Duth	33.79	11.20	34.08	12.49	28.51	79.01	7.54	—	—
Wheat	*Triticum aestivum* L.	10.50	1.89	83.86	1.85	6.30	92.27	1.90	0.14	0.34
Wheat bran		15.41	10.76	64.79	3.45	11.80	74.93	5.59	0.18	0.82

poorer quality than the better animal proteins such as those of fish meal, meat meal, milk and eggs. Proteins of oilseed cakes have a low glutamic acid, cystine and methionine and a variable but usually low lysine content. The meals usually have a high phosphorus content, which tends to aggravate their generally low calcium content. They may provide good amount of B-vitamins but are poor sources of carotene and vitamin A.

The high temperatures and pressures of the expeller process may result in a lowering of digestibility and in denaturation of the protein, with a consequent lowering of its nutritive value. For ruminants such a denaturation may be beneficial owing to an associated reduction in degradability. The high temperatures and pressures also reduces most of the deleterious substances which might be present in oilcakes such as gossypol and goitrin. Solvent extraction does not involve pressing or any high temperature and thus the protein value of the meal remains unaffected.

Groundnut or Peanut Oil meal

1. It is the most widely used high protein feed
2. The meal is usually made from the kernels (a grain or seed) ground to a meal with occasional use of whole pod when it is known as undecorticated groundnut meal
3. Its composition and feeding value vary considerably, depending on the quality of the nuts, the method of fat extraction used and the amount of hull included
4. It has about 45% protein and 10% oil in expeller variety
5. It is deficient in lysine, methionine and cystine
6. The cake is satisfactory as a source of protein for all kinds of livestock and poultry
7. Liable to contain a toxic factor—*Aflatoxin* a metabolite of the fungus *Aspergillus flavus* particularly in warm rainy season
8. The cake tends to become rancid specially in warm moist climate. It should not be stored longer than 6 weeks in the summer or 3-4 months in winter

Linseed meal

1. The meal is produced from flax seeds and the oil being a drying one used in paints, linoleum and soft soap
2. The cake is satisfactory for all classes of livestock except for poultry where if fed in more than 5%, it has a depressing effect on the growth. The toxicity can largely be eliminated by soaking the meal in water for 24 hours or by adding pyridoxin, one of the B vitamins
3. The meal has a very good reputation as a feed for ruminant animals due to high content (3-10%) of mucilage. The compound is capable of absorbing large amounts of water which results higher retention time in the rumen and give a better opportunity for microbial digestion. The lubricating character of the mucilage also protects the gut wall against mechanical damage and together with the bulkiness, regulates excretion, preventing constipation without causing looseness.
4. It is a satisfactory source of protein (about 35%) for almost all livestock. D.C.P. is about 30% with low T.D.N. (about 65%).
5. Immature linseed contains a small amount of a cyanogenetic glycoside, *linamarin*, and an associated enzyme, *linase*, which is capable of hydrolyzing it with the evaluation of hydrogen cyanide (HCN). Normal processing conditions however, destroy linase and most of the linamarin and the resultant meals are quite safe.

Mustard Cake (*Sarson*)

1. Widely used in many parts of India for cattle feeding.
2. Nutritive value is much less than that of groundnut cake. D.C.P. and T.D.N values are 27% and 74% respectively. It should preferably be mixed with other, more well-liked feeds. The deoiled type can be used for poultry upto 10 percent of the ration and for pigs the amount may go as high as 20 percent.
3. The calcium and phosphorus content are much higher, being about 0.6 percent and 1.0 percent.

Cottonseed Cake

1. It is an excellent high protein feed (about 40%) for ruminants but low in cystine, methionine and lysine.

2. The cake can also be used in pig and poultry rations if the free gossypol does not exceed 0.03 percent.
3. The free gossypol content of cottonseed meal decreased during processing. Expeller variety has about 200 to 500 mg free gossypol/kg, while deoiled type has about 1000 – 5,000 mg/kg.
4. In pig ration if the percentage of cottonseed meal exceeds 9%, it will kill the growing swine due to the presence of gossypol.
5. The cakes are available in two forms, (i) Whole pressed cottonseed cakes (i.e. undecorticated and (ii) Dehulled (decorticated, without hulls) cottonseed cakes containing less of fibers and more of proteins than the whole pressed type.
6. Today, glandless cottonseed, free of gossypol, is being grown in developed countries.
7. Gossypol is found bound to free amino groups in the seed protein or in a free form which can be extracted with solvents. The free gossypol is the toxic form. Gossypol toxicity can be prevented by addition of ferrous sulphate and other iron salts.

Coconut meal (*Copra meal*)

1. This is the by-product from the production of oil from the dried meats of coconuts and is available in many areas of the world
2. The crude protein content is low (20-26%), and poor in lysine and histidine
3. The oil content of coconut meal varies from 2.5 to 6.5%, the higher oilmeals tends to get rancidity and thus will cause diarrhoea. Hence low oil content type should be preferred
4. Due to poor quality of protein and high fiber, its use should be restricted in swine and poultry rations. If it is fed to monogastric, it should be supplemented with lysine and methionine
5. The lipid component of copra meal is very low in unsaturated fatty acids, hence the feeding of copra meal produces firm body fat in swine. Also dairymen use copra meal to produce a pleasant flavoured, rather hard (highly saturated) butterfat
6. The maximum safe amount for dairy cows seems to be 1.5 to 2 kg daily
7. The cake has the valuable property of absorbing upto half its own weight of molasses, and as a result is popular in compounding.

Sesame meal (*Til cake*)

1. Sesame oil meal is produced from what remains following the production of oil from sesame seed and the meal is extensively used for all classes of livestock including poultry
2. Protein content varies from 40-50% depending upon the variety used and the type of oil extraction. The protein is rich in arginine, leucine and methionine but is low in lysine
3. There are 3 varieties of til cakes, white, black and red grown at different seasons and in different parts of our country. Nutritive value is highest in white variety and lowest in the red variety cakes
4. Til cake is richest among all oil cakes in calcium content, being 2·3 percent but because of its high content of phytic acid, it appears to bind calcium so the amount of calcium in diets containing sesame meal should be increased
5. It has been used upto 15 percent, mixed with equal amount of groundnut cake in chicks ration.

Soybean oil meal

1. Soybean oil meal consists of fat extracted soyoeans which have been ground to a meal and sometimes pelleted, has the highest nutritive value of any plant protein source, making up approximately, two thirds of the need of developed countries like U.S.A. and Canada
2. Most soybean oil meal is deoiled type
3. There are two grades : 44% and 49% protein
4. The protein contains all the indispensable amino acids, but the concentrations of cystine and methionine are sub-optimal
5. The cake is used for all kinds of livestock including poultry
6. As with most other oil seeds, soybeans have a number of toxic, stimulatory and inhibitory substances. For example, (i) a *goitrogenic material* is found in the meal and its long term use may result in goiter in some animal species, (ii) it also contains *antigens*, which are specially toxic to young pre-ruminants, (iii) a *trypsin inhibitor*, affects in digestibility of proteins specially in monogastric animals, (iv) a *haemogglutinin*, agglutinates red blood cells in rats, rabbits, and human beings but not in sheep and calves. Fortunately, these inhibitors and other factors like saponins are inactivated by proper heat treatment during processing
7. Soybeans also contain *genistein*, a plant estrogen, which may account, in some cases for part of its high growth inducing properties
8. Currently, there is interest in feeding whole soybeans after appropriate heat processing to inactivate the trypsin inhibitors (110°C for 3 minutes). This product is known in the feed trade as full fat soybean meal, it contains about 38% C.P., 18% fat and 5% C.F.

Pulse Protein

Pulses are the seeds of leguminous plants. They are used primarily for human consumption,

Table 10.4

Name	*Latin name*	*Crude Protein %*	*General comments*
Beans—includes Kidney bean, Navy bean, Mung bean, Common bean, Dry bean,	*(Phaseolus spp.)*	20—28	Many of these beans contain components which are harmful, if they are not processed properly.
Cowpeas	*(Vigna sinensis)*	18—29	Cooking or germinating seeds improves feeding value greatly.
Field pea	*(Pisum sativum)*	22—29	Highly palatable feed for all types of livestock.
Soybeans	*(Glycine max)*	39—45	Used primarily for production of vegetable oil and oilseed meal. Should be cooked before feeding to non-ruminants.

but they may be fed to livestock at a time when it is available at a reasonable price. A listing of some important pulses used as livestock feed is given below :

All of the pulses contain components which possess antinutritional properties. Fortunately processing procedures, such as cooking, germination, and fermentation, can reduce risks of feeding pulses to livestock. Chemical factors present in various leguminous seeds are given in tabular form as below :

Table 10.5

Antinutritional factor	*Mode of action*	*Comments*
Antivitamin factors	These factors render certain vitamins physiologically inactive	1. Soybeans contain a rachitogenic factor & antivitamin B_{12} factor. 2. Kidney beans contain an antagonist to Vit. E. 3. Cooking of the grains destroys these factors.
Cyanogens	Upon hydrolysis these compounds release HCN	1. All legumes contain some cyanogens.
Lathyrogens	Nervous disorders and weakness in humans.	1. Peas of the genus Lathyrus contain this. 2. Soaking & heat treatment will destroy the factor.
Phytohaemagglutins	Agglutinates RBC	1. Found in all legumes. 2. Heat treatment is effective.
Protease inhibitors	Combine with trypsin forms inactive complex. Causes hypertrophy of the pancreas.	1. Found in all legumes seeds. 2. Heat treatment : autoclaving at 15 lb/sq in for 15-20 minutes. 3. Soaking followed by steaming. 4. Germination will cause detoxification.
Goitrogens	Enlargement of thyroid in rat and chicks.	1. A number of feed ingredients including mustard oil cake, rapeseed cake, plant of the cabbage family e.g., cabbage, kale, turnips, cauliflower contain this factor. 2. Administration of iodides and heat treatment in some cases will help detoxification.

Brewer's Grains and Yeast. In brewing, barely is first soaked and allowed to germinate. During this process, which is allowed for 6 days, there is development of a complete enzyme system for hydrolysing starch to dextrins and maltose. After this the grain or malt is dried, care being taken not to inactivate the enzymes. The sprouts are removed and are sold as *malt culms* or coombs. The dried malt is then passed through a process known as "mashing". The object of mashing is to promote enzymatic action on proteins and starch, the latter being converted to dextrins, maltose and small amount of other sugars. Water is sprayed onto this mixture and the temperature of the mash increased to about 65°C. After the mashing process is complete the sugary liquid or "wort" is drained off, leaving *brewer's grains* as residue and are sold wet or dried as food for farm animals. Dried grains contain 18 per cent crude protein and 15 per cent crude fiber.

The wort is then fermented in an open vassel with yeast for a number of days, during which time most of the sugars are converted to alcohol and CO_2. The yeast is filtered off, dried and sold as *brewer's yeast.* Dried yeast is rich protein concentrate containing about 42 per-cent crude protein. It is highly digestible and may be used for all classes of farm animals. It is a valuable source of B group of vitamins, is relatively rich in phosphorus but has a low calcium content.

B. ANIMAL PROTEINS

Protein supplements derived from animal tissues are obtained primarily from inedible tissues, such as meat packing, from surplus milk by-products or from marine sources.

Many such compounds are difficult to process and store without some spoilage and nutrient loss. If not properly dried or heated to destroy disease producing bacteria they may be a source of infection. On the other hand, protein availability will be reduced and some nutrients are lost if the feed is heated excessively.

These materials are given to animals in much smaller amounts than the oilseed derivatives so far discussed, since they are not used primarily as sources of protein but to make good deficiencies of certain indispensable amino acids from which non-ruminant animals may suffer when they are fed on all vegetable protein diets. Due to high cost, large scale use of animal proteins become uneconomic.

Meat meal or Meal scrap.

1. It is obtained from mammal tissue exclusive of hair, hoof, horn, stomach contents and hide trimmings by proper drying and grinding to which no other matter has been added, but which may have been preliminarily treated for the removal of fat and dried blood.
2. The product is normally used for swine and poultry.
3. Rich in crude protein (50-55%) and ash (21%) with high calcium about 8% and 4% phosphorus—but low in methionine and tryptophan.
4. Good sources of vitamins of B complex, specially riboflavin, choline, nicotinamide and B_{12}.

Meat and Bone meal or scrap

1. The product is similar to meat scrap except it contains more bone, and consequently is higher in calcium and phosphorus and lower in protein, about 40%.
2. Used primarily in rations of swine and poultry.

Blood meal

1. The meal is prepared by passing live steam through the blood until the temperature reaches 100°C. The treatment causes sterilization and the blood gets clotted. It is then drained, pressed to express occluded serum, dried by steam heating and ground.
2. It has got high protein value, 80%, but the protein is lower in digestibility and quality

than most other animal protein feeds. Poor in calcium and phosphorus content.

3. The meal is unpalatable and its use has resulted in reduced growth rates in poultry and it is not recommended for young stock. For older birds rates of inclusion are limited to about 1 to 2 percent.

Feathermeal

1. Poultry feathers are not digested by single stomach animals. However, when feathers are either processed under low pressure (130°C) for 2½ hours or under high pressure (145°C) for 30 minutes and dried at about 60°C and ground to pass a 20 mesh screen, the product is highly digestible.
2. The product is extremely high in protein, usually containing well over 80%.
3. Concentrates of dairy cattle may contain as high as 10%.
4. The product is used primarily in rations for swine and poultry.
5. Since feathermeal is deficient in several essential amino acids, it is customary to use the product upto 5% or less in the ration of poultry.

Hatchery by-product meal

1. Hatchery refuse consisting of infertile eggs, dead embryos, shells of hatched eggs and unsaleable chickens, can be made into a useful feed by cooking, drying and grinding.
2. Its high level of calcium (15-25%) limits its inclusion in ordinary diets but upto 5% level it can go with broiler type rations. It has got variable percentages of protein (45-55%) and fat (10-13%) depending upon the type of materials used.
3. It is used primarily in rations of swine and poultry.

Fish meal

1. Fish meal consists of fish or fish by-products which have been dried and ground into a meal.
2. There are several types depending on the type of fish and method of preparations.
3. Small scale production is made under rural condition in the following way : the fish or fish waste is ground or chopped, boiled for a short time and squeezed in cloth to get rid of water and excess oil. The residue is then dried in the sun.

   Another simple way is to dry fish materials directly under the sun on sea shore with an admixture of salt after removing alimentary tracts. The product is known as *'White fish meal'* and is made from fish which contains minimum fat.
4. The protein content of fish meal is usually around 60% with a digestibility of betwen 93 and 95 percent. Fish meal protein has a high content of lysine, methionine, and tryptophan. It has about 20 percent mineral content which is high in calcium (8%) and phosphorus (3.5%).
5. They are a good source of vitamins of the B complex, particularly choline, B_{12} and riboflavin, and have an enhanced nutritional value because of their content of growth factors collectively known as *Animal Protein Factor* (APF).
6. For pigs and poultry fish meal has become a standard ingredient and is added to about 10% of the ration to make up for deficiencies of essential amino acids. Response from fish meal is greater than other protein sources in ruminants have been achieved but high cost makes it uneconomical.

7. Care must be taken to check the presence of urea, which is added as adulterant by uncrupulous businessmen with inferior type of fish meal to raise the nitrogen content.
8. Fish meals containing high levels of fat are considered to be of low quality. If they are incorporated into poultry feeds, they tend to impart a fishy flavour to poultry products. Also, problems of rancidity are greater in high-fat fish meals.

C. NON-PROTEIN NITROGEN (NPN) FEEDSTUFFS

Feedstuffs which contain nitrogen in a form other than proteins or peptides are termed non-protein nitrogen (NPN). Organic NPN compounds would include ammonia, amides, amines, amino acids. Inorganic NPN compounds would include a variety of ammonium salts and ammoniated by-products. Of these urea dominates for feeding of animals with a functioning rumen as a substitute of protein feeds. Since microorganisms in the rumen of ruminant animals degrade dietary protein to synthesize microbial protein, similarly they degrade urea into ammonia which microbes utilise as the nitrogenous portion of the amino acids. For complete synthesis of amino acids, which will be utilized as polymer of proteins microbes needs carbon skeleton of amino acids. This will come from readily available carbohydrates. Thus for utilisation of urea or any other NPN compounds simultaneous ingestion of soluble carbohydrate is a must.

Crude protein is determined by multiplying the nitrogen content of a feed stuff by 6.25. Thus, urea having average of 45% nitrogen would have a crude protein equivalent of 281 percent.

Some of the non-protein nitrogenous sources being used successfully for ruminants are given below :

Table 10.6

Some NPN sources for Ruminants

	Formula	N_2 (%)	Protein equivalent (%)
Ammonium acetate	$CH_3\ CO_2\ NH_4$	18	112
Ammonium bicarbonate	$NH_4\ H\ CO_3$	18	112
Ammonium carbamate	$NH_2\ CO_2\ NH_4$	36	225
Ammonium lactate	$CH_3\ CHOH\ CO_2\ NH_4$	13	81
Biuret	$NH_2\ CONHCO\ NH_2\ H_2O$	35	219
Urea	$(NH_2)_2\ CO$	42-45	262-281
Oilseed meals*		5.8-8.0	36-50

* Includes cottonseed, soybean, linseed, coconut and similar oil cakes.

FACTORS AFFECTING UREA UTILISATION

The efficiency of urea utilisation is dependent on the composition of the ration and practical feed management.

A. Composition of Ration

1. Urea can effectively be used in high T. D. N. concentrates (greater than 75% T. D. N. on dry basis) when the crude protein level is below 12-13%. With low energy feeds (less than 60% feed on dry basis) urea may be fed when crude protein level is below 7%. Energy source must be provided by the feed so that carbon skeletons can be available for amination. Soluble carbohydrates are, by far, the most important precursors for these skeletons.
2. Minerals of the feed affect the utilisation of urea since many of them are constituents of key co-factors involved in the production of microbial protein. Additional sulphur in the form of sulphate must be provided as a precursor for the sulphur containing amino acids.
3. Feed additives have generally been shown to have little effect on urea utilisation.
4. Low levels of antibiotics generally added to feed are not sufficient to reduce urea utilisation significantly.

B. Managerial Factors

1. Animals started on a feed containing urea should be given an initial period of adaptation for the following purposes :
   (*i*) The microbial population of the rumen is altered slowly, thus reducing the stress on the animal.
   (*ii*) The rate of urea hydrolysis is reduced.
   (*iii*) Microorganisms develop a greater ability to synthesise protein.
   (*iv*) Animals have an opportunity to adjust to the taste of the feed.
2. Mixing of urea is an important factor in its ultimate conversion to protein. If it is improperly mixed, a serious threat of urea toxicity arises.
3. Frequency of feeding can affect the efficiency of urea utilisation. Urea should never be used in a feeding programme where feed containing urea is fed infrequently or fed two or three times weekly.

METHODS OF FEEDING UREA

Urea can be provided by different methods and systems, with consideration given to the following factors : (*i*) protein needs of the animal as dictated by the type of production ; (*ii*) availability and cost of urea ; (*iii*) availability of energy sources and amount of plant protein being used (*iv*) cost of processing and mixing.

1. Urea Mixed in Concentrates

Most of the urea fed to growing and lactating dairy cattle is incorporated into the concentrate portion of the ration. Generally speaking, urea is not employed in amounts higher than 3% of the total concentrate feed or 1% of the total dry matter in the ration, which comes to be 1/3 of the total nitrogen in the ration. In most of the compounded feed industry the percentages of urea as incorporated in concentrate feeds of cattle and buffaloes are always on the lower side (1.5 to 2.0). This is because of the inclusion of very many poor quality agro-industrial by-products having poor TDN values.

The maximum safe limit is 136 gm of urea per animal over 360 kg body weight, 91 gm for animals between 225–360 kg, 45 gm. for those between 135–225 kg Smaller animals should not be fed urea.

Young calves below 6 months also not be fed urea in any form.

Urea should never be mixed with raw soybean as it contains *urease* and thus it will liberate ammonia and carbon dioxide which will be lost before consumption.

While mixing urea to concentrates, utmost care should be taken for uniform distribution otherwise chances of toxicity may be observed in those cases where excessive amounts of urea are consumed.

2. Liquid Supplements

This is a homogenous mixture of urea in the liquid molasses along with minerals and vitamins. Normally, it is prepared by completely dissolving 2.5 parts of urea in equal amount of water. The mixture is fortified with vitablend AD_3 at the rate of 25 grams per 100 kg of liquid feed. Common salt @ 1 part and mineral mixure @ 2 parts are sprinkled over 92 parts of sugarcane molasses. (2.5 parts urea + 2.5 parts water + 1 part salt + 2 parts mineral mixture + 92 parts molasses = 100). Special attention is required for the uniform mixing of urea solution in the liquid molasses. Undiluted urea-molasses liquid feed containing 65% or more dry matter can be safely stored for a long period. Animals started on a feed containing liquid molasses supplement should be given an initial period of 15 days as adaptation.

For initial 3 days feed your animals by substituting ¼th of the grain mixture with that of 500 ml of liquid feed after feeding concentrate part of the ration.

In the next 3 days substitute half of grain mixture with that of 1 kg. liquid feed.

From 7th day entire concentrate mixture may be substituted by offering liquid feed *ad libitum*. Animals should first be fed about 1 kg dry matter in the form of forage.

It is important to provide fresh drinking water at all times.

3. Urea Mixed with Silage

Another way of feeding urea to cattle—especially dairy cattle—is through the addition of urea to crops which are being ensiled. If chopped, whole maize plant is being ensiled at 35% to 40% dry matter, urea is then added at a level of 0.5% of wet material. This level should increase the crude protein level of the silage on a dry matter basis about 5 points.

4. Urea Added to Dry Roughages

To-day the availability of wheat and paddy straw in India is around 50 and 100 million tonnes per year respectively. Knowing fully well about the extremely poor nutritive value (DCP% = 0, TDN% = 38 to 40), the farmers have no other alternative but to use these straws as sole dry roughage.

A newer method of adding urea has not only enhanced the palatibility and the nutritive value of straw but also partially solved the crisis of quality dry roughages in the country. The following formula has been suggested by the National Dairy Research Institute at Karnal in India for enrichment of straw quality by adding urea.

Ingredient			Quality
Straw	...	...	100 kg of 90% DM
Urea	...	...	4 kg
Clean water	...	...	50 litres

According to this ratio, it is better to prepare 10, 25 or 50 quintals stack at a time.

The method

For a stack of 25 quintals, at first about one quintal of straw is spread over a circle of about 2 metres radius. Base can also be a rectangular shape. While treating paddy straw, small bundles should be used (as it makes a good stack that loose paddy straw). To this amount of straw sprinkle 4 kg of urea solution already dissolved in 50 litres of clean water either by hand or by gardener's sprinkler. The straw layer is then pressed thoroughly by trampling with feet, in order to make the stack more compact and to drive out unwanted air from the stack.

Another straw layer of one quintal is then spread over the previous layer, sprinkled with urea solution of 4 kg in 50 litres of water and pressed thoroughly. The procedure is repeated till the desired quintals of straw are treated with urea. At last the stack should preferably be covered by polythene sheet or by banana leaf or by untreated straw. Dome shape of straw is preferred. The idea of covering the stack is to restrict the minimum leakage of ammonia gas from the stack and to prevent the entry of outside air into the stack.

Precautions Against Fungal Spoilage

1. Dirty water should not be used for dissolving urea.
2. Urea solution should be sprinkled, uniformly over the straw layer.
3. Stack should be made thoroughly compact by trampling.
4. The stack should be properly covered from all sides.

A period of 3 weeks is needed for the physiochemical reaction to complete inside the stack. During this period the urea is first hydrolysed to ammonia which then penetrates into the straw fibres break the lignocellulosic bonds. Once the bonds are broken, it will be easier to hydrolyse the cellulose and hemicellulose by the rumen microbial enzymes. After removing the quantity of urea treated straw to be fed to animals, the opening is again closed properly with the untreated paddy straw. The treated straw is exposed for an hour to remove the smell of ammonia gas before being offered to animals. Comparative nutritive values are given below:

		DCP(%)	TDN(%)
Untreated straw	...	Zero	38–40
Urea treated straw	...	4–5	48–50

The treated straw can be chaffed, mixed with a little of green fodder and then fed to the animals. The experiments have shown increased palatability of treated straw as compared to untreated straw.

Quantity of Treated Straw to be Fed

1. *For dry animals*: 5 to 6 kg of treated straw can meet all the requirements for energy and protein.
2. *For milk yielding animal*: 4 to 5 kg of treated straw can either reduce concentrate by $\frac{1}{2}$ to 1 kg or increase milk yield by 1–$1\frac{1}{2}$ kg.

5. Urea in Salt Blocks

Another simple way of supplying protein precursors to livestock on pasture is through the use of urea in salt licks or blocks. Numerous combinations of salt and urea are in use.

One such preparation developed by the National Dairy Development Board, Anand in India is one of the latest innovations. The block known as "Urea molasses block" contains molasses, urea, minerals like calcium, phosphorous, iron, cobalt, manganese, copper, salt with small amounts of oil cakes. It has been claimed that animal's body derives 40–50% more nutrients from kadvi, straw and other crop residue, and also increases the consumption of such crop residues. The solidified blocks are placed in front of the animals in a special dispensor so that they can lick as and when necessary for them to obtain any or all of the nutrients embedded inside the block.

GUIDELINES FOR USING UREA IN FEEDS

Urea and its use as Cattle feed

While various products have been and are being studied as non-protein nitrogen of sources, the principal NPN source in use today in livestock (ruminant) feeding is urea. It is produced by combining natural gas with water and air. It has a chemical formula of $CO(NH_2)_2$. Consequently urea in pure form contains 46.67% nitrogen. Commercial urea contains an inert conditioner to keep it flowing freely, which reduces its nitrogen content between 42–45% equivalent to 262–281 protein per cent. Urea is hydrolysed by the urease activity of the rumen microorganisms resulting production of ammonia and carbon dioxide.

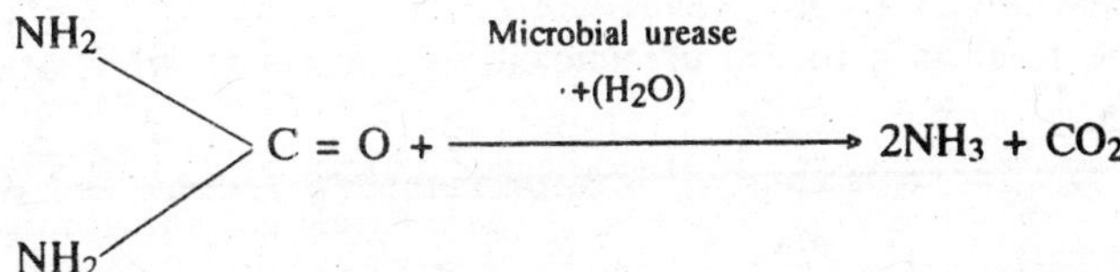

As ammonia is liberated in the rumen, it apparently reacts with organic acids of fermentation to form ammonium salts of organic acids such as ammonium acetate and ammonium propionate. These in turn are metabolized by rumen microbes to form their body protein. The ease and speed with which this reaction occurs when urea enters the rumen, may give rise to two problems owing to excessive absorption of ammonia from the rumen. Thus wastage of nitrogen may occur, and there may be a danger of ammonia toxicity. This is diagnosed by muscular twitching, ataxia, excessive salivation, tetany, bloat and respiration defects.

It is to be noted that for proper utilisation of urea for the purpose of microbial body proliferation, a readily available source of energy is a must. Starch is the most satisfactory, being fermented at a moderate rate. Molasses is somewhat less valuable as it is fermented too rapidly, while cellulose is least valuable as it is fermented too slowly. A level of 1 kg of starch per 100 gm of urea is often suggested as a guideline.

How to compute how much urea is in a feed?

The level of urea in a feed may be determined in the following ways:

a. Per cent of urea in the feed

When the per cent of urea is given, one can calculate the amount of protein furnished by urea by multiplying the per cent urea by 281% (the protein equivalent of urea). For example, if a 40% supplement contains 5% urea, then 14% protein is furnished by urea (281 % × 5% = 14%). To determine the per cent of the total protein furnished by urea, divide the per cent of protein as urea by the per cent of protein in the supplement (14% ÷ 40% = 35%). In this case, slightly more than one-third of the protein in the supplement is furnished by urea.

b. Per cent protein as urea

When the urea in the supplement is expressed in per cent protein as urea, one can determine the amount of urea by dividing this value by 281%. For example, if a 35% protein supplement has 12% protein as urea, it contains 4.3% urea (12 ÷ 281 = 4.3%). Slightly more than one-third of the protein in the supplement is furnished by urea (12% ÷ 35% = 34.3%).

A. Urea is best utilised in well-balanced, high energy rations.

Urea is not well utilised in supplements to low quality roughages. The explanation is that the carbohydrates in grasses and hays appear to be so slowly available that the bacteria have difficulty in using the energy from roughages to make use of urea in preparing bacterial protein.

Other components of balanced feed include essential minerals and vitamins.

B. Factors essential for optimum use of urea

1. **Mix the urea thoroughly.**
2. **Feed urea only to mature cattle, buffaloes, sheep and goat. Never feed it to monogastrics.**
3. **Provide a readily available energy source, such as molassess or grain.**
4. **Supply adequate and balanced levels of minerals.**
5. **Achieve a nitrogen-sulphur ratio not wider than 15 : 1.**
6. **Incorporate lucerne meal as a source of unidentified factors to stimulate the microbial synthesis of protein.**
7. **Include adequate salt for palatability; 0.5% in complete rations and 3.5% in protein supplements.**
8. **Provide the proper level of vitamins particularly of vitamin A.**
9. **Accustom animals gradually to urea containing feeds (over a period of 5-7 days), feed at equal intervals.**
10. **Limit the intake of urea to recommended maximum level as below**

Sheep **: 1% of the dry matter in the ration (or one-third of the total nitrogen in the ration or 3% of the concentrate portion of the ration).**

Beef Cattle **: Urea may constitute upto one-third of the total protein of the ration. Total protein refers to the protein intake of the entire ration—including forage, grain and protein supplements.**

Dairy Cattle **: Lactating cows producing less than 20 litres of milk per day urea could constitute upto 2 percent of the concentrate mixture or upto 1 percent of the total hay. It was further recommended that no more than one-third of the protein requirements be met through the use of urea. For lactating cows yielding more than 20 litres of milk urea should not be fed. At this level of production, the microbes are unable to synthesise enough protein to meet the needs, thereby placing a premium on dietary protein which escapes ruminal fermentation (undegraded protein).**

Bulls, heifers and low-producing cows **:**

1.5 to 2.0% of the concentrate mixture may be used as urea.

N.B.—Young calves and monogastric amimals should never be given urea.

C. Toxicity

When urea is fed at excessive levels, large amounts of ammonia are liberated in the rumen.

Eventually, the pH of the ruminal fluid increases, thus facilitating the passage of ammonia across the rumen wall. If the levels of ammonia abosrbed are greater than the capacity of the liver to convert ammonia to urea, ammonia accumulates in the blood which when exceeds 1 mg/100 ml in cattle, the animal is under toxic condition. Such a condition may arise due to followings :

a. Poor mixing of urea in feed
b. Error in ration formulation
c. Inadequate period of adaptation
d. Low intake of water
e. Feeding of urea in conjunction with poor quality roughages
f. Rations that promote a high pH in ruminal fluid.

Symptoms of ammonia toxicity may include tetany, respiratory difficulty, bloat, excessive salivation, ataxia, convulsions and bellowing. If not promptly treated, death will follow in 30 minutes to 2.5 hours. The common treatment consists of drenching 20-40 litres of cold water which inihibits ureolytic activity of the rumen. Another way of curing is by drenching 4 litres of dilute acetic acids like vinegar along with cold water.

Biuret

The compound is produced by heating urea. The formula of the colourless crystalline compound is $NH_2CO.NH.CO.NH_2$. It contains 30 percent nitrogen, equivalent to 188 per cent of crude protein. A considerable period of adaptation is necessary for ruminants before the compound is effectively utilised. The compound is expensive and at present not produced in this country and moreover it is utilised by the ruminant less efficiently than urea. The advantage is that biuret is not toxic even at higher level.

Poultry litters

The composition varies, but on an average it contains about 5 percent nitrogen equivalent to about 31 per cent crude protein. The nitrogen is in the form of ureates. In concentrate diets, levels of inclusion may be as high as 35 per cent. The inclusion of poultry manure necessitates an allowance for extra energy and proper calcium and phosphorus inclusion.

SINGLE-CELL PROTEIN (SCP)

Single-cell protein (SCP) is obtained from single-cell organisms, such as yeast, bacteria and algae, that have been grown on specially prepared growth media. Production of this type of protein can be attained through the fermentation of petrolium derivatives or organic waste or through the culturing of photosynthetic organisms (algae) in special illuminated ponds. Microbes grow very fast. While 1,000 kg of livestock can produce a maximum of 1 kg protein in 24 hours, 1000 kg of yeast in the same period of time may increase to 5,000 kg of which half is edible protein

		Time required to double the biomass
Yeast and bacteria	...	20 min —2 hours
Algae	...	1 hour—2 days
Grass	...	1 to 2 weeks
Broilers	...	2 to 4 weeks

Growing pigs	...	4 to 6 weeks
Growing cattle	...	1 to 2 months

1. *Bacteria*

Among various types of bacteria, *Methanomonas methanica* Sohngen has been more thoroughly investigated for single cell protein production. The bacteria are cultivated as a submerged culture in a water solution of mineral salts and as a source of nitrogen (ammonia or urea). Air and methane is bubbled through the liquid and stirred. A batch of culture is harvested after 3 days and yields about 12 grams wet bacteria per litre, the protein of which contains 70-80% balanced amino acids.

2. *Algae*

Three species of unicellular algae viz., *Chlorella vulgaris, Spirulina maxima* and *Scenedesmus obliquus* are of interest in the production of single cell protein. For growth algae requires CO_2, sunlight, nitrogen and minerals.

Algae meal, which is non-toxic is not fed to ruminants due to high cost but fed to pigs up to 10%. The protein value is comparable with that of meat and bone meal.

3. *Yeast and Mould*

While brewer's and distiller's yeast are usually *Saccharomyces cerevisiae,* yeast propagated specifically for animal feed is usually *Torulopsis utilis* (Torula yeast or fodder yeast) which grows very fast and can be grown on a variety of materials including press liquor obtained from paper industry and fruit wastes. Dried yeast is a valuable product and lacks the bitter taste of brewer's yeast.

Another type of yeast, *Candida lipolytica* are grown on paraffin fraction of petroleum oil. Yeasts grown on crude oil or paraffin extracted from oil are now commercially produced at several plants close to refineries. The fermentation takes place in an oil-water emulsion supplied with ammonia and mineral salts in presence of generous supply of oxygen.

IDENTIFYING FEEDS FROM THEIR COMPOSITION

Students of feeds and feeding very often talk about the proximate composition and nutritive value of innumerable feed stuffs. This might seem initially to be due to extra-ordinary callibre. But actually they relate individual feeds to a certain general feed group on the basis of distinguishing chemical composition characters.

It should be realised that in many instances there is considerable overlapping of different feed groups with respect to their content of the various nutritive fractions. Even so, information such as is presented in Table 89 will surely guide a student to identify feeds from their composition.

The first criterion of putting the feeds in two categories on is the basis of their respective moisture content, (1) Air-dry and (2) High moisture feed.

I. If a feed contains over 80% dry matter (DM), it should be regarded as an air-dry feed,

Mineral products	Energy rich concentrates
Hays	Protein rich concentrates
Straws	(both plant and animal
Other dry roughages	origin)

II. On the otherhand, if a feed contains less than 80% DM, it should be regarded as a high moisture feed e.g.,

High moisture grains	Fresh forages
Molasseses	Wet by-products
Haylages	Root crops
Silages	Fresh whole or skimmed milk.

I. Air-dry roughages vs. Air-dry concentrates

1. An air-dry non-mineral feed may be grouped either as roughages or as concentrates based on the crude fiber and/or TDN content. Generally all air-dry roughages will contain over 18% CF and less than 60% TDN. On the other hand air-dry concentrates will usually contain less than 18% CF and over 60% TDN.

2. Air-dry roughages may further be divided on the basis of their composition as (i) Legume hays, (ii) Non-legume hays and (iii) Low-quality air-dry forages.

The hays are characterised by having CF from 18-34%, TDN from 40-60% and a significant amount of carotene whereas the low-quality dry roughages are higher in fiber and lower in TDN with little or no carotene and a protein value under 6.0% except for groundnut hulls which is about 6.6%.

The legume hays contain over 10.5% CP and over 0.9% calcium while non-legume hay have values for CP and calcium less than the former.

Energy rich concentrates vs. Protein rich concentrates

Air-dry concentrates having more than 18% CP are classed as protein rich concentrates and those with less than 18% CP as energy feeds.

The protein rich concentrates may be either of animal or plant origin. When the amount of protein content, is above 47% then it is of animal origin and if it is less than 47% then it is of plant origin. The latter may be either deoiled meals which will run under 1.0% EE or expeller type where the ether extract will usually be more than 4.0%

II. High Moisture Feeds

A. High moisture grains

Among high moisture feeds, if the composition of a feed shows that it contains DM between 60-80%, the feed in that case may be either high moisture grain or molasses. Protein and crude fiber values in this case will help to identify the feed. High moisture grains will have more than 7% CP and some fibers but molasses has got less than (3% cane 6% beet) 7% CP and no CF.

In recent years in developed countries like U.S.A., Canada a considerable quantity of some grains mostly maize (corn) and Jowar (sorghum) are harvested when the moisture content varies between 22-40% and it is commonly referred to high moisture grains—not that it is extremely high in moisture content, but that it is simply somewhat higher than that normally harvested for air-dry preservation.

High moisture grains have been found to be equal to and in some instances superior to air-dry grains as a feed for most classes of livestock on a dry matter basis. The improvement in efficiency is believed to be due to the fact that in early harvested grain, the starch and protein components are not in the crystalline states as with dry grains. Another factor is that early harvested grain would require considerably less wetting in the rumen for microbial digestion. Other advantages of the use of high moisture grain are as below :

1. Harvesting of such grains can begun 2-3 weeks earlier than usual harvesting time thus decreases the risk of potential losses caused by poor weather and bird eating.
2. Harvesting losses are 5-10% less than regular practice.
3. Handling costs for high moisture grains are reduced because they are ready for feeding when they come from special silo meant for preservation of grains. For best results, the silo should be as nearly airtight as it can be made. The acid preservation of high moisture grain involves the addition of 1-1.5% propionic acid (or a mixture of propionic acid with either acetic or formic acid) to high moisture cereal grain to inhibit mould or spoilage, thereby alleviating artificial drying or the necessity to store in an airtight silo.

B. Haylages

Haylage, sometimes called low-moisture silage, is a form of preserved forage with characteristics between those of hay and silage. It is made from grass and/or legume to a moisture level of about 45-55% when harvested or wilted to this level if the harvested forage is having higher moisture percent before ensiling. It must be preserved by processes somewhat different from those for wilted or unwilted silage. The silos should be well constructed and as airtight as possible so that the oxygen present is soon used up, the CO_2 that is produced is trapped and held within the silo. These conditions prevent the forage from spoiling by moulding, oxidising, heating etc. *Air exclusion is the key to the success or failure of making low moisture silage.*

Advantages

1. Properly made haylage has a pleasant aroma and is a palatable high quality feed. Animals usually receive more DM and net feed value than silage made from the same cut.

2. If forage is mowed with the intention of making hay and the weather becomes unfavourable for drying, the partially dried forage can be made into haylage.

Disadvantages

1. With haylage, fine chopping, good packing and complete sealing against air entrance inside the silo is a must and more critical than with silage.

2. The danger of excessive heating which lowers protein digestibility is more acute in haylages than silages.

However, being easy to prepare and preserve in a gas type silo or other special silos as mentioned above, and capped with plastic until feeding is initiated, haylage is gaining popularity as a dairy feed. Nutritive value depends on the stage of the growth of the crop when cut and on the percentage or dry matter in it.

C. Wet by-product feeds

Wet by-product feeds might be confused with fresh forages on the one hand, and root crops, on the other, based on their content of DM. However, the fresh forages can usually be differentiated from the wet by-products on the basis of carotene content. Root crops likewise be differentiated from wet by-products in that the latter will contain over 3% crude fibre on a wet basis while the root crops will have lower values.

D. Root crops

Occassionally root crops might be confused with fresh milk on the basis of DM content, but when crude fibre content is taken into consideration (root crops always have some amount of CF) the confusion can be cleared out.

III Identifying Individual Feeds

With more experience it is possible to distinguish between two feed ingredients of the same feed group on the basis of their composition. For example fresh whole milk can be distinguished from fresh skimmed milk on the basis of fat content.

Ghani, expeller and deoiled type of oilcakes can be differentiated again on the basis of oil and protein content.

Meat scrap might be distinguished from meat and bone meal on the basis of higher bone content and so on the basis of higher calcium and phosphorus contents for the latter product.

USE OF UNCONVENTIONAL LIVESTOCK FEEDS IN INDIA

The importance of utilising the unconventional feeds to augment the existing resources of conventional livestock feed was recognised more than 30 years ago. India is facing a shortage of animal feeds and fodder which in terms of nutrients works out to 77 per cent D.C.P. and 62 per cent S.E. for feeding the livestock population. Moreover, this condition aggravates due to natural calamities like drought and flood. Recent studies indicated that quite a large number of agricultural by-products and industrial waste materials could be used for feeding livestock. Some of the unconventional livestock feeds used in India are described below:

A. *Vegetable protein sources*
B. *Animal protein sources*
C. *Energy sources*
D. *Other miscellaneous unconventional feeds*

A. VEGETABLE PROTEIN SOURCES

1. Sunflower Meal

Indian work on Sunflower seed oil meal is limited but studies abroad indicate that decorticated sunflower seed oil meal in combination with other protein supplement is good for poultry. Recent move by the Government to locate areas for cultivation of sunflower seed is, therefore, welcomed by the animal nutritionists.

Table 10.7

Identifying feeds from their Composition (*figures are on as fed basis*)

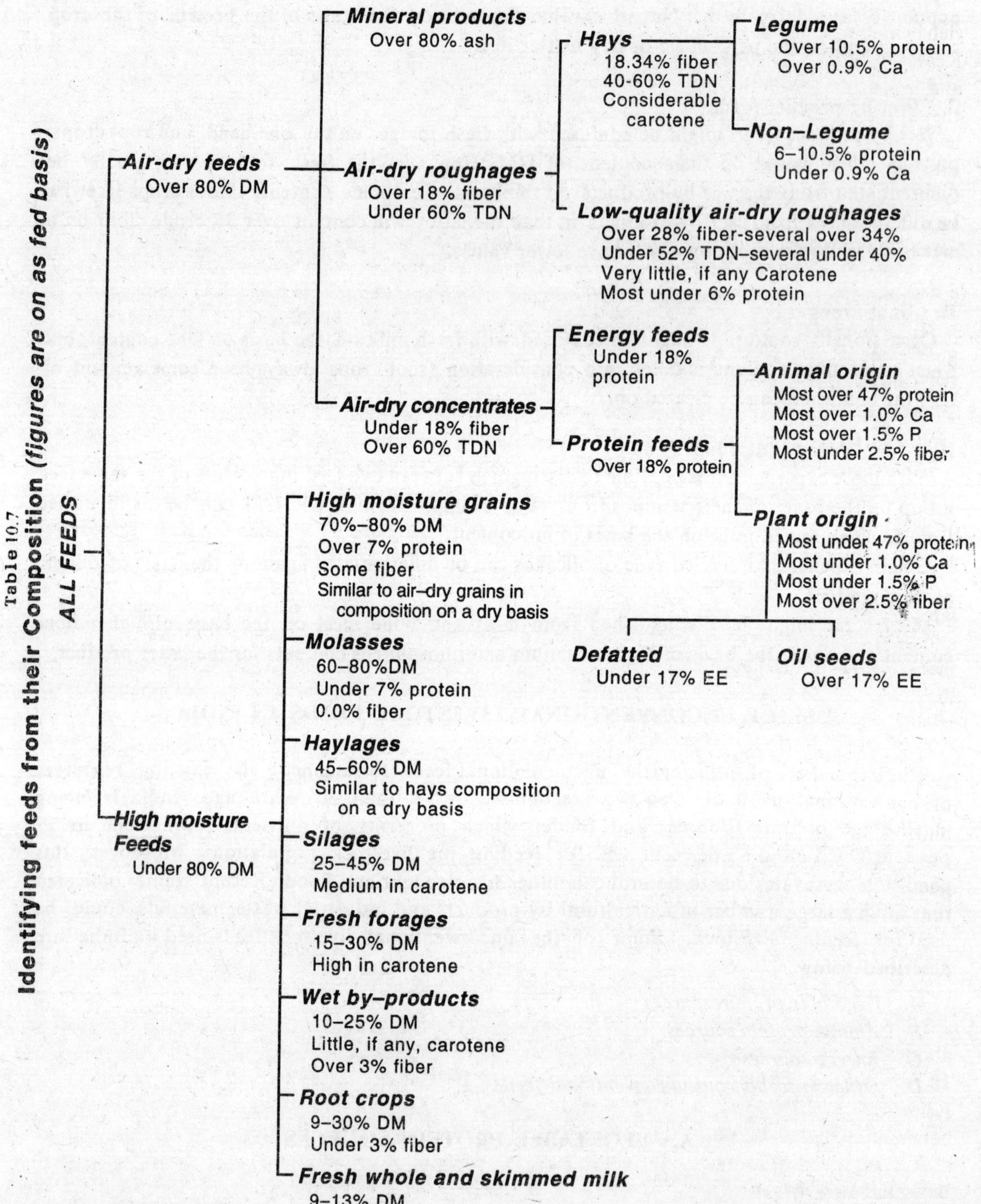

Source : Feeds and Feeding (4th edn.) – by Arthur E. Cullison and Robert S. Lowrey; Prentice–Hall, Inc. New Jersey U.S.A. 1987

Good quality sunflower meal contains about 40–44 per cent high grade protein especially rich in methionine, but that made from unhulled seed has only 20 per cent protein. It has 2200-2610 Kcal of ME/kg. The expeller variety of sunflower meal or cake tends to produce soft pork and it also makes the butter soft if fed in large amounts in cows because of the character of the oil it contains. This can be used in cattle ration and safely included at 20 per cent level. Its effect is said to resemble linseed cake in dairy ration. Sunflower seed meal is a satisfactory substitute to groundnut cake in starter rations and it can replace 100 per cent GNC without any adverse effect on weight gain and feed efficiency. The meal can also be satisfactorily used in layers' ration. Studies indicated that it could be used in total replacement of groundnut cake without any adverse effect on egg production and egg weight.

2. Guar Meal

Guar is a drought resistant legume, and the meal, a by-product from the preparation of guar gum, is a potential source of protein. ME content is 2022-2274 Kcal of ME/kg. The two undesirable characteristics of guar meal are as below:

(i) Residual guar gum (Galactomannan)—may be as high as 18 per cent of the guar meal. It is polysaccharide in nature which is neither digested nor absorbed.

(ii) Trypsin inhibitor.

It contains about 40-45 per cent protein and is a good source of amino acids. It is richer in lysine (2.55 per cent), cysteine (1.16 per cent) and glycine (4.61 per cent) than groundnut cake but comparable in respect of methionine content. It is also fairly rich in trace minerals.

Earlier experiments showed that it could be used in chick ration only up to 6.5 per cent; later it was found that up to 20 per cent guar meal could be used in chick ration if it is toasted and mixed with 0.1 per cent to 0.2 per cent cellulose enzyme. Substitution of 50 per cent guar meal (toasted) in replacement of groundnut cake was shown to give comparable performance in layers. High protein level in the mash is beneficial for its utilisation (i.e., depress the adverse effects of guar meal) in poultry.

Guar meal is not palatable to cattle since its inclusion at only 5 per cent level was refused at the initial phase by cows, although if accustomed, cows can accept rations containing as high as 15 per cent raw guar meal. Toasted guar meal, however, has not that acute palatability problem. Further, trypsin inhibitor factor is depressed. Higher levels of guar meal may cause diarrhoea, particularly in young calves. It is, therefore, always advisable to incorporate guar meal in the ration very gradually and once accustomed may be used as high as 10-15 per cent level in cows and 5-10 per cent level in calves.

3. Niger Cake

This is chiefly produced in Andhra Pradesh, Madhya Pradesh, Maharashtra and Orissa.

Niger cake compares well with other oil seed cakes in its chemical composition. It contains about 36 per cent crude protein and 5.98 per cent mineral matter, but contains about 14 to 18 per cent crude fibre. Its protein digestibility is about 80 per cent. It is richer in available lysine (400 mg/100 gms) and methionine content than groundnut cake. ME value varies between 2700-2800 Kcal/kg.

It is suggested that niger cake can completely replace groundnut cake on protein equivalent basis for the growing chicks and the two oil cakes have a complementary effect on chick growth with better efficiency in economics of feeding. The same is also true for layers, particularly if the fibre content of the ration is adjusted. Unfortunately not much studies have been made with the extracted variety of niger cake which is comparatively cheaper. Therefore, its suitability in feeding value will go a long way in economics of poultry rations.

The use of niger cake in cattle ration is also encouraging. Its inclusion in the cattle ration as high as 10 to 15 per cent is not uncommon. Unconfirmed reports suggest that higher levels may cause depression in total solids of milk. It is, therefore, advisable to include this along with other oil cakes like groundnut cake, copra cake, mustard cake, etc.

4. Karanja Cake

Pioneer work on the use of Karanja cake as livestock and poultry feed was first studied by L. Mandal and G.C. Banerjee at B.C. Krishi Viswavidyalaya in West Bengal, India.

Karanja seed grows widely in almost all the states of India especially in Mysore, Andhra Pradesh, Maharashtra, M.P., Bihar, West Bengal and Assam. So long the residual oil cakes are used as manure for paddy and rabi crops as a source of nitrogen.

Karanja cake is less palatable. It contains probably some polyphenolic compounds which have a deleterious effect on growth and production. The deoiled variety of karanja cake contains about 30 per cent crude protein and 60 per cent NFE, and only 6.66 per cent crude fibre. Its ME value as determined by Mandal and Banerjee as 2.20-2.34 Kcal/gm. Unfortunately, the expeller variety of karanja cake is not suitable for chickens since it results in high mortality, low feed consumption and poor growth whereas the deoiled variety is much better in growth response. It is moderately rich in all essential amino acids such as lysine (5.60 gm/100 gm of protein) methionine (0.99 gm/100 gm of protein).

Extracted karanja cake can be included in the ration replacing til cake to the extent of 30 per cent on protein equivalent basis in starters and growing chicks (18 week) with distinct economic advantage.

5. Neem Cake

The potential production of neem seed is estimated at 4.15 lakh tonnes. This can give 3.3 lakh tonnes of cake and 83,000 tonnes of oil every year provided this potentiality is fully utilized.

Neem cake contains 34 per cent protein while processed cake shows 48 per cent protein. Fibre content is only 4.4 per cent. The amino acid content in terms of lysine and methionine is also comparable to groundnut cake protein.

Neem cake as such is unpalatable and, therefore, it should be mixed with other well liked feed stuffs.

It is observed, however, that if this cake is introduced gradually then it can be included in the cattle ration about 15–20 per cent level. A few animals, however, may be reluctant to consume feeds at this level. 1 per cent inclusion, however, is a safe level.

Recent studies in poultry indicate that mixing of deoiled neem seed cake beyond 5 per cent level in replacement of groundnut cake causes high mortality in chicks. It is, however, of interest to note that Gupta et al. (1975) recommended use of processed neem seed meal at 20 per cent level in chicks and layers without any harmful effect.

6. Rubber Seed Cake

The total availability of rubber seed cake is about 1.5 lakh tonnes. The rubber pod contains three seeds which burst at maturity scattering its contents.

Rubber seed meal contains some cyanogenetic components. A good quality rubber seed cake contains about 30 per cent protein and 9-10 per cent ether extract. Fibre content of decorticated variety is, however, 5 per cent. D.C.P. content in cattle on fresh basis would be

18.6 per cent and T.D.N. 54 per cent, and for pigs 16.7 per cent D.C.P. and 78.8 per cent T.D.N. The material can successfully be used in the feed of cattle and pigs. It is suggested that rubber seed cake may be used at 10 per cent and 20 per cent level in concentrate mixture of pigs and calves without any deleterious effect on growth. It can be used in lactating cows at 20 per cent level in concentrate mixture. Rubber seed cake can also be used at a maximum level of 10 per cent in poultry ration without any adverse effect.

7. Sunnhemp Seed (*Crotolaria Juncea*)

The seed is grown throughout India but in most cases this is used as manure. In some parts, however, this is fed as fodder. After crushing this can be fed to cattle but feeding as such is not palatable. This can, however, be mixed with other palatable feed stuffs in a concentrate mixture and fed to cattle.

The nutritive value in terms of D.C.P. and T.D.N. is 30 per cent and 71 per cent respectively. Sunnhemp contains about 4.7 per cent lysine and 1.7 per cent methionine (on protein basis) and inclusion of this in chick ration at 80 per cent level resulted in improved growth rate.

8. Dhaincha Seed

This is a leguminous seed and is excellent in protein quality. It contains 30-33 per cent protein, and 8.32 per cent and 1.019 g/16 g N lysine and methionine respectively.

The seed cannot be used as such, as it contains deleterious factors like gum, trypsin inhibitor and tannin. Enzymic treatment as in the case of guar meal can improve the feeding value of this material. Recent studies indicated that deleterious factors can be removed by microbial fermentation. The growth rate of chicks fed on fermented dhaincha seed was almost similar to that of control. With the majority of seeds, the gum content and trypsin inhibitory activity increased while the tannin content decreased.

Fermentation by fungi decreases the gum content and trypsin inhibitory activity appreciably and increases the crude protein content of the seed.

Studies with dhaincha seed in cattle is limited. However, autoclaved dhaincha seed may be used in cattle in limited quantities.

9. Cassia Tora Seed

Available in plenty in Gujarat. Feeding this as part of the ration for milch cows has given encouraging results. Boiled cassia tora seeds up to the level of 15 per cent in the concentrate ration can safely be fed to milch cows. Cassia tora seeds (unboiled), however, can be incorporated up to the level of 10 per cent in concentrate mixture for cows without affecting milk yield and composition.

10. Kapok Seed Cake

It can be used as one of the components of cattle feed concentrate. D.C.P. and T.D.N. being 26 per cent and 69 per cent approximately.

11. Kidney Bean Chuni

Kidney bean chuni, a by-product from pulse, is a good source of cattle feed. It consists chiefly of broken kidney grains and kidney bean hulls. It contains 20.5 per cent crude protein, 7.8 per cent ether extract, 10.9 per cent crude fibre, 5.8 per cent NFE, 7 per cent ash, 0.52 per cent calcium and 0.34 per cent phosphorus. The D.C.P. and T.D.N. of the kidney bean chuni are 16.3 and 66.9 kg respectively per 100 kg dry matter. The much higher balance of nitrogen indicates that kidney bean chuni can be used as one of the protein supplements in the rations of young and milch animals.

12. Corn Gluten Meal

This feed consists chiefly of the dried residue from maize after the removal of the larger part of the starch and bran by the process employed in the wet milling manufacture of maize starch. Occasionally it may include maize oil meal. It contains protein from 50 to 60 per cent.

13. Safflower Meal

The meal is produced after removal of most of the hull and oil from safflower seed. In decorticated form it has about 40-45 per cent protein while the value goes down to about 18-20 if not decorticated. The 18-20 per cent protein safflower meals contains about 60 per cent hulls which limits its energy value and utilization in non-ruminants. Even the decorticated type contains about 14 per cent fibre. Safflower meal is low in lysine and methionine. It is always desirable that whenever safflower meal is fed to non-ruminants like pigs, it should be used in conjunction with other lysine rich protein concentrates.

B. ANIMAL PROTEIN SOURCES

1. Incubator Waste or Hatchery By-product Meal (HBPM)

It is a mixture of egg shells, infertile and unhatched eggs which have been cooked, dried and powdered.

Broiler chicks when fed at levels of 3 or 6 per cent of the total ration with dried incubator waste proved a satisfactory substitute for meal or soyabean oil meal. Properly processed HBPM containing infertile eggs and eggs with dead embryos is found to replace 33 per cent fish neal and is a good supplement for increasing body weight of chicks.

2. Liver Residue Meal

This can profitably be used as animal protein supplement in place of fish meal. Liver residue can be favourably introduced in poultry rations at 10 per cent level or at 5 per cent level along with the same level of fish meal as an animal protein supplement. A good quality of liver residue meal should contain about 65 per cent protein, 5 per cent lysine, 1.2 per cent methionine and 1 per cent cystine apart from other amino acids.

3. Frog Meal

It is a leftover of the frog leg industry. It is suggested that it can replace fish meal twice by weight in poultry rations for growth as well as for egg production.

4. Dried Poultry Manure

So long poultry manure was considered as a fertiliser and was being exclusively used for that purpose. Droppings from poultry fed with high energy rations are likely to be rich in nitrogen and energy. Poultry droppings contain 60-90 per cent of urinary nitrogen as uric acid and 9-13 per cent as ammonium salts. The digestibility of nitrogen in pure droppings ranges from 70-85 per cent.

The composition varies, but on an average it contains about 5 per cent nitrogen, equivalent to about 31 per cent crude protein. Properly dried poultry manure can be used at 10-15 per cent level in chick and broiler rations with good results. If the fibre content is high, it is preferable to use the same at lower levels. The inclusion of poultry manure necessitates an allowance for extra energy and proper calcium and phosphorus inclusion.

Dried poultry manure can also be used in cattle ration with definite economic advantage. It is, however, not palatable and hence should be used with other palatable feed stuffs.

5. Cow Dung Meal (Cow Manure)

Attempt was made to replace cereals in poultry ration by dried cow-dung meal. It can be used at 10 per cent level satisfactorily in growing ration in replacement of maize. Sun dried sheep dung meal is recommended at 5 per cent level in starter mash. Sun dried manure is as effective as oven dried cow-dung manure. In layers 10 per cent inclusion of air on oven dried cow manure satisfactorily supported egg production, egg weight, body weight, hatchability and feed consumption.

6. Shrimp Shell Powder (Prawn Waste)

It is the waste product of shrimp processing industry. The crude protein content varies from 32 per cent to 43 per cent according to the source of supply. The soluble ash content is high. The calcium content is high (9.3 per cent) whereas the phosphorus is low (1.3 per cent). The salt content is only 3.7 per cent (chloride content expressed as sodium chloride). Depending on protein content, it is likely to replace fish meal at the maximum level of 5 per cent in broiler chickens.

7. Crab Meal

It is the well ground dried waste of the crab containing shell, viscera and part or all of the flesh. It usually contains 30 per cent protein (25 to 30 per cent) and 3 per cent salt, but must not contain less than 25 per cent crude protein and more than 7 per cent salt. It contains about 12 per cent fibre, 13 to 16 per cent calcium, 1.5 to 3.5 per cent phosphorus.

It can satisfactorily replace fish meal when the content and the ratio of calcium and phosphorus in the ration is adjusted.

8. Poultry By-product Meal

It is the ground product obtained after dry rendering or wet rendering process from parts of the carcass of slaughtered poultry, such as heads, feet, undeveloped eggs and intestines exclusive of feathers. It must not contain more than 16 per cent ash and not more than 4 per cent acid insoluble ash. It is an excellent source of protein (50-58 per cent) for chickens. It is also fairly rich in energy (2900 Kcal ME/kg), fat 10-13 per cent, calcium 3 per cent and phospho us 2 per cent. It is fairly rich in minerals and provides unidentified growth factors. It can be used in broiler and layers rations. It is a good substitute of fish meal.

9. Hydrolysed Poultry Feathers

It is the product resulting from the treatment under pressure of clean, undecomposed feathers from slaughtered poultry. A minimum of 80 per cent of its crude protein must consist of "digestible protein". It is rich in protein (80-86 per cent), fairly rich in energy and is said to possess unidentified growth factor which is inorganic in nature. But the protein is severely deficient in methionine, lysine, histidine and tryptophan. This product, therefore, should be used judiciously with other protein supplements to balance the amino acid deficiencies. Feather meal can replace 2 per cent fish meal and 2 per cent dried whey in poultry ration satisfactorily.

10. Squilla Meal

It is obtained from the fisheries industries and appears to be one of the promising by-products. This product is very rich in protein (37.6 per cent). Calcium content is very high, about 10 per cent while comparatively it contains low phosphorus, being 2.0 per cent only.

11. Processed Fish Ensilage

Fish ensilage contains 31.18 per cent crude protein, 4.66 per cent ether extract, 10.63 per cent crude fibre, and 32.29 per cent total carbohydrates. The mineral contents namely Ca and P present are 3.20 and 1.97 per cent respectively. The nutritive value in terms of D.C.P., T.D.N. and S.E. work out to 19.41, 53.79 and 57.82 per cent respectively. The nitrogen balance is positive.

C. ENERGY SOURCES

1. Sal Seed Meal

Sal seed meal or sal seed cake is a by-product obtained after the extraction of oil from sal seed for industrial use. The maximum potential yield of sal seed all over the country would be 56, 80, 000 tonnes. Sal seed is a good source of fat which can be used as substitute extender for cocoa, butter and soap industry. The meal left over is a good source of carbohydrate and contains fairly good amount of tannins. It is interesting to note that the extracted sal seed meal in addition to a small amount of oil, contains substantial amount of starch which can be a good source of energy and can be incorporated in animal feed.

Sal seed meal contains abount 8–9 per cent protein, 12–16 per cent oil and 2-3 per cent fibre. Sal seed is very rich in N.F.E. fraction (70–72 per cent) while meal contains about 85 per cent. It is rich in tannin content which varies from 8–12 per cent. Due to this large tannin content the energy present in the meal is not released for utilisation in the animals. Besides tannic acid, there might be certain other alkaloids or some other substances which might prove detrimental to growth and production.

Sal seed meal does not have D.C.P. Protein is not available to the animals. T.D.N. is about 55 per cent of maize. Its use as a source of T.D.N. should be limited to a maximum level of 20 per cent of concentrate mixture for maintenance and growth. However, ISI has recommended use of sal seed meal at 10 per cent level in cattle concentrate mixture after having taken all points into consideration from all aspects.

Further work on supplementation of sal seed meal on milk producing cows is still in progress. However, with the available information it shows that there is depression of milk yield without affecting its composition when sal seed meal is used at 20 per cent level of the concentrate mixture, while substitution of sal fruits up to 20 per cent in the ration is found to be most economical for milk production.

Sal seed and sal seed cake can be used in growing chick ration up to 5 per cent and in laying up to 10 per cent level. The use of greater percentage in chick shows growth depressing effect and in layers lower egg production. Further discolouration of yolk (greenish) is also evidenced.

Verma and Panda (1972) determined ME value of sal seed and sal seed meal which are found to be 2,718 and 2,653 Kcal/kg respectively when the oil content was 16.10 per cent and

8.58 per cent for sal seed and seed meal respectively. Sarkar and Banerjee, however, found 2.64 and 2.34 Kcal/gm when the oil content was 13.64 per cent and 1.31 per cent respectively for sal seed and sal seed cake.

D.C.P. was 1.52 per cent and T.D.N. 65.34 per cent with pigs at 10 months of age and D.C.P. 1.55 per cent and T.D.N. 58.96 per cent at 14 months of age.

Growth studies on pigs by replacing 50, 75 and 10 per cent ragi in the concentrate mixture by deoiled sal seed meal for 8 months indicated progressive decrease in growth rate with the increase in the percentage of deoiled sal seed meal in the concentrate mixture.

Research works are in progress to remove tannins from sal seed meal. Panda et al (1968) showed that washing sal seed cake overnight in cold water could remove 60 per cent tannic acid. Boiling for half an hour also had the same result. Patel et al. (1972) found that 65 per cent of tannins could be removed by decinormal caustic soda. Treatments with calcium hydroxide at 0, 1, 1.5 and 2.0 per cent level have been tried without any significant improvement. Passing of steam at 15 lbs pressure for 1 hour, however, eliminated tannic acid to the extent of about 70 per cent as found by Sarkar and Banerjee (1973) at Bidhan Chandra Krishi Viswavidyalaya. Studies with such processed sal seed meal have shown very encouraging results and much greater percentage could be used.

2. Cassava (Tapioca) Root

It is a very good source of energy and rich in carbohydrates. Tapioca roots contain a glucoside, linamarin, which when acted upon by an enzyme liberates HCN (0.03 per cent in the flesh). Varieties considered poisonous contain much higher HCN. It is low in protein (2 per cent) and rich in NFE (85 per cent). Reports from Philippines suggest the possibility of making cassava silage from chopped, freshly dug tubers.

In India, dried tapioca roots are sold in the name of tapioca chips, and the meal in the name of tapisoca flour. This can be used safely upto 10 per cent level in chick and broiler feeds. In laying, ration upto a maximum of 20 per cent can be included with supplementation of methionine (0.15 per cent) or when proper care is taken of protein quality due to replacement of cereals from the diet. In ruminants this may be used in higher percentage with economic advantage provided it is mixed with other palatable feed stuffs.

3. Tapioca Starch Waste

This is a by-product obtained during the manufacture of starch from tapioca roots. Like chips it is also low in protein and fat. It is, however, rich in fibre, about 10-12 per cent. This is mostly used in the ration for cattle and buffaloes. It has 2.00 per cent D.C.P. and 64 per cent T.D.N. on DM basis for ruminants. Tapioca waste can be used safely upto 30 per cent level of the concentrate mixture with a considerable economy for maintaining body weight, milk yield and butterfat production. Tapioca waste can replace at least 50 per cent of maize as a source of energy for growing pigs without affecting the carcass characteristics.

4. Tapioca Thippi

During manufacture of sago, first the tapioca roots/tubers are deskinned and soaked in water. The tubers are then fed into the crusher adding equal amount of water for extraction of milk. The milk thus obtained is allowed to pass through a sieve to remove the fibrous material. This fibrous material in pulp form when dried is known as Tapioca thippi.

Studies in chicks at Bidhan Chandra Krishi Viswa Vidyalaya by Sarkar and Banerjee showed that it contained low protein and fat but fibre content was 8-9 per cent. This could replace unaffected. The use of 15 per cent level in a 4 week trial showed that the gain in body weight was lower by only 19.8 gm and FER higher by 0.28 when compared with the control ration. The ME as determined by Sarker and Banerjee was 2.45 Kcal/gm. Tapioca thippi can be used in cattle and pigs in the same way as tapioca starch waste.

5. Tapioca Milk Residue

Tapioca tubers after deskinning and soaking in water are fed into the crusher and milk is obtained. The heavier starch particles are collected for sago preparation while the lighter starch particles which cannot get together to form the crystals of sago are collected by a different process and dried. This dried second grade starch is known at tapioca milk residue.

It is a by-product of tapioca root in preparation of sago. It contains about 3-4 per cent protein, 3–4 per cent fat, about 2.5 per cent fibre and 66-70 per cent starch. This material can be used at a maximum level of 20 per cent in chick without any adverse effect on growth and feed efficiency. The ME value is 8.99 Kcal/gm. This can also be used in cattle in the same way as tapioca chips.

6. Palm Flour

Palm flour of good quality is obtained when the trees are cut before flowering, usually at the age of sixty years. The pith of the tree is cut into small pieces, dried and powdered to get the palm flour. This is low in protein and very rich in NFE. Fibre content is about 8.0 per cent. This can be used as a source of energy and can be used at a level of 17.5 per cent in chick ration in complete replacement of rice polish. In layer's ration it can be included upto 11.5 per cent replacing rice polish completely without affecting production and feed consumption.

Not much studies have been done with palm flour in cattle, but the proximate composition suggests that this can be used in cattle also for growth and production with economic advantage.

7. Tamarind Seed Powder

This is mostly used in textile and paper industry. It is a fairly good source of protein and energy. About 0.5 million tonnes of Tamarind seed are available in India. It is not very much palatable. It contains 15-20 per cent protein and about 5 per cent fibre. This has 13 per cent D.C.P. and 64 per cent T.D.N. It can be used in cattle as a component of concentrate mixture.

Tamarind seeds contain tannin, but overnight soaking in cold water reduces the tannin content. Increasing level of tamarind seed in chick ration from 10 to 30 per cent have revealed progressive decline in the growth ratio and FER.

8. Triticale

This is a cross between wheat and rye. This can be used favourably for egg and meat type growing chicks replacing maize to the extent of 50 per cent and 100 per cent respectively, in terms of weight gain and FER. In broiler chicks, triticale effected a better weight gain compared to that in laying strain. ME is 2043-3357 Kcal/kg for different varieties.

9. Mango Seed Kernel

This is a by-product available after extraction of juices from mangoes or from the leftovers of fruits after the same has been consumed by human beings. The availability of this by-product can be grossly estimated to be more than 1 million tonnes per year. It contains about 8 per cent protein. It is very rich in NFE, about 75-80 per cent, and low in fibre, about 3 per cent. This has 6 per cent D.C.P. and 70 per cent T.D.N.

This can be used as one of the ingredients of concentrate mixture upto a level of 40 per cent in bullocks, 20 per cent level for growing cattle and 10 per cent level to cows without affecting growth, milk production and fat content.

This can also be used in poultry in more or less the same way as sal seed meal. The tannin content, however, is less (5-7 per cent) than sal seed meal (9-13 per cent).

10. Oak Kernel

Large quantities of oak kernels are available from the oak forests. Experiments conducted so far have pointed out that this material cannot be used in either poultry or cattle ration exclusively or in appreciable amount. Oak kernels contain tannin which may be the factor for lower D.C.P. intake on higher level of oak kernel in cattle ration. Results suggest that oak kernel may be used to replace maize in cattle ration with only two thirds efficiency.

Oak kernel was used in starter's mash at levels 0, 2, 5 and 10 per cent replacing equal quantity of maize. There was no significant difference in growth rate of chicks on 0, 2 and 5 per cent levels of oak kernel. Higher (10 per cent) level showed adverse effect such as poor growth, low feed efficiency and low nitrogen retention probably due to high content of tannin.

D. OTHER MISCELLANEOUS UNCONVENTIONAL FEED

1. Sea Weed Meal

India has got a long coastal belt—where different varieties of sea weeds are available in plenty. Experiments indicated that some weeds are rich in protein while others are in minerals. Experiments so far suggest that it could be used at 15 per cent level in concentrate mixture without any adverse effect on growth and milk production. The nutritive value of sea weed meals has a wide variation, being 9 to 19.93 per cent crude protein and 23 to 44.62 per cent total ash; while the extracted variety of sea weed meal contains more protein but less minerals. Observations revealed the possibilities of utilising sea weeds as cattle feed.

2. Babul Pods (*Acacia arabica*)

It grows extensively over a wide area in India. Babul was tried on growing calves and milch animals to effect economy in feed cost. It contains about 14 per cent protein, 10.0 per cent D.C.P. and 74 per cent T.D.N. It can be used as a component of concentrate mixture in cattle ration.

3. Rain Tree Pods

It is found in Bengal, Assam, Orissa, Bombay, Southern India as shed tree. The pods are palatable. As a component of concentrate mixture it can be included in the cattle ration. It contains about 8-9 per cent D.C.P. and 64 per cent T.D.N.

4. Jack Fruit Waste

The waste from ripe fruits is more palatable than the waste from raw fruits. It contains 7.9 per cent protein, 14.1 per cent crude fibre, 0 80 per cent calcium and 0.10 per cent phosphorus. This is a rich source of energy, being 65.3 per cent nitrogen-free extract. The nutritive value of jack fruit waste has been estimated in cattle, the T.D.N. value being 19.9 per cent. The material is very poor in D.C.P. content which is only 1.2 per cent.

5. **African Payal** (*Salvinia molesta*, **Mitchell)**

This material as such is not relished by cattle and hence affects the feed consumption. The chemical composition of african payal shows crude protein 13.2 per cent, nitrogen-free extract 46.9 per cent; while the crude fibre content is very high, being 23.5 per cent. Among the minerals, calcium is 1 35 per cent with low phosphorus content (0.35 per cent).

6. **Sugar Cane Bagasse**

Sugar cane bagasse is the fibrous residue of sugar cane stalks after the juice has been pressed out in factories and mainly two varieties are available viz., (1) fine bagasse and (2) coarse bagasse. The chemical compositions of fine and coarse varieties depend on the place of production being crude protein 2.23–4.74 per cent and 1.76–3.32 per cent, crude fibre 36.52–42.1 per cent and 40.49–43.22 per cent, ether extract 0.52–1.68 per cent and 0.53–0.87 per cent, ash 2.60–3.49 per cent and 1.81–2.58, per cent nitrogen-free extract 51.95–54.8 per cent 50.39–54.54 per cent. The in-vitro dry matter digestibility of various samples of sugar cane bagasse range between 19-40 per cent.

7. **Sugar Beet Pulp**

It is a by-product of cane sugar. Its chemical composition reveals that it cannot be considered as a concentrate because of its high ADF (44.37 per cent), CF (25.98 per cent) and lignin (6.69 per cent) contents. It might be better classified as a good roughage as its D.C.P. is 3.46 per cent and T.D.N. is 58.11 per cent.

8. **Sugar Cane Tops**

These include the growing point of the cane, a few of the upper nodes, and accompanying leaves. On large farms the tops and dry leaves are burned off before the cane is processed for disposal, while on small farms the tops are cut for livestock feed. The feeding value of fresh cane tops is not very promising: 0.5 to 1.5 per cent crude protein, 0.5 per cent fat, and 9 per cent crude fibre. The material serves as a roughage in conjunction with concentrates. In South Africa, cattle fed 6 to 7 kg of sugar cane tops per 100 kg live weight, along with groundnut meal, gained 0.6 kg per day.

Sugar cane tops as worked out by Bharatiya Agro-industries Foundation, can be very well ensiled alone as well as with 0.5 per cent urea. The silage is well acceptable to cross-bred cattle and contain 4.0 per cent D.C.P. and 47.8 per cent T.D.N.

9. **Petro-Protein**

It is high in protein which is about 52.37 per cent. It contains 11.7 per cent ether extract, 26.48 per cent NFE, 9.45 per cent ash, 0.41 per cent calcium and 1.81 per cent phosphorus. The digestibility co-efficients of crude protein and ether extract range from 89.9-99 per cent (average 95.7 per cent) and 58.6-69.0 per cent (average 61.9 per cent), respectively. Petro-protein is estimated to contain a significant amount of T.D.N. on dry matter basis Calcium balance is found to be negative. It seems to be very good source of protein and phosphorus and thus it can replace groundnut.

NUTRIENTS OF FEEDING STUFF AND ANIMAL BODY

A nutrient is a substance that promotes the growth, maintenance, function, and reproduction of a cell or an organism. The principal nutrients of all feeding stuffs are water, organic and mineral matters. The organic in turn is composed of crude protein, ether extract, crude fibre and nitrogen free extract. The occurrence of these nutrients in feeds and their role as constituents of feed in the nutrition of animal body may briefly be stated as follows.

WATER

Water is one of the most vital of all nutrients. In fact animals may live for more than 100 days without organic food but they die in 5–10 days when deprived of water. In general it makes up about two thirds of the fat free animal body weight (the water content of the fat free adult body is relatively constant) for many species averaging 73 per cent of total body weight. As a result of this constant relationship, the composition of the animal body can be estimated with reasonable accuracy if either the fat or water content is known. Body water can be estimated with various dyes, deuterium oxide, or tritium by administering through intravenously and determining the amount of dilution of the test compound; fat content of the tissues may be calculated by the formula:

$$\text{Per cent fat} = 100 - \frac{\text{per cent water}}{0.732}$$

The greatest amount of water in the body tissues will be found as *intracellular fluids*, which may account for 40% or more of total body weight. Most of the intracellular water is found in muscle and skin with lesser amounts in other tissues. Extracellular water is found in interstitial fluids, which occupy spaces between cells, blood plasma, and other miscellaneous fluids such as lymph, synovial, and cerebrospinal fluids. *Extracellular water* accounts for the second largest water "compartment," or roughly one-third of the total body water of which about 6% is blood plasma water.

Most of the remaining body water will be found in the contents of the GI tract and urinary tract. The amount present in the GI tract is quite variable, even within species, and is greatly affected by the type and amount of feed consumed. As indicated, body water tends to decrease with age and has an inverse relationship with body fat. Body water is apt to be higher in lactating cows than in dry cows (usually less body fat also), and extracellular water is greater in young male calves than in female calves of the same age. An embryonic calf is composed of 90 per cent or more water, a new born calf is slightly more than 70 per cent and a steer (bullock) in adult comprises only 45–60 per cent water.

Table 10.8

Average water content of bovine and human body at various ages

Bovine	% H_2O	Human	% H_2O
Embryo	90	Embryo	93
New born calf	80	New born infant	72
6–12 mo calf	65	2 mo infant	70
Adult steer	55	Adult	60

Animals can lose most of their fat, about half of their protein, and many other constituents of their body tissues, but a loss of one tenth of the water in the body is lethal. Dehydration involves the loss of water and electrolytes. Dehydration associated with the loss of 10% of water content of the body is considered severe and a 20% loss results in death, whereas animals are capable of living even after a loss of 40% of their dry body weight caused by starvation.

Water Sources

Water available to an animal's tissues comes from five sources, viz. (1) drinking water; (2) water present in all feeds (green succulent fodder contains on an average 70 per cent moisture while dry roughage and concentrates contain about 10 percent moisture), (3) metabolic water produced by oxidation of carbohydrate, fat and protein nutrients, (4) water liberated from polymerization (combination of some molecules into one organic macro molecule compound) reactions such as condensation of amino acids to peptides, and (5) preformed water associated with the tissues which are catabolized during a period of negative energy balance.

Metabolic Water

Metabolic water is produced inside the body by metabolic processes of tissues mainly by oxidation of nutrients which comprises to about 5 to 10 per cent of the total intake. The three main kinds of nutrients produce different amounts of water. One molecule of glucose on oxidation gives six molecules of water.

$$C_6H_{12}O_6 + 6O_2 \longrightarrow 6CO_2 + 6H_2O$$

By calculation from this equation it can be noted that the metabolism of glucose yield 60 per cent of its weight as water. Similarly protein produces 40 per cent (i.e. each gram of protein yields 0.4 gram of water) and fat yields 1.1 gram water (which is more than 100% of its weight) from each molecule. For some domestic animals metabolic water is the major source of water. In such cases and also in animals consuming less food than required, the production of metabolic water becomes more important, since depot fat and tissue protein are catabolized to supply energy. In other cases, this water may form the major if not the only source of supply; for example in the incubating chick and in hibernating animals.

Table 10.9

Production of metabolic water
(Yield in gm Water from 1 gm of substance oxidised)

Substance	*Water*
Glucose	**0.60**
Starch	**0.56**
Tributyrin	**0.77**
Tristearin	**1.11**
Protein (average)	**0.42**

Metabolic water is also produced by the dehydration synthesis of body proteins, fats and carbohydrates.

Bound Water

Bound water differs from free water in that it is combined with the constituents of protoplasm by either physical or chemical means. Therefore, bound water does not separate easily from protoplasm by freezing at low temperature or by evaporation at high temperature or under dry conditions. Bound water is of special interest in connection with the ability of plants and animals to resist low temperature and drought.

Functions of Water

1. CELL RIGIDITY AND ELASTICITY. The body must have a definite form which it can retain and yet, within limits, it must be able to change its shape by confirming to some extent to the force applied at any particular point. This is made possible by the liquid contents of the cell. In particular, the cerebrospinal fluid acts as cushion for the nerves.

2. SOLVENT ACTION. By its solvent action it serves as a universal medium in which the intra- and extra-cellular chemical reaction take place. Probably no chemical reaction inside the body can take place without water.

3. HYDROLYTIC REACTIONS. Hydrolysis is an important chemical process involved in digestion and other metabolism. In this process the H and OH ions of water are introduced into bigger molecules and the latter is broken down into smaller units.

4. IONIC AND OTHER REACTIONS. The process of living depends upon a continuous series of chemical reactions and many of these reactions require a medium in which to act; in the animal body this medium is water. The dielectric constant of water being very high, oppositely charged ions can co-exist in water without much interference.

5. LUBRICATION. Water acts as a lubricant to prevent friction and drying. In joints, pleura, conjunctiva, etc., the aqueous solution practically free from fat acts as a lubricant against rubbing and drying.

6. TRANSPORT. Water acts as a vehicle for various physiological processes, such as:

(a) For absorption of food material from intestine.
(b) For reabsorption from kidney tubules.
(c) For the transport of various foodstuffs from place to place.
(d) For the drainage and excretion of the end products of metabolism.
(e) For the manufacture of various secretions, such as digestive juices, etc.
(f) For carrying the hormones (water soluble) to their places of activity.

7. HEAT REGULATION. Body temperature is regulated by water in following ways:

(*a*) *Heat absorption.* Due to high specific heat of water more heat is required to raise the temperature of 1 gm. of water to 1°C than most of the known solids and liquids. By virtue of this property water can absorb large quantity of heat.

(*b*) *Heat conduction and distribution.* Heat conducting power of water being very high, it acts as a very good agent in carrying away heat from the site of production and distributing it throughout the body. By the above two properties water acts as an important buffer.

(*c*) *Heat loss.* Water helps heat loss through urine and stool and by evaporation from skin, lungs, etc. Water has got the highest latent heat of evaporation, 589 cal. per gm which means that to change 1 gm of liquid water to 1 gm of water vapour without any change in tempera-

Table 10.10

CLASSIFICATION OF NUTRIENTS BY ANALYSIS

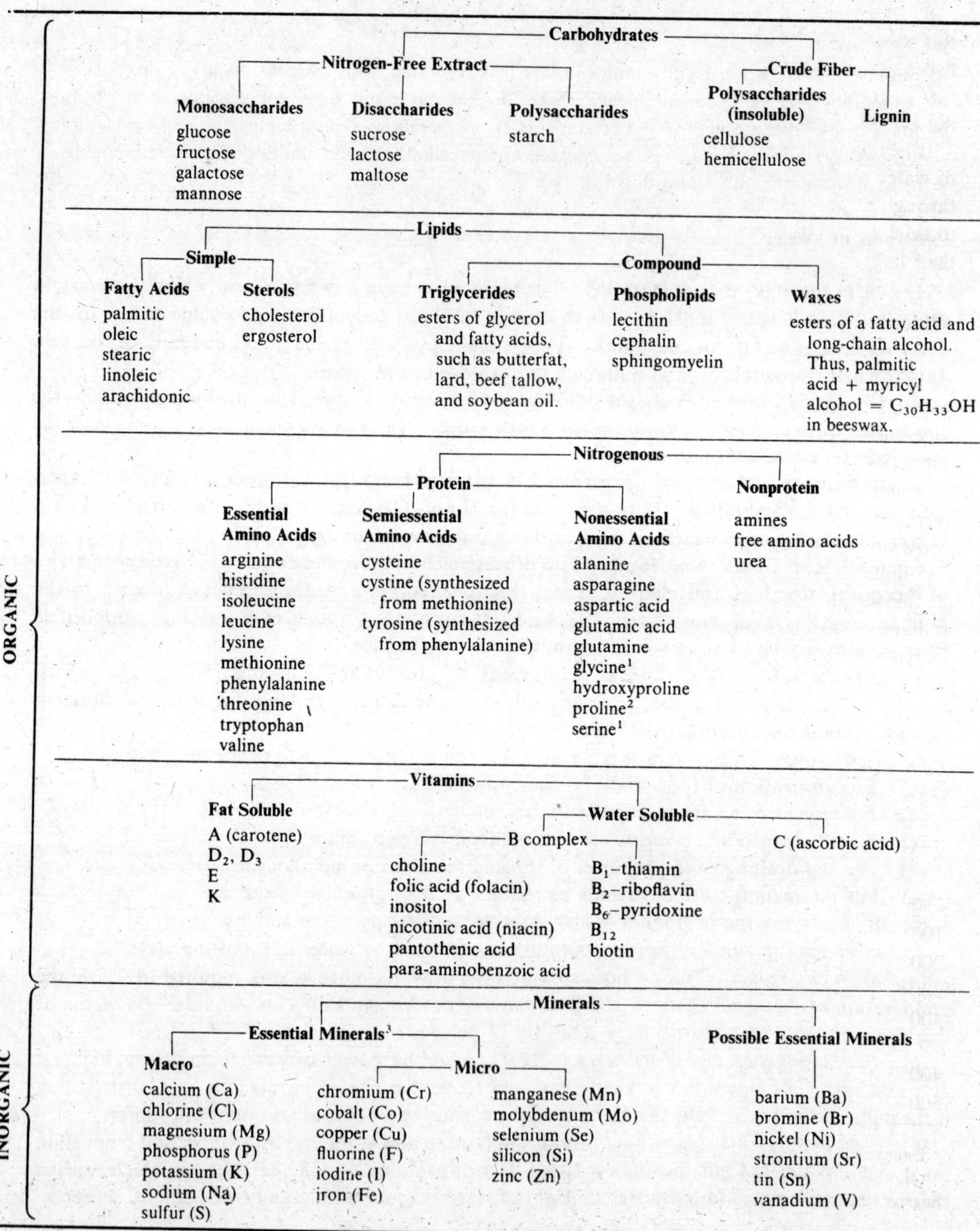

ORGANIC

- **Carbohydrates**
  - **Nitrogen-Free Extract**
    - **Monosaccharides**: glucose, fructose, galactose, mannose
    - **Disaccharides**: sucrose, lactose, maltose
    - **Polysaccharides**: starch
  - **Crude Fiber**
    - **Polysaccharides (insoluble)**: cellulose, hemicellulose
    - **Lignin**
- **Lipids**
  - **Simple**
    - **Fatty Acids**: palmitic, oleic, stearic, linoleic, arachidonic
    - **Sterols**: cholesterol, ergosterol
  - **Compound**
    - **Triglycerides**: esters of glycerol and fatty acids, such as butterfat, lard, beef tallow, and soybean oil.
    - **Phospholipids**: lecithin, cephalin, sphingomyelin
    - **Waxes**: esters of a fatty acid and long-chain alcohol. Thus, palmitic acid + myricyl alcohol = $C_{30}H_{33}OH$ in beeswax.
- **Nitrogenous**
  - **Protein**
    - **Essential Amino Acids**: arginine, histidine, isoleucine, leucine, lysine, methionine, phenylalanine, threonine, tryptophan, valine
    - **Semiessential Amino Acids**: cysteine, cystine (synthesized from methionine), tyrosine (synthesized from phenylalanine)
    - **Nonessential Amino Acids**: alanine, asparagine, aspartic acid, glutamic acid, glutamine, glycine[1], hydroxyproline, proline[2], serine[1]
  - **Nonprotein**: amines, free amino acids, urea
- **Vitamins**
  - **Fat Soluble**: A (carotene), D_2, D_3, E, K
  - **Water Soluble**
    - B complex: choline, folic acid (folacin), inositol, nicotinic acid (niacin), pantothenic acid, para-aminobenzoic acid, B_1–thiamin, B_2–riboflavin, B_6–pyridoxine, B_{12}, biotin
    - C (ascorbic acid)

INORGANIC

- **Minerals**
  - **Essential Minerals**[3]
    - **Macro**: calcium (Ca), chlorine (Cl), magnesium (Mg), phosphorus (P), potassium (K), sodium (Na), sulfur (S)
    - **Micro**: chromium (Cr), cobalt (Co), copper (Cu), fluorine (F), iodine (I), iron (Fe), manganese (Mn), molybdenum (Mo), selenium (Se), silicon (Si), zinc (Zn)
  - **Possible Essential Minerals**: barium (Ba), bromine (Br), nickel (Ni), strontium (Sr), tin (Sn), vanadium (V)

[1]Under some conditions, glycine or serine synthesis may not be sufficient for most rapid growth; either glycine or serine may need to be supplied in the diet.
[2]When diets composed of crystalline amino acids are used, proline may be necessary to achieve maximum growth.
[3]Required by at least one animal species.

ture, 589 cal. are required. By this means the body is able to rid itself of 589 cal. of heat for every gm of water it evaporates.

8. RESPIRATORY FUNCTION. Although CO_2 and O_2 are only slightly soluble in water, yet this solubility is of immense importance for the gaseous exchange in the tissues and lungs. The fishes derive oxygen almost exclusively from dissolved oxygen in water.

9. REFRACTIVE MEDIUM. The aqueous humour helps to keep up the shape and tension of the eye ball and acts as a refractive medium for light.

It is, therefore, apparent that the animal should be given liberal quantities of water. Deficiency of water on the other hand, delays digestion, assimilation and excretion of waste products through urine. If the deficiency of water in an animal be continued long then its blood tends to thicken with a rise in temperature. Animals, like men, can stand lack of food much longer than lack of water.

Water Requirements

In a given environmental situation water requirements are highly related to dry matter intake with the result that an increased consumption of dry matter will increase water consumption and vice versa. Water intake of adult cattle is 3–5 kg for every kg of dry matter intake; for suckling calves it is much higher, being 6–7 kg per kg dry matter. Milking cows require additional amounts of water to the tune of 4–5 kg of water for each kg of milk produced. Egg laying, likewise, increases water requirement.

At an environmental temperature which causes no heat stress, water intake tends to be about 3–5 units/unit of dry feed intake in adult cattle.

Consumption is increased during late pregnancy. The presence of mineral salt, particularly sodium chloride in the diet, ingestion of high protein diets, pentosans, fibre and silage in diet increase water requirement.

Table 10.11

Estimated daily Water Intake of Various Groups of Cattle

Body weight (kg)	*Litres per day by temperature**	
	20°C	*30°C*
	Dairy heifers	
50	3.6	5.3
100	11.0	16.3
200	20.0	26.5
300	27.3	37.0
400	35.2	46.2
	*Lactating dairy cows***	
400	26.5	27.0
500	31.0	32.0

* Estimates include both the free water consumed and water contained in the feed.

** Not including allowance for production.

Source: NDRI Handbook (Production), 1980, p. 13.

Considering all the factors, the water requirement for each animal can be calculated on daily basis. Further amount of water when calculated for cleaning of animals, floors, containers etc., the total requirement may reach to about 100 litres per cow per day. For all practical purposes, domestic animals may be offered water *ad libitum* at least twice a day.

Water Losses

Losses of water from the animal body occur by way of (1) urine, (2) faeces, (3) vaporisation from lungs and skin, (4) sweat glands during warm or hot weather.

Urine

Amount is highly variable, depending upon many factors. The kidneys regulate the volume and composition of body fluids, excreting more or less water depending upon intake, outgo through other channels viz., faeces, respiration, sweat etc. along with the amounts of catabolic products and environmental temperature. Other factors which have an important effect on urinary losses include: dry matter in the diet, N_2 consumption, urinary N_2 production and consumption of fat, K, P and Cl.

Faeces

Faecal water losses are normally considerably higher in ruminants than in many other species, being about equal to urinary losses, whereas in man the faecal loss is about 7–10% of urinary water. There are appreciable differences between species in the percentage of water found in faeces. Goat and sheep usually excrete faeces with less water than other species. It is about 50–70% water with an average of 65% against cattle which would be on the order of 68–80% water depending on the diet.

Water vapourised (respiration) from the body

Represents a rather large amount of the total water loss through lungs. Respiratory water loss ranges from about 23 ml/m^2 of body surface per hour at 27°C to 50 ml at 41°C.

Sweat Losses

(Respiration) mainly depends upon environmental temperature and on type of physical labour that the animal has to perform. Under field condition on moderate climate sweating rates varies from 2.99 to 5.06 $g/m^2/5$ minutes.

Water Quality

Water quality is of great importance in many areas. Excess salt will cause greater excretion. Domestic ruminants can tolerate about 1.5–1.8% total dissolved solids (TDS). Higher TDS will reduce production. Surface waters in particular those from closed lakes, may be very high in some other mineral elements are mentioned along with *safe upper limit* in mg/litre given in bracket Arsenic (0.2), Cadmium (0.05), Chromium (1.0), Cobalt (1.0), Copper (0.5), Fluoride (2.0), Lead (0.1), Nitrate (100.0) and Zinc (25.0).

Toxins of various types produced by micro-organism as well as from industrial pollution, will become an increasing problem for liver in many areas. For maximum production all species of domestic animals should always be provided with plenty of water which is safe for human consumption although it appears that animals can tolerate slightly higher salinity than humans.

CARBOHYDRATES

Carbohydrates literally means *hydrate of Carbon.* When sugars are heated for a long time in a test tube, a black residue (Carbon) and droplets of water condensed on the sides of the tube will be obtained.

Carbohydrates are all compounds of carbon, hydrogen and oxygen. Generally but not always the hydrogen and oxygen in carbohydrates are present in the proportion of two hydrogen atoms to one oxygen atom as in H_2O, from which fact the term "carbohydrates" (carbon hydrate) was derived and thus carbohydrates were originally represented with an empirical formula $C_x(H_2O)_n$. Glucose has the molecular formula $C_6H_{12}O_6$ and can be written as carbon hydrate, $C_6(H_2O)_6$.

Today we retain the name but are not bound to the empirical formula. Many substances not carbohydrates contain hydrogen and oxygen in the proportion of H_2O such as acetate ($C_2H_4O_2$) and lactic acids ($C_3H_6O_3$). Also some carbohydrates, such as deoxyribose ($C_5H_{10}O_4$), rhamnose ($C_6H_{12}O_5$) do not contain hydrogen and oxygen in the proportion of H_2O.

Carbohydrate thus may well be defined as polyhydroxy (more than one OH group) aldehyde or polyhydroxy ketone as in monosaccharides; their polymers as oligo and polysaccharides; their reduction products as polyhydric alcohols; oxidation products as aldonic, uronic and saccharic acid; substitution products as amino sugars.

Carbohydrates are the major constituents of most plants comprising from 60—90 percent of their dry mass (mostly as cellulose). They form the woody framework of plants as well as the chief reserve food stored in seeds. In contrast, animal tissue contains very small (less than 1%) amount but without which life will be at stake. Humans, the special animals not only utilise carbohydrates for their food (about 60-75% by mass of the average diet), but also for their clothing (cotton, linen, rayon), shelter (wood), fuel (wood), and paper (wood).

The amount of carbohydrate present in an adult human body is about 300-350 gm. Of this 110 gm is stored as glycogen in the liver. Another 200-250 gm is present as glycogen in cardiac smooth and skeletal muscle and about 15 gm makes up the glucose in the blood and extracellular fluid.

Biological importance

1. The principal function of carbohydrate in the form of glucose and glycogen is to furnish energy for the body. More than 50% of the energy value of the diet is provided by the carbohydrates.

$$\text{Glucose} + 2\text{ ATP (or glycogen} + 1\text{ ATP)} \xrightarrow{\text{Anaerobic}} 2\text{ lactic acid} + 4\text{ ATP}$$

$$\text{Glucose} + 2\text{ ATP (or glycogen} + 1\text{ ATP)} \xrightarrow[O_2]{\text{Aerobic}} 6\,CO_2 + 6\,H_2O + 40\text{ ATP}$$

2. It is said that fats and proteins are burnt (oxidised) in the flame of carbohydrates. It means certain products of carbohydrate metabolism (in Kreb cycle) are absolutely essential for oxidation of fats and proteins.

3. Some carbohydrates have highly specific functions, e.g., ribose in the nucleo protein (in RNA, DNA, ATP) etc., galactose in certain lipids and the lactose of milk.

4. When the intake of carbohydrate is more than what is required by the body, the excess is utilised for the transformation of fats or even for the carbon skeleton of proteins.

5. In plants simple sugars, specially glucose and ribose are involved in energy transformation and tissue synthesis. Less soluble forms, such as starch serves as energy reserves in roots, tubers and seeds. The rather insoluble fractions like celluloses and hemicelluloses provide structural support for living plants.

CLASSIFICATION OF CARBOHYDRATES

Carbohydrates are classified according to their acid hydrolysis products. Three major categories are recognised.

1. The monosaccharides, or *simple sugars*, can not be broken down into smaller molecules by hydrolysis.
2. The disaccharides yield two monosaccharide molecules upon hydrolysis.
3. The polysaccharides yield many monosaccharide molecules upon hydrolysis.

This method of classifying carbohydrate is shown as below :

Table 10.12

Structural classification of carbohydrates

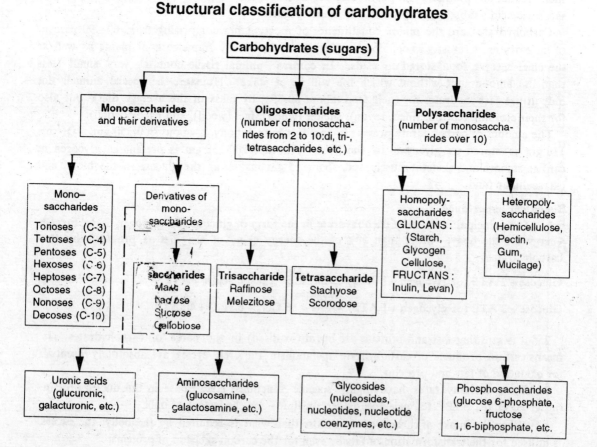

Carbohydrates (sugars)

- **Monosaccharides** and their derivatives
  - Mono–saccharides
    - Torioses (C-3)
    - Tetroses (C-4)
    - Pentoses (C-5)
    - Hexoses (C-6)
    - Heptoses (C-7)
    - Octoses (C-8)
    - Nonoses (C-9)
    - Decoses (C-10)
  - Derivatives of mono-saccharides
    - Uronic acids (glucuronic, galacturonic, etc.)
    - Aminosaccharides (glucosamine, galactosamine, etc.)
    - Glycosides (nucleosides, nucleotides, nucleotide coenzymes, etc.)
    - Phosphosaccharides (glucose 6-phosphate, fructose 1, 6-biphosphate, etc.
- **Oligosaccharides** (number of monosaccharides from 2 to 10:di, tri-, tetrasaccharides, etc.)
  - **saccharides**: Ma[illegible]e, [illegible]ose, Sucrose, Cellobiose
  - **Trisaccharide**: Raffinose, Melezitose
  - **Tetrasaccharide**: Stachyose, Scorodose
- **Polysaccharides** (number of monosaccharides over 10)
  - Homopoly-saccharides: GLUCANS : (Starch, Glycogen Cellulose, FRUCTANS : Inulin, Levan)
  - Heteropoly-saccharides (Hemicellulose, Pectin, Gum, Mucilage)

Table 10.13

Chemical Classification of Carbohydrates

MONOSACCHARIDES				POLYSACCHARIDES	
Pentoses ($C_5H_{10}O_5$)	Hexoses ($C_6H_{12}O_6$)	Disaccharides ($C_{12}H_{22}O_{11}$)	Trisaccharides ($C_{18}H_{32}O_6$)	(Homopolysaccharides) ($C_6H_{12}O_6)_n$	(Heteropolysaccharides)
Arabinose Occur in pectins, plum and cherry gums. ***Ribose*** Found in every living cell, e.g., ATP, ADP, riboflavin, RNA, nucleic acid of all living cells, certain enzymes. ***Xylose*** Derived from pentosans of fruits–plums, cherries and grapes, also present in hemicellulose, xylan of hay, oat hulls and many kinds of wood.	***Fructose*** Source : Fruit juices. Honey. Hydrolysis of cane sugar and of inulin (from the Jerusalem artichoke). Can be changed to glucose in the liver and intestine and so used in the body. ***Galactose*** Source : Hydrolysis of lactose. Can be changed to glucose in the liver and metabolized. Synthesized in the mammary gland to make the lactose of milk. A constituent of glycolipids and glycoproteins. ***Mannose*** Source : Hydrolysis of plant mannosans and gums. A constituent of prosthetic polysaccharide of albumins, globulins, mucoproteins. A sugar frequently occurring in glycoproteins. ***Glucose*** Source : Fruit juices. Hydrolysis of starch, cane sugar, maltose, and lactose. The "sugar" of the body. The sugars carried by the blood, and the principal one used by the tissues. Glucose is usually the "sugar" of the urine when glycosuria occurs.	***Lactose*** Made up of glactose and glucose. β [1, 4] linkage. Occurs in milks May occur in urine during pregnancy and milk products [1, 4]. ***Maltose*** Obtained due to digestion by amylase or hydrolysis of starch. Germinating cereals and malt. The compound is 2 mols. of glucose α [1, 4 linkage]. ***Sucrose*** Consists of glucose and sucrose α[1, 5] linkage. Found in cane and beet sugar, sorghum, pineapple, carrot roots. ***Cellobiose*** Does not exist naturally as free sugar, but is the basic repeating unit of cellulose. Composed of two β-D – glucose residue linked through a β-(1,4) bond which can not be split by mammalian digestive enzymes but by microbial enzymes.	***Raffinose*** Made up of one mole of Glucose + Fructose + Galactose Found in sugar beets and is concentrated in sugar beet molasses. Also found in higher plants and fungi. The sugar is not well utilized as food by man. ***Gentianose*** Occurs in gentian root. When hydrolyzed, it yields fructose and two molecules of glucose. The order of linkage is fructose–glucose–glucose.	***Cellulose*** Subunits : D–glucose Linkages : β–(1–4) glycosidic bonds Branching : none; linear chains Molecular weight : 50,000 to 2,000,000 Function : structural element of plant cell walls; forms microfibrils several hundred angstroms in length ***Glycogen*** Subunits : D–glucose Linkages : α–(1–4) glycosidic bonds α–(1–6) glycosidic bonds Branching : about 9% Molecular Weight : from several hundred thousand to about 100,000.00 Function: nutritional glucose reservoir in animals. It is also known as animal starch.	***Hemicellulose*** Found in cell walls of all plants, trees and also in certain seeds, soluble in alkali. Composed of a main chain of xylose units with side chains arabinose, uronic acids, glucose, galactose, arabinose. The composition varies in different species of plants and trees. More digestible than cellulose. ***Chitin*** Subunits : 2–acetamido–2–deoxy–D–glucose Linkages : β–(1–4) glycosidic bonds Branching : none; linear chains Molecular Weight : difficult to estimate because of tightly–bound noncarbohydrate material, especially proteins and inorganic salts. Function : structural element in lower plants (e.g., fungi) and in invertebrates, especially arthropods where it serves as exoskeletal material.
			Starch (Amyloses and Amylopectins) ***Amyloses*** Subunits : D–glucose Linkages : α–(1–4) glycosidic bonds Branching : None : Linear chains Molecular Weight : 4000 to 40,000 Function : Nutritional reservoir for glucose in plants ***Dextrin*** Intermediate products of the hydrolysis of starch and glycogen. Having lower molecular w[illegible] are highly branched. These are generally soluble i[illegible] wa[illegible] [illegible]ns mucilage	***Amylopectins*** Subunits : D–glucose Linkages : α-(1–4) and α-(1–6) glycosidic bonds Branching : About 4% Molecular Weight : 50,000 to 1,000,000 Function : Nutritional reservoir for glucose in plants.	***Pectin*** Composed of galacturonic acid, chain with arabinose, glactose and xylose. Occurs in primary cell wall. Soluble in hot water. "Pectin" is a group term, different pectins are known of which some are insoluble. Large amount of pectins are used in the fruit conserving industry. In rumen pectin is hydrolyzed by microbial enzyme polygalacturonidase, which in turn yields xylose in rumen. Pectin forms jel with sugar.

For the most part, the mono and disaccharides are sweet tasting, crystalline solids, readily soluble in water and insoluble in non-polar or organic solvents.

Another way of classifying carbohydrates is on the basis of sugar and non-sugar groups. The term 'sugar' is applied to those carbohydrates which contain less than 10 monosaccharide units, while non-sugar comprise members of the carbohydrate family having more than 10 monosaccharide units.

1. Monosaccharides

Monosaccharides or simple sugars are those that can not be hydrolysed into simpler form, seldom found free in nature. Rather, they constitute the building block of more-complex carbohydrate molecules. They may be subdivided into trioses, tetroses, pentoses, hexoses or heptoses, depending upon the number of carbon atom they possess; and as aldoses or ketoses, depending upon whether the aldehyde or ketone group is present. Examples are :

	Aldoses	*Ketoses*
Trioses ($C_3H_6O_3$)	Glyceraldehyde	Dihydroxyacetone
Tetroses ($C_4H_8O_4$)	Erythrose	Erythrulose
Pentoses ($C_5H_{10}O_5$)	Ribose	Ribulose
Hexoses ($C_6H_{12}O_6$)	Glucose	Fructose

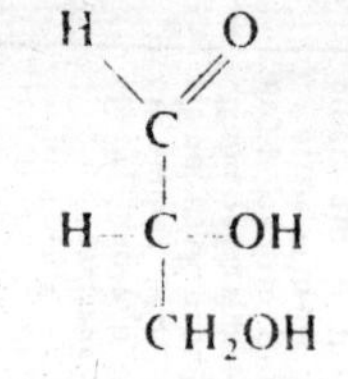

Glyceraldehyde

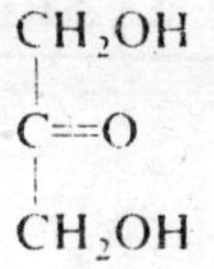

Dihydroxyacetone

(a) *Trioses*

Both of these compounds are found in plant and animal cells and play an important role in carbohydrate metabolism.

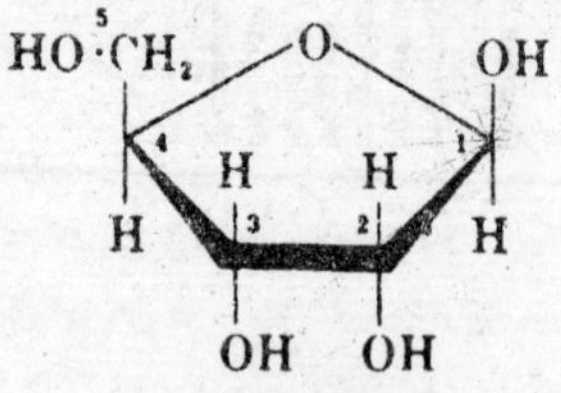

D-Ribose
(β-D-ribofuranose)

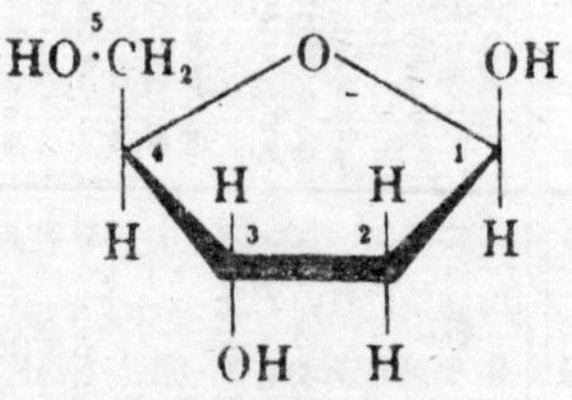

2-Deoxy-D-ribose
(β-2-deoxyribofuranose)

(b) *Pentoses*

Both sugars are found in the nucleic acid of all living cells. Ribose is also an intermediate in the pathway of carbohydrate metabolism and is a constituent of several of the coenzymes.

(c) *Hexoses*

1. GLUCOSE. The majority of carbohydrates taken in by the body are eventually converted to a glucose in series of a metabolic pathways. Glucose is the circulating carbohydrate of animals ; the blood of cow, sheep, goat, pig and laying chicken contain, 40-70 ; 30-50 ; 46-60 ; 80-120 and 130-290 mg per 100 ml respectively.

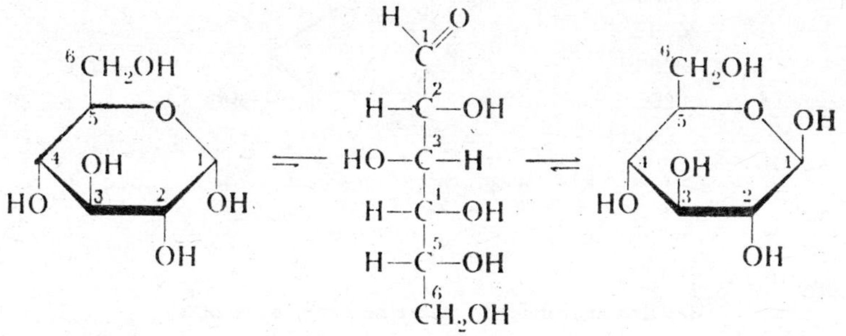

α-D(+)-Glucose ⇌ D(+)-Glucose ⇌ β-D(+)-Glucose

Glucose is the most abundant sugar found in nature. It is commonly found in fruits, especially in ripe grapes, and for this reason it is often referred to as *grape sugar*. It is also known as *dextrose*, a name that derives from the fact that the sugar is dextrorotatory. Commercially, glucose is made by the hydrolysis of starch. Glucose is only 75 per cent as sweet as table sugar (sucrose) but it has the same caloric value.

2. GALACTOSE. It is formed by the hydrolysis of lactose (milk sugar), a disaccharide composed of a glucose unit and a galactose unit. It does not occur in nature in the uncombined

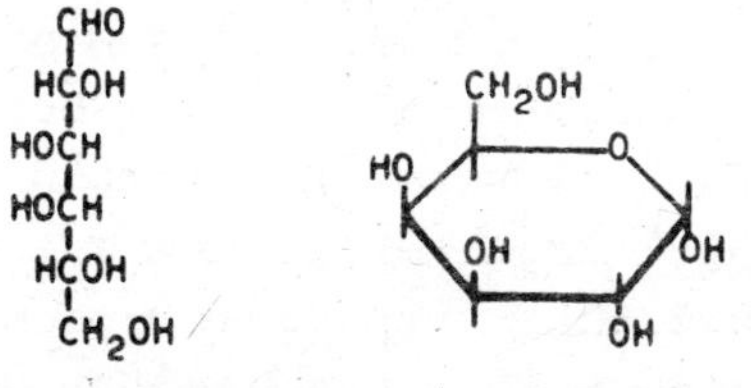

D GALACTOSE

state. The galactose needed by the human body for the synthesis of lactose (in the mammary glands) is obtained by the conversion of D-glucose into D-galactose. In addition, galactose is an important constituent of the glycolipids which occur in the brain and in the Myelin sheath of nerves.

3. FRUCTOSE. Fructose is the only naturally occurring ketohexose. In the free state it occurs predominantly in the pyranose form whereas in nature the furanose form predominates (as in sucrose and insulin). This sugar is also referred to as *levulose* because it has an optical rotation which is strongly levorotatory (−92°). It is the sweetest sugar, and it is found, together with glucose and sucrose, in sweeter fruits and honey.

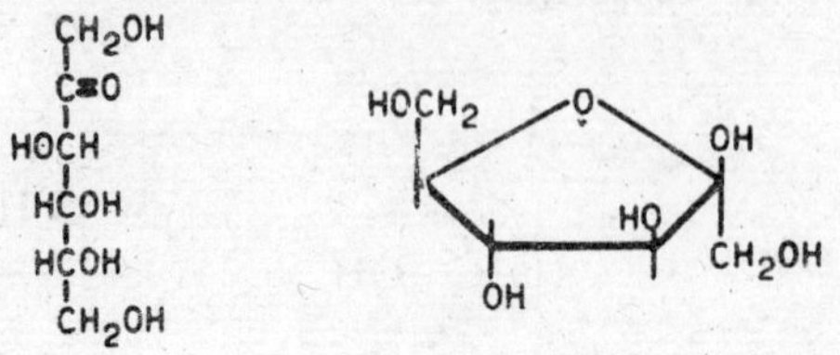

$$\begin{array}{c} CH_2OH \\ | \\ C{=}O \\ | \\ HOCH \\ | \\ HCOH \\ | \\ HCOH \\ | \\ CH_2OH \end{array}$$

D-FRUCTOSE

Table 10.14

Relative sweetness in water of some compounds

Less sweet that sucrose		*More sweet than sucrose*	
Lactose	0.16	Fructose	1.1
Liquid glucose	0.23	Cyclamate	30.0
Sorbitol	0.54	Saccharin	350.0
Glucose (dextrose)	0.75		

Sucrose (Household sugar) = 1

II. Disaccharides

Disaccharides are compound sugars composed of two monosaccharides. The manner in which two monosaccharide molecules are joined together is of particular interest, e.g., both cellobiose and maltose contain two molecules of glucose, but they differ in the manner in which the glucose units are joined. In maltose it is alpha 1, 4-Glucosidic linkage while in cellobiose it is beta 1, 4-Glucosidic linkage. Humans lack necessary enzyme to hydrolyse beta glucosidic enzyme and so cannot utilise cellulose as a source of glucose. The microbes present in ruminants can secrete necessary enzymes and thus can utilise cellulose materials. The termite also contains such microbes whose enzymes (*Cellulase*) catalyse cellulose hydrolysis of the wood or straw.

1. *Sucrose* : Sucrose is known as beet sugar, cane sugar, table sugar or simply as sugar. It is probably the largest selling pure organic compound in the world. As its names apply, sucrose is obtained from sugar canes and sugar beets (whose juice contain 14-20% sugar) by evaporation of the water and recrystallisation. The dark brown liquid that remains after crystallisation of the sugar is sold as molasses.

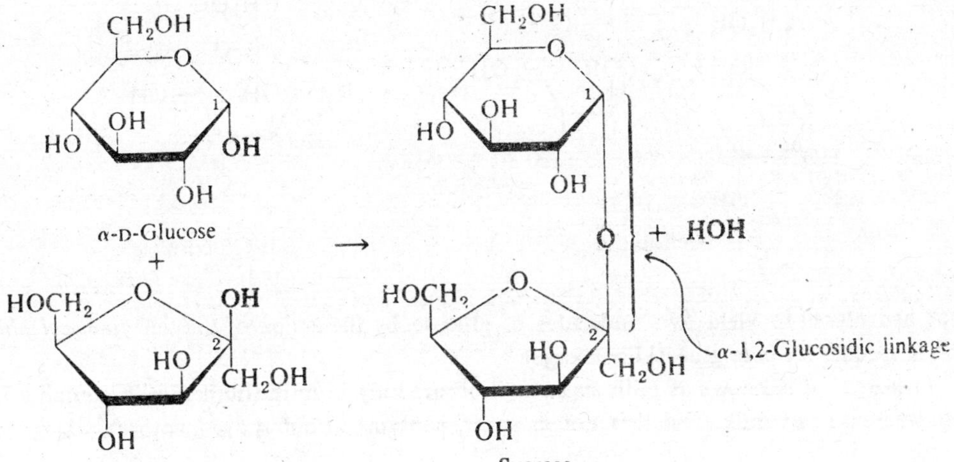

Sucrose

The presence of the 1, 2-glucosidic linkage makes it impossible for sucrose to exist in the alpha or beta configuration or in the open chain form. This is a direct result of the fact that the potential aldehyde group of the glucose moity and the ketone group of the fructose moity have been tied up in the formation of the 1, 2 (head-to-head) linkage. As long as the sucrose molecule remains in tact, it can not uncyclise to form the open chain structure. Sucrose, therefore, does not undergo reactions that are typical of aldehydes and ketones, and it is said to be a *non-reducing* sugar.

2. *Maltose* : It does not occur in free state but occurs in animals as the principal sugar formed by the enzymatic (ptyalin) hydrolysis of starch. It is fairly abundant in germinating

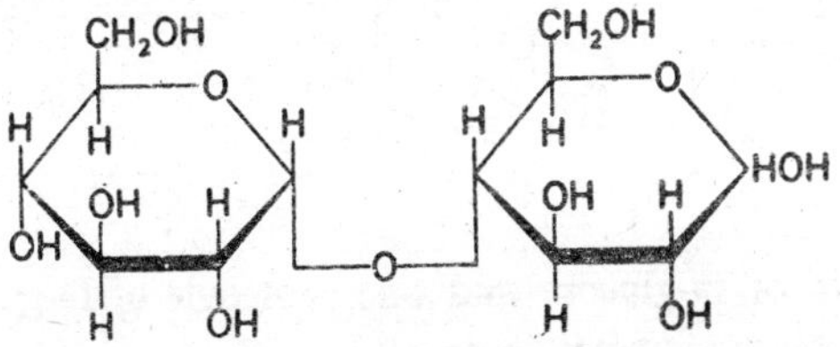

Maltose

grain where it is formed by the enzyme (diastase) breakdown of starch. In the manufacture of beer, maltose is liberated by the action of malt (germinating barley) on starch, and for this reason it is often referred to as *malt sugar*.

3. *Cellobiose* : Cellobiose is obtained by the partial hydrolysis of cellulose. It may be

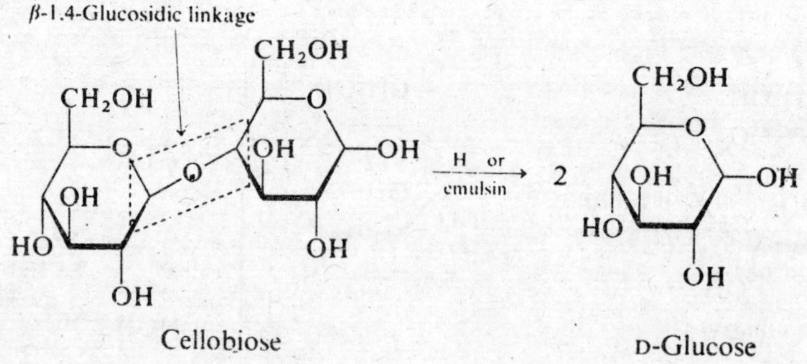

β-1.4-Glucosidic linkage

Cellobiose $\xrightarrow[\text{emulsin}]{\text{H or}}$ 2 D-Glucose

further hydrolysed to yield two molecules of glucose by the action of the enzyme *cellobiase* (which is specific for beta glucosidic linkage).

4. *Lactose* **:** **It is known as milk sugar as it occurs only in milk (human milk contains 7.5% lactose whereas cows milk, which is not as sweet, contains about 4.5% lacotose). Lactose is**

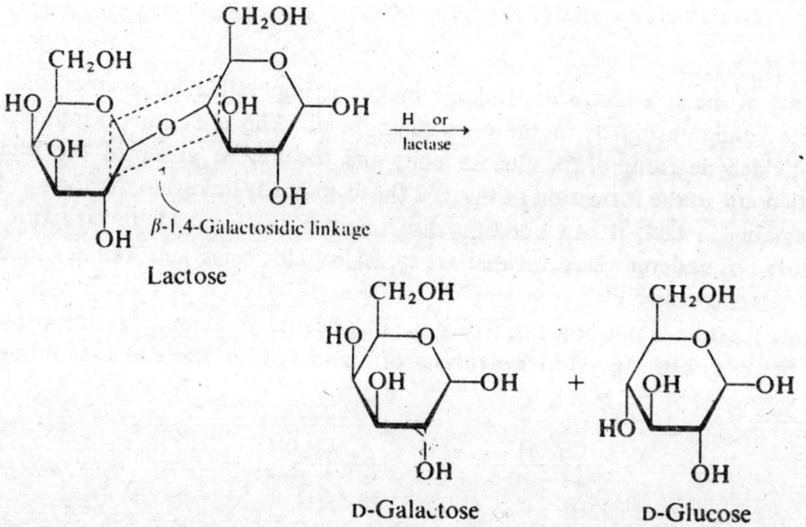

β-1.4-Galactosidic linkage

Lactose $\xrightarrow[\text{lactase}]{\text{H or}}$ D-Galactose + D-Glucose

composed of one molecule of D-glucose and one nolecule of D-galactose which are obtained upon hydrolysis of lactose by the enzyme ***lactase.***

III Polysaccharides

These are the most abundant carbohydrates found in nature. They serve as reserve food substances and as structural components of plants. The members of this group are condensation products joined together by glycosidic linkages. Biochemically the three most important members are starch, glycogen and cellulose. These are homopolysaccharides since

each of them yields only one type of monosaccharide (glucose) upon complete hydrolysis.

Heteropolysaccharides on the other hand yield more than one particular type of components (sugar acids, amino sugars or non-carbohydrates) etc. as in hemicelluloses, gums, mucilages etc.

Starch: This is the most important source of carbohydrates in the human diet. We often think of potatoes as a "starchy" food, yet other plants contain a much greater percentage of starch (e.g., potatoes 15%, wheat 55%, maize 65% and rice 75%).

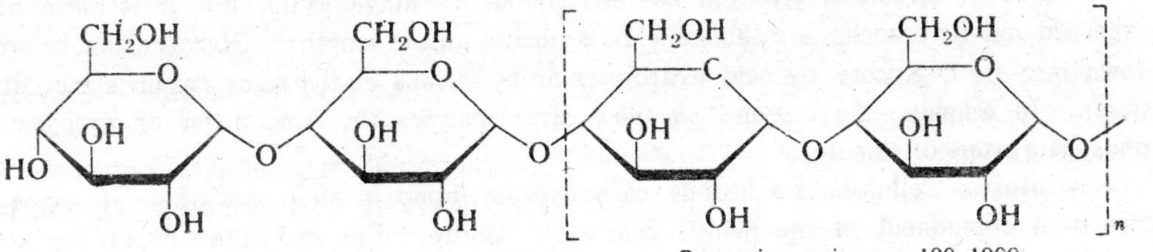

Repeating unit; n = 100–1000

Amylose

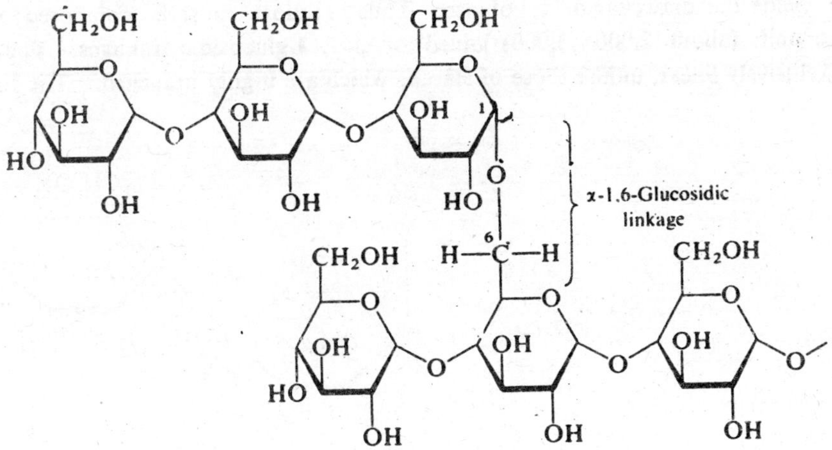

α-1,6-Glucosidic linkage

Amylopectin

Starch is a mixture of two polymers, *amylose* (10-20 percent) and *amylopectin* (80-90 percent). Amylose is a straight chain polysaccharide composed entirely of D-glucose units joined by an α - 1, 4-glucosidic linkage, as in maltose. Thus amylose might be thought of as polymaltose. Amylopectin is a branched chain polysaccharide composed of glucose units which are linked primarily by α - 1, 4—glucosidic bonds, but that have an occasional α - 1, 6-glucosidic linkage responsible for the branching. It has been estimated that there are over 1,000 glucose units in amylopectin, and that branching occurs about one over 25 units.

The complete hydrolysis of starch (amylose and amylopectin) yields glucose, in three succesive stages, which is as follows :

$$\text{Starch} \xrightarrow[\textit{amylase}]{H_+ \text{ or}} \text{Dextrins} \xrightarrow[\textit{amylase}]{H_+ \text{ or}} \text{Maltose} \xrightarrow[\textit{maltase}]{H_+ \text{ or}} \text{Glucose}$$

Glycogen: It is the polysaccharide of the animal body and is often called animal starch. The amount of glycogen in animal tissues is relatively small, 1.5-4.0 per cent in the liver and 0.5-1.0 per cent in the muscle. Fasting animals draw upon these glycogen reserves to obtain that glucose needed to maintain a proper state of metabolic balance.

In terms of structure, glycogen is quite similar to amylopectin, but it is more highly branched and its branches are shorter (12-18 glucose unit in length). Glycogen can be broken down into its D-glucose by acid hydrolysis or by means of the same enzymes that attack starch. In animals, the enzyme *phosphorylase* catalyses the breakdown of glycogen into phosphate esters of glucose.

Cellulose: Cellulose is a fibrous carbohydrate found in all plants where it serves as a structural component of the plant's cell wall. Cotton fibre and filter paper are almost entirely cellulose. Wood is about 50% cellulose. Most of straw contains 20—40% cellulose.

Complete hydrolysis of cellulose yields only D-glucose, whereas partial hydrolysis of cellulose yields the disaccharide cellobiose. Thus cellulose must be composed of chains of D-glucose units (about 2,000—3,000) joined by β 1, 4-glucosidic linkages. The chains are almost exclusively linear, unlike those of starch, which are highly branched. The linear nature

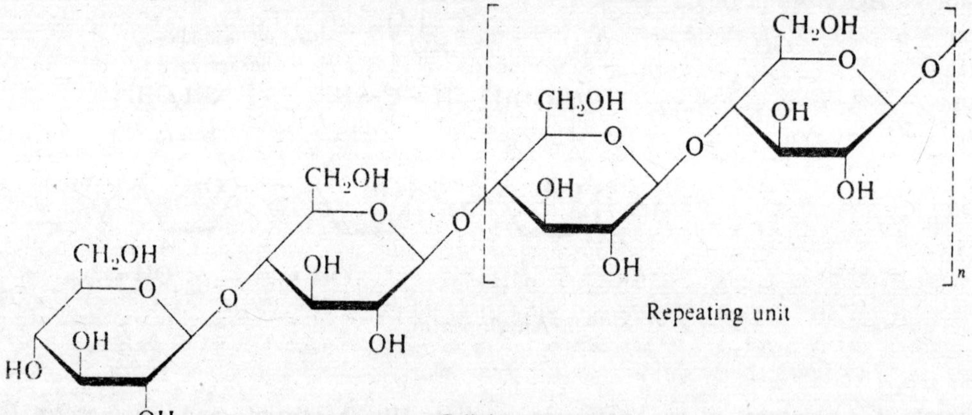

CH₂OH O OH HO OH O CH₂OH O OH OH O CH₂OH O OH OH O CH₂OH O OH OH O n

Repeating unit

Cellulose

of the cellulose chain allows a great deal of hydrogen bonding between hydroxyl groups on adjacent chains. As a result, the chains are closely packed into fibres, and there is little interaction with water or with any other solvent.

The uniform structure of cellulose, being polyglucan with β-1-4 linkage, is associated with high insolubility and refractoriness to many reagents that will dissolve most other polysaccharides. The insolubility of cellulose has not necessarily indicated low digestibility.

While cellulose may have chemical uniformity as β-glucan, nutritionally it is quite variable, principally because as forage ages, the lignin-to-cellulose ratio rises and digestibility declines. Native celluloses also vary widely in fermentation rate, which may be limited by crystallinity or some kind of cross-linking. Most forage or vegetable celluloses are apparently uncrystalline, as they exist in the plant cell wall but may become crystallized when the branched hemicelluloses and three-dimensional lignin components are removed by chemical treatments. This allows cellulose chains to come together. Drying may be an important part of the process to elicit such crystallization. Thus it is possible through de-lignification to obtain a cellulose that is both more potentially digestible, but which ferments at a slower rate than the available part of native carbohydrate.

Cellulose yields, D-glucose upon complete acid hydrolysis, yet human and the carnivorous animals cannot utilise cellulose as a source of glucose. Our digestive juices lack the enzymes that hydrolyse beta glucosidic linkages. Ruminants can do so as they contain microorganisms in the digestive tracts whose enzyme *(Cellulose)* catalyse cellulose hydrolysis.

Hemicellulose: **These are the most complex plant carbohydrates which are present not only in the cell walls of all plants and trees but also found in certain seeds. Hemicellulose and lignin together form the incrusting material of the secondary wall thickening of plant cells, thus the cell walls gets strengthened.**

Hemicellulose is much less resistant to chemical degradation than cellulose, soluble in mild alkali as well as in mild acid.

Basically it is a polymer of D-xylose made up of β 1, 4 linked xylose units (a pentose sugar) with side chains of other sugars or compounds derived from sugars. Hemicelluloses obtained from leaves and stems of most plants have main chain of xylose units linked with side chains of arabinose and uronic acids like glucuronic and galacturonic acids. (These acids are formed form glucose and galactose respectively upon oxidation. The sugar acids contains their aldehyde group). In many plant seeds the xylose chain is linked up directly with glucose or mannose. The composition of hemicelluloses thus are found variable among plant parts and with species. Hemicellulose *A* is less bonded, often higher in xylan and relatively richer in stems than leaves. Hemicellulose *B* contains more branched fractions often high in arabinose or in various urononic acids.

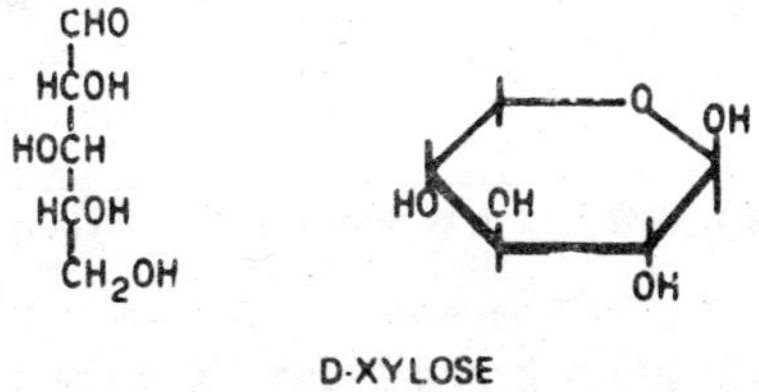

CHO
HCOH
HOCH
HCOH
CH_2OH

D-XYLOSE

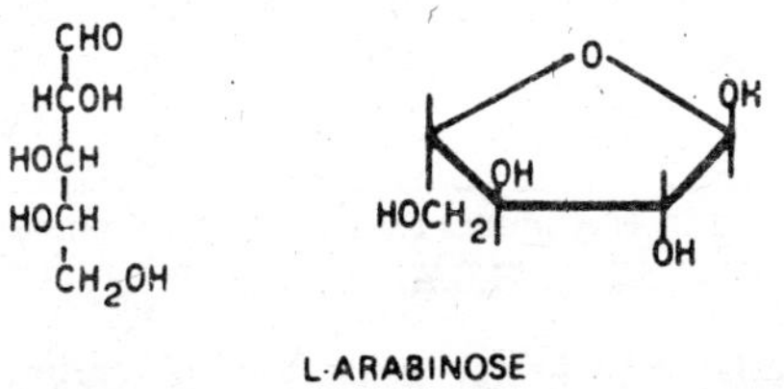

CHO
HCOH
HOCH
HOCH
CH_2OH

L-ARABINOSE

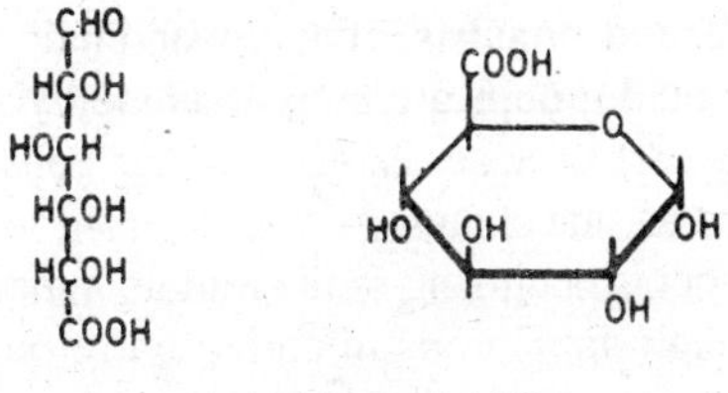

CHO
HCOH
HOCH
HCOH
HCOH
COOH

D-GLUCURONIC ACID

CHO
HCOH
HOCH
HOCH
HCOH
COOH

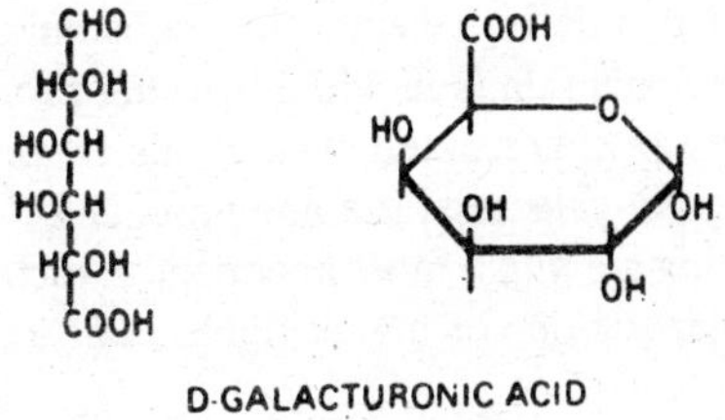

D-GALACTURONIC ACID

The compound may constitute up to 20% of the crude fibre in diets of herbivorous animals. The enzyme *hemicellulases* are produced by some rumen bacteria and ciliate protozoa. All enzymes so far identified appear to be of the endo type which randomly attack the glycosidic chain.

The hemicellulose is neither chemically nor nutritionally uniform. Containing a variety of sugars and linkages it is very much bonded with lignin through its arabinoxylan components. Although hemicellulose is water insoluble polysaccharide but delignification results in a soluble gum-like material which has similar properties to pectin. Since both hemicellulose and pectin have some common sugars and linkages that is why probably both of them individually known as acid soluble polysaccharides.

Once the pentose and uronic acid containing polymers of hemicellulose or pectin is lignified, it will render them insoluble and partially indigestible, whereas the soluble unlignified fraction is completely digestible. This distinction is also relevant to alkali treated grasses and straws where freed hemicellulose becomes pectin-like in its physical and digestive behaviour.

Cellulose and hemicellulose are not digested to sugars but to VFA and gases. These are absorbed at the site of their formation ; that is, they are absorbed through the walls of the rumen and colon in ruminants. In pig, rabbit, guinea pig, dog and poultry through caicum. In human through small and large intestine. In horse VFA's are absorbed through caecum and colon.

Non-ruminants digest relatively more hemicellulose than cellulose as compared to ruminants that digest about equal amounts of both carbohydrates.

Table 10.15

Comparative Digestibilities of fiber fractions by various non-ruminants

Species	*Body wt. kg*	*Feed*	*Hemicellulose %*	*Cellulose %*
Elepnant	1930—3400	Lucerne	49—68	56
Horse	388— 460	Lucerne	55—72	45—66
Zebra	340— 386	Timothy	54—58	39—48
Ass	136— 277	Timothy	53—59	39—45
Pig	48— 89	Lucerne	22—54	9—59
Man	64— 89	Veg+fruit	94—98	15—55
Dog	11— 12	Cereal	30—54	7—22

Source : Nutritional Ecology of the Ruminants by Van Soest, 1982. O & B Books, Inc. Corvallis, Oregon 97330. U.S.A.

A relatively better utlisation of legume compared to grass hemicellulose is made by non-ruminants.

Pectin : It is a cementing substance in plant cell and consists of a linear chain of D-galacturonic acid units in which varying proportions of the acid groups are present as methyl esters. The chains are interrupted at intervals by the insertions of L-rhamnose residues. Other constituent sugars, e.g., D-galactose, L-arabninose, D-xylose are attached as side chains.

Pectins are much more abundant in dicots than in monocots occurring in the middle lamella and intercellular regions of higher plants. The compound although not fibrous in nature but grouped as part of crude fiber. Mammals do not have the necessary enzymes to hydrolyze pectins and their digestibility is performed by microbial enzymes. Inspite of this fact it is highly digestible by most species including human.

Pectin possess considerable water holding (gel) capacity and thus used to reduce diarrhoea in infants and calves and also in jam making.

Plant Gums : These are excretions of certain plants and trees formed at the site of injury or by deliberate incision made at bark or leaves. Gums occur naturally as salts of calcium and magnesium. These are viscous fluids which become hard when dry. The compound is regarded as polysaccharide since the complex substance on hydrolysis yields arabinose, galactose, rhamnose, glucuronic and galacturonic acids. *Gum arabic* is produced by trees of the genus *Acacia* is a well known commercial gum.

Mucilages : These are complex colloidal carbohydrate materials found in bark, seeds, roots and leave of a variety of plants and function as a water holding compound, thus prevent dessication. The mucilage of lucerne and linseed are well known example which produce arabinose, galactose, rhamnose and galacturonic acid on hydrolysis.

CRUDE FIBER AND NITROGEN FREE EXTRACT

The chemical classification of carbohydrates has already been discussed. In the case of ruminant animals, a more relevant classification of the carbohydrates is to divide most of the broad family into nitrogen-free extract (NFE) and crude fiber.

Crude Fiber (CF)

What is Crude Fiber ?

Crude fiber (CF) is also known as Dietary fiber and includes a variety of polysaccharide substances, viz., cellulose, hemicellulose, lignin plus gums, pectins and mucilages. The last three components are not fibrous while lignin is also not at all a carbohydrate component.Inspite of all such shortcornings, CF includes all these plant fractions. A widely accepted definition is *"the sum of lignin and the polysaccharides that are not digested by the endogenous secretions of the digestive tract"* For the purpose of easy estimation the dietary fiber has also been defined as *non-starch polysaccharides and lignin.* Crude fiber is available only in vegetative kingdom.

Tow sorts of fiber can be distinguished : (1) water-insoluble fiber and (2) water-soluble fiber.

Water-soluble fiber corresponds chemically with the non-starchy water-soluble polysaccharides. These polysaccharides can be extracted by cold and hot water and precipitated by ethanol or acetone. Water-soluble fiber-includes β-(1→3) glucan from barley, arabinoxylan from rye, highly methylated pectin from fruits, galactomannan from leguminosae such as guar gum, polysaccharides from algae such as alginate.

Water-insoluble fiber consits of insoluble cell material and is composed of cellulose, hemicellulose (except for the portion present as cereal 'primary' cell walls, which are mainly arabinoxylan, are readily soluble in water or in dilute alkali) pectic substances (which also can sometimes be extracted by hot water, but, very often the use of chelating agents such as EDTA or ammonia oxalate diluted in hot water, is needed to extract them), protein and lignin. In plant kingdom the proportions of these CF components vary widely, depending on the origin, age and environment where plant materials are grown.

This portion of carbohydrates composed of cellulose, hemicellulose and lignin, even though the latter is not a true carbohydrate, it is included as it is almost always associated with cellulose. The component (CF) serves as the structural and protective parts of plants. It is high in forages and low in grains.

After removal of the fat and water, the feed sample is boiled for 30 minutes, with weak H_2SO_4 (1.25%) and then for another 30 minutes with weak NaOH (1.25%). This removes the proteins, soluble sugars and starchs leaving lignin, cellulose and other complex carbohydrates along with the mineral matter. The loss on ignition of the remaining material is defined as crude fiber. This procedure is based on the supposition that carbohydrates which are readily dissolved also will be readily digested by all classes of livestock, and that those which are not soluble under such conditions are not readily digested. Unfortunately it is not so as the treatment dissolves much of the lignin, a non-digestible component. Hence crude fiber is only an approximation of the indigestible material in feedstuffs which is a rough indicator of energy value. Also, the C.F. value is needed for the computation of Total Digestible Nutrient (TDN) of feedstuffs.

Essentially, animal kingdom are uncapable of degrading cellulose or hemicellulose. However, the microscopic life which are habitats of first three sections of the ruminant's stomach and of the caecum and colon of other species, secrete appropriate enzymes capable of hydrolysing the chemical bonds holding the cellulose or hemicellulose molecules together with lignin. Large intestines of many animals including human beings also contain similar microbes thus aid in CF digestion to some extent. In all cases, the end products are volatile fatty acids and gases which are absorbed from the site of production.

Table 10.16

Digestibility of CF by Various Species

Species	*Where digested*	*% Digested*
Ruminants	Rumen, Colon	50–90
Horse	Caecum, Colon	34–40
Pig	Caecum, Colon	3–25
Rabbit	Caecum	16–18
Guinea pig	Caecum	43–40
Dog	Caecum	10–30
Human	Small and large intestine	25–35
Poultry	Caeca	20–30

Factors affecting Utilisation of C.F.

1. *Age of the animal*

In general, young animals are less able to digest cellulose than adults.

2. *Nutritional habits of the animal*

It is easy to demonstrate increasing digestibility of CF with an increasing length of time that fiber has been a part of the diet.

3. *Nutrient make up of the diet*

4. *Species of animals*

5. *Age of feeds rich in CF*

6. *Preparation of Feedstuffs*

Inportance of Dietary Crude Fiber

The concept regarding the role of fiber in human and animal feeds have undergone a considerable revolution in the past decade.

IN HUMAN : The dietary fiber in food undergoes little or no hydrolysis by digestive enzymes in the small intestine. It then passes through the large intestine essentially unchanged. Some components of dietary fiber are degraded by bacteria in the large intestine to form VFA (acetic, propionic and butyric acids), CO_2 and CH_4. The importance of VFA in non-ruminants are not very clear and thus regarded as non-nutritive substance. The caloric yield to the body by this fermentation accounts for only 5% of the caloric equivalent of the total fiber ingested and is of no practical significance. As such the importance of CF lies in their functions which they do physically. Various components of dietary fiber act in different ways in the body. The following overall effect have been postulated :

1. Dietary fiber holds water so that stools are soft, bulky and readily eliminated. Coarse bran is effective but fine bran has little effect. The large, bulky stool also represnts a dilution of colon content so that any potentially toxic substances such as carcinogens that might be present would thus be less harmful.

2. Fiber generally increases motility of the small intestine and colon and decreases transit time. This could result from the stimulation of the mucosa by mechanical effect or perhaps by the by-products of bacterial fermentation. If transit time is shortened, then there could be less time for exposure of the mucosa to harmful toxicants.

3. Pectins, mucilages and gums retard gastric emptying. This can have two benefits : increased satiety so that less food is eaten, thus helping to keep energy intake within the requirement ; and a smoother response by the blood circulation to glucose and hence lesser insulin requirement.

4. Lignin, pectin, mucilages and gums bind bile acids and thereby prevent normal absorption of bile acids containing cholesterol. This tend to lower the serum cholesterol level and thereby scientists believe that a low-fiber diet is associated with the increased incidence of colon cancer, coronary heart disease, atherosclerosis, gallstones, appendicitis and other ailments.

IN RUMINANT : In ruminants diet lacking in fiber but having high proportion of grains, the normal fermentation pattern will be changed and thereby will affect the production. Changed fermentation pattern are as follows :

1. Low pH of the rumen
2. Reduction in the number of cellulolytic and fiber digesting bacteria
3. Large number of lactic acid and propionic acid bactéria and in some instances a virtual disappearence of the ciliate protozoa
4. Substantial fall in acetate and a rise in the ratio of propionate to butyrate in rumen liquor
5. A reduced hydrogenation of dietary unsaturated acids
6. An increased ruminal synthesis of lipid
7. An increased flow of soluble carbohydrate to the intestine
8. In milking cows, milk fat content and total yield are depressed by up to 60%
9. The proportion of saturated fatty acids in milk fat is decreased and that of unsaturated fatty acids including polyunsaturated acids are increased
10. Increase deposition of body fat and an increase of up to 0.5% unit in milk protein content.
11. Development of acidosis, rumen parakeratosis and lack of bulk promotes flabby muscle tone and thereby causing displacement of abomasum.

Nitrogen-free Extract (NFE)

The relatively soluble carbohydrates are classified as the nitrogen-free extract (NFE) and include the mono-and disaccharides plus the starches and perhaps a part of the hemicelluloses, based on their relative solubility and digestibility and some cellulose and pentosans along with a limited amount of lignin.

There is no practical method for exact determination of the NFE portion of feedstuffs. Rather, it is determined mathematically by subtracting all other from 100 :

$$\text{NFE}\ \% = 100 - \left(\begin{array}{c} \text{Moisture}\ \% + \text{Crude protein}\ \% + \text{Ether extract}\ \% \\ + \text{Crude fiber}\ \% + \text{Ash}\ \% \end{array} \right)$$

For feeding purposes this calculation has proved satisfactory, although it is not too accurate.

Lignin

The term lignin is not a single substance but a class of substances which are indigestible and

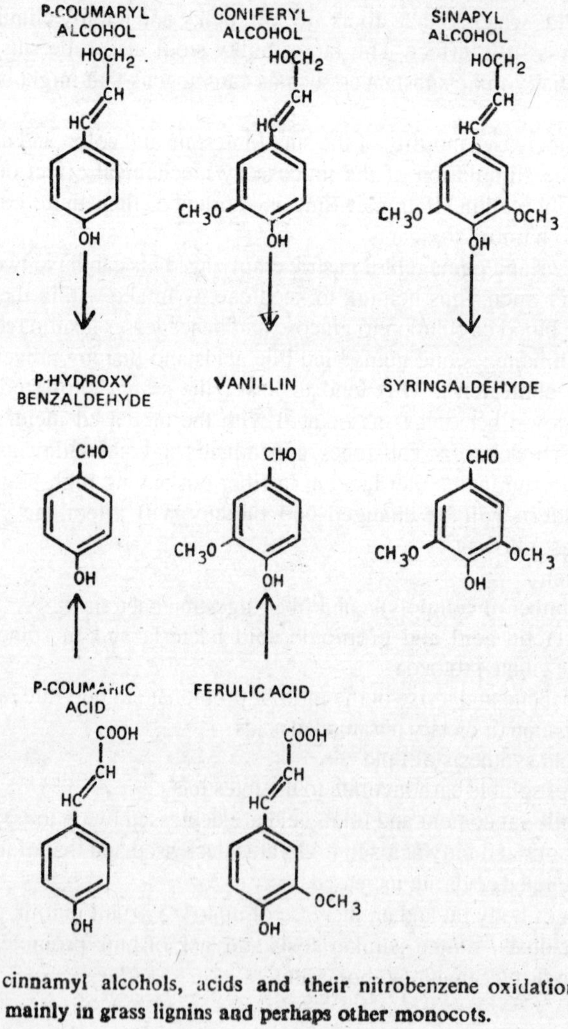

P-COUMARYL ALCOHOL — CONIFERYL ALCOHOL — SINAPYL ALCOHOL

P-HYDROXY BENZALDEHYDE — VANILLIN — SYRINGALDEHYDE

P-COUMARIC ACID — FERULIC ACID

The relation between cinnamyl alcohols, acids and their nitrobenzene oxidation products. Ferulic and P-Coumaric acids occur mainly in grass lignins and perhaps other monocots.

major components of the cell wall of certain plant materials, such as wood, hulls, straws and overfipe hays.

True lignin appears to be a polymerised product of (1) phenylpropanoid alcohols, (2) ferulic and (3) para coumaric acids, which vary in proportion among generic plant sources. The second and third compounds occur mainly in grass lignins and perhaps other monocot. Thus having high molecular weight with carbon to carbon bonds and ether linkages are resistant to the hydrolytic action of acids and alkalis. Like other phenolic compounds lignin is very liable to oxidation.

The lignins of grass and legumes always contain some nitrogen (1.5 – 2.0%). *The lignins of woody trees, on the other hand, contain no nitrogen.* Grass lignins are considerably more soluble in alkali than are lignins from wood or from non-grass forage.

Influence of lignin on digestibility

Lignin is the main factor limiting digestibility in forages. Physical incrustation and entrapment of plant fibres within lignified cell walls renders them inaccessible to enzymes that would normally digest them.

An alternative mechanism is the presence of lignin-carbohydrate linkages resistant to cellulolytic enzymes but are easily cleaved by alkali. That is why alkali treatments of graminaecious straws without washing increase digestibility without alteration of lignin content.

Delignification and Improvement of Straw

It was observed as early as 1880 that delignification increased the digestibility of cellulose. Since that time various methods have been applied to increase digestibility of wood, straw and other highly lignified materials. Chemical removal involves either destruction or extruction of lignin. Lignin is largely soluble in alkali with high temperature and pressure or with bisulphite treatment, as lignosulphonic acid, Neutral systems may involve oxidative delignification and bleaching with chlorine or chlorine dioxide. However, alkali treatments (NaOH) without washing as described earlier is a feasible system, the additional advantages include (1) no waste residues, (2) simpler & (3) low cost.

Biological delignification

Lignin destruction may be possible by the use of lignin-destroying fungi or bacteria which are all aerobic in nature. The process requires a considerable amount of time—weeks to months. Some control over the culture to avoid microbial destruction of the already released carbohydrate would seem necessary, while some lignin-destroying organisms may depend on freed carbohydrate for growth. The method thus requires standardisation.

OTHER METHODS FOR PARTITIONING CARBOHYDRATES

Since 1960 efforts to find alternative schemes of greater precision to evaluate forages have shown promise. Dr. P.J. Van Soest in 1965 developed a method which makes use of the concept that the dry matter of plant origin consists of two principal parts: *Cell wall* and *Cell contents.*

Table 10.17

Division of Forage Organic Matter by System of Analysis Using Detergents (Van Soest, 1966)

Fraction	*Components*	*Nutritional available*	
		Ruminant	*Non-ruminant*
Cell contents (*soluble in neutral detergent*)	Lipids	Virtually complete	Highly available
	Sugars, organic acids, and water soluble matters	,,	,,
	Starch	,	,,
	Non-protein nitrogen	,,	,,
	Soluble protein	,,	,,
	Pectin	,,	,,
Cell wall (Fibre insoluble in neutral detergent)			
(1) *Soluble in acid detergent*	Hemicellulose	Partial	Very low
(2) *Insoluble in acid detergent* (acid detergent fibre)	Cellulose	,,	,,
	Lignin	Indigestible	Indigetible
	Lignified nitrogen compounds	,,	,,
	Heat damaged protein	,,	,,
	Silica	,,	,,

Plant cell contents consist of sugars, starch, soluble carbohydrates, pectin, non-protein nitrogen, protein, lipids and miscellaneous other water-soluble materials, including minerals and several vitamins. True digestibility is almost complete, averaging 98 per cent.

The cell walls of feeds of plant origin are not uniformly nutritious, in the sense that their principal components consist of cellulose, hemicellulose, silica, lignin, etc., singly or in such combinations as nitrogen-hemicellulose or lignocellulose differ widely in nutrition availability depending on the kind and maturity of the plant as well as on the age and species of the animal fed. Nitrogen-hemicellulose are not at all digestible. Chemical procedure to estimate various organic components are given below after Van Soest method.

Van Soest and Moore at U.S.D.A. have found high correlation of the *in vivo* digestibility of the cell contents, of the cell wall, and of the lignin with the *in vitro* data. Their formula for predicting the *in vivo* apparent digestibility of cattle feed (as dry matter) is:

$$0.98\ \text{NDS} + \text{W}\ (147.3 - 78.9 \log \text{lignin}) + 12.9 \text{ per cent}$$

in which 12.9 per cent is the constant percentage of the weight of the feed due to metabolic dry matter. NDS and lignin are expressed as percentages of a unit weight of feed. If the constants of this equation are, in fact, constants for feeds in general, it means that we will have a valid, entirelv in *in vitro* method of describing the nutritionally available energy of feedstuffs.

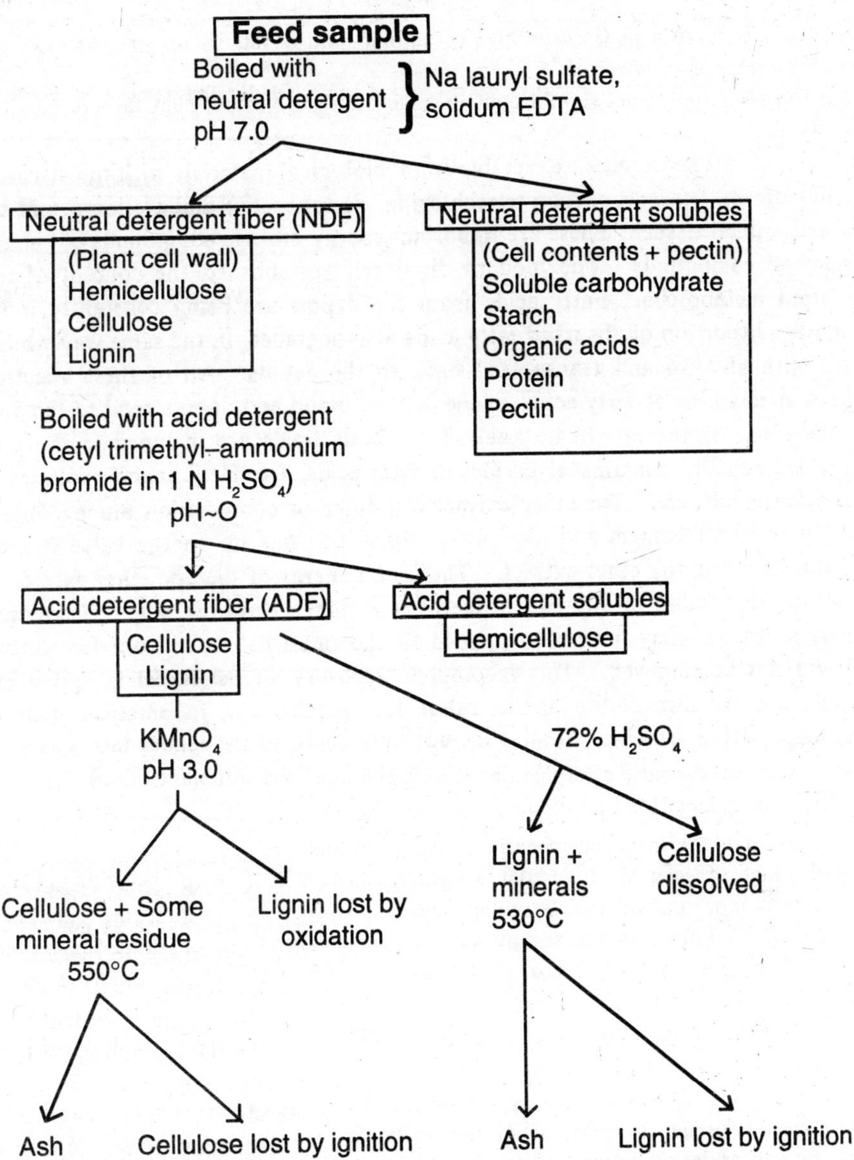

Fig. 10.5 The Van Soest method of partitioning fiber in feeds.

LIPIDS

The term lipid refers to any compound that is soluble in ether or benzene or in chloroform, but only sparingly soluble in water. In routine feed analysis, all kinds of lipids are determined together as the ether extract.

Fats are esters of glycerol that are solid at room temperature while oils are glycerol esters that are liquid at body temperature. 98% of animal lipid is fat. *Waxes are esters of fatty acids with alcohols other than glycerol.*

Ration for adult ruminants should contain no more than 3–5 per cent fat and 15–20% fat for non-ruminants.

Lipids include all substances extractable from biological materials with the usual fat solvents (ether, chloroform, benzene, carbon tetrachloride, acetone, etc.) and are important constituents of plant and animal tissue. These are important energy storage compounds of animal kingdom and structural compounds. The modern discoveries established the concept of the dynamic state of lipid metabolism. Fatty acids from the depots are being constantly mobilised and transported. A portion of absorbed fatty acids also degraded in the same way while others are combined with glycerol and transported back to the depots. All of these reactions are so balanced that mixtures of fatty acids in the depots, blood and organs tend to remain at equilibrium condition. In the proximate analysis of foods lipids are included in the ether extract portion which actually contains glycerides of fatty acids, free fatty acids, cholesterol, lecithin, alkalies, volatile oils, etc. The ether extract will differ in composition among different foods particularly in sterol content and also wax. Since this has no energy value it will affect the energy value of the entire ether extract. The useful energy of dietary ether extract is its gross energy minus that found in subsequent faecal excretion. However, when faeces are extracted with ether, soaps that may have been formed in the intestinal tract from free fatty acids and calcium will not be removed. This incomplete recovery of the faecel fat gives erroneously high value, for the digestibility of the ration fat, particularly in practical diets containing relatively high calcium content. Lipids include fatty acids, soaps, neutral fats, waxes, cholesterol and other types of steroids, phosphatides, prostaglandins, fat soluble vitamins like A, D, E, K, and the very abundant chlorophylls in green forages.

Chemically lipids are made up of carbon, hydrogen and oxygen.

The percentage of each by molecular weight is: carbon 77%, hydrogen 12% and oxygen 11%. Because there is more carbon and hydrogen and less oxygen in the molecule, fats and oils supply approximately 2.25 times as much energy as an equal weight of carbohydrates or protein. One gram of typical carbohydrate yields 4.2 kcal of gross energy when completely oxidized while a gram of typical fat yields 9.45 kcal,.

Body fat when in excess are stored mainly in adipose tissue, approximately 50% of which are found under the skin, i.e., subcutaneous fat.

Apart from adipose tissue, fats are also present in the cytoplasm as well as the cell wall throughout the body. Nervous tissues are particularly rich in lipids.

Excess fat accumulation, however, can be deterimental. It puts constant strain on the heart, forcing it to pump blood further. It contributes to circulatory diseaseas and shortens our lives. Exercise discourages fat accumulation by consuming energy. On the otherhand deficiency of fats and particularly essential fatty acids will hamper absorption of fat soluble vitamins, will affect productivity of the animals and in extreme cases it may prove to be fatal.

CLASSIFICATION OF LIPIDS

Unlike polysaccharides and proteins, lipids are not polymers – they lack a repeating monometric unit. Lipids have been classified in several different ways. The present classification is one the basis of whether they are *saponifiable* or *nonsaponifiable*. (Saponification is the alkaline hydrolysis of lipids, particularly of glyceride, that yields sodium or potassium salts of fatty acids i.e., soaps.)

The saponifiable and non-saponifiable lipids are further subdivided according to their hydrolysis products.

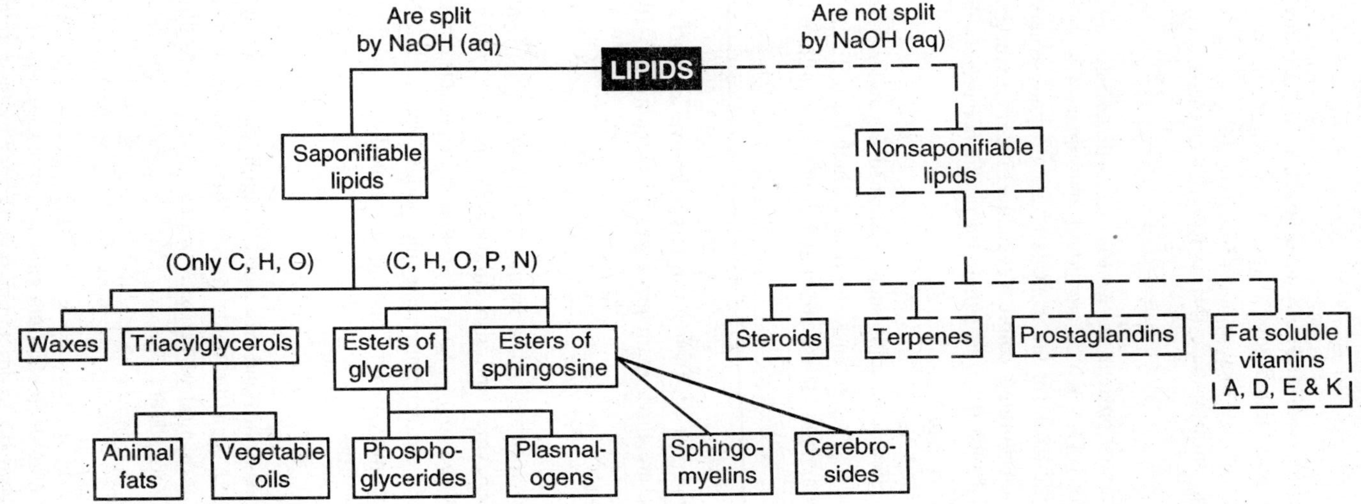

Another way of classifying lipids is on the basis of chemical nature of individual lipids : (1) Simple lipids areesters of fatty acids with various alcohols. Fats and oils and waxes are simple lipids. Fats & oils are esters of fatty acids with glycerol, and waxes are esters of a fatty acids with alcohols other than glycerol; (2) Compound lipids are esters of fatty acids containing groups in addition to an alcohol and fatty acids. They include Phospholipids (phosphatides) are fats containing phosphoric acid and N. Glycolipids are fats containing carbohydrate and, often, N, and lipoproteins are lipids bound to proteins in blood and other tissues; (3) Derived lipids include substances derived from the previous groups as in serial 1 and 2 above by hydrolysis – that is, fatty acids, glycerols and other alcohols; (4) Miscellanious lipids such as Sterolswhich are lipids with complex phenanthrene – type ring structures, whereas terpenes are compounds that usually have isoprenes type structures.

Chemical Properties of Triacylglycerol

1. ***Hydrolysis***

The ester links between glycerol and fatty acids present in all triacylglycerols get separated (hydrolysed) by enzymes as present in digestive tract, or by treating the compound with superheated steam, or by boiling with acids or alkalies. In alkali hydrolysis using NaOH or KOH, the fatty acids liberated will combine with the base (Na or K) to form soaps.

2. ***Additive reactions***

The unsaturated fatty acids present in neutral fat will exhibit all the additive reactions (hydrogenation, halogenation). Oils which are liquid at ordinary temperatures on hydrogenation become solidified. This is the basis for the vanaspathi manufacture, where oils like sunflower oil, cotton seed oil and other unsaturated edible vegetable oils are hydrogenated and converted to saturated fats. Unlike animal fats, these vegetable oil products have no cholesterol.

3. ***Oxidation***

Fats very rich in unsaturated fatty acids such as linseed oil undergo spontaneous oxidation at the double bond forming aldehydes, ketones and resins which form thin transparent coating on the surfaces to which the oil is applied. These are called drying oils and are used in the manufacture of paints and varnishes.

4. ***Rancidity***

The process of development of off-flavours in fats is known as rancidity and the fat is said to have become rancid. There are three main processes of rancidity: (a) Hydrolytic, (b) Oxidative and (c) Ketonic.

(a) Hydrolytic Rancidity

Naturally occurring fats, specially those from animal sources are contaminated with enzyme like *lipase*. The action of enzymes and also atmospheric moisture and temperature bring about partial hydrolysis of the fat and some degree of oxidation of unsaturated fatty acids at the double bond, all of which develop a characteristic taste and odour. Vegetable oils containing substances like vit E, phenols, hydro-quinine, tannins and other antioxidants and therefore, prevent development of rancidity for longer time.

(b) Oxidative Rancidity

Very common for all types of fats and oils. The oxidation takes place at the unsaturated linkage. Certain metals, e.g., copper hasten the oxidation. Further addition of oxygen to the unsaturated linkage also results in the formation of peroxide which on decomposition, yields aldehydes and ketones having pronounced off odour.

(c) Ketonic Rancidity

This type is most frequently encountered as a result of fungus contamination such as by *Aspergillus niger* and blue green mould, *Penicillium glaucum* on coconut or other oilseeds. The tallowy odour developed may be due to aldehydes and ketones formed by the action of the enzymes present in fungi on oil or fat.

Characterisation of fats

1. *Saponification Number*

Number of milligrams of KOH required to saponify the free and combined fatty acids present in 1 gram of fat. It is a measure of the extent of unsaturated fatty acids present in fats or oils. Higher value indicates that the fat is made up of low molecular weight fatty acids and vice versa.

HOW DETERGENTS WORK ?

Soap Water is a very poor cleansing agent because it can't penetrate greasy substances, the "glues" that bind soil to skin and fabrics. When just a little soap is present, however, water cleans very well, especially warm water. Soap is a simple chemical, a mixture of the sodium or potassium salts of the long-chain fatty acids obtained by the saponification of fats or oils.

Detergents Soap is just one kind of detergent. All detergents are surface-active agents that lower the surface tension of water. All consist of ions or molecules that have long hydrocarbon portions plus ionic or very polar sections at one end. The accompanying structures illustrate these features and show the varieties of detergents that are available.

Although soap is manufactured, it is not called a synthetic detergent. This term is limited to detergents that are not soap, that is, not the salts of naturally-occurring fatty acids obtained by the saponification of lipids. Most synthetic detergents are salts of sulfonic acids, but others have different kinds of ionic or polar sites. The great advantageof synthetic detergents is that they work in hard water and are not precipitated by the hardness ions — $Mg2^+$, $Ca2^+$, and the two ions of iron. The anions of the fatty acids present in soap from messy precipitates with these ions. The anions of synthetic detergents do not have this property.

In part *(a)* we see the hydrocarbon tails of the detergent work their way into the hydrocarbon environment of the grease layer. ("Like dissolves like" is the principle at work here.) The ionic heads stay in the water phase, and the grease layer becomes pincushioned with electrically charged sites. In part *(b)* we see the grease layer breaking up, aided with some agitation or scrubbing. Part *(c)* shows a magnified view of grease globules studded with ionic groups; being like-charged, these globules repel one another. They also tend to dissolve in water, so they are ready to be washed down the drain.

$$\begin{array}{l} CH_2-O-\overset{O}{\overset{\|}{C}}-R \\ | \\ CH-O-\overset{O}{\overset{\|}{C}}-R' \\ | \\ CH_2-O-\overset{O}{\overset{\|}{C}}-R'' \end{array} + 3NaOH\,(aq) \xrightarrow[\text{heat}]{} \begin{array}{l} CH_2-OH + NaO-\overset{O}{\overset{\|}{C}}-R \\ | \\ CH-OH + NaO-\overset{O}{\overset{\|}{C}}-R' \\ | \\ CH_2-OH + NaO-\overset{O}{\overset{\|}{C}}-R'' \end{array}$$

Glycerol Mixture of salts0

2. *Iodine Value*

It is defined as the number of grams of iodine absorbed by 100 g of fat. Since iodine is taken up only by the double bonds, a high iodine number indicates a high degree of unsaturation of the fatty acids in the fat.

3. *Reichert-Meissl Value*

This is defined as the number of millilitres of 0.1 N alkali (sodium or potassium hydroxide) required to neutralize the steam volatile water soluble fatty acids present in 5 grams sample of fat. The test determines the amount of butyric acid and caproic acid which are readily soluble in water and a part of caprylic acid which is slightly soluble in H_2O.

SAPONIFIABLE LIPIDS

Fats and Oils

Like Carbohydrates, the fats contain the elements carbon, hydrogen and oxygen but they are relatively much richer in carbon and hydrogen as shown below.

	Carbon	Hydrogen	Oxygen
Fat	77	12	11
Starch	44	6	50

Because of this large proportion of hydrogen in addition to carbon and the fact that much more atmospheric oxygen instead of internal oxygen must be used to oxidise them, fats produce much more heat than carbohydrates or protein. The burning of 1 gram of hydrogen produces 34.5 kcal while one gram of carbon gives only 8 kcal.

Fats and Oils are the most abundant lipids found in nature. Both types of compounds are called *"Triacylglycerols"* because they are *esters* compound of *three fatty acids* joined to *glycerol*, a trihydroxy alcohol. Formerly these compounds were called triglycerides.

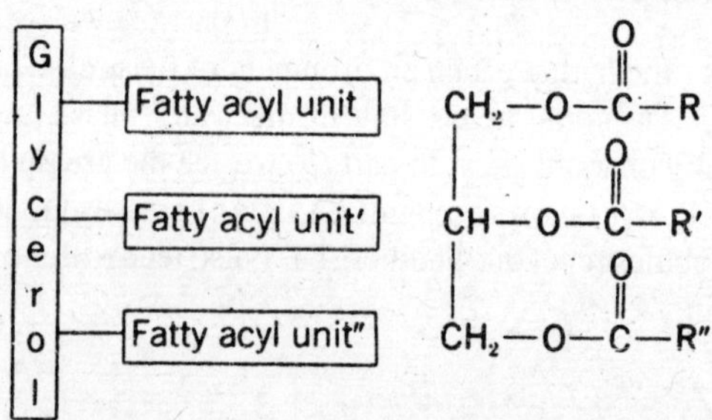

Components of neutral fats (triacylglycerols)

Further classification of triacylglycerols is made on the basis of their physical states at room temperature. It is customary to call a lipid a *fat* if it is a solid at 25°C, and an *oil*, if it is a liquid at the same temperature. These differences in melting points reflect differences in the degree of unsaturation of the constituent fatty acids. Furthermore, lipids obtained from animal sources are usually solids, whereas oils are generally of plant origin. Therefore, we commonly speak of *animal fats* and *vegetable oils*.

Acylglycerols are esters of one, two, or three fatty acids with the trihydroxy alcohol, glycerol. As mentioned earlier, these are designated as simple or mixed acylglycerols depending upon the number of different fatty acids present in the molecule. Tristearin, for example,

$$\begin{array}{l} C_{17}H_{35}-\overset{O}{\overset{\|}{C}}-O-\overset{H}{\overset{|}{C}}-H \\ C_{17}H_{35}-\overset{O}{\overset{\|}{C}}-O-\overset{|}{C}-H \\ C_{17}H_{35}-\overset{O}{\overset{\|}{C}}-O-\underset{H}{\underset{|}{\overset{|}{C}}}-H \end{array}$$

Glyceryl stearate
(Tristearin)
(a simple triacylglycerol)
mp 71°C

$$\begin{array}{l} C_{11}H_{23}-\overset{O}{\overset{\|}{C}}-O-\overset{H}{\overset{|}{C}}-H \\ C_{15}H_{31}-\overset{O}{\overset{\|}{C}}-O-\overset{|}{C}-H \\ C_{17}H_{33}-\overset{O}{\overset{\|}{C}}-O-\underset{H}{\underset{|}{\overset{|}{C}}}-H \end{array}$$

Glyceryl lauropalmitooleate
(a mixed triacylglycerol)

$$\begin{array}{l} C_{17}H_{31}-\overset{O}{\overset{\|}{C}}-O-\overset{H}{\overset{|}{C}}-H \\ C_{17}H_{31}-\overset{O}{\overset{\|}{C}}-O-\overset{|}{C}-H \\ C_{17}H_{31}-\overset{O}{\overset{\|}{C}}-O-\underset{H}{\underset{|}{\overset{|}{C}}}-H \end{array}$$

Glyceryl linoleate
(Trilinolein)
(a simple triacylglycerol)
mp 9°C

indicates a simple triacylglyceride containing only stearic acid in the molecule, whereas 1-oleo-2-stearo-3 palmitin is a triacylglycerol containing oleic, stearic and palmitic acids.

Triacylglycerols are a form of stored energy in animal tissues (adipose cells) and are commonly referred to as neutral fat.

Fatty acids

Fatty acids are integral parts of lipids, and may be divided into : (1) saturated acids ; (2) unsaturated acids ; (3) branched chain acids ; (4) cyclic acids

Table 11.18
Common fatty acids of natural fats and oils

Molecular Formula	Common Name	No. Carbon Atoms	No. Double Bonds	Structural Formula	Melting Point (°C)	Common Source
A. Saturated Fatty Acids						
$C_2H_4O_2$	Acetic	2	0	CH_3COOH	16.6	Major end product of carbohydrate fermentation by rumen organisms, Vinegar.
$C_3H_6O_2$	Propionic	3	0	CH_3CH_2COOH	-22.0	An end product of carbohydrate fermentation by rumen organisms
$C_4H_8O_2$	Butyric	4	0	$CH_3(CH_2)_2COOH$	-7.9	In certain fats in small amounts (especially butter). An end product of carbohydrate fermentation by rumen organisms.
$C_6H_{12}O_2$	Caproic	6	0	$CH_3(CH_2)_4COOH$	-3.4	An end product of carbohydrate fermentation by rumen organisms, butter.
$C_8H_{16}O_2$	Caprylic	8	0	$CH_3(CH_2)_6COOH$	16.3	In small amounts in many fats (including butter), especially those of plant origin
$C_{10}H_{20}O_2$	Capric	10	0	$CH_3(CH_2)_8COOH$	31.2	In small amounts in many fats (including butter), especially those of plant origin, e.g., Coconut oil.

(Contd.)

Molecular Formula	Common Name	No. Carbon Atoms	No. Double Bonds	Structural Formula	Melting Point (°C)	Common Source
$C_{12}H_{24}O_2$	Lauric	12	0	$CH_3(CH_2)_{10}COOH$	43.9	Spermaceti, cinnamon, palm kernel, coconut oils, laurels
$C_{14}H_{28}O_2$	Myristic	14	0	$CH_3(CH_2)_{12}COOH$	54.1	Nutmeg, palm kernel, coconut oils, myrtles
$C_{16}H_{32}O_2$	Palmitic	16	0	$CH_3(CH_2)_{14}COOH$	62.7	Common in all animal and plant fats
$C_{18}H_{36}O_2$	Stearic	18	0	$CH_3(CH_2)_{16}COOH$	69.9	Common in all animal and plant fats
$C_{20}H_{40}O_2$	Arachidic	20	0	$CH_3(CH_2)_{18}COOH$	75.4	Peanut (arachis) oil
$C_{22}H_{44}O_2$	Behenic	22	0	$CH_3(CH_2)_{20}COOH$	79.9	Seeds
$C_{24}H_{48}O_2$	Lignoceric	24	0	$CH_3(CH_2)_{22}COOH$	84.2	Cerebrosides, peanut oil
B. Unsaturated Fatty Acids						
$C_{16}H_{30}O_2$	Palmitoleic	16	1	$CH_3(CH_2)_5CH{=}CH(CH_2)_7COOH$	0.5	Milk fat
$C_{18}H_{34}O_2$	Oleic	18	1	$CH_3(CH_2)_7CH{=}CH(CH_2)_7COOH$	13.4	Olive oil, animal tissues
$C_{18}H_{32}O_2$	Linoleic	18	2	$CH_3(CH_2)_3(CH_2CH{=}CH)_2(CH_2)_7COOH$	11.0	Occur in many seed oil, e.g., maize, groundnut, cotton seed, soybean oils etc., animal body tissues and also in fish oils.
$C_{18}H_{30}O_2$	Linolenic	18	3	$CH_3(CH_2CH{=}CH)_3(CH_2)_7COOH$	-11.2	Vegetable oil like linseed oil, animal body tissues and also in fish oils.
$C_{20}H_{32}O_2$	Arachidonic	20	4	$CH_3(CH_2)_3(CH_2CH{=}CH)_4(CH_2)_3COOH$	-49.5	Groundnut oil, Lecithin, Cephalin.
C. Branched Chain Acid :						
C_3H_7COOH	Isobutyric	4	0	$(CH_3)_2CH\ CH_2OH$	-47.0	Rumen bacteria
C_4H_9COOH	Isovaleric	5	0	$(CH_3)_2CHCH_2CO_2H$	-37.6	Rumen bacteria
D. Cyclic Acid						
$C_{18}H_{32}O_2$	Chaulmoogric acid	18	1	CH = CH H / CH₂—CH₂ ring, C—$(CH_2)_{12}COOH$	68.5	Chaulmogra oil

- Fatty acids are water-insoluble long-chain hydrocarbons with one carboxyl group at the end of the chain. The chains may be saturated, unsaturated, cyclic or branched.

- Fatty acids are detergent-like due to their amphipathic nature; that is, they have nonpolar (CH_3) and polar (-COOH) ends and, in biphasic systems, will orient with the polar end associated with water and the nonpolar end associated with the hydrophobic phase.

- The melting point of fatty acids is related to chain length and degree of unsaturation. The longer the chain length, the higher the melting point, and the greater the number of double bonds, the lower the melting point

- **Saturated fatty acids** have no double bonds in the chain.
  a. Their general formula is

$$CH_3—(CH_2)_n—COOH$$

  where n specifies the number of methylene groups between the methyl and carboxyl carbons.

  b. The systematic name gives the number of carbons, with the suffix-*anoic* appended. Palmitic acid, for example, has 16 carbons and has the systematic name hexadecanoic acid.

- **Unsaturated fatty acids** have one or more double bonds.
  a. The most commonly used system for dsignating the positiion of double bonds in an unsaturated fatty acid is the delta (Δ) numbering system.
    1) The terminal carboxyl carbon is designated carbon 1, and the double bond is given the number of the carbon atom on the carboxyl side of the double bond. For example, palmitoleic acid has 16 carbons and has a double bond between carbons 9 and 10. It is designated as 16:1:Δ^9, or 16:1:9.
    2) The systematic name gives the number of carbon atoms, the number of double bonds (unless it has only one), and bears the suffix *enoic*. Thus, palmitoleic acid is Cis-Δ^9- hexadecenoic acid; linoleic acid, which has 18 carbons and two double bonds, is all (i.e., all double bonds are cis)cis-Δ^9,Δ^{12}-octadecadienoic acid.

    The following lists shows the position of the double bonds in some unsaturated fatty acids :

Oleic ($C_{18:1}$)

$$CH_3.(CH_2)_7.\overset{H}{\overset{|}{C}}{=}\overset{H}{\overset{|}{C}}.(CH_2)_7.COOH \quad (10)\ (9) \qquad (\Delta^9)$$

Linoleic ($C_{18:2}$)

$$CH_3.(CH_2)_4.\overset{H}{\overset{|}{C}}{=}\overset{H}{\overset{|}{C}}.CH_2.\overset{H}{\overset{|}{C}}{=}\overset{H}{\overset{|}{C}}.(CH_2)_7.COOH \quad (13)\ (12)\quad (10)\ (9) \qquad (\Delta^{9,12})$$

Palmitoleic ($C_{16:1}$)

$$CH_3.(CH_2)_5.\overset{H}{\overset{|}{C}}{=}\overset{H}{\overset{|}{C}}.(CH_2)_7.COOH \quad (10)\ (9) \qquad (\Delta^9)$$

Linolenic ($C_{18:3}$)

$$CH_3.CH_2.\overset{H}{\overset{|}{C}}{=}\overset{H}{\overset{|}{C}}.CH_2.\overset{H}{\overset{|}{C}}{=}\overset{H}{\overset{|}{C}}.CH_2.\overset{H}{\overset{|}{C}}{=}\overset{H}{\overset{|}{C}}.(CH_2)_7.COOH \quad (16)\ (15)\quad (13)\ (12)\quad (10)\ (9) \qquad (\Delta^{9,12,15})$$

Arachidonic ($C_{20:4}$)

$$CH_3.(CH_2)_4.(\overset{H}{\overset{|}{C}}{=}\overset{H}{\overset{|}{C}}.CH_2)_4.CH_2.CH_2.COOH \qquad (\Delta^{5,8,11,14})$$

  b. Double bonds in naturally occurring fatty acids are always in a *cis* as opposed to a *trans* configuration.

(Contd.)

$$-CH_2-\overset{H}{\underset{}{C}}=\overset{H}{C}-CH_2)- \qquad -CH_2-\overset{H}{C}=\underset{H}{C}-CH_2)-$$

Cis *Trans*

- **Source**

1. **Nonessential fatty acids.** All nonessential fatty acids can be synthesized from acetyl coenzyme A (acetyl CoA) derived from glucose oxidation. They are nonessential in the sense that they do not have to be obligatorily included in the diet. However, the bulk of nonessential fatty acids in humans may in fact be obtained from the diet, particularly in the case of the high-fat diets of affluent societies.
2. **Essential fatty acids.** Fatty acids of the linoleic ($18:2:\Delta^{9,12}$) and linoenic ($18:3:\Delta^{9,12,15}$) families, which are the precursors of the prostaglandins, must be obtained from the diet. There are no mammalian enzyme systems that can introduce a double bond beyond the ninth carbon atom (9-10 position) of a fatty acid chain, and all double bonds that are introduced are separated by three-carbon intervals. ;This rule, combined with the fact that fatty acid elongation only occurs by two-carbon additions, makes it impossible to synthesize do novo certain polyunsaturated fatty acids.

ESSENTIAL FATTY ACIDS

It is fact that excess of the absorbed carbohydrates are readily changed into fat and that essential lipid constituents such as phospholipids and cholesterol can be made in the body naturally led to to the view that lipids as such are not required in the diet.

Some fifty years ago it has been first observed that the following fatty acids are dietary essentials : linoleic, linolenic and arachidonic acid. Deficiency symptoms of these fatty acids have been observed in mice, poultry, dogs, guinea pigs, swine and human infants. Suggestive evidence that calves, lambs and kids need these acids in their rations has also been reported. Depending on the type of animals, numerous manifestations of these deficiencies are seen ; among them, dermatitis, reduced growth, increased water consumption and retention, necrosis of tail, impaired reproduction and increases in metabolic rate.

Two functions of the essential fatty acids (EFA) have been postulated : (1) precursors of the prostaglandins—a group of hormone like compounds widely distributed in reproductive organs and other tissues of humans and animals. The prostaglandins are biosynthesized from arachidonic acid and have a wide variety of metabolic effects including the following : lower blood pressure, stimulate smooth muscle contraction etc. (2) The other function of EFA is that they are widely distributed in phospholipids and cholesterol esters which inturn constitute a significant part of all cell membranes and lipid transport moieties.

Among the three EFA, linoleic acid (C 18 : 2) and linólenic acid (C 18 : 3) apparently can not be synthesized by animal tissues, or at least not in sufficient amounts to prevent pathological changes, and so must be supplied in the diets. Arachidonic acid (C 20 : 4) can be synthesized from linoleic acid, and therefore, is required in the diet only if linoleic acid is not available or insufficient.

It has long been a puzzling question as to how ruminants derive their essential fatty acids when on the one hand the dietary intake of essential fatty acids (which are all unsaturated) gets destructed by hydrogenation (saturation of double bonds by hydrogen) in the rumen and on the other hand animal body can not synthesise these acids from any source.

The answer is as follows :

(1) For young ruminants, which are born with very little linoleic acid in its tissue lipids but are noted to have higher values during the first few days after birth. No doubt that the maternal origin is the major source but some may be available to the young ruminant as a result of microbial synthesis in the undeveloped rumen.

(2) Adult or young animals with a functioning rumen meet their needs firstly from the digestion of microbial lipids which takes place in the small intestine. In the abomasum dead bodies of millions of microbes are disintegrated. The lipid portion is thus enters the small intestine. In one estimate of it has been noted that at least 140 grams of microbial lipid per 20 hours are available for intestinal digestion by an adult cow. Of the lipid composition of mixed rumen bacteria phospholipid amounts to about 30 percent while the rest 70 percent comprises free fatty acids mostly linoleic and linolenic. There is evidence that rumen bacteria takes up linoleic acid from the rumen and incorporates it into their cell membranes.

(3) Ruminants apparently are able to utilize essential fatty acids much more efficiently

Table 10.19 **Fatty Acid Components of Some Common Fats and Oils**

		Average Composition of Fatty Acids (%)							
Type	Fat or Oil	Myristic Acid	Palmitic Acid	Stearic Acid	Oleic Acid	Linoleic Acid	Iodine Number	Saponification Value	Others
Animal Fats	Butter	8-15	25-29	9-12	18-33	2-4	26-42	210-230	a
	Lard	1-2	25-30	12-18	48-60	6-12	46-70	195-203	b
	Beef tallow	2-5	24-34	15-30	35-45	1-3	30-48	190-200	b
Vegetable Oils	Olive	0-1	5-15	1-4	67-84	8-12	79-90	187-196	
	Peanut	—	7-12	2-6	30-60	20-38	84-100	188-195	
	Corn (Maize)	1-2	7-11	3-4	25-35	50-60	103-128	187-196	
	Cottonseed	1-2	18-25	1-2	17-38	45-55	97-112	190-198	
	Soybean	1-2	6-10	2-4	20-30	50-58	120-141	189-195	c
	Linseed	—	4-7	2-4	14-30	14-25	175-202	187-195	d
	Coconut	13-18	7-10	1-4	5-8	1-3	8-11	191-195	
	Safflower	—	6-7	2-3	12-14	75-80	140-150	188-194	
Marine Oils	Whale	5-10	10-20	2-5	33-40	—	—	—	e
	Fish	6-8	10-25	1-3	—	—	—	—	e

a Also, 3-4% butyric acid, 1-2% caprylic acid, 2-3% capric acid, 2-5% lauric acid.
b Also, linolenic acid, 1%.
c Also, linolenic acid, 5-10%.
d Also, linolenic acid, 45-60%.
e Large percentages of other highly unsaturated fatty acids.

than non-ruminants through selective retention of these substances in their essential role. In ruminants these acids are selectively incorporated into cholesterol esters and phospholipids, while in non-ruminants this selectivity is only partial. Thus ruminants tissue represent species metabolic adaptation.

(4) Even after ruminal hydrogenation, the digesta of these diets contain linoleic acid equivalent to about 0.8% of gross energy intake escape rumen (*Rumen bypass*) to satisfy the animal requirement.

As a result of which we can find no well-authenticated case of essential fatty acid dificiency in adult ruminants or young animals with a functioning rumen.

The dietary supply of linoleic acid for both young and adult ruminants is normally assured when it contributes 1 – 2% of total energy intake. For milk-fed ruminants it is suggested that the dietary concentration of linoleate should be no less than that recommended for non-ruminant animals (i.e., 1% of energy content or 6 grams of linoleate per litre of milk or milk substitutes).

Excessive amounts of unsaturated fatty acids in the diet may induce a vitamin E shortage due to the fact that vitamin E is utilised to prevent unsaturated acids from oxidation.

Waxes

A wax is an ester of a long chain alcohol (usually monohydroxy and a fatty acid. The acids and alcohols normally found in waxes have chains of the order of 12—34 carbon atoms in length. They are not easily hydrolysed as the tracylglycerols and therefore are useful as protecting coatings.

Plant waxes are found on the surfaces of leaves, stems, flowers, and fruits and serve to protect the plant from dehydration and from invasion by harmful micro-organisms. (You can polish an apple to a high luster because of the waxes present in its skin).

Animal waxes also serve as protective coatings. They are found on the surface of feathers skin and hair and help to keep these surfaces pliable and water repellant.

Phospholipids :

Phospholipids have the useful property of attracting both water soluble and fat soluble substances. In combination with protein, they are constituents of cell membranes and

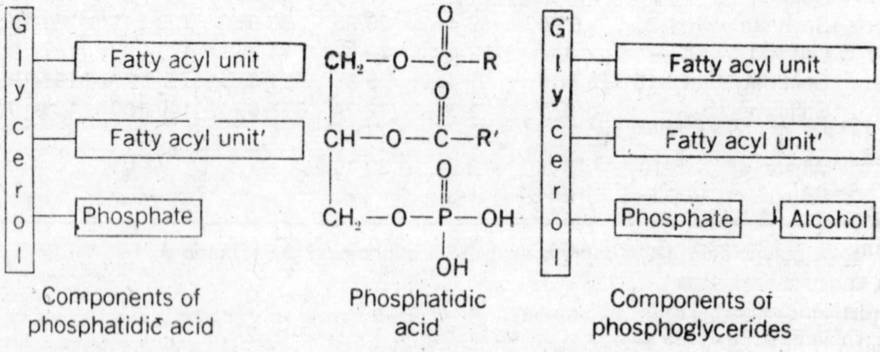

Components of phosphatidic acid
Phosphatidic acid
Components of phosphoglycerides

membranes of subcellular particles where they serve as a liaison between fat soluble and water soluble materials that must penetrate the membrane and interact once they have gained entry. In this structural role, phospholipids are not generally available as an energy source. Even a starved animal will retain the phospholipid necessary to maintain the integrity of tissue cells. It is thought that phospholipids take part in fat metabolism by promoting the transportation of lipids in the blood stream as lipoprotein complexes.

Phospholipids differ chiefly in the specific compound attached to the phosphate group of the phosphatidic acid core. The fatty acids present in the molecule are usually saturated in the α-position (palmitic or stearic) and unsaturated in the β-position (oleic or linolenic).

Phosphatidic Acid

Phosphatidic acids are compounds consisting of glycerol, two fatty acids, and a phosphate group and, as the structure suggests, they easily give rise to triacylglycerols or to phospholipids. Because they are active intermediates in the biosynthesis of other lipid compounds, the phosphatidic acids do not accumulate in tissues in significant amounts.

There are 3 common phospholipids found in animal body which are :

(a) PHOSPHATIDYL CHOLINE (LECITHIN)—A choline melecule is attached with the phosphate group of phosphatidic acid.

(b) PHOSPHATIDYL ETHANOLAMINE (CEPHALIN)—In place of choline if an ethanolamine molecule is attached with the phosphate group of phosphatidic acid, then it becomes phosphatidyl ethanolamine or commonly known as cephalin.

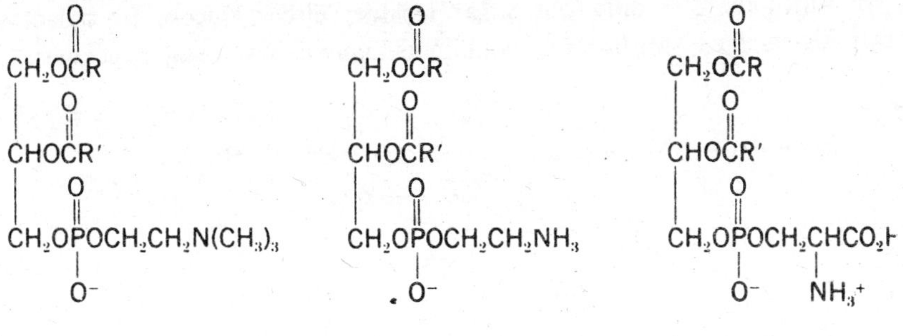

$$\begin{array}{l} CH_2OC(=O)R \\ | \\ CHOC(=O)R' \\ | \\ CH_2OP(=O)(O^-)OCH_2CH_2N(CH_3)_3 \end{array}$$

Phosphatidylcholine (lecithin)

$$\begin{array}{l} CH_2OC(=O)R \\ | \\ CHOC(=O)R' \\ | \\ CH_2OP(=O)(O^-)OCH_2CH_2NH_3 \end{array}$$

Phosphatidylethanolamine

$$\begin{array}{l} CH_2OC(=O)R \\ | \\ CHOC(=O)R' \\ | \\ CH_2OP(=O)(O^-)OCH_2CH(NH_3^+)CO_2H \end{array}$$

Phosphatidylserine

(c) PHOSPHATIDYL SERINE (CEPHALIN LIKE COMPOUNDS)—Here is a serine molecule is attached with the phosphate group.

Sphingosine Lipids :

Sphingolipids, or sphingomyelins, are derivatives of the basic compound sphingosine also known as 4-Sphingenine.

In sphingolipids the amino group of the sphingosine is attached to a fatty acid and the terminal alcoholic group to phosphocholine.

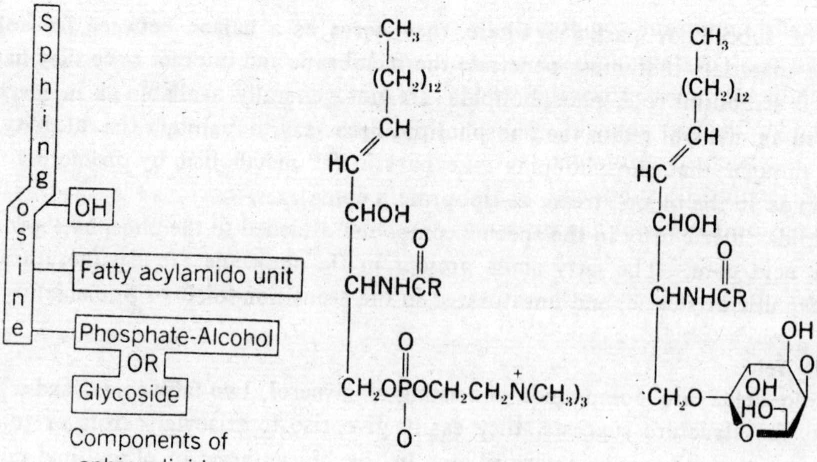

Components of sphingolipids

Sphingomyelin

Cerebrosides

Sphingomyelins occur in large amounts in brain and in the myelin sheath of nerve tissue and derive their name from the structure.

Glycolipids (Cerebrosides)

Glycolipids, as their name implies, are sugar containing lipids. The simplest glycolipid is *Cerebroside,* in which there is only one sugar residue, either glucose or galactose. More complex glycolipids, such as *gangliosides,* contain as many as seven sugar residues. In animal

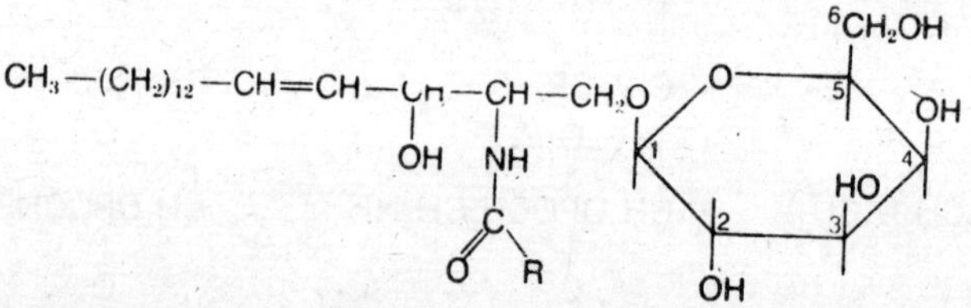

The structure of galactocerebroside (galactolipid).

cells, glycolipids, like sphingomyelin are derived from sphingosine. The sugar molecule(s) is attached with the primary hydroxyl group of sphingosine instead of phosphoryl choline as in sphingomyelin. The compound is abundant in the myelin sheath of nerves and in brain tissue.

NONSAPONIFIABLE LIPIDS

Steroids

The steroids constitute a large group of cyclic compounds that have a common basic structural unit of a phenanthrene nucleus linked to a cyclopentane ring. They include a number

of biologically important compounds as the sterols, the bile acids, the adrenal hormones and sex hormones. They are often found in association with fat. They may be separated from fat after the fat is saponified, since they occur in the "unsaponifiable residue". All of the steroids have a similar nucleus resembling phenanthrene (rings A, B and C) to which a cyclopentane ring (D) is attached. However, the rings are not uniformly unsaturated, so the parent (completely saturated) substance is better designated as cyclopentaneperhydrophenanthrene The positions of the steroid nucleus are numbered as is shown.

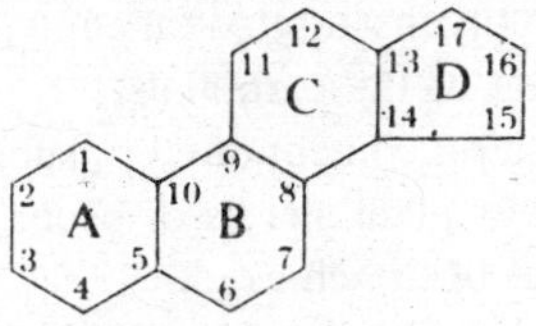

Perhydrocyclopentanophenanthrene

The individual compounds belonging to the steroid group differ in the number and positions of their double bonds and in the nature of the side chain at carbon atom 17. Methyl groups are frequently attached at positions 10 and 14 (constituting Carbon atoms 19 and 18). If the compound has one or more hydroxyl groups and no carbonyl or carboxyl groups, it is *sterol*, and the name terminates in -ol. If it has one or more carbonyl or carboxy-groups, it is a *steroid*.

CHOLESTEROL IN ANIMAL PRODUCTS

Cholesterol is widespread in animal tissue as an essential constituent of all membranes. Further, it is a precusor of steroid hormones, vitamin D and bile acids. Esters of cholesterol predominate in plasma and adrenals, whereas nearly all cholesterol present in brain and nerve tissue is in free form; milk and meat contain small amounts and egg yolk contains fairly high amounts, one whole egg on an average contains 250 mg of cholesterol.

Cholesterol in animal tissues originates mainly from biosynthesis and to a lesser extent from dietary cholesterol absorbed from the intestine. The liver is the major site of cholesterol synthesis, but synthesis also occurs in the intestinal mucosa, arterial wall and other tissues. Acetyl-CoA is the major precursor for biosynthetic cholesterol. The rate of the synthesis occurring in the liver is inversely proportional to the amount of cholesterol present in the body derived from biosynthesis and from dietary input as well. A reaction catalysed by hydroxymethylglutaryl-CoA reductase is the rate-limiting step among the various reactions leading from acetyl-CoA to cholesterol. Many other factors influence cholesterol synthesis in animals; for example, a high level of fat in the diet increases this synthesis and this may be explained as follows. High inputs of saturated fat furnish acetyl-CoA in excess of that required for energy production and body fat synthesis, and the excess acetyl-CoA will be available for cholesterol formation. Thus, the body cholesterol pool will enlarge and the plasma cholesterol level increase. However, if the saturated fats are replaced with polyunsaturated fats, the plasma cholesterol level falls because of a shift of cholesterol from the plasma into the tissues. This is because the presence of polyunsaturated fats in the plasma lipoproteins leads to a decrease in their capacity to carry cholesterol.

The influence of dietary factors on plasma cholesterol levels, well established by experiments with laboratory rodents, seems to be valid in all monogastric species and deserves particular interest because of the correlation of blood cholesterol level and the incidence of atherosclerotic diseases in human beings. An elevated blood cholesterol level is one of the risk factors indicating a susceptibility to atherosclerotic heart disease. Cholesterol is the principal constituent of the plaques which form in the walls of blood vessels causing them to narrow and become rigid, thus reducing the blood flow.

In order to avoid dietary risk factors in human nutrition, it has been recommended (1) to decrease the intake of saturated fat, (2) to increase the intake of polyunsaturated fat by substituting saturated fat with polyunsaturated fat, and (3) to lower cholesterol consumption. For this reason Australian authors have proposed to increase the polyunsaturated fat content of body and milk fat of ruminants by including 'protected' fats in the diet of these animals.

In an attempt to decrease the cholesterol content of eggs, substances which impair the absorption of cholesterol from the intestine, such as plant sterols or pectin, were added to the mash of laying hens, but practical results have not yet been achieved.

Metabolism of Body Cholestrol

Without cholesterol domestic animals including human being cannot live, since it is the most abundant steroid in the diet and precursor of most other animal steroids as has already been mentioned. Regulation of biosynthesis due partly by dietary intake; a high intake depresses synthesis by the liver, and low intake or reduced absorption results in increased synthesis. The total body pool is due to (1) synthesis by liver, (2) dietary intake, (3) reabsorption from small intestine. The sources for reduction of total body cholesterol are (1) conversion to bile acids, (2) secretion of cholesterol into intestinal lumen via bile duct, part of which are reabsorbed while rest are excreted through faeces as dietary fibres or compound like cholestyramine, a non-absorable resin, binds with cholesterol and ultimately excreted through faeces, (3) used for steroid hormone synthesis (progesterone, estrogen, adrenal cortical hormones, testosterone or (4) stored as a component of pathologic deposits in bile ducts (gall stone) and also in arteries (atherosclerotic). Further conjugation of bile acids with taurine or glycine results in the excretion of these conjugated bile acids in the bile as taurocholic and glycocholic acid, respectively.

The turnover of cholesterol in humans is summarised in the figure below. The liver of an adult man contains about 3–5 g and the blood pool is 10–12 g. Daily synthesis is 1–1.5 g of which about half is converted to bile acids. Secretion of cholesterol and bile acids into the intestinal lumen via the bile duct approximates 2 and 20–30 g/day, respectively, but due to reabsorption by the enterohepatic circulation, less than 1 g of each is lost in the faeces. Thus compounds that reduce absorption of cholesterol and bile acids may have a profound effect on the body pool of cholesterol and on its biosynthesis.

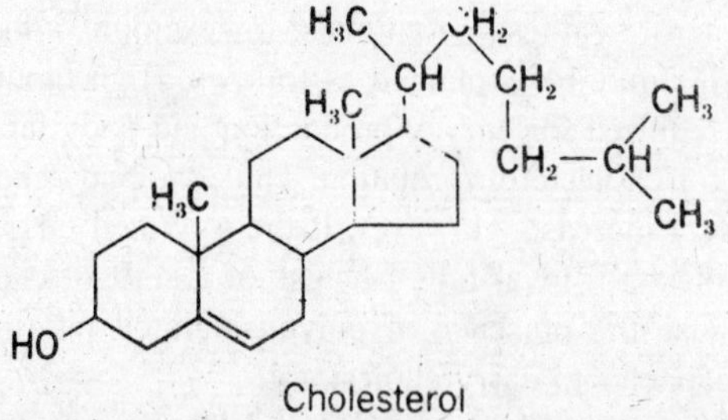

Cholesterol
(Greek: *chole*, bile; *stereos*, solid; -ol, alcohol)

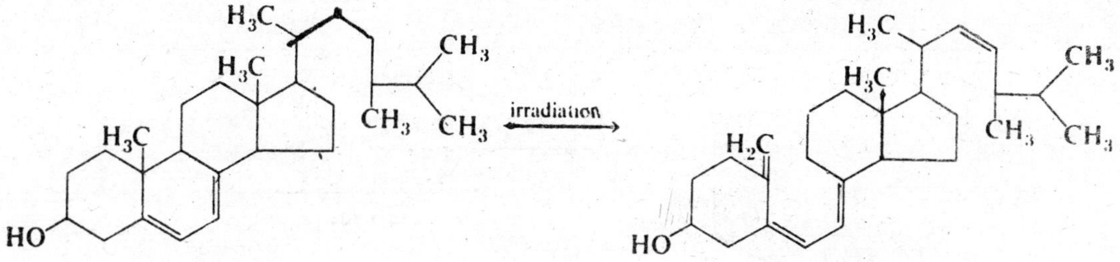

Ergosterol

Vitamin D_2 (ergocalciferol)

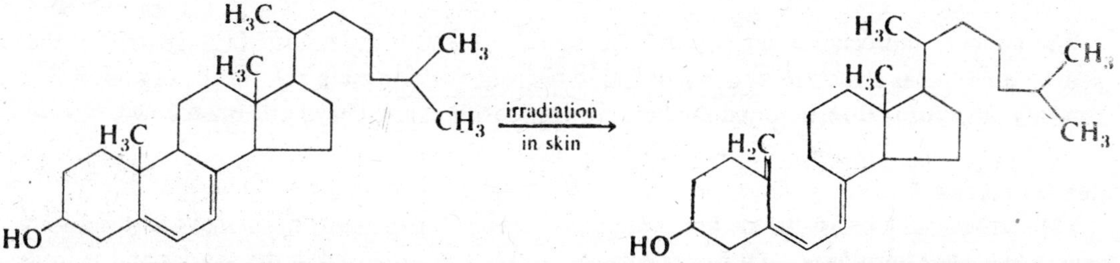

7-Dehydrocholesterol

Vitamin D_3 (cholecalciferol)

Ergosterol

Ergosterol occurs in ergot and yeast. It is important as a precursor of vitamin D_2. When ergosterol is irradiated with ultraviolet light, it changes into vitamin D_2.

Bile acids

Human liver contains 3 different bile acids—cholic, deoxycholic and chemodeoxycholic. The last one is microbial in origin and is absorbed from intestinal contents. The bile acids have a five carbon side chain at carbon 17 terminating in a carboxyl group which is bound by an amide linkage to amino acids glycine and taurine

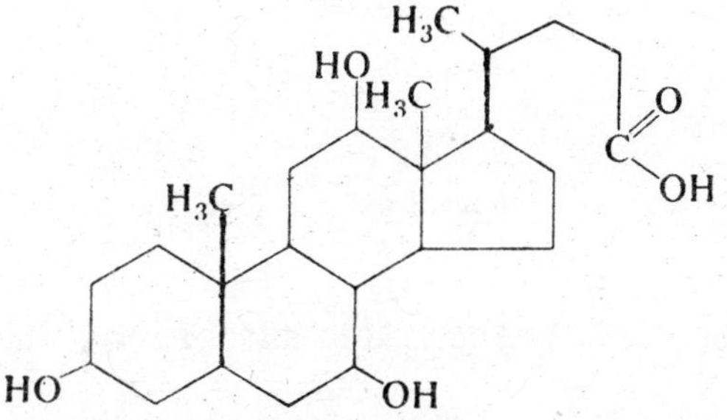

Cholic acid
(a bile acid)

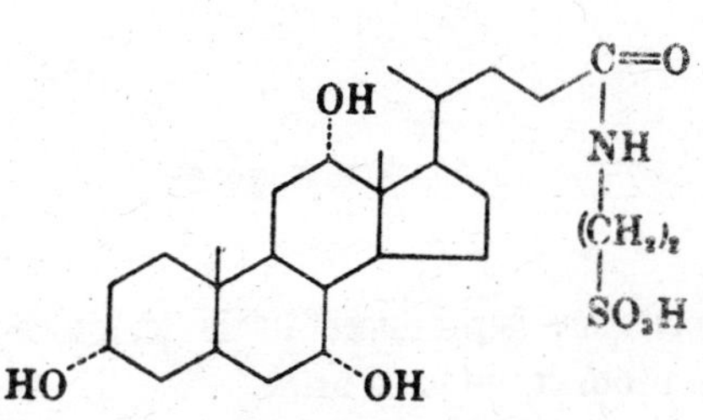

Taurocholic acid

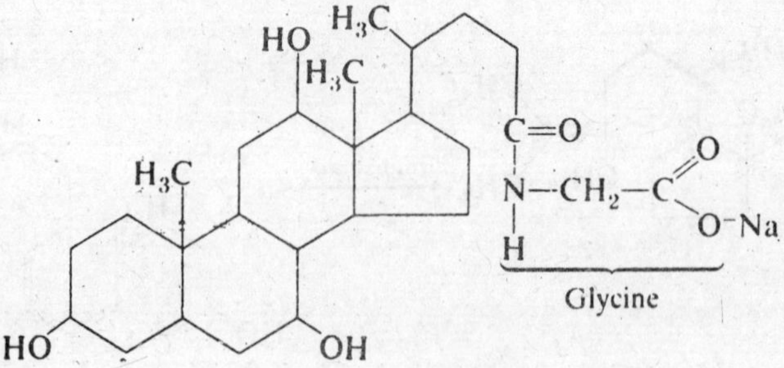

Sodium glycocholate
(a bile salt)

The amides, taurocholic and glycocholic acids, are excellent emulsifying agents, as they possess a nonpolar structure and a changed side chain. Their main role in the organism is to emulsify fats during digestion and facilitate their absorption and enzymatic breakdown.

Sex Hormones

The estrogen and progesterone are commonly known as female sex hormones and the androgens as male sex hormones. Of the estrogens, estradiol is produced in the ovaries and estrone and estriol formed as a result of enzymatic transformations of estradiol. Progesterone, which is also produced in the ovaries, is related more closely to the androgens in structure.

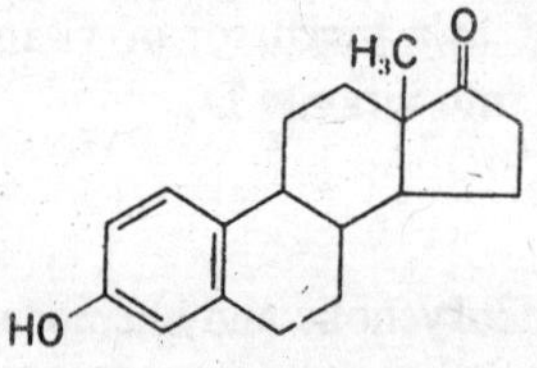

Estrone

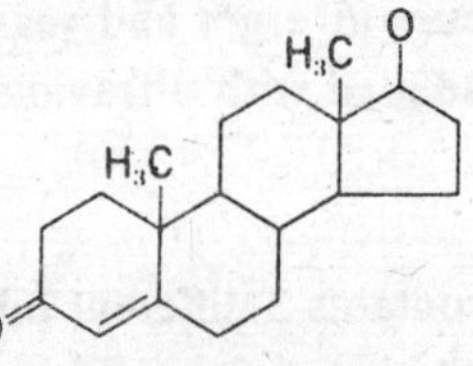

Testosterone

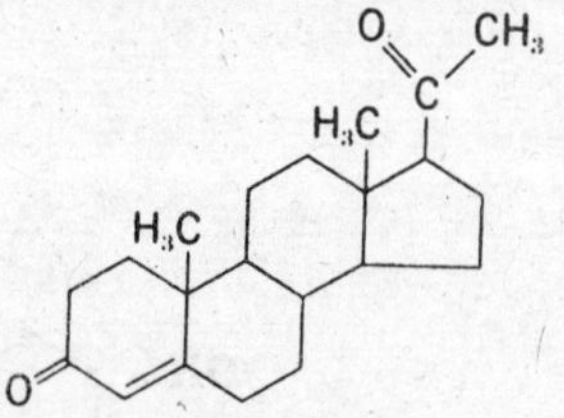

Progesterone

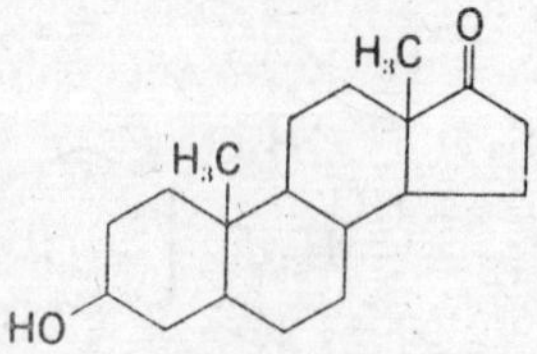

Androsterone

Testosterone is produced in the testes and biochemically transformed to androsterone, which is the product found in urine.

PROSTAGLANDINS

Prostaglandins were discovered in the mid-1930s by a Swedish scientist, Ulf von Euler (Nobel prize, 1970), but they did not arouse much interest in medical circles until the late 1960s, largely through the work of Sune Bergstrom. It became apparent that these compounds, which occur widely in the body in almost all the cells, affect a large number of processes. Their general name comes from an organ, the prostrate gland, from which they were first obtained. About 20 are known, and they occur in four major subclasses designated as PGA, PGB, PGE, and PGF. (A subscript numerals 1, 2, 3, is generally placed after the third letter to designate the number of double bonds that occur outside the five-membered ring of the molecule). The structures of some typical examples are shown here.

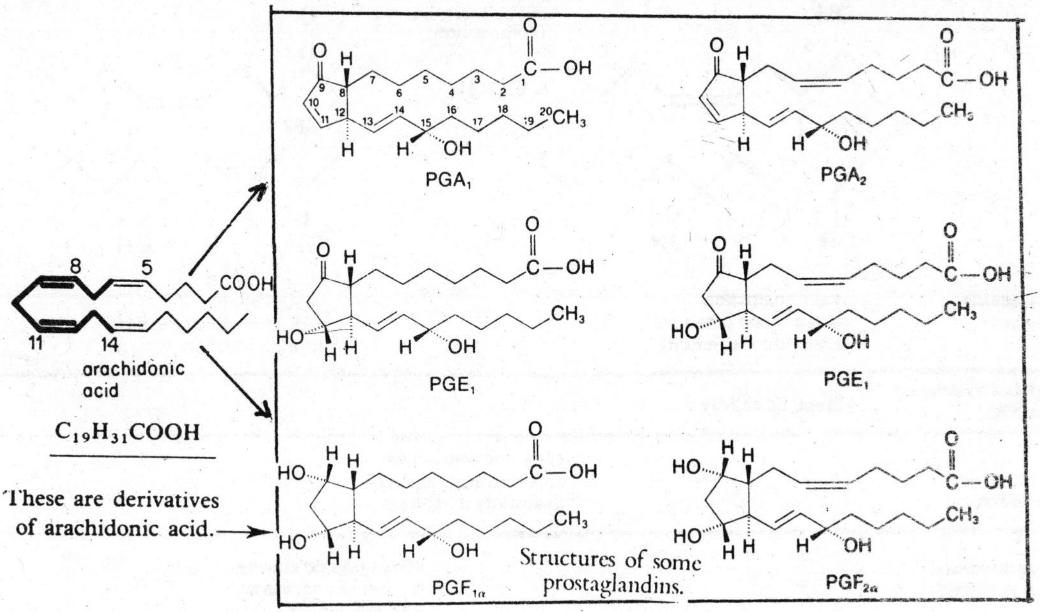

arachidonic acid

$C_{19}H_{31}COOH$

These are derivatives of arachidonic acid.

PGA$_1$ PGA$_2$ PGE$_1$ PGE$_1$ PGF$_{1\alpha}$ PGF$_{2\alpha}$

Structures of some prostaglandins.

Prostaglandins are made from C-20 fatty acids such as arachidonic acid. By coiling a portion of this acid, it results one ring closer, to form prostaglandins. Thus these are unsaturated hydroxy acids with one five membered ring in a 20 carbon skeleton.

Recent research has shown that these substances are not confined to the male genital tract but can be detected in several tissues of both the sexes and are found to function as regulators of metabolism.

The prostaglandins are like hormone in many ways, except that they do not act globally, that is over the entire body. They do their work within the cells where they are made or in nearby cells, move through diffusion in the interstitial fluid rather than by circulation in the blood. Thus they are known as *local hormones*. They work together with other established hormones to modify the chemical messages that other hormones bring to cells, in some cells, the prostaglandins inhibit enzymes and in others they activate them. In some organs, the prostaglandins help to regulate the flow of blood within them. In others, they affect the transmission of nerve impulses.

Some prostaglandins enhance inflammation in a tissue, and it is interesting that aspirin, an inflammation reducer, does exactly the opposite. This effect is caused by aspirin's ability to inhibit the work of an enzyme needed for the synthesis of prostaglandins.

In experiments that use prostaglandins as pharmaceuticals, they have been found to have an astonishing variety of effects. One prostaglandin regulates body temperature, another stops the flow of gastric juice while the body heals an ulcer. Other possible uses are to treat high blood pressure, rhematoid arthritis, asthma, nasal congestion and some viral diseases. Certain prostaglandins especially I_2 inhibit platelet aggregation, whereas E_2 and A_2 promote this clotting process.

The prostaglandins have also been used extensively as drugs in the reproductive area. F_2 and E_2 have been used to induce parturition and for the termination of unwanted pregnancy. There is also evidence that E series of prostaglandins may play some role in infertility in male animals.

The compound has a very short life, soon after their release these are rapidly taken up by cells and get inactivated.

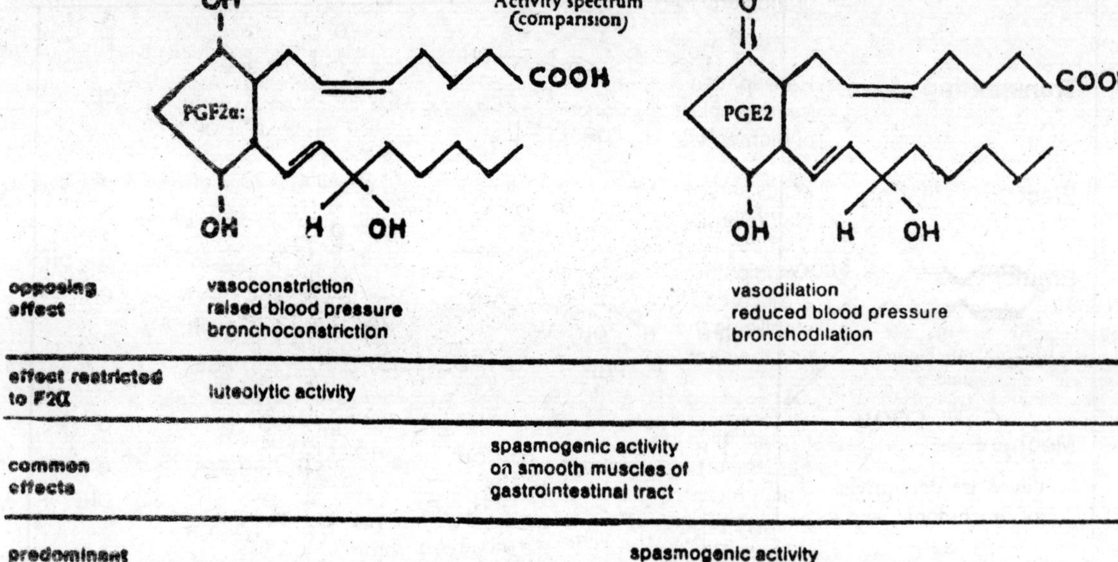

However, the following problems are inherent in the incorporation of fats in feeds :

1. **Animal fats can become rancid**
2. **Fats at higher percentage may get deposited around vital organs.**

Lipids in Feeds and Forages

Ruminant diets are normally quite low in lipid because of its low content (1 – 4%) in most plant food sources other than oil cakes. These dietary characteristics have allowed adaptations, so that the rumen is intolerant to high levels of fat that may upset rumen fermentation. However, in new born ruminant which ingests milk at about 30% fat in the dry matter, represents 50% or more of caloric intake.

Lipids are present in plants may be grouped from quantitative point of view as (1) storage compounds in seeds (chiefly triacylglycerides), (2) leaf lipids (galactolipids), and a miscellaneous group including waxes, carotenoids, chlorophyll, essential oils and other ether soluble substances. The fatty acids associated with galactolipids, and of many of the triacyl-

Table 10.20

Biological Functions of Lipids

Function	*Characterization of the function*	*Lipids exercising the function*
Substrate-energetic	The oxidation of lipids in the organism is attended by a release of energy greater than (2.5 times) that from other energetic substrates (proteins and carbohydrates). Energy generated by combustion of 1 g of lipids amounts to 39.1. KJ or 9.3 KCal	Acylglycerides, free fatty acids
Structural	Lipids are components of the cell membranes and form a lipid basis thereof	Phospholipids (phosphoglycerides, sphingomyelins), cholesterol and its esters
Transporting	Participation in the transport of materials (for example, cations) across the lipid layer of biomembranes	Phospholipids
Electric insulating	Lipids serve as a specific electro-insulating material in the myelin sheath of nerve tissues	Sphingomyelins, glycosphingolipids
Emulsifying	Amphipathic lipids are emulsifiers. They are located at the oil/water interface surface stabilizing thereby emulsions and preventing their separation into layers.	Phosphoglycerides, bile acids (sterols) are emulsifiers for the intestinal acylglycerides. Phosphoglycerides stabilize the solubility of cholesterol in blood
Mechanical	Protection of internal organs from eventual damage on exposure to mechanical action (lipids of connective tegmental tissues of internal organs and lipids of panniculus adiposus)	Triacylglycerides
Heat-insulating	Conservation of heat by the lipids of subcutaneous adiposus tissue owing to their low heat conduction	Triacylglycerides
Dissolving	Dissolution of certain lipid materials in other lipids under physiological conditions	Bile acids (sterols) are solvents for fat-soluble vitamins in the intestine
Hormonal	Regulation of a large variety of physiological functions with the involvement of steroid hormones (lipids) and prostaglandins (hormone-like lipids)	Steroids (sex hormones, corticosteroids). Derivatives of unsaturated fatty acids
Vitaminogenic	Special function with the participation of fat-soluble vitamins (lipids)	Isoprenoids, unsaturated fatty acids

glycerides of seeds are mostly unsaturated and contain high amounts of linoleic and linolenic acids. In forages the amount of galactolipids decreases with the age of the plant.

Effect of Storage & Handling

It is well known that the ether extract and carotenoid content of forage decline with storage. The decline is a result of slow oxidation and polymerisation of the unsaturated oils to form resins. The polymerised products are indigestible, generally insoluble in fat solvents, and in the analytical scheme become associated with the cutin fraction of crude lignin.

Miscellaneous Lipid Components

Roughly half of the ether-soluble matter of forages is composed of galactolipids, the remaining portion being made up of a variety of substances. These are grouped into (I) pigments, such as chlorophyll, carotenoids, the related xanthophylls, saponins, etc., (ii) waxes, (iii) essential oils include anything that is steam volatile, including terpenes, aldehydes, ketones, etc.

PROTEINS

The term protein is taken from the Greek work *proteus* which roughly translated means first. The terminology was suggested in 1840 by Mulder, who clearly recognised that protein was necessary for life in a more fundmental way than could be attributed to either carbohydrate or lipid: "Without it no life is possible."

Nearly half of the dry weight of a typical animal cell is protein. Structural components of the cell, antibodies, and many of the hormones are proteins, but as much as 90 per cent of cellular proteins are the enzymes upon which fundamental cellular function depends. There may be up to 1000 different enzymes in a single cell.

Table 10.21

Elements	Per cent	Elements	Per cent
1. Carbon	50	4. Nitrogen	16
2. Hydrogen	7	5. Sulphur	0 to 3
3. Oxygen	23	6. Phosphorus	0 to 3

All proteins contain C, H, O, N, and generally sulphur with occasional occurrence of phosphorus. Approximately average composition of protein is as given in the Table 10.21.

Amino acids—Building Blocks of Protein

As each flower constitutes a garland, as each brick constitutes an unit of any big wall, similarly each amino acid constitutes an unit of any protein. The amino acids are chemical compounds which contain both an acidic carboxyl (—COOH) and a basic amino ($-NH_2$) group. The common amino acid has a general structure,

$$R-\overset{\displaystyle H}{\underset{\displaystyle NH_2}{\overset{|}{\underset{|}{C}}}}-COOH$$

Most amino acids occurring naturally in proteins are of the α type, having the amino group attached to the carbon atom adjacent to the carboxyl group and can be represented by the general formula as below, where R—, called the amino acid side chain or residue, represents a great variety of structures. Complete hydrolysis of naturally occurring proteins produces approximately 20 different α amino acids. Out of these 20 amino acids any number of amino acids may be present in a particular protein molecule. Thus, the amino acid present, their position in the molecule, and the spacial arrangement of the molecule all determine the properties and characteristic of the protein.

Properties of amino acids

All amino acids are amphoteric in nature, i.e., have both basic property due to $—NH_2$ group and also have acidic property due to —COOH group and thus in solution as in blood, amino acids are mostly present as uncharged molecules (one positive and one negative charge—so in total there is no charge effect, hence it is called uncharged or dipolar ions). Such a structure is known as "Zwitter ions" (from the German Zwitter, a hermaphrodite):

$$\begin{array}{c} H \\ | \\ R—C—COO^- \\ | \\ NH_3^+ \end{array}$$

In a strongly acid solution an amino acid exists largely as cation, while in alkaline solution it exists largely as anion. There is a pH value at which it is electrically neutral; this value is known as *isoelectric point*. Because of their amphoteric nature amino acids act as buffers, resisting changes in pH. All the amino acids except glycine are optically active.

ESSENTIAL AMINO ACIDS

Physiologically all (about 20) amino acids found in animal tissues are essential. Under this circumstance you can ask yourself how many of these amino acids the body cannot synthesise from other nitrogenous compounds in sufficient amount required by the animal. From this question you may realise that animal body can synthesise some amino acids in sufficient amount, can synthesise some which are not sufficient to maintain their body requirements and some amino acids cannot at all be synthesised. We infer "essential amino acids" of the last two categories. Different animals have different capacity of synthesising amino acid types. So, the list of essential amino acids is different from species to species.

W.C. Rose first found on experiment with rats that ten of the amino acids cannot be synthesised rapidly enough by the animal (rat) body to permit normal growth. These are listed in Table 10.22 as "essential amino acids" for rats.

It is to be borne in mind that all amino acids found in the body are physiologically essential; out of them some are dietary essential. The dietary non-essential acids have got no less physiological importance. One research philosopher mentioned, "Some are so essential that the body ensures an adequate supply by synthesis." However, if the diet does not supply adequate quantity of the "non-essential" ones, they will have to be synthesised from other non-

Table 10.22

Requirement for each individual amino acid when all other amino acids of nutritive importance are provided (figures are % of total diet except for human which are in (g/kg body weight/day)

Amino acids	Growing pigs[2]	Human[3]			Young rat[2]	Fish	Growing chickens[1]			Layers
		Infants (4-6 mths)	Child (10-12 yrs)	Adult			0-6 weeks	6-14 weeks	14-20 weeks	
Isoleucine	0.63	83	28	12	0.5	0.9	0.60	0.50	0.40	0.50
Leucine	0.75	135	42	16	0.75	1.6	1.00	0.83	0.67	0.73
Lysine	0.95	99	44	12	0.7	2.0	0.85	0.60	0.45	0.64
Methionine + Cystine	0.56[4]	49[5]	22[5]	10[5]	0.6[4]	1.6	0.60[4]	0.50[4]	0.40[4]	0.55[4]
Phenylalanine + Tyrosine	0.88[6]	141	22[7]	16[7]	0.8[6]	2.1	1.00[6]	0.83[6]	0.67	0 80[6]
Threonine	0.56	68	28	8	0.5	0.9	0.68	0.57	0.37	0.45
Tryptophan	0.15	21	4	3	0.15	0.2	0.17	0.14	0.11	0.14
Valine	0.63	92	25	14	0.6	1.3	0.62	0.52	0.41	0.55
Histidine	—	33	NA	NA	0.3	0.7	0.26	0.22	0.17	0.16
Arginine	—	—	—	—	0.6	2.4	1.00	0.83	0.67	0.68
Glycine & serine	—	—	—	—	—	—	0.70	0.58	0.47	0.50
No. of Essential amino acids	8	9	9	9	10	10	11	11	11	11
Total Protein requirement		gm per kg body weight								
	16-20%	2.0	1.5	0.8	20%	40%	20%	16%	14%	15%

1. Data for chickens obtained from 1984 NRC publication on Poultry.
2. Data for rats and pigs obtained from 1972 and 1978 NRC Publication respectively. On the basis of recent findings regarding sufficient synthesis of Histidine and Arginine by the pig, data given for pit in original source have been neglected.
3. Food and Nutrition Board: Recommended Dietary allowances, 9th ed. National Academy of Sciences-NRC, 1980.
4. About 1/2 of the requirements can be met by cystine.
5. About 3/4 of the requirement can be met by cystine.
6. About 1/3 to 1/2 of the requirement can be met by tyrosine.
7. About 3/4 of the requirement can be met by tyrosine.

NA Not available.

protein nitrogenous substances or it will come from the essential amino acids that are present. Thus, provision in the diet for adequate quantities of either non-protein nitrogen or of non-essential amino acids must be made to meet the needs of non-essential amino acids. For essential amino acids there is no other alternative except to supply these acids through diet.

The number and types of amino acids which are essential for a particular species are not exactly the same for other species. The requirement varies depending on the age and species of animal, as shown in Table 10.22

For ruminants the situation is quite different. The micro-organisms which are common inhabitants in the rumen can utilise any kind of nitrogenous substance present in the animal ration, and converts them into different essential and non-essential amino acids which are deposited as microbial protein and later on utilised by animal body. Thus the problem of essential amino acids arises only in non-ruminants like man, pig, horse, poultry, etc., but not for sheep, goat or cattle except during their very young age when their rumen is not developed to carry this function.

Classification of Amino Acids

About two dozen amino acids have so far been definitely established as occurring in proteins, and most proteins contain a large proportion of these amino acids while others may be rich in one or other type of amino acids as in silk protein which is specially rich in glycine, about 40 per cent.

Amino acids have been classified in various ways. One system classifies them as aliphatic, aromatic and heterocyclic amino acids, depending upon the presence of chain and ring structure. Another system classifies them according to the number of amino and carboxyl groups present in the molecule as monoamino monocarboxylic acids, monoamino dicarboxylic acids, etc. Again they are classified according to reaction in solution as neutral, acidic and basic amino acids. From the nutrition point of view these acids are further classified as essential or non-essential type based on whether the body can or cannot synthesise the particular type of acid as per requirement. Lastly, the amino acids are also classified into three groups according to their catabolic fates as (*i*) *Glucogenic*, (*ii*) *Ketogenic*, and (*iii*) *Glucogenic and/or Ketogenic* based on the major end products formed from degradation of carbon skeletons of various amino acids.

Glucogenic and Ketogenic Amino Acids

After absorption of amino acids mostly from the jejunum portion of the small intestine these are largely utilised as such for the synthesis of various protein and other non-protein nitrogenous compounds. A significant portion of absorbed amino acids, after shaking off of their amino (NH_2) group either by deamination or by transamination, are also utilised as a carbon skeleton for the synthesis of other non-nitrogenous compounds as glucose (the process is known as *Gluconeogenesis*) or some other ketones. The physiological conditions which encourage the acids to follow such glycogenic and/or ketogenic pathway are either fasting or at diabetes mellitus condition or at situations when the animals are on low levels of dietary carbohydrates.

If amino acids are fed one at a time to a starving phlorizinised dog it has been observed that some give rise to glucose in the urine, while others give rise to acetoacetic acid. A few give rise to neither. In such an animal about 60 gms of glucose are formed and excreted in the urine for each 100 gms of protein metabolised; this means, 60 per cent of protein is potentially glucogenic. Thus it has been proved that amino acids differ in yielding products from the degradation of their carbon skeleton and accordingly amino acids are classified into three groups.

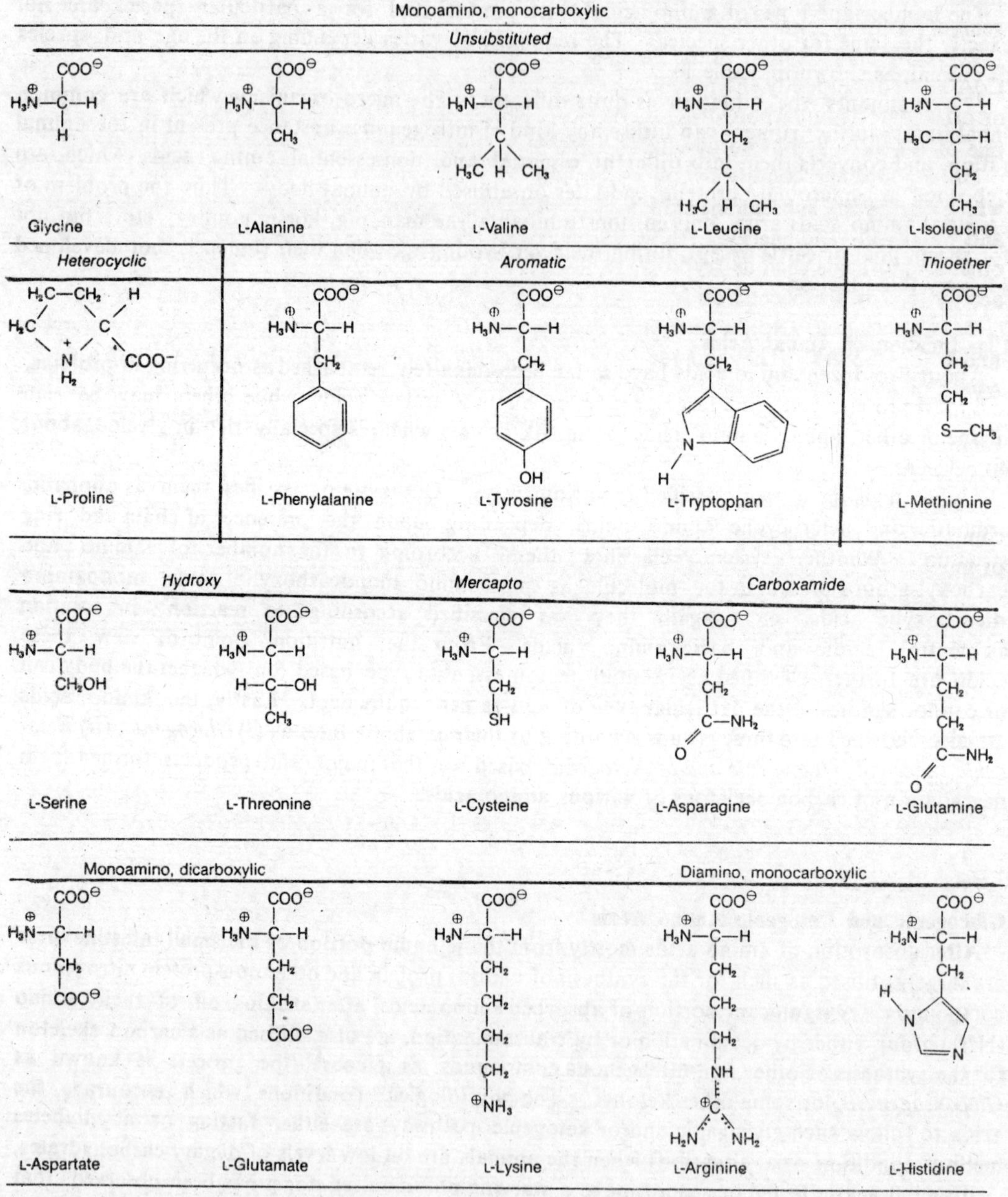

Monoamino, monocarboxylic

Unsubstituted

Glycine | L-Alanine | L-Valine | L-Leucine | L-Isoleucine

Heterocyclic

L-Proline

Aromatic

L-Phenylalanine | L-Tyrosine | L-Tryptophan

Thioether

L-Methionine

Hydroxy

L-Serine | L-Threonine

Mercapto

L-Cysteine

Carboxamide

L-Asparagine | L-Glutamine

Monoamino, dicarboxylic

L-Aspartate | L-Glutamate

Diamino, monocarboxylic

L-Lysine | L-Arginine | L-Histidine

Structures of the common amino acids.

Fig. 10.6

1. GLUCOGENIC OR ANTIKETOGENIC AMINO ACIDS. Amino acids belonging to this group, just after deamination, initially form keto acids and immediately change into glucose which may be stored temporarily as glycogen in the liver. The term *Glucogenic* is often used to designate those acids which give rise to TCA cycle intermediates or pyruvate and therefore are on the general pathway to carbohydrate synthesis.

2. KETOGENIC AMINO ACIDS. *Ketogenic* refers to those amino acids which give rise to acetyl CoA and consequently the potential fatty acid producers. During starvation, diabetes mellitus or other defects in carbohydrate metabolism acetyl CoA accumulate and will be converted into one of the three ketone compounds—aceto acetic acid, acetone and β-hydroxybutyric acid.

Under ordinary conditions ketogenic amino acids after deamination will yield keto acids which during the subsequent oxidation (through the stage of acetoacetic acid) to carbon dioxide and water will yield energy. Although leucine is the only truly ketogenic amino acid, several other amino acids such as tryptophan, lysine, tyrosine, etc., are also catabolised to form some acetyl CoA or acetoacetic acid.

3. GLUCOGENIC AND/OR KETOGENIC. Amino acids of this group can give rise to both glucose and ketone bodies. They include isoleucine, lysine, phenylalanine, tyrosine, threonine and tryptophan.

Limiting amino acid

The essential amino acid of a protein that shows the greatest percentage deficit in comparison to amino acids contained in the same quantity of any standard protein, viz., egg or milk.

Table 10.23
Amino acids

Name	% in egg protein	% in wheat Protein	% deficiency in wheat
Arginine	6.4	4.2	—34
Histidine	2.1	2.1	0
Lysine	7.2	2.7	—63
Tyrosine	4.5	4.4	—2
Tryptophan	1.5	1.2	—20
Phenylalanine	6.3	5.7	—10
Cystine	2.4	1.8	—25
Methionine	4.1	2.5	—39
Cystine + Methionine	6.5	4.3	—34
Threonine	4.9	3.3	—33
Leucine	9.2	6.8	—26
Isoleucine	8.0	3.6	—55
Valine	7.3	4.5	—38

Here lysine is the first order and isoleucine is the second order limited amino acids.

Table 10.24
Limiting amino acids

Ingredients	Order of limitations				
	First	Second	Third	Fourth	Fifth
Soyabean	Methionine	Threonine	Valine	Lysine	Isoleucine
Meat and bone	Tryptophan	Methionine	Isoleucine	Threonine	Histidine
Maize	Lysine	Tryptophan	Isoleucine	Threonine	Valine
Milo	Lysine	Threonine	Methionine	Isoleucine	Tryptopan
Wheat	Lysine	Isoleucine	Methionine	Valine	Arginine
Barley	Lysine	Threonine	Methionine	Isoleucine	Valine

Protein and Amino Acid Anomalies in Diets of Non-ruminants

Inadequate protein nutrition is the most common of all nutrient deficiencies. Signs of protein deficiencies include reduced feed intake and utilization, reduced growth rate, infertility, reduced serum protein concentration, accumulation of fat in the liver and carcass, reduced synthesis of certain enzymes and hormones resulting depression of most metabolic activities which may lead even to early death.

The term '*protein requirement*' should now be replaced by various essential and non-essential amino acid requirements. This is absolutely true for non-ruminants since unlike ruminants this group is unable to obtain essential amino acids other than dietary source.

Amino Acid deficiency

Amino acid *deficiency* is a condition in which the dietary supply of one or more of the essential amino acids is less than that required for the efficient utilization of other amino acids and other nutrients. Diets are in general unlikely to be completely devoid of any one or more amino acids but may be deficient in respect of required quantity. The amino acid which provides the lowest proportion of the theoretical requirement is referred to as the *first limiting amino acid* (lysine).

Deficiency is therefore judged against a control diet adequate in the supply of all essential amino acids.

Amino Acid Imbalance

The term *amino acid imbalance*, is normally restricted to circumstances where the composition of essential amino acids in the diet results in a further poorer animal performance than would be expected in case of amino acid deficiency where the effect depends on the extent of deficiencies of limiting amino acid(s).

The term is often used generically but three specific categories of imbalance have been identified viz. *imbalance, antagonism* and *toxicity*. The categorisation distinguishes particular dietary conditions that impair performance and not implying common mechanism within a category.

1. Amino Acid Imbalance

Imbalance is produced by the addition to a diet *low in total protein* of either the second-limiting amino acid, or more usually a group of amino acids which does not include the first-limiting amino acid. The adverse effect on performance can be avoided by supplementation with the first-limiting amino acid.

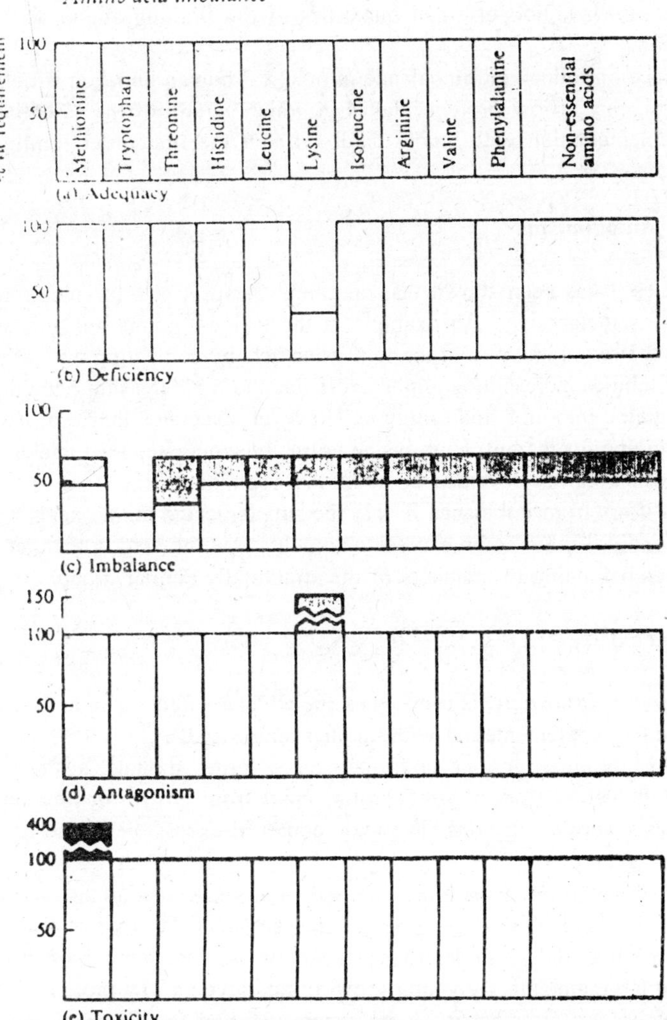

Fig. 10.7 Diagrammatic representation of: (a) idealized amino acid-adequate diet in which all amino acids are present in amounts sufficient to satisfy but not exceed requirements; (b) idealized amino acid-deficient diet, in which one amino acid, lysine, is limiting; (c) amino acid imbalance induced by addition of all amino acids except tryptophan to a protein-deficient diet in which tryptophan is the first-limiting and threonine the second-limiting amino acid; (d) amino acid antagonism induced by addition of lysine to an adequate diet which increases the requirement for arginine; and (e) toxicity induced by addition of a large excess of methionine (□, represents amino acid(s) added). (Adapted from Austic, 1978.)

Feed intake is depressed via the same mechanism described for an amino acid deficiency.

Note that in this case a deficient protein source has been made more deficient by the addition of other amino acids (except first limiting amino acid) thus resulted growth retardation much greater than that caused by original deficient diet.

In such cases, the addition of small quantities of the limiting amino acid alone can prevent growth retardation.

The significance of amino acid imbalance in practical human nutrition is not yet clear. It seems possible, however, that at low protein intakes in which certain of the essential amino acids may be limiting, supplementation with amino acids without the first order limiting acid could have detrimental effects.

2. Amino Acid Antagonism

In special cases it has been shown that one amino acid affects the requirement of another by interfering with its metabolism. An example is the lysine-arginine antagonism, wherein dietary lysine increases the requirement of arginine. Lysine acts by competing with arginine for reabsorption in the renal tubules increasing arginine excretion and by increasing renal arginase activity and thus splitting arginine into urea and ornithine. However, excessive intake of lysine does not affect absorption of arginine for the gut. High lysine normally suppresses feed intake and growth depression in chicks, which can be reversed by additional arginine.

Antagonism differs from imbalance in that the supplemented amino acids need not be limiting amino acid. Secondly it refers to an excessive amount of amino acid in the diet which affects only those amino acids belonging to members of the structurally similar group.

3. Amino Acid Toxicity

The term, *amino acid toxicity*, is used when the adverse effect of an amino acid in excess cannot be overcome by supplementation with another amino acids.

Ingestion of methionine, tyrosine or tryptophan in large amounts, up to about 2–3 times the requirement is followed by serious irregularities apart from growth depression. A dietary excess of tyrosine causes severe eye lesions. The toxic action of excess methioine has been attributed to inhibition of ATP synthesis.

The effect of the inclusion of the gross amounts of an individual amino acid within a diet varies among amino acids. Threonine, even in very large amounts (50 g/kg of the DM of the diet), is tolerated well and causes only a moderate depression of feed intake and growth. Tyrosine, however, when ingested in large amounts by young growing rats given a low protein diet, not only depress severely feed intake and growth but causes severe eye and paw lesions, and in great excess is lethal. Methionine is the most toxic and in amounts exceeding 20 kg/kg of the dry matter of the diet may produce severe histopathological changes.

NON-PROTEIN NITROGENOUS COMPOUNDS

A considerable variety of nitrogenous compounds which are not classed as proteins occur in plants and animals. In plant analysis these compounds have been frequently classed together as non-protein nitrogenous compounds to distinguish them from "true proteins" determined in routine chemical analysis. In general above 50 per cent of the total non-protein is the free

amino acid, followed by the amides. Among others, amines, purines, pyrimidines, nitrates,

Table 10.25

Non-protein nitrogenous constituents formed from amino acids in animals

Biological compound	*Amino acid precursor*	*Physiological function*
Purines and pyrimidines	Glycine and aspartic acid	Constituents of nucleotides and nucleic acids
Creatine	Glycine and arginine	Energy storage as creatine phosphate in muscle
Glycocholic and taurocholic acids	Glycine and cysteine	Bile acids, aid in fat digestion and absorption
Thyroxine, epinephrine and norepinephrine	Tyrosine	Hormones
Ethanolamine and choline	Serine	Constituents of phospholipids
Histamine	Histidine	A vasodepressor
Serotonin	Tryptophan	Transmission of nerve impulses
Porphyrins	Glycine	Constituent of hemoglobin
Niacin	Tryptophan	Vitamin
Melanin	Tyrosine	Pigment of hair, skin, and eyes

and alkaloids are noteworthy. In addition many members of the vitamin B complex and some types of lipids contain nitrogen in their structure.

Formerly, the protein requirements were stated in terms of digestible true protein, and as a rule, no allowances were made for the nutrient value of the non-protein portion of the nitrogenous matter. It was later generally accepted that the "amide" had half the nutrient value of true protein and when calculating rations the sum of the digestible true protein and crude protein was halved and the result was called "Protein Equivalent". This was used in place of true protein. However, recent researches have shown that the non-protein nitrogenous compounds play in ruminant system almost an identical role as the true protein. As mentioned earlier, the amides and the amino acids are the only ones which occur to any considerable extent, and they are present in large amounts in only a few of the common feeds. In fast growing plants such substances are abundant and may make up as much as one-third of the total nitrogen. The developing seed is high in non-protein nitrogen at the start but low at maturity. Commonly fed concentrate grain mixture and mature hays contain relatively little non-protein nitrogen.

In addition to the non-protein nitrogen compounds which occur in feed as in free state, there are a number of other non-protein nitrogenous constituents which are formed either as intermediary or end products of various amino acid metabolism. Some of such non-protein nitrogenous compounds that originate from amino acids are listed with their physiological functions in Table 10.25

CRUDE PROTEIN (CP)

The protein part of feeding stuff as determined in the routine analysis is really made up of two component parts; one is the true protein occuring in larger proportions, the other is constituted of non-protein nitrogenous compounds. The term crude protein includes both the types as a whole.

The estimation of crude protein in the feeding stuff is determined by the standard Kjeldhal procedure which gives the estimation of the feed coming from the protein and non-protein nitrogenous compounds. The percentage of nitrogen (N_2) is then expressed in terms of crude protein (CP), calculated as mentioned in next page.

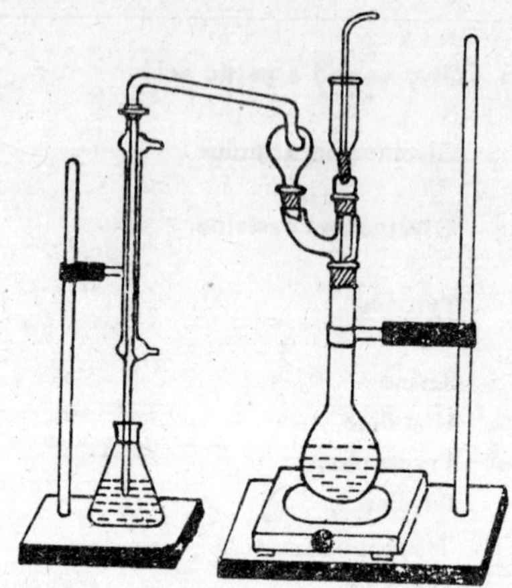

Fig. 110.8. Macro-Kjeldahl distillation apparatus for distilling nitrogen content.

$$\text{Per cent CP} = \text{Per cent } N_2 \times 6.25$$

The factor 6.25 is used on the assumption that proteins contain 16 per cent nitrogen. (100/16=6.25).

So, when we express the total nitrogen content in terms of CP, we make two assumptions: (1) all food protein contain 16 per cent nitrogen, (2) all the nitrogen of the food is present as true protein. Both of these assumptions are unsound. Different food proteins have different

Table 10.26

*Factors for converting nitrogen to CP

Food protein	*Per cent N_2*	*Conversion factor*
Cotton seed	18.87	5.30
Soybean	17.51	5.71
Maize	16.00	6.25
Wheat	17.15	5.83
Egg and Meat	16.00	6.25
Milk	15.68	6.38

*From D.B. Jones; 1931. U.S.D.A. Circular 183.

Table 10.27

CLASSIFICATION OF PROTEINS

Type	*Chemical Properties*	*General Comments*
Fibrous proteins :		
Collagen	Insoluble in water; highly resistant to enzymic digestion; becomes gelatinous upon boiling in water or dilute acids or bases; high content of proline and hydroxyproline; no cystine, tryptophan, or cysteine present.	Constitutes about 30% of total protein in the body. Fibrous connective tissue.
Elastins	Properties similar to collagen except it will not become gelatinous upon boiling : bound together by a deriva–tive of lysine (desmosine)	Present in tendons, arteries, and elastic tissue.
Keratins	Highly indigestible and insoluble : autoclaving will increase solubility : high–cystine content	Protein present in hair, wool, feathers, hoofs, claws, beaks and horns.
Globular proteins :		
Albumins	Readily soluble in water : coagulate upon heating.	Present in egg and serum.
Globulins	Low solubility in water : solubility increases with the addition of neutral salts : coagulates upon heating.	Abundant in nature : examples are serum globulins and numerous plant globulins
Glutelins	Insoluble in water : soluble in dilute acids or bases.	Present in plant material.
Histones	Soluble in water : hydrolysis yields large quantities of arginine and lysine.	Are combined with nucleic acid.
Prolamines	Insoluble in water, absolute alcohol or neutral solvents : soluble in 80% ethanol.	Zein in maize is a prolamine.
Protamines	Strongly basic : low molecular : contains high amounts of arginine : has no sulfur amino acids, tyrosine, or tryptophan	Associated with nucleic acids.
Conjugated proteins :		
Nucleoproteins	Combination of proteins and nucleic acids.	Present in germs of seeds and in glandular tissue.
Mucoproteins	Resistant to heat and not easily preci–pitated. Contain N–acetyl–hexosamine.	Can be found in egg white, serum and human pregnancy urine.
Glycoproteins	Contain less than 4% carbohydrate	Found in mucin. Includes many albumins and globulins.
Lipoprotein	Water–soluble : conjugated with various lipids.	Brain and nerve tissue are excellent sources
Lecithoproteins	Combination of protein and lecithin	Found in tissue fibrinogen
Hemoproteins	Contain hematin and protein Porphyrin structure	Hemoglobin is a hemoprotein
Metalloproteins	Proteins that are complexed with metals.	One example is transferrin, a metalloprotein that can bind with copper, iron, and zinc.

nitrogen contents and therefore different factors should be used in the conversion of nitrogen to protein for individual foods.

The second assumption that the whole of the food nitrogen is present as protein is also false, since many simple nitrogenous compounds such as amides, amino acids, glycosides, alkaloids, ammonium salts may be present in the food.

From practical point of view, as all ruminants can utilise nitrogen from protein and non-protein equally and hence the two assumptions that are made to calculate CP will not affect the ruminants. In the diet of pigs and poultry, cereals and oilseed meals predominate, and in these there is little non-protein nitrogen. Hence in practice there is little to be gained from attempting to distinguish between the two types of nitrogen.

True Proteins

True proteins are sometimes determined to know the actual nitrogen substances present as only protein. This is done by boiling the feeding stuff with suspension of copper hydroxide in glycerol (Stutzer's reagent) followed by filtration. All the true protein remains on the filter paper and can be determined in the usual manner, while the non-protein nitrogen compounds pass through into the filtrate.

Table 10.28

Biological Functions of Proteins

Protein function	Characterization of protein function	Example(s) of proteins exercising the function
Enzymic, or catalytic	A most essential protein function is in exercising the acceleration of chemical conversions (synthesis and degradation of materials; transfer of electrons, atoms and molecules from one compound to another)	*Fumarate hydratase*: catalyzes the reversible conversion fumarate + $H_2O \Rightarrow$ malate *Cytochrome oxidase*: participates in the transfer of electrons onto oxygen
Hormonal, or regulatory	Regulation of intracellular metabolism and integration of cellular metabolism throughout the whole organism	*Insulin*: participates in the regulation of metabolic processes involving carbohydrates, proteins, fats, and other materials *Luteotropin*: participates in the regulation of progesterone synthesis in the ovarian corpus luteum
Receptory	Selective binding of various regulators (hormones, mediators, and cyclic nucleotides) on the surface of cell membranes or inside the cells (cytosolic receptors)	*Cytosolic receptor of estradiol*: binds estradiol inside the cells, for example, those of endometrium *Glucagon receptor*: binds the hormone glucagon on the surface of a cell membrane, for example, that of liver *Regulatory subunit of protein kinase*: binds cAMP inside the cells
Transport	Binding and transport of materials between tissues and through the cell membranes	*Lipoproteins*: responsible for the transport and distribution of lipids in the organism tissues *Transcortin*: responsible for the transport of

(Contd.)

Protein function	Characterization of protein function	Example(s) of proteins exercising the function
		corticosteroids (hormones secreted by the adrenal cortex into the blood) *Myoglobin* : responsible for the transport of oxygen in muscle tissues
Structural	Involvement in the buildup of various membranes	*Structural proteins* of mitochondria, cytoplasmic membranes, etc.
Supportive, or mechanical	Functionally close to the structural function. Provides for the strength of supporing tissues and intervenes in the formation of extracellular structures	*Collagen*, as a structural element of supporting framework of osseous tissues and tendons *Fibroin* : intervenes in the formation of silkworm cocoon capsule β–*Keratin* : structural basis for wool, nail, and hoof
Reserve, or trophic	Utilization of proteins as reserve material for nutrition of developing cells.	*Prolamines and glutelins* : as reserve material in wheat grains *Ovalbumin* : as reserve protein of hen's egg (consumed in developmental growth of zygote)
Substrato-energetic	Functionally close to the trophic function. Protein is used as a substrate (in degradation) for energy supply. On degradation, 1 g of protein releases 17.1 kJ or 4.08 Kcal of energy	*All proteins* (dietary or intracellular) : decompose to end products (CO_2, H_2O, urea)
Mechano-chemical, or contractile	Contraction (mechanical process), by making use of chemical energy	*Myosin* : fixed filaments in myofibrils *Actin* : moveable filaments in myofibrils
Electroosmotic	Involvement in the buildup of electric charge difference (electrochemical gradient) and ion concentration gradient across the cell membrane	Na^+, K^+– *AT Pase* : an anzyme mediating in the buildup of Na^+ and K^+ ion concentration gradient and electrochemical gradient across the cell membrane
Energy converting	Conversion of electric and osmotic energy to chemical energy	*ATP–synthetase* : performs the synthesis of ATP owing to the electric potential difference or ion osmotic concentratiion gradient across the cell membrane
Cogenetic	Auxiliary genetic function of proteins (the Latin prefix "co" implies a co–operative action). The proteins themselves are not genetic (hereditary) material, but assist the nucleic acids in the accomplishment of self–reproduction and genetic information transfer	*DNA–polymerase* : an enzyme participating in the replication of DNA *DNA–dependent RNA–polymerase* : an enzyme involved in the information transfer from DNA to RNA

(Contd.)

Protein function	Characterization of protein function	Example(s) of proteins exercising the function
Gene–regulatory	Ability of certain proteins to participate in the regulation of template functions of nucleic acids and genetic transformation transfer	*Histones*: proteins participating in the regulation of replication and, in part, of transcription of certain portions of DNA *Acidic proteins*: participate in the regulation of transcription of certain portions of DNA
Immunologic, or antitoxic	Antibodies participate in the defense reactions against foreign antigens of microorganisms (toxins produced by them) via formation of antigen–antibody complexes	*Immunoglobulins IgA, IgM, IgG*, etc. : perform defense functions *Complement*: a complex series of enzymic proteins that interact to combine with antigen–antibody complex
Toxigenic	Certain proteins and peptides produced by organisms (primarily by microorganisms) are poisonous for other living organisms	*Botulinus toxin* : a peptide secreted by *Bacillus botulinus*
Detoxicating	Proteins, owing to their functional groups, are capale of binding toxic compounds (heavy metal ions and alkaloids) rendering them harmless	*Albumins* : binding agents for heavy metal ions and alkaloids
Hemostatic	Participation in thrombosis and arrest of bleeding (hemostasis)	*Fibrinogen* : a protein of blood serum, polymerizable as a network (structural basis for thromb formation)

DEGRADABLE AND UNDEGRADABLE PROTEIN

The protein intake of a ruminant becomes available for maintenance and production in two ways. In the first place it is broken down (degraded) by the microbes in the rumen and used in their own protein synthesis. Later in the digestion process the microbes are themselves digested and the protein they contain becomes available to the animal for their own protein synthesis. On the other hand, some protein is resistant to microbial breakdown (undegraded) and passes unchanged into the small intestine where it is digested and absorbed in the usual way.

At a low level of productivity a cow can meet her protein needs from the microbial protein, i.e., provided by digesting the bacteria and protozoa. In these circumstances, therefore, the diet only needs to contain a supply of degradable protein. High-yielding cows, however, cannot meet all their protein needs from that supplied by the microbes as in general the digestibility of bacterial protein is lower, 0.74 and thus the Net Protein utilisation (NPU) is about 0.59.

About 20% of bacterial nitrogen comprise nucleic acid. This fraction ot the crude protein is essentially wasted as these are degraded to form urea in the post-ruminal section of the gastro-intestinal tract. There is thus a great demand of undegradable protein in the diet of high yielders. This is also true for young ruminants where the rumen has not developed at all.

The protein in silage and barley is highly degradable (85%), and, therefore, supplies only a small amount of undegradable protein. On the other hand some high protein concentrates, e.g. soybean meal. fish meal etc., contain a higher proportion of undegradable protein, and these feeds should be used as protein supplements in the concentrate mixes of high yielding cows. In U. K. some feed manufacturers use this knowledge as a sales feature for their compound feeds and high protein supplements.

The feeding standards for dairy cows and the protein content of feeds may in the future, be given in these terms. For further information on degradable protein one may refer "Evaluation of Protein Quality for Ruminants'' written in this book.

Methods to Increase Utilisation of Crude Protein in Ruminants.

In plants, the protein is largely concentrated in the actively growing portions, especially the leaves and seeds. In animals, proteins are much more widely distributed than in plants.

Crude protein refers to all nitrogenous compounds (true protein + non-protein N_2) in a feed. It is determined by finding the N_2 content and multiplying the result by 6.25. The nitrogen comes from true protein as well as from non-protein nitrogen fraction. In fresh herbage as much as 30% of the N_2 may be in NPN form. Seeds such as maize grain or soybean seed also contain NPN which may be as high as 30—40% at the immature stage while levels reach as low as of 4-5% at maturity. Thus the amount and chemical nature of nitrogenous compounds in the diet may be extremely variable.

The amount of protein, its digestibility and the balance of essential amino acids are important factors that must be considered in balancing rations. In general, animal proteins are superior to plant proteins for monogastric animals due to the presence of all essential amino acids in proper ratio. Fortunately, the amino acid content of proteins varies from various plant and animal sources. Thus, the deficiencies of one protein source may be improved by combining it with another. It is for this reason that a combination of protein feeds in a ration is usually recommended when the person formulating the ration does not have access to specific amino acid values of the feeds to be used.

Amino Acid Availability in Non-ruminants.

Amino acid availability is critical in the nutrition of non-ruminants since they do not have the ability to systhesise certain essential amino acids. Therefore, non-ruminant nutritionists not only calculate total protein intake by a non-ruminant but also the proportion of each amino acids present in that. In recent years requirement of all essential amino acids in nonruminant species are calculated instead of total protein requirements. A deficiency, and sometimes an excess, of a particular amino acid can severely affect production though total protein levels appear to be adequate.

Amino Acid Availability in Ruminants

Since the great bulk of dietary protein fed to ruminants is subject to microbial attack in the rumen, methods of protecting a portion of protein from ruminal degradation, are matter of current investigations. It has been estimated that 20 percent of the nitrogen found in the crude protein fraction of the ruminal microorganisms is actually nitrogen from nucleic acids. This fraction of crude protein is essentially wasted as the nucleic acids are, for the most part degraded to form urea in the postruminal section of the gastrointestinal tract. Moreover, the true protein fraction from ruminal microorganisms is not as digestible as the dietary protein in many cases.

It has been observed that when amino acids and high quality proteins such as casein have been infused in the abomasum by-passing ruminal degradation, it always lead in improved N_2 retention, more rapid wool growth, greater milk production, and so forth. Qualitatively, ruminants have the same essential amino acid requirments as non-ruminants on a tissue level. Therefore, if certain essential amino acids are deficient in microbial protein, maximum performance cannot be achieved.

Many factors influence the rate of protein degradation such as (1) secretion of urea into the rumen via saliva and of ammonia through the rumen epithelia, (2) absorption of ammonia and other nitrogenous compounds by rumen epithelia, (3) recycling of bacterial and protozoal proteins in the rumen, (4) protein solubility and (5) flow rate through the rumen. The last two factors are most important.

Dietary proteins are degraded in proportion to their solubility in the ruminal fluid, For this reason, it may not be advantagious to feed ruminants high protein feeds which are highly soluble. Zein, a protein present in maize, is extremely insoluble, thus 40-60% is escaping ruminal breakdown. On the other hand, casein is highly soluble and is almost totally degradable in the rumen.

Various methods of protecting protein from ruminal degradation are described below :

1. *Heat treatment*

When protein feeds are heated, free amino groups within and between forms cross linkages which not only reduces the solubility but also reduce the surface of the protein for enzymatic attack.

2. *Treatment of proteins with tannins*

Tannins form hydrogen bonds with proteins, thereby protects protein from enzymatic degradation. As the treated protein travels down the digestive tract, the acidity of the fluids is altered and the tannin-protein complex dissociates.

3. *Treatment with formaldehyde*

The aldehyde reacts with free amino groups and N-terminal groups to form Schiff bases and cross-linkages between protein chains thus reduces the solubility of the protein and protects it from enzymatic degradation. Once the treated protein enters into a highly acid medium in the abomasum, the reaction is reversed and the protein is degraded.

4. *Encapsulation of amino acids*

The theory of encapsulating specific amino acids appears to be an easy, efficient means of ruminal bypass but yet the technique has not proven to be entirely successful.

5. *Use of amino acid analogues*

Only one analogue, methionine hydroxy analogue (MHA) produced variable but promising result. The compound is less soluble in ruminal fluids than methionine and thereby much of it escapes degradation in the rumen.

MINERALS

Animal body contains about 3 per cent minerals, which are constant constituents of animal tissues. These may be defined as those elements which remain mostly as ash when plant and animal tissues are burned. In animal body there are about 30-40 mineral elements which occur largely in the various parts of their body. Calcium and phosphorus account for three-fourths of the mineral elements in the body (49 per cent calcium, 27 per cent phosphorus and 24 per cent other elements). A predominant part of the mineral material in the animal body is located in the skeletal tissue (bones and teeth). In the four human bodies analysed in the laboratories of H.H. Mitchell of U.S.A., an average of 98.3 per cent calcium, 87.9 per cent of the phosphorus and 86.0 per cent of the total mineral matter (ash) was found in the skeleton. Out of 30-40 mineral elements which are found in animal body, a large number of these are not essential for body processes. Their presence in a tissue may be purely adventitious, due to their ingestion with the food, their imbibition in water, or their inhalation with air during respiration. In fact the essentiality of any mineral element is known from its metabolic role in the animal body from the criteria as mentioned below:

(1) it is present in all healthy tissues of all animals;
(2) its concentration from one animal to the next is fairly constant;
(3) its withdrawal from the body induces reproducibly the same structural and physiological abnormalities regardless of the species studied;
(4) its addition either prevents or reverses these abnormalities.
(5) the abnormalities induced by deficiency are always accompanied by pertinent, specific biochemical changes; and
(6) these biochemical changes can be prevented or cured when the deficiencies are prevented or cured.

Elements which do not meet these exacting requirements occur more or less constantly in highly variable concentrations in living tissues. They include aluminium, antimony, mercury, cadmium, vanadium, silicon, rubidium, silver, gold, lead, bismuth, titanium and others.

In general, *purified diet experiment* is conducted to know initially about the essentiality of any element. In such experiments, the animals are fed with ration made up of all pure ingredients such as for protein—purified uncontaminated casein, for carbohydrate—purified uncontaminated starch, for oils or fats—purified stripped lard or purified oil of maize or any other vegetable oil in stripped condition by which oil is made free of any other factor as oil soluble vitamins or any other compounds. For minerals and vitamins, individual purified items are added except that particular one about which we are interested to know the essentiality. Thus due to absence of that item in the ration, the experimental animal will develop some deficiency symptoms within a reasonable period of feeding purified diet. If the missing element is really an essential one, upon addition of it in ration where it was missing, the deficiency symptoms will be cured.

Twenty-one such elements have uptil now been proved to be essential and there is some

Table 10.29.

The essential mineral elements and their approximate concentration in animal body

Macro-elements				Trace of micro-elements	ppm mg/kg	Possibly essential mineral elements
Principal cations	(%)	*Principal anions*	(%)			
Calcium	1.5	Phosphorus	1.0	Manganese	0.2–0.5	Arsenic
Magnesium	0.04	Chlorine	0.11	Iron	20.80	Barium
Sodium	0.16	Sulfur	0.15	Copper	1.5	Bromine
Potassium	0.3			Iodine	0.3–0.6	Cadmium
				Zinc	10.50	Strontium
				Fluorine	2.5	
				Vanadium	50–500 ppb	
				Cobalt	0.02–0.04	
				Molybdenum	1–4	
				Selenium	1.7	
				Chromium	0.08	
				Tin	1.5–2.0	
				Nickel	?	
				Silicon	?	

evidence that six other elements may also be essential. Table 10.29 **gives an idea of the amount of such essential mineral elements present in the animal body.**

Many of the essential or non-essential elements may be toxic if their amounts are higher than usual level which cause disorder in normal metabolic disturbances. Selenium is an example of an essential mineral which is toxic at quite low levels in the diet while fluorine is another example of a mineral believed to be essential which in excess amounts produces toxicity. When any specific mineral is present at too high a level it may cause a metabolic deficiency of another mineral element by inhibiting the absorption of the latter; such is the case where a high level of molybdenum causes a conditioned copper deficiency. This fact is sufficient enough to emphasise that an imbalance of mineral elements—as distinct from a single deficiency—is equally effective to cause mineral deficiency. Supplementation of any diet with minerals should be done with proper care. In modern age the use of radioactive isotopes has advanced our knowledge of mineral nutrition and it is hoped that in the near future we may know much more through this type of experiment.

Over 80 per cent of the total mineral matter is found in the skeleton, giving strength and rigidity to the bones and teeth; the remaining mineral elements occur in the tissues and in the blood where they are frequently in orgahic combination and play an essential part in many of the body functions.

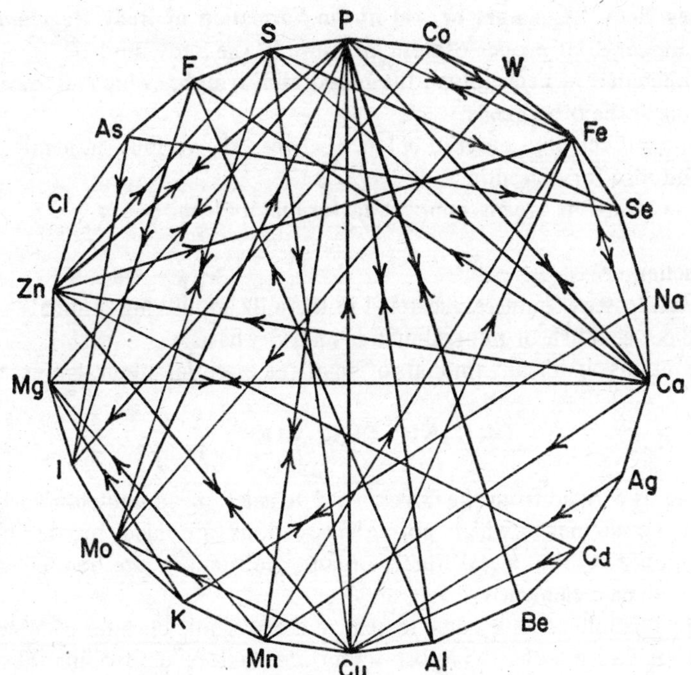

Fig. 10.9 Mineral interrelationships in animal metabolism. The arrows indicate antagonism between elements. For example, calcium is antagonistic to manganese. Magnesium and calcium are mutually antagonistic. (*Adapted from drawing by A. D. Tillman, Oklahoma University.*)

Minerals are necessary in the animal body in general for the following reasons:

A. In Tissue Growth and Repair

1. For the formation of new bones and tissues in growing animals. Bones and teetn are high in mineral matter.

Composition of fresh bone

Water	45 per cent		Calcium	36 per cent
Ash	25 ,,	⟶	Phosphorus	17 ,,
Protein	20 ,,		Magnesium	0.8 ,,
Fat	10 ,,		Others	46.2 ,,
				100 ,,

2. For the formation of hair, hoofs and horn.

3. A small amount is present in all soft tissue, which quantitatively may be small but are vital for life processing.

4. Blood cells also contain a small amount of minerals ror the normal functioning of blood cells. Haemoglobin of R.B.C. contains Fe^{++}, without which blood will not be able to carry oxygen or carbondioxide.

B. Minerals Act as Body Regulators or Aid in the Formation of Body Regulators

1. For the maintenance of proper osmotic pressure in the body fluids.
2. For the maintenance of neutrality of the blood and lymph, which is essential for the normal action of the blood cells.
3. To maintain a proper physiological balance between the various mineral ingredients in the blood and also for digestion.
4. As co-enzyme, minerals are also important for metabolism.

C. In Milk Production

1. To make good, losses of minerals secreted in the milk in milking animals. Cow's milk contains 5.8 per cent ash or mineral matter on a dry basis.

Milk normally contains significant amounts of all of the essential minerals—except iron.

ORGANIC CHELATES

The word "chelate' is derived from the Greek word "Chele" meaning "claw" which is a good descriptive term for the manner in which polyvalent cations are held by the metal binding agents. Prior to union with the metal these organic substances are termed as "ligands". Ligand + mineral = chelate element.

Recently, animal nutritionists have come to realize that organic chelates of mineral elements which are cyclic compounds may be the most important factors controlling absorption of a number of mineral elements. A particular element in chelated form may be released in ionic form at the intestinal wall or might be readily absorbed as the intact chelate. Chelates may be of naturally occurring substances such as chlorophyll, cytochromes, haemoglobin, vitamin B_{12}, some amino acids, etc., or may be of synthetic substances like ethylenediaminetetracetic acid (EDTA).

Chelates show exceptionally high stability. The bonds between the ligand and the metal ions are of "coordinate" type and occur because of peculiarities in the electron shell of the transition metals. Sometimes the chelates are so stable that the metal ion is released with great difficulty resulting in difficulties in availability by the animal or plant tissues.

In biological systems there are three types of chelates:

Type I. Chelates that Aid in Transport and to Store Metal Ions

Chelates of this group behave as a carrier for proper absorption, transportation in the circulatory system and passing across cell membranes to deposit the metal ion at the site where needed.

(a) Among amino acids, cysteine and histidine are particularly effective metal binding agents and may be of primary importance in the transport and storage of mineral elements throughout the animal body.

(b) Ethylenediaminetetracetic acid (EDTA) and other similar synthetic ligands also may improve the availability of zinc and other minerals.

Type II. Chelates Essential in Metabolism

Many chelates of animal body are holding metal ions in such a cyclic fashion which are absolutely necessary to be in that form to perform metabolic function. Vitamin B_{12}, cytochrome

1. 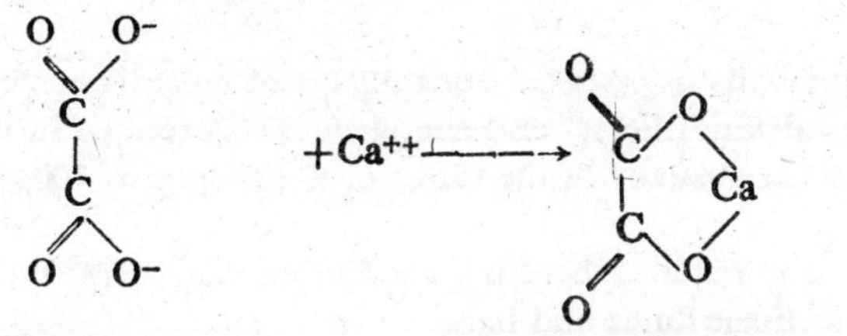 Oxalic acid + Ca^{++} ⟶ Insoluble Calcium Oxalate

Oxalic acid   *Insoluble Calcium Oxalate*

2. 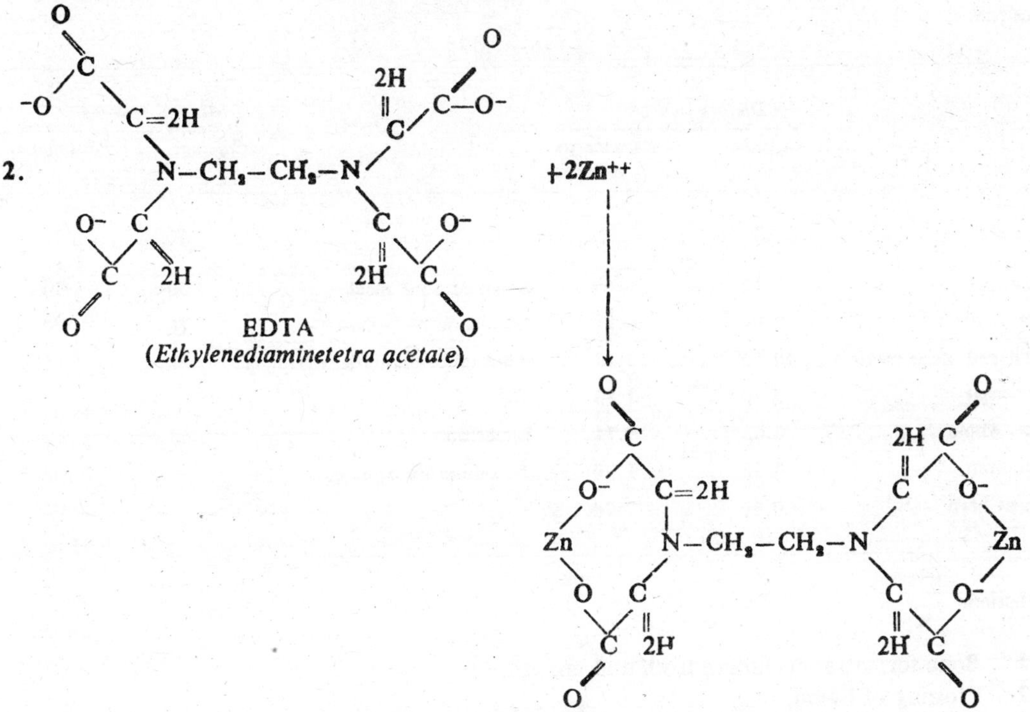 EDTA + $2Zn^{++}$

EDTA
(*Ethylenediaminetetra acetate*)

Chelates as example number 1 interfere with absorption while Chelates like number 2, serve to transport and to store metal ions.

enzymes and haemoglobin are some of the examples of this type. Haemoglobin molecule without its content of ferrous form of iron will be of no use in transporting oxygen.

Type III. Chelates Which Interfere with Utilisation of Essential Cations

There are some chelates found in the body which might have accidentally formed and are of no use to the subject. Rather, those chelates may be detrimental for the proper utilisation of the element. Phytic-acid-Zn chelate or oxalic acid calcium chelate are examples of this type.

CALCIUM (Ca^{++} at. wt. 40)

Calcium is present in the body in larger amounts than any other cations. 99 per cent of body calcium occurs in the skeleton and teeth, the remaining 1 per cent is vital for any normal animal body and is widely distributed throughout the body as essential constituents of most living cells and tissue fluids. In all species most of the calcium (dietary and endogenous) is excreted in the faeces. Blood serum inorganic calcium levels are usually in the range of 9–12 mg per 100 ml although that of laying hens contains more.

Calcium like phosphorus present in bone is not static; there is a continuous and very rapid interchange of these elements between blood, tissue fluids and bone.

Sources

Table 10.30

	Dietary sources			*Mineral sources*	
	Calcium	*Phosphorus*		*Calcium*	*Phosphorus*
	%	%		%	%
Milk	0.12	0.09	Steamed bone meal	30	14
Egg, whole	0.05	0.21	Dicalcium phosphate	26	20
Meat and Bone meal	10.60	5.10	Rock phosphate (defluorinated)	27	13
Fish meal	5.50	2.80			
Rice, whole	0.02	0.14	Limestone	38	—
Rice bran	0.10	1.70	Disodium Phosphate	—	9
Wheat bran	0.10	1.20			

Functions

1. Bone formation including teeth and growth.
2. Clotting of blood.
3. Regulation of heartbeat and working of muscle.
4. Maintenance of acid base equilibrium.
5. Control of irritability of neuromuscular system.
6. Maintenance of selective permeability of cell membrane.

Symptoms of Calcium Deficiency

1. Rickets in young and osteomalacia in adults leading to fragility of bones and fracture.
2. Milk fever in parturient can be due to sudden depletion of calcium.
3. Reduction in milk yield.
4. Thin shelled eggs with poor hatchability.

Absorption

It is believed that calcium is absorbed by active process (active transport) in the small intestine, more readily in the upper than in the lower portions. Several factors influence the degree of absorption, some of which are as discussed in the next page.

1. *Concentration of Calcium in the Diet.* The ratio of Ca to P in the diet has an important bearing on the degree of absorption and thus on blood levels on both elements. With a marked excess of either in the diets, the faecal excretion of both increases. At any rate, a ratio of Ca : P in the diet within the limits of 1:2 to 2:1 allows the optimum utilisation of both elements. (Find out the Ca : P ratio in your daily diet.)

2. *Intestinal pH.* Calcium salts particularly phosphates and carbonates are quite soluble in acid solution. Calcium chloride and acid phosphate are probably absorbed from the duodenum before the gastric juice acidity is neutralised. Subsequently absorption of calcium may be favoured by the presence of organic acids (lactic, citric, amino acids, etc).

3. *Protein in the Diet.* Certain calcium salts are much more soluble in an aqueous solution of amino acids than in water. Calcium absorption increases with increased protein intake. Lysine and Arginine are two amino acids found to be most potent in promoting absorption.

4. *Presence of Free Fatty Acids.* When fat absorption is impaired, much free fatty acid is present. These free fatty acids react with free calcium to form insoluble calcium soaps.

5. *Phytic Acid, Iron and Oxalates.* Phytic acid forms insoluble salts with calcium and makes it insoluble. In rats a sufficiently high iron intake will result in a low phosphate rickets. This is due to formation of ferric phosphate complex which is highly insoluble. The net result is an upset in the Ca : P ratio. Oxalates, in certain foods precipitates calcium in the intestine as insoluble calcium oxalates. No practical problem is generally observed since few foods are high in oxalates.

6. *Vitamin D and Parathyroid.* Vitamin D promotes the absorption of calcium by enhancing the active transport of calcium across the ileum. Parathyroid hormone has also some effect in increasing calcium absorption through the intestine.

Metabolism

Almost all the calcium in the blood is present in the plasma portion where it exists in fractions. The distribution is shown as below:

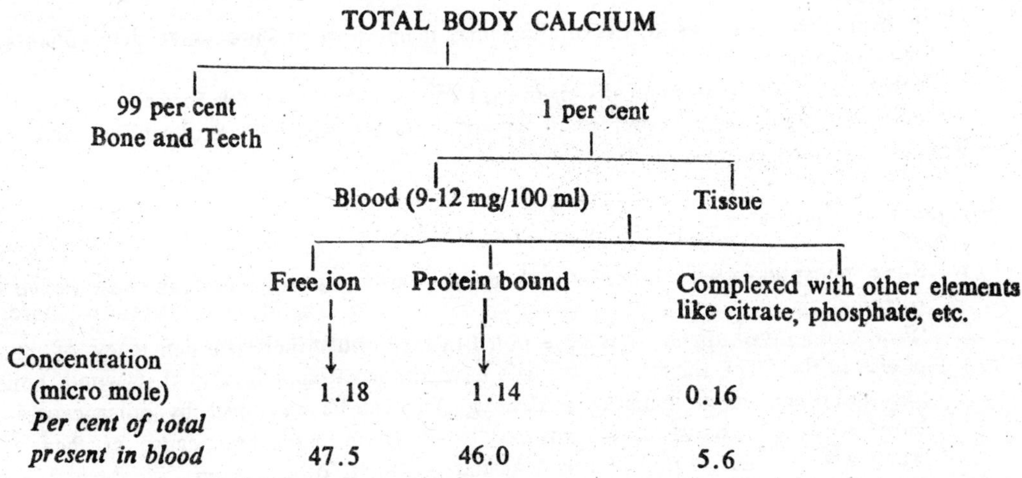

All of these forms of calcium in the serum are in equilibrium with one another. In the usual determination of calcium all three forms are measured together, although we are most interested to know the ionized amount, as it is the free ionized calcium in the body fluids that is necessary for blood coagulation, heart and skeletal muscle components, nerve transmission, etc. Ultracentrifugal method is used to determine the ionized amount.

The hormone of parathyroid gland causes the mobilization of bone calcium to the blood serum and the hormone of thyroid gland—calcitonin causes the deposition of calcium ions, in the bone; thus the two hormones maintain of calcium concentration of blood at uniform concentration.

Sources

Legumes like alfalfa, sterilised bone meal and milk products are major sources of calcium. Shell grit, oyster shell, dicalcium phosphate are the chief sources of calcium for poultry.

PHOSPHORUS (P at. wt. 31)

Phosphorus is found in every cell of the body, but most of it (about 80 per cent of the total) is combined with calcium in the bones and teeth. About 10 per cent is in combination with proteins, lipids and carbohydrates, and in other compounds in blood and muscle. The remaining 10 per cent is widely distributed in various chemical compounds. The amount of phosphorus present in blood serum is usually within the range of 4-12 mg per 100 ml.

Functions

1. Constituents of bone and teeth.
2. A constituent of the high energy compound ATP and thus is necessary for energy transductions essential for all cellular activity.
3. The oxidation of carbohydrate leading to the formation of ATP also requires phosphorus since phosphorylation is an obligatory step in the metabolism of any type of monosaccharides.
4. Phospholipids are constituents of all cellular membranes and are active determinants of cellular premeability.
5. DNA and RNA, the genetically significant compounds responsible for cell reproduction and therefore for growth and for all type of protein synthesis these phosphorylated compounds are absolutely necessary.

Symptoms of Phosphorus Deficiency

1. Since phosphorus is required for bone formation, a deficiency can cause rickets or osteomalacia.
2. 'Pica' or depraved appetite has been noted in cattle when there is a deficiency of phosphorus in their diet; the affected animals have abnormal appetite and chew wood, bones, rags and other foreign materials. Although Pica can be developed by other causes—a blood serum analysis of phosphorus may be run to know the exact cause of Pica, i.e., whether Pica is due to phosphorus deficiency or due to other reasons.
3. In chronic phosphorus deficiency animals may have stiff joints and muscular weakness.
4. Low dietary intakes of phosphorus have also been associated with low fertility and low-milk yield in cows and with stunted growth in young animals.

Phosphorus deficiency is usually more common in cattle than in sheep or goat as the latter group tend to have more selective grazing habits and choose the growing parts of plants which happen to be richer in phosphorus.

Absorption

In vitro studies indicate an active transport (molecules move from a low concentration to area of high concentration and this process requires extra metabolic energy). Excess of magnesium, iron, aluminium, by forming insoluble phosphates, made phosphorus unavailable. Remember, when there is either excess of calcium or excess phosphorus the larger amount interferes with the absorption of the smaller one.

Much of the phosphorus present in cereal grains is in the forms of phytates, which are salt of phytic acid, a phosphoric acid derivative. Insoluble calcium and magnesium phytates occur in cereals and other plant products. In ruminants like sheep and cattle there is no problem to hydrolyze insoluble phytates as rumen microbes produce phytase, an enzyme which changes the insoluble form into soluble form and thus renders the phosphorus available. In pigs some of the phytate phosphorus is made available in the stomach by the action of plant phytase enzymes present in the food. Chicks can utilise only 10 per cent as effectively as disodium phosphate.

Metabolism

The metabolism of phosphorus is in large part related to that of calcium, as heretofore. The Ca : P ratio in the diet affects the absorption and excretion of these elements. If either elements is given in excess, excretion of the other is increased. The Ca : P ratio considered most suitable for farm animals other than poultry is generally within the range 1 : 1 to 2 : 1. The proportion of calcium for laying hens is much larger, since they require great amount of this element for egg shell production.

Parathyroid hormone, when it becomes more, increases the serum calcium and lowers the serum phosphorus and vice versa.

Out of the total 4-12 mg of phosphorus per 100 ml of blood 43 per cent are present as free HPO_4^-; 20 per cent as $NaHPO_4^-$; like calcium, magnesium, etc.

Source

Grains, grain by-products, concentrates like oil cakes, brans, sterilized bone meal, milk products are the major sources of phosphorus.

POTASSIUM (K^+ at. wt. 39)

Potassium is the chief cation of the intra-cellular fluid and plays a very important part along with sodium, chloride and bicarbonate ions, in the osmotic regulation of the body fluids. Nerve and muscle cells ase specially rich in potassium.

Functions

1. Maintenance of acid-base equilibrium
2. Maintenance of osmotic pressure
3. Nerve transmission

4. Heart beat relaxation
5. Activates certain enzymes
6. Potassium ion is necessary for carbohydrate and protein metabolism but the mechanism by which it acts is not clear
7. It also aids in the uptake of certain amino acids by the cell.

Deficiency Symptoms

Overall muscle weakness characterized by:

1. Weak extremities
2. Poor intestinal tone with poor intestinal distension
3. Cardiac weakness
4. Weakness of the respiratory muscle.

The potassium content of plants is generally very high. The amount present in grass dry matter, for example, being frequently above 2.5 per cent; so that it is normally ingested by animals in larger amounts than any other element. Consequently it is extremely unlikely that potassium deficiency could occur in farm animals under natural conditions. Fortunately dietary excess of potassium is normally rapidly excreted from the body, chiefly in the urine. High intake interferes with the absorption and metabolism of magnesium in the animal.

SODIUM (Na^+ at. wt. 23)

The value of salt has been recognized for centuries. The common expression "worth his salt" and even the word "salary" all derive from the high value placed upon salt throughout history. Unlike potassium, sodium is present in the extracellular fluid. The sodium concentration within the cells is relatively low, the element being replaced largely by potassium and magnesium. Only one-third of the total body sodium is present in the skeleton, rest all in body fluids.

Functions

1. Maintains body fluid pH
2. Regulates body fluid volume
3. Takes active part in nerve functions (transmission) and muscle contraction
4. Functions in the permeability and carrier of the cells

Deficiency Symptoms

1. Growth failure and reduces the utilisation of digested protein and energy
2. Dehydration—decreases plasma and body fluid volume
3. Vascular disturbances—decrease cardiac output, decrease arterial pressure and increase hematocrit
4. Corneal keratinization
5. Nervous disorder
6. In hens egg production is adversely affected as well as growth. Experiments carried out on rats fed on low sodium diets resulted in reproductive disturbances
7. Salt (NaCl) deficiency is maintained by an intense craving for salt, a lack of appetite, a

generally haggard appearance, lustreless eyes and a rough haircoat. In milking cows there is a rapid loss of weight and a decline in milk production. In high producing cows collapse may be sudden and death may rapidly ensue.

Sodium metabolism is regulated primarily by aldosterone, a hormone of the adrenal cortex which promotes the reabsorption of sodium from the kidney tubules. In the absence of this hormone, sodium excretion is increased and symptoms of deficiency ensue.

Sources

All animal products, especially meat meals and foods of marine origin are richer sources; vegetable origin have comparatively low sodium contents. The commonest source is common salt.

SULPHUR (S at. wt. 32)

Sulphur is present in all cells of the body, primarily in the cell proteins containing amino acids, cystine, cysteine and methionine. The hormone insulin, the two vitamins biotin and thiamine also contain sulphur. In addition to these other organic compounds such as heparin, glutathione, conzyme-A, lipoic acid, taurocholic acid also contain sulphur. Wool is rich in cystine and contains about 4 per cent sulphur. Keratin, the protein of hair, hoofs, etc., is rich in sulphur containing amino acids. Small amounts of inorganic sulphates, with sodium and potassium are present in blood and other tissues.

Sources and Metabolism

The main (if not the only) sources of sulphur for the body are the two sulphur containing amino acids as mentioned above. Elemental sulphur or sulphate is not known to be utilised. Organic sulphur is mainly oxidised to sulphate and excreted as inorganic sulphate. The metabolic importance of some sulphur-containing compounds reside in the easy interconvertibility of disulphide and sulphydryl groups in oxidation reduction reactions.

Deficiency of this element in the body is not usually considered, since the intake is mainly in the form of protein and a deficiency of sulphur would indicate a protein deficiency. However, in ruminant diets in which urea is used as a partial nitrogen replacement for protein nitrogen, sulphur may be limiting for the synthesis of cysteine, cystine and methionine. There is evidence that sodium sulphate can be used by the micro-organisms more efficiently than elemental sulphur.

MAGNESIUM (Mg^{++} at. wt. 24)

About 70 per cent of the total magnesium is found in the skeleton, the remainder being distributed in the soft tissues and fluids. The normal magnesium content of blood serum in cattle is within the range of 1.7 to 4 mg magnesium per 100 ml blood serum, but the levels below 1.7 frequently occur without clinical symptoms of disease.

Functions

1. An essential component of bone.
2. Magnesium ion activates enzymes like phosphatases and the phosphorylation reaction

involving ATP. Among the later groups are glucokinase, phosphoglucokinase, creatine transphosphorylase, arginine transphosphorylase, etc.

3. Controls the irritability of neuromuscular system.

Symptoms of Deficiency

Symptoms due to a simple deficiency of magnesium in the diet have been reported for a number of animals. In rats fed on purified diets the symptoms include tetany which is exhibited by (a) redness of exposed skin surface, (b) hyperirritability, (c) cardiac arhythmia, (d) marked vasodilation.

In adult ruminants a condition known as *hypomagneseamic tetany* associated with low blood levels of magnesium has been recognised since the early thirties. The condition is known as *Grass tetany* or *Grass staggers* characterized by (a) convulsions, (b) hyperirritability, (c) twitching of the facial muscles, (d) staggering gait and ultimately tetany. Tetany is usually preceded by a fall in blood serum magnesium to amount 0.5 mg per 100 ml.

Symptoms can be reversed by injecting magnesium sulphate at an early time. but in practice this is sometimes difficult.

The exact cause of grass tetany is yet unknown, although a dietary deficiency may be a factor. Some research workers consider that the condition may be caused by a cation-anion imbalance in the diet. Others suggest that soils which are heavily fertilized with $(NH_4)_2SO_4$ and when cattles are pastured on such soils develop the disease as ammonium interferes with absorption of magnesium. Still others suggest that excessive ruminal ammonia production may be the cause.

Experimental magnesium deficiency has been produced in dogs, rabbits, guinea pigs and chicks. In most cases the deficiency diseases are similar to those of rats and cattle. Magnesium deficient chicks grow slowly for about one week, then growth stops and they become lethargic.

Source

Green fodders, pericarp of cereal grains, bran, cotton seed cake and linseed cake are good sources of magnesium. When hypomagneseamic tetany is likely to occur it is generally considered that about 50 gm of magnesium oxide should be given to cows per day as a prophylactic measure.

TRACE ELEMENTS

IRON (Fe at. wt. 56)

About 65 per cent of the total body iron is present in the form of haemoglobin (which contains about 0.34 per cent of the element). Myoglobin accounts for another 4 per cent, 1 per cent in the form of various heme enzymes that control intracellular oxidation, 0.1 per cent in the form of transferrin in the blood plasma, 15 per cent stored in the form of ferritin or hemosiderin and 10–15 per cent probably in other forms. Broadly, iron is utilized in the body for (a) transport of oxygen to the tissues, (b) for maintenance of oxidative enzyme system within the tissue cells and (c) it is also concerned in melanin formation. Without all these important functions life would cease within a few seconds.

Absorption from Gastrointestinal Tract

Iron is present in most of the animal feed as in ferric iron (Fe^{+++}). It is reduced in the acid medium of the stomach to ferrous form (Fe^{++}), the form necessary for absorption. The metal is absorbed almost entirely in the upper part of the small intestine, mainly in the duodenum. By an active process it is absorbed probably as a complex with amino acids and

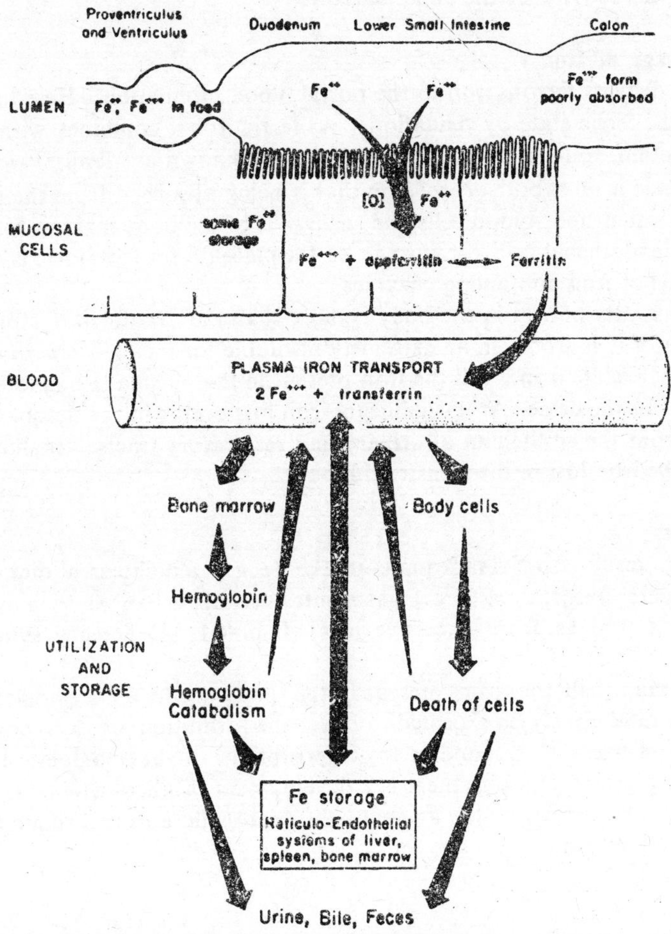

Fig. 10.10 Iron metabolism in Chicken.

is then carried to the mucosal cells of the intestine where it combines with a protein, *apoferritin*, to form *ferritin*.

Absorption is related to the requirements of the animal body. It is greatly increased if the body stores are reduced or the rate of formation of red blood cells are increased. In such cases, the iron portion of ferritin is more utilised and thus the mucosal cell becomes rich in apoferritin, which are further utilised to bind more and more of digested iron. When all the available apoferritin has become bound to iron form as ferritin, any additional iron that arrive at the binding site is rejected, returned back to the lumen of the gut and passes away for excretion. This means that the reserve ferritin present in mucosal cells correlates with body's need for iron. Thus, the two most important factors which control iron absorption are:

1. The state of iron stores in the body.
2. The state of the activity of the bone marrow.

Transport and Storage of Iron

Mucosal ferritin delivers ferrous iron to the portal blood circulation. Here the iron is again converted back to the ferric state by oxidation. As ferric iron it combines with a plasma β_1 globulin (carrier protein) to form a ferric-protein complex known as *Transferrin.* It serves a complex function since it must both *accept* iron that is being absorbed from the intestinal tract or from the degenerated red blood cells and *deliver* it to the bone marrow for haemoglobin synthesis, to reticuloendothelial cells for storage, to the placenta for foetal needs and to all other cells for the synthesis of iron containing enzymes.

When the total quantity of iron in the body is more than the apoferritin storage pool can accommodate, some of it is stored in an extremely insoluble form called *hemosiderin.*

The body does not excrete iron. All the iron present in the plasma is bound to protein and this does not appear in the urine. An insignificant iron loss occurs in the desquamation of cells from the skin and from the epithelium of urinary and respiratory tracts. In human being the more important is the iron loss in the menstrual blood.

Deficiency Symptoms

A deficiency may result from inadequate intake (e.g., a high cereal diet, low in animal protein) or inadequate absorption, (e.g., gastrointestinal disturbances such as diarrhoea or intestinal disease) as well as from excessive loss of blood. Deficiency symptoms may be narrated as below:

1. Since more than half the iron present in the body occurs as haemoglobin, a dietary deficiency of iron would clearly be expected to effect the formation of this compound. The red blood cells contain haemoglobin and in any interruption of haemoglobin formation will result in anemia. In pigs and chickens there is a development of microcytic (small red cell) and hypochromic anemia while in calves the anemia is of microcytic normochromic type.
2. Skin colour may be redden.
3. Decrease growth rate.

Sources of Iron

Green leafy materials, most leguminous plants and seed coats are excellent sources. Bone meal, glandular meal, liver and meat meal are other good sources.

ZINC (Zn at. wt. 65)

Zinc has been found in every tissue in the animal body. The element tends to accumulate in the bones rather than the liver, which is the main storage organ of many of the other trace elements. Most of the zinc in blood is present in the erythrocyte. The element is poorly absorbed from the intestine, virtually all zinc in food being excreted in the faeces, and only small amount in the urine. The amount excreted in urine is not influenced significantly by the intake or by the concentration in the blood plasma, suggesting that the zinc contained in the urine is derived from metabolic processes in the kidney. Traces are present in bile and somewhat more in pancreatic juice and milk.

Biochemical Functions

Zinc is an integral part of the enzyme *carbonic anhydrase*, which is present in especially high concentration in the red blood cells. This enzyme is responsible for rapid combination of carbon dioxide with water in the red blood cells of the peripheral capillary blood and for rapid release of carbon dioxide from the pulmonary capillary blood into the alveoli of the lungs.

Zinc is also a component of *lactic dehydrogenase* and, therefore is important for the interconversions of pyruvic acid and lactic acid. Also, zinc is a component part of some *peptidases* and therefore is important for digestion of proteins in the gastrointestinal tract. High concentrations have been found in the skin, hair and wool of animals.

Deficiency ymptoms

1. Retarded growth
2. Disorders of the bones
3. Skin diseases
4. Disorders of the feathers and hair coat
5. Reduced efficiency of feed utilisation
6. Delayed sexual maturity, sterility and loss of fertility
7. Severe zinc deficiency also causes loss of appetite in swine, poultry and cattle
8. Parakeratosis (a skin disease characterized by sore and itchiness), a naturally occurring disease of pigs, cattle, has been shown to be due to zinc deficiency.
9. Leg abnormality in poultry is a common feature of zinc deficiency. The defect is characterised by stiff and unsteady gait, shortening and thickening of the leg bones, apparent failure of cartilage cell development in the epiphyseal plate region of the long bone.

Sources

The element is fairly well distributed. Wheat standard middlings,safflower seed oil meal, molasses, fish meal with solubles are rich sources. Yeast is another very good source.

COPPER (Cu at. wt. 64)

Although Boutigny demonstrated the presence of copper in animals in 1833, its importance in nutrition was not recognised until Hart et al. (1928) of the University of Wisconsin showed that addition of both copper and iron is necessary for haemoglobin formation in rats suffering from anemia produced by feeding a milk diet. The role of copper appears to be that of a catalyst since it is not a part of the haemoglobin molecule. Soon after demonstration of the essential role of copper in haematopoiesis, several enzymes with oxidase functions were shown to contain copper. Among these are *tyrosinase, ascorbic acid oxidase* as well as uricase, which contains 550 micro gram of copper per gram of enzyme protein.

In the blood, copper is distributed approximately equal between erythrocytes and plasma, except in late pregnancy, when the concentration rises in the plasma. It is present in erythrocyte in the form of *erythrocuprein.* About 96 per cent of the plasma copper is firmly bound to an α-2 globulin as *ceruloplasmin,* the form in which copper is transported in the body. *Cerebrocuprein* is another form of copper protein isolated from human brain by Porter and Folch (1957). It differs from erythrocuprein in that the copper of cerebrocuprein reacts directly with diethyl dithiocarbamate.

Interest in copper nutrition was markedly increased when in the 1930's certain diseases of sheep and cattle in various parts of the world were shown to be due to copper deficiency. The first that copper deficiency is responsible for a disease known as *"salt sick"* in cattle came from Florida (U.S.A.). In 1933 a report from Holland showed that copper deficiency was responsible for the disease of sheep and cattle characterised by diarrhoea, loss of appetite and anemia, called *"Lechsucht"*. Bennetts and Chapman (1937) in Australia showed that a disease of lambs called *"enzootic ataxia"* was due to a copper deficiency and could be prevented by feeding copper to the ewes during pregnancy. These studies led to an extensive mapping of the copper deficient areas in most parts of the world. In all copper deficient areas the situation was markedly similar, as follows: (*a*) Sheep and cattle failed to thrive unless supplied with extra copper, either directly or indirectly; (*b*) blood and liver of the copper deficient animals contained copper levels which were greatly below normal, and (*c*) the forages and the soils contained low levels of copper.

Copper Content of the Body

A normal adult human contains approximately 100-150 mg of copper, or 1.5-2.0 ppm. Similar concentrations of copper occur in the bodies of the adult animal species. The body of the new born calf apparently is much richer in copper than that of any of the other species. By far the largest concentration of copper is in the liver. The liver copper level reflects the dietary intake; with high copper levels it may be increased manifold.

Deficiency Diseases

1. *Spontaneous fracture of bone.* Bone defects in grazing cattle and sheep on copper deficient pastures are characterized by spontaneous fracture and a condition very similar to rickets in young calves and osteoporosis in older animals.

2. *Demyelination of the central nervous system.* Severe ataxias have occurred in lambs and calves in various parts of the world and is known as *Sway back* or *Swing back* or *Gingin rickets* or *Enzootic neonatal ataxia.* The last name has been widely accepted throughout the world. Two types of neonatal ataxia are now recognised in lambs: (1) a common acute form occurs in new born lambs and (2) a delayed type often occurs in which clinical symptoms are not observed for several weeks or sometimes months after birth. In both diseases the symptoms are characterised by spastic paralysis, incoordination of the hind legs, a stiff and staggering gait and an exaggerated swaying of the hind quarters. Some lambs are completely paralyzed or ataxic at birth and die immediately.

3. *Pigmentation and structure of hair and wool.* A syndrome consisting of achromotrichia, alopecia and dermatitis is the most sensitive index of copper deficiency in the rabbit occurring even before a pronounced anemia. In sheep, copper deficiency produces a lack of black wooled sheep, and characteristic loss of *"crimp"* from the fibers of all wool. This has been found in Merino sheep, which normally have a crimpy wool, grow relatively straight when allowed to graze on copper-deficient fields. Copper content of the wool is decreased but

more interesting is an increase in sulphydryl groups and a decrease in disulphide linkages, which likely accounts for change in protein structure and change from crimpy to straight wool.

4. *Fibrosis of the myocardium.* A disease condition in cattle in Australia known locally as "*falling disease*", characterised by sudden death, usually without any preliminary signs. The anemia associated with 'falling disease' is of the macrocytic hypochromic type. The disease appears to be interrelated with complicating factors since it disappears spontaneously in each summer in spite of continued very low copper intake.

5. "*Scouring*" (*diarrhoea*) *in cattle.* Severe diarrhoea has been observed in many parts of the world. In Holland it was called "*scouring disease*", and in New Zealand, "*peat scours*". Scouring is known to be accentuated in areas containing excess molybdenum and low amounts of copper. In high molybdenum areas it has been believed to be due to molybdenum toxicosis and is referred to as "*teart*".

6. *Aortic rupture.* Recently in the University of Missouri (U.S.A.), it has been found that copper deficiency in chicks produces dissecting aneurysm of the aorta and various bone deformities, all in all resembling lathyrism.

7. *Decreased reporductive capacity and milk production.* Many experimental reports are accumulating to show the above effect on copper deficiency states.

Source

Under normal conditions the diet of farm animals is likely to contain adequate amounts. Copper level of the soil is an index of the copper content of the corps. Liver and glandular meal contains about 90 ppm. Among other good sources, cron distillers dried solubles, dried whey, peanut meal, cotton seed meal and fish meal are noteworthy.

MANGANESE (Mn at. wt. 55)

Kemmerer, Elvehjem and Hart (1931) were probably the first to demonstrate manganese to be an essential element in nutrition. A diet composed exclusively of milk cause poor growth and poor reproduction in mice which were corrected by supplementing the diet with manganese. It was soon found that manganese is also required by the rat and that high mortality, testicular degeneration and poor lactation accompany manganese deficiency. Interest in manganese nutrition was greatly stimulated by the discovery of Wilgus, Norris Heuser (1936) that a deficiency of this element was responsible for a crippling disease of chickens known as "*perosis*" or "*slipped tendon*".

The highest concentration of manganese is in bone followed by pituitary gland, pineal gland, lactating mammary gland, liver, gastrointestinal tissue, kidney and pancreas. Blood contains about 12-18 micro gram, about 2/3rd of which is in the blood cells. An interesting observation has been that lactating gland of the rabbit contains about ten times as much manganese as the non-lactating tissue, significance not known.

Absorption of Manganese

Absorption and final excretion of manganese appears to depend upon formation of natural chelates, (the word 'chelate' is taken from the Greek word *chele* meaning "claw") which is a fairly good descriptive term for the manner in which polyvalent cations are held by the metal binding agents. A metal chelate is formed as a ring structure produced by attraction between the positive charges of certain polyvalent cations and any two or more sites of high electronegative activity in a chemical compound. The bonds are known as "coordinate" bonds and occur because of peculiarities in the electron shells of the transition metals, specially chelates with bile salts. It is excreted in the faeces primarily via the bile and is probably reabsorbed as bile bound manganese. It appears likely that each manganese atom may recirculate several times before it is finally excreted. Therefore, manganese in the gastrointestinal tract represents a manganese pool which is in more rapid equilibrium with the tissues than it is with the outside environment. Excretion rate is effected by the presence of diet and not by the presence of other metal ions.

Biochemical Functions

1. Manganese has been reported to be effective in the *in vitro* activation of the following enzymes: Arginase, cysteine desulphydrase, thiaminase, deoxyribonuclease, enolase, intestinal prolinase and glycyl-L-leucine dipeptidase.

It is also thought to be required for (1) oxidative phosphorylation in mitochondria; (2) fatty acid synthesis (as a manganese chelate of acetoacetyl-S-coenzyme-A); (3) acetate incorporation into cholesterol and mucopolysaccharide synthesis.

2. Manganese metabolism is believed to be involved in amino acid metabolism, not only because of its activation of some of the hydrolysing enzymes (i.e., arginase), but also because it forms chelates with amino acid in which pyridoxal may participate. These complexes of amino acid, pyridoxal and manganese are transported in the body more rapidly than are amino acids alone. This links protein metabolism to manganese turnover.

3. Wakil *et al.* (1957) have demonstrated that manganese is an activator in the synthesis of fatty acids *in vitro*. It has also been found that manganese is involved in mucopolysaccharide synthesis and bone matrix cell maturation in chicks. Lastly it is believed that manganese also has a direct effect upon calcification.

Deficiency Diseases

Symptoms of manganese deficiency in mammals (rats, mice, rabbits) are similar but not identical. The nature and severity of symptoms depend upon the previous nutritional history of the experimental animals, specially the carryover of manganese from the mother and the manganese content of the diet prior to being placed on manganese deficient diets. Manganese deficiency in these animals is characterised by reduced growth, slightly reduced mineralisation, defective structure of the bones and decreased reproductive performance in both males and females.

In chicks the most dramatic manganese deficiency syndrome occurs which is termed as "*perosis*" and is characterized by gross enlargement and malformation of the tibiometatarsal joint, twisting and bending of the distal end of the tibia, and the proximal end of the tarsometatarsus, thickening and shortening of the leg bones and slippage of the gastrocnemius or Achilles tendon from its condyles. The disease is markedly aggravated by high intakes of calcium and phosphorus which is due to the absorption of manganese by precipitated calcium phosphate in the intestinal tract. Thus manganese is rendered into unabsorbable form.

Source

Whole rice is wonderful, contains about 420 ppm, this quality deteriorates when the rice is made polished (18 ppm). All other cereals contain moderate amounts, except for maize which is low in the element. Most green foods contain adequate amounts.

IODINE (I at. wt. 127)

As early as 1820, a Swiss physician, J. Francois, Coindet, first recommended iodine as a remedy for goiter—a disease results in a swelling of the thyroid gland. As far as is known the role of iodine in the animal body is related solely to its function as a constituent of thyroxine and other related compounds synthesized by the thyroid gland. Hence, a deficiency of iodine first causes the structural and then physiological abnormalities of thyroid gland and thereby affect entire animal body.

The adult animal body contains less than 0.6 parts per million of iodine, one third of which is concentrated in the thyroid gland, the rest is present in all tissues; next to the thyroids, ovary, muscle and blood tend to have the highest concentration.

Absorption and Formation of Thyroid Hormone

The element is absorbed as iodide from any portion of the alimentary tract, most readily perhaps from the small intestine. On reaching the thyroid gland iodide is quickly oxidized to iodine and bound to the tyrosine molecules of thyroglobulin a glycoprotein. In the thyroglobulin molecule, iodine is present primarily as (*i*) 3-monoiodotyrosine; (*ii*) 3,5-diiodotyrosine; (*iii*) 3,5,3,5-tetraiodothyronine (thyroxine) and (*iv*) 3,5,3-triiodothyronine. On hydrolysis of thyroglobulin, thyroxine and other iodinated compounds are released into the blood stream.

Metabolic Functions

The functions of thyroxine and thyronine and therefore of iodine are as follows:

1. Exercises control of the rate of energy metabolism or level of oxidation of all cells (calorigenic effect).
2. Influences physical and mental growth and differentiation or maturation of tissues.
3. Affects other endocrine glands, especially the hypophysis and the gonads.
4. Influences neuromuscular functioning.
5. Affects circulatory dynamics.
6. Thyroxine has an effect on the integument and its outgrowths, hair, fur, and feathers.
7. Influences the metabolism of food nutrients, including various minerals and water.

In cold blooded animals thyroid hormone action is manifested mainly by (1) an effect on the differentiation and function of the nervous system, (2) an effect on the skin and its derivatives, and (3) a role in metamorphosis.

Symptoms of Deficiency

Iodine deficiency is characterised by endemic goiter, resulting in cretinism and myxedima. Iodine deficiency greatly retards general growth, including a delayed osseous development which results in dwarfism in humans known as "*cretinism*". Severe deprivation of iodine is accompanied by a delay in almost all developmental processes. There is retarded mental development in the young and mental dullness and apathy in both young and old. *Myxedima* is characterized by a dropsy-like swelling (edema), specially of the face and hands, slow pulse rate, dryness and wrinkling of the skin, falling of hair and dulling of mental activity.

Sources

Foods of marine origin are very rich in iodine. Among common animal feeds, fish meal, meat and bone meal, molasses are the richest sources. Synthetic iodized salts are more commonly used by the farmers.

COBALT (Co at. wt. 59)

The first evidence that cobalt is an essential mineral nutrient for ruminants came from a group of Australian investigators, (Lines, 1935; Marston, 1935; Underwood and Filmer, 1935).

A number of disorders of cattle and sheep characterized by an emaciation and listness typical of mal-nutrition have been recognized for many years and have given a variety of local names, some of which are descriptive of the disease and some of which merely reflect the district or area in which the deficiency occurs. Thus the disease was known as *bush sickness* in New Zealand, *coast disease* in South Australia, *wasting disease* in western Australia, *nakuruitis* in Kenya, *pining* in Great Britain etc. The most appropriate scientific designation for all these conditions is *enzootic marusmus.* All these names clearly indicate the occurrence of cobalt deficiency in many areas of the world including Australia, New Zealand, U.S.A., Canada, middle and northern Europe, and many parts of Asia.

Progress in understanding the mode of action of cobalt in the animal organism was slow until after the discovery that the anti-pernicious anemia factor in liver, subsequently designated

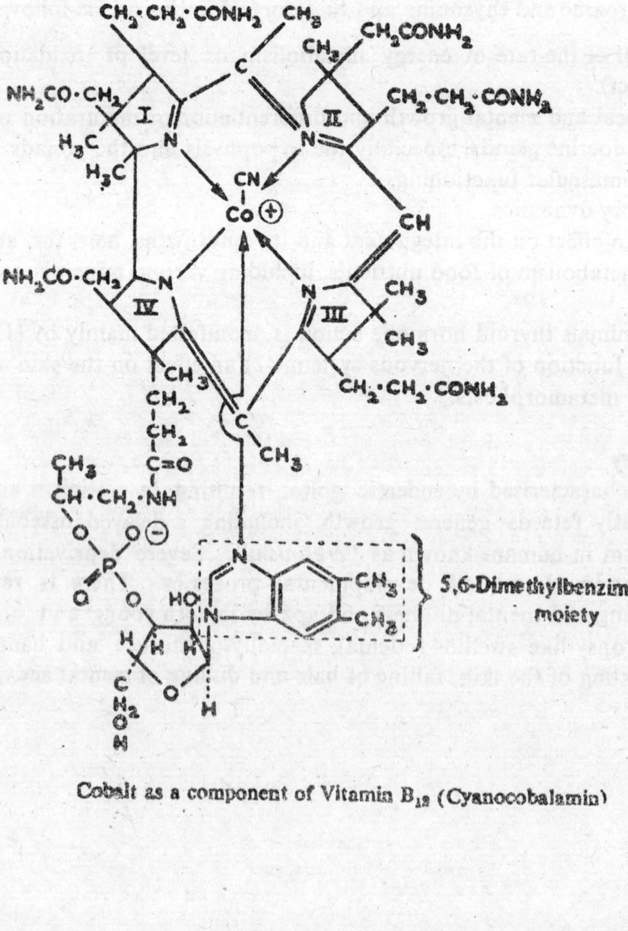

Cobalt as a component of Vitamin B_{12} (Cyanocobalamin)

vitamin B_{12}, is a cobalt compound containing almost 4 per cent of the metal. Within three years of that discovery complete remission of all signs of cobalt deficiency in lambs was secured with parenteral injections of vitamin B_{12}. Thus it has been proved that cobalt deficiency in ruminants is actually a vitamin B_{12} deficiency brought about by the inability of the rumen micro-organisms, in the lack of dietary cobalt, to synthesize sufficient vitamin B_{12} to meet the need of ruminant tissues for the vitamin. The other function of cobalt in animal nutrition has so far been demonstrated as the activating ion in certain enzyme reactions.

Deficiency Symptoms in Ruminants

The syndrome of cobalt deficiency in sheep, goat and cattle is essentially that of starvation. There is a gradual wasting of the animals. With this, there develops the usual straggly, rough wool in sheep, severe anemia with almost complete appetite failure. As the condition becomes more advanced, the animal is dull, listless, and because of the anemia all the exposed skin surface around the eyes and mouth take on a blanched or pale anemic look. The oxygen carrying capacity of the blood is markedly reduced and the blood volume may be severely reduced. There is a total absence of body fat, on the other hand the liver becomes fatty. As the cobalt deficiency state progresses the concentration of cobalt and vitamin B_{12} decline to subnormal levels in the liver and kidneys (which are the main sites of vitamin B_{12} storage). The levels of vitamin B_{12} in the blood serum also decline significantly below those of normal animals.

Prevention and Control

Cobalt deficiency in ruminants can be cured or prevented through treatment of the soils or pastures with cobalt-containing fertilizers. It has been found that single dressings of cobalt sulphate at the rate of 4 oz. to 8 oz. per acre raised the cobalt content of pasture from 0.04 to 0.19 and 0.39 ppm respectively.

The provision of salt licks containing about 0.1 per cent cobalt is a satisfactory procedure.

Sources

Although all plants and animal materials commonly used in the feeding of farm animals contain cobalt in trace amounts, but in general the legumes are richer sources. This also depends on the amount of cobalt in the soil. Cereal grains are poor in cobalt. Among animal feeds except the livermeal which may contain 0.2 ppm or more, the rest are mostly poor sources of cobalt. The cobalt content of milk and milk products is even lower, although it is possible to increase the cobalt of cow's milk several-fold by heavy supplementation of the cow's diet with cobalt salts. Normal pastures have a cobalt content in the dry matter within the range 0.1 to 0.25 mg/kg.

Cobalt Toxicity

Cobalt salts are not particularly toxic to animals, and there is wide margin between the levels which may be administered to prevent deficiency conditions. Unlike copper, cobalt is poorly retained by the body tissues and the excess will always be eliminated from the body. The toxic level of cobalt for cattle is 40 to 50 mg. cobalt per 100 lb. body weight daily. Sheep are less susceptible to cobalt toxicosis.

MOLYBDENUM (Mo at. wt. 96)

Although molybdenum has been known for several decades to be toxic when consumed in excessive amounts, knowledge of its nutritional essentiality stemmed from the fact that two enzymes of the animal tissues, (1) xanthine oxidase and (2) liver aldehyde oxidase contain molybdenum as an essential part of the molecule. Xanthine oxidases catalyse the oxidation of many different substrates including purines, aldehydes pterins and reduced diphosphopyridine nucleotide (NADH). The level of these enzymes in the tissues have been shown to be affected by the levels of dietary molybdenum.

A nutritional role of molybdenum has also been demonstrated in young lambs, where addition of the element as molybdate to a diet low in molybdenum increased liveweight gains. Similar growth stimulating effect have been observed in chicks and poults. Although in animal body about 1 to 4 ppm of molybdenum has been found but yet the amount required per day in the diets of the animal have not been worked out.

The effects of excess molybdenum in cattle, however, have been known for almost 30 years. A condition in cattle known for a long time in England as "*teartness*" has been identified as a molybdenum poisoning. It occurs when the forage contains 0.002 per cent or more of the element. Recently, potentially toxic levels in soils and forages have also been found in Canada and in New Zealand where the clinical toxicity is known as "peat scours".

The chief symptoms of molybdenum poisoning are extreme diarrhoea and consequent weight losses, and a decreases in production. The diarrhoea due to molybdenum poisoning can be restored by the administration of copper sulphate. The interrelationship between molybdenum and copper is as follows:

In the normal metabolism of both ruminant and monogastric animals, there is an antagonism between molybdenum and copper which is markedly affected by the sulphur content of the diet. It was shown that sheep on a low molybdenum diet (less than 0.1 ppm dry weight) rapidly accumulated copper in their livers resulting in a typical copper toxicity. Conversely, when the diet is high in molybdenum (5 ppm) sheep may develop a clinical copper deficiency. Sulphate administration also results in an increased excretion of molybdenum in the faeces, suggesting a reduction in the rate of molybdenum absorption from the gut.

Sources

Molybdenum (ppm)

Cabbage	1.00	Peas	1.40
Liver and glandular meal	1.80	Alfalfa meal (dehydrated)	0.35
Soyabeans, whole	2.50	Cereals	trace or nil.

CHROMIUM (Cr at. wt. 24)

The amount of chromium in body tissue is maximum at birth, falls quite rapidly during the early years of life and then levels off throughout the rest of life.

Schwarz and Mertz of Maryland in U.S.A. as early as in 1959 have reported that chromium in the trivalent form (Cr^{+++}) is needed for the normal glucose utilization. The importance lies in the fact that trivalent chromium acts as a cofactor with insulin at the cellular level, through the formation of a complex with membrane sites, insulin and chromium.

In the metabolism of lipids chromium might have got a significant rolo since it has been observed that when chromium is added to low chromium diets it reduces the level of serum cholesterol.

Similarly chromium also involves in protein metabolism. Rats fed diets having deficiency in protein and chromium showed an irregularities during incorporation of certain amino acids, such as methionine, serine, etc., into the protein of their hearts.

FLUORINE (F at. wt. 9)

Fluorine as fluoride is present in various tissues of the body, particularly in bone and teeth. Normal bone contains 0.01 to 0.04 per cent of fluorine as an integral part of the molecule and thus is an essential mineral.

Physiological Functions

(1) By combining with calcium phosphate, fluorine hardens tooth enamel and so helps to guard against tooth decay.

(2) It enhances growth in rats: 2.5 ppm of fluoride in the diet produce an optimal rate of growth in this species.

(3) In adults the osteoporosis is retarded by fluorine.

Absorption and excretion. About 90 per cent of the dietary fluorine is absorbed from the small intestine although large amounts of dietary calcium, aluminium and fat will depress its uptake. Excess amount of plasma fluorine which could not be deposited in bones and teeth is excreted in the urine, with the result that the level of fluoride in blood plasma is quite constant. At the time of low intake, the plasma level is maintained from the release of fluorine from bones and teeth.

Deficiency symptoms. Excess of fluorine are more of a concern than are deficiencies in livestock production because of its presence at moderate concentrations in the forages and in drinking water; also because of its presence at high (3-4 per cent) levels in variety of natural phosphate sources.

The only reported fluorine deficiency have been noted in children in the form of excessive dental caries.

Supplementation. No need has ever been felt for supplementing livestock with fluorine since most, if not all, livestock rations seem to contain adequate amount of fluorine. In case of real necessity, addition of 1 ppm to the drinking water should suffice.

Toxicity. The element at higher concentration is very much toxic to all classes of livestock. It has been estimated that a level in the diet above 20 mg per kg of the dry matter or from 8 to 9 mg of fluorine per kilo of body weight given to cattle causes a condition described as "Fluorosis". in which the following symptoms have been noted.

1. Teeth become pitted and worn until the pulp cavities are exposed.
2. Drastic reduction in appetite
3. Disturb osseous metabolism
4. Causes fatty degeneration

5. Inhibit certain enzymes concerned with carbohydrate and lipid metabolism (e.g., glucose-6-phosphate dehydrogenase, ATPases, lipase, alkaline phosphatase).

Note. Mineral mixture containing rock phosphate might carry more than 0.1 per cent fluorine. Their use should be made after defluorination.

SELENIUM (Se at. wt. 34)

It has been confirmed in 1935 by the scientists of South Dakota Experiment Station, U.S.A. that selenium of forages causes toxicity by promoting alkali disease or blind staggers in cattle. Interest in selenium was enhanced greatly by the discovery in 1957 that selenium in traces (0.05 to 0.2 ppm) is an essential nutrient despite its toxicity in larger intakes. Animals grazing on certain soils suffered from retarded growth and reproduction troubles which could be overcome by the feeding of traces of the element. M.L. Scott and associate of Cornell University have confirmed that selenium at a level of approximately 0.15 ppm is required for prevention of dietary liver necrosis in vitamin E deficient rats, exudative diathesis in vitamin E deficient chicks, and also for pancreatic degeneration of chicks.

Types of Selenium Compounds

The most common inorganic forms of selenium are selenic acid, selenates and selenites, which are the selenium analogues of sulphuric acid, sulphurous acid, sulphates and sulphites. Plants and micro-organisms have been shown to be able to replace the sulphur in cystine, and methionine with selenium. thereby producing selenocystine and selenomethionine.

In ruminants a large percentage of the ingested selenium appears to be incorporated by the rumen micro-organisms into the selenoanalogues of cystine and methionine. These may be absorbed by the animals and deposited in the tissues in the form of selenoamino acids.

Absorption, Transport and Excretion of Selenium Compounds. Inorganic selenite and selenocystine are absorbed for the intestine by passive processes whereas selenomethionine is absorbed by an active transport mechanism.

After absorption the compound gets binded with α_2 and β_1 globulin fractions of the plasma. From this selenium binding protein, selenium is then transferred to erythrocytes (RBC). Uptake by the erythrocytes is influenced by adequate intracellular reduced glutathione.

Selenium intake in excess of that which can be bound by proteins are methylated. In mammals this methylation occurs in two steps: (1) formation of dimethyl selenide; and (2) further conversion of dimethyl selenide to trimethyl selenonium ion which is water soluble and represents the normal excretory product of moderate excess of dietary selenium. At the time of excess intake, the transformation of dimethyl to trimethyl stops at certain stage and then the dimethyl selenide, being a volatile compound is excreted through expired air imparting a garlic odour to the breath.

Physiological Functions

1. Acts as non-specific antioxidant,
2. Protects against peroxidation in tissues and membranes,
3. Participates in the biosynthesis of ubiquinone,
4. Participates in hydrogen transport along the respiratory chain.

5. Prevents degeneration and fibrosis of the pancreas in chicks.
6. Selenium influences the absorption and retention of vitamin E and of triglycerides in at least three ways:
   (a) It is required to preserve the integrity of the pancreas, which in turn allows normal fat digestion, normal lipid-bile salt micelle formation, and thus normal vitamin E absorption.
   (b) Since selenium is an integral part of the enzyme, *glutathione peroxidase* (0.34 per cent of selenium), this converts reduced glutathione to oxidized glutathione and at the same time destroys peroxides by converting them to harmless aocohols.

$$\underset{\text{(A)}}{2GSH} + \underset{\text{Peroxide}}{H_2O_2} \longrightarrow GSSG + 2H_2O$$

Thus a portion of reduced glutathione (A) is spent to destroy the toxic compound peroxide. In the same way it also destroys fatty acid hydroperoxides (general structure ROOH) through reactions catalyzed by the glutathione peroxidase as below.

$$2GSH + ROOH \longrightarrow GSSG + ROH + H_2O$$

This prevention of attack by peroxides upon the polyunsaturated fatty acids of the lipid membranes of cells thus greatly reduces the requirement of Vitamin E.

Oxidised glutathione is again regenerated by the activity of the enzyme glutathione reductase

$$GSSG \xrightarrow[\text{NADPH + H}^+ \longrightarrow \text{NADP}^+]{\text{(Glutathione reductase)}} 2\ GSH$$

   (c) Selenium acids in some unknown way in the retention of vitamin E in the blood plasma.

Note. Vitamin E reduces selenium requirement in at least two ways:

(a) By maintaining body selenium in an active form or by preventing its loss from the body.
(b) By preventing a chain reactive auto-oxidation of the lipid membranes thereby inhibiting the production of hydroperoxides. This reduces the amount of selenium containing glutathione peroxidase needed to destroy the peroxides formed in the cells.

Toxicity

Selenium poisoning afflicts grazing animals if the forage contains 5 ppm or more of the element, or if the plants consume by the animals are grown on soil containing more than 0.5 ppm of selenium. Within plants grown on seleniferous soil, the highest concentration of selenium is in the leaves; less is found in the stem and still less in the seed.

The mechanisms by which selenium experts its toxic effects in animals appear to be through its competition with sulphur compounds or because of its strong affinity for sulphur in the formation of sulphur-selenium complexes.

The symptoms of selenium poisoning disease *Alkali disease* (blind staggers) which occur in horses cattle and sheep are as follows:

1. Dullness and lack of vitality,
2. Emaciation and roughness of haircoat,
3. Loss of hair,
4. Grating of teeth,
5. Stiffness of the joints and lameness,
7. Paralysis of the swallowing and respiratory mechanism.

Note: Certain species of plants contain 10-30 mg/kg of selenium and are potentially dangerous for the grazing animals.

Sources: Selenium is widely distributed in the animal body and is found in highest concentration in the kidney cortex, pancreas, pituitary and liver. The amount of selenium in feedstuffs is highly variable, due largely to differences in soil selenium content in the areas where feed is grown. Fish meal contains a good amount of selenium (1.2 to 5 μg/gram).

Relationship to Vitamin E

Some of the disorders of animals induced by dietary means are responsive either to selenium or to Vitamin E, indicating that a close relationship exists between the two nutrients. However, certain diseases are apparently caused by a deficiency which responds specifically to one nutrient but not to the other. The role of selenium in hydroperoxide destruction through glutathione peroxidase activity, serves to clarify the interrelationships between vitamin E and cystine as a precursor of glutathione.

If vitamin E prevents fatty acid hydroperoxide formation, and the sulphur containing amino acids (as precursors of glutathione) and selenium are involved in peroxide breakdown, all of these nutrients would obviously lead to a similar biochemical results, i.e., lowering in the tissues of the concentrations of peroxides or products induced by them. Certain tissues or subcellular components that are inherently low in glutathione peroxidase would not be affected by selenium, but would still be protected by Vitamin E, which acts as an antioxidant by a mechanism not involving glutathione peroxidase.

VITAMINS

When animals are maintained on a chemically defined diet containing only purified proteins, carbohydrates, and fats, and the necessary minerals, it is not possible to sustain life. Additional factors present in natural foods are required, although often only minute amounts are necessary. These "accessory food factors" are called vitamins. A vitamin is now generally accepted to be an organic compound which (*a*) is component of natural food but distinct from carbohydrates, fat, protein, and water; (*b*) is present in normal foods in minute amounts; (*c*) essential for development of normal tissue and for normal health, growth and maintenance; (*d*) when absent from the diet or not properly absorbed or utilized, causes a specific deficiency disease or syndrome; and (*e*) cannot be synthesized by the host and therefore must be obtained either from the diet or from the micro-organisms of the intestinal tract. The latter characteristic distinguishes a vitamin from a hormone; it is possible, however, that a substance may be a vitamin in one species and a hormone for ano her. Ascorbic acid, for example, is a vitamin for man, monkeys, and guinea pigs, but may be called a hormone in all other animals since they are capable of producing it by biosynthesis.

The vitamins have no chemical resemblance to each other, but because of a similar general function in metabolism they are considered together.

Early studies of the vitamins emphasized the more obvious pathologic changes which occurred when animals were maintained on vitamin deficient diets. Increased knowledge of the physiologic role of each vitamin has enabled attention to be concentrated on the metabolic defects which occur when these substances are lacking, and we may therefore refer to the

Table 10.31

Some typical differences between fat and water soluble B vitamins

	Fat soluble vitamins	*Water soluble B vitamins*
1.	**Chemical composition**	
	The group contains only carbon, hydrogen and oxygen.	Along with carbon, hydrogen and oxygen the group also contains either nitrogen, sulphur or cobalt.
2.	**Occurrence**	
	Fat soluble vitamins can occur in plant tissue in the form of a provitamin, which can be converted into vitamin in the animal body.	No provitamins are known for any water soluble B vitamins.
	Vitamins are not universally distributed rather are completely absent from some tissues.	Water soluble B vitamins are universally distributed in every living tissues.
3.	**Physiological action**	
	The members of this group are required for the regulation of the metabolism of structural units and each member appears to have one or more specific and independent roles.	Water soluble B vitamins almost collectively concerned with the transfer of energy in every cell.
4	**Absorption**	
	Absorbed from the intestinal tract in the presence of fat and thus related with factors which govern fat absorption.	In general, the absorption is a simple process as there is a constant absorption of water from the intestine.
5.	**Storage**	
	Any of the fat soluble vitamins can be stored wherever fat is deposited. The amount to be stored depends upon the intake.	Water soluble B vitamins are not stored in the same way or to the same extent.
6.	**Excretion**	
	Members of this group are excreted usually through faeces.	The water soluble B vitamins may also be present in the faeces (though sometimes only because of bacterial synthesis) but their chief pathway of excretion following metabolic use is through urine.

biochemical changes as well as to the anatomical lesions which are characteristic of the various vitamin deficiency states.

Before the chemical structures of the vitamins were known it was customary to identify these substances by letters of the alphabet (A, B, C, etc.). This system is gradually being replaced by a nomenclature based on the chemical nature of the compound or a description of its source or function.

The vitamins are generally divided into two major groups: fat soluble and water soluble. The fat soluble vitamins, which are usually found associated with the lipids of natural foods, include vitamins A, D, E, and K. The vitamins of the B complex and vitamin C comprise the water soluble group.

Vitamin C is the only member of the water soluble group that is not a member of the B family and its functions and characteristics are so different from the B vitamins that it requires special discussion. Consequently while making a differential study between fat and water soluble vitamins (Table 10.31)the consideration of Vitamin C has been excluded.

Table 10.32

Summary of the metabolic activities of vitamins

Vitamin	*Metabolic activity*	*Deficiency symptoms*
Lipid Soluble		
Vitamin A (Retinol, Retinal and Retinoic acid)	1. Oxidation-reduction activity, visual cycle 2. Necessary for normal synthesis of chondrotin sulphate	Cattle and pigs—skin conditions, xerophthalmia. Poultry—retarded growth, high mortality.
Vitamin D (D_2=ergocalciferol D_3=cholecalciferol)	1. Absorption of calcium from intestine 2. Necessary for calcification of bone matrix	Young animals—rickets; old animals—osteomalacia.
Vitamin E (α-tocopherol)	1. Inhibits autoxidation of unsaturated fatty acids	Most animals fail to reproduce; young cattle and lambs—muscle degeneration—chick—cerebral degeneration.
Vitamin K (Phylloquinine)	1. Necessary for the hepatic synthesis of proconvertin	Chicks—delayed clotting time of blood.
Water Soluble		
Thiamine (B_1)	1. Decarboxylation of pyruvic acid 2. Transketolase reaction of hexose-monophosphate shunt	Emaciation, weakness, and nervous disorders (polyneuritis of chicks and Chastek paralysis of foxes)
Riboflavin (B_2)	1. Biosynthesis of flavin nucleotide (FAD, FMN) 2. Used in oxidation-reduction reactions	Pigs—retarded growth, skin, conditions, eye diseases; chicks—curled toe paralysis.

Table 10.32(*Contd.*)

Vitamin	*Metabolic activity*	*Deficiency symptoms*
Nicotinamide	1. Component of pyrimidine nucleotides (DPN and TPN) 2. Necessary for biological oxidation-reduction	Pigs—Poor growth, enteritis, dermatitis; dogs—black tongue
Vitamin B_6 (Pyridoxine, Pyridoxal Pyridoxanine)	1. Amino acid metabolism 2. Active transport across cell membrane	Pigs—anemia and convulsions Chicks—slow growth, convulsions
Pantothenic acid	1. Component of acetylcoenzyme A 2. Acyl carrier protein	Pigs—slow growth, skin conditions, "goose step": chicks—slow growth, dermatitis
Folic acid	1. Co-factor in "active methyl" or one carbon metabolism	Rare in farm animals but will cause anemia and poor growth
Choline	1. Necessary for synthesis of lecithin 2. Lipid metabolism	Slow growth, fatty livers
Biotin	1. Necessary for the incorporation of CO_2 into organic compounds	Dermatitis and weight loss
Vitamin B_{12} (Cyanocobalamin)	1. Glutamic acid metabolism 2. Certain alcohols and synthesis of nucleic acids	All animals—slow growth wasting sickness in cattle
Vitamin C (Ascorbic acid)	1. Oxidation-reduction reactions	Farm animals do not require this vitamin, but deficiency in man, monkey and guinea pig produces Scurvy

FAT SOLUBLE VITAMINS

VITAMIN A

Vitamin A was the first of the accessory food factors to be identified as a component of specific foods. In 1913 McCollum and Davis reported that rats failed to grow on diets containing carbohydrates, protein fats, and salts. Addition of eggs promoted growth and established that the missing factor was a fat soluble substance. Finally vitamin A was isolated in large amounts from fish liver oils by Karrer in 1931. It was not until the late 1940's however, that synthetic vitamin A became available on the commercial market.

Structure, Absorption and Properties

Vitamin A (retinol) is a fat-soluble, long-chained alcohol that is almost colourles in pure form. Quite often, it is administered in an esterified form with either acetate or palmitate. Several of the carotenoids found in plants can be converted with varying efficiencies into vitamin A. Four of these carotenoids – α-carotene, β-carotene, γ-carotene, and cryptoxanthine (the main carotenoid of maize) – are of particular importance due to their provitamin activity. Of the four, β-carotene has the highest vitamin A activity.

β-CAROTENE

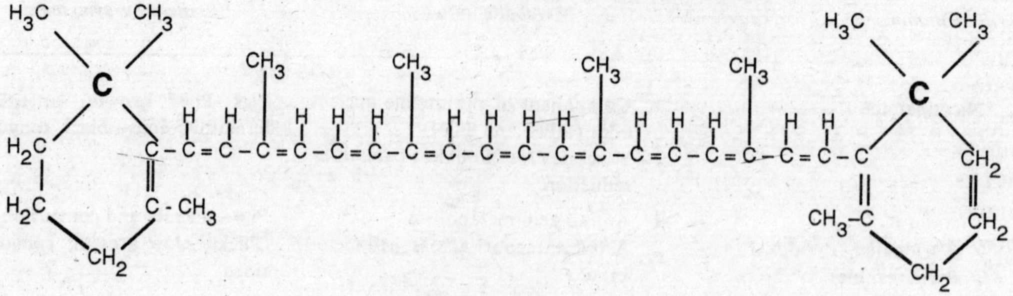

VITAMIN A

(Carotenase enzyme)

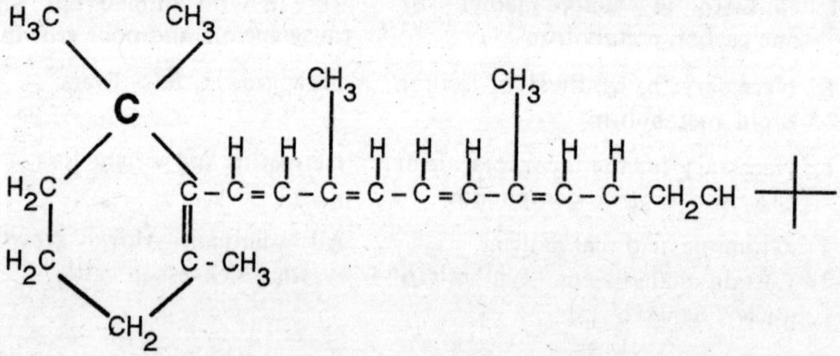

Table 10.33

CONVERSION OF BETA-CAROTENE TO VITAMIN A FOR DIFFERENT SPECIES[1]

Species	*Conversion of mg of Beta-Carotene to IU of Vitamin A*		*IU of Vitamin A Activity (calculated from carotene)*
	(mg)	(IU)	(%)
Standard (rat)	1	1,667	100
Cattle	1	400	24.0
Dairy cattle	1	400	24.0
Sheep	1	400-500	24.0-30.0
Swine	1	500	30.0
Horses			
Growth	1	555	33.3
Pregnancy	1	333	20.0
Poultry	1	1,667	100
Mink	Carotene not utilized		–
Man	1	556	33.3

[1]*Adapted from the Atlas of Nutritional Data on United States and Canadian Feeds, NRC–National Academy of Sciences, 1972 p. XVI, Table 6.*

Vitamin A is measured in international units (IU) or, less frequently, United States Pharmacopeia Units (USP), both of which are of equal value. One IU has the activity of 0.300 mcg of crystalline retinol (equivalent to 0.344 mcg of vitamin A acetate or 0.550 mcg of vitamin A palmitate). One IU of vitamin A is equal in activity to 0.6 mcg of β-carotene, the reference compound for the carotenoids. From the structure of β-carotene, it would appear that 1 molecule of carotene could be split into 2 molecules of vitamin A. However, in physiological systems, this 2:1 conversion ratio has not been demonstrated. So, in the standardization procedure, vitamin A is evaluated with β-carotene on a 1:1 basis. Different species of animals convert β-carotene to vitamin A with varying degrees of efficiency. The conversion rate of the rat has been used as the standard value, with 1 milligram of β-carotene equal to 1,667 IU of vitamin A. Based on this standard, the comparative efficiency of each animal species is as shown.

The alcohol retinol is converted *in vivo* to an aldehyde Retinal, isolated from the retina and is the form in which the vitamin functions in dark adaptation. A synthetic derivative, retinoic acid, possesses some vitamin A activity and is believed to be normal metabolite in the *in vivo* degradation of the vitamin.

The general term vitamin A includes a number of isomeric compounds which have various degrees of vitamin A activity (Page 520). The *cis-trans* isomers of retinol result from configurational differences at the double bonds in the side chain as illustrated below. Retinal and retinoic acid also exist in *cis-trans* isomeric forms.

Retinol and Retinal are interconvertible and Retinoic acid is a normal *in vivo* metabolite of retinol and retinal. It appears that retinoic acid cannot be converted to retinal or retinol since the acid will promote growth and maintenance in rats but is ineffective in preventing night blindness or in supporting normal reproduction.

Vitamin A molecule contains a β ionine ring with an unsaturated side chain. The molecule is derived by the cleavage of the mid-point of the polyene connecting the β ionine in one side

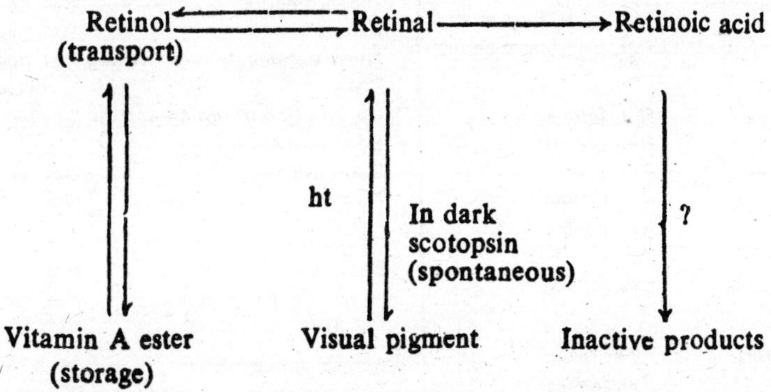

and in other side may be β ionine as in β carotene, or α ionine or some other rings as found in other carotinoids.

Absorption. For absorption of the vitamin A group, fat must be present in the ration. The fat is necessary for the release of bile and pancreatic enzymes, and bile acids and phospholipids are required for micelle formation (without micelles the fat is poorly absorbed, as are the fat-soluble vitamins). Provitamin A carotenoids, vitamin A and esters remain in the micelle. The retinal esters are hydrolyzed by a specific esterase; the ester is poorly absorbed. Retinol may be absorbed by a car-

Isomeric forms of vitamin A.

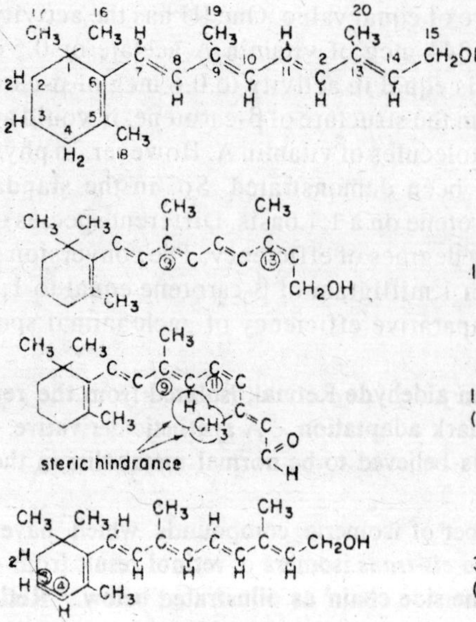

	Relative Biological Activity	
	CHICKS	RATS
Trans-Retinol	100	100
13-*cis* Retinol	50	75
11-*cis* Retinol (neo-b-retinene)	?	47
3-Dehydro-retinol (vitamin A_2, retinol$_2$)	?	40

steric hindrance

Table 10.34 Viatmin A deficiency signs in animals.

Abnormality	Animals studied
General	
Anorexia	Rat, fowl, farm animals
Growth failure and weight loss	Rat, fowl, farm animals
Xerosis of membranes	Rat fowl
Roughened hair or feathers	Rat, birds, farm animals
Infections	Rat, birds, farm animals
Death	Rat, birds, farm animals
Eyes	
Night blindness	Rat, farm animals
Xerophthalmia	Rat, bovine
Keratomalacia	Rat
Opacity of cornea	Rat, bovine
Loss of lens	Rat, bovine
Papilloidema	Bovine
Constriction of optic nerve	Bovine, dog
Respiratory system	
Metaplasia of nasal passages	Fowl
Pneumonia	Rat, bovine
Lung abscesses	Rat
GIT	
Metaplasia of forestomach	Rat
Enteritis	Rat, farm animals
Urinary system	
Thickened bladder wall	Rat
Cystitis	Rat
Urolithiasis	Rat
Nephrosis	Rat
Liver	
Metaplasia of bile	?
Degeneration of Kupffer cells	Rat
Nervous system	
Incoordination	Rat, bovine, pig
Paresis	Rat, pig
Nerve degeneration or twisting	Rat, dog, rabbit, bovine, bird, pig
Constriction of optic foramina	Bovine, dog
Bone formation	
Defective modeling	Dog, bovine
Restriction of brain cavity	Dog
Reproduction	
Degeneration of testes	Rat
Abnormal estrus cycle	Rat, bovine
Resorption of fetuses	Rat
Congenital abnormalities	
Anophthalmia	Pig, rat
Microophthalmia	Pig, rat
Cleft palate	Pig, rat
Aortic arch deformation	Rat
Kidney deformities	Rat
Hydrocephalus	Rabbit, bovine
Miscellaneous	
Increased cerebro-spinal fluid pressure	Bovine, pig
Cystic pituitary	Bovine

rier-mediated mechanism at low concentrations and by passive cellular diffusion at higher concentrations. The absorption of β carotene is much lower than that of the retinoids. Before transport from intestine, some β carotene may be cleaved by carotenoid 15–15′ dioxygenase to retinal. The retinal is reduced to retional by alcohol dehydrogenases esterified with palmitate. Chylomicrons carry mostly retinylester, with retinoic acid going into teeth portal vein.

In the liver, hepatocytes continue the β carotene cleavage with eventual formation of additional retinyl palmitate. Chylomicrons carry mostly retinyl ester, with retinoic acid going into the portal vein. In the liver, liver cells continue the β carotene cleavage with eventual formation of additional retinyl palmitate.

Almost no absorption of vitamin A occurs in the stomach. In the small intestine, vitamin A and β-carotene are emulsified with bile salts and products of fat digestion are absorbed in the intestinal mucosa. Here, much of the conversion of β-carotene to vitamin A takes place. From the intestines, vitamin A is carried through the lymph system by a lipoprotein carrier to the liver where it is stored. From the liver, vitamin A enters the bloodstream as a free alcohol, whereupon it travels to the tissues for use. While the liver is the main storage site for vitamin A, adipose tissue and the kidneys can also serve as rservoirs for excess vitamin A. In some animals, notably buffalo, swine and sheep, carotene is not absorbed without conversion of Vitamin A in the bloodstream. But other animals, such as the cow, have the ability to absorb and store this precursor. Grass-fed cattle have large stores of carotene in their body fat, which is evidenced by a deep yellow colour.

When feed is handled and stored properly, its vitamin A potency can be maintained for relatively long periods of time. Vitamin A is extremely heat labile, and contact with steam will immediately inactivate it. As storage temperature increases, the rate of destruction of vitamin A is accelerated. It is also sensitive to certain acids and rancid fats: Minerals such as iron oxide, charcoal, sulfur, ground limestone, bone meal, manganese, and iodine, all contribute to the destruction of vitamin A in feed. In addition to the destructive influences of minerals, many feed ingredients reduce the potency and shelf life of vitamin A in feed; among them, dried whey, meat scraps, and dried milk are noteworthy.

Through the use of antioxidants, either natural or synthetic, a substantial amount of the vitamin A fraction can be protcted from oxidation.

Vitamin A and Vision

In the retina of the eye there are structures called rods, which are concerned with vision in dim light, and cones, which are concerned with vision in bright light and are responsible for colour vision. The characteristic pigments of rods and cones are the conjugated carotenoid proteins known respectively as rhodopsin and iodopsin. According to Wald they differ only in their opsin, or protein, moieties. The carotenoid common to rhodopsin and iodopsin is a *cis* isomer of retinal.

Rhodopsin, which is essential to night vision, is a bright red pigment that bleaches on exposure to light, becoming the yellow compound retinal (or retinene) through the loss of the protein opsin. Upon reduction, retinal yields retinol, which is colorless

In the dark, rhodopsin can be regenerated. Through the action of alcohol dehydrogenase and

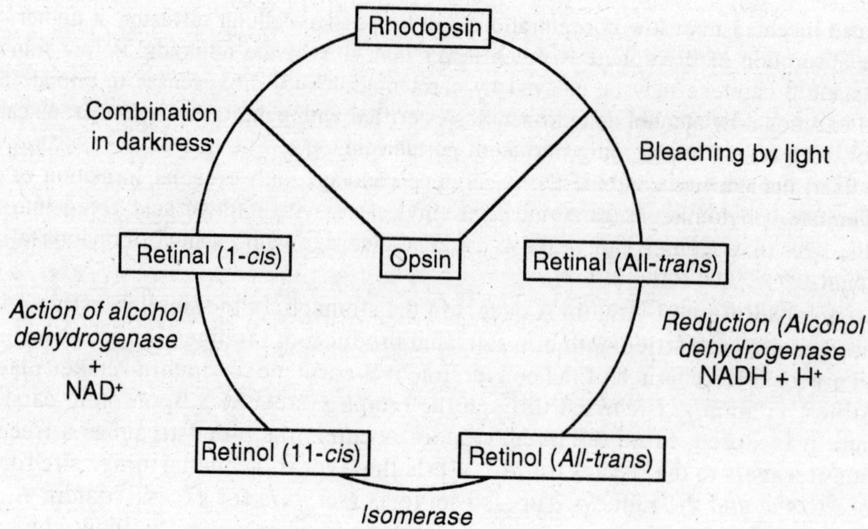

Fig. 10.11 **The Rhodopsin-Vitamin A cycle**

NAD, the 11-*cis* isomer of retinol oxidizes to the corresponding isomer of retinal. Then in the absence of light the 11-*cis*-retinal combines with the ε-amino group of a specific lysine residue in opsin to form rhodopsin or visual purple.

Some vitamin A is lost in the rhodopsin-vitamin A visual cycle, and consequently a deficiency of the vitamin eventually results in a lessened ability to see in dim light. This condition, commonly known as *night blindness.*

Vision also can be impared due to a condition called *xerophathalmia*, another manifestation of a vitamin A deficiency. The conjunctivita (the covering of the eye) dries out, the cornea becomes inflamed, and the eye becomes ulcerated.

Vitamin A and Carotene

Plant kingdom is devoid of vitamin A as such. It is not possible to trace of vitamin A in any fruits, vegetables or any part of vegetable origin, but it is the pigments carotinoids, which are present as precursor of vitamin A i.e., vitamin A will be formed from various carotinoids after their consumption by animals or human beings inside their body systems. Carotene derives its name from the carrot, from which it was first isolated over 100 years ago, is the yellow coloured, fat soluble substance that gives the characteristic colour to carrots and butter made from cow but not from buffalo (since buffalo milk does not contain carotene as the compound before reaching the udder completely converted into vitamin A, which is colourless. Carotenes are abundantly present in all green plants and grasses, although the yellow colour is masked by the green colour of chlorophyll. Quite often vitamin A is administered in an esterified form with either acetate or palmitate.

2. VITAMIN A IN REPRODUCTION. In rat experiment, it has been found that Retinol or Retinal is required for maintenance of the placenta in the second half of the gestation period (22 days).

At about the 16th day necrosis of the periphery of the placental disk occurs with resorption of the fetus. In male there is failure of spermatogenesis. The damage can be reversed in both sexes by retinol.

3. SYNTHESIS OF MUCOPOLYSACCHARIDES (MPS). Mucus epithelial cells are distributed throughout the body as in respiratory tract, alimentary tract, reproductive tract, etc. Vitamin A is concerned in the synthesis of MPS by doing activation of sulphate molecule which is an important element of MPS. In its absence keratinization of epithelial cells take place which thus affects.

(a) *Respiratory*—due to keratinized tissue, cold and sinus trouble tend to be more severe
(b) *Alimentary tract*—leads of diarrhoea
(c) *Genito-urinary tract*—accounts for the high incidence of kidney and bladder stones through interference with elimination of urine
(d) *Reproductive tract*—directly interferes with normal reproduction.

4. DEVELOPMENT OF BONE. It is concerned with normal development of bone through a control exercised over the activity of osteoclasts and osteoblasts of the epithelial cartilage.

A failure of the spinal and some other bone to develop normally results in turn a pressure on the nerves and in their degeneration. Blindness in calves results from a constriction of optic nerve caused by a narrowing of the bone canal through which it passes. Avitaminosis can result in deafness in dogs, owing to an injury to the auditory nerve.

In practice severe deficiency symptoms are unlikely to occur an adult animals except after prolonged deprivation. Grazing animals generally obtain sufficient amount of provitamin—carotinoids, from pasture grass and normally build up liver reserves.

In poultry on a diet deficient in vitamin A, the mortality rate is usually high. Early symptoms include retarded growth, weakness, ruffled plumage and a staggering gait Yellow maize, dried grass or other green feed, or alternatively cod or other fish liver oils or vitamin A concentrate, can be added to the diet.

5. GROWTH. Because of stimulant for building new cells of epithelial in nature and for bones where it controls the osteoclastic and osteoblastic activity, vitamin A definitely interferes with growth.

Sources of Vitamin A. Plant kingdom contains no vitamin A. It is the precursor like different carotinoids which are the potent forms of vit-A present in the plant kingdom. All yellow vegetables and fruits and the leafy green vegetables supply provitamin A in the diet. Preformed vit-A supplied by milk, fat, liver, egg yolk, and certain fish oils are all excellent sources.

Synthetic vitamin A can be obtained in pure form.

VITAMIN D

The history of vitamin D started in 1809 with Bardsley, who found that cod liver oil could cure rickets. The relationship between sunlight and rickets was recognised in 1809 by Palm. The great expansion in the understanding of vitamin D occurred in the late 1910s and early 1920s with experimental rickets, teeth development and its distinction from vitamin A due to its stability.

The disease rachitis, now commonly called rickets, is known to mankind since ancient times. In 1950 Infant rickets was described by Glisson in England. The desease was prevalent especially among the children of the lower classes of people in England (and other sections of the world) for centuries. Infection was early postulated as a cause of the disease. Around

London the abundance of fog was held responsible by some to be a contributing factor. In other words, the lack of sunshine due to the fog was a predisposing factor.

In 1918 Mellanby produced the first clear-cut experimental rickets in dogs by feeding only milk. Rickets developed regularly on such diets. In 1919 Huldschinsky demonstrated marked clinical improvement in severely rachitic children by applying ultraviolet rays on their bodies. In 1931 Angus and co-workers isolated crystalline vitamin D upon ultraviolet irradiation of ergosterol. This was named calciferol and is referred to as vitamin D_2. Later on vitamin D_3 was isolated by irradiation of 7-dehydrocholesterol. It is now established that small amounts of 7-dehydrocholesterol is associated with skin of animals, and thus ultraviolet light, from the sun or from artificial sources, is able to activate and yield vitamin D_3 to the body.

Vitamin D is not actually a vitamin and in normal conditions its inclusion in the diet is probably unnecessary for full health. Rather, vitamin D is hormone, a steroid derivative, that is synthesized in the skin, undergoes a series of activating biochemical reactions, and acts on specific intracellular receptor sides in a wide variety of tissues.

Vitamin D is sterioid that is acid- and light unstable. The two major vitamin D compounds are D_2 from ergosterol in plants yeast and fungi while D_3 from 7-dehydrocholesterol, which is present in the skin and undergoes photochemical transformation in which the bond between C9 and C10 in ring B is broken to yield cholecalciferol or vitamin D_3. 7 dehydrocholesterol is converted in the skin to previtamin D_3 producing 10 mg within 10–15 minutes exposure of hands and face in main by ultraviolet (UV) at 282 nm. Cholecalciferol when hydroxylated in liver at position 25, it yields 25 hydroxy vitamin D_3 or calcifediol. The same compound is then converted in kidney to 1, 25-dihydroxyvitamin D_3 or calcitriol. It is likely that growth hormone and prolactin are major physiological regulators of calcitriol production and are particularly important during conditions of growth, pregnancy and lactation.

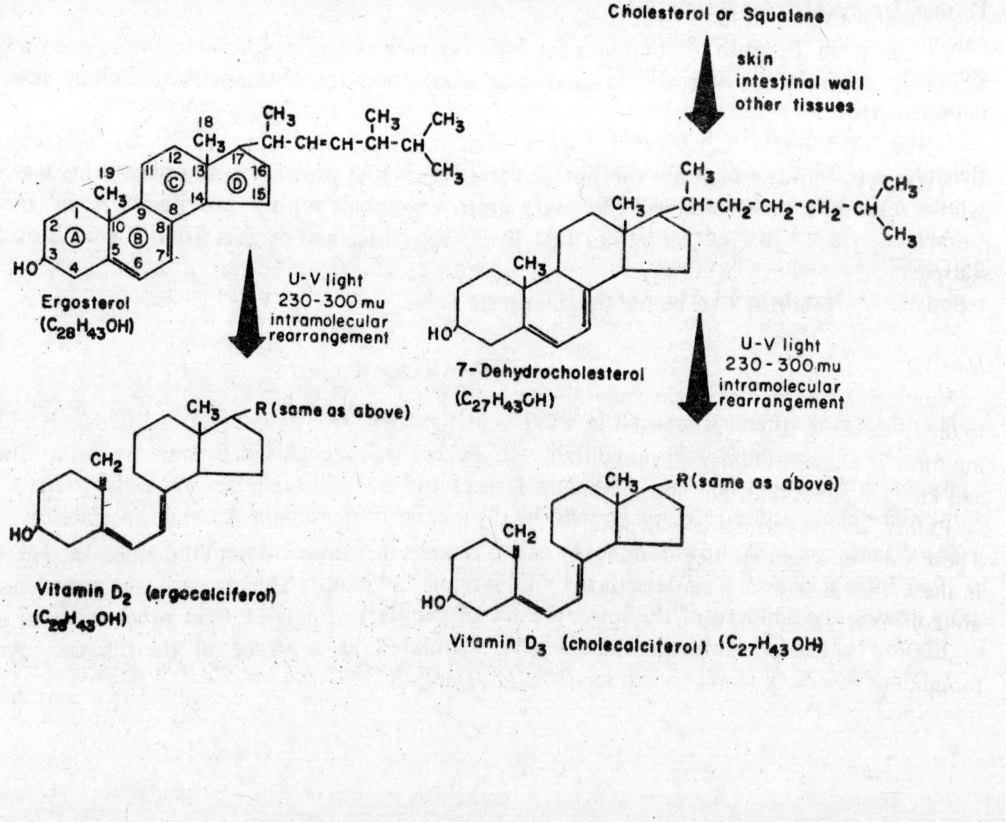

Cholesterol or Squalene

skin
intestinal wall
other tissues

Ergosterol
$(C_{28}H_{43}OH)$

U-V light
230-300 mu
intramolecular
rearrangement

7-Dehydrocholesterol
$(C_{27}H_{43}OH)$

U-V light
230-300 mu
intramolecular
rearrangement

R (same as above)

Vitamin D_2 (ergocalciferol)
$(C_{28}H_{43}OH)$

R (same as above)

Vitamin D_3 (cholecalciferol) $(C_{27}H_{43}OH)$

The value of other forms of vitamin D cannot be accurately assessed at present, since small amounts may occur in natural sources and their value, if any, is not established. Vitamin D_4 is activated 22-dehydroergosterol. Vitamin D_5 is activated 7-dehydrositosterol. The structures of vitamin D_2 and D_3 are given below: (both differ in side chain only).

Absorption. As with vitamin A, fat digestion products are required for optimal intestinal absorption of vitamin D because bile acids are required for micelle formation. Absorption probably occurs in both the jejunum and ileum. It is transported then in chylomicrons to the liver and fat tissue and stored with DBP (vitamin D-binding protein) in the liver. Subsequent transport from the liver or skin uses α_2-globulin DBP as a carrier, except previtamin D. The first major step in vitamin D metabolism is 25 hydroxylation in the hepatocytes; it may also occur in lung, kidney, and intestine.

This may increase with deficiency. The second important step is 1 α hydroxylation by the kidney and placenta, a step tightly regulated by hormones. Low serum calcium causes release of parathyroid hormone (PTH), which lowers intracellular phophate and in turn stimulates 1 α hydroxylation of 25 vitamin D. It is suppressed also by 1, 25 $(OH)_2$ vitamin and serum calcium. 24 hydroxylation, which probably occurs in the kidney, is regulated also but opposite to 1 α hydroxylation in relation to 1, 25 vitamin D levels. 24 hydroxylation is a preliminary step to biliary excretion, which is the major pathway. Chronic alcohol consumption can cause an increased loss of 25 vitamin D into bile.

Metabolic Functions

1. The active form of vitamin D is the metabolite 1, 25 $(OH)_2$ vitamin D, which acts as a hormone, controlling calcium and phosphorus homeostasis. Calcium absorption is increased by 1, 25 vitamin D.

How it is done ? 1, 25 vitamin D binds to a cytosol (the unsaturated aqueous phase of the cytoplasm between the structured organelles) receptor protein (RP). This complex compound (RP + 1, 25 vitamin D) then binds to DNA causing mRNA transcription for calcium binding protein (CaBP). High dietary calcium decreases the production of 1, $25(OH)_2D_3$ by the kidney, and low dietary Ca stimulates it. Regulation of 1, $25(OH)_2D_3$ synthesis is related also to serum concentration, through the action of parathyroid hormone (PTH) which catalyzes the conversion of 25-OH-D_3 to 1, 25-$(OH)_2D_3$. Thus, 1, 25-$(OH)D_3$ appears to be the ideal compound for treatment of diseases related to parathyroid insufficiency. Various analogs of this very expensively isolated and purified compound are receiving attention for use in clinical problems of Ca homeostasis in humans and animals.

Although it is generally agreed that the kidney is the principal site of production of 1, $25(OH)_2D_3$, a number of other cell types, including bone, placenta, intestine, and yolk sac have been reported to make the conversion of 25-OH-D_3 to 1, 25 $(OH)_2D_3$.

How Vitamin D3 is changed into 1, $25(OH)_2D_3$?

Vitamin D absorbed from the small intestines or made in the skin by ultraviolet radiation is carried to the liver where it is hydroxylated to produce 25-hydroxyvitamin D_3 (25-OH-D_3), the main circulating form of vitamin D. Significant hydroxylation also occurs in other tissues, including lung, intestine and kidney. There does not appear to be a direct action of 25-OH-D_3 on any target tissue.

Rather, further formation is needed; metabolism of 1, $25(OH)2D_3$ occurs exclusively in the kidney. These final products are delivered by the blood to the target tissues of intestine, bone and elsewhere in the kidney where they carry out their functions. Thus the metabolically active forms of vitamin D are considered to hormones

2. Bone formation is another/important function of 1, 25 vitamin D which increases receptors for/epidermal growth factor and stimulate transforming-growth factor B(TGF). TGFB stimulates bone

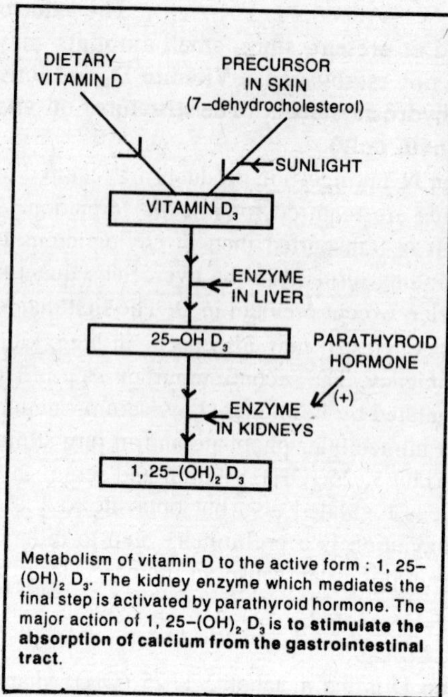

Metabolism of vitamin D to the active form : 1, 25-$(OH)_2$ D_3. The kidney enzyme which mediates the final step is activated by parathyroid hormone. The major action of 1, 25-$(OH)_2$ D_3 is to **stimulate the absorption of calcium from the gastrointestinal tract.**

Fig. 10.12

resorption and cartilage induction.

3. Vitamin D is also involved to facilitate the clearance of phosphate in the kidney.

4. Addition of vitamin D reduces oxidation of citric acid and a high citrate concentration is found in kidney, bone and blood but not in liver. As citrate has nothing to do with bone growth, the high citrate level which is also accompanied by more citrate excretion has no known physiological role.

5. It has been found that vitamin D increases the activity of the enzyme phytase in the rat intestine. This enzyme hydrolysed food phytic acid (grains primarily), yielding inorganic phosphate. However, the increased enzyme activities do not liberate sufficient inorganic phosphate to account for the antirachitic action of vitamin D.

6. It has been found by De Luca that vitamin D stimulates incorporation of phosphorus into phospholipids of intestinal mucosa.

7. Vitamin D also affects differentiation of some cells, i.e., myleocytes to monocytes or macro phages. It inhibits growth of some carcinomas, specially breast cancer and malignant melanoma.

8. Available evidence also indicates that vitamin D promotes absorption from the GI tract of Be, CO, Mg, Sr, Zn and perhaps still other elements.

Deficiency Symptoms

1. In young animal vitamin D deficiency results in rickets and retarded growth. Rickets includes skeletal deformities characterized by (*i*) enlarged junctions between bone and cartilages, (*ii*) curvatures of the bones and in severe cases, (*iii*) weakening of muscular tissue and particular susceptibility to infection.

2. In older animals vitamin D deficiency causes osteomalacia, where there is reabsorption of bone already laid down.

3. In poultry, a deficiency of vitamin D causes the bones and beak to become soft and rubbery; growth is usually retarded and the legs may become bowed.

Vitamin D_2 and D_3 have the same potency for cattle, sheep and pigs, but vitamin D_2 has about 1/35th of the potency of D_3 for poultry. One μg of vitamin D_3 is equivalent to 40 international units (IU).

Sources

In its active from vitamin D is not well distributed in nature except in some dried roughages. In animal kingdom it is abundant in fish liver on entire body oil. Milk is a very poor source of vitamin D. Fresh green alfalfa forage has zero vitamin D value whereas sun cured hay contain on an average 200 I.U. per 100 gms.

VITAMIN E

The earliest indication that natural food contain material specifically concerned with reproduction is found in a report by Mattil and Conklin (1920). They indicated that rats fed on a milk diet supplemented with yeast (B vitamin) and iron were unable to bear young. In 1922 Bishop and Evans announced the existance of a factor X in certain foods for normal rat. reproduction. In the year 1936, Evans and his colleagues isolated pure Vitamin E from the unsaponifiable fraction of wheat-germ oil. The active substance was later termed by Evans as "vitamin E", and now at least eight compounds with E activity are known to occur in a variety of plant and animal tissues. These are called "tocopherols". The name tocopherol was derived from the Greek *tokos* (childbirth) and phero (to bear), but the influence of tocopherols is vastly greater than influencing reproduction in rats.

The synthesis of α-tocopherol was accomplished in 1938 by Smith in U.S.A. and Karrer in Switzerland

Chemistry of Tocopherols

In reality vitamin E is a group of vitamins. There are about eight naturally occurring tocopherols and toco-trienols with vitamin E activity have so far identified. They differ from each other in the number and position of the methyl groups round the ring of the molecule. All have the same physiological properties, although α-tocopherol is the most active and this is the main tocopherol in animal tissue and that is why tocopherol in this form is now synthesised commercially.

Among tocopherols the four compounds so far identified are α-tocopherol (5,7,8-trimethyl tocol), β-tocopherol (5,8-dimethyl tocol) γ-tocopherol (7,8-dimethyl tocol) and δ-tocopherol (8-methyl tocol). Relative to α-tocopherol the biological activities of β-and γ-tocopherols are 40 and 8 per cent respectively.

Among toco-trienols, (three double bonds in the side chain) α,β,γ and δ-are noteworthy. The structural formulae are given in previous page. Except α-toco-trienol which has got 20 per cent biological activity of α-tocopherol, other toco-trienols have very little activity. There is no evidence of inter-conversion between the different tocopherols.

Tocopherols are yellow, oily liquid, remarkably stable to heat (even at above 100°C) and acids but not to alkalies. It oxidizes very slowly.

Tocopherols are largely found in wheat germ oil and in other grain oil portion. In animal body the compound is mostly found in body fat. There is some evidence that all α-tocopherol in heart muscle is localised in the mitochondria.

Tocopherols are potent antioxidants and function at least in part in protecting other nutrients, such as vitamin A and polyunsaturated fatty acids from destructive oxidation. It also pro-α Tocopherol

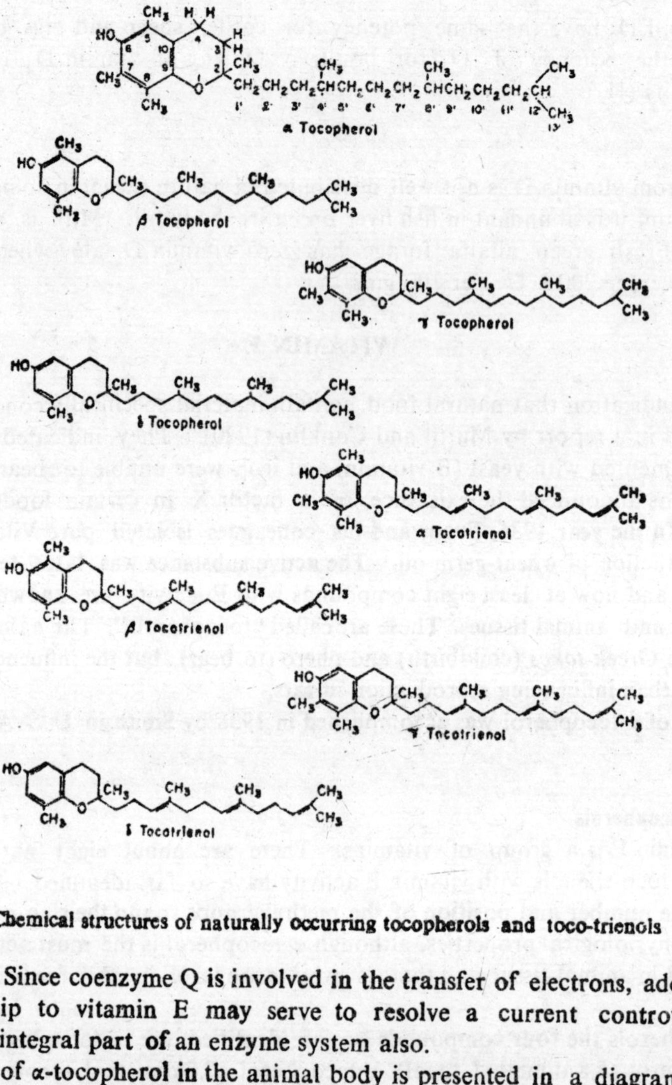

β Tocopherol

γ Tocopherol

δ Tocopherol

α Tocotrienol

β Tocotrienol

γ Tocotrienol

δ Tocotrienol

Chemical structures of naturally occurring tocopherols and toco-trienols

tects coenzyme Q. Since coenzyme Q is involved in the transfer of electrons, additional studies on this relationship to vitamin E may serve to resolve a current controversy—whether α-tocopherol is an integral part of an enzyme system also.

The degradation of α-tocopherol in the animal body is presented in a diagramatic sketch as below. α-tocopherol is converted to tocopheryl quinone, its biological activity is then lost and the reaction is not ordinarily reversible. α-tocopheroxide apparently is reversibly converted to α-tocopherol to a limited extent in the presence of adequate ascorbic acid.

Absorption. Fat digestion produces are important in the absorption of the vitamin Es, the amount absorbed being proportional to the amount of lipids in the diet. The per cent absorption can range from 10 to 70%. The absorbed vitamin E is transported from intestine in chylomicrons; one of its storage sites are Ito cells in the liver. Further transport to most other tissues occurs by way of the lipoproteins, VLDL and LDL. There are many distribution pools with various biological half-lives, a relatively short-term pool in the plasma and liver, and a longer one in adipocytes (a major storage site) and muscle. The isomers have varying half-lives, with the α isomer lasting much longer than the γ. The major excretory route is through the bile in the faeces.

Table 10.35

Pathology of vitamin E deficiency

Condition	*Animal*	*Tissue affected*	*Prevented by*	
			Vitamin E	*Selenium*
I. Reproductive failure	*Female:* Rat, Hen, Turkey	Vascular system of embryo	Yes	No
Embryonic degeneration	Ewe		No*	Yes**
Sterility	*Male:* Rat, Guinea pig, Hamster, Dog, Cock	Male gonads	Yes	No
II. Liver Blood, Capillaries, etc. Brain				
Liver necrosis	Rat, Pig, Mice, Chick	Liver	Yes	Yes
Erythrocyte destruction	Rat, Chick, Premature infant	Blood (RBC hemolysis)	Yes	No
Blood proteins loss	Chick, Turkey, Pigs	Serum albumin	Yes	Yes
Encephalomalacia	Chick	Cerebellum (Purkinje cells)	Yes	No
Exudative diathesis	Chick, Turkey, pigs	Capillary walls	Yes	Yes
Kindney degeneration	Rat, Monkey Mink	Tubular epithelium	Yes	Yes
Steatitis	Mink, Pig, Chick	Depot fat	Yes	Yes
III. Nutritional Myopathies				
Nutritional muscular dystrophy	Rabbit, Guinea pig Duck, Chick, Turkey	Skeletal muscle	Yes	No or only partially
Stiff lamb	Lamb, Kid	Skeletal muscle	Yes	Yes
White muscle disease	Calf, Sheep, Mouse, Mink	Skeletal and heart muscle	Yes	Yes
Myopathy of gizzard	Turkey poult	Gizzard, heart, skeletal muscle	Yes	Yes
Cardiac muscle abnormlaites	Cattle, Lambs, Poultry, Rats, Monkey, Rabbits	Heart	Yes	Yes

*Not in selenium-deficiency diets

**When added to diets containing vitamin E

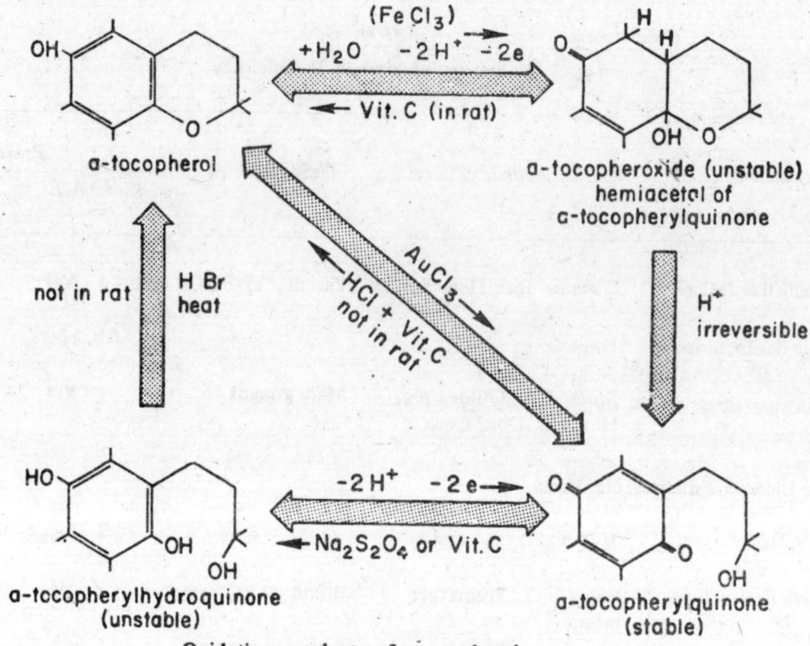

(FeCl3) +H2O −2H+ −2e
Vit. C (in rat)
α-tocopherol
α-tocopheroxide (unstable) hemiacetal of α-tocopherylquinone
not in rat
H Br heat
AuCl3
HCl + Vit. C not in rat
H+ irreversible
−2H+ −2e
Na2S2O4 or Vit. C
α-tocopherylhydroquinone (unstable)
α-tocopherylquinone (stable)

Oxidation products of α-tocopherol

Biochemical Functions

1. It is well established that vitamin E acts as an antioxidant in the cellular level. Thus for an example it prevents the oxidation of unsaturated fatty acids, mostly present in all cell wall components.

2. Vitamin E also participates in normal tissue respiration possibly (*i*) aid in some unknown way the function of cytochrome reductase system and (*ii*) to protect the lipid structure of mitochondria from oxidation destruction.

3. Aids the normal phosphorylation of creatine phosphate, ATP—which are all high energy phosphate compounds of the body.

4. It is also involved in the synthesis of ascorbic acid (vitamin C) and ubiquinine (coenzyme) and in the metabolism of nucleic acid (DNA) probably by regulating the incorporation of pyrimidines into the nucleic acid structure and sulphur amino acid.

Pathology of Vitamin E Deficiency

Early experiments showed the importance of vitamin E only in rat reproduction, but further studies showed that reproduction is only affected in some species but not in all species. The effect of vitamin E deficiency has been found in various nature in different animals. Some of the vitamin E deficiency has been found cured by adding selenium to the diet. How a mineral can substitute a vitamin deficiency is a mystery. Table 10.35 is a list of pathology of vitamin E deficiency in different species, it also shows where selenium can replace vitamin E.

Sources

Table 10.36

Food or feed stuff	α-tocopherol (mg/100 gms.)	Food or feed stuff	α-tocopherol (mg/100 gms.)
Wheat	145	Rice, brown	1-2
Sunflower seed, whole	13	Sweet potatoes	4-10
Clover, dehydrated	10	Bone meal	0.05
Alfalfa meal, dehydrated	7-25	Fish meal	0.8-2.0

NOTE: Encephalomalacia—Damage to the brain, edema and hemorrhage cerebellum.
Muscular dystrophy—wasting way of muscle.
Steatitis—Inflammation of addipose tissue.
Exudative diathesis—Blood serum oozed into the tissues.

VITAMIN K

Vitamin K was identified in 1935 by Dam as a factor present in green leaves which prevented a hemorrhagic syndrome observed in chicks maintained on a low fat diet. The new fat soluble vitamin was designated as vitamin K for the Danish word, *Koagulation*. The purified compound was isolated from alfalfa by Dam and associates in 1939.

It is now well established that vitamin K is an essential metabolite for humans and for all laboratory and farm animals. The dietary vitamin K requirement of animals depends upon many modifying factors. Among these are factors affecting (1) the availability of the vitamin from various foods and foodstuffs; (2) its stability in foods and/or the innate stability of the vitamin K supplement being fed; (3) its gastrointestinal microbial synthesis, including the site of synthesis in the tract; (4) its absorbability which depends upon the level of dietary fat, adequate bile secretion, competition for absorptive and/or transport mechanisms by high levels of other fat-soluble vitamins and freedom from coccidiosis or other intestinal disturbances; (5) its destruction in the gestrointestinal tract, such as possible destruction by action of Coccidia, *Capillaria*, or other parasites; and (6) interference with its metabolic activity, such as by sulphaquinoxaline, dicoumarol, warfarin, etc.

Chemical Nature

A number of compounds are known to have vitamin K activity. Naturally occurring compounds come from two sources: (1) Phylloquinone (K_1) series occurs in all green leafy materials, (2) Prenylmenaquinone (K_2) series occurs in the intestine by the microbial syinthesis. Among so many synthetic compounds, Menadione (K_3) is noteworthy. It is about 3.3 times as active biologically as the naturally occurring vitamins. This property may be due to the fact that menadione is slightly water soluble which aids rapid absorption than the other two natural compounds which are fat soluble. The chemical structure of above three compounds are given below.

Vitamin K_1 (green leafy vegetables)

Phylloquinone

Vitamin K_3

(menadione)

Vitamin K_2 (intestinal bacteria)

Menaquinone-4

Dicoumarol

Absorption. The absorption of vitamin K requires bile and pancreatic juices and probably occurs by a passive mechanism, but K_1 may also have an active transport process in the distal small intestine. Vitamin K is transported from the intestine to the rest of the body in chylomicrons and later in very low density lipoproteins (VLDL) and low-density lipoproteins (LDL). The highest concentrations occur in the liver, spleen, and lungs, but even with a lower concentration the muscle is the largest storage site. Vitamin K has a short half-life, 2–3 hours, excreted primarily as lactones and glucuronides in the faeces through bile with a much smaller amount appearing in the urine.

Biochemical Function

Schematically it may be elaborated as follows:

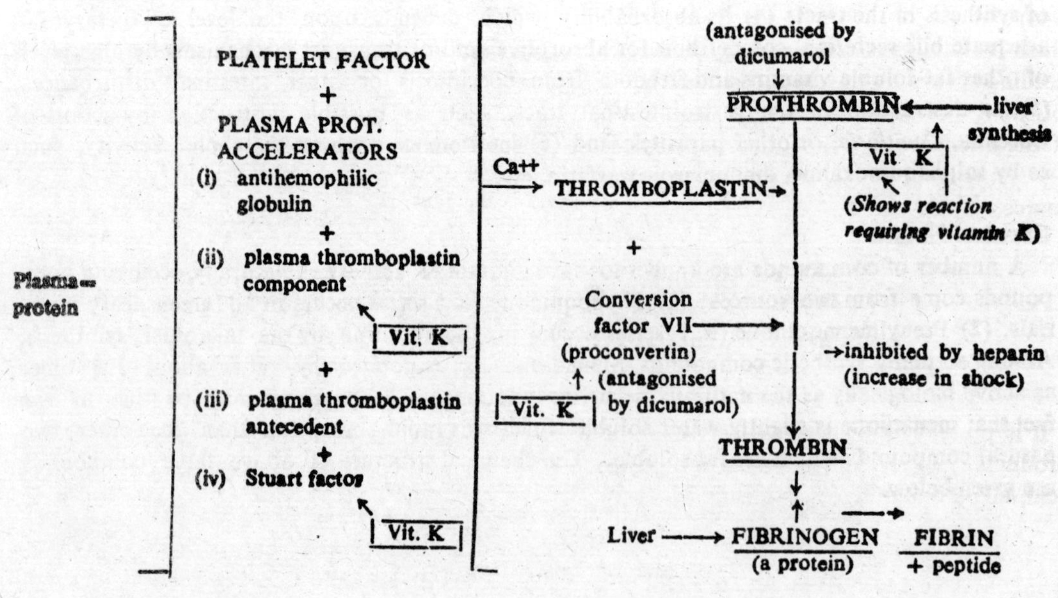

The site of the metabolic action of vitamin K is in the liver. The main function has been attributed in its participation in the blood clotting mechanism. R.E. Olson (Science, 1964) has proposed that vitamin K is needed for the formation of the specific mRNA which directs the synthesis of prothrombin and several other plasma proteins concerned with blood clotting. A simplified form of blood clotting reactions are as follows:

(1) Platelet factor + Plasma protein accelerators $\xrightarrow{Ca^{++}}$ Thromboplastin

(2) Plasma thromboplastin + Prothrombin + Conversion factor = Thrombin

(3) Fibrinogen $\xrightarrow{+\text{Thrombin}}$ Fibrin + Peptide (a glycoprotein enzyme) (responsible for clot)

Apart from this important biochemical function, vitamin K has been found to be involved in electron transport and oxidation phosphorylation.

Deficiency Symptoms

A. AVIAN SPECIES. Symptoms of vitamin K deficiency occur most frequently in chicks or poults about 2–3 weeks after they are placed on vitamin K-deficient diet. Sulphaquinoxaline in the feed or in the drinking water increases the incidence and severity of the symptoms. Gross deficiency of vitamin K results in such a prolonged blood clotting time that severely deficient chicks may bleed to death from slight bruise or other injury. Borderline deficiencies often cause small haemorrhagic blemishes. Haemorrhages may appear on the breast, legs, wings, in the abdominal cavity and on the surface of the intestines. Chicks show an anemia which in part may be due to loss of blood, or to the development of a hypoplastic bone marrow.

B. RUMINANTS. Although vitamin K is synthesized in the rumen of cattle and other ruminants in adequate amounts under normal conditions but deficiency symptoms occur when spoiled sweet clover forage is fed. Link and associates of the University of Wisconsin (Link 1944) showed that when sweet clover hay undergoes spoilage with certain molds, the coumarin which it contains is converted to dicumarol, an anti-vitamin of K and at the same time a bleeding syndrome develops throughout the animal body. This disease is called *"sweet clover poisoining"* or *"bleeding disease"* and has been shown to be caused by the antivitamin K action of the dicumarol.

Source

Milligram of Vit-K_1 per 100 gms. edible portion

Cabbage	250	Grass meal	20
Cauliflower	275	Soyabeans	190
Spinach	334	Wheat bran	80

It is present in most green leafy materials, some of which are shown above. Among animals products egg yolk and fish meal and generally good sources. The vitamin is destroyed by light, acid, alkali and different oxidising agents.

ASCORBIC ACID (VITAMIN C)

Historically the disease scurvy (marked by weakness, anemia, spongy dental gums, and mucocutaneous haemorrhages), become widely recognized when man learned to build ships capable of long sea voyages, and it is probably true that on long-term explorations more deaths were caused by scurvy than any other single factor. Vitamin C deficiency not only was prevalent on long sea voyages because fresh foods were unavailable, but also was epidemic over parts of the world during times of famine and war.

Of the mammals, only man, the monkey, Indian fruit bat, and the guinea pig require the vitamin from dietary source, other species possess the necessary enzymes to synthesize ascorbic acid. Thus farm animals do not require a dietary source of this vitamin.

Ascorbic acid was first isolated by Szent-Gyorgyi (1928) from-orange juice, cabbage juice and adrenal cortex; he named the compound hexuronic acid in recognition of the six carbon atoms in the molecule.

Chemical Nature and Metabolism

Vitamin C is chemically known as L-ascorbic acid. Highly soluble in water and slightly soluble in alcohol. Stable in dry crystalline state but oxidised quickly in solution. The acid is a derivative of hexose, it can be classified as carbohydrates. It occurs in two active forms: asoorbic acid (reduced form) and dehydro ascorbic acid (the oxidized form). If the latter is oxidised further to diketogulonic acid, the compound loses its biological activity.

```
        O                          O
        ‖                          ‖
    ┌── C ──┐                  ┌── C ──┐                 COOH
    │       │                  │       │                  |
 HO─C       │     −2H       O═C       │                 C═O
    ‖       O   ═══════                │     ───────→      |
 HO─C       │     +2H       O═C       O                 C═O
    │       │                  │       │                  |
  H─C ──────┘                H─C ──────┘               H─C─OH
    |                          |                          |
 HO─C─H                     HO─C─H                     HO─C─H
    |                          |                          |
  CH₂OH                      CH₂OH                      CH₂OH
```

Ascorbic acid — Dehydroascorbic acid — Diketogulonic acid

```
     ┌──────────┐                                  ┌──────────┐
    C═O         │                                 C═O         │
     |          │     L-gulonolactone              |          │   spontaneously
 HO─C─H         O        oxidase                  C═O         O ──────────→ Vit. C
     |          │     ──────────→                  |          │
 HO─C─H         │       (enzyme)              HO─C─H          │
     |          │                                  |          │
   H─C──────────┘                                H─C──────────┘
     |                                             |
 HO─C─H                                       HO─C─H
     |                                             |
   CH₂OH                                        CH₂OH
 L-gulonolactone                          2-keto-L-gulonolactone
```

Species capable of synthesising vitamin C can do it from glucose, via glucuronic acid and gluconic acid lactone.

The enzyme *L*-gulonolactone oxidase is deficient in man, monkey, Indian fruit bat and guinea pig and hence vitamin C cannot be synthesised by these mammals. On the other hand farm animals have the ability to synthesise this vitamin in their body as per requirement. Thus we can say that vitamin C is essential for all groups of animals but it is not a dietary essential for any farm animals.

Absorption, Metabolism, Excretion. Absorption occurs by two mechanisms. Both forms can be absorbed by passive diffusion, but only ascorbic acid is absorbed by a sodium-dependent carrier-mediated mechanism. In guinea pigs, one of the few animals that require vitamin C, most absorption occurs in the ileum. The per cent absorption decreases with increasing intake, ranging from 90 to 20%, with the maximal per cent absorption occurring at amounts below 180 mg and the lowest at levels or above 2 g.

Vitamin C is stored in all tissues, with the highest concentrations in the adrenal and pituitary glands, and lower levels in the liver, spleen, and brain. Humans have about 100 days of storage, but this can change with the season, being lower in the winter.

Biochemical Functions

1. Vitamin C is essential for the collagen (an albuminoid which is the main supportive protein of all connective tissue, predominantly found in the gums) formation.
2. It aids for the conversion of folic acid to its active form tetrahydrofolic acid.
3. Vitamin C is also involved in the hydroxylation of proline, lysine and aniline—which are important for normal physiology of the animal.
4. It aids iron to stay in reduced state, which is very important for the body.
5. Participates in the synthesis of steroid hormones by the adrenal cortex.
6. It involves in the metabolism of lipids as blood cholesterol level appear to fall with the administration of ascorbic acid and rise due to deficiency of vitamin.
7. It aids for the conversion of tryptophan to serotonin.

Deficiency Symptoms

Deficiency symptoms for farm animals is unknown. For man, monkey and guinea pigs extensive study has been made. The classical manifestation of severe ascorbic acid deficiency is termed scurvy. The gross lesions observed are those related to degeneration of the collaginous intracellular substance. The disease is characterised by weakness, swollen tendor joints, delayed healing of wounds, spongy haemorrhagic friable gums, loose teeth, and small haemorrhages which may appear anywhere throughout the body, particularly near the bones and joints and under the skin and mucus membrane due to increased fragility of the capillaries.

Source

Vitamin C, unlike the vitamin B, is not universally distributed, being absent from eggs and seeds and in general from bacteria, yeasts and protozoa. The outstanding dietary sources of vitamin C are fresh fruits and leafy vegetables. Interestingly enough, for poor man green chilli is a good source. The richest fruit source known is a west Indian cherry called acerola (4.0 mg./gm.). Well-known sources include all citrus fruits and tomatoes. Less regard but good additional sources, include cabbage, sweet potatoes, white potatoes. Other sources are seasonal such as berris, melons, guavas, pineapple etc.

Animal products as a whole are poor sources. Cereal grains have no vitamin C. Raw cow's milk is a fair source; but some is lost is pasteurisation.

THE VITAMINS OF THE B COMPLEX

The vitamins included under this complex all have the property of being soluble in water and most of them are components of enzyme systems.

Complete agreement has still not been reached concerning which substances should be considered as B vitamins, but those listed here under B complex are generally accepted as members of the B complex. Many writers include choline, inositol and *p*-aminobenzonic acid with the B vitamins.

It is possible that the requirements of different animal species vary. In recent years it has become apparent that the activity of the intestinal flora in synthesizing vitamins of the B group explains species differences. In general we can say that microbial synthesis of the B complex in the digestive tract can supply part of the requirements of all monogastric animals. For ruminants the entire requirements of B vitamins are synthesised by the microbes in their digestive tract. Deficiency symptoms in farm animals do occur only in pigs and poultry.

THIAMINE (VITAMIN B_1)

The disease beriberi had been known for several centuries before its dietary origin was recognized. Beriberi is characterized by extensive damage to the nervous and cardiovascular system and may be accompanied by severe muscle wasting (dry beriberi) or edema (wet beriberi). In the late nineteenth century, Eijkmann, working in a hospital laboratory in Batavia, Dutch East Indies, discovered that a polyneuritis (characterized by a peculiar head retraction obviously of neurological origin) in chickens with symptoms similar to beriberi in humans was produced by feeding an experimental diet of polished rice. It did not occur when brown rice was substituted for polished rice or when rice polishings were added to the polished rice diet.

In 1926, Jansen and Donath, successors of Eijkmann succeeded in crystalizing vitamin B_1 in pure form. The identification of the structure of the vitamin and its synthesis was accomplished in 1936 by Williams and co-workers in the same laboratory.

Chemistry of Thiamine. Thiamine (aneurine, vitamin B_1) is a complex nitrogenous base composed of a pyrimidine and a thiazole ring; it is available commercially in hyrdochloride form.

CH_3
NH_2 $C{=}C{-}CH_2{-}CH_2OH$
N $-CH_2{-}N^+$
Cl^- C–S
$CH_3{-}C$ –H H
N

Thiamine Chloride

Due to the presence of a hydroxyl group at the end of the side chain thiamine easily forms esters with phosphorus of ATP. In the esterified form the molecule becomes active and this active molecule is known as cocarboxylase (thiamine pyrophosphate or TPP). The structure of thiamine pyrophosphate is shown below:

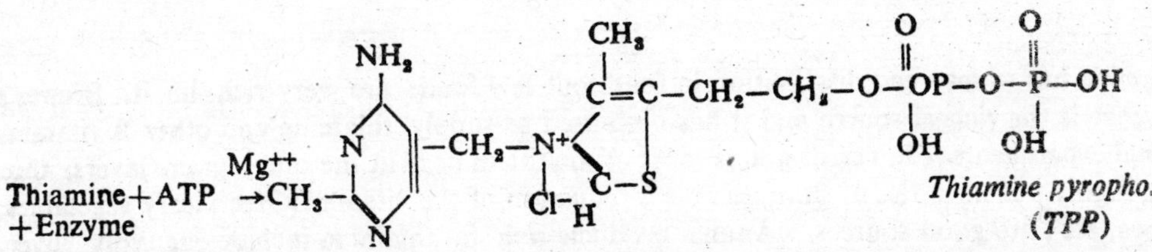

$$\text{Thiamine} + \text{ATP} + \text{Enzyme} \xrightarrow{Mg^{++}} CH_3\text{–(pyrimidine ring with } NH_2\text{)–}CH_2\text{–}N^+\text{(thiazole ring: } C(CH_3)\text{=C–}CH_2\text{–}CH_2\text{–O–}\overset{O}{\overset{\|}{P}}(OH)\text{–O–}\overset{O}{\overset{\|}{P}}(OH)\text{–OH; C–S; C–H)} \; Cl^-$$

Thiamine pyrophosphate
(TPP)

Absorption. Some antinutrients to thiamin exist. The most important antithiamin is the enzyme thiaminase that is found in some raw fish and in tea, coffee and blueberries. Tannins found in tea and red wine may also destroy thiamin.

Thiamin can be absorbed passively in the small intestine at high levels (less than 5 mg/day) and by an active carrier-mediated mechanism probably in the jejunum. The large intestine may absorb thiamin also by a passive pathway. In the intestine, thiamin is phosphorylated by thiaminokinase to TPP and secreted into the portal blood. It is in this form (TPP) that most of the thiamin is stored with about one half in muscle and one tenth in the brain (as TTP). The pool in the brain is slow to turn over, being metabolized to thiamin monophosphate. Most of the thiamin in the plasma is free as the alcohol. Many thiamin metabolites are excreted in the urine.

Deficiency Diseases. Deficiency ot thiamine in humans (onset of beriberi) occurs first as a numbness of the legs, later with pain in the calf muscle, severe exhaustion, finally emaciation and paralysis. The patient has difficulty in breathing, there is an abnormal enlargement of the right side of the heart and a decrease in the rate of the heart beat. The most characteristic feature of the disease is the so called "*peripheral neuritis*". This is often accompanied by contractions of the feet and severe weakness of the wrists. The brain may be affected. Under these conditions the desease has been termed "*cerebral beriberi*" or "*Wernicke's encephalopathy*".

Symptoms in animals, termed *polyneuritis*, are particularly characterized by unthrifitiness, paralysis convulsions and in birds (pigeons, chicks etc.) there is a characteristic paralysis of the neck muscles which causes the head to be drawn back against the back of the bird so that the break is pointed straight up in a "*star-grazing*" attitude.

Paralysis appears to be due to accumulation in the brain and muscles of lactic acid. This results from the fact that the pyruvate which builds up during cocarboxylase deficiency is quickly converted to lactic acid.

Evidence indicates that the myelin sheath of the nerves and the white matter of the brain are the tissues most seriously affected. The exact cause of the deterioration of this tissue has not yet been shown.

Vitamin B_1 is not stored to any great extent in the animal body. Symptoms begin to appear, therefore, within a very short time following consumption of deficient diets. The severity of the symptoms is in direct proportion to the degree of the deficiency.

Biochemical Function

Thiamine, in the form of the thiamine diphosphate (thiamine pyrophosphate or TPP) is the coenzyme for the decarboxylation of keto acids such as pyruvic acid. The decarboxylation reaction with pyruvic acid is as follows:

$$\underset{\textit{Pyruvic acid}}{CH_3\text{–}\overset{O}{\overset{\|}{C}}\text{–}COOH} \xrightarrow[(TPP)]{\nearrow CO_2} \underset{\textit{Acetaldehyde}}{CH_3\text{–}\overset{O}{\overset{\|}{C}}\text{–}H}$$

Source

Thiamine has widespread distribution in food, but few foods are very rich in it. **Brewer's dried yeast** is the richest source and it has been used to supply thiamine and other B vitamins in animal experiments. In cereal grains most of the thiamine is in the outer grain layers, thus making highly polished rice or flour there is a reduction of the vitamin. Green leafy vegetables, bean, pea, etc , are good sources. Animal products rich in thiamine include egg yolk, liver, kidney etc. The synthetic vitamin is obtainable and is usually marketed as the hydrochloride .

RIBOFLAVIN (VITAMIN B_2)

In the early days of vitamin research it was believed that the antiberiberi factor represented a single vitamin. After thiamine was isolated, however, it became clear that at least two factors were involved, a heat labile fraction which was the true antiberiberi vitamin and a heat stable fraction essential for rat growth. The latter fraction for sometime was thought to be only one substance and was named vitamin B_2 in Great Britain and Vitamin G in the United States. Subsequently the heat stable fraction was shown to be not one vitamin but a mixture of several vitamins (later indentified as riboflavin, pyridoxin, nicotinic acid, and pantothenic acid). The orange-yellow colour of riboflavin and its natural fluorescence in solution undoubtedly aided in its discovery since its presence in extracts from foods and other biological materials could be confirmed with the naked eye.

The vitamin was first isolated from egg white and called "*ovoflavin*". Compounds later isolated by other groups from milk and liver were designated "*lactoflavin*" and "*hepatoflavin*" respectively. The name riboflavin was adopted only after the compound was shown to contain ribose in the molecule and has since been changed to riboflavin (IUPAC, 1960).

Riboflavin was synthesized independently by Kuhn *et al.* (1935) at Heidelberg and Karrer *et al.* (1935) at Zurich.

Riboflavin consists of a dimethyl-isoalloxazine nucleus combined with ribose. The vitamin is an orange-yellow crystalline substance, very slightly soluble in water or acid solution. In neutral or acid media it is stable to heat. It is highly soluble in alkaline solution.

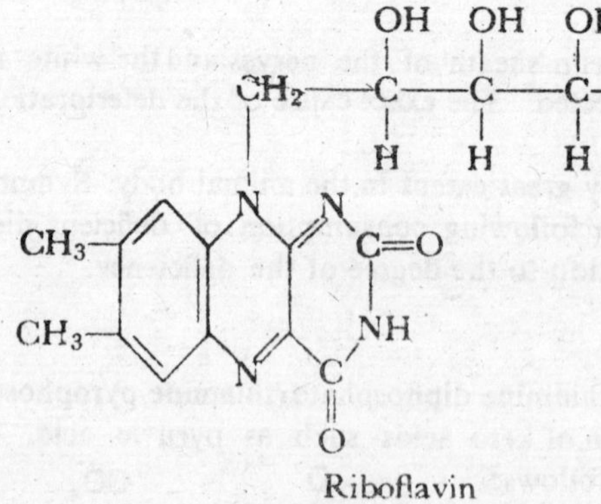

OH OH OH
CH_2—C—C—C—CH_2OH
H H H
N N
CH_3 C=O
CH_3 NH
N C
O

Riboflavin

Absorption. Before absorption, riboflavin must be released from dietary protein by acidic gastric conditions, and phosphatases are required for its release from the covalently linked forms. It is absorbed by a passive and active mechanism that is saturated at consumption of 25 mg/day. There is little storage of riboflavin, and this occurs mainly in the plasma complexed with proteins (for transport) and intracellularly with flavoprotein complexes and covalent flavoproteins. The amount of riboflavin excreted in the urine provides a fairly accurate measure of riboflavin intake.

Deficiency Symptoms

Riboflavin forms the prosthetic part of over a dozen enzymes in the animal body. Among these are cytochrome reductase, diaphorase, xanthine oxidase, l-and d-amino acid oxidases, histaminase, and others, all of which are vitally associated with oxidation reduction involved in cell respiration. These are essential enzymes for growth and tissue repair in all animals. Many tissues may be affected by riboflavin deficiency. It appears, however, that the two most severely affected tissues are the epithelium and the myelin sheaths of some of the main nerve trunks.

Ariboflavinosis in humans produces a cheilosis (severe dermatitis and fissures at the corners of the mouth), angular somatitis, glossitis and seborrheic dermatitis. The seborrheic dermatitis is usually found in the nasolabial region near the inner and outer canthi of the eyes, behind the ears, and on the posterior surface of the serotum. The eyes are also affected. Ocular manifestations include photophobia, indistinct vision, itching burning and circumcorneal capillary engorgement with invasion of the superficial strata of the eye by small capillaries.

While there are other disease disorders which will also produce each of these symptoms, and therefore, one symptom taken alone is not necessarily suggestive of ariboflavinosis, the occurrence of a number of these symptoms together makes up a syndrome which, with a history of poor dietary intake of foods rich in riboflavin, can be used as a diagnosis of ariboflavinosis. If the symptoms disappear after treatment with riboflavin, the diagnosis is confirmed.

Severe riboflavin deficiency in chicks causes a marked swelling and softening of the sciatic and branchial nerves. The sciatic nerves usually show the most pronounced effects. They may reach a diameter four to five times normal size. The affected nerves show degenerative changes in the myelin sheaths of the main peripheral nerve trunks. These changes cause a continual stimulation of the sciatic nerve which produces a contraction of the toes and development of the typical symptoms of riboflavin deficiency in the chick known as "*curled-toe paralysis*".

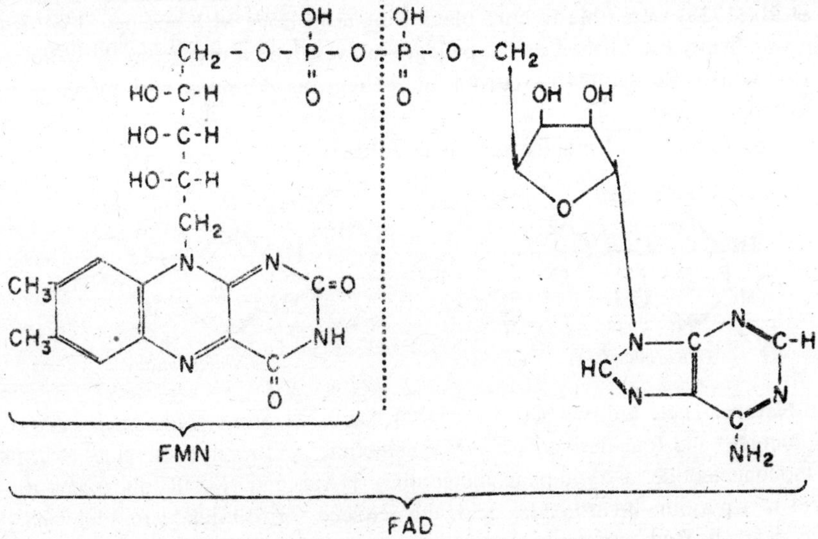

OH OH
CH2 - O - P - O - P - O - CH2
HO - C - H O O OH OH
HO - C - H
HO - C - H
CH2
CH3 N N C=O
CH3 NH N C H
N C N C-H
O HC N
N C
NH2
FMN
FAD

Flavin mononucleotide (FMN) and flavin adinine dinucleotide (FAD).

Metabolic Function

Riboflavin in the form of flavin monouncleotides (FMN) and flavin adinine dinucleotide (FAD) acts as the prosthetic group of several enzymes involved in biological oxidation-reduction reactions. These enzymes serve as bridges over which hydrogen atoms can pass between two other molecules. In its reduction and oxidation riboflavin alternately accepts and releases two hydrogen atoms. Reactions catalyzed by flavoproteins may be divided into three groups:

1. Reactions in which enzyme removes hydrogen, not from the primary substrate but from an intermediate carrier *e.g.*, from reduced pyridine nucleotide.
2. Reactions in which the enzyme removes hydrogen directly from substrate such as succinic and choline which are transformed to fumaric and betaine aldehyde respectively.
3. Catalyze the reactions of molecular oxygen *e.g.*, xanthine oxidase and oxygen to produce uric acid.

Source

Riboflavin is widely distributed throughout the plant and animal kingdoms, with very rich sources in anaerobic fermenting bacteria. Milk, liver, kidney and heart are excellent sources. Many vegetables are also good sources, but the cereals are rather low in riboflavin content.

NIACIN AND NIACINAMIDE

The terms niacin and niacinamide have replaced the older terms nicotinic acid and nicotinic acide amide (nicotinamide). The latter names were found to be undesirable because of confusion and the unwanted belief by many that they were physically related to nicotine.

Funk had isolated nicotinic acid from rice polishings as early as 1914, but he did not realize that it was a vitamin. In fact he was searching for an antiberiberi factor but discarded it when it was ineffective against beriberi! However, the discovery of niacinamide as component of coenzyme II (NADP) concerned in hydrogen transport (oxidation-reduction system) by Warburg and Christian (1935) suggested that the substance was of metabolic importance. When Elvehjem et al. (1938) were able to cure black tongue in dogs with niacinamide isolated from liver, niacin was firmly established as the pellagra-preventive factor (from the Italian *pelle agra* means rough skin). Subsequently curing of pellegrous humans with niacin in their ration became a common practice.

The structure of niacin and niacinamide is as follows:

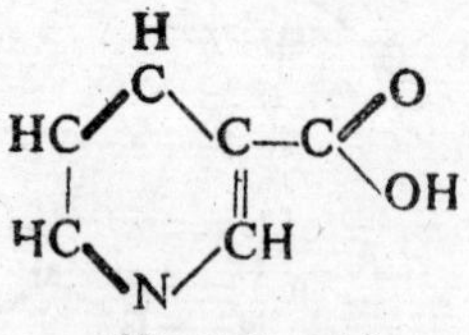

```
        H                                  H
        C                                  C
   HC /   \ C—C =O                    HC /   \ C—C =O
    |      ||   \OH                    |      ||   \NH2
   HC \   / CH                        HC \   / CH
        N                                  N
```

(Nicotinic acid) 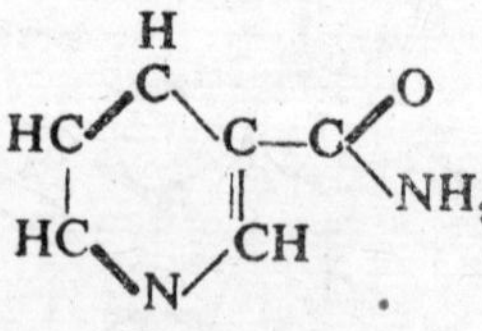 *(Niacinamide)*

Chemical Nature. There are two active forms of niacin: nicotinic acid (niacin) and nicotinic acid amide (nicotinamide) and four derivatives: NMV (nicotinic acid mononucleotide), NaMN (nicotinic) acid amide mononucleotide, a tryptophan metabolite), NAD, and NADP (phosphate on the ribose). Nicotinic acid is a pyridine-3-carboxylic acid; the reduced form is labile to acid, and the oxidized form is labile to alkali. Both are stable to heat and are stable as solids. Tryptophan can be converted to niacin with an efficiency of about 60 tryptophan molecules for 1 niacin molecule. This ration varies with individuals and certain conditions (e.g., estrogen administration increase the efficiency of conversion).

Absorption, Metabolism. Nicotinic acid is absorbed passively in the intestine after hydrolysis of either the protein or the nucleotide and coenzymes, but nicotinamide is not readily absorbed. The storage of niacin occurs in all tissues, but the total is low. The usually storage forms are NAD or NADP, but some is stored in the liver as niacin. The liver is also the primary site of nicotinic acid formation from tryptophan. Tryptophan is converted to quinolinate and then to NaMN.

NaMN and NMN are metabolized eventually by different routes to NAD and then to NADP. Nicotinamide is converted to nicotinic acid after conversion of NAD with the production of adenosine-5′- pyrophospho-5 ribose (ADPR). With a normal intake of niacin, most of the metabolites are excreted in the urine as 1-methyl-nicotinamide (20–30%) and 1-methyl-3-caroxamido-6-pyridone (40-60%). These metabolites are made in the liver through a pathway that utilizes methionine. A high intake of nicotinic acid results in an increase in the 1-methyl and glycine conjugates, whereas a high intake of nicotinamide increase the excretion of unmetabolized nicotinamide.

Biochemical Function

Two well defined coenzymes containing nicotinamide are: **(1) Diphosphopyridine nucleotide (DPN), or coenzyme I (Co I), or NAD (nicotinamide adenine dinucleotide); (2) Triphospho-**

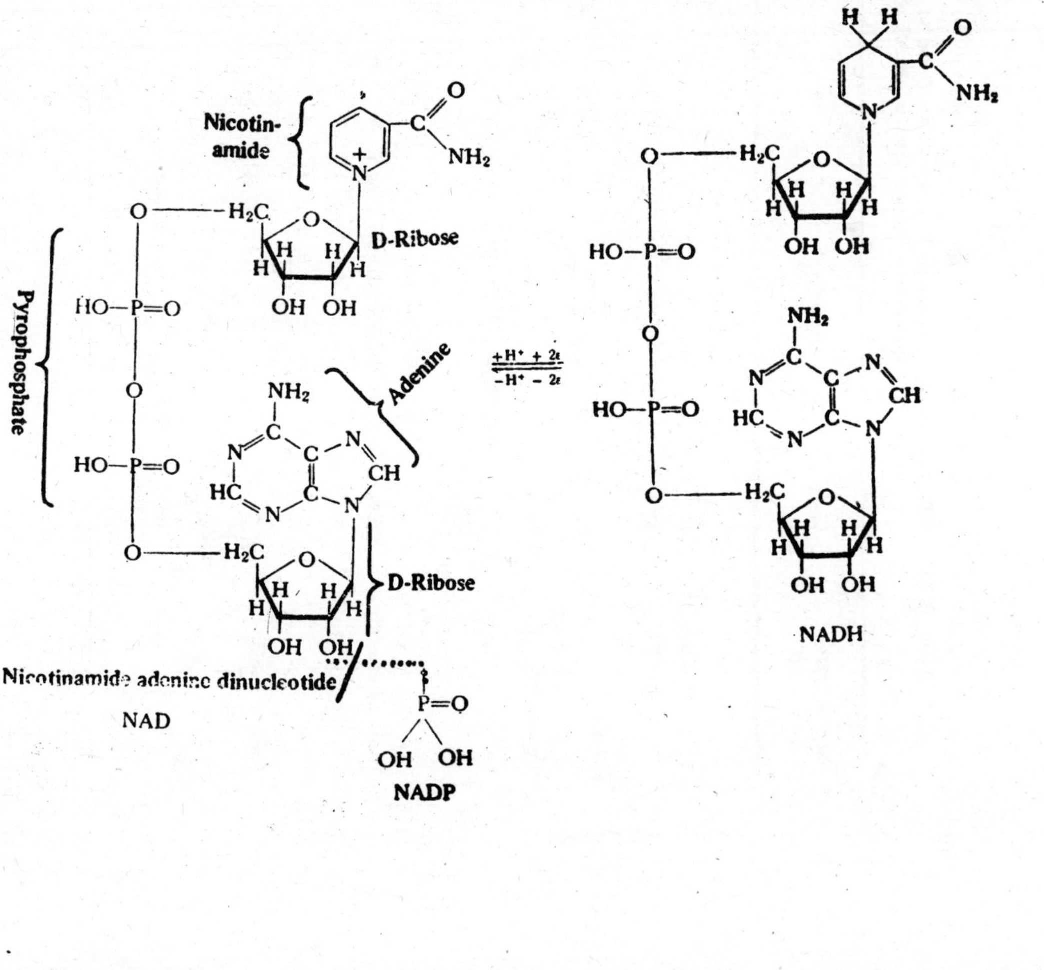

Nicotinamide

D-Ribose

Pyrophosphate

Adenine

D-Ribose

Nicotinamide adenine dinucleotide

NAD

NADP

$\underset{-H^+ - 2e}{\overset{+H^+ + 2e}{\rightleftharpoons}}$

NADH

Table 10.37

Many of the substances belonging to vitamin B group as are found to act as coenzymes or prosthetic groups of enzymes are summarised below. Details already discussed in the text.

Growth factor or vitamin	*Structure*	*Related prosthetic group or coenzyme*	*Function*
Thiamin (B_1)	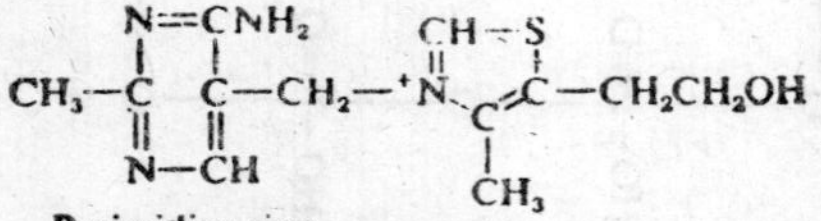 Pyrimidine ring (N=C(NH$_2$), CH$_3$–C, N–CH) –CH_2–$^+$N– Thiazole ring (CH=S, C–CH_2CH_2OH, C–CH_3) Pyrimidine ring · Thiazole ring	**Thiamin pyrophosphate**	**Transfer of some aldehyde groups, e.g., pyruvate dehydrogenase system, transketolase.**
Lipoic acid	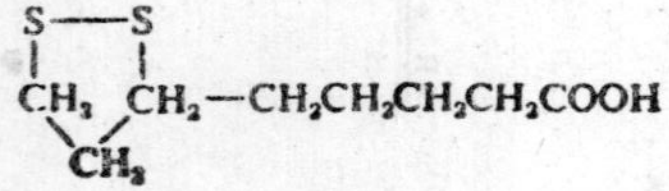 S—S ring: CH_2, CH_2, CH–$CH_2CH_2CH_2CH_2COOH$	**Enzyme-bound lipoic acid**	**Acceptance of some aldehyde groups and their oxidation to acyl complexes, e.g., pyruvate dehydrogenase complex.**
Pantothenic acid	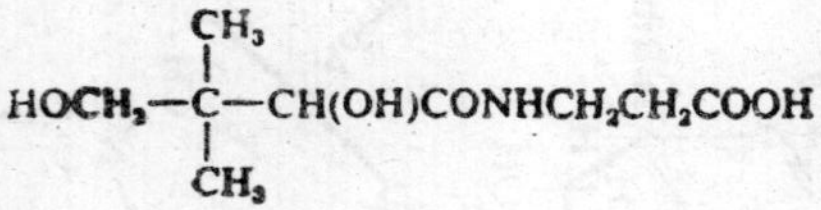 $HOCH_2-C(CH_3)_2-CH(OH)CONHCH_2CH_2COOH$	**Coenzyme A**	**Acyl transfer and alteration, e.g., pyruvate dehydrogenase system, fatty acid oxidation.**
Nicotinic acid (niacin)	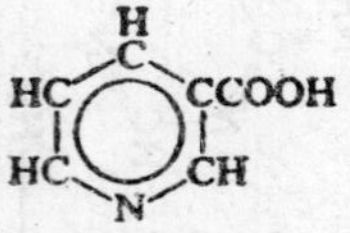 Pyridine ring with CCOOH (Nicotinic acid (niacin)); 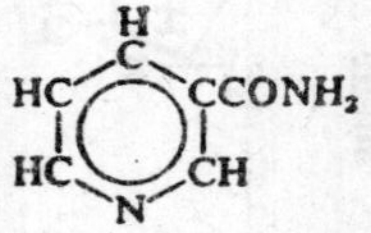 Pyridine ring with $CCONH_2$ (Nicotinamide)	**NAD, NADP**	**Transfer of H = $e^- + H^+$**

Growth factor or vitamin	Structure	Related prosthetic group of coenzyme	Function
Riboflavin	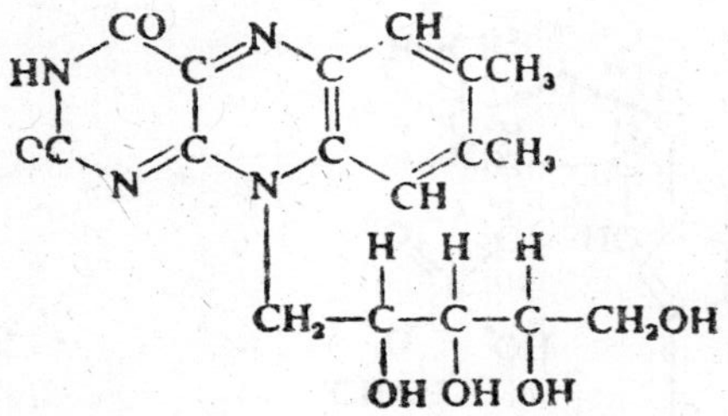	FMN, FAD	Transfer of H ≡ $e^- + H^+$
Pyridoxal and derivatives (B_6)	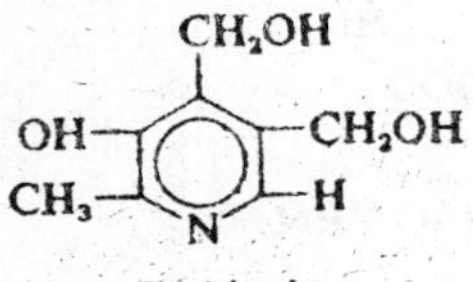 Pyridoxine; 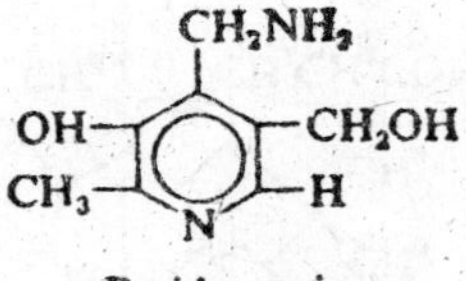 Pyridoxamine	Pyridoxal phosphate	Transfer of amino groups, generally by the formation of Schiff's bases, e.g., aminotransferases, serine hydroxymethyltransferase.
Folic acid	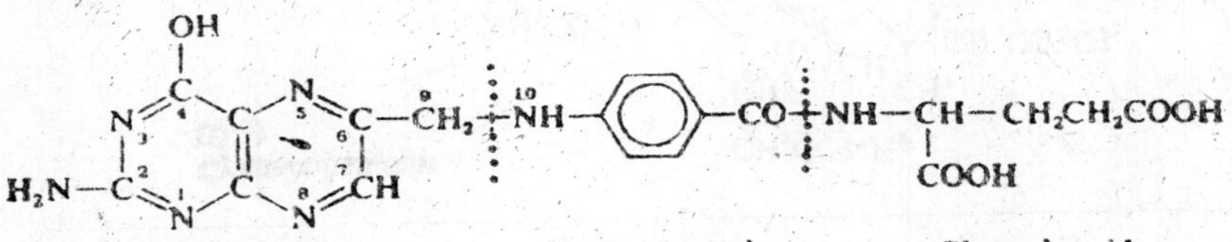 Pterin residue; *p*-Amino-benzoic acid residue; Glutamic acid residue	Tetrahydrofolic	Transfer and interconversion of C_1 units at level of oxidation of formate, formaldehyde and methanol, e.g., in purine synthesis, serine transhydroxymethylase, methionine synthesis.

Growth factor or vitamin	*Structure*	*Related prosthetic group of coenzyme*	*Function*
Cyanocobalamin (B_{12})	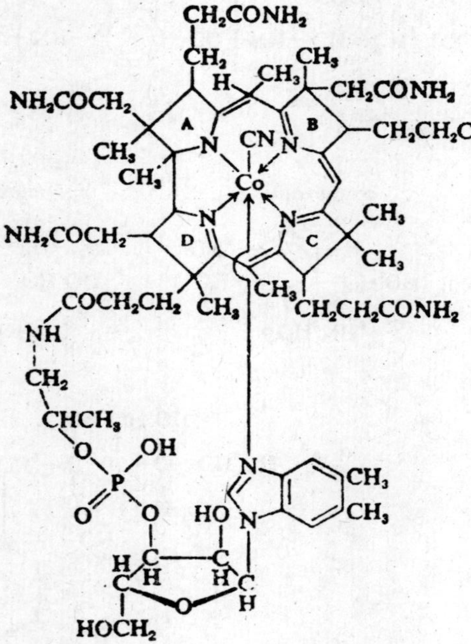	Cobamide coenzymes	1. **Molecular rearrangements and formation of methyl groups.** 2. The isomerisation of methylmalonyl CoA to succinyl CoA in fat metabolism requires a vitamin B_{12} coenzyme. This reaction is extremely important in the overall process of gluconeogenesis, especially in ruminants. 3. Vitamin B_{12} catalyzes the production of folacin from conjugated folates and aids in the formation of folacin coenzymes. 4. It sustains nerve function through its involvement in carbohydrate metabolism (it is known that vitamin B_{12} maintains glutathione in its biologically active reduced state).
Biotin	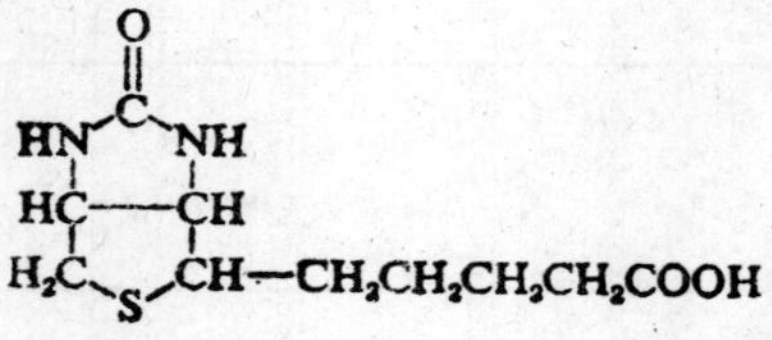		

pyridine nucleotide (TPN), or coenzyme II (Co II), or NADP (nicotinamide adenine denucleotide phosphate).

The primary action of the two coenzymes is to remove hydrogen from substrate as part of dehydrogenase enzymes and transfer hydrogen and/or electrons to the next coenzyme in the chain or to another substrate which then becomes reduced. The enzymes are thus alternately oxidized and reduced.

Deficiency Symptoms

In chicks, a deficiency produces an enlargement of the tibiotarsal joint, a bowing of the legs, poor feathering and slight dermatitis. A disease characterized by inflammation of the mouth cavity known as "*black tongue*" in fowls is well known. The symptoms of nicotinic acid deficiency in turkeys and ducks while similar are much severe. In swine niacin deficiency is known as "*pig pellagra*" and results in moderate slowing of growth, poor hair and skin condition, occasional vomiting and diarrhoea with foul smelling faeces, particularly involving the large instestine. The large intestine thickens, is very red and appears weak and rotten. Another characteristic symptom is that of high white cell count in the blood.

Sources

Niacin is found most abundantly in yeast. Lean meats, liver, and poultry are good sources. Milk, tomatoes and varieties of leafy green vegetables contribute sufficient amounts of the vitamins to prevent disease although they are not excellent sources.

Niacin requirements are influenced by the protein content of the diet because of the ability of the amino acid tryptophan to supply much of the niacin required by the body which later on is converted to amide. *Sixty mg. of tryptophan are considered to give rise to one mg. of niacin.* Thus if the diet is adequately supplied with protein rich in tryptophan, then the dietary requirement for the niacin should be very low. Moreover, bacterial activity in the intestine contributes niacin which fulfils part of the requirement.

PYRIDOXINE (VITAMIN B_6)

Pyridoxine was first defined by Gyorgy (1934) as "that part of the vitamin B complex responsible for the cure of a specific dermatitis in rats that developed on synthetic rations containing vitamin B_1 (thiamin) and vitamin B_2 (riboflavin)." The dermatitis of pyridoxine deficiency in rats is a characteristic scaliness around the peripheral parts of the body such as paws and mouth; these areas eventually become denuded as the scales slough off. Hence the vitamin was first indentified as the rat antidermatitis factor. Other names applied to principle included rat acrodynia factor, and *vitamin H*. The term adermin was used by some in European literature.

The vitamin was isolated by Kerestezy (1938) and the synthesis of the vitamin was accomplished by Harris and Folkers in United States. It was not until 1945, however, that the multiple nature of the vitamin was recognized and the other compounds of the complex identified as pyridoxal and pyridoxamine.

Chemical Nature

Three closely related compounds, pyridoxol, pyridoxal, and pyridoxamine, constitute the group originally known as vitamin B_6. Pyridoxine, the previous designation for alcohol form of the vitamin, now is accepted as the group name and is the accepted alternate designation for pyridoxol (IUPAC, 1966). Commercially the vitamin is available in hydrochloride form.

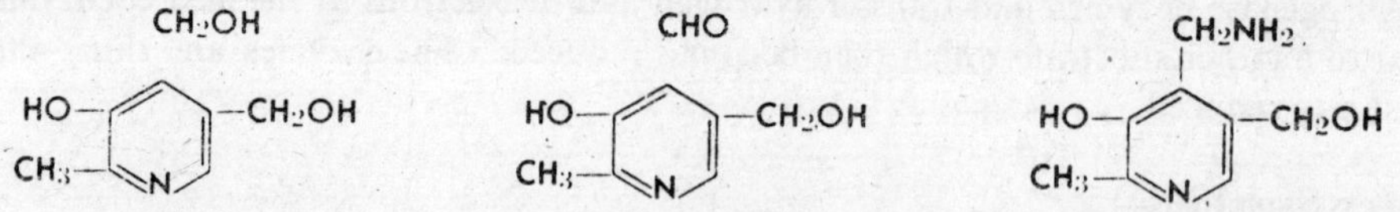

CH_2OH | CHO | CH_2NH_2
HO— —CH_2OH | HO— —CH_2OH | HO— —CH_2OH
CH_3— N | CH_3— N | CH_3— N

pyridoxine | pyridoxal | pyridoxamine

Metabolic Function

Of the three related compounds, the actively functioning one appears to be pyridoxal, in the form of the phosphate. Pyridoxal phosphate and other members are essential to amino acid metabolism in several roles: as a coenzyme for decarboxylation, deamination of serine and threonine, transamination, transulfuration, desulfuration of cysteine, the activity of kynureninase, and the transfer of amino acid into cells. Vitamin B_6 bound to protein is not easily absorbed, but the vitamin in the free form is absorbed rapidly from the intestine.

Deficiency Disease

In chicks, a deficiency causes acute convulsion, flatter on the pan, usually starts kicking and generally die. In adult birds with mild deficiency hatchability and egg production are reduced.

A number of symptoms have been reported for pigs which are anorexia, roughness of hair coat, fatty infiltration of the liver, goose step type of gait, convulsions, etc.

In rat characteristic skin lesions appear in the peripheral parts of the body such as paws, nose, ears, tails, etc.

Sources

Good sources of the vitamin include yeast and certain seeds, such as wheat and maize, liver and to a limited extent milk, eggs, and green leafy vegetables.

PANTOTHENIC ACID

Pantothenic acid was isolated and synthesised long before its metabolic role was identified. The vitamin was purified from liver and yeast along with pyridoxine and the two vitamins were separated by adsorption chromatography. Pyridoxine was absorbed on a column of Fuller's earth and subsequently eluted; pantothenic acid was not absorbed and was recovered in the filtrate leaving the column. For this reason, pantothenic acid was designated the *filtrate factor* and pyridoxine, the eluate factor.

At about the same time several groups of investigators were searching for the identification of the vitamin known to be necessary for growth of lactic acid bacteria, prevention of dermatitis in chicks, and prevention of greying of hair in rats. Pantothenic acid was isolated by R.J. Williams and his associates (1938) and synthesised by a group at Merk and Company in 1940. Later tests with the purified vitamin proved it to be the factor required by bacteria chicks, and rats for preventing the dissimilar deficiency symptoms.

Chemical Nature

The pantothenic acid molecule is a condensation product of alanine and a hydroxyl and methyl substituted butyric acid, pantoic acid.

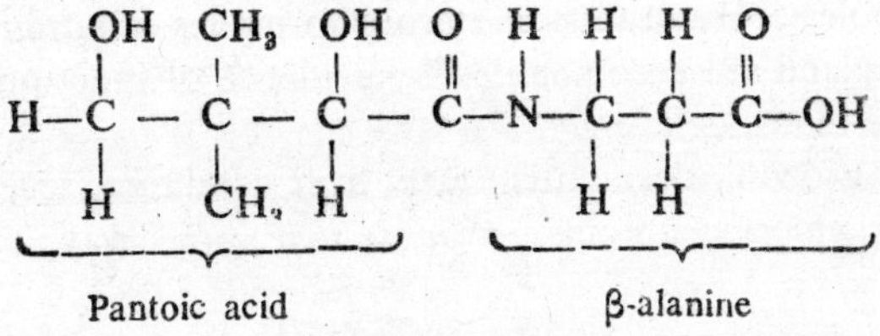

```
 OH  CH3  OH  O  H  H  H  O
 |    |    |  ||  |  |  |  ||
H—C — C — C — C—N—C—C—C—OH
 |    |    |        |  |
 H   CH3   H        H  H
 \_____________/  \___________/
   Pantoic acid     β-alanine
```

Pantothenic acid

Absorption. Absorption is almost complete at normal with subsequent transport from intestine through the portal vein as the free vitamin. Most of the pantothenic acid is stored as CoA (80%), with the highest levels found in the liver. Excretion in the urine is as pantothenate.

Biochemical Functions

Pantothenic acid is the prosthetic group of coenzyme A, an important coenzyme involved in many reversible acetylation reactions in carbohydrate, fat, and amino acid metabolism. The complete enzyme system consists of a specific protein (apoenzyme) combined with the coenzyme moiety. Coenzyme A may act as an acetyl donor or acetyl acceptor. It facilitates condensation

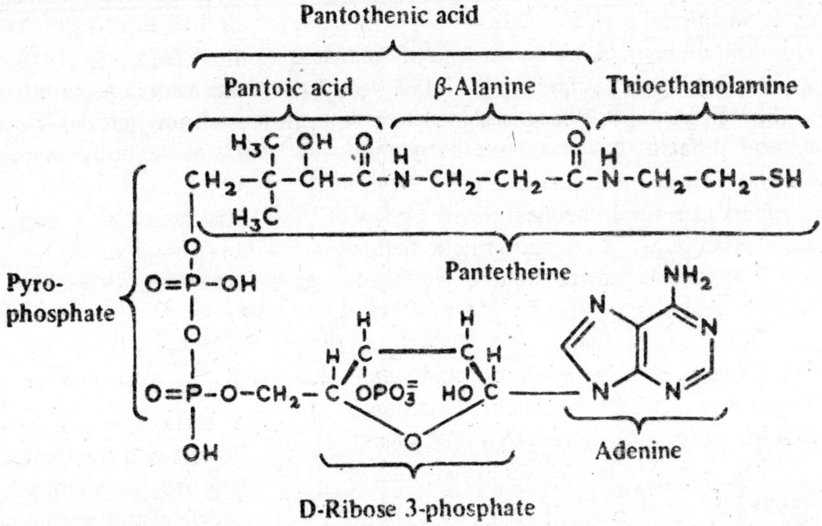

```
                         Pantothenic acid
          Pantoic acid      β-Alanine      Thioethanolamine
           H3C OH  O              O  H
              |  |  ||  H           ||  |
          CH2—C—CH—C—N—CH2—CH2—C—N—CH2—CH2—SH
           |  |
           | H3C
           O                 Pantetheine              NH2
Pyro-      |
phosphate O=P—OH                                    Adenine
           |
           O        H         H
           |        H C———C H
          O=P—O—CH2—C OPO3⁼ HO C ——— N (adenine)
           |            \ O /
           OH
                    D-Ribose 3-phosphate
```

Structure of coenzyme A.

reactions such as the formation of citrate from oxaloacetate in the Krebs cycle. Coenzyme A also acts as a receiver of acetyl radicals formed in the β-oxidation of fatty acids, and from pyruvate and citrate, and transfer them elsewhere. It conjugates not only with acetyl, but also with acyl groups and with malonyl, the later compound malonyl CoA, being of primary importance in the biosynthesis of fatty acids. Pantothenic acid, through coenzyme A, is of fundamental importance in the metabolism of all cells.

Deficiency Symptoms

Affects mainly on three tissues: (1) Nerve—lesions and demyelination. Norris found Riboflavin deficiency causes excessive swelling of nerves but Pantothenic deficiency causes degeneration of sheath, probably both maintain the normal condition of the nerve. (2) Adrenal gland—Acetyl CoA is precursor of cholesterol and thus of steroid hormones of adrenal gland. The anatomic changes of the adrenal gland are accompanied by evidence of functioning inefficiency. (3) Skin —severe dermatitis like biotin deficiency.

In chicks, retarded growth, dermatitis, fatty liver condition, severe edema, subcutaneous haemorrhage are the common symptoms. "*Goose step walk*," a typical nerve disease is found in case of pigs.

Sources

Excellent food sources include egg yolk, kidney, liver and yeast. Skimmed milk, sweet potatoes and molasses are fair sources.

FOLIC ACID (FOLACIN)

A deficiency disease found to be folic acid deficiency was first described by Wills (1931) as a "tropical macrocytic anemia" observed in pregnant women patients in Bombay, India, whose diet consisted primarily of white rice and bread. Since the anemia responded to yeast and could be produced in monkeys maintained on similiar monotonous diet it was apparent that the anemia was of nutritional origin.

The development of our present knowledge of folic acid resulted from studies of the nutritional needs of animals, on the one hand, and of bacterial requirements on the other. It is no wonder that this compound has been assigned to a wide variety of designations, since so many test animals and different bacteria have been employed. Also, a variety of symptoms were used as deficiency criteria in animals. Further complications surely resulted from the fact that the vitamin occurs in several chemical forms. A few of the names previously applied to this vitamin include vitamin M (a haematopoietic factor for monkeys), vitamin B_6 (chick growth factor), factor R (bacterial growth factor), vitamin B_{10} and vitamin B_{11}.

The name folic acid was proposed by Mitchell et al. (1941) for a compound isolated from spinach and shown to be necessary for growth of *Streptococcus faecalis* R. Eventually the structure and synthesis of pteroylglutamic acid were determined by investigators working at Lederle laboratories and Parke Davis Company. A few years later it was clear that all the factors were a form of the vitamin now known as folic acid or pteroylglutamic acid.

Chemical Nature

The vitamin consists of a pteridine nucleus, *p*-aminobenzoic acid, and glutamic acid, hence the name pteroylglutamic acid. The portion of the molecule containing pteridine and *p*-aminobenzoic acid is designated pteroic acid. At one time both *p*-aminobenzoic acid and pteroylglutamic acid were considered to be vitamins, but it is now apparent that the species requirement is for one or the other of the two. Pteroylglutamic acid is the vitamin for most mammals, whereas *p*-aminobenzoic acid is essential to certain bacteria that are able to synthesise the larger molecules.

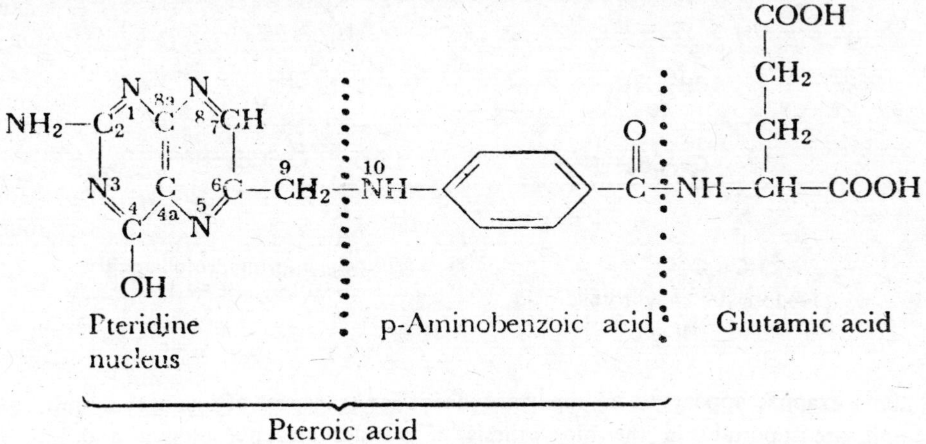

Pteridine nucleus | p-Aminobenzoic acid | Glutamic acid

Pteroic acid

Pteroylglutamic acid

Biochemical Function

The active form of the vitamin is tetrahydrofolic acid (FH_4), which is formed by reduction of the second ring of the pteridine nucleus with the addition of hydrogen at positions 5, 6, 7 and 8. It is formed from folic acid or dihydrofolic acid (FH_2) by action of a reductase and NADH or NADPH serving as carrier. Loss of hydrogen from positions 5 and 6 results in reformation of FH_2.

Just as coenzyme A is carrier for acetyl groups, FH_4 is carrier for the single carbon groups, may be either formyl (—CHO), formate (H. COOH), or hydroxymethyl (—CH_2OH). These are metabolically interconvertible in a reaction catalysed by a NADP—dependent hydroxymethyl dehydrogenase.

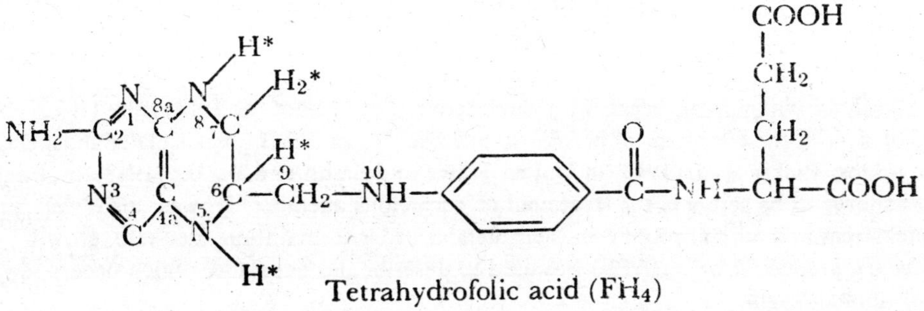

Tetrahydrofolic acid (FH_4)

The one carbon moiety is attached at position 10 or in unstable ring formation at positions 5 and 10 (see following examples).

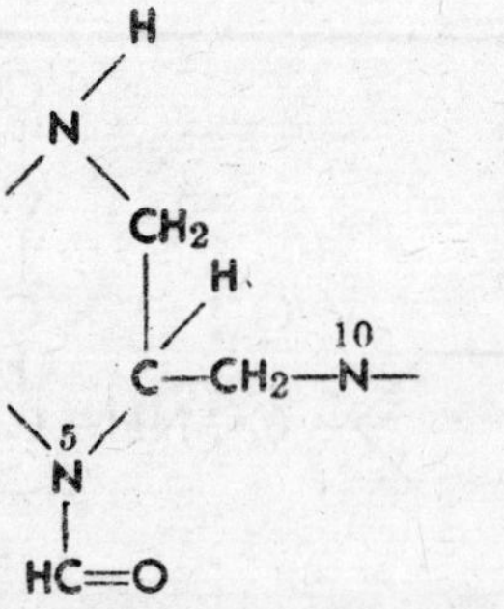

N[5]-formyltetrahydrofolic acid (N^5-formyl FH_4)

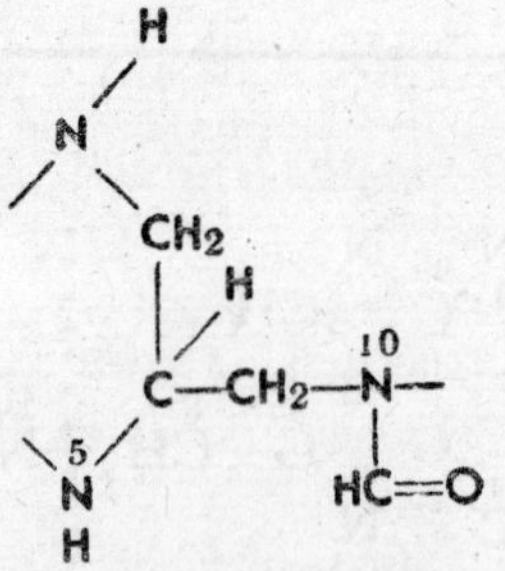

N[10]-formyltetrahydrofolic acid (N^{10}-formyl FH_4)

The above example appears to be important means for transport of one carbon units. Single carbon units are important in the biosynthesis of purines and pyrimidines and in certain methylation reactions, emphasises the fundamental role of folic acid in growth and reproduction of cells. Because the blood cells are subject to relatively rapid rate of synthesis and destruction, it is not surprising that interference with red blood cell formation would lead to anemia, an early sign of a deficiency of folic acid.

Some specific reactions in which FH_4 participates are conversion of glycine to serine, methylation of ethanolamine to choline, methylation of homocysteine to methionine, etc.

Deficiency Symptoms

The clinical pathology of folic acid deficiency, glossitis, gastrointestinal disturbances, diarrhoea, and reduced erythropoiesis appears to be due to inhibition of mitosis in actively dividing cells such as those of epithelial tissues and bone marrow.

In pigs, macrocytic anemia, lipopenia, megaloblastic arrest, etc., develops. In chicks, poor growth, very poor feathering, depigmentation, anemic appearance and perosis develops.

Sources

Fresh leafy green vegetables, cauliflower, kidney, and liver are rich sources of folic acid.

VITAMIN B_{12}

The search for vitamin B_{12} began with the discovery by Minot and Murphy (1926) of the efficacy of liver in the treatment of pernicious anemia. Crystalline B_{12} was isolated independently by two groups, Rickes et al. (1948) in United States and Smith and Parker (1948) in England, and was shown to be active in the treatment of pernicious anemia. It was also well known that chicks required animal protein in their diets in order to maintain adequate growth. The term "*animal protein factor*" (APF) was used to describe this substance which occurs only in foods of animal origin.

Chemical Nature

Vitamin B_{12} has been isolated in several different biologically active forms. Cyanocobalamin, the principal form of the vitamin contains a cyanide group attached to the central cobalt. The cyanide ion may be replaced by a variety of anions, e.g., hydroxyl (hydroxy cobalamin or B_{12} a) or nitrite nitrocobalamin (or B_{12} c). The biological action of these derivates appears to be similar to that of cobalamin, although hydroxy cobalamin is more active in enzyme systems requiring B_{12} and therefore is used more often than any other forms in experimental studies.

Metabolic Function

At least five different vitamin B_{12} coenzymes (cobamide coenzymes) have been identified. The form most frequently encountered in mammalian cells contains a 5-deoxyadenine nucleoside in place of the cyanide group of the vitamin molecule.

The mechanism by which the cobamide coenzyme functions is not clear. Many of its functions appear to be closely linked with FH_4 in the metabolism of one carbon groups; it has been suggested that the cobamide coenzyme is required for the interconversion of one carbon units by oxidation reduction reactions. Evidence suggests that the vitamin participates in nucleic acid synthesis, possibly in the conversion of ribose to deoxyribose and in the formation of the methyl group of thiamin. Changes in bone marrow leading to arrested erythrocyte production in pernicious anemia may be related to this function of the vitamin.

Though the mode of actions of folic acid and vitamin B_{12} are referred to similarly in many books, it is believed that they act as coenzymes at different stages in the synthesis of nucleic acids, folic acid and vitamin B_{12} both being required for the formation of deoxyribonucleic acid (DNA) and vitamin B_{12} alone being necessary for the production of ribonucleic acid (RNA). Though folic acid can often substitute for vitamin B_{12} in the maturation of red blood cells it cannot substitute for vitamin B_{12} in maintenance of central nervous system integrity because here the major requirement is for production of RNA rather than DNA.

Deficiency Symptoms

In humans, pernicious anemia is the prime symptom. The disease develops either due to lack of vitamin B_{12} in the diet or may be due to lack of a heat labile protein known as "*intrinsic factor*" which is required to "*carry*" vitamin B_{12} across the intestinal mucosa and into the blood stream. The ultimate effect of these two kinds of deficiency results in a lower level of vitamin B_{12} in the body and pernicious anemia crops up.

In chicks and other animals, B_{12} deficiency usually is characterised by poor growth and reproductive failures, with only a slight or no anemia. When pigs are reared indoors on all-plant diets vitamin B_{12} should be included in the diet of pigs.

Sources

The origin of vitamin B_{12} in nature is probably the result of microbial synthesis. There is no convincing evidence that the vitamin is produced in the tissues of higher plants or animals. Microbes of the family Actinomycetaceae can synthesise it, although yeast and most fungi apparently do not.

Vitamin B_{12} (animal protein factor) is widely distributed in foods of animal origin; meat, milk, eggs, fish. Its presences in these tissues is a result of ingestion of B_{12} in the food or in some instances from intestinal or rumen synthesis. The best sources are fermentation residues which serve as animal feeds like dried brewer's yeast. However, cobalamin is also found in fishmeal and meatmeal.

Plant products are absolutely devoid of vitamin B_{12}.

BIOTIN

Biotin was first described as the factor protective against "egg white injury". Rats fed large amounts of raw egg white developed an eczema-like dermatitis, paralysis of the hind legs, and a characteristic alopecia around the eyes, aptly termed *spectacle eye*. Cooked egg white was shown to be non-toxic to rats. This member of the group of B vitamins, has been known by a variety of names including bios factor, vitamin H, and coenzyme R. Duvigneaud and co-workers characterised biotin and published its structure in 1942. Harris and others announced the synthesis of *d*-biotin in 1943. Numerous improvements in synthesis of biotin have been made and at present biotin is readily available to the research worker.

Chemical Nature

From the structure it can be said that biotin is a relatively simple monocarboxylic acid. Unlike all other members of the B vitamins, biotin is very slightly soluble in water and alcohol. In the free state biotin has the structure shown below:

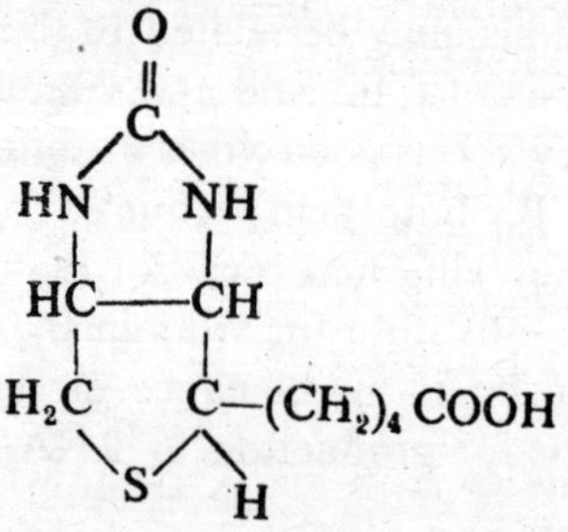

```
           O
           ‖
           C
         /   \
      HN       NH
       |        |
      HC ——— CH
       |        |
     H2C       C—(CH2)4 COOH
        \     / \
          S       H
```

Biotin

Biochemical Functions

In biological systems, biotin functions as the coenzyme for carboxylases, enzymes which catalyse carbon dioxide "fixation" or carboxylation. An important example is acetyl-CoA carboxylase, the enzyme which catalyses the reaction of carboxylation in the first step of non-mitochondrial pathway for the synthesis of fatty acids. Biotin also appears to be necessary for synthesis of dicarboxylic acids.

Deficiency Symptoms

Experimental biotin deficiency in man, which has been induced by feeding a biotin deficient diet together with large quantities of raw egg white, results in a syndrome characterised by a scaly dermatitis, greyish pallor, extreme lassitude, anorexia, muscle pains, insomnia and a slight anemia.

In chicks biotin deficiency results in dermatitis similar to that occurring in pantothenic acid deficiency. The bottoms of the feet become rough, contain fissures, which show some haemorrhaging. The toes may become necrotic and slough off.

Sources

Richest sources of biotin are royal jelly, liver, yeast, molasses peanuts and eggs. Most fresh vegetables are fairly good sources. Intestinal synthesis of biotin contributes a major portion, if not all of the daily requirements for rats and many other mammals.

ANTIBIOTICS, HORMONES AND OTHER GROWTH STIMULATING SUBSTANCES

The constant effort to exploit our domestic animals to produce more human foods economically has stimulated search for new additives which will increase the efficiency and rate of growth of animals. These efforts have led to the present use of antibiotics, hormones and other organic and inorganic elements in animal production.

ANTIBIOTICS

Antibiotics are chemical substances, produced by micro-organisms, which in small concentration have the capacity of inhibiting the growth of other micro-organisms, and even of destroying them. They were originally developed for medical and veterinary purposes to control specific pathogenic organisms, but from the work of Stockstad and associates of the American Cyanamid Company (1949), it was discovered that certain antibiotics could increase the rate of growth of young pigs and chicks when included in their diet in small amounts. Soon after this report a wide range of antibiotics have been tested and the following have been shown to have growth promoting properties: penicillin, oxytetracycline (Terramycin), chlortetracycline, bacitracin, streptomycin, tyrothricin, gramicidin, neomycin, erythromycin and flavomycin. Increased weight gain is most evident during the period of rapid growth and then decreases. Differences between control and treated animals are greater when the diet is slightly deficient or marginal in protein, B-vitamins or certain mineral elements.

Mode of Action of Antibiotics

1. Antibiotics "spare" protein, amino acids and vitamin on diets containing 1 to 3 per cent less protein, but balance experiments have often failed to show increased nitrogen retention. However, it has been suggested that some antibiotics have a sparing effect on B. vitamins as found in rats and chickens. The materials act by increasing the absorption of these vitamins.
2. Intestinal wall of animals fed antibiotics is thinner than that of untreated animals, which might explain the enhanced absorption of calcium shown for chicks.
3. Reduce or eliminate the activity of pathogens causing "subclinical infection".
4. Reduce the growth of micro-organisms that compete with the host for supplies of nutrients.
5. Antibiotics alter intestinal bacteria so that less urease is produced and thus less ammonia is formed. Ammonia is highly toxic and suppresses growth in non-ruminants.
6. Stimulate the growth of micro-organisms that synthesise known or unidentified nutrients.

Antibiotics in Pig Feeding

The good effects of feeding the antibiotic feed supplement is observed with animals given all-vegetable protein diets than those receiving animal protein supplements. The optimum level for most antibiotics in the diet is within the range of 5–15 mg/kg and there is no advantage in exceeding these low levels. Under normal condition of health adding Aureomycin or Terramycin supplement to rations for growing or fattening pigs increases the growth by about 15% reducing the feed intake by 2.5%. A mixture of two or more antibiotics is no more effective than a single effective antibiotic. The greatest increase in the rate of gain from an antibiotic feed supplement occurs during early growth, i.e., the suckling pigs gain more body weight.

Antibiotics in Poultry Feeding

Penicillin is more effective than other antibiotics especially to young and growing chicks. It increases the growth rate and this effect is most marked upto 1 month of age. As with pigs, the effect diminishes with age. Growth stimulation has been greatest when the antibiotic penicillin supplement has been added to a ration containing no protein supplements of animal origin or to a ration low in vitamin B_{12}. Under hygienic conditions growth increases are small. In "old" (infected) buildings increases of 10–15% in the growth rate of fowls are likely to be obtained with similiar increases in efficiency of feed utilisation. About 5 gm. of procaine penicillin per ton of ration for poultry is needed; but to control diseases, a higher level of 50 gm. or more per ton for feed is used.

Use of a combination of antibiotics has been no more effective than that of a single effective antibiotic. In layers, egg production has not been increased by adding antibiotics to a ration which is nutritionally complete. But, if hens are fed on only vegetable product ration, an antibiotic vitamin B_{12} feed supplement may increase both egg production and hatchability.

Antibiotics in the Diet of Ruminant Animals

The addition of Aureomycin supplement to calf rations has increased the growth rate of dairy calves specially when there had been much trouble from disease in the herd. It has reduced the incidence of scours and other infectious diseases. Most of the growth improvement occurs before the calves are 8 weeks old. Feeding daily 30 milligrams of Aureomycin or Terramycin per calf is the dose.

As far as mature animals are concerned, the results are conflicting. It has been assumed that the inclusion of antibiotics in the diet could be harmful by suppressing the activity of cellulolytic organisms and thus impairing cellulose digestion. In cows neither the milk production nor the fat percentage has been increased. It is similarly of no use in sterile animals and irregular breeders.

Following points should be kept in mind while using antibiotics for animal feeding:

1. Antibiotics should be used only for (a) growing and fattening pigs for slaughter as pork or becon; (b) growing chicks and turkey poults for killing as table poultry.
2. Antibiotics should not be used in the feed of ruminant animals (cattle, sheep and goats), breeding pigs and breeding and laying poultry stock.
3. While adding antibiotics at the recommended level, care should be taken that they are thoroughly and evenly mixed with the feed.
4. For best results, antibiotics should be used with properly balanced feeds. Also, the feeds containing antibiotics should be fed only to the type of stock for which they are intended.
5. Antibiotics are not a substitute for good management and healthy living conditions, or for properly balanced rations.

The use of antibiotic feed supplements or the fortified ration or the medicated feeds is governed by strict State laws in some countries (U.S.A., Canada and U.K.) where they are used for livestock and poultry so that farmers will not run unnecessary risk in using them.

Table 10.38

Antibiotics used as feed additives for growth promotion

Product	*Animal*	*Dose (mg/lb feed)*
Bacitracin and derivatives	Poultry	2–25
	Swine	5–25
	Beef	17–35*
Arsanilic acid, Sodium arsanilate	Poultry	22–45
	Swine	22–45
Chlortetracycline	Poultry	5–25
	Swine	5–25
	Beef	25–70*
	Sheep	10–25
Dynafac	Poultry	45–90
	Swine	200*
	Sheep	200*
	Beef	300–400*
Erythromycin	Growing chicks and turkeys	2.3–9
	Beef	37*
Furazolidone	Poultry	3.5–5.0
	Swine	75
Oleandomycine	Broilers and turkeys	0.5–1·0
Oxytetracycline	Poultry	25
	Swine	
	(10–30 lb)	12–25
	(30–200 lb)	3.5–5
	Beef	2.5–75*
	Sheep	5–10
Penicillin	Poultry	1.2–25
	Swine	5–25
Roxarsone	Poultry	11–22
	Swine	11–33
Tylosin	Poultry	2–25
	Swine	5–10

*mg/head/day

SOURCE: Hafez, E.S.E. and A. Dyer, *Animal growth and Nutrition* (1969), Published by Lea and Febiger, Philadelphia.

Table 10.38 as summarised by Prof. Carlson of Washington State University illustrates the exhaustive list of antibiotics used for various livestock with an appropriate dose.

Extensive use is being made of synthetic and purified estrogens, androgens, progestogens, growth hormones and thyroxine or thyroprotein (iodinated casein) to stimulate the growth and fattening of meat-producing animals. There is concern, however, about possible harmful effects of any residues of these materials in the meat or milk for the consumers.

Hormones related to animal growth on the basis of their effect in body can be grouped into two major categories *viz.*, ANABOLIC and CATABOLIC. Somatotropin, thyroxine and androgens are anabolic while estrogen and glucocorticoids belong to catabolic group.

The hormones of the anabolic class by nature exert their effect on both skeleton and protein metabolism. Somatotropin stimulates growth of endochondral bone and epiphysis of long bones while in protein metabolism it aids in nitrogen retention and overall protein synthesis. Thyroxine also stimulates growth of long bones as well as protein synthesis. Testosterone at low dose increases the epiphyseal diameter, promotes muscle growth by augmenting nitrogen retention.

The hormones belonging to catabolic group similarly exert their effect on both skeleton and protein metabolism. Estrogen inhibits skeletal growth although in ruminants it increases nitrogen retention. Glucocorticoids decrease growth of epiphysis and also aid in degrading protein and amino acids and thereby inhibit protein synthesis in extrahepatic tissue.

It is thought that the hormone alters the metabolism so as to increase muscle and bone formation at the expense of fat deposition. Since the energy required to synthesise protein or bone is less than that required to synthesise the same weight of fat, and the amount of water in muscle is greater than in body fat, it follows that a given amount of food will produce a higher live-weight increase due to hormone treatment.

It is an established fact that milk production in the cow will increase following the feeding of thyroprotein or L-thyroxine. The most effective daily dose appears to be about 15 gm per cow in the case of thyroprotein and 100 mg/cow daily for L-thyroxine. The addition of thyroxine or thyroprotein to the diet has increased milk production from 15 to 20 per cent above control animals, if a concomitant increase in energy intake was maintained. If additional feed is not given then the response is muted. A problem which has encountered is that sudden withdrawal of thyroprotein will cause milk production to drop below that of normal control cows, resulting no appreciable increase in the total milk produced in an entire lactation. University of Tennesse investigators found gradual withdrawing of thyroprotein caused milk production to drop only to the expected level or to that of controls. The indications are that feeding thyroprotein for short periods in successive lactation periods does not impair production; feeding the hormone for long periods in successive lactations may have an adverse effect on milk production but adequate proof for this is lacking. Some dairymen have experienced an increase in teat and other injuries and general excitability in thyroprotein fed herd. This is reasonable to expect. The overall seriousness of the problem will vary with a particular situation. During periods of extremely high environmental temperature, , there should be some caution exercised in the artificial induction of a hyperthyroid state.

Some workers have reported increased rates of gain and improved feed efficiency as a result of feeding thyroprotein or thyroxine to growing pigs from the time of weaning to market weight. As in the cow, administration of thyroprotein to lactating cows has been recommended by some investigators, with additional energy intake, lactation would probably be increased.

Studies with fattening lambs have shown that feeding 2-5 mg of stilbesterol daily increased the average daily gain about 20 per cent and reduced the feed per unit of gain. These substances either be given at the rate of 10 mg/day in beef cattle or can be implanted under the skin in the form of pellets in a single dose of 75 gm and 10 mg in sheep. Synthetic oestrogens should never be given to female animals, as otherwise there will be derangement of the breeding behaviour.

The widest application of the use of synthetic estrogenic hormones has undoubtedly been in the field of beef cattle and fat lamb production. The use of synthetic stilbesterol, hexoestrol has attracted more attention in recent years and these are in commercial use as growth promoters in many countries. Optimal amounts of oral dose or implantation of various hormonal compounds as reported by the National Research Council Committee are given in Table 10.39

Table 10.39

Products	*Animal*	*Dosages*	*Method of use*
1. Diethylstilbesterol	Cattle	[illegible]/day	In feed
	Sheep	2 mg/day	
(Thyroprotein)	Cattle	24 to 3[illegible] mg	Subcutaneous
	Poultry	12 to 15 mg	
2. Diethylstilbesterol plus testosterone	Cattle	24 mg+120 mg	Subcutaneous
3. Testosterone propionate+estradiol benzoate	Heifers	200 mg+20 mg	Subcutaneous
4. Thiouracil	Swine and Poultry	0.2% of diet	In feed
5. Iodinated casein (thyroprotein)	Lactating cows	15 mg/day	In feed
	Lactating sows	200 mg/kg diet	In feed
		25–50 mg/kg diet	In feed

SOURCE: *Animal Nutrition*, L. Maynard and J.K. Loosli, 6th edition.

The whole question whether hormones should be used as growth promoters is still debatable, but it seems logical that with any feeding system the economic advantages, however great, should never take precedence over any potential risk to human health. These substances may induce cancer in human beings if taken over a prolonged period through products of the treated animals. The use of such substances in poultry rearing has been prohibited by law in U.S.A.

OTHER GROWTH STIMULATING SUBSTANCES

A number of other compounds have been studied as feed additives in hopes of increasing the growth rate and health of animals or enhancing feed utilisation. Further study is necessary:

1. ARSENICALS: In 1949 it was reported that organic arsenicals had growth promoting properties similar to those of antibiotics when added to the diets of chicks. Arsanilic acid. sodium arsanilate are common compounds used.

2. TRANQUILLISERS: Certain tranquillisers such as natural alkaloid of *Rauwolfia*, reserpine, hydroxyzine chloropromazine have been shown in certain trials to improve daily liveweight

gain to livestock. The compounds act by reducing hypertension and nervousness specially in summer or under any stress condition.

3. COPPER SULPHATE: At 0.1 per cent level of the diet in fattening pigs, improves the rate of gain and feed conversion efficiency between weaning and becon weight. Sheep are particularly susceptible to copper poisoning, and there are several instances of death through sheep eating copper-fortified pig meals.

4. LIVE YEAST CULTURE: Conflicting results have been obtained regarding rate of gain, milk yield or the efficiency of feed utilisation in cattle.

5. DRIED RUMEN CULTURE: Although it was claimed that feeding the dried culture improves rumen development in calves and feed utilisation in older ruminants, but no confirmation has yet been made.

6. ANTHELMINTICS: Under some practical feeding conditions anthelmintics have also been used. The compounds act by reducing parasitic infections. Out of many commercial products, DDVP (2,2 dichlorovinyl dimethyl phosphate, has both anthelmintics and separate growth stimulatory effect in cattle.

BIOENERGETICS

In this universe, neither energy nor chemical elements can be created or destroyed and the animal system is no exception to this. However, the form of energy and the nature of the chemical compounds present in the animal or ingested in the food are subject to changes through the processes of metabolism in the animal. Nutritional requirement and its efficiency as a growth promoter or as a media for high production in animal system depends upon the nature and the extent of such metabolic transactions.

Bioenergetics or *Biochemical thermodynamics* is the study of the energy changes accompanying biochemical reactions. These reactions, as occurring in every cell are accompanied by an exchange of energy in the system.

What is Energy?

The term 'Energy' is a combination of two Greek words: *en,* meaning 'in' and *ergon*, meaning 'work'. The Greeks put the two words together to form *energon*, meaning 'active'. Hence energy is that force or power that enables the body to carry on life sustaining activities. Death is the cessation of this activity. Thus energy is the capacity to do work and is derived from mechanics.

Basic Units of Energy

In contrast to matter which has a mass and a space, energy neither occupies space nor has weight. There is no such thing, for example, as '3 cubic feet' or '4 kg' of energy. *Energy can only be measured by its effects* upon matter. In general greater the effect, the greater the amount of energy. For example, under similar conditions, a stick of dynamite causes more damage to a house (matter) than a firecracker does. The dynamite releases more energy.

The calorie has so long been used as a unit of energy since last two centuries. It is actually a unit of heat since one calorie is the amount of heat required to raise the temperature of one gram of water from 14.5 to 15.5°C at atmospheric pressure. This is also the specific heat of water. In nutritional and physiological studies, the unit of measure is the large calorie or kilocalorie, which is equal to 1000 small calories. Thus a kilocalorie (kcal) is the amount of heat required to raise 1 kg of water to 1°C. 1000 kcal is equal to 1 megacalorie (Mcal) or the Therm. In popular writings, particularly those concerned with human and animal calorie requirements, the term calorie is frequently used erroneously in place of the kilocalorie.

The International Union of Pure and Applied Chemistry (IUPAC) voted to adopt the energy unit as Joule (J) for measuring all forms of energy. The electrical energy required to increase the temperature of water from 14.5°C to 15.5°C has been determined, and average out to 4.1855 joules per 15° calorie. Thus it has been accepted that one small calorie = 4.185 J. The joule is defined as "the amount of work done by giving a force of 1 newton to displace the point of application of force through a distance of 1 meter. One newton is the force that will give a mass of 1 kg an acceleration of 1m/sec². By analogy with current practice the units employed would be kilojoule (kJ) and the megajoule (MJ). The advantages of expressing unit of energy as joule is that in the metric system of measurement this unit is suitable for expressing mechanical, chemical or electrical energy as well as in explaining the concept of heat. At present the system has been approved for use in about thirty countries, which has created pressure to replace the calorie with joule as a unit of energy. This pressure has resulted in controversy among nutritional scientists about the pros and cons of discarding the calorie and adopting the joule.

In nutritional work, kilocalories are often rounded off to the nearest 50, which would be approximately to the nearest 200 kilojoules.

Comparisons of physiological fuel values are as follows:

Table 10.40

	Kilocalories/gram	*Kilojoules/gram*
Protein	4	17
Fat	9	38
Carbohydrate	4	17

The Kinds and Forms of Energy

Energy exist in two kinds, *Kinetic* and *Potential*. Potential energy is energy which is stored, or inactive. A stick of dynamite represents a great deal of potential energy. When released, potential energy is capable of causing an effect on matter. However, when it does so it is no longer potential energy. It is kinetic energy, the energy which is in the processes of causing an effect on matter. Kinetic energy can also be measured by determining how much matter it moves in a given period of time, and how far and how fast it moves it.

In addition to the two kinds of energy (potential and kinetic), five more forms are also recognised. These are *chemical, electrical, mechanical, radiant* and *atomic energy.* The last of these atomic energy, has little direct relationship to the normal functioning of living organisms.

CHEMICAL ENERGY. It is the energy possessed by chemical compounds present in every cell. This energy is the most fundamental form of energy in the life processes. Every thought, every nerve impulse, every muscle movement, indeed every activity of any sort shown by living organisms is ultimately traceable to the release of chemical energy. Thus it may be said that animal body is a chemical engine. At rest it transduces the chemical energy present in feed into mechanical work as in the beating of heart and the movements of the diaphragm in respiration.

ELECTRICAL ENERGY. The energy generated in the biological system is due to the movement of electrons. Electrons actually do not flow through the cell in the same manner that they flow along a copper wire. Electrochemical reactions, combinations of electrical and chemical energy, play a large part in the functioning of the brain and the rest of the nervous system.

MECHANICAL ENERGY. The energy directly involved in moving matter. This movement involves the conversion of potential chemical energy into kinetic chemical energy, resulting in the contraction of muscles. Since in many organisms the muscles act upon the bones, which serve as levers, the total movement of such an organism demonstrates kinetic mechanical energy.

RADIANT ENERGY. The energy travels in waves. It includes radio waves, infra-red, ultra-violet rays, X-rays, gamma and cosmic rays. Ultra-violet light present in sunlight or artificially produced radiant energy is necessary for converting sterol molecules into vitamin D. It is only this radiant heat by which all classes of livestocks maintain their heat balance.

The Transformations of Energy

All forms of energy are interrelated and interconvertible and the process to some extent goes on continuously Metabolism involves the conversion of chemical energy to other forms of energy for the body's work. This chemical energy is changed to electrical energy as in brain and nerve activity, mechanical energy as in muscle contraction, thermal energy as in regulation of body temperature and to other types of chemical energy as in the synthesis of new compounds. In all these activities of the body, heat is given off.

Measurement of Energy

The amount of energy locked up by the bonds that hold a molecule of feed stuff together cannot be determined by direct means. However, the amount of heat energy given off or absorbed when a molecule is formed or decomposed during a chemical reaction is determined by a metal instrument, which is called a *Bomb calorimeter* because its shape resembles that of a bomb. The instrument (Fig 110) consists of an insulated water jacket containing a known amount of water into which a thermometer, a stirrer to keep the temperature of the water uniform, and a reaction chamber are immersed. The reaction or combustion chamber is known as a bomb. The bomb is a sturdy metal chamber into which the firmly palleted, or otherwise homogeneous substance to be burned, is placed. It is equipped with a valve through which oxygen is introduced to develop a 25 to 30 atmosphere pressure. The combustible substance is ignited in the presence of oxygen pressure by means of magnesium fuse wire sealed within the bomb and connected to an outside switch. As the feed burns, heat produced leads to a rise in temperature of the surrounding water. Thus heat production can be accurately measured from the change in mercury level of the attached thermometer immersed in the water of the jacket. This value, when multiplied by the water equivalent of that instrument, gives the number of calories produced by the burning of the sample.

Gross Energy (GE)

This is the total energy of the feed and is mostly determined by bomb calorimeter and sometimes by multiplying the percentage of carbohydrates, proteins and fats with 4.15, 5.65 and 9.40 respectively (Atwater and Bryant, 1899—Gross energy value, kcal/gram). Since none of

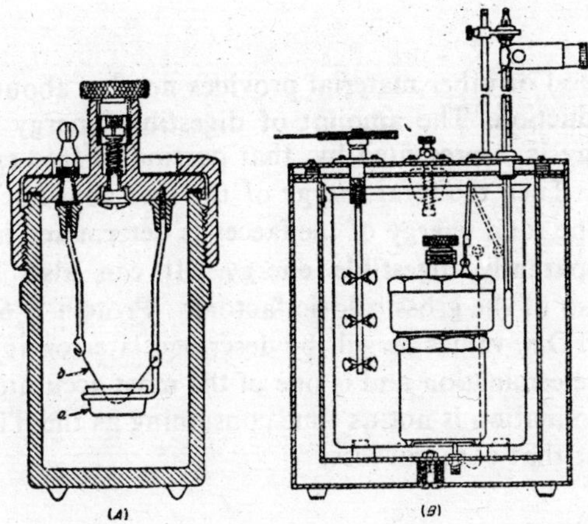

Fig. 10.13 Cross section of a Bomb Calorimeter.
A. Bomb : (*a*) Cup, (*b*) Fuse wire
B. Insulated calorimeter with bomb in place.

the foodstuffs is completely absorbed; some potential energy, therefore, never enters the body and is excreted in the faeces. Since gross energy includes both digestible and non-digestible components, gross energy has little physiological significance especially in animals that consume large quantities of crude fibre.

Table 10.41

Feed energy utilisation by cow

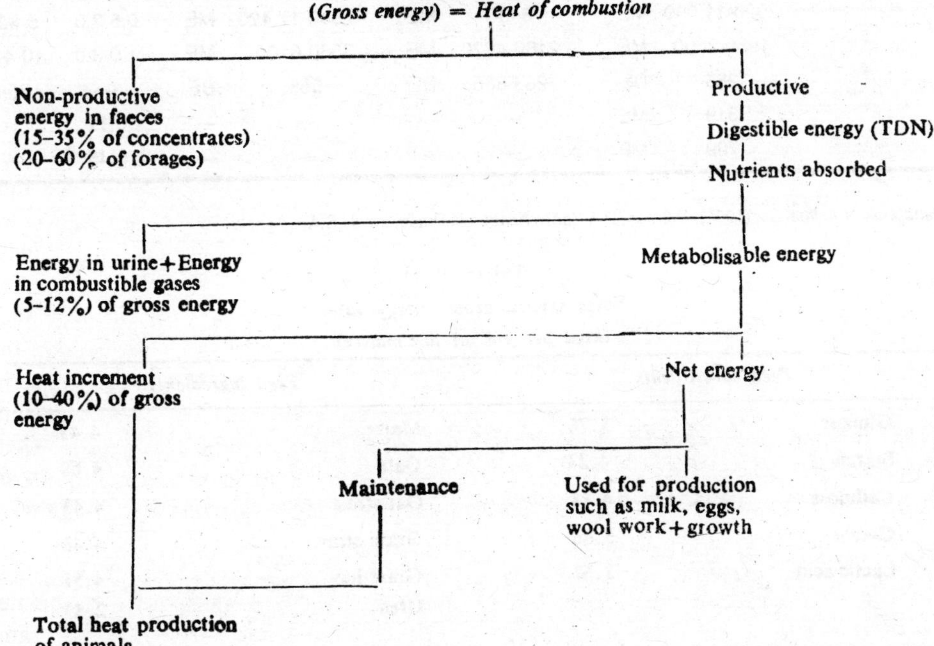

Digestible Energy (DE)

The gross energy of a food or other material provides no clue about the amount of energy available for livestock production. The amount of digestible energy is more useful for this purpose. Digestible energy is represented by that portion of feed energy consumed which is not excreted in the faeces. Then the total energy of the feed consumed (GE) is first measured in a bomb calorimeter. The total energy of the faeces is determined in the same way and the difference is called the apparently digestible energy. It can also be calculated from the digested nutrients by the use of the gross caloric factors: Protein 5 65; Carbohydrates 4.15; and Fat 9.45 or from the TDN values as will be described later on in this Chapter.

The method is a direct determination and is one of the most accurate analyses performed in the laboratory. The determination is not as time consuming as the TDN method. It does not account for any loss except that of faecal loss.

Metabolisable Energy (ME)

All of the digestible energy is not available for productive purposes and other energy losses

Table 10.42

Average Energy Requirements of Selected Species

Common Name	Energy Requirement (Growth) (kcal/day)		Energy Requirement (Pregnancy) (kcal/day)		Energy Requirement (Lactation) (kcal/day)		Output (kg/day)	Urine Output (ml/day)
Beef cattle	4200-31,000	ME	12,600-24,000	ME	15,900-27,500	ME	13-35	17-45/kg bw
Dairy cattle	1800-31,980	ME	13,000-25,600	ME	40,190-48,380	ME	13-35	17-45/kg bw
Horse	7430-19,200	DE	8700-19,950	DE	15,240-30,020	DE	20	—
Goat	2100-3300	ME	3100-4100	ME	3400-4300	ME	0.5-3.0	10-40/kg bw
Swine	2020-11,090	ME	6430	ME	15,840-17,420	ME	0.5-3.0	5-30/kg bw
Sheep	1980-2600	ME	2160-4620	ME	3580-6100	ME	1.0-3.0	10-40/kg bw
Rabbit	283	DE	283-635	DE	588	DE	—	65/kg bw
Chicken	319	ME	—	—	—	—	0.11	—
Turkey	769	ME	—	—	—	—	0.45	—

Source : *Handbook of Animal Sc.* (1991), Putman, P.A. (ed)., Academic Press, Inc. U.S.A.

Table 10.43

Some typical gross energy value

(kcal per gm. of dry matter)

Feed constituents		*Feed ingredients*	
Glucose	3.76	Maize	4.43
Starch	4.23	Oats	4.68
Cellulose	4.18	Oat straw	4.43
Casein	5.86	Grass straw	4.43
Lactic acid	3.62	Grass hay	4.51
		Urea	2.53

Table 10.44

Ranges in loss of dietary gross energy (%)

	Simple stomached animal	*Non-ruminants herbivores*	*Ruminants*
Faeces	2–40	10–70	10–60
Gases (Less than)	0.5	3–7	5–12
Urinary	1–3	3–5	3–5
Heat increment	5–30	10–35	10–40
Net use ⟶	25–50	15–50	10–35

occur. When energy losses in the urine and combustible gases (primarily methane, CH_4) are subtracted from the digestible energy, the remaining energy is called the metabolisable energy. Generally the energy losses in the combustible gases and urine account for about 8 and 3 to 5% of the gross energy of the feed respectively. Losses are usually greater in ruminants than non-ruminants.

The method significantly represents the useful energy of a feed and is not affected by plane of nutrition nor by the activity of the animal. The urinary and faecal loss are determined by bomb calorimeter while for methane production suitable factors may be employed. The draw-back of this method is that comparison of high and low fibre containing feeds cannot be made by this method.

Net Energy (NE)

This is the net remainder of the useful energy after all the losses accounted for faeces, urine, methane and heat increment are subtracted. By this NE represents that part of the feed energy which is actually retained and utilised by the body for its growth or production. As such this is the ideal method of expressing the nutritive energy of a feed. The disadvantages are that it is very difficult to have a respiratory chamber or animal calorimeter for the estimation of heat increment. Moreover, it is also a hard job to keep the animals in fast condition required for estimation of heat increment and that heat increment may not be a loss in cold season.

However, a few years ago a relatively simpler slaughter technique was developed at the University of California for determining the net energy requirement for growing and finishing cattle and the net energy value of feeds for this class of cattle. The system includes separate estimates for energy depending on whether it was used for maintenance (NE_m) or for body weight gain (NE_g). The formula suggested to find out the NE_m) is as follows:

$$NE_m = 77 \text{ kcal}/W_k{}^{0.75}$$

Using this formula it has been observed that the average net energy required for maintenance for a beef cattle ranges between 72 to 82 kcal per unit of metabolic size ($W_{kg}{}^{0.75}$).

For determining the net energy for weight gain, Lofgreen and Garrett* observed that the relationship between NE_g and weight gain could be expressed by the following equations:

*Lofgreen, G.P. and W.N., Garrett Jr., *Animal Science*, 27 (1968): 793.

$$NE_g = (52.72a + 6.84a^2)\ (W_{kg}^{0.75}) \text{ for steers}$$

$$NE_g = (56.03a + 12.65a^2)\ (W_{kg}^{0.75}) \text{ for heifers}$$

where NE_g is in kilocalories, a is daily weight gain in kilograms, and W_{kg} is the body weight in kilogram.

The NE_g for any feed is determined after feeding it at two levels and estimating the energy deposited as a result of the intake of feed between two levels. Any two levels of feeding above that required for maintenance can be used to determine the NE_g of a ration.

Heat Increment (HI)

The increase in heat production after the ingestion of feed has been the subject of much investigation and thought, and a variety of names for the effect have been suggested, for example, specific dynamic action (SDA), specific dynamic effect (SDE), heat increment (HI), calorigenic effect of feed and thermogenic effect of feed.

The cause of heat increment of nutrients is unknown. Several theories have been proposed: (1) the absorbed amino acids excite body cells to a high level of energy metabolism, (2) the energy expense of digestion, absorption, excretion and secretion, (3) energetic inefficiency of the reactions by which absorbed nutrients are metabolised. For example, when glucose is oxidised in the formation of ATP, the efficiency of free energy capture, is only about 44 per cent. The rest amount, i.e., 56 per cent being lost as heat. It seems probable that many or all of these factors contribute to the heat increment. The HI may be expressed in absolute terms (kcal/of feed dry matter) or relative as a proportion of the gross or metabolisable energy.

HI ean be reduced somewhat by feeding higher levels of grains. Perhaps this is why we have observed cows on low grain ration eating larger quantities of hay during extreme cold weather (one of nature's provisions for keeping warm).

Control of Energy in Animal Metabolism

The energy in any system may be uncontrolled and destructive, as in an atomic bomb used for warfare; or it may be controlled and constructive, as in an atomic reactor used for research and industry. In the animal body also the energy produced in its many chemical reactions, if "exploded" at once, could be destructive. The mechanism by which energy is retained in the animal system is by *chemical bonding*. The chemical bonds that hold the elements of the compounds together consist of various quantum of energy. So long the compound remains constant, energy is being exerted to maintain the atomic constellation that is characteristic for that molecule. It is in this way that potential energy is stored in the compound. When such compounds are broken into various products, energy is released and it becomes free energy. By nature free energy immediately involves in the bonding of other atoms.,

Bonds which are involved in exchanging energy are: *Covalent bonds, hydrogen bonds* and *phosphate bonds.*

COVALENT BOND. When two atoms share a pair of electrons, they are joined by a covalent bond. Common examples of such bonds are those shared between neighbour carbon atoms in the core of an organic compound (–C –C –C).

HYDROGEN BOND. This type of bonding takes place between a hydrogen donor group and an acceptor group. Commonly found in peptide linkage. Bonds are weak and can be broken easily. They are less rich in energy than covalent bonds.

HIGH-ENERGY-PHOSPHATE BOND. Phosphate bonds attach the phosphate radical to a compound. Since the phosphate radical is highly labile, more energy is required to bind it and similarly more free energy is released when the phosphate bond is broken. Most of the phosphate bonds are referred to as high energy bonds and are expressed by ~ sign. An example of such high energy compound is adenosine triphosphate (ATP) $A—PO_4 \sim PO_4 \sim PO_4$ (Fig.111).

Examples of low energy phosphate bonds include those formed by the phosphorylation of glucose (glucose-6-phosphate, glucose-1, phosphate) which activates glucose for participation in cell metabolism.

Mechanism of controlling the reaction rate is also an important aspect of energy metabolism as it is this mechanism by which the release of required amount of energy from energy rich compounds is obtained at the time of need at particular cell or tissue. For example some of the chemical reactions that break down proteins if left to themselves (as in sterile decomposition) would span several years. Such reactions must be accelerated or else it might take years to get the necessary energy from a meal. At the same time, they must be regulated so that too fast a reaction will not produce energy in a single explosion. Enzymes, coenzymes and hormones control numerous biological oxidation of the cells.

The Role of ATP

When fuel molecules are broken down within living organisms, the energy released must be channelled in a useful direction. If it is not captured immediately, the energy is lost for useless work within the cell causing damage to the cells.

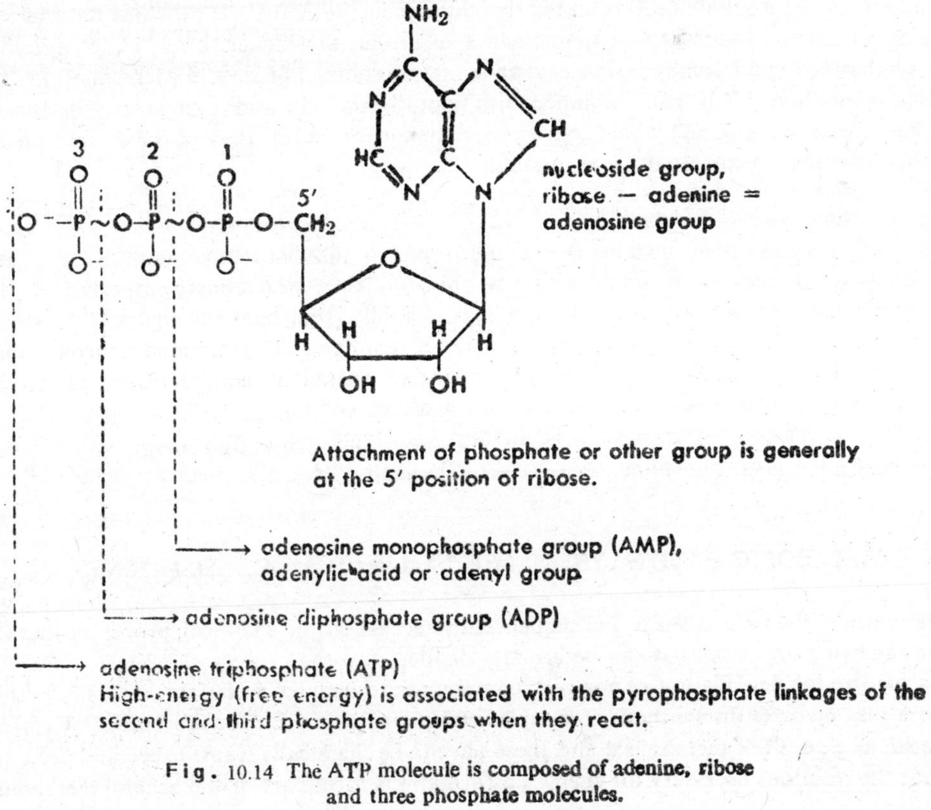

nucleoside group,
ribose — adenine =
adenosine group

Attachment of phosphate or other group is generally at the 5′ position of ribose.

adenosine monophosphate group (AMP), adenylic acid or adenyl group

adenosine diphosphate group (ADP)

adenosine triphosphate (ATP)
High-energy (free energy) is associated with the pyrophosphate linkages of the second and third phosphate groups when they react.

Fig. 10.14 The ATP molecule is composed of adenine, ribose and three phosphate molecules.

None of the energy released is used directly to power chemical reactions. All such energy is stored in small "packages" of energy known as *high energy phosphate bonds*. In this way the energy is available in a common form for all metabolic processes of the cells.

In most living systems, high energy bonds are found in the form of a compound known as adenosine triphosphate (ATP). It is composed of one molecule of adenine and ribose to which are attached three phosphate groups Fig.]10:14 The last two phosphate groups are jointed to the main body of the molecule by high energy bonds (represented as ~). Upon hydrolysis of the bond which is between the terminal carbon atom and the first phosphate group (which is not a high energy bond) an energy exchange of —1 to —5 kilocalories per mole occurs. When either of the two terminal phosphates are hydrolysed, about —5 to—15 kcal/mole are liberated. These are referred to as high energy bonds. There are also other high energy compounds in nature and a large percentage of those are associated with a terminal phosphate group.

For living organisms there are two advantages to having energy stored in high energy phosphate bonds. First, the energy in such bonds is readily available to the cell for immediate use. The process of extracting the energy from the monophosphate bond is a one-step reaction. Second, and perhaps most important, the amount of energy in a high energy phosphate bond is approximately that amount which is the most useful for producing biochemical reactions. This means that there is less wastage of energy. As a result, biochemical reactions within living organisms are quite efficient. They do not release more energy than can be used at any one time.

By virtue of its role in energy transfer mechanisms, ATP is involved in the oxidation and also in synthesis of all proteins, fats and carbohydrates in the body. It provides the energy of muscular contraction so vital to the maintenance of life in the higher forms. ATP is involved in the synthesis of and in many instances is an actual component of several coenzymes involved in tissue respiration. It is also combined with pantothenic acid and cysteamine in the very important coenzyme A (CoA) which acts as an activator of substrates in most intermediary metabolic reactions occurring in living tissues.

Storage of High-energy Phosphate

The ATP yield is a rather unstable compound, rapidly utilised in other physiological reactions of the body and is present in small amounts only in tissue. For storage, especially in liver and muscle, any surplus high-energy phosphate is rapidly transferred from ATP to creatine phosphate, the major form of storage in all domestic animals. The terminal pyrophosphate linkage of ATP is hydrolysed and a bond of similar free energy of hydrolysis, a phosphoguanidine linkage, is created by transfer of the phosphate to creatine, forming phosphocreatine. Any increase in the concentration of ATP favours the synthesis of phosphocreatine. When ATP concentration falls, phosphocreatine returns the high energy phosphate to yield ATP from ADP.

METABOLIC PATHWAYS IN THE UTILISATION OF NUTRIENTS

Metabolism is the term given to the sequence, or succession, of chemical processes that take place in the living organism. It can be broadly divided into the processes namely *Catabolism* process involve the degradation of complex compounds to simpler materials and *Anabolism*—processes that involves the synthesis of complex compounds from simpler substances. Waste products arise as a result of metabolism and these have to be chemically transformed and ultimately excreted; the reactions necessary for such transformations form part of the general metabolism.

CARBOHYDRATE METABOLISM

Glucose enters the cell from the intestinal fluid in the free state and is then actively transported across most cell membranes under the influence of the hormone insulin. Intestinal mucosa and brain do not require insulin for glucose transport. Free glucose cannot enter into other cellular metabolic activities; thus upon entrance into the cell, it is immediately phosphorylated, a process which requires ATP and which results in the formation of glucose-6-phosphate. Three chief pathways are open to the phosphorylated glucose:

(1) Glycolysis, (2) Glycogenesis (formation of glycogen), (3) Metabolism by way of the pentose phosphate shunt. The pathway followed is determined by the metabolic condition existing within the cell; primarily, the available amounts of glucose, ATP, NADP and oxygen determine the pathway of glucose degradation.

Glycolysis

The pathway of glycolysis was elucidated by G. Embden and O. Meyerhof during the period between 1920 and 1940 and thus the processes of glycolysis is also termed as Embden-Meyerhof

Embden-Meyerhof of Glycolysis

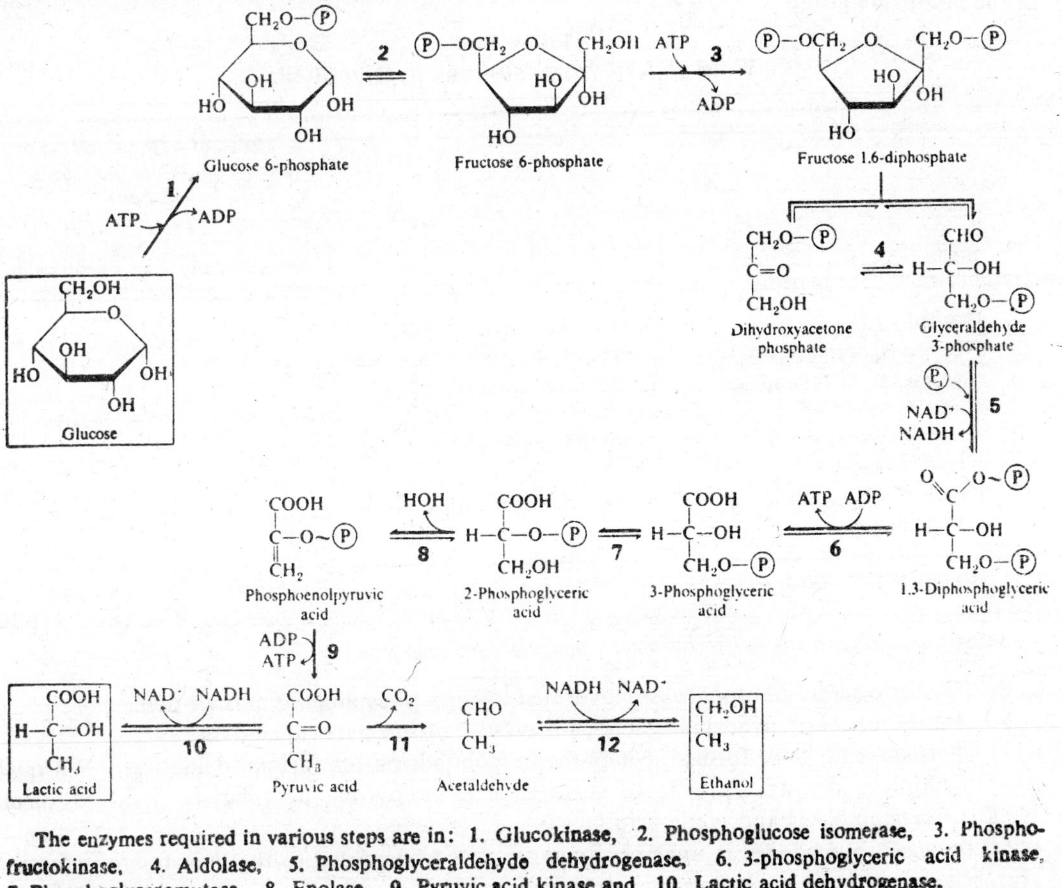

Glucose →(1; ATP → ADP) Glucose 6-phosphate ⇌(2) Fructose 6-phosphate →(3; ATP → ADP) Fructose 1.6-diphosphate

Fructose 1.6-diphosphate → Dihydroxyacetone phosphate (CH_2O–Ⓟ, C=O, CH_2OH) ⇌(4) Glyceraldehyde 3-phosphate (CHO, H–C–OH, CH_2O–Ⓟ)

Glyceraldehyde 3-phosphate ⇌(5; P_i, NAD^+ → NADH) 1.3-Diphosphoglyceric acid

1.3-Diphosphoglyceric acid ⇌(6; ATP ADP) 3-Phosphoglyceric acid ⇌(7) 2-Phosphoglyceric acid ⇌(8; HOH) Phosphoenolpyruvic acid

Phosphoenolpyruvic acid →(9; ADP → ATP) Pyruvic acid (COOH, C=O, CH_3)

Pyruvic acid ⇌(10; NAD^+ NADH) Lactic acid (COOH, H–C–OH, CH_3)

Pyruvic acid →(11; CO_2) Acetaldehyde (CHO, CH_3) ⇌(12; NADH NAD^+) Ethanol (CH_2OH, CH_3)

The enzymes required in various steps are in: 1. Glucokinase, 2. Phosphoglucose isomerase, 3. Phosphofructokinase, 4. Aldolase, 5. Phosphoglyceraldehyde dehydrogenase, 6. 3-phosphoglyceric acid kinase, 7. Phosphoglyceromutase, 8. Enolase, 9. Pyruvic acid kinase and 10. Lactic acid dehydrogenase.

glycolytic pathway. The principal reactions involved in glycolysis are depicted below. Reactions corresponding to numbers are described below:

1. Free glucose is phosphorylated to form glucose-6-phosphate which requires ATP.

2. Glucose-6-phosphate is isomerised to fructose-6-phosphate.

3. Fructose-6-phosphate is further phosphorylated by ATP at the first carbon to form fructose-1, 6-diphosphate.

4. Fructose-1, 6-diphosphate is split into two molecules of glyceraldehyde-3-phosphate, and dihydroxyacetone phospnate. From this point, carbohydrate metabolism proceeds from glyceraldehyde-3-phosphate, but, because this compound and dihydroxyacetone phosphate are interconvertible, in effect, two molecules of glyceraldehyde are formed from one hexose unit.

5. Glyceraldehyde-3-phosphate is then oxidised to glyceric acid-1, 3-diphosphate. The hydrogen thus released is taken up by NAD which may be reoxidised by the mitochondrial electron transport system leading to the synthesis of 3 moles of ATP. In the absence of oxygen (anaerobic glycolysis), NADH is utilised in the formation of lactic acid from pyruvic acid.

6. Glyceric acid-1, 3-diphosphate reacts directly with ADP to form ATP and glyceric acid-3-phosphate.

7. Glyceric acid-3-phosphate is converted to glyceric acid 2-phosphate, essentially migration of the phosphate group.

Table 10.45

Yield of ATP from Glucose in Glycolysis

	Steps		*Moles of ATP gained (+) or loss (-) per initial glucose unit Steps*	
			Anaerobically	***Aerobically***
1.	Glucose + ATP	Glucose -6 phosphate + ADP	-1	-1
2.	Fructose-6 phosphate + ATP	Fructose-1, -6-diphosphate + ADP	-1	-1
3.	Glyceraldehyde-3-phosphate (2 moles)	1,3-diphosphoglyceric acid	-	+6
4.	1,3-diphosphoglyceric acid + 2 ADP (2 moles)	3 phosphoglyceric acid (2 moles) + 2 ATP	+2	+2
5.	Phosphenol pyruvic acid + 2 ADP (2 moles)	Pyruvic acid (2 moles) + 2 ATP	+2	+2
	Net gain in ATP via Glycolysis		**+2**	**+8**

Note that Glycolysis can proceed in both aerobic and anaerobic conditions

8. Glyceric acid-2-phosphate is dehydrated to form phosphoenol pyruvic acid..

9. Phosphoenol pyruvic acid reacts with ADP, to form pyruvic acid and ATP.

10. Pyruvic acid, thus formed, enters the mitochondrion for further oxidation. When the oxygen supply is low, as in prolonged muscular activity, pyruvic acid may be used to oxidize NADH, forming NAD and lactic acid.

Lactic acid, so produced in anaerobic condition, is transported to the liver for resynthesis to glycogen since there is no enzymatic mechanism in muscle cells for the conversion of lactic acid to glycogen.

Metabolic fates of pyruvate.

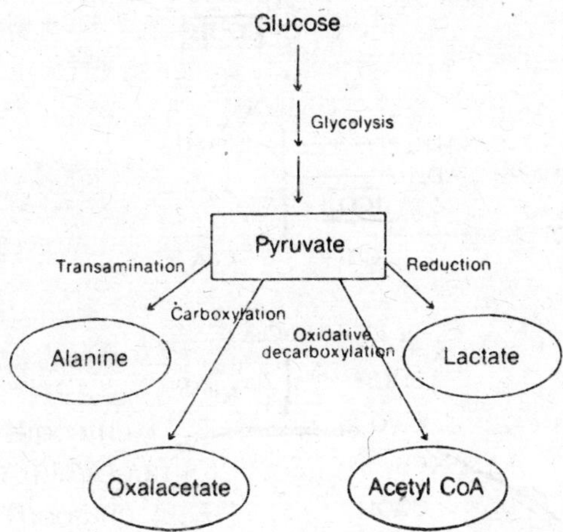

Glycolysis may thus proceed in the presence or absence of oxygen. From the standpoint of energy yield to the cell, however, aerobic glycolysis is the more efficient mechanism.

The Tricarboxylic Acid Cycle

The chemical energy that is not liberated when glucose is broken down anaerobically, to lactate, is released during the third stage of nutrient degradation when pyruvate is oxidised in the mitochondria to CO_2 and H_2O via the tricarboxylic acid, TCA cycle. In a quantitative sense, this cycle is the most important phase in the oxidation of foodstuffs, since approximately 90 per cent of the energy released from food is the result of TCA cycle oxidation.

Although metabolites may enter the cycle at any point, the cycle is usually visualised as beginning with the condensation of acetyl CoA with oxaloacetate to form citric acid. The subsequent series of reactions comprising the cycle uses up two moles of H_2O and results in the release of two moles of CO_2 and four pairs of hydrogens and electrons. The over-all reaction in the degradation of acetate may be expressed as:

$$\underset{\text{Acetic acid.}}{CH_3COOH} + 2H_2O \longrightarrow 2CO_2 + 2H^+$$

The individual reactions of TCA cycle are depicted diagrammatically in next page. A description of the reactions corresponding to numbers in the diagram follows:

1. Pyruvic acid is converted to an active form of acetic acid, acetyl coenzyme A (acetyl CoA). In the process of forming acetyl CoA, pyruvic acid is decarboxylated and two hydrogen ions are released and are picked up by NAD^+.

2. Condensation of oxaloacetate and acetyl CoA form citrate. CoA is split off hydrolytically in the process.

3 & 4. Isomerisation of citrate to yield isocitrate. *Cis*-aconitic acid may be formed as an intermediary. Water assists in the isomerisation but is not used up in the process.

5. Dehydrogenation and decarboxylation of isocitrate to form α-keto-glutaric acid . NAD or NADP may serve as hydrogen acceptor.

6 & 7. Oxidative decarboxylation of α-keto-gluterate to form succinate. Succinyl CoA is

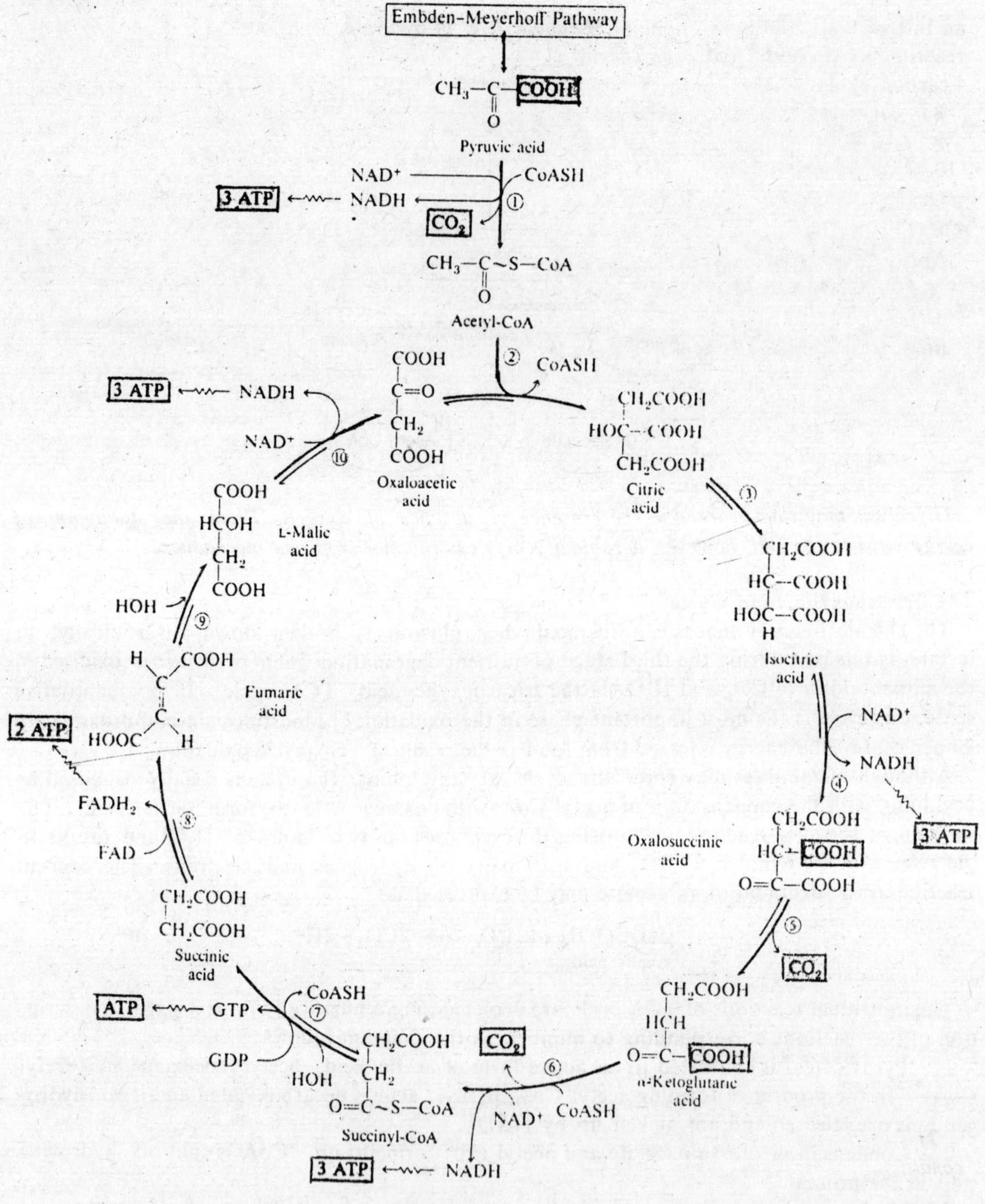

The Krebs cycle.

Fig. 10.15 Enzymes required in various steps are in: 1. Pyruvate oxidase, 2. Citrate condensing enzyme, 3 and 4. Aconitase, 5. Isocitrate dehydrogenase. 6. α-keto glutarate dehydrogenase, 7. Succinyl thiokinase. 8. Succinate, dehydrogenase, 9. Fumerase, and 10. Malate dehydrogenase.

an intermediary and both Thiamine pyrophosphate (TPP) and lipoic acid are required for this reaction. NAD is the hydrogen acceptor. The loss of a second CO_2 molecule results in a 4 carbon chain.

8. Dehydrogenation of succinate to form fumerate. FAD is the hydrogen acceptor.
9. Addition of water to fumerate to form malate.
10. Dehydrogenation of malate to form oxaloacetate.

Oxaloacetate now is available to condense with another mole of acetyl CoA and thus to repeat the cycle.

Note: During the conversion of

(i) NAD into NADH there is a genesis of 3 moles of ATP.

(ii) FAD into $FADH_2$ there is a genesis of 2 moles of ATP.

(iii) GDP into GTP there is a genesis of 1 mole of ATP.

Table 10.46

Yield of ATP from pyruvic acid in TCA cycle

Steps		*Moles ATP formed*
Pyruvic acid	acetyl CoA	3
Isocitric acid	α-keto-glutaric acid	3
α-keto-glutaric acid	succinyl CoA	3
Succinyl CoA	succinic acid	1
Succinic acid	fumeric acid	2
Malic acid	oxaloacetic acid	3
Total ATP per molecule	pyruvic acid	15
Total from 2 mols-of pyruvate (15×2)=		30

The total ATP production from the oxidation of one mole of glucose aerobically is then:

	Moles ATP
1 mole of glucose to 2 moles of pyruvate	8
2 moles of pyruvate to CO_2 and H_2O	30
Total per mole of glucose	38

The entire process of citric acid cycle takes place inside the mitochondria under only aerobic condition.

Hexose Monophosphate Shunt of Glucose Catabolism

The principal catabolic route for carbohydrates is the glycolysis pathway, followed under aerobic conditions, by the TCA pathway. The glycolytic enzymes are present in the soluble fraction of cell but the route from pyruvate is located in the mitochondria. There is however, an alternative route by which the oxidation of carbohydrates can take place. Quantitatively, it usually accounts for only a very small percentage of the oxygen taken up by the cell.

The discussion of this pathway is brief, for even indirectly it is not important for ATP production in skeletal muscle. It is, however, a way of converting glucose ultimately of CO_2 and H_2O without going through the citric acid cycle. Its most important function is in generating NADPH, which is needed to furnish hydrogen for reduction steps whenever the body synthesises fatty acids and steroids.

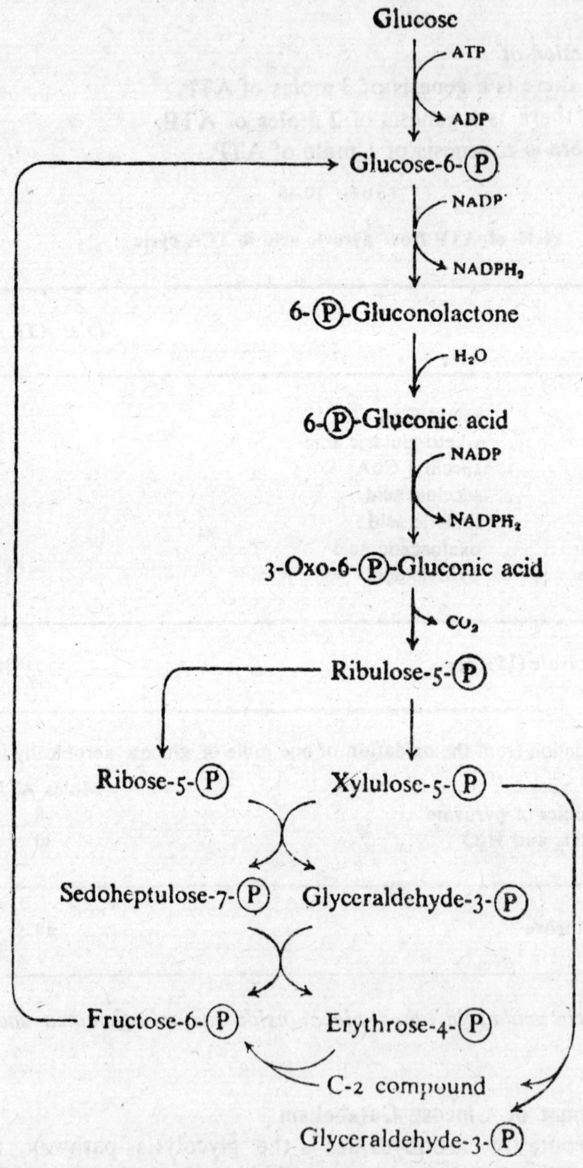

Reactions of the pentose phosphate pathway, sometimes called the hexose monophosphate shunt, or alternate pathway.

Starting from glucose-6-phosphate, the balanced equation representing the net effect of this pathway is

$$6 \text{ glucose 6-phosphate} + 12 \text{ NADP}^+ \xrightarrow[\text{Shunt}]{\text{Hexose monophosphate}}$$

$$5 \text{ glucose 6-phosphate} + 6 \text{ CO}_2 + 12 \text{ NADPH} + 12 \text{ H}^+ + \text{Pi}$$

There are of course several intermediate steps, some of them using enzymes of the glycolysis pathway. Among the intermediates are certain 5-carbon sugars (e.g., ribose) needed by the body to make nucleotides and nucleic acids. We should remember that this shunt is an important way to produce NADPH for fat synthesis.

GLYCOGEN, GLYCOGENESIS, GLYCOGENOLYSIS AND GLUCONEOGENESIS

What is Glycogen?

Glycogen is a highly branched, very large polymer of glucose molecules linked along its main line by α-1,4-glycosidic linkages, branches arise by α-1,6-glycosidic bonds at about every tenth residue.

It occurs in the cytosol (the soluble portion of the cytoplasm that includes dissolved solutes but that excludes the particulate matter) as granules, which also contain the enzymes that catalyze its formation and use. Glycogen is known as animal starch, resembles that of amylopectin but glycogen is more highly branched with branch points occurring every 8–12 glucose residues (shorter than amylopectin).

Glycogen Storage

1. Glycogen is the storage form of glucose. Its polymeric nature allows the sequestering of energy stores with much less of a problem from osmotic effects than glucose would cause.

2. Muscle and liver are the major sites for the storage of glycogen, and although its concentration in the liver is higher, the much greater mass of skeletal muscle stores a greater total amount of glycogen.

3. Liver can mobilize its glycogen for the release of glucose to the rest of the body, but muscle can only use its glycogen for its own energy needs.

Glycogenesis (Glycogen Synthesis)

Glycogenesis (synthesis of glycogen) and glycogenolysis (break-down of glycogen) occur by separate enzyme pathways. Glycogen is synthesized exclusively from glucose-1-phosphate and uridine triphosphate (UTP).

Glucose-1-phosphate is derived from glucose-6-phosphate by the action of phosphoglucomutase. The reaction proceeds by way of an intermediate, glucose-1,6-diphosphate

This glucose-1-phosphate then reacts with UTP in presence of UDP-glucose pyrophsphorylase to form Uridine diphosphate glucose as below.

The reaction is although reversible, but the hydrolysis of inorganic pyrophosphate (PP_i) by cellular pyrophosphatases renders it essentially irreversible. The compound UDP-glucose is an activated form of glucose, the carbon-1 carbon of the glucosyl unit esterified to the diphosphate.

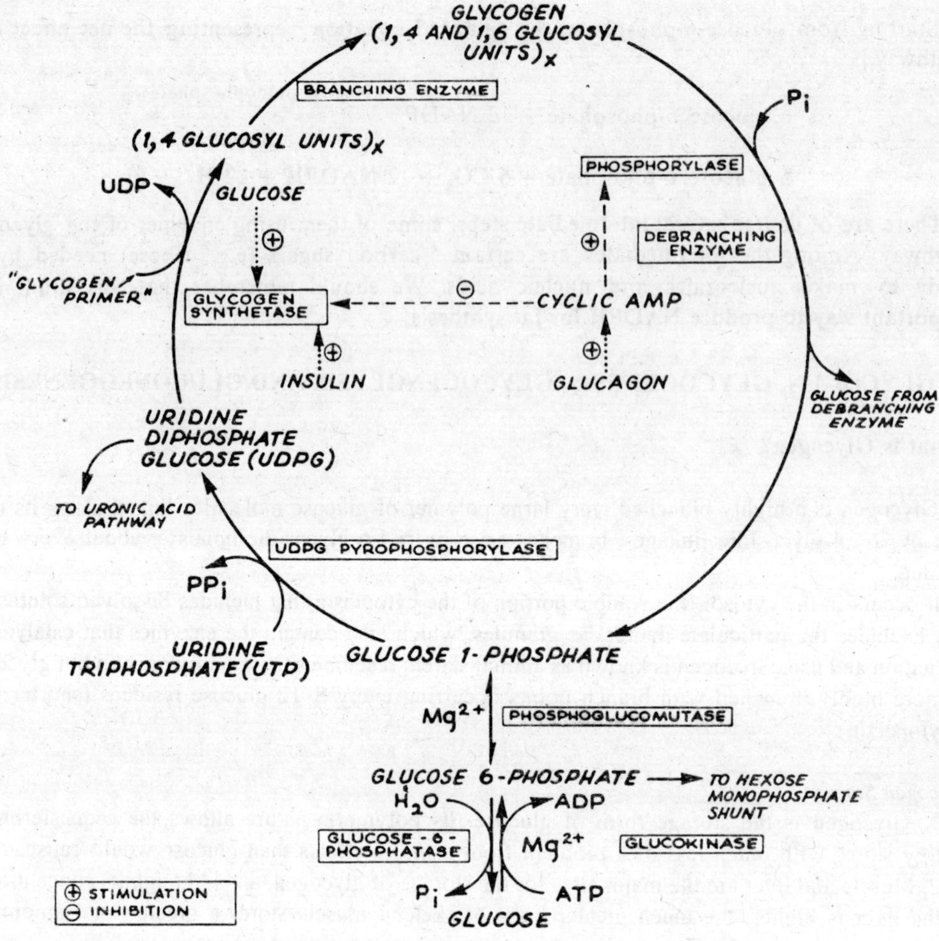

Fig. 10.16. Pathway of glycogenesis and of glycogenolysis in the liver.

Formation of Amylose Chain

The synthesis of new glycogen requires the presence of existing glycogen chains and glucosyl residues from UDP-glucose. The residues are successively transferred to a C-4 terminus of an existing glycogen chain in α-1,4-glycosidic linkages to form a growing chain.

UDP-glucose + (glycogen)n residues = UDP + (glycogen)n + residues

Note: 1. The reaction is catalyzed by glycogen synthetase also known as UDP-glycogen transferase.
2. This is the rate-limiting step in glycogen synthesis.

Formation of Branch Chains and Further Growth

Segments of the amylose chain are transferred onto the C-6 hydroxyl of a pre-existing glycogen chain, forming α-1,6 linkages.

The enzyme responsible is glucosyl 4 : 6 transferase (branching enzyme). In branch formation, seven residue segments of the amylose to terminal chains are transferred to a C-6 hydroxyl of a glucosyl residue that is four residue away for an existing branch. The initial terminal branch must be at least eleven residues in length before a segment is transferred from it. (Fig. 10.17).

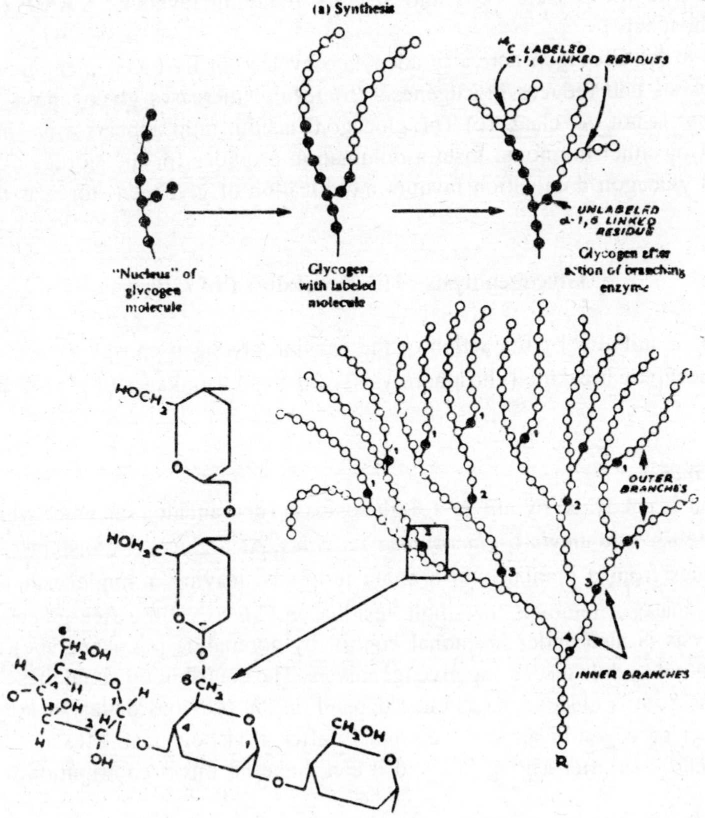

Fig. 10.17 The Glycogen molecule.

Open circles are glucose residues linked by α-1, 4-glucosidic bonds and solid circles are glucose residues linked by α-1, 6 bonds. Segments at the branch point is enlarged to show structure.

Regulation of Glycogenesis

1. The rate limiting step in glycogen formation is the addition of activated glycosyl units (derived from UDP-glucose) to an existing chain by glycogen synthetase—which again exists in two forms, e.g., dependent (D) and independent (I) forms.
   Interconversion of the D and I forms takes place by phosphorylation and is catalyzed by cyclic adenosine monophosphate-dependent. (C-AMP-dependent) protein kinase. The phosphorylated form is the inactive (D) form.

2. *Hormonal Regulation*
   In Muscle: (a) Epinephrine promotes glycogenolysis and inhibits glycogenesis. The hormone stimulates the formation of (cyclic AMP) CAMP by activating adenylate cyclase. Thus in an emergency when epinephrene is released and acts upon the muscle cell membrane.

glycogenolysis is activated via the phosphorylation and simultaneously glycogenesis is retarded.

(b) Insulin increases glycogenesis and decreases glycogenolysis by heightening the entry of glucose into the muscle cells and also by reducing levels of CAMP (cyclic adenosive monophosphate).

In the Liver: (a) Glucagon activates adenylate cyclase in liver cell membranes and thus turns on glycogenolysis and reduces glycogenesis (b) Insulin increases glycogenesis in the liver by a mechanism that is not yet clear. (c) The glucagon: insulin ratio appears more important than the absolute level of either hormone. Insulin domination provides for the storage of glycogen after a meal whereas glucagon domination favours mobilization of glycogen stores as the blood glucose level declines.

Glycogenolysis (The Breakdown of Glycogen)

The process is initiated by the action of the enzyme glycogen phosphorylase, which is specific for the phosphorylytic breaking (phosphorolysis) of the α-1,4-linkages of glycogen to yield glucose 1-phosphate.

Removal of Branches

The reaction is catalyzed by amylo-1,6-glucosidase (debranching enzyme) which contains both *glucosyl transferase* and *amylo-6-glucosidase activities*. As a glucosyl transferase, it transfers three glucosyl residues from a branch onto a chain terminus, leaving a single residue on C-6. As an amylo-6-glucosidase, it removes the single residue on C-6 to yield a free glucose molecule.

Glycogenolysis is also under hormonal control by adrenaline (epinepherene) and glucagon as mentioned pointwise while discussing glycogenolysis. The contribution about these hormones which can make to the body's glucose needs must depend on the previous dietary history, but it is usual to find that liver glycogen disappears completely after a 24 hour fast. Muscle glycogen does not usually disappear even after a long fast and it can make no direct contribution to blood glucose.

Gluconeogenesis

Gluconeogenesis is the synthesis of glucose from noncarbohydrate precursors including the glycolysis products, lactate, pyruvate, citric acid cycle intermediates, most of the amino acids which are glucogenic (The only amino acids that cannot be converted to oxaloacetate in animals are leucine and lysine because their breakdown yields only acetyl-CoA, which cannot be converted to oxaloacetate) and in ruminants the propionic acid. First, all these substances are converted to oxaloacetate which is the starting material for gluconeogenesis. Similarly, fatty acids cannot serve as glucose precursors in animals because most fatty acids are degraded completely to acetyl-CoA.

For the most part gluconeogenesis is confined to the liver. Under normal circumstances, the liver is responsible for 85–95% of the glucose that is made. The only other tissues capable of gluconeogenesis are the epithelial cells of the small intestine and kidney to some small extents (not more than 5% of total glucose formation).

Glucose occupies a central role in metabolism, both as a fuel and as a precursor of essential structural carbohydrates and other biomolecules. The brain and red blood cells are almost completely dependent on glucose as an energy source. Yet the liver's capacity to store glycogen is

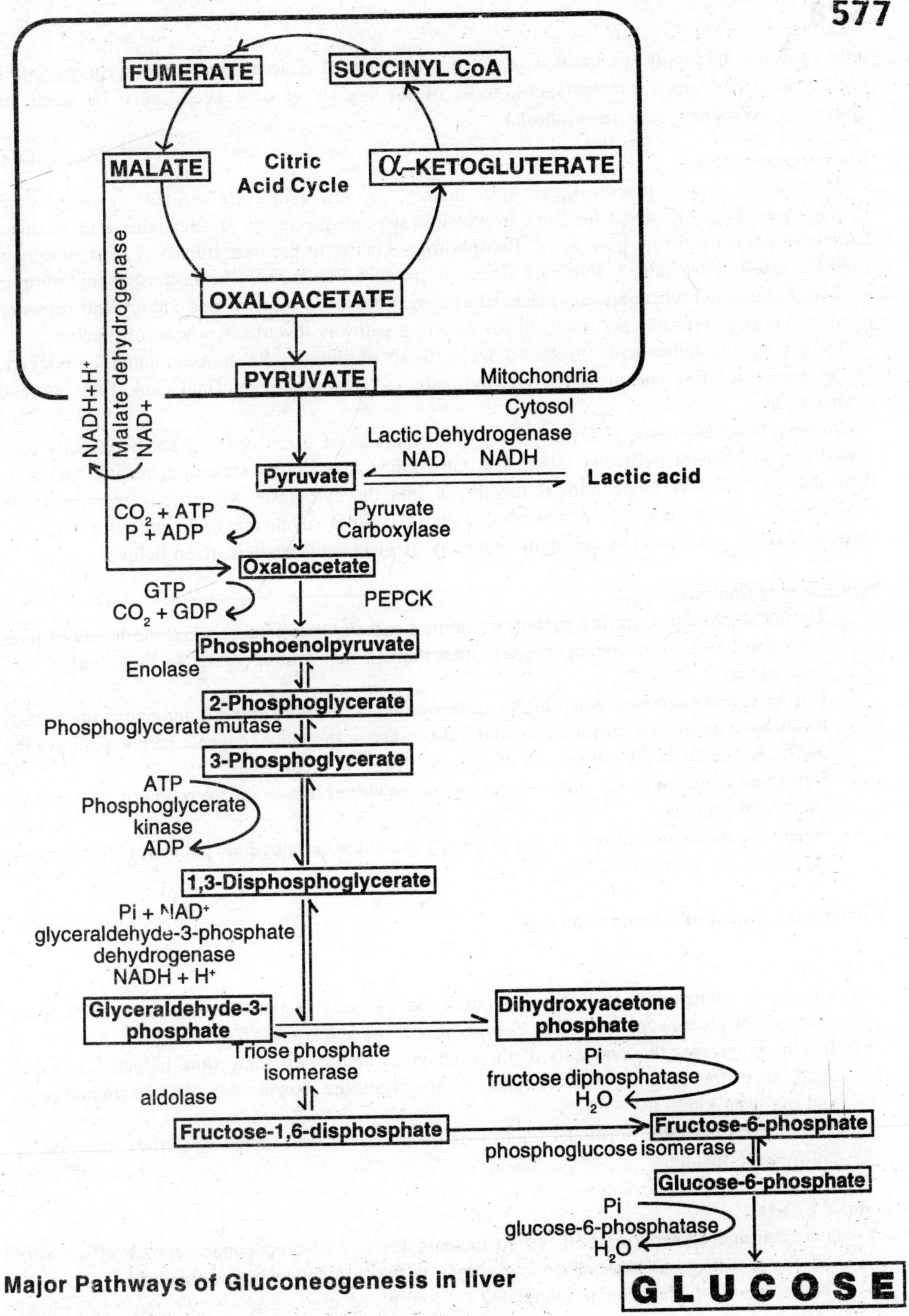

Major Pathways of Gluconeogenesis in liver

Fig. 10.18

only sufficient to supply the brain with glucose for about half a day under fasting or starvation conditions. Under such circumstances, most of the body's glucose needs must be made by gluconeogenesis (new glucose synthesis).

Gluconeogenic Pathway

Most of the steps in gluconeogenesis are mainly the citric acid cycle and the reverse of steps in glycolysis (Page), except for three irreversible steps in glycolysis (1. Hexokinase to produce. Glucose-6 phosphate from glucose; 2. Phosphofructokinase, to produce fructose-1, 6-diphosphate from fructose-6-phosphate; 3. Pyruvate kinase, to produce Pyruvic acid from Phosphoenol pyruvic acids in Glycolysis) where special teams of enzymes produced by liver and kidney and presence of high-energy phosphates get involved for directing pathway towards synthesis of glucose.

The glycogenic amino acids produce a net synthesis of glucose after transamination by converting in one of the five end products, viz. pyruvate, α-ketoglutarate, succinyl CoA, fumerate and oxaloacetate.

During gluconeogenesis, pyruvate in the mitochondrias of every cells cannot be directly converted to phosphoenol pyruvate, rather are transformed into oxaloacetate and malate. Malate is then able to cross the mitochondrial membrane into the cytoplasm where it is reconverted to oxaloacetate. Oxaloacetate is then converted to phosphoenol pyruvate due to the presence of special type of enzymic reaction. The schematic pathway of gluconeogenesis is given below:

Importance of Gluconeogenesis

1. During starvation or during periods of limited carbohydrate intake, when the levels of liver glycogen are low, gluconeogenesis is important in maintaining adequate blood sugar concentrations.
2. During severe exercises, when high *catecholamine* (adrenaline and nor adrenaline hormones) levels have mobilized carbohydrate and lipid reserves, the gluconeogenic pathway allows the use of lactate from glycolysis and of glycerol from fat breakdown.
3. During metabolic acidosis, gluconeogenesis in the kidney allows the excretion of an increased number of protons.
4. Gluconeogenesis also allows the use of dietary protein in carbohydrate pathways after disposal of amino acid nitrogen as urea.

Hormonal Control of Gluconeogenesis

1. *Slow Effects*

a) Glucagon, epinephrine, and glucocorticoids can all cause increased synthesis of the bypass enzymes of gluconeogenesis. The change in enzyme levels takes 24 to 48 hr.
b) Insulin suppresses the synthesis of these enzymes and at the same time induces increased synthesis of the three allosteric enzymes of glycolysis (i.e. hexokinase, phosphofructokinase, and pyruvate kinase).
c) The major short-term hormonal control of the gluconeogenic pathway is thus the ratio of glucagon to insulin.

2. *Rapid Effects*

a) Glucagon and epinephrine both act to increase the rate of gluconeogenesis, an effect over and above that of substrate control; glucagon is the major physiologic regulator.
b) The secretion of glucagon is stimulated by low blood glucose levels, whereas high blood

glucose levels shut down glucagon secretion.

c) A high blood glucose level stimulates insulin secretion, which reduces gluconeogenesis by lowering cAMP levels in the liver. Insulin does not slow down the basal rate of gluconeogenesis, but only the elevated rate due to glucagon action.

d) Glucocorticoids have a rapid effect on the pathway by causing peripheral protein breakdown, which provides additional amino acid substrates for gluconeogenesis.

GLUCOSE METABOLISM IN RUMINANTS

The greatest part of the carbohydrates ingested by ruminants is fermented in the reticulorumen; the volatile fatty acids formed serve in these animals as the main source of energy, unlike monogastric species in which it is the glucose originating from food that fulfils this function. Nevertheless, glucose participates also in ruminants in important metabolic processes. However, the small amount of glucose absorbed from the intestine of ruminants is insufficient and the prevailing amount of glucose used by these animals is produced in their tissues by biosynthesis (gluconeogenesis) mainly in the liver and to a small extent in the kidneys. Of the glucose present inruminants 40–60% originates from propionic acid about 20% from protein (amino acids absorbed from the digestive tract) and the remainder from branched volatile fatty acids, lactic acid and glycerol. Gluconeogenesis is of prime importance in ruminants. The various enzymes needed for gluconeogenesis are abundantly present in the liver, particularly those needed for the conversion of propionic acid to glucose. These enzymatic activities are very low in the livers of suckling animals, which process their food like monogastric animals. The enzymatic activities increase during weaning.

Metabolic Functions of Glucose in Ruminants

Glucose fulfils the following functions in the ruminant body :

(1) Although it is a minor source of energy in the whole ruminant body, glucose is the main source of energy in nervous tissue, particularly in the brain, and also in red blood corpuscles.

(2) Glucose is required for the metabolism of muscles and for the production of glycogen, serving as an energy store in muscles and liver.

(3) The requirement for biosynthetically formed glucose increases during lactation and in late pregnancy. Glucose is the main precursor of lactose and glycerol (as a component of milk fat) and serves as a supply of nutrients for the fetus. Indeed the amounts of glucose required by lactating and late-pregnant ruminants increase considerably beyond that required by non-producing animals. The amounts of glucose utilized by one animal during 24 hours are : ewe, neither lactating, nor pregnant : 100 g; pregnant ewe : 180 g; lactating ewe : 320 g; dry cow : 500 g; and high producing cow : 4–6 kg.

(4) Apart from its function as a precursor of glycerol, glucose is necessary for the formation of NADPH, which in turn is required for the synthesis of long-chain fatty acids by reduction of acetate NADPH originates from glucose oxidation via the pentose-phosphate pathway.

It is important to note that in ruminants the pathway most common in monogastric species for the conversion of glucose into long-chain fatty acids is almost non-existent. Ruminants are adapted to the very economic utilization of glucose, and their tissues lack the enzymes which in monogastric animals allow the conversion of glucose into long-chain fatty acids.

Control of Glucose Metabolism

As mentioned above, glucose provides a relatively small part of the energy requirement of ruminants which under normal conditions is mainly covered by acetate about 70% on the average, and when energy requirements increase long-chain fatty acids are used as an additional energy source. Despite this, ruminants utilize almost as much glucose on a body-weight basis as do other species; this may be concluded from the similar turnover rates.

The rate of gluconeogenesis in ruminants increases after feed ingestion when the supply of propionic acid and other glucose precursors is increased, and this rate decreases after feed estriction. This is in contrast with monogastric species where hepatic glucose production increases markedly during gasting. Glucose entry rate in fasting ruminants is about 60–65% of that in fasting non-ruminants, but that in fed ruminants falls by only 10–20% below the entry rate in fed monogastric species.

Insulin and glucagon are regulators of glucose disposal and production also in ruminants and they control glucose homeostasis, particularly in the blood. The role of both hormones in ruminants is less important than in species absorbing large amounts of glucose. Insulin reduces glucose production from propionic acid and other glucose precursors and enhances its utilization by peripheral tissues. Glucagon counteracts the effects of insulin; it promotes gluconeogenesis from glucose precursors and the release of glucose from liver glycogen. The secretion of insulin and of glucagon responds to circulating metabolites (glucose, volatile fatty acids) and to food intake. The relationship between both hormones seems to be of greater importance in maintaining glucose homeostasis than is the absolute plasma concentration.

In addition to insulin and glucagon, which influence glucose metabolism in inverse directions, growth hormone seems to be involved in the maintenance of glucose homeostasis and acts similarly to glucagon. Whether the effects of growth hormone on glucose availability are direct (promoting gluconeogenesis) or indirect (sparing glucose utilization) has not yet been ascertained.

LIPID METABOLISM

Function of Body Lipids

Animal systems contain a group of substances which are insoluble in water, but soluble in ether, chloroform, benzene are collectively known as lipids. The main groups of lipids of nutritional interest are the fatty acids, glycerides, phospholipids, cerebrosides, cholesterol and other alcohols which include vitamins A, D, E and K. From the stand point of the quantity present in the animal body and its food, the fatty acids are the most important lipid fraction. Some of the important characteristics of lipid are given below:

1. Much of the excess carbohydrate of the diet is converted to fat prior to its utilisation for supply of energy.
2. Some organs prefer fat as a fuel in preference to carbohydrate.
3. The calorific value of fat is about 2.25 times that of carbohydrate and protein i.e., 9.3 kcal per gram.
4. Lipids supply essential fatty acids, linolenic and linoleic acids and are carriers of fat soluble vitamins, A, D, E and K.
5. Phospholipids, cholesterol and glycolipids are essential components of various structural constituents of various organs in the body.

6. Amino acids can be synthesised from fatty acids and ammonia in the liver.
7. Being a poor heat conductor the subcutaneous fat helps in heat regulation.
8. The depot fats act mechanically in protecting the vital organs and also act as cushions and packing tissues.

Fat Transport from Lymph to Tissues

The main site of absorption of lipids by intestinal mucosa is the proximal jejunum. Investigation with electron microscope determined that the surface of the upper intestinal mucosal cell, which originally thought to be tiny pores, actually contains millions of small protoplasmic processes, termed micro-villi (Fig 10.19) These are continuous with the intestinal epithelial cell and greatly increase the absorptive surface of each mucosal cell.

It is now believed that practically all of the triglycerides (with the exception of the very small amount of fatty acids of carbon atom less than 10-12 which are absorbed directly into the portal circulation), and other lipids as well, enter the lymph from these micro-villi of the intestine on their way to the liver and to other tissues. As mentioned earlier along with the discussion on absortion of fat digestion that triglycerides which are synthesised in the mucosa from dietary fatty acids appear in the lymph as *chylomicrons.* These are complex compounds containing triglycerides, phospholipid, cholesterol and its esters, and protein. Protein, free cholesterol and phospholipid (lecithin) form an outer coating for the triglyceride. Chylomicrons are formed in the smooth endoplasmic reticulum of the mucosal cell which are then discharged into the intercellular space and appear in the lacteals, from which they are collected

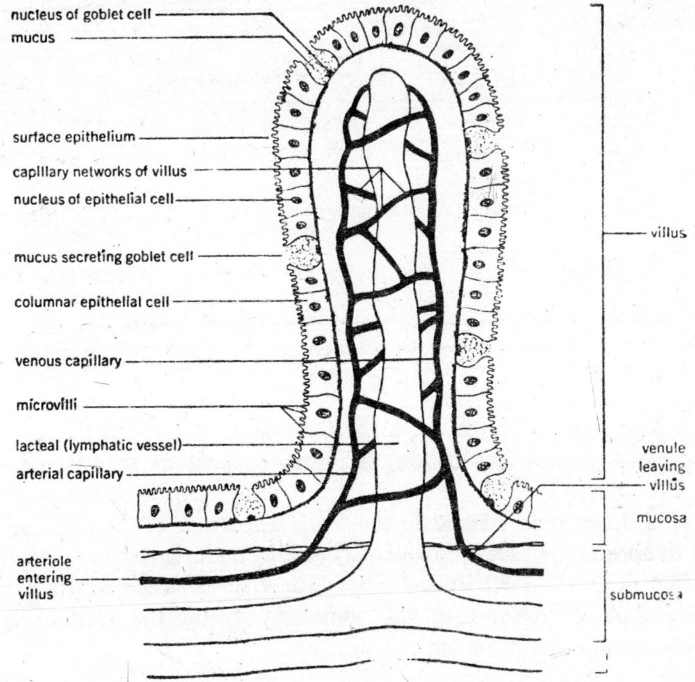

Fig. 10.19 Structure of a villus, present throughout the small intestine. The centre is largely occupied by lacteal (lymphatic vessel) for absorption of fat and fat soluble materials (except fatty acids having less than 10–12 carbon atoms).

into thoracic duct; and finally enter the blood system through the subclavian vein.*

The presence of large amounts of chylomicrons in blood makes the plasma milky (lipemic) in appearance for several hours following the ingestion of a fat-containing meal. Normally this alimentary hyperlipemia is moderate because very soon the rate of entry of chylomicron lipid into the plasma is balanced by its rate of exit—by uptake of the lipid by the tissues of the body.

Although most of the fatty acids in the chylomicron triglycerides are derived from the diet; endogenous fatty acids may be incorporated in significant amounts. In plasma the "triglycerides of chylomicrons" are quickly hydrolysed by the *lipoprotein lipase,* also known as clearing factor.

After the hydrolysis of chylomicrons with a concomitant clearance of blood serum from milky apperance, the lipid components, glyceride, phospholipid, cholesterol for the sake of solubility in water continues with a water soluble protein and forms *lipoproteins* in the liver which are then transported in the plasma. Lipoproteins are thus macromolecules with a central core of triglycerides surrounded by cholesterol and its esters, phospholipid, mainly phosphotidyl choline and sphingomyelin, and a little protein the apoproteins. The phosphate

Table 10.47 Composition of lipoprotein isolated from normal subjects.

LIPOPROTEIN CLASS[a]	DENSITY RANGE (G/ML)	ELECTRO-PHORETIC MOBILITY	COMPOSITION (WEIGHT %)				
					CHOLESTEROL		
			PROTEIN	TRIGLYCERIDE	FREE	ESTER	PHOSPHOLIPID
Chylomicrons	<0.94	Origin	1–2	85–95	1–3	2–4	3–6
VLDL (Beta lipoprotein)	0.94–1.006	Prebeta	6–10	50–65	4–8	16–22	15–20
LDL (Beta lipoprotein)	1.006–1.063	Beta	18–22	4–8	6–8	45–50	18–24
HDL (alpha lipoprotein)	1.063–1.21	Alpha	45–55	2–7	3–5	15–20	26–32

[a]VLDL denotes very-low-density lipoprotein, LDL low-density lipoprotein, and HDL high-density lipoprotein.
From Schaefer and Levy (1985) (ref. 6).

groups of phospholipids are in contact with the aqueous phase and their charge may stabilise the colloid. Lipoproteins then may be looked upon as transporters which carry triglycerides and cholesterol.

The three types of lipoprotein formed in the Golgi apparatus of the liver are designated as very low density lipoprotein (VLDL), low density (LDL) and high density (HDL) on the basis of their separation in ultra centrifuge. They are also classified as pre-β, β and α form in accordance to their mobility relative to the globulins during the electrophoresis of serum. Each has its own structure and chemical composition.

*Chylomicrons do not enter the portal blood directly because they are too large to pass through the endothelial membranes of blood capillaries. Therefore absorbed triglyceride, cholesterol cholesterol ester, and phospholipid enter the body primarily through the lymph system.

FAT STORAGE AND DYNAMIC STATE

In adult animals fat is stored mostly in adipose tissue. Approximately 50 per cent of the adipose tissue is found under the skin, the balance is located around certain organs, notably the kidneys, the membranes surrounding the intestines, in the muscles, etc. Adipose cells have the ability to store fat in a central vacuole surrounded by cytoplasm; other cells store only small amounts of fat as inclusions in their cytoplasm. The cells of the adipose tissue are equipped with a special enzyme system, which can take up fat from the tissue fluid and store it up in the cell and in time of necessity, the same enzyme system will help to mobilise the depot fats. In this connection it is noteworthy that adipose tissue forms 10–12 per cent of body weight, but 70–80 per cent of this is fat, mostly triglycerides. This tissue is known to be one of the most metabolically active body tissue. Fatty acids form the depots are being constantly mobilised and transported. Absorbed fatty acids merge with these form the depots. Some of the acids of this pool are constantly being converted into others. Some are degraded, while others are combined with glycerol and transported back to the depot. All of these reactions are so balanced that mixtures of fatty acids in the depots, blood, and organs tend to remain qualitatively and quantitatively constant.

VOLATILE FATTY ACIDS AND ENERGY METABOLISM IN RUMINANTS

Energy metabolism involves a very large number of metabolites, many of which may be used by the body cells as fuel for respiratory oxidation.

Glucose is usually considered to be the main fuel. This is certainly true in the non-ruminants, and even in the ruminant where other metabolites may substitute : glucose still holds a central position and is vital for certain key functions such as brain metabolism, nourishment of foetus, requirement for lactation.

In non-ruminant only simple carbohydrates such as starch etc. are digested in the alimentary tract for releasing glucose as major end product. This simplifies energy metabolism as glucose is absorbed directly and is deposited in liver and in various tissues of the body as liver and muscle glycogen. The excess amount of course will be stored as depot fat. Under normal circumstances there is little need to synthesise glucose by gluconeogenesis until the animal needs to draw on its energy reserves.

In the ruminants the situation is entirely different. Ruminant species absorb very little glucose from the alimentary tract due to lack of production as end products of carbohydrate digestion. The rumen micro-organisms ferment greater part of dietary carbohydrates including soluble sugars, such as starches, insoluble carbohydrates as cellulose, hemicelluloses into short chain fatty acids (VFA) and they do this by means of microorganisms in the rumen which have powerful enzymes for converting all carbohydrates mostly into acetic, propionic and butyric acids and to some extent isobutyric, valeric, isovaleric with traces of various higher acids. Similarly during lipid digestion, a large portion of glycerol is fermented to propionic acid.

All these acids are absorbed directly through the rumen wall in the free form, apparently without active transport to the liver.

Only one of them, namely propionate, is capable of being converted into glucose, whereas acetate and butyrate serve as substrates for the production of energy (ATP) and acetate in particular may be used with glucose for the synthesis of fat in adipose tissue. *In ruminants glucose cannot be converted to fat as it lacks in necessary* two key enzymes, ATP citrate lyase (splitting citrate into oxaloacetate and malate) and NADP— malate dehydrogenase (converting malate to pyruvate, Thus the ruminant rely entirely on acetate or butyrate for fat synthesis

As mentioned earlier, glucose which is obtained mostly from propionate metabolism in ruminants are vital for the species for (i) lactose synthesis in milk production, (ii) for the supply of energy to the foetus, (iii) for the synthesis of triacylglycerides in adipose tissue, (iv) for the respiration of brain cells. Should a supply of glucose fail then a metabolic disorder known as *Ketosis* will occur.

On the other hand, an excess input of energy which might lead mearly to a transient hyperglycaemia in the non-ruminant can provoke a special condition in ruminant species. Excessive supplies of fermentable carbohydrate such as starch can upset the balance of fermentation in the rumen leading to the accumulation of lactic acid and a metabolic disorder known as *acidosis.*

Thus ketosis and acidosis are the result of imbalances between input and output of energy and are man-made problems imposed upon the ruminants.

Normal Energy Metabolism

Factors Controlling Input of Energy

1. *The Production of VFA*

As already stated, most carbohydrates eaten by ruminants are fermented to a mixture of volatile fatty acids (VFA's) by the rumen microbes. On roughage diets the most important VFA's are acetic, propionic and butyric acids produced in the approximate proportions of 65% acetic, 20% propionic and 15% butyric acids. Because the molecules are of different sizes, on a weight basis the proportions are closer to 50% for acetate, 25% propionate and 25% butyrate. The percentages depend on the nature of the feed. Those quoted above refer to a typical hay diet containing about 35% cellulose and 5% starch. In contrast ration, which contains 5% cellulose and 45% starch, given entirely different proportions of VFA's when fermented in the rumen. The predominant VFA then moves from acetic to propionic acid. Should the diet contain large quantities of starch appreciable quantities of lactic acid will also be produced and absorbed. This acid is normally found in low concentration within the rumen, but if it too is absorbed through the rumen wall it serves as a useful precursor of glucose in the liver. However, as mentioned earlier, excess is potentially toxic and may cause acidosis.

An exception to the general rule that ruminants do not absorb glucose as an end product of digestion needs mention. Some grain diets, specially those on ground maize, may partially escape fermentation within the rumen and pass through into the abomasum and small intestine for enzyme digestion with pancreatic amylase. Glucose, the end product of this digestive process is absorbed and metabolised in much the same way as in non-ruminants.

In spite of this exception the bulk of the digestible energy fed to the ruminant is fermented into VFA's. In fact the VFA contribution approximates 70% of the total energy input.

A. Acetate : This is the predominant VFA produced in the rumen by the fermentation of forage diets. It is absorbed through the rumen wall into the portal circulation, and although a little may be used for oxidation or fat synthesis in the liver most passes through and into the systemic circulation. It is also known that some acetate is synthesised within the liver so that in general circumastances the concentration of acetate in systemic blood is relatively high (about 10 mg/100 ml) compared with non-ruminants.

It is used by a wide variety of tissues as a source of energy. The initial reaction in this case is conversion of acetate to acetyl coenzyme A in the presence of acetyl-coenzyme synthetase.

$$\underset{\text{Acetic acid}}{\begin{array}{c}CH_3\\|\\COOH\end{array}} + \underset{\text{Coenzyme A}}{\begin{array}{c}H\\|\\S-CoA\end{array}} \xrightarrow[+ATP]{\textit{Acetyl-CoA Synthetase}} \underset{\text{Acetyl CoA}}{\begin{array}{c}CH_3\\|\\CO\sim S-CoA\end{array}} + H_2O$$

The acetyl-coenzyme A is then oxidised via the TCA cycle yielding 12 moles of ATP per mole. Since two high energy phosphate bonds are used in the initial Synthetase—mediated reaction the net yield of ATP is 10 moles per mole of acetate.

Acetate does not appear to contribute to the net synthesis of glucose although it serves as a component for fat synthesis both in adipose tissue and also in mammary gland.

B. Propionate :

It is the most important precursor of glucose, contributes as much as 30 – 54% of the total body glucose. The acid after absorption through rumen wall is taken up to liver for the

CH3	ATP AMP	CH3	ATP AMP	CH3	
CH2	+CoA	CH2	Propionyl - CoA cocarboxylose	CH-COOH	
Cooh	+Thiokinase	CO-CoA	+CO	CO-CoA	
Propionic acid		Propionyl-CoA		Methylimalonyl-CoA	

	CH2-COOH	CH2-COOH		CH-COOH	
Isomerization	CH2-CO-CoA	CH2-COOH	H2	CH-COOH	-H2O
Methylmalonyl-CoA mutase	Succinyl-CoA	Succinic acid		Fumaric acid	

CH2-COOH		CH2-COOH		CH	
CHOH-COOH	-H2	CO-COOH	+ATP	C-OPO3H2	GLUCOSE
MALIC ACID		Oxaloacetic acid	Phosphoendpyruvate carboxylase	COCH Phosphoenolpynuvate	

Conversion of propionic acid to glucose (gluconeogenesis)

conversion. A small portion of propionate is changed into lactic acid in the rumen wall, which also later on converted into glucose in the liver.

There exist two pathways for the oxidation of propionic acid : (1) oxidation after conversion to glucose, and (2) direct oxidation of propionic acid.

(1) The mechanism of the conversion of propionic acid to glucose by gluconeogenesis is also utilized when glucose serves other purposes than energy supply by its oxidation, such as in the formation of glycogen or lactose. The enzyme which catalyses the conversion of methylmalonyl-CoA to succinyl-CoA requires coenzyme B_{12}. Vitamin B_{12}, which contains cobalt, is synthesized by rumen microorganisms; since this vitamin is essential for gluconeogenesis, ruminants are particularly affected by cobalt deficiency. The reactions leading from succinie acid to oxaloacetic acid are

identical with the respective intermediate stages of the tricarboxylic acid cycle. The liver of ruminants contains highly active enzymes needed for the conversion of oxaloacetic acid to phosphoenolpyruvic acid and of the latter to glucose. The pathway leading from phosphoenolpyruvic acid to glucose is the reverse of glycolysis. The yield of ATP obtained by the oxidation of propionic acid via glucose is 17 mol of ATP per mol of propionic acid,

C. Butyrate :

Butyrate contributes **relatively** small proportion of total **VFA** and partly metabolised by

Butyrate oxidation is via acetyl CoA as follows :

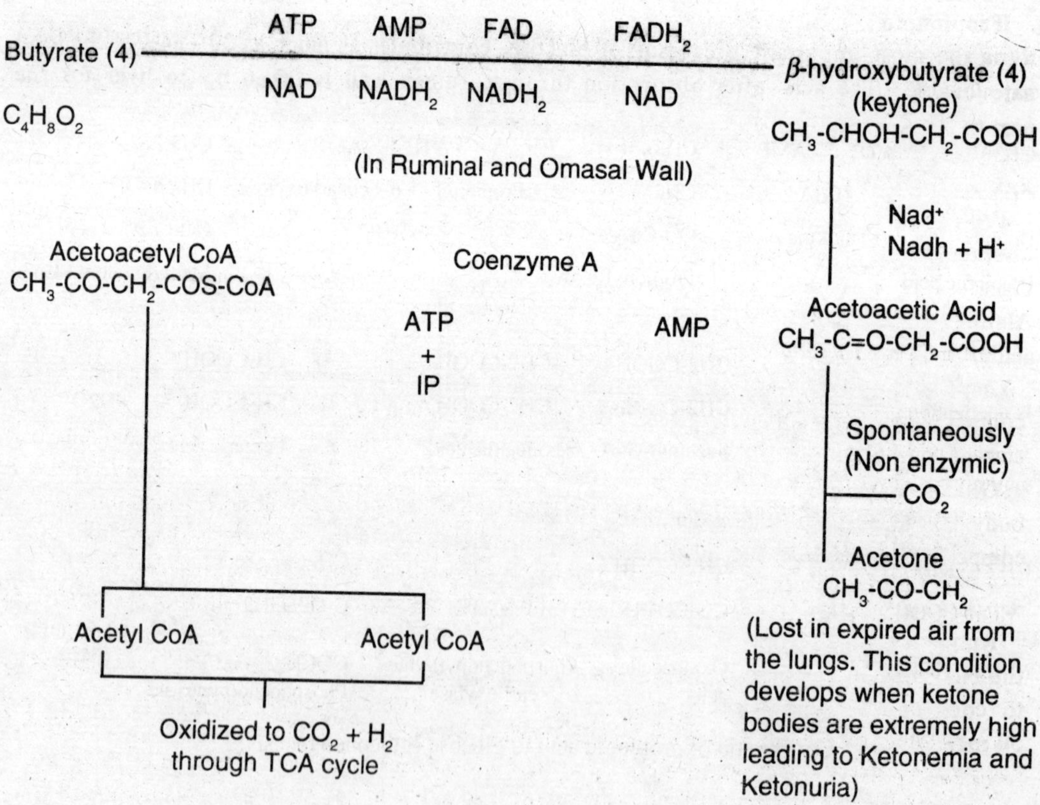

rumen epithelium to ketone bodies principally acetoacetate and (D –) β hydroxybutyrate which is interconverted in the liver.

In normal circumstances ketones are valuable metabolites. Although not used by the liver cells they are utilised almost preferentially by tissues such as cardiac and skeletal muscle as respiratory fuel for energy production. Net gain of ATP per mole of butyric acid is 25 ATP.

Excess ketone bodies are excreted in the urine or may be recycled through the rumen. Acetoacetic acid is relatively unstable and is non-enzymetically decarboxylated to acetone, giving rise to the "*Sweet breath*" of ketotic ruminants. In rumen acetone can be reduced to isopropyl alcohol.

The absorption of all the VFA'S is facilitated by the papillae which consist of elongated projections from the rumen mucosa thus considerably increasing its surface area and absorptive capacity. This may be important as absorption of VFA's is not an active process but passive along a concentration gradient, the rate being proportional to concentration within the rumen. It is also pH dependent being specially rapid under acidic conditions within the rumen fluid. VFA's which have escaped absorption in the rumen may be absorbed in the reticulum, omasum, or even lower down the alimentary tract.

Another minor source of VFA's is the large intestine in ruminants. This receives feed materials and secretions which have escaped digestion and absorption higher up the alimentary tract. It contains microbes very similar to those found in the rumen. In horse, the main site of VFA production is the caecum.

It is clear that the VFA's are vital part of energy metabolism in the ruminant. They provide a source of energy to the rumen bacteria and also to the rumen wall and, although only propionate can be used to synthesise a supply of glucose, taken together they contribute the major part of total energy input of the ruminant.

2. *Gluconeogenesis*

Propionate produces 50% of glucose requirements while glucogenic amino acids contribute another 25%, and lactic acid 15%. The glucogenic amino acids may be derived either from the digestion of microbial protein in the intestines, or from the catabolism of body proteins. Alanine and the glutamine/glutamic acid couplet are said to be the most important amino acids.

Lactic acid on the other hand may arise either from propionate in the rumen wall or by incomplete oxidation of glucose under anaerobic condition in body tissues or from fermentation of excess carbohydrates in the rumen.

Glucose in the blood may also come from the liver glycogenolysis. The last source is from body fat in adipose tissue which during lipolysis results in glycerol and free fatty acids. Both compounds are transported in the blood to the liver where glycerol is converted to glucose.

3. *Ketones*

Ruminants also utilise ketones as one of the energy sources. The normal concentration in the blood is between 5 and 10 mg percent. At times when mobilisation of body fat is required to compensate carbohydrate deficiency for energy, ketone concentration may rise to some 50 mg/100 ml or more thus causes a threat to ketosis.

Factors Controlling Output of Energy

It has already been mentioned that the foetus, and the lactating mammary gland impose obligatory demands for glucose on the adult cow.

Glucose is the major source of energy supplied to the foetus *in utero.* In sheep on advanced stage of pregnancy requirement may range between 8-9 g glucose/kg body weight daily. A single foetus may require 32 g of glucose daily depending on the size. In certain circumstances the total glucose requirement may amount to 70% of the glucose entry rate for the mother cow.

Lactose may impose even large burdens on glucose supply. Fortunately, there is a *"fail safe"* mechanism i.e., as blood glucose falls milk yield tends to fall in parallel. However, mammary gland has no power of gluconeogenesis for lactose synthesis so it must be supplied with preformed glucose. Between 1 and 1.5 kg of lactose may be secreted in milk daily in early lactation. Glucose is also needed for the synthesis of glycerol which is a vital component of the milk fat and also for oxidative purposes in the mammary gland itself, so that in all 70-90% of the animals total glucose entry may be taken up by lactation.

Endocrinological Control of Energy Metabolism

If the animal becomes hyperglycemic then the pancreas is stimulated to secrete insulin. This has several effects. It will tend to reduce blood sugar level by storing glucose in the liver and muscle as liver and muscle glycogen. *Insulin secretion in the ruminant is also stimulated by a rise in VFA concentration.* This is hardly surprising in view of the important part VFA's play in the energy metabolism in ruminants.

If the animal becomes hypoglycaemic, there will be increase in glucagon secretion. Moreover, hypoglycaemia will stimulate glucoreceptors in the hypothalamus to send impulses to the adrenal medulla for increased secretion of epinephrene. The combined effect of these will cause (1) more hepatic glycogenolysis, (2) will mobilise glycerol and FFA's from adipose tissue—the glycerol being used for gluconeogenesis and the FFA's as an alternative fuel for oxidation. In extreme cases it will also stimulate amino acid release from muscle for the production of glucose via gluconeogenesis.

FAT SYNTHESIS

Fat synthesis are continually renewed in order to provide not only of various multicomponent lipids (triacyl-glycerides, phospholipids, etc.), but also to meet the energy requirement of animals. The amount of energy that higher vertebrates can store in the form of carbohydrate is strictly limited and thus most of the surplus energy taken in as carbohydrate when food is plentiful is stored as fat (except in ruminants). Although carbon residues of the amino acids are readily transformed into citrate cycle intermediates, which may in turn be converted into fat, significant amounts are unlikely to be derived from dietary protein in normal circumstances.

Fat synthesis occurs in two stages: (1) fatty acid synthesis, and (2) Biosynthesis of triacylglycerides and incorporation of fatty acids.

Liver, mammary gland, and adipose tissue are the three major sites of biosynthesis of fatty acids and triacylglyceredes. In mouse and rat about half of the synthesis occurs in the liver, but in chicken and pigeon nearly all occurs in the liver; in the pig it is adipose tissue while in cow and sheep both liver and adipose tissue are important, although the latter predominates. In liver and adipose tissue the major product is palmitic acid. In the mammary gland, shorter chain fatty acids are produced.

In ruminants, a major portion of the energy absorbed from the gastrointestinal tract (GI) for lipid synthesis is in the form of VFA (acetic, propionic and butyric acids). Although it has been believed that acetate is the primary substrate for fatty acid synthesis in ruminants, recent work indicates that lactate may also be an important substitute. The relative potency of substrates in inducing lipogenesis in ruminant adipose tissue as has been recently ranked as follows:

Glucose > Propionate > Lactate > Acetate

Fatty Acid Biosynthesis

Acetyl CoA (coenzyme A) stands at a major metabolic crossroads. It can be made from carbohydrate, from virtually all amino acids, and from fatty acids.

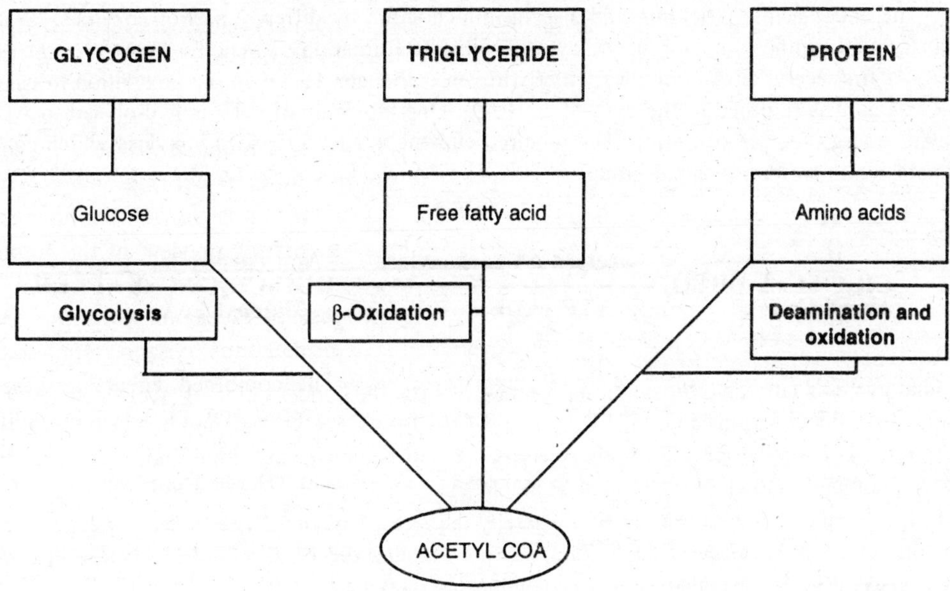

Once synthesized, it can be shunted into the citric acid cycle where its chemical energy can be used to make ATP, or its acetyl group can be made into other compounds that the body needs. Note that whenever acetyl CoA molecules are made within mitochondria but are not needed for the citric acid cycle or for respiratory chain, or for elongation of fatty acids further from palmitic acid (16 carbons long), they are forced to come out of mitochondria into the cytosol (soluble portion of the cytoplasm that excludes the particulate matter) where necessary enzymes are found for the synthesis of fatty acids.

Thus body segregates its sequences of catabolism of fatty acids (beta-oxidation of fatty acids which takes place only inside the mitochondria) from those of anabolism (synthesis of fatty acids take place outside the mitochondria). Further elongation of fatty acids more than 16 carbon are made either in the endoplasmic reticulum or inside the mitochondria.

Biosynthesis of fatty acids exhibits a number of specific features:

1. Fatty acid biosynthesis, as distinct from oxidation, is localised in the soluble portion of the endoplasmic reticulum.

2. The source for the synthesis is acetyl-CoA.
3. NADPH (manufactured by the pentose phosphate pathway of glucose catabolism) is used to reduce fatty acid biosynthesis intermediates and not NADH.
4. The involvement of one unique enzyme complex *Fatty acid synthetase,* having multifuntional *six enzymes* (1. Acetyl-CoA-ACP transcyclase, 2. Malonyl-CoA-ACP transacyclase, 3. Beta-ketoacyl-ACP synthase, 4. Beta-ketoacyl-ACP reductase, 5. Beta-hydroxyacyl-ACP dehydrase and 6. Enoyl-ACP reductase) joined together by another protein, known as *Acyl carrier protein* (ACP). The ACP, which is not an enzyme but situated in the centre of this enzyme complex (fatty acid synthetase) and like the boom of a construction crane, it brings one intermediate compound of fatty acid synthesis to one enzyme and then to another and at each stop a chemical reaction is catalyzed which all contributes to chain lengthening from 2-carbon compound of Acetyl CoA upto 16 carbon length of palmitic acid.
5. Further lengthening of fatty acids takes place through the addition of two-carbon units inside the endoplasmic reticulum and also in mitochondria by different sets of enzymes.

Fatty acid synthesis begins in the cytosol with the formation of malonyl CoA from the acetyl CoA. At first acetyl CoA combines with hydrogen carbonate, HCO_3 for carboxylation in catalytic amounts as it is returned to the cytosol as HCO_3. One molecule of ATP is hydrolysed to ADP to provide energy for carboxylation. The required enzyme is acetyl CoA carboxylase which contains vitamin biotin as its prosthetic group.

$$\underset{\text{Acetyl CoA}}{CH_3\overset{\overset{O}{\|}}{C}\text{-SCoA}} + HCO_3^- \xrightarrow[\text{ATP} \quad \text{ADP}]{\text{acetyl CoA carboxylase}} \underset{\text{Malonyl CoA}}{\overset{\text{New carboxylate group}}{^-OOC\text{-}CH_2C\text{-}SCoA}} + Pi + H^+$$

First cycle of fatty acid biosynthesis commence from the condensation of Acetoacetyl ACP and Malonyl ACP and for this as in STEP 1, Acetyl-CoA forms Acetyl-ACP and in STEP 2b Malonyl-CoA forms Malonyl-ACP (i.e. both Acetyl-CoA and Malonyl-CoA joins individually with the enzyme complex known as Fatty acid Synthetase).

STEP 3 is the condensation reaction whereby the Acetyl-malonyl-ACP is decarboxylated resulting formation of Acetoacetyl ACP. The reaction is catalyzed by the third synthetase enzyme-β-ketoacyl-ACP synthetase also known as condensing enzyme.

STEPS 4–6 are the dehydration and reduction which ultimately results in formation of Butyril-ACP. It will recycle six times following steps 4–6 for forming palmitoyl-ACP. For the sake of removing ACP for the last intermediate compound (acyl carrier protein), another enzyme from cytosol, palmitoyl thioesterase, is necessary and thereby Palmitate production is completed.

The overall reaction that occurs in the synthesis of palmitate is 8 Acetyl-CoA + 7 ATP + 14 NADPH + $14H^+$ + H_2O ⟶ 1 Palmitate + 7 ADP +$7P_i$ + 8CoASH + 14 $NADP^+$.

Elongation of Fatty Acids

Fatty acids longer than 16 carbons can be formed through the addition of two-carbon units by elongation systems. There are two elongation systems.

1. The most active system is found in the endoplasmic reticulum. It adds malonyl-CoA onto palmitate in a manner similar to the action of fatty acid synthetase, except that CoASH is involved rather than the ACP. Stearic acid (18 carbons) is a common product of this elongation system.

2. A mitochondrial elongation system uses acetyl CoA units, rather than malonyl CoA units, to elongate fatty acids for the synthesis of structural lipids in this organelle.

Desaturation of Fatty Acids

The two most common mono-unsaturated fatty acids in mammals are palmitoleic acid and oleic acid. The double bonds are introduced between carbons 9 and 10 by fatty acid oxygenase in the endoplasmic reticulum.

Synthesis of Triacylglycerides

The biosynthesis of triacylglycerides does not involve direct reaction of free glycerol with free fatty acids rather triacylglycerides are synthesized from fatty acyl-CoA esters and glycerol-3-phosphate. The initial step in this process is catalyzed by glycorol-3-phosphate dehydrogenase for converting dihydroxy acetone phosphate into glycerol-3-phosphate. Two moles of "activated" fatty acids (in the form of fatty acyl CoA) are introduced once with glycerol-3-phosphate and then with Lysophosphatidic acid.

OXIDATION OF FATTY ACIDS

Knoop (1905) proposed that fatty acids were oxidised physiologically by β-oxidation. The catabolism of fatty acids to CO_2 and H_2O occurs by means of the sequential combination of the multienzyme systems, the β-oxidation cycle and the TCA cycle. The β-oxidation cycle first converts the fatty acid into 2-carbon units, acetyl CoA. The TCA cycle then converts the acetyl moiety of acetyl CoA to CO_2 and H_2O. The steps in the oxidation of fatty acids are given below correspond to the numbers in the sketch.

1. Activation of the fatty acid by formation of a corresponding fatty acid-CoA ester. ATP is required as the source of energy. The products are fatty acid-CoA ester, AMP, and inorganic pyrophosphate (PPi).
2. Dehydrogenation of the fatty acid-CoA ester to form the α-β-unsaturated acyl CoA. The enzymes involved in this reaction contain FAD and Cu or Fe.
3. Hydration of the α-β-unsaturated acyl CoA to form β-hydroxyacyl CoA.
4. Dehydrogenation of the β-hydroxy-acyl CoA to form β-keto acyl CoA. NAD is the hydrogen acceptor.
5. Thiolytic cleavage of the β-keto-acyl CoA to yield acetyl CoA and a fatty acyl CoA having 2 fewer carbon atoms.

This cycle, then, is repeated as indicated by the side line representing subsequent removal of C_2 fragments as acetyl CoA and will pass through TCA cycle for energy liberation.

Calculation of Energy Yield from Palmitic Acid

Then palmitic acid is degraded enzymetically, one energy rich ATP is required for the primary activation and 8 acetyl S CoA is ultimately formed. Each time the helical cycle is traversed, 1 mole of $FAD\,H_2$ and 1 mole of DPNH are formed: which may be reoxidised by the electron transport chain. Since the chemical formula of palmitic acid is $C_{16}H_{32}O_2$ and in the final turn of the helix, 2 moles of acetyl CoA are produced, the helical scheme must be

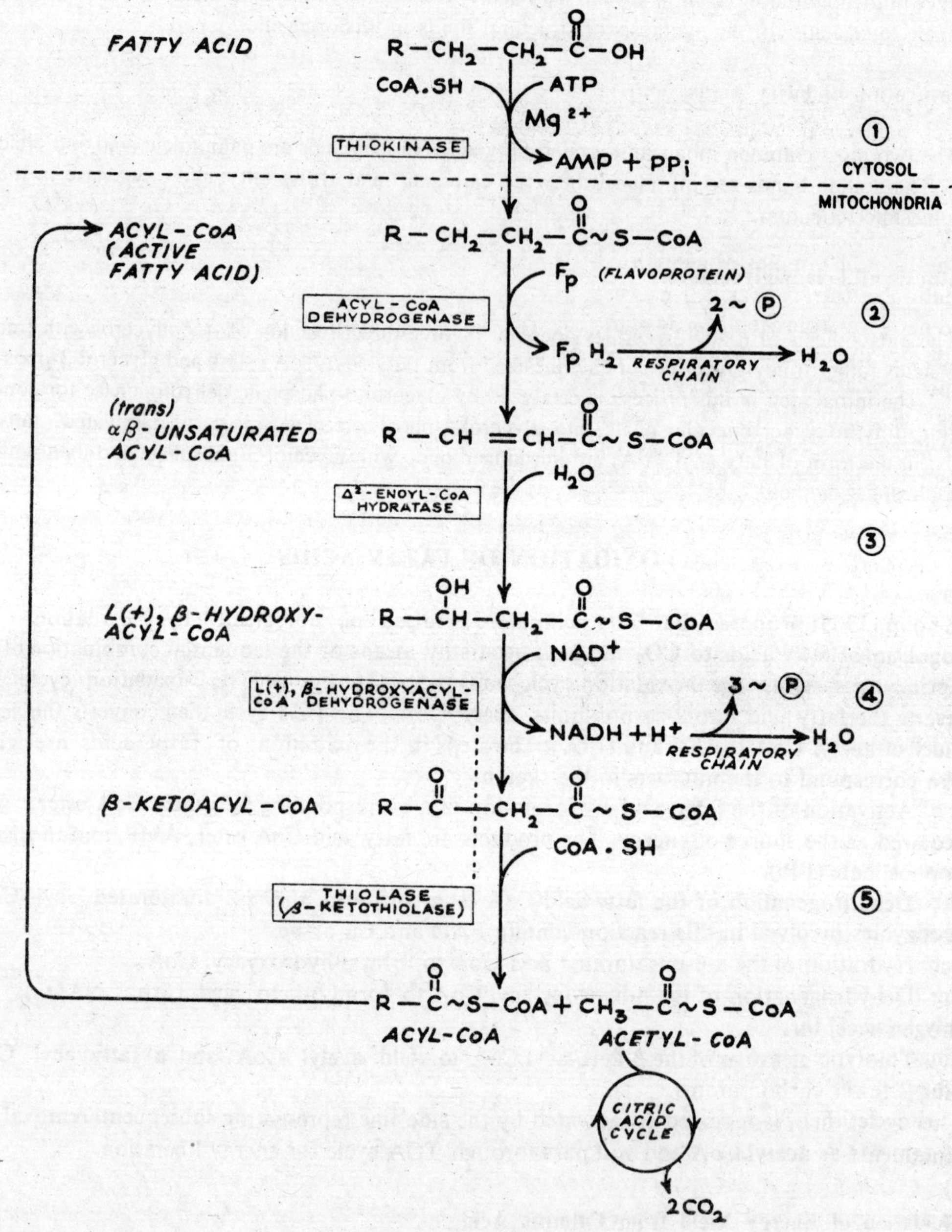

β-Oxidation of fatty acids.

traversed only *seven* times to degrade palmitic acid completely. In this process, in total there will be a production of 7 moles of reduced flavin and 7 moles of reduced pyridine nucleotide are formed. The sequence can be divided into two steps:

Step 1

7 moles of flavin system	=	+ 14 ATP
7 moles of DPN$^+$ system	=	+ 21 ATP
		35
1 mole ATP for primary activation	=	− 1 ATP
Total gain	=	34 ATP

Step 2

The total of 8 moles of acetyl CoA formed will each further give rise to at least 12 ATP on oxidation in the citric acid, i.e., there will be $8 \times 12 = 96$ energy rich bonds.

So net gain from Step 1 = 34 and from Step 2 = 96 in total $(34 + 96) = 130$ energy rich bonds or $130 \times 7.6 = 988$ kcal. As the caloric value of palmitic acid is 2340 kcal per mole, the process captures as high energy phosphate at least 41% ($988/2340 \times 100$) of the total energy of combustion. The remaining energy is lost probably as heat. It hence becomes clear why a food fat is an effective source of available energy. In this calculation we neglect the combustion value of glycerol, the other component of a triglyceride.

PROTEIN METABOLISM

Avenues through which Nitrogen is Excreted

1. FAECAL NITROGEN. The faecal nitrogen includes the undigested or unabsorbed feed nitrogen along with nitrogen from endogenous sources, called *metabolic faecal nitrogen* and comprises substances originating in the body, such as residues of the bile and other digestive juices, epithelial cells abraded from the alimentary tract by the feed materials passing through it and bacterial residues. Strictly speaking, the nitrogen in bacterial residues must be considered to have come, at least in part from the feed. The fact that the division of faecal nitrogen is made is due to the fact that the two components have their separate origins. When one is really interested to find out the amount of two fractions separately, it is customary to deduct the amount of metabolic faecal nitrogen from the total faecal nitrogen. The amount of metabolic faecal nitrogen in faeces is directly proportional to the dry matter consumption and the body size of the animal. Upon feeding a nitrogen free diet, it has been observed that animal excretes nitrogenous compounds through faeces. This amount is the metabolic faecal nitrogen. Using this procedure the amount of metabolic faecal nitrogen has beed found to be approximately 1 gram for rats, pigs and man per kg. of feed dry matter consumed, and 5 gram for ruminants. The latter figure is smaller with rations low in roughage, but greater where roughage alone is fed.

2. URINARY NITROGEN: Through urine a number of nitrogenous compounds are excreted originating from a variety of sources. These are discussed below:

(*i*) *Creatinine:* It is derived from the breakdown of creatine phosphate present in muscle brain and blood. Creatinine is the anhydride of creatine. It is formed largely in muscle by the irreversible and nonenzymatic removal of water from creatine phosphate.

Excretion of creatinine is a constant physiological phenomenon. It is related to the muscle bulk and is higher in animals having more body weight. Amount of excretion is in no way related with the dietary intake.

(*ii*) *Urea* $CO(NH_2)_2$*:* More than 80 per cent of urinary nitrogen is excreted in the form of urea. The compound is derived mainly (*a*) from deamination of unused amino acids; (*b*) by conver-

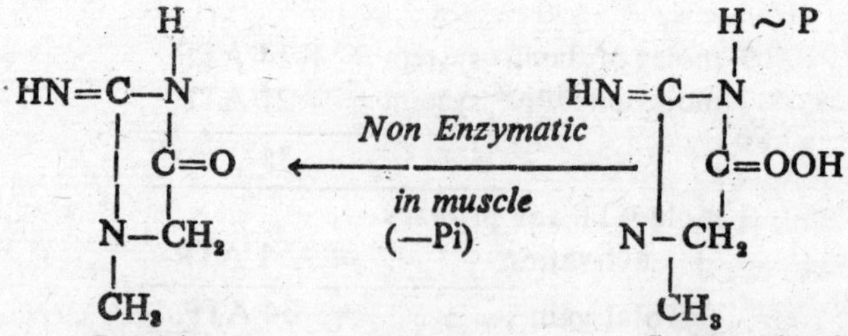

```
        H                                      H ~ P
        |                                      |
HN=C—N                                HN=C—N
   |   |          Non Enzymatic           |    |
   |  C=O   ←———————————————————————   |   C=OOH
   |   |            in muscle             |    |
  N—CH₂              (—Pi)              N—CH₂
   |                                       |
  CH₃                                     CH₃
```

Creatinine   *Creatine Phosphate*

sion of absorbed ammonia from rumen fermentation; (*c*) from salts like ammonium carbonate, lactate, etc., (*d*) from the amino acid arginine—it breaks down into urea and ornithine, (*e*) from catabolism of pyrimidine bases. The end product of metabolism of these compounds in liver is urea. Urea formation helps to maintain the reaction of blood constant as in it one acid (carbonic acid) and two molecules of ammonia remain neutralised.

(*iii*) *Ammonia:* With a mixed diet in an adult animal, a small amount of ammonia is always excreted through urine as free ammonia. The compound is mainly formed (1) from deamination of amino acids, both exogenous and endogenous. Although deamination takes place chiefly in the liver, recent observations indicate that some free ammonia is also formed in the kidney largely from glutamine, which serves as a method of transfer of NH_2^- groups in a non-toxic form between tissues, (2) Ammonia is also formed in large quantities in rumen, part of which is directly diffused through the ruminal wall into the circulatory system.

(*iv*) *Uric acid and Allantoin:* The amount in urine depends partly on the purine content of the diet and rest on the rate of the turnover of purines in cellular nucleic acids. Uric acid is the catabolite of purines. Allantoin is the hydroliylic end product of uric acid which is highly water enzyme, *uricase* for conversion of uric acid to Allantoin. So they excrete uric acid.

(*v*) *Amino acids:* Under normal conditions small amounts of amino acids are always excreted through urine.

(*vi*) *Other avenues of N loss:* Gaseous NH_3 losses from the alimentary tract can occur. Excretion and secretion from the skin contain urea and other N compounds. Protein is also lost through growth and removal of wool, feathers, horn, hair. During milk production a good amount of nitrogenous compounds are excreted and similarly faetal growth requires a good deposition of protein.

Endogenous Urinary Nitrogen (EUN)

From the discussions made so far under 'Urinary nitrogen', it may be observed that the total urinary nitrogen has got two sources: (*i*) the "inescapable" losses in tissues turnover of nitrogenous constituents: and (*ii*) the other highly variable contribution depending on effects of dietary protein level. Thus when the absorbed dietary protein is in excess of the requirement, it will exert pressure on kidney for a way out in the forms already discussed. Endogenous urinary nitrogen (EUN) comprises the first category. On protein free diets the animal will continue to excrete EUN and the amount of nitrogen in the urine may fall progressively for several days before stabilising at a lower level. This minimum nitrogen excretion is referred to as the *endogenous urinary nitrogen value* (EUN). At the time of conduction of experiments for obtaining EUN value, all care must be taken to feed the animals with diet balanced in all respects particularly the energy content because at lower level of energy, extra tissue will be broken down to meet the energy deficiency. Another important point that should be kept in mind that experimental animals will hardly continue to consume normal quantum of feed for a along time required for the experiment without any nitrogen (protein) in their ration. Thus it is very difficult to find out the EUN value although theoretically the procedure seems to be very simple. However, when the values are determined, the amount denotes the minimum amount of protein that should be put back (fed) to the system for filling up the daily loss of nitrogenous material. This is the amount that we say as the basal metabolism and in fact there is a relationship between the two conceptions (EUN and basal metabolism), viz., 2 mg endogenous urinary nitrogen per kcal basal metabolic rate (BMR) for non-ruminants. The value is about 2.0 mg of nitrogen per kcal of BMR in ruminants. Brody and coworkers confirmed about a relationship between endogenous urinary nitrogen with that of body weight of the animal and accordingly a formula is also suggested by them which is as follows:

$$\text{EUN mg per day} = 146\ W_{kg}^{0.72}$$

Total nitrogen excreted through urine in excess of the endogenous portion is known as *exogenous urinary nitrogen.* This term implies that portion of nitrogen which is comming from dietary source alone and not from the body itself that might be resulting due to catabolism incident to the maintenance of the vital processes as already discussed.

Interpretation of Nitrogen Balance Trial

If all nitrogen losses are accounted for, and are debited against the nitrogen intake, the balance represents the amount of nitrogen retained by the animal. Whenever the nitrogen intake exceeds excretion, a *positive nitrogen balance* exists. Some of the conditions that cause this include (1) growth, (2) recovery from fasting, starving or extended illness and (3) pregnancy mostly related to foetus growth. *Negative nitrogen balance* is that condition in which the excretion of nitrogen exceeds the intake. An individual with a negative nitrogen balance is losing nitrogen from tissues more rapidly than it is being replaced—an undesirable state of affairs. Conditions that result include (1) fasting, (2) starvation, (3) high fever, (4) prolonged illness, (5) low protein diets, (6) diets optimum in protein per cent but the protein is of extremely poor quality or protein lacking in essential amino acids (affects all monogastric), (7) the caloric content of the diet if inadequate, the tissues will be broken down to supply energy, (8) injury, immobilisation etc., cause excessive breakdown of tissues. In all such conditions the liver is the major gland which is affected the most. As much as 50 per cent of its total nitrogen, and skeletal muscle may also lose considerable nitrogen. Some enzymes may decrease in activity while others may increase. In extreme protein restriction, certain peptide hormones may not be synthesised in adequate quantities and endocrine disorder may appear.

In case of animals where growth has ceased and no more protein is stored either in the form of growth, milk or foetus development, and the intake and output of nitrogen are the same, in that case the animal is in a state of *nitrogen equilibrium.* Established nitrogen equilibrium in any subject shows the following facts:

(1) That the animal is no more growing and therefore not storing any protein,
(2) That the protein in the diet is sufficient in quality and quantity,
(3) That the diet is adequate in energy,
(4) That the animal is not suffering from any wasting disease.

Body Protein Reserves

So far protein is concerned, although the body does not store in the sense that it stores carbohydrate, fat or fat soluble vitamins but certain "reserves" are available from practically all body tissues for the purpose of meeting emergent situations. It has been said earlier that when an animal is first placed on a nitrogen-free diet, the quantity of nitrogen in its urine may fall progressively for several days before stablising at a lower level, and when nitrogen is re-introduced into the diet there is a similar lag in the re-establishment of the previous status. This suggests that the animal possesses a protein reserve which can be drawn upon in times of emergency and restored in times of excess. In times of emergency, among all the tissues, liver is very much affected. Based upon the studies made so far with laboratory experimental animals, about one fourth of the body protein especially the liver followed by kidney, heart and skeletal muscles are depleted and repleted. Thus, due to this property, the vital functions may be protected upto 30-50 days of total starvation. It should be apparent that the use of these reserves eventually requires restoration of tissues of their normal protein composition.

Not only growing and producing animals, but also adult, non-producing animals can show a positive nitrogen balance when they obtain amounts of protein exceeding requirements. Moderate amounts of excess protein can be taken up by animals independently of their function and age, while amounts exceeding a certain limit are oxidized and excreted. Small protein surpluses are deposited as protein reserves in various organs such as liver, muscles, etc. Protein reserves form up to 5–7% of the total body protein; they are labile, drawn upon in periods of starvation or reduced protein intake, and restored in times of plenty, thereby contributing to the free amino acid pools of the body during depleting processes. However, less metabolic importance should be attributed to the existence of protein reserves than to energy reserves which are stored in larger amounts and in specific organs.

The Disposal of Excess Body Amino Acids

Sources of Free Amino Acids

(1) As discussed earlier, body proteins are continually being broken down and reconstituted in the cells. The use of isotopically labelled compounds have made it abundantly clear about high rates of protein turnover in plasma protein, intestinal mucosa, pancreas, liver and kidney white muscle, brain, skin and connective tissue have low rates of turnover. On an average the half life of 'whole body' protein is 17-20 days.

(2) In the small intestine of all ruminants and non-ruminants the nitrogenous digestion products enter the blood stream mostly as amino acids along with small amounts of ammonia and simpler peptides.

Amino acid arising from cellular protein mix freely with those entering from outside the cells as absorbed through small intestines and this constitutes the *amino acid pool.* Eventually the amino acids are disposed of in one of the following ways:

Disposal

1. A portion is utilised for the resynthesis of tissue proteins and other nitrogen containing tissue constituents. Such a synthesis includes the formation of the protein and other nitrogenous compounds of milk, replacement of tissues and nitrogenous compounds used up in the

normal 'wear and tear' of body processes. Synthesis of essential body proteinous compounds always take a priority over deaminisation.

2. Some fraction of the pool of amino acids enters into other pathways either involving movement out of the cell or catabolism in the cell itself. Oxidative deamination and transamination methods result in a loss of amino acids to the system. Oxidative deamination in details will be explained along with discussions of protein digestion in ruminants, the other method of sorting out of amino group from amino acids is transamination, is discussed below.

Transamination *is an interconversion of keto and amino compounds.* The keto acid corresponding to the amino acid is produced, and one of the three α-keto acids, is converted to its analogous α-amino acid.

$$\alpha\text{-amino acid} + \text{pyruvic acid} \xrightarrow[\text{transaminase}]{\text{alanine}} \alpha\text{-keto acid} + \text{alanine}$$

$$\alpha\text{-amino acid} + \alpha\text{-ketoglutaric acid} \xrightarrow[\text{transaminase}]{\text{glutamate}} \alpha\text{-keto acid} + \text{glutamic acid}$$

$$\alpha\text{-amino acid} + \text{oxaloacetic acid} \xrightarrow[\text{transaminase}]{\text{aspartate}} \alpha\text{-keto acid} + \text{aspartic acid}$$

These three amino acids are further collected in the form of only one amino acid, glutamic acid.

$$\text{alanine} + \alpha\text{-ketoglutaric acid} \xrightarrow[\text{transaminase}]{\text{glutamic-pyruvic}} \text{pyruvic acid} + \text{glutamic acid}$$

$$\text{aspartic acid} + \alpha\text{-ketoglutaric acid} \xrightarrow[\text{transaminase}]{\text{glutamic-oxaloacetic}} \text{oxaloacetic acid} + \text{glutamic acid}$$

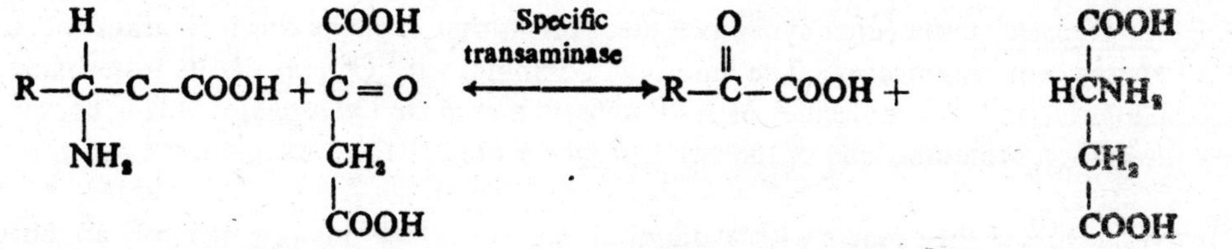

$$\underset{\text{L-Amino acid}}{R{-}CH(NH_2){-}C{-}COOH} + \underset{\text{Oxaloacetic acid}}{HOOC{-}C(=O){-}CH_2{-}COOH} \xrightleftharpoons{\text{Specific transaminase}} \underset{\text{Keto acid corresponding to original amino acid}}{R{-}C(=O){-}COOH} + \underset{\text{Apartic acid}}{HOOC{-}CH(NH_2){-}CH_2{-}COOH}$$

$$\underset{\text{Alanine}}{H_2N{-}CH(CH_3){-}COOH} + \underset{\alpha\text{-Ketoglutaric acid}}{HOOC{-}C(=O){-}CH_2{-}CH_2{-}COOH} \xrightleftharpoons{\text{Specific transaminase}} \underset{\text{Pyruvic acid}}{HOOC{-}C(=O){-}CH_3} + \underset{\text{Glutamic acid}}{HOOC{-}CH(NH_2){-}CH_2{-}CH_2{-}COOH}$$

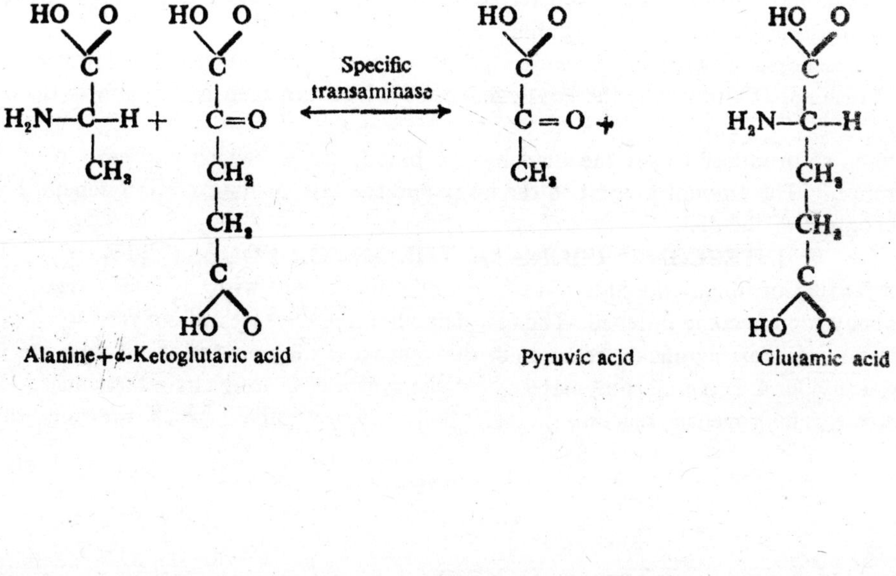

Alanine+α-Ketoglutaric acid   Pyruvic acid   Glutamic acid

The reverse of the collection reactions can also occur. Glutamic acid acts as a "universal" donor of an amino group to keto acids (Page 597). The enzyme glutamic-pyruvic transaminase (GPT) is released from the liver into the blood in cases of severe liver damage.

The enzyme glutamic-oxaloacetic transaminase (GOT) is abundant in heart muscle. In myocardial infarction, the damaged heart muscle releases its transaminase into the blood.

Oxidative deamination *is the conversion of an amino acid into a keto acid with the release of an ammonium ion.*

$$\text{glutamic acid} + NAD^+ + H_2O \xrightarrow[\textit{Glutamate dehydrogenase}]{} \alpha\text{-ketoglutaric acid} + NADH + NH_4^+$$

Method of Excretion of Circulatory NH_3 (Urea Cycle)

In ruminants, urea is one of the main microbial fermentation products of proteinous feed formed inside rumen, the large quantum of which are utilised by the microbes for the synthesis of their body protein and a good amount enters in the circulation by diffusion through ruminal wall. Apart from this urea, the liver of all mammals synthesise urea out of the excess ammonia formed by deamination of amino acids on the liver, which if allowed to accumulate in the system by virtue of their toxic property could be fatal for the species concerned. However, a very small amount of ammonia is otherwise utilised for the formation of some non-essential amino acids, purines, pyramidines, creatine and to other non-protein nitrogenous substances. The major portion thus remains unutilised and that is why all mammals have evolved biochemical reactions to remove excess ammonia rapidly in the form of urea—a comparatively non-toxic substance finally excreted out through urine.

Technique

The Krebs-Henseleit cycle (urea cycle) is a mechanism that explains the formation of urea. This is an energy requiring process. The ammonia combines with CO_2 (available from oxidation in the Kreb's cycle) and two molecules of ATP to form a *carbamyl phosphate*. (The compound provides the carbon atom and one of the two nitrogen atoms of the urea molecule at the final stage).

Carbamyl phosphate then reacts with a diamino acid *ornithine* in presence of an enzyme *ornithine transcarbamylase* resulting in the production of an amino acid *citrulline*, the other product being inorganic orthophosphate (Fig.10.19)

A second amino group is then transferred from aspartic acid to carbamyl keto group of citrulline, to form the amino acid arginine.

In the presence of an enzyme, *arginase*, and magnesium, arginine yields one molecule of urea and of ornithine. Ornithine is thereby regenerated which can then participate in the next turn of the cycle.

The urea so produced leaves the liver by the blood stream, which carries it to the kidney for excretion. The amount present in the body and the rate of its excretion depend largely on protein content of the diet.

INTERCONVERSIONS OF THE MAJOR FOODSTUFFS

Upon feeding of liberal amounts of carbohydrate diet along with sufficient rest, domestic animals may soon become fattened. The fact demonstrates the eases of conversion of carbohydrate into fat. A most significant reaction in this respect is the conversion of pyruvate to acetyl CoA, as acetyl CoA is the starting material for the synthesis of long chain fatty acid. However, the pyruvate dehydrogenase reaction is essentially nonreversible, which prevents the direct

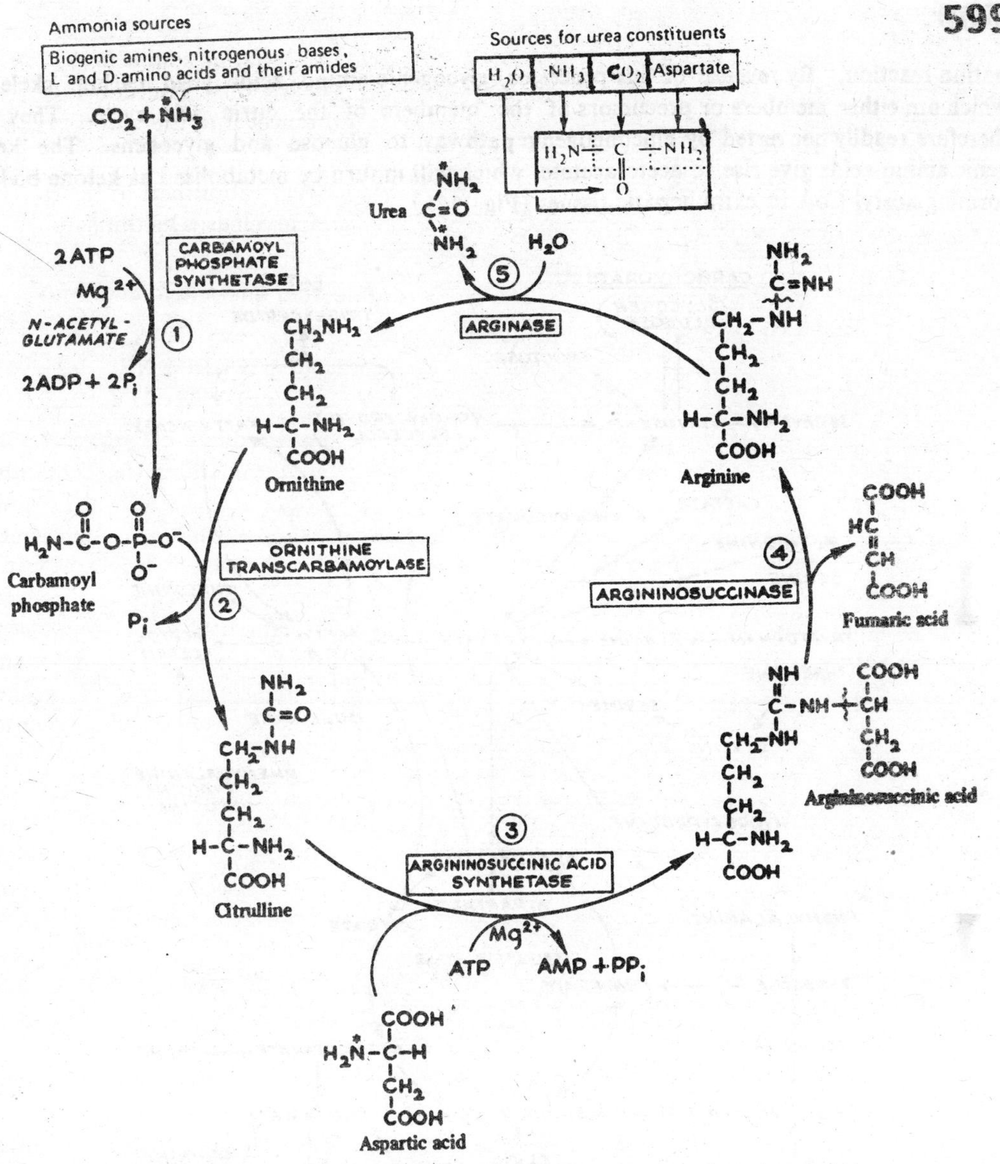

Ammonia sources

Biogenic amines, nitrogenous bases, L and D-amino acids and their amides

$CO_2 + \overset{*}{N}H_3$

Sources for urea constituents

H_2O | NH_3 | CO_2 | Aspartate

Urea

2ATP, Mg^{2+}, N-ACETYL-GLUTAMATE, CARBAMOYL PHOSPHATE SYNTHETASE (1), 2ADP + $2P_i$

Ornithine

Carbamoyl phosphate

ORNITHINE TRANSCARBAMOYLASE (2), P_i

Citrulline

ARGININOSUCCINIC ACID SYNTHETASE (3), ATP, Mg^{2+}, AMP + PP_i

Aspartic acid

Argininosuccinic acid

ARGININOSUCCINASE (4), Fumaric acid

Arginine

ARGINASE (5), H_2O

Fig. 10.20 Urea cycle.

conversion of acetyl CoA, (formed from the oxidation of fatty acid) to pyruvates. As a result there is no net conversion of long chain fatty acids to carbohydrates. Only the terminal 3-carbon of a fatty acid having an odd number of carbon atoms is glycogenic, as this portion of the molecule will form propionate upon oxidation. Nevertheless, it is possible for levelled carbon atoms of all fatty acids to be found ultimately in glycogen after reversing the citric acid cycle; this is because oxaloacetate is an intermediate both in the citric acid cycle; and in the pathway of gluconeogenesis.

Many of the carbon skeleton of the non-essential amino acids can be produced from carbohydrate via the citric acid cycle. In it the amino group is added with the help of transamination reaction. By reversal of this processes, glycogenic amino acids yield carbon skeleton which are either members or precursors of the members of the citric acid cycle. They are therefore readily converted by gluconeogenic pathway to glucose and glycogens. The ketogenic amino acids give rise to aceto acetate, which will in turn be metabolised as ketone bodies, forming acetyl CoA in extra hepatic tissues (Fig. 10.21)

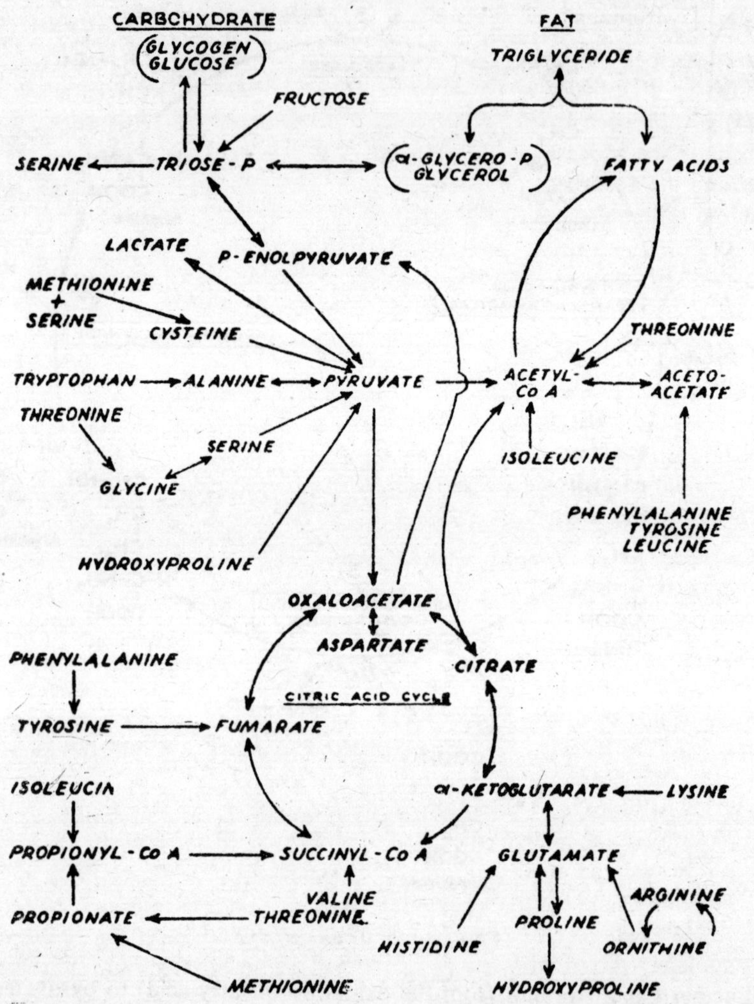

Fig. 10.21. Possible interconversion of fat, carbohydrate and amino acids.

For the same reasons that it is not possible for a net conversion of fatty acids to carbohydrate to occur, it is also not possible for a net conversion of fatty acids to glucogenic amino acids to take place. Neither it is possible to reverse the pathways of breakdown of ketogenic amino acids, all of which fall into the category of "*essential amino acids*".

Conversion of the carbon skeleton of glucogenic amino acids to fatty acids is possible by formation of pyruvate and acetyl CoA. However, under most natural conditions, e.g., starvation, a net break down of protein and amino acids is usually accompanied by a net breakdown of fat. The net conversion of amino acid to fat is therefore not a significant process except in animals receiving a high protein diet.

DIGESTIVE PROCESSES

The function described by the term "Digestion" includes all the changes which food undergoes within the digestive tract to prepare it for absorption and use in the body of an animal. Since digestion occurs within the digestive tract, we can say that it is separated from tissue metabolism by the process of absorption. Absorption occurs through the wall of the alimentary tract and the absorbed nutrients are then carried by the portal blood system and the lymphatic system to different parts of the body for tissue metabolism.

Digestion———→Absorption———→Metabolism

The processes by which food is digested can be categorised by:

(i) *Mechanical*—such as chewing and gastro-intestinal motility;

(ii) *Secretory*—such as the large volume of saliva secreted by three salivary glands of the mouth region; secretion of gastric juice by the stomach;

(iii) *Chemical*—such as hydrochloric acid in the true stomach; various digestive enzymes and the chemical activity of the rumen micro-organisms.

DIGESTION AND ABSORPTION OF CARBOHYDRATES IN NON-RUMINANTS

When food is chewed, it is mixed with saliva, which contains the enzyme *ptyalin* (it is absent in the saliva of cat, dog, horse and all ruminant animals) secreted mainly by the parotid glands. The enzyme acts on the polysaccharides, starch and glycogen and certain of their derivatives, hydrolysing these to the disaccharide maltose, but the food remains in the mouth only for a short time and probably not more than 3 to 5 per cent of all the starches that are eaten will have become hydrolysed into maltose by the time the food is swallowed.

Even though food does not remain in mouth long enough for ptyalin to complete the breakdown of starches info maltose, the action of this enzyme continues long after the food has entered the stomach, until the contents are mixed well with stomach secretion. Then the activity of the salivary amylase is blocked by the acid of the gastric secretions. Nevertheless, before the food becomes completely mixed with the gastric secretions as much as 30 to 40 per cent of the starches will have been changed into maltose.

Digestion of carbohydrates in the small intestine is mainly performed by the pancreatic secretion which like saliva, contains a large quantity of α-amylase capable of splitting starches into maltose and isomaltose. Also, a minute quantity of amylase is secreted in the intestinal juices. Therefore, immediately after the chyme empties from the stomach into the duodenum and mixes with pancreatic juice, the starches that have not already been split are digested by amylase. In general, the starches are almost totally converted into maltose and isomaltose before they have passed beyond jejunum. Indeed, pancreatic amylase is a more powerful enzyme than salivary amylase as the former can digest uncooked starch.

The epithelial cells of the small intestine contain four enzymes, *lactase, sucrase, maltase* and *isomaltase*, which are capable of splitting the disaccharides lactose, sucrose, maltose and isomaltose respectively, into their constituent monosaccharides. There is much reason to believe that these enzymes are located in the brush border of the cell lining, the lumen of the intestine and that the disaccharides are digested as they come in contact with this border. The digested products are then immediately absorbed into the portal blood. Lactose splits into a molecule of glucose and galactose. Sucrose spilts into a molecule of glucose and a molecule of fructose. Thus, the final products of carbohydrate digestion in non-ruminants are monosaccharides which are directly absorbed into the blood.

SUGAR ABSORPTION. It has been known for over 60 years that the small intestine absorbs certain hexoses faster than others. If the rate of absorption of glucose is taken as 100, the absorption rate of certain other sugars are as follows (data from Cori, using the rat as experimental animal):

Galactose—110
Glucose—100
Fructose—43
Mannose—19
Xylose—15
Arabinose—9

It was established that galactose and glucose were actively absorbed against a concentration gradient and that fructose, mannose, xylose and arabinose do not enjoy active transport.

Despite the inability of fructose to qualify structurally for active transport and its consequent slower rate of absorption than galactose and glucose, it does enjoy a faster rate of movement than mannose, xylose and arabinose. It has been shown that this is due to the conversion of fructose to both lactic acid and to glucose in the intestinal mucosal cell, each of which can then pass through the cell into the blood. The absence of fructokinase and/or glucose-6-phosphatase from intestinal mucosal cells accounts for species difference in the ability to convert fructose. Whereas both enzymes are present in guineapig mucosa, preparations from either rats or humans have shown no evidence of glucose-6-phosphatase and therefore these species are believed to be unable to convert fructose in the intestinal mucosal cell.

Although the exact mechanism of transport is not known, the current consensus is that there is a carrier on the lumenal border of the epithelial cell membrane to which the sugar becomes attached. Sugars which are actively transported inhibit each other; this suggests that there is a shared common carrier and pathway for these sugars. The sugar-carrier complex is not mobile unless Na^+ is present and moves with it.

DIGESTION AND ABSORPTION OF CARBOHYDRATES IN RUMINANTS

Ruminant's ration largely consists of carbohydrates rich in cellulose, hemicellulose and other carbohydrates which are not attacked by the digestive enzymes secreted by ruminants. When animals are on soft green pasture during rainy season, about 35 to 46 per cent of the dry matter consists of cellulose and hemicellulose, while in more mature herbage, hay and straw, the proportion of complex carbohydrates are generally higher.

When these carbohydrates reach the rumen, these are then subject to breakdown by enzymes secreted by microorganisms inhabiting the rumen. The important end products of the process were for a long time thought to be monosaccharides, but it is now established that once these are formed they are immediately fermented to a mixture of organic volatile fatty acids (V.F.A.) viz., acetic, propionic and butyric acids apart from gases like CO_2 and

Table 10.48

Type of common bacteria and protozoa involved in degradation of carbohydrate components of plants

Organisms	*Substrates*	*Products*
A. Bacteria		
Bacteroides succinogenes	Cellulose, cellobiose, glucose, CO_2	Succinate, acetate formate
Ruminococcus	Cellulose, cellobiose xylan, CO_2	Succinate, lactate, acetate, ethanol, H_2
Butyrivibrio	10-12 carbohydrates, varying among strains including xylan	Butyrate, lactate, ethanol, formate, CO_2 and sometimes acetate and propionate.
Eubacterium	Glucose, and 4-6 other sugars	Formate, lactate, acetate, butyrate, CO_2, H_2
B. Protozoa		
Holotrichs		
Isotricha prostoma I. intestinalis	Many sugars bacteria	Stored starch (?) H_2, CO_2, lactic, acetic, butyric
Dasytricha ruminantium	Many sugars, cellobiose	
Entodiniomorphs		
Entodinium spp.	Starch, bacteria Protozoa (?)	Stored starch, H_2, CO_2, lactic, acetic and butyric acids
Dipliodinium spp.	Starch, bacteria, cellulose, hemicellulose	

CH_4. Furthermore it is now well established that starch and soluble sugars entering the rumen are also broken down in the same manner.

The major carbohydrate components of pasture grass plants are, on a dry weight basis consist of pectin (upto 10 per cent), hemicellulose (12–17 per cent) and cellulose (20–30 per cent). Protein probably makes up a further 1–30 per cent of the dry matter of forages.

The bacteria and protozoa mainly responsible for fermentation in the digestive tract are largely strict anaerobes although there may be a small number of facultative anaerobes. Rumen contents of adult animals under normal feeding conditions contain about 10^{11} bacteria per ml. and up to 10^6 protozoa per ml.

With normal diets the predominant acid is acetic followed by propionic acid and butyric acid. By changing the ratio to (a) high ratio of concentrates, (b) finely ground forages, pelleted or unpelleted, (c) lack of physical fibrousness, (d) green forage low in fibre and high in soluble carbohydrates, (e) pelleted concentrates, (f) heated concentrates (high in starch) will bring relatively high ratio of propionic acid to acetic acid. The condition favours body fattening and lowers milk fat test. Propionic acid after reaching the liver is either oxidised or converted to glucose (ruminants can not utilise glucose for direct synthesis of fatty acids, mostly it is from acetic acid). Oxidation of acetic acid by liver tissue is less rapid, hence the body can utilise acetic acid either for milk formation or for other purposes. Butyric acid is mostly converted to ketone bodies in rumen epithelium and any butyric acid reaching the liver is also metabolised to ketone bodies or is oxidised in the TCA cycle after conversion to acetyl CoA.

The rate of gas production in the rumen is most rapid immediately after a meal and in the cow, may exceed 30 litres per hour. Carbon dioxide is produced partly as a byproduct of

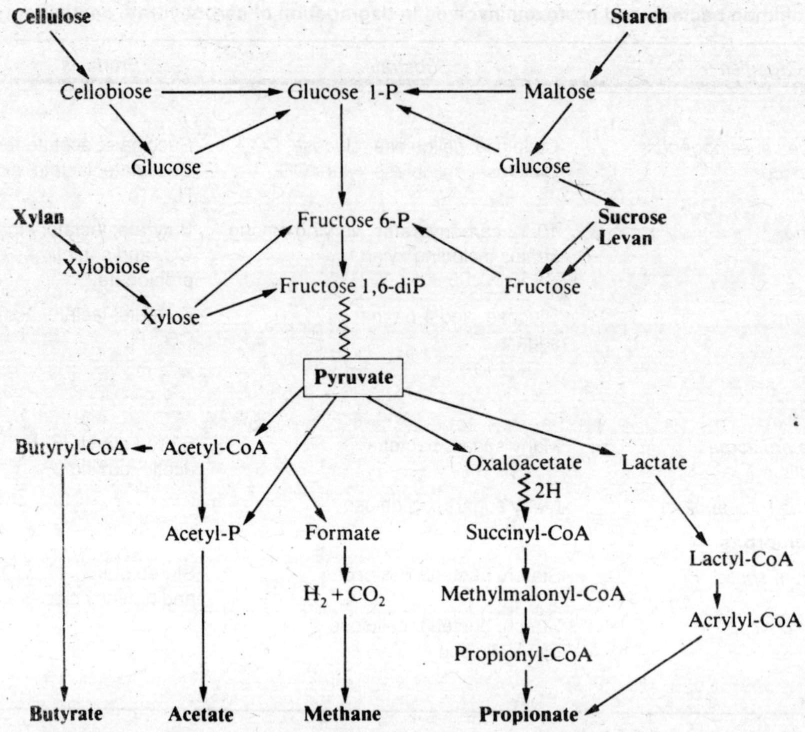

Fig. 10.22 Metabolic pathways for the production of VFA.

fermentation and partly by the reaction of organic acids with the bicarbonate present in the saliva. The major precursor of methane appears to be formic acid through carbon dioxide and hydrogen.

$$HCOOH \longrightarrow CO_2 + H_2$$

$$4H_2 + CO_2 \longrightarrow CH_4 + 2H_2O$$

About 4.5 g being formed for every 100 g. of carbohydrate digested by the ruminants.

The extent to which cellulose is digested in the rumen depends particularly on the degree of lignification of the plant material. Lignin is itself resistant to bacterial attack and appears to hinder the breakdown of cellulose with which it is associated. Thus, in young pasture grass containing only 5 per cent lignin in the dry matter, 80 per cent of the cellulose may be digested but in older herbage with 12 per cent lignin the proportion of celluiose digested may be less than 50 per cent.

The fatty acids are absorbed into the portal blood system mainly through the rumen wall, but some of them may pass in the reticulum omasum or even in abomasum and from there the acids are absorbed. Small amounts of lactic acid may also be absorbed from the entire digestive tract. Present evidence indicates that little glucose is absorbed as such when the ration is very much rich in starch or other carbohydrates. Most of the gas produced is lost by eruction; if gas accumulates it causes the condition known as bloat, in which the distention of the rumen may be so great that animal may die due to high pressure of the diaphragm towards heart.

DIGESTION AND ABSORPTION OF PROTEINS IN NON-RUMINANTS

The dietary proteins are derived almost entirely from animal and vegetable portions of the diet. You may recall that proteins are formed of long chains of amino acids bound together. The way each amino acid is linked with other amino acid is termed as *peptide linkage*. A typical linkage may be shown as follows:

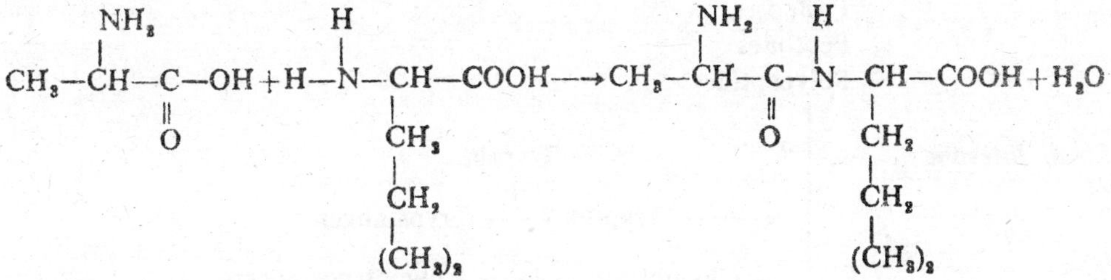

Alanine + Leucine = Alanylleucine + Water

$$\underset{\text{(Alanine)}}{CH_3-\overset{NH_2}{\overset{|}{CH}}-\underset{O}{\underset{\|}{C}}-OH} + \underset{\text{(Leucine)}}{H-\overset{H}{\overset{|}{N}}-\underset{\underset{(CH_3)_2}{\underset{|}{\underset{CH_2}{\underset{|}{CH_2}}}}}{\underset{|}{CH}}-COOH} \longrightarrow \underset{\text{(Alanylleucine)}}{CH_3-\overset{NH_2}{\overset{|}{CH}}-\underset{O}{\underset{\|}{C}}-\overset{H}{\overset{|}{N}}-\underset{\underset{(CH_3)_2}{\underset{|}{\underset{CH_2}{\underset{|}{CH_2}}}}}{\underset{|}{CH}}-COOH} + \underset{\text{(Water)}}{H_2O}$$

The characteristics of each type of proteins are determined by the type of amino acids in the protein molecule and by the arrangement of these amino acids. When we talk of digestion of protein, we mean the sequential attack on protein by a series of hydrolytic enzymes and this renders the protein molecule into its unit structure, i.e., amino acids. We are to know the site of digestion of protein, what enzymes does that, in what condition it is performed, the way in which different enzymes attack the protein mole. This is what we will learn in protein digestion.

Digestion of protein starts in the stomach of the non-ruminants like man, pig, horse etc. In all non-ruminants, stomach functions as a reservoir, a place where a great mass of food may be received to be fed slowly into the intestine. It also possesses an important digestive function. The wall of the stomach is replete with glands. It has been estimated that there are about 350,000,000 such glands present in human stomach. The ducts of these gastric glands open into the stomach cavity.

Three types of cells have been described in the gastric gland. (1) Mucous neck cells secrete mucous; (2) chief cells secrete pepsin; (3) parietal cells liberate hydrochloric acid. Thus the gastric juice is composed of water, mucin, pepsin, hydrochloric acid and a gastric lipase.

Perhaps the most unusual component of the gastric secretion is the hydrochloric acid which has the following functions:

(a) Brings satisfactory pH for enzyme action
(b) Preliminary action on protein as swelling etc.
(c) Possibly renders some hydrolysis of protein
(d) Activates pepsinogen enzyme which after activation changes into active enzyme *Pepsin*
(e) Germicidal action on microbes
(f) Probably aids iron absorption.

The enzyme pepsin is capable of digesting any kind of protein of the diet. It does not complete the process of protein digestion all the way to amino acids but simply splits the polypeptide chain and converts protein into proteoses, peptones and some small polypeptide chains which then enters the small intestine.

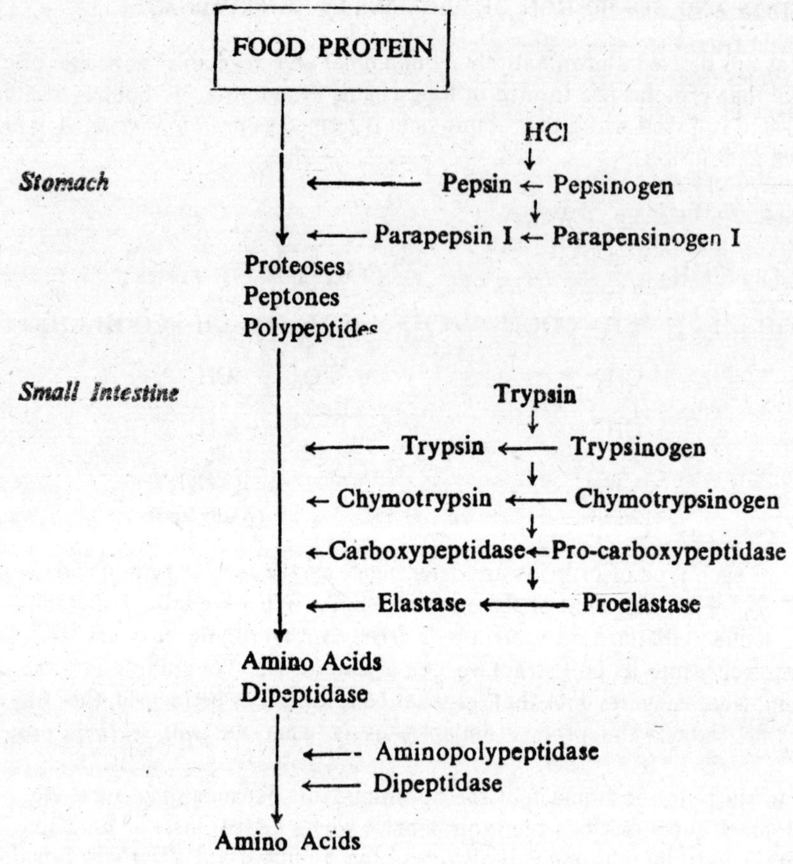

Note: In stomach, the main enzyme pepsin originates from pepsinogen and thus perapepsin I originates from parapepsinogen I and so on. In all cases, HCl cause these changes by activating the zymogen, i.e., precursor of these enzymes (here pepsinogen is the zymogen and pepsin is the active enzyme).

In the small intestine all the zymogens are activated by trypsin.

Upon entering the small intestine these partial breakdown products of protein come in contact with pancreatic and bile secretion thereby in an alkaline environment the pancreatic enzymes complete the protein digestion.

The pancreatic juice contains apart from carbohydrate and fat digesting enzymes, inactive protein digesting enzymes (*trypsinogen*, *chymotrypsinogen*, and *procarboxypeptidases*). The juice is an aqueous, isotonic fluid with a high bicarbonate ion concentration and a basic pH (about 8.0). In the intestine trypsinogen is converted into active *trypsin* by a substance called *enterokinase* from the intestinal mucosa and by previously formed trypsin. In turn trypsin is able to convert chymotrypsinogen to active *chymotrypsin*, and the procarboxypeptidases to active *carboxypeptidases*. These active enzymes continue the protein digestion begun in the stomach by pepsin. Trypsin splits bonds of the polypeptide chain next to basic amino acids (such as lysine and arginine), thus producing smaller polypeptides and dipeptides. Chymotrypsin also splits particular amino acid bonds (which involve aromatic amino acids such as tyrosine and phenylalanine) to produce smaller polypeptides and dipeptides. The carboxypeptidases free the terminal amino acid from the carboxyl (acid) end of the polypeptide chain. *Aminopeptidase* and *dipeptidase* enzymes originating from the mucosal epithelium of the small intestine complete the digestion of the small polypeptides and dipeptides to free amino acids. The amino peptidase enzymes liberate the terminal amino acid from the amino end of the polypeptide, and the dipeptidases split the dipeptides into their component amino acids.

Pancreatic nucleases (*ribonuclease, deoxyribonuclease*) perform the digestion of dietary nucleic acids (which are not proteins but non-protein nitrogenous substances) present in every plant and animal cell, thereby release purines and pyrimidins, ribose or deoxyribose and phosphoric acids.

There is a difference in the rate of absorption of different amino acids. By the word "different" we mean mainly three classes of amino acids—(1) **neutral,** (2) basic, and (3) acidic. You might have noticed the characteristics of 20 common amino acids which have previously been discussed. All neutral amino acids have one $-NH_2$ group but one $-COOH$ group, all basic have two or more $-NH_2$ groups but one $-COOH$ group, while acidic amino acids have two $-COOH$ groups with one $-NH_2$ group.

It has been postulated that these groups of acids utilise three different carrier systems (some unidentified compound which aids transferring amino acids from the lumen to the other side of the intestinal cell, imagined as a boat carrying passengers from one side of the canal to the other side).

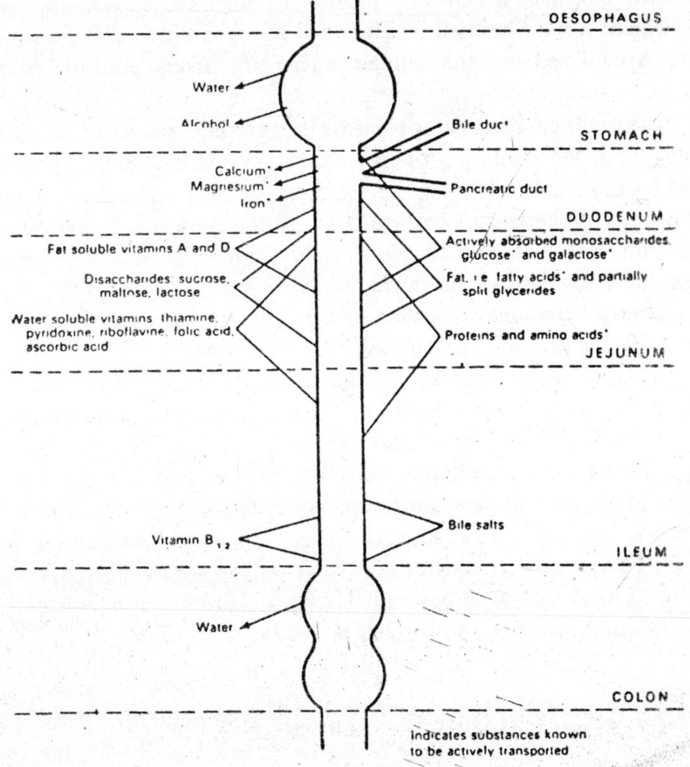

Fig. 10.23 Site of absorption of feedstuffs in the alimentary canal in non-ruminants.

Among all neutral amino acids, which utilises same carrier also has some competition, e.g., leucine is more inhibitor for glycine than others and so on. Like neutral, basic utilises a common carrier but they also have some competition among themselves, e.g., arginine or cystine inhibits lysine. Both neutral and basic amino acids are actively transported, i.e., they require extra energy for their transfer across the wall.

The absorption of acidic amino acids like glutamic and aspartic acid is still not entirely clear. It has been suggested that they are not actively transported since relatively small amounts were recoverable in the portal blood after feeding, but Wilson (1962) proposed that this might have been the result of transmission during absorption and that the system requires further investigation.

Some neutral acids compete with other basic or acidic acids but the reverse is not true.

DIGESTION AND METABOLISM OF PROTEINS AND NON-PROTEIN NITROGENOUS COMPOUNDS IN RUMEN

Digestion and absorption of proteins in ruminants is unique by itself due to the presence of compound stomach. As early as 1938, it was recognised that microorganisms were responsible for proteolytic activity within the rumen, a fact subsequently confirmed by other workers. Unlike simple stomached animal, there is no free proteolytic enzyme source in the rumen wall. Microorganisms, which are normal inhabitants of the rumen, digest the dietary protein by releasing proteolytic enzymes which are mostly intracellular, associated with the cell wall fraction from which it is liberated. Thus all the proteins and non-protein nitrogenous compounds are hydrolysed by the rumen micro-organisms comprising both bacteria and protozoa.

Proteolysis. The bulk of the dietary nitrogen entering the rumen, under ordinary conditions of feeding, is in the form of protein. Since there is no extracellular, free proteolytic enzyme secreted by any part of the rumen, the feed proteins are entirely depended on rumen microbial enzyme for further simplification, i.e., proteolysis which involves at first conversion into free amino acids, followed by a change into ammonia. The rate of proteolysis being closely related to the solubility of the protein in the rumen fluid.

In spite of a strong proteolytic activity in the rumen, the amino acid concentration in the rumen fluid is low because of the presence of microbial deaminases, the activity of which increases with increasing protein content of the ration. The enzyme is directly responsible for the process of deamination. *Deamination* is the removal of the amino group from an amino acid which may be oxidative or non-oxidative as explained below:

Oxidative Deamination. A deamination reaction proceeds with a simultaneous oxidation as in the conversion of (1) an α-amino acid to an α-keto acid and (2) the amino group to ammonia. The reaction is catalysed by *amino acid oxidase*, an enzyme which contains the oxidising co-enzyme, FAD. The reduced coenzyme is further reoxidised by molecular oxygen (not by the respiratory chain) to form hydrogen peroxide (H_2O_2). Under the influence of *catalase*, H_2O_2 is then finally decomposed to water and oxygen.

1.
$$\begin{array}{c} CH_3 \\ | \\ CHNH_2 \\ | \\ COOH \\ \text{Alanine} \end{array} + FAD + H_2O \rightleftharpoons \begin{array}{c} CH_3 \\ | \\ C=O \\ | \\ COOH \\ \text{Pyruvic acid} \end{array} + NH_3 + FADH_2$$

2. $FADH_2 + O_2 \longrightarrow FAD + H_2O_2$

3. $H_2O_2 \xrightarrow{\textit{Catalase}} H_2O + 1/2O_2$

Non-oxidative Deamination. By this process a significant contribution to the total ammonia production results in the rumen. The amino acids which are mostly affected are hydroxy amino acids, serine, threonine and homoserine. These acids are deaminated by a specific enzyme *amino acid dehydrase,* which catalyse to form an intermediary unstable compound by primary dehydration. This unstable compound then reacts with water to produce an α-keto acid and ammonia as below:

$$\underset{\text{Serine}}{HO{-}CH_2{-}\underset{\displaystyle NH_2}{\underset{|}{CH}}{-}COOH} \xrightarrow{-H_2O} CH_2{=}\underset{\displaystyle NH_2}{\underset{|}{C}}{-}COOH$$

$$\underset{\text{Ammonia + Pyruvic acid}}{NH_3 + CH_3{-}\overset{\displaystyle O}{\overset{\|}{C}}{-}COOH} \xleftarrow{+H_2O} \underset{\text{Amino acid}}{CH_3{-}\underset{\displaystyle NH}{\underset{\|}{C}}{-}COOH}$$

The dietary nitrogenous compounds of the ruminants also contain appreciable amounts of nitrogenus materials other than the proteins (Fig. 10.24.)Pasture plants, for example, contain about 20-30 per cent of their total nitrogen as non-protein nitrogen (NPN) and silage contains a much more greater proportion. Most of the compounds of the NPN fraction such as amino acids and peptides, nucleic acids, nitrate and various amines are also rapidly degraded in the rumen and thus form mainly ammonia with less volatile fatty acids and other compounds. According to some recent studies, the volatile acids formed from the microbial breakdown of amino acids and other non-protein nitrogenous compounds appear to be C_2, C_3, C_4 and C_5 acids, the latter being principally branched chain acids which though absorbed, are probably not available for resynthesis of amino acids. This means that microbial action is wasteful of the carbon chains as well as of ammonia. Apart from NPN derived from natural feeds, various other ammonium compounds such as urea may be added to the diet of the ruminants upto a certain quantity. The strong *urease* activity of the rumen bacteria converts entire urea into ammonia. Thus for a wide variety of diets it appears that ammonia forms an important intermediate in the conversion of feed nitrogen to microbial nitrogen (Fig. 10.24.).

Excessively high rates of ammonia production may result, particularly if large amounts of urea or proteins, such as casein, which are very soluble in rumen fluid, are eaten rapidly. The ingestion of rainy season grasses, particularly the leafy parts, also tends to cause rapid ammonia production in the rumen. If the rate of production exceeds the rate at which the bacteria can utilize the ammonia, the concentration of the ammonia in the rumen increases and thereby maximum amount will then be absorbed through portal blood and ultimately to liver where the excess ammonia will be converted into urea and finally excretion through urine will be the only way to get rid of ammonia toxicity. Thus excess ammonia production is definitely not only a great loss of the nitrogenous compounds of the feed material but also will exert an undue pressure on liver and kidney for the exit of the excess gas in the form of urea.

Ammonia Production. The preceding sections have shown that in the rumen, protein is rapidly hydrolyzed to amino acids which are then deaminated to ammonia. It has been further shown that more soluble proteins give rise to larger concentration of rumen ammonia. The rate of deamination is somewhat slower than proteolysis and thus immediately after feeding there may be increased concentration of amino acids and peptides in the rumen, but eventually, virtually all amino acids are deaminated; ammonia concentration being its maximum approximately three hours after feeding.

Ammonia may also be formed in the rumen from sources other than amino acids. Many proteins contain amide nitrogen and amidase activity is present in many proteolytic rumen bacteria. Many urea derivatives, for example, biuret and some amides such as guanidine acetate, are metabolised by rumen becteria but there is no evidence that ammonia is liberated. Rumen bacteria liberate ammonia from adenine, guanine, hypoxanthene, xanthene, uric acid, uracil and thymine. Another source of ammonia in the rumen is urea from feed source or from saliva or back flow of ammonia through rumen wall directly inside the rumen. Whatsoever may be the source, the ultimate end product of the microbial enzymatic action is ammonia.

Fate of Ammonia. 1. Considerable protein is utilised by the rumen microbes for their rapid proliferation. During this build up process, microbes utilise ammonia and fix it as excellent body protein composing of essential and non-essential amino acids in presence of soluble carbohydrates, particularly starch. When the organisms numbering in billions and billions are carried through to the abomasum and small intestine, their cell proteins are then digested by the usual gastric enzymes of the abomasum and are absorbed as units of amino acids mostly in the region of the small intestine. The output of the microbial protein from the rumen is, however, a function of the amount of nitrogen and energy available for microbial growth and the anaerobic nature of the ruminal fermentation.

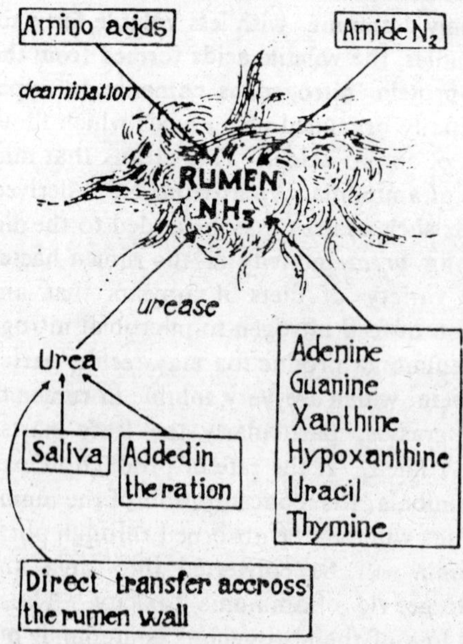

Fig. 10.24. Schematic presentation of the possible ways and means of formation of ammonia in rumen.

Several groups of workers have studied the growth of micro-organisms in relation to energy supply under anaerobic conditions both *in vitro* and *in vivo*. Yield were found to be higher in *in vivo* than *in vitro* and a value of about 30 gram of bacterial crude microbial protein per 1000 gram of organic matter digested in the rumen was obtained.

2. A portion of total ammonia of the rumen is absorbed directly from the rumen to the systemic blood which in the liver is mostly converted into urea. A small fraction may also be utilised for the synthesis of non-essential amino acids or some other compounds.

The rate of ammonia absorption is dependent on ruminal pH, as ammonia is being absorbed much more rapidly in the unionised form. Lowering the pH of the rumen due to carbohydrate fermentation would thus decrease the rate of absorption. This could particularly account for the increased, nitrogen retentions found when carbohydrates are fed with a nitrogen source which is readily converted to ruminal ammonia.

3. A portion may flow to other compartments of the compound stomach such as reticulum, omasum and abomasum.

Urea Recycling. It is now well established that blood urea enters back into the rumen directly by transfusion through rumen wall and also indirectly through saliva. Blaxter has estimated that about 20 per cent of the nitrogen absorbed as ammonia is recycled in sheep on normal nitrogen intakes. The process would be of greatest value to animals on low nitrogen intakes.

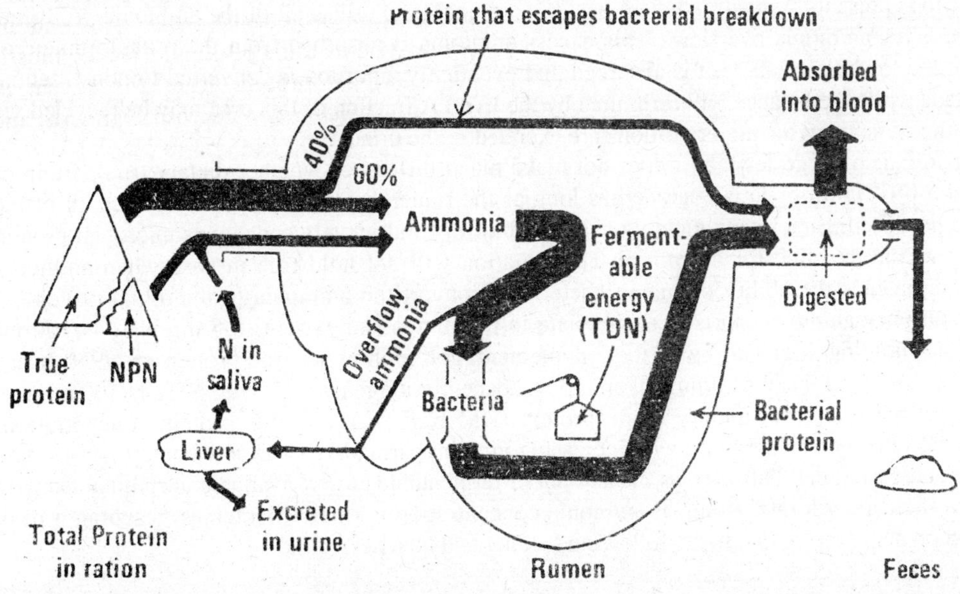

Fig. 10.25 Schematic summary of nitrogen utilization by the ruminant (adapted from Satter and Roffler, 1978).

Utilisation of Ammonia by Rumen microbes

A schematic summary of nitrogen utilisation by ruminants is shown in Fig 10.25 Ingested true protein are generally partially degraded by ruminal microbes and the balance by escaping degradation pass to the lower gut (also called by-pass protein) for further digestion or excreted in the faeces. The amount of true protein that escapes degradation may vary considerably, but with most management and feeding conditions an escape rate of 40 per cent for dietary protein probably represents an acceptable average. The remaining 60 per cent of dietary protein is degraded in the rumen almost entirely to ammonia.

Dietary NPN, salivary nitrogen and possibly a small amount of urea entering across the rumen wall (recycling) are converted almost totally to ammonia. Several other nitrogen sources also contribute to ruminal ammonia production.

The amount of ammonia that can be utilised by bacteria will depend on the number of bacteria and how rapidly they are growing. In other words, it will also depend on the amount of readily available energy present in the feed. The function of carbohydrate in converting NH_3 to microbial protein is to make energy and carbon skeletons available for microbial synthesis. Carbohydrates differ widely in ways they fulfil their function. The least effective carbohydrate seems to be cellulose and the most effective is starch. Starch is also superior to molasses or even simple sugars. The effectiveness of starch has been shown to be increased by cooking which makes it gelatinized and thus becomes more susceptible to microbial breakdown. The process release energy at a rate more nearly parallel to ammonia release from urea which all again permits rumen microorganisms to use the NH_3 more effectively. Ration high in grain or digestible dry matter is thus more useful than high forage rations. Therefore, more ammonia (NPN) can be slowly utilised (Fig10.25 where an increase in total digestible nutrients (TDN) 'opens the gate' and allows more ammonia use by supporting greater production of bacterial numbers.

Fig.10.25 presents a situation where bacteria are unable to utilise all of the ammonia produced, and there is an 'ammonia overflow'. This excess ammonia is absorbed from the reticulorumen, or passed to the lower gut, where it is absorbed and eventually a portion is converted to non-essential amino acids while the balance will form urea by the liver. A fraction of this urea may be recycled via saliva to the rumen, but the major portions are excreted in the urine.

Fig.10.25 also suggestes that it does not make much difference whether dietary true portein or dietary non-protein nitrogen is degraded as long as the rumen bacteria are able to utilise all of the ammonia produced. Either way, dietary or recycled nitrogen ultimately ends up as microbial protein presented to the intestine for absorption.The situation will not hold true in case when ammonia production exceeds the ability of rumen bacteria to convert the ammonia to microbial protein. It appears that once ammonia starts to accumulate in the rumen and exceeds 5-8 mg NH_3–N/100 ml rumen fluid, nothing is gained by further supplementation with either true protein or NPN. It has been further observed that mean ruminal ammonia concentration reached 5-8 mg NH_3–N/100 ml at an approximately 13 per cent dietary crude protein (DM basis). Above this protein concentration, ruminal ammonia increases rapidly with increasing protein, particularly with low energy rations than with high energy rations. This is so as the amount of fermentable energy available to ruminal bacteria influences their growth rate. Ruminal ammonia concentration normally fluctuates, reaching a peak concentration about one to two hours following feeding and then decreases.

Some significant average values and factors of protein digestion in ruminants are given below :

1. In a typical ruminant ration 85 per cent of the dietary nitrogen is in true protein form and 15 per cent in natural NPN form.
2. The amount of nitrogen recycled into reticulorumen is equal to 12 per cent of the dietary nitrogen intake.
3. 40 per cent of the true dietary protein escapes rumen digestion (by pass protein) and goes to the

intestine while rest 60 per cent true protein and all of the dietary NPN along with recycled nitrogen (through saliva and amount entering across the ruminal wall) contributes total ruminal ammonia pool.

4. 90 per cent of all ruminal ammonia produced is incorporated into microbial nitrogen when the ration fed does not exceed 13 per cent dietary crude protein (DM basis).
5. No ruminal ammonia derived from total dietary crude protein if fed in excess of the 'upper limit' will be utilized by microbes for their body building.
6. Metabolizable protein conprises the amount of total amino acids absorbed in the small intestine which actually come from (a) dietary by pass protein, and (b) dead bodies of ruminal microbes. From the total metabolizable protein, 87 per cent of the dietary by pass protein are absorbed, while it is 80 per cent in case of microbial true protein.
7. The rumen microorganisms synthesize all essential and non-essential amino acids for their body building purposes. Hence the mixture of amino acids eventually enters the animal's blood after the digestion of dead bodies of these microbes bear no relationship to the protein quality of original diet.
8. The digestibility of bacterial protein is lower, 0.74 compared to 0.91 for protozoal protein and thus has an NPU of about 0.59. The portion digested and absorbed has a 'Biological Value' (per cent of the absorbed N_2 retained by the body) of 0.8, whether it is bacterial or protozoal origin.
9. A value of 30 g microbial nitrogen (or about 200 gram microbial protein) synthesized for each kg organic matter apparently digested in the rumen has been accepted.
10. The rate of growth of microbes in the rumen is always greater than the rate at which microbes flow from the rumen to abomasun. This is because :
    (a) Protozoa are retained and only a small proportion move down the tract. Those retained apparently lyse (the process of cell destruction through the action of any antibody dissolving microbe) in the rumen and are fermented.
    (b) Protozoa, by their predatory (materials taken by force) action, engulf and digest quite a proportion of the bacterial pool.
    (c) Bacteria and protozoa spontaneously lyse either due to the action of infective agents, lack of substrate or a change in environment conditions such as a lowering of rumen fluid pH.
    (d) Bacteria may also lyse through perturbations which cause bacteriophages to become lysogenic.

The net effect of these interactions is a considerable recycling of nitrogen within the rumen. Up to 50% of the microbes that were produced were lysed in the rumen of sheep on straw based diet.

Periodic fasting of animals may also result in lysis of a high proportion of the microbial pool in the rumen. It has been noted that 60% of rumen bacteria died and 30% lysed where bacteria were without substrate for two hours.

11. Sulfur, like nitrogen, is an essential element for microbial synthesis as it contributes to microbial sulfur containing amino acids. Recommended S/N ratio has been found to be 1 : 10 in urea based diets.
12. There is positive correlation between increased dilution rate and increased microbial growth. Rumen dilution rate is defined as the proportion of total rumen volume leaving the rumen per hour. Several factors such as type of diet, (feed particle size, density, wettability, salt content etc.), rumen osmotic pressure and volume, salivary flow, level of intake and environmental conditions have been found to alter rumen ditution rate.
13. Since the amount of ammonia produced in the rumen from various protein sources is inversely correlated with the N_2 retention, it has been suggested that suitable processing of high protein concentrates may improve their usefulness to the animal. Out of the methods,

(i) Post-ruminal infusion,
(ii) Heat treatment of the proteins
(iii) Tannic acid treatment
(iv) Chemical treatments including Formaldehyde.
(v) Protection of amino acids
  (a) By using amino acid analogue
  (b) By using encapsulated amino acids

Otherwise select feed proteins having very low solubility while computing rations for high yielders. billion dead microbes along with undergraded dietary protein (by pass protein) are brought to the abomasum. Af first the gastric juice which is highly acidic due to the presence of HCl, convert the proenzyme pepsinogen into pepsin by H^+ and also simultaneously denatures the protein and make the peptide bonds more susceptible to enzymatic hydrolysis. Pepsin catalyses the hydrolysis of only certain peptide bonds and as a result peptides (not amino acids) are formed. About 15% of the ingested proteins are thus partially hydrolyzed in.

14. High concentrations of rumen ammonia obviously do not necessarily indicate ammonia toxicity ; high rumen ammonia concentration commensurate with high rumen pH, however, would indicate toxicity because the free NH_3 concentration would be much higher at high pH. Ammonia exists as free NH_3 at high pH but as the ammonium ion (NH_4^+) at lower pH. Because tissue membranes are permeable to the lipid soluble NH_3 form but impermeable to the charged NH_4+ form, more ammonia is absorbed at high pH than at low pH.

The significance of this is that a large ammonia pool can be maintained in the rumen for microbial protein sysnthesis by maintaining low rumen pH. Readily available starch, such as cooked starch in *Starea*, is rapidly fermented to volatile fatty acids, which help to maintain low rumen pH.

15. High concentration of ammonia in the rumen does not stop normal bacterial growth, it is only that the cxcess amount of free NH_3 are absorbed through the rumen wall and most of these get lost through urine.

16. It is apparent that the rate at which energy is released from the carbohydrate material is crucial for conversion of ammonia to microbial protein. If it is released too slowly, as from cellulose, or if it released too rapidly as from glucose, ammonia conversion to microbial body in either case be poor. Starch has been considered the ideal source for supplying not only energy but also for carbon skeleton as well as production of VFA and thereby lowering pH value of rumen contents. Cooked starch gives more encouraging results than uncooked form.

17. Various types of microorganisms are present in the rumen, viz., Bacteria (5.4 to 31.4) x 10^{10}/ml ; Protozoa (0.3 to 19.7) x 10^6/ml ; Oscillospira (6.1 to 8.5) x 10^4/ml ; Yeast (0.0 to 10.0) x 10^3/ml and Bacteriophage which exceeds bacteria in the ratio of 2:1 to 10:1. Rumen protozoa which are mostly of ciliate types although are present in small numbers than bacteria, but because of their greater size can occupy little less than 50% of the biomass.

Absorption of Amino Acids. It has been emphasised earlier that rumen amino acid concentrations are very low, except soon after feeding a diet containing much of soluble protein. In general when a continuous normal feeding programme is followed, the concentrations of all free amino acids are very low and the rate of dissimilation by rumen microorganisms are so high that it would be surprising if significant absorption takes place. Interestingly enough, a definite transport of glycine across rumen epithelium and an increase in blood glycine following glycine addition to the rumen, has been demonstrated in goat and sheep.

It is very unlikely that there is any significant absorption of amino acids in general from the rumen and in most circumstances it must be negligible. But when we consider the fact that the life of microorganisms are very short, they are continuously flowing along with partially digested feeds through the gastro-intestinal tract in profuse amounts. In this way several billion dead microbes are brought to the abomasum, where like in monogastric animals, proteolytic enzymes are secreted by the numerous glands of abomasum, and as they reach the small intestine, pancreatic secretion and the proteolytic enzymes of the small intestine present in brush border of epithelial walls act on these dead microbes and bring about a complete protein digestion resulting in amino acids as end products.

Table 10.49

The Average Amino acid composition of bacterial and protozoal protein isolated from rumen of sheep compared with animal proteins (g amino acid/100 g. protein)

Amino acids (AA)	*Milk*	*Beef*	*Bacterial protein*	*protozoal-protein*
Threonine	5.0	4.6	5.37	5.07
Valine	7.4	5.3	5.49	5.24
Isoleucine	5.8	5.1	4.68	5.80
Leucine	10.2	8.0	6.47	7.18
Phenylalanine	5.4	4.5	3.98	5.29
Histidine	3.0	3.7	1.49	1.79
Lysine	8.2	9.1	6.99	10.14
Arginine	4.0	6.7	4.09	4.58
Methionine	2.9	2.7	1.78	1.65
Aspertic acid	8.5	9.6	12.10	12.62
Serine	5.9	4.5	4.24	4.10
Gultamic acid	23.0	17.3	11.18	13.81
Glycine	2.2	5.6	4.85	3.61
Alanine	3.8	6.4	6.12	3.48
Tyrosine	4.5	3.8	3.90	4.49

Due to peristaltic movement the abomasal contents enter the duodenum and jejunum. Here the pancreatic digestive juices which contain zymogens : chymotrypsinogen and trypsinogen as well as procarboxypeptidases gets activated resulting into chymotrypsin, trypsin and carboxypeptidases. All these three enzymes have a broad range of hydrolytic capabilities of protein. Intestinal secretion of dipeptidase hydrolyzes dipeptides to liberate individual amno acids. The rate of hydrolysis appears to be regulated to the rate of absorption so that there is never a large excess of amino acids in the intestinal lumen.

For absorption of amino acids there are 4 distinct carrier systems situated throughout the microvilli of the small intestine, viz. (1) neutral amino acids, (2) basic amino acids, (3) acidic amino acids, and (4) glycine and imino acids. Absorption of individual amino acids into the mucosal cell from the lumen is associated with absorption of Na^+ from the serosal surface. While the amino acid transport is against gradient (up hill), the absorption of Na^+ is along gradient (down hill).

These amino acids are then absorbed through the microvilli of the small intestine for growth, tissue repair, maintenance of body protein reserves and for products like milk etc.

Table 10.50 **Protein Solubility and degradation in the rumen of selected feedstuffs**

Feedstuff	Crude protein % DM	Protein solubility % of CP	Total ruminal degradation %
Urea	280	100	100
Dried milk	27	93	96
Maize silage	9	55	77
Linseed meal	39	51	76
Groundnut meal	52	40	70
Wheat bran	18	35	68
Maize gluten feed	28	32	66
Wheat grain	14	30	65
Distilled dried grains	30	26	63
Oat grains	13	26	63
Lucerne	19	18	62
Corn gluten meal	21	18	59
Barley grain	13	17	59
Soybean meal	52	13	56
Maize	10	12	56
Cotton seed meal	45	7	53
Milo grain	12	5	52
Sugar beet pulp	10	4	52
Brewer's grains	25	3	51

Digestion of Nitrogenous Compounds in Small Intestine

Apart from ammonia which is not present in any significant amount in the small intestine, the nitrogenous component entering the duodenum consists mainly of proteins which might have escaped digestion upto abomasum or may be the products resulted from partial digestion of protein in abomasum originally derived from microbial protein and partly from endogenous secretion into the abomasum. Nucleic acids also account for an appreciable proportion of the nitrogen in the duodenal ingesta. In the small intestine the undigested protein is again digested to yield amino acids, some of which may also be deaminated to form ammonia. The ammonia thus formed is absorbed to the systemic blood through the epithelial lining of the small intestine. The enzymes required are secreted firstly by the pancreatic juices viz., trypsinogen, and chymotrypsinogen. The proteolytic enzyme *enterokinase* secreted by the unidentified cells of the duodenum catalyses the activation of trypsinogen to trypsin. Secondly several other proteolytic enzymes like amino *polypeptidase*, *dipeptidase* etc. are also released by the brush borders of the epithelial cells of the small intestine. These enzymes are responsible for final hydrolysis of the peptides into amino acids.

USE OF UREA AS A PROTEIN REPLACER

J.K. Loosli and associates of Cornell University produced first time a specific evidence that microbial action in the rumen can synthesise all of the 10 essential amino acids required for rat growth from urea. Since than the non-protein nitrogen (NPN) utilisation is considered to be of great practical importance; several investigations have been made with ruminants receiving urea on the influence of rumen function, growth and nitrogen balance and now there are many excellent reviews on various aspects of NPN utilisation.

Several studies have shown that urea can replace satisfactorily upto about 30 per cent of the protein in practical rations for matured ruminants and lactating cows. This replacement has become possible since in practice, ruminants natural feed also contain about 30 per cent of the nitrogen as non-protein nitrogenous substances such as amino acids, amides and amines. This means that urea can be added at the rate of 3 per cent of the concentrate mixture. For the efficient utilisation of urea, simultaneous feeding of soluble carbohydrate, preferably of starch at the rate of 1 kg for every 100 gram of urea is a must for the sake of providing necessary energy requirement of the microbes.

How Urea is Utilised by Ruminants?

$$\text{Urea} \xrightarrow[\textit{from microbes}]{\textit{urease}} \text{ammonia } (NH_3) + CO_2 \quad (1)$$

$$\text{Carbohydrate} \xrightarrow[\textit{from rumen microbes}]{\textit{enzymes}} \text{VFA + Keto acids} \quad (2)$$

$$NH_3 + \text{Keto acids} \xrightarrow[\textit{from microbes}]{\textit{enzymes}} \text{amino acids} \quad (3)$$

$$\text{Amino acids} \xrightarrow[\textit{from microbes}]{\textit{enzymes}} \text{microbial protein} \quad (4)$$

$$\text{Microbial protein} \xrightarrow[\textit{and small intestine}]{\textit{enzymes in abomasum}} \text{free amino acids} \quad (5)$$

Free amino acid absorbed from small intestine ——→ for building body protein in the ruminants (6)

Apart from these, addition of required amount of sulfur and phosphorus in the ration, containing urea will initiate in the synthesis of sulphur containing amino acids, so essential for the normal body components of the microbes.

Urea entering the rumen is rapidly hydrolysed by bacterial *urease* to ammonia which is then converted into amino acids (3) and finally utilised by the microbes for their synthetic activities.

Urea or any other NPN, if ever, has no technical advantage over feed protein of matured ruminants, and therefore, the use of such compounds has to be justified by economic considerations.

DIGESTION AND ABSORPTION OF LIPIDS IN NON-RUMINANTS

In the usual diet, components of lipids comprises mostly of neutral fats but some phospholipid, cholesterol, cholesterol ester, and fat-soluble vitamins are also present. Almost no digestion of the lipid occurs in the mouth and stomach. Although gastric juice contains a lipase, there is very little hydrolysis of triglyceride in the lumen of the stomach because the pH optimum of *gastric lipase* ranges from 5.5 to 7.5 whereas the pH of the gastric contents is quite acidic.

However, as the amount of digestion in the stomach is mostly confined with the digestion of minute milk fat globules or of egg fat globules, the action is regarded as insignificant in adult animals.

The pre-requisite of fat digestion requires a drastic physical change which involves the conversion of water insoluble fats into partly water soluble forms. The principal steps include (1) emulsification, (2) enzymatic hydrolisation and formation of micelles, (3) absorption mostly in the forms of 2-monoacyl glycerides and free fatty acids in the intestinal epithelium, (4) resynthesis of fat molecules in the epithelium and finally (5) transportation of fat molecules mostly in the forms of chylomicrons and other low density lipoproteins through lymphatic channels.

Of the lipids being ingested are thus enter the duodenum from the stomach almost without any change at a slow rate (in human it is about 10 gm. of lipid per hour) along with the acid chyme. Mere presence of fats in the lumen of the duodenum stimulates the production of a digestive hormone, *Cholecystokinin* (previously termed as *pancreozymin*) which after originating from the duodenum reaches the gall bladder and pancreas through blood circulation and causes contraction of gall bladder as well as forces the pancreas to secrete pancreatic enzymes.

In the intestinal lumen under the influence of peristaltic action on the one hand and of the contact of bile, fat globules exist in the duodenum as a spherical coarse particle as emulsion in the semi-liquid intestinal contents. (*Emulsion is a colloidal dispersion of one liquid in another immiscible or partially miscible, liquid, size of the globules varies from* 300 – 1000 m μ, *scatter light, require energy for formation.*)

As we know, the nonpolar compounds (compounds which have got no charge on the molecule) are insoluble in water and therefore no attraction for water molecules which are charged and thus polar, that is why fats are also totally insoluble in water. The important non-polar groups in lipids are primarily the hydrocarbon tails of the fatty acids, or fatty acyl moities, and the fused hydrocarbon rings of the steroids. However, lipids also contain polar groups, such as the three ester linkages of triacylglyceride, which because of a great mass of non-polar hydrocarbon, has lost the water soluble property. Similarly although cholesterol has got a polar carbinol group, it is highly insoluble in water because of the massive fused hydrocarbon ring. The carboxyl part of the bile salt is highly soluble in water, whereas rest of the fused hydrocarbon portion being non-polar is soluble in fats. These substances tend to occupy the inter-face between water and the non-polar lipid droplet and inhibit coalescence because of the repulsion forces of approaching polar groups. These stabilised dispersions of non-polar lipids in aqueous solutions are the *emulsions*.

Bile

The secretory and excretory activities of the liver continually produce bile which is stored in gall bladder and also travels directly through hepatic ducts. Bile from gall bladder is drained by the cystic duct, which joins with the hepatic duct to form the common bile duct.

Bile is an aqueous solution, greenish, or greenish yellow in colour with bitter taste. It contains no enzyme but electrolytes such as sodium and bicarbonate that contains bile salts. The acid side chains of the sodium salts are conjugated with taurine or glycine to form taurocholic or glycocholic acids, bile pigments, cholesterol, neutral fats and lecithin. Approximately 94 percent of the bile salts that are released into the duodenum are reabsorbed in the ileum. They may then be returned to the liver by the blood stream and resecreted. This cycle is known as *enterohepatic circulation.*

The rate of bile secretion is chemically, neurally and hormonally controlled. Chemical substances that increase bile flow are called *Choleretics.* Shortly after ingestion of a meal, the gall bladder contracts and bile is released into the duodenum. The contraction of the gall bladder is stimulated primarily by the hormone *Cholecystokinin,* which is released from the duodenal mucosa in response to the presence of fat and protein breakdown products in the chyme. Vagal stimulation may also cause weak contractions of the gall bladder.

Table 10.51

Composition of Hepatic and of Gall bladder bile

(Percent of Total bile)

	Hepatic Bile (as secreted)	Bladder Bile
Water	97.00	85.92
Bile acid	1.93	9.14
Mucin and pigments	0.53	2.98
Cholesterol	0.06	0.26
Fatty acids and fats	0.14	0.32
Inorganic salts	0.84	0.65
pH	7.1 – 7.3	6.9 – 7.7

Functions served by Bile

1. It emulsifies fat thus by increasing number of fat globules it increases surface area to be acted upon by lypolytic enzymes.
2. Provides optimum pH for the enzymes to hydrolyse.
3. Activates the enzyme lipase.
4. An important vehicle of excretion. It removes many drugs, toxins, bile pigments and various inorganic substances such as copper, zinc and murcury.

Pancreatic secretion

Pancreas secrete its various digestive enzymes almost entirely by means of hormonal stimulation such as (1) *secretin,* which stimulates the production of watery fluid, high in bicarbonate but low in enzyme content & (2) *pancreozymin,* stimulates the production of secretion high in enzymes and low in bicarbonates.

So far lipid digestion is concerned, pancreatic lipase is the most significant contribution of pancreas.

Hydrolysis of lipids in the small intestine

In the presence of bile, the pancreatic lipase hydrolyses the triacylglyceride droplets into fatty acids and monoglycerides. The fatty acids in the 1 – and 3 – positions of the triacylglycerides project into the aqueous phase of the intestinal contents and are readily acted upon by the pancreatic lipase. The 2 – monoacylglycerides can not be hydrolysed as such, but may be broken down only if they are isomerised to 1 – monoacylglycerides. The specificity of *pancreatic lipase* for the primary ester linkages of glycerides is not altered by the degree of unsaturation or chain length of the fatty acids involved. Using isotopically-labelled monoglycerides, it has been shown that unhydrolised monoacylglycerides are absorbed intact. 50-78% of the dietary triacylglyceride molecules are hydrolised to 2 – monoacylglycerides and absorbed in this form. A portion of the released monoacylglycerides and the unsaturated fatty acids aid in the formation and stabilisation of smaller emulsion droplets while most of the monoacylglycerides and unsaturated fatty acids, together with the conjugated bile salts, sponteniously form *mixed micelles.* It is estimated that each emulsion particle gives rise to nearly 1 million micelles.

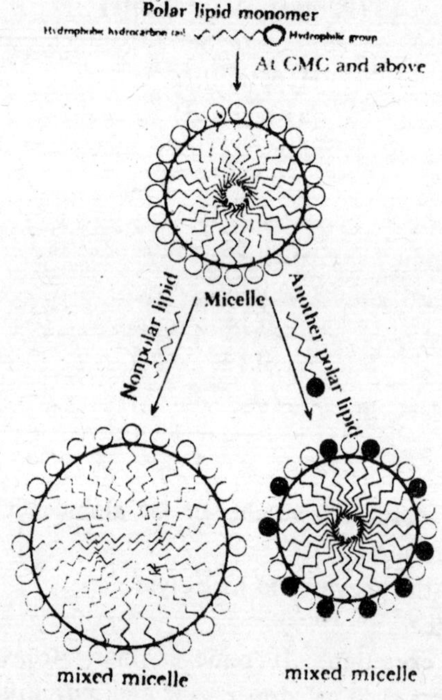

Fig. 10.26. Formation of Micelles.

Formation of Micelles & Mixed Micelles

When polar free fatty acids and or polar bile salts are present in the aqueous medium of the small intestine, these will dissolve into small extent monomerically in water. When larger quantities of these polar compounds (20-50 bile salt molecules) are introduced at a characteristic concentration known as *critical miceller concentration* (CMC), they will form *micelles* of the size between 30 to 100 Å in diameter. Upon incorporation of some other polar lipids, the same micelles become *mixed micelles*.

These tiny mixed micelles become highly dispersed in the aqueous medium of the intestinal lumen. They solubilise the non-polar fatty acids such as palmitic and stearic acids. In this

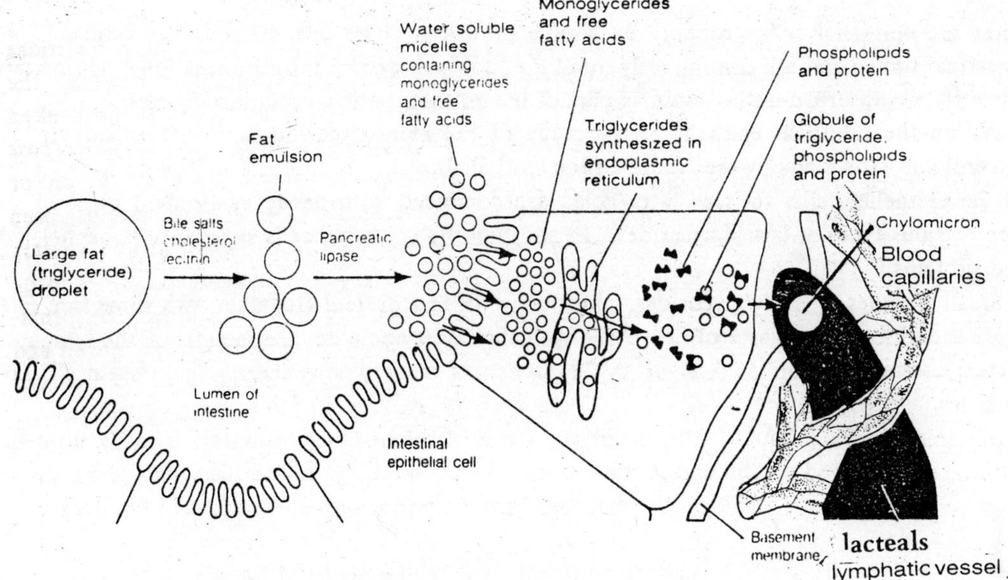

Fig. 10.27 Processes of fat digestion, absorption and chylomicron formation.

form the fatty acids and the monoglycerides are readily brought into contact with the microvilli. Each intestinal epithelial cell contains approximately 1000 microvilli which increase the surface area of the intestinal epithelial membrane by 15 to 25 fold. Monoacylglyceride and fatty acids

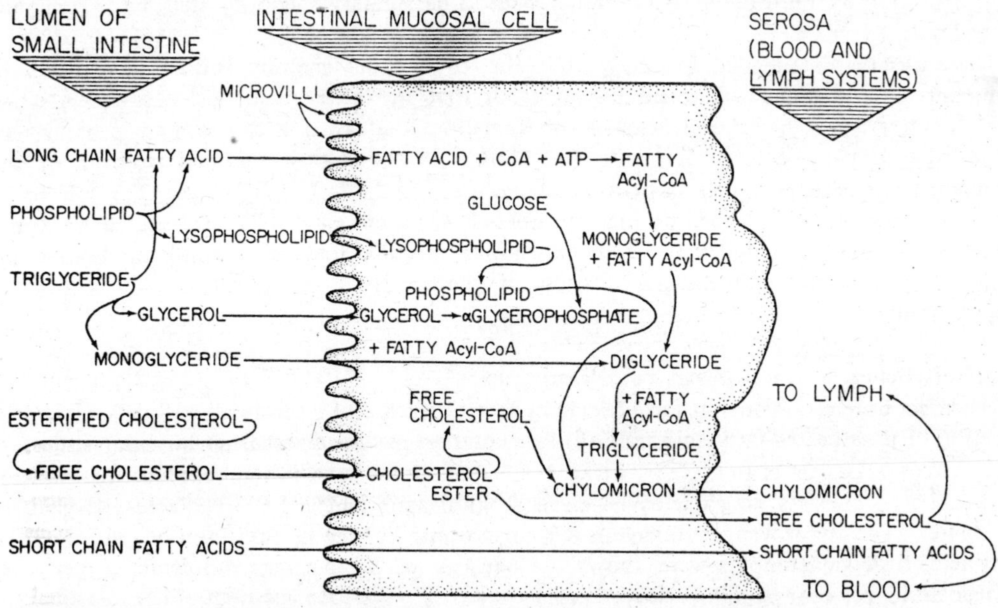

Fig. 10.28. Schematic diagram of the major conversions that occur in transport of lipids across the intestinal mucosal cell during absorption.

enter the epithelial cells probably by simple diffusion. The bile salt micelles return to the intestinal lumen and are continuously re-utilised for subsequent micell formation. Ultimately bile salts are absorbed in the ileum as part of the enterohepatic circulation process.

Within the intestinal epithelial cells, many of the monoglycerides are further digested to glycerol and fatty acids by the *lipase* of the epithelial cells. Within the endoplasmic reticulum of the epithelial cells, the free fatty acids are combined with newly synthesised glycerol and form various types of triacylglycerides. In addition the epithelial cells synthesise phospholipids and proteins.

Small globules of triacylglycerides, phospholipids, and protein (together with some free fatty acids and absorbed cholesterol) leave the epithelial cells and enter the lacteals of the lymphatic system as minute droplets known as *Chylomicrons* or very low density lipoprotein (VLDL) particles.

While free glycerol (about 22-50 percent) by virtue of being soluble in water, is easily absorbed into the portal blood system and carried to the liver. Similarly unesterified fatty acids, shorter than 10-12 carbons are also directly absorbed into the portal vein and carried to the liver.

DIGESTION AND ABSORPTION OF LIPIDS IN RUMINANTS

Until recently, little was known about the metabolism of lipids in ruminants. It is however recognised that this group of animal differed from other mammals and in particular from other herbivores in that (1) the depot fat of ruminant animals contain high levels of stearic and oleic acids, (2) presence of branched chain and odd numbered fatty acids in tissues and milk of ruminants, (3) dietary unsaturated fatty acids known to be readily assimilated into their depot fats by non-ruminants did not appear to be similarly incorporated into ruminant tissue lipids.

These observations tended to imply that the endogenous metabolism of fatty acids in ruminants differ in some fundamental ways from that in other mammals. However, when one considers that it had been known for sometime that carbohydrates and proteins are subjected to drastic bacterial fermentative changes in the highly modified stomach of the ruminants, it is perhaps a little surprising that only within the last decade or so the effects of the rumen bateria and protozoa on ingested lipids have been extensively investigated. These investigations have indicated that the aforementioned peculiar features of ruminant lipid composition are associated with the assimilation of the products of microbial modification of dietary lipids.

Effect of Rumen Microorganisms on Dietary Lipids

The effect of microorganisms includes (1) hydrolytic release of esterified fatty acids, (2) hydrogenetion of unsaturated fatty acids and (3) fermentation of free glycerol during lipolysis.

(1) HYDROLYSIS OF PLANT LIPIDS IN RUMEN. Plant lipids have a high content of galactolipids. The consists of galactosyl-1-glycerol linolenate and α-1,6, digalactosyl-1-glycerol linolinate. The glycerol sugar linkage is a β-galactosidic linkage in α-position of glycerol. The fatty acids from galactolipids were shown to consists of 96 per cent linolenic, 2 per cent linoleic and 2 per cent palmitic acid.

It has been shown that mixed microorganisms of the sheep rumen produced enzymes including galactosidases which liberate galactose from galactolipids. It has also been established that these cell free extracts of bovine rumen bacteria hydrolyses only mono and digalactosyl glycerol, indicating that hydrolysis of fatty acids must have taken place before bacterial galactosidase action.

(2) HYDROGENATION OF UNSATURATED ACIDS. The unsaturated fatty acids after their release from glycerol molecule are subjected to saturation by the microbial action. The mechanism of the reaction and the source of hydrogen is not yet known. It is possible that microbial activation of molecular hydrogen by a hydrogenase enzyme is involved. It has been found that anaerobic condition is necessary for hydrogenation and that greater activity resulted when hydrogen is in gas phase.

(3) FERMENTATION OF GLYCEROL AND GALACTOSE. Both glycerol and galactose released from lipids in the rumen are readily fermented to yield volatile fatty acids of which propionic acid is the main product of glycerol fermentation. Glycerol-fermenting bacteria isolated from sheep rumen contents were identified as *Selenomonas ruminantium* var *lactilyticus*; they did not show lipolytic activity. Galactose can be fermented by various rumen microorganisms including several bacterial species and the protozoan *Dasytricha ruminantium.* The main changes in the principal dietary lipids which are effected by microorganisms in the rumen are summarised as shown below.

All short chain fatty acids and volatile fatty acids produced from the hydrolysis and fermentation of lipids are largely absorbed through the rumen wall. Long chain fatty acids, mostly saturated are not absorbed in the rumen, so they pass along with rumen contents more or less continuously through the omasum into the true stomach or abomasum where also the dead bodies of million microorganisms reach and disintegrate before the digesta enters the small intestine. The extent of microbial lipids is not known though rough calculation indicate that the microbial lipids may provide upto 25 per cent of the total amount of fatty acids (about 12 grams per day in sheep) reaching the small intestine of sheep fed on hay and concentrates

Fate of Dietary Lipids in the Rumen

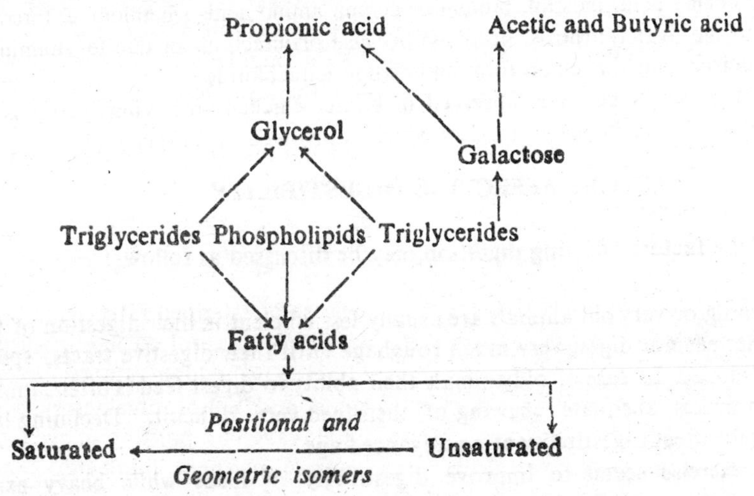

and it has also been concluded that at least 140 grams of microbial lipid per 24 hours are available for intestinal digestion by an adult cow.

Of the total fatty acids entering the duodenum and jejunum of the sheep, the proportion of free fatty acid is lower than the corresponding value of rumen contents and this is accompanied by an increase in the proportion of C_{18} unsaturated compounds as esterified condition. Such lipids could be derived from the phospholipids of the bile, tissue fluid lipoprotein, shed epithelial cells and other secretion entering the intestinal lumen.

The absorption of lipids from the small intestine involves the process of emulsification by bile and hydrolysis of lipids from microbial and other endogenous sources of (pancreatic) lipase. These are the two important steps preliminary to the production of soluble micells consisting largely of bile salts, free fatty acids and monoglycerides. These are then taken up by the microvilli of the intestinal mucosal cells and are converted into the triglyceride of chylomicra.

Hydrolysis and fermentation in the rumen result in a considerable loss of glycerol from feed lipids and so only traces of monoglycerides are normally present in the small intestine of the ruminants. The glycerol required for the synthesis of triglyceride in the intestinal mucosa is evidently almost entirely of endogenous origin.

FATTY LIVERS

Fat normally constitutes about 5% of the wet weight of the liver, but the fat content in the liver can rise to 30% or even 50% in pathologic condition. Fatty livers are a symptom of deranged fat metabolism; it may be associated with an over-production of fat in the liver and an increased transport of fat to the liver, on the one hand, or to an under-utilization of fat by the liver and a defective release of it from the liver on the other.

Fatty liver may arise from: 1. High fat or high cholesterol diet; 2. Increased liver lipogenesis due to excessive carbohydrate intake or excessive intake of certain B-vitamins (biotín, riboflavin, thiamin); 3. Increased mobilization of lipids from adipose tissue due to diabetes mellitus; 4. Hypoglycemia; 5. Increased hormone output (growth hormone, adrenal corticotrophic hormone, adrenal corticosteroids); 6. Decreased transport of lipids from liver to other tissues due to deficiencies of choline, pantothenic acid, inositol, protein or certain amino acids (methionine, threonine); 7. Cellular damage to the liver (cirrhosis, necrosis) because of infections or due to vitamin E-Se deficiency, or liver poisons such as chloroform and carbon tetrachloride.

A "fatty liver and kidney syndrome" observed in broiler chickens receiving diets based on cereals has been attributed to deficiency of biotin which is involved in fat metabolism.

FACTORS AFFECTING DIGESTIBILITY

For convenience, the factors affecting digestion may be discussed as follows:

A. Animal Effects

1. AGE. Very young or very old animals are usually less efficient in their digestion of feeds. The young can neither eat nor digest very much roughage until their digestive tracts, specially their rumens are developed. In case of old animals their ability to digest feed is often impaired by poor teeth, which makes adequate chewing of their feed very difficult. Declining health might further adversely affect digestibility at an advanced age.

2. WORK. Light exercise seems to improve digestibility of feeds while heavy exercise depresses it.

3. INDIVIDUALITY. Animals have been shown to differ in their digestion of the same kind of feed as much as 25 per cent. However, most animals vary about 4-5 per cent.

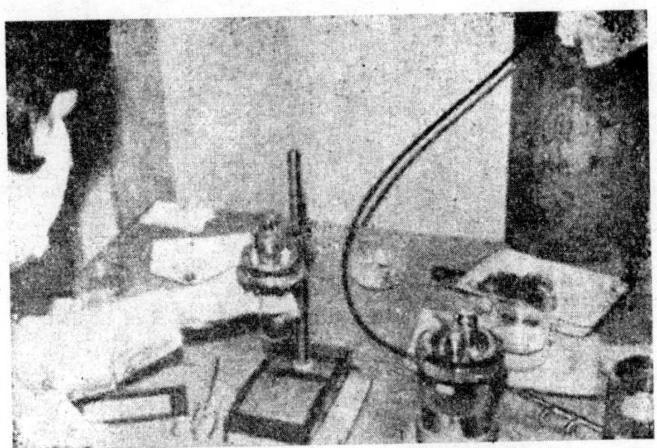

Plate 17. The assembly of feed sample in pelleted from inside the crucible of the bomb (Chapter 10).

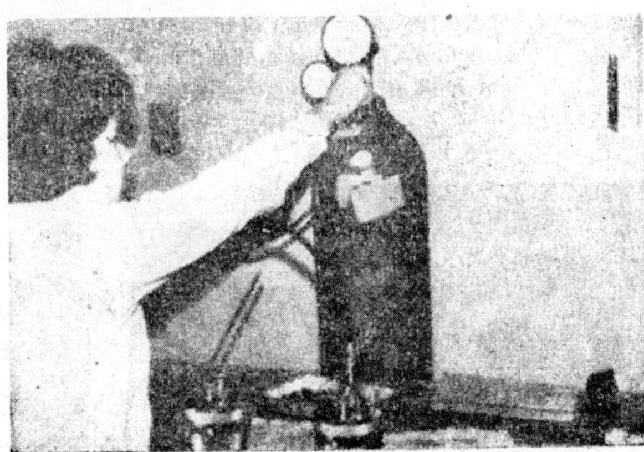

Plate 18. The inflow of oxygen gas inside the bomb as required for proper burning of the sample (Chapter 10).

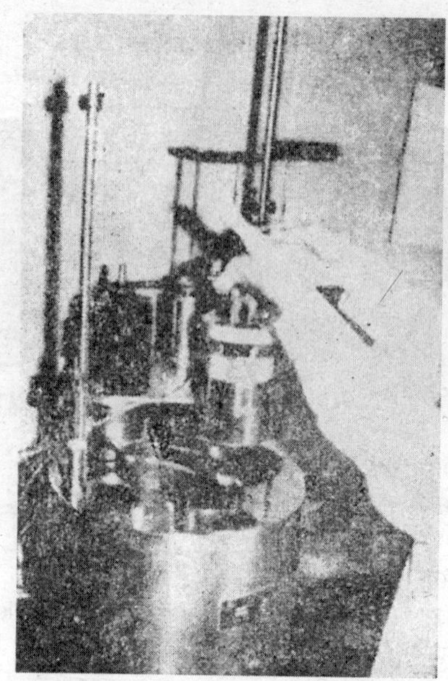

Plate 19. Placement of the bomb (sample inside) underneath the water of the insulated jacket (Chapter 10).

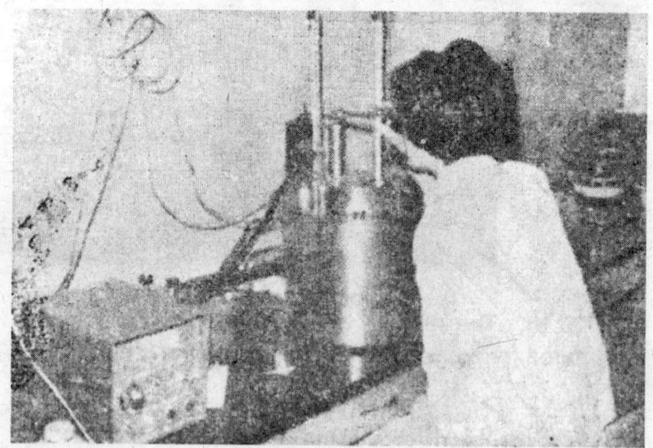

Plate 20. Rise of temperature of water as seen in the thermometer due to heat from the burning sample (Chapter 10).

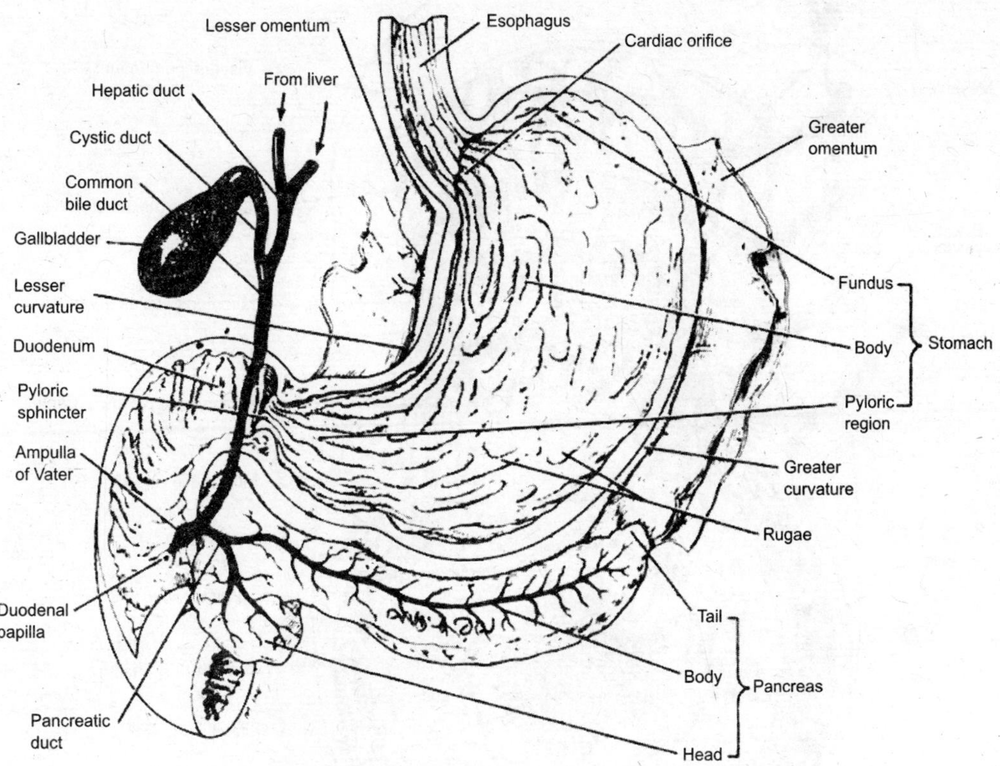

Plate 21. Frontal section of a typical memmalian monogastric stomach and duodenum showing the pancreatic and bile duct.

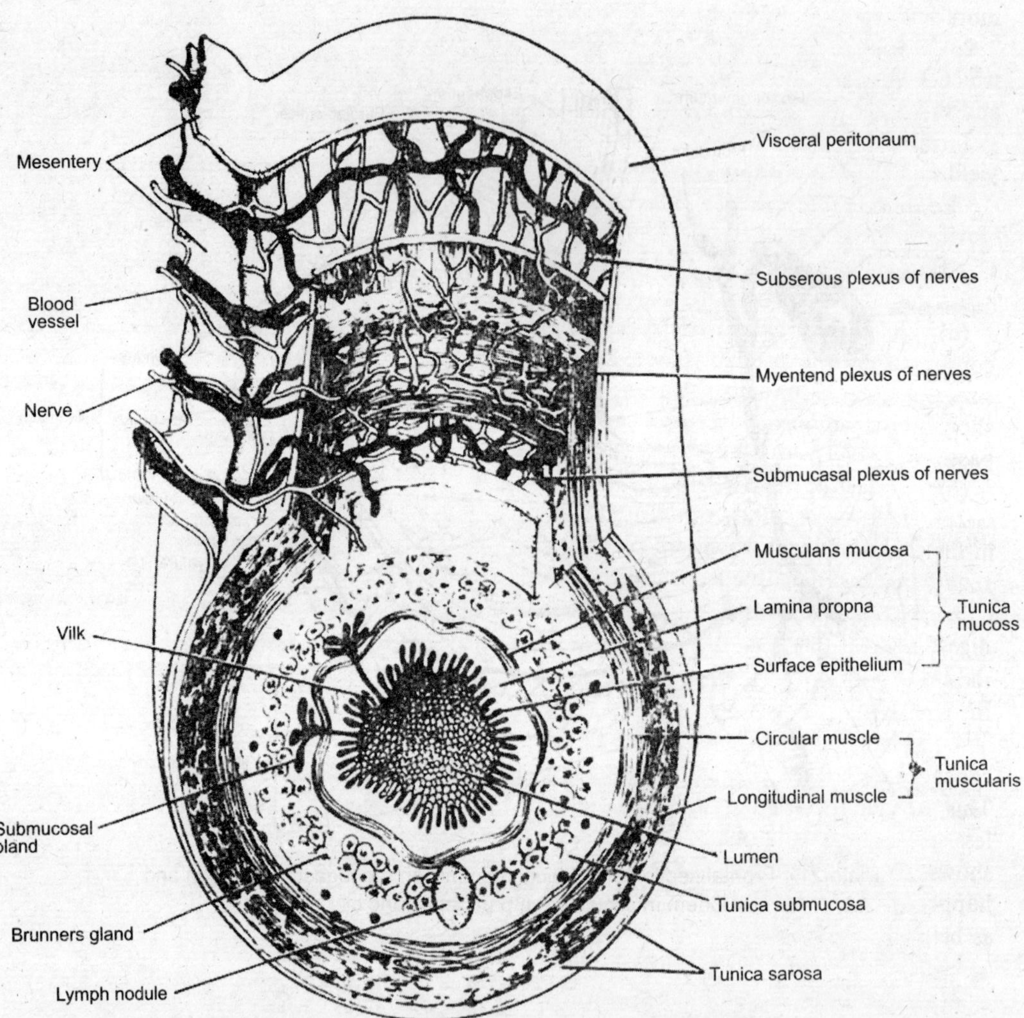

Plate 22. Representing the layers of the well of the stomach, small intestine and colon.

B. Plant Effect

1. VARIETY. Differences have been reported between varieties within the same species, i.e., two varieties of lucerne. However, there may be more actual difference in the feeding value of the two lots of the same variety of hay than there is between hay of two entirely different kinds. Thus, other factors such as soil fertility, method of harvesting, etc., are much more important than the variety.

2. STAGE OF MATURITY. Hay that is cut late has considerably lower digestibility than that which is cut early, if the early-cut hay is cured well. The percentage of protein, digestibility and the content of minerals and vitamins all decrease as hay crops advance in maturity.

3. SOIL FERTILITY BALANCE. The supply of mineral nutrients in the soil affects both the yield and the composition of forages.

4. HARVESTING. Loss of leaves, fermentation, bleaching and leaching all contribute to a lower value of hay.

C. Preparation of Feed

1. DEGREE OF FINENESS

(*a*) *Roughage.* If particle size becomes too fine, digestibility is decreased while total consumption will probably rise. The results of feeding roughage, which is of small particle size, are changes in the concentration of acetic and propionic acid produced in the rumen, as shown by consequent decreases in milk-fat percentages; probably due to increased rate of passage.

(*b*) *Grain.* If the particle size is too small, the feed is less digestible and less palatable.

2. LEVEL OF FEEDING. Increased levels of feeding result in decreased digestibility. However, in the case of animals which are kept for meat, milk or work, levels of feeding well above the requirements for maintenance are needed for production.

3. NUTRIENT BALANCE. When several feeds are fed in a ration, one feed may influence the digestibility of the other, or it gives "associative effects". For example, protein may increase the breakdown of the higher, more complex carbohydrates because of its favourable effect upon the rumen micro-organisms.

4. EFFECT OF PELLETING. Pellets or cubes are made by grinding, pressing and extruding concentrates consist of finely ground feed and/or hay or other roughage in special machines. This process reduces the bulkiness of feeds. Since a given weight of pelleted feed takes up less space, animals may eat more pelleted feed than ground feed. Review of the literature shows that the feeding of pelleted roughage does not increase digestibility. What actually happens upon consumption of ground and pelleted feed by the ruminants may be summarised as below:

1. Reduced time of prehension and mastication,
2. Less of saliva secretion,
3. Decrease in rumination,
4. Increase in rate of fermentation in the rumen,
5. Decreased in pH in the rumen,
6. Increase rate of passage of feed particles from the rumen,
7. Decrease in ratio of acetate to propionate in rumen,
8. Increase in concentration of rumen VFA one to 4 hours after feeding,
9. Increased dry matter intake,
10. Decrease in dry matter and crude fibre digestibility,
11. The finer the grinding of the forage prior to pelleting, the greater the effect.

5. TREATMENT OF STRAWS, HULLS, SAWDUST, etc., TO INCREASE DIGESTIBILITY. Products having very poor feeding value when treated by soaking, cooking, boiling, steaming with and without pressure, roasting, fermenting with yeast, hydrolysing and treating with chemicals such as NaOH, $Ca (OH)_2$, HCl, Na_2S, $NaHCO_4$ and H_2SO_4 followed by washing and drying did not appear to influence digestibility.

6. MOLASSES. May improve the palatibility of the ration, but large amounts tend to depress cellulose digestion. Levels above 7 per cent seem to depress digestibility while lower levels improve it. Most benefits will be received with lower amounts of molasses.

7. SALT AND WATER. Adequate amounts tend to favourably improve digestibility.

8. ADDITION OF ANTIBIOTICS. Feeding antibiotics to farm animals have been found to stimulate growth. The benefits have been postulated to be caused by: (*i*) the inhibition of toxin producing bacteria, (*ii*) the reduction in total numbers of intestinal bacteria and lowering of competition between host and micro flora for nutrients, and (*iii*) the selective inhibition of micro-flora permits increased growth of other micro-organisms that synthesise unidentified essential nutrients, promote digestion or detract from it. The antibiotics have not been found to exert any effect on the digestibility of dry matter, the ether extract, crude fibre or nitrogen-free extract.

D. The Following Factors, while of Less Practical Importance Have Been Observed in Laboratory Work to Affect the Digestion of Cellulose Which Comprises a Large Per Cent of Roughages

1. Ash from lucerne crops improves cellulose digestion; probably due to the presence of cobalt in the lucerne which is needed for vitamin B_{12} synthesis.
2. Many minerals in varying amounts are needed for optimum cellulose digestion, especially cobalt, phosphorus, calcium, chlorine, magnesium, sodium, potassium, sulfur and others in trace amounts.
3. Protein, in quantities up to 15 per cent of the ration, increases cellulose digestion.
4. Rumen fluid has properties which cannot be substituted in the laboratory; it improves cellulose digestion.
5. Plant enzymes, when included in the substrate, improve cellulose digestion.
6. Other factors such as urea and maize extract, stilbesterol and others have shown to be beneficial to rumen micro-organisms in the breakdown of cellulose.

What Can Be Done to Improve Digestion of Feed in the Dairy Herd?

The following ten points are suggestions which might be made to improve the quality of the feed and its digestibility, thus improving the efficiency of production on the farm. Undoubtedly there are other factors which have been overlooked.

1. The basis of selection of dairy cows should include their efficiency of digestion; however, a practical method of doing this is not readily available. If a cow is a high producer, she should provide ample profits, although she might not be quite as efficient in feed digestibility as another cow of slightly lower production.
2. Providing feed of the highest nutritive value is probably the best means of improving digestibility. One should try to:

(*a*) Test soil prior to seeding pastures and forage crops; provide the mineral balance needed by the soil.

(*b*) Use only the highest quality seed for establishing the stand: use recommended varieties and certified seed.

(*c*) Cut hay crops early when possible; while less tonnage may be received, more digestible dry matter will probably be obtained.

(*d*) Avoid excess exposure of hay to rain and sun to keep leaching, bleaching and shattering to a minimum.

(*e*) Provide adequate storage of high quality hay; keep it out of the weather.

3. If finely ground roughage is fed, such as dehydrated alfalfa pellets, it is advisable to provide at least 3-4 kg of coarse roughage to the milking cow in order to avoid butterfat depression.

4. Evaluate the quality of roughage available to the milking herd and determine the approximate amount of energy needed, which should be provided through concentrates.

5. Avoid unnecessary fine grinding of concentrates which are unpalatable and costly to grind.

6. When feeding increases amount of grain (probably 10 kg or more), observe cows individually to avoid throwing.

7. Provide ample salt and plenty of fresh water.

8. Avoid prolonged exposure of animals to adverse weather; provide shade and shelter.

9. Feed, milk and care for the herd on schedule with a reasonably quite atmosphere.

10. Use good common sense in the application of the above recommendations.

EVALUATION OF ANIMAL FEED QUALITY

The evaluation of feeds used for the nutrition of our domestic animals is a matter of very great importance. This problem, therefore, is given much emphasis in all textbooks on animal nutrition. The estimation of livestock requirements and the extent to which different feeding stuffs supply those needs are essential to the efficient feeding of millions of cattle and other animals. The criteria by which the relative values of different feeds may be assessed are:

A. Chemical Analysis

1. Proximate analysis (Weende system of feed analysis)
2. The Van Soest method of analysis.

B. Digestibility trials

1. Conventional type of digestion trial
2. In-vivo digestibility methods.

C. Estimation of energy content

1. Carbon Nitrogen balance technique
2. By bomb calorimeter
3. By calculating TDN from digestion trial
4. From chemical composition.

D. Evaluation of protein quality

(a) *For non-ruminants*

1. Protein efficiency ratio
2. Biological value (BV)
3. Net protein utilisation (NPU)

(b) *For ruminants*

1. D.C.P. estimation by digestion trial
2. Nitrogen balance experiment.

A. CHEMICAL ANALYSIS

Chemical analysis is the starting point for determining the nutritive value of any feed. The methods of chemical analysis that have been described have a history of more than 100 years. Millions of feed samples have been analysed by these methods. Thus, much data has been published on feeds expressed as crude protein, ether extract, crude fibre, ash and nitrogen-free-extract. By these methods we can have first hand information about the potentiality of the feed to fulfil the required nutrients. The procedure is simple, economic and rapid. From the results of analysis we can merely know the gross chemical composition of a feeding stuff without any idea of its efficiency of being utilised in animal system.

1. Proximate Analysis

The methods used in the analysis are called feed analysis, agricultural analysis or proximate analysis. Also since many of the techniques were first worked out at Weende, a village near the University of Goettingen in Germany, where early research in animal nutrition was conducted, it is also called Weende system.

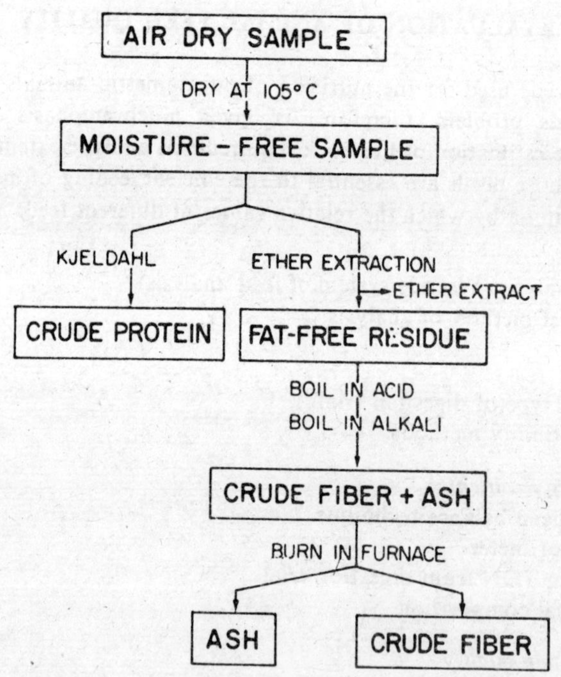

Fig. 10.29 Flow diagram for the proximate analysis.

Proximate analysis is a system for approximating the nutritive value of a feed or material for feeding purposes without actually using the feed in a feeding trial and was developed at

Weende in the middle of 1800 A.D. The principle of the analysis is to separate the feed components into groups or fractions in accordance with their feeding value. The various fractions are:

1. Water or Mo'sture
2. Crude protein
3. Ether extract
4. Crude fibre
5. Nitrogen free extract
6. Mineral matter or Ash.

The basis of the scheme is that the feedstuff contain organic and inorganic constituents. The former comprises oi carbohydrátes, crude fibre and nitrogen free extract, fats and oils, proteins and other nitrogenous compounds along with other numerous organic compounds.

The inorganic matter comprises ash composed of various minerals but the proximate analysis gives no indication about the kinds of minerals present. Rice straw contains about 16 per cent ash, but 85 per cent of this ash is silica which is of no value to the animal. On the other hand, meat and bone meals have about 30 per cent ash mainly of calcium and phosphorus which are so essential for animal body. It was originally assumed that crude fibre represented the indigestible portion of the feed material and as such was considered as non-nutritive residue. But since the crude fibre is partially digestible in herbivora, this assumption has been proved to be wrong.

Further, the nitrogen-free-extract includes pentosans and small amount of other complex polysaccharides along with some soluble lignin which are by no means completely digestible, thus overestimates the digestibility of nitrogen-free-extract.

Table 10.52

The fractions of proximate analysis

Procedure	*Fraction*	*Major components*
Drying at approximately 100°C to constant weight	Moisture	Water and any other vo'atile compounds
Ignite at 500°C to 600°C	Ash	Mineral elements
N_2 by Kjeldhal digestion	Crude protein	Proteins, amino acids, Non-protein N_2
Extraction with pet. ether	Ether extract	Fats, oils, waxes
Residue after boiling with acid and alkali	Crude fibre	Cellulose, hemicellulose, lignin
Remainder; i.e., 100 minus sum of the other fractions	N-free extract	Starch, sugars, some cellulose, hemicellulose and some lignin.

Table 10.53

Limitations of the proximate analysis

Component	*Supposed to contain*	*Contains*	*Missing*	*Excess*
Crude Fibe	I- brous matter	Cellulose, part of lignin	Hemicellulose, part of Lignin and acid insoluble ash	None
Nitrogen-free-extract	Soluble carbo-hydrates	Soluble carbo-hydrates, hemi-cellulose, part of lignin and acid insoluble ash	None	Hemicellulose, Lignin and Acid insoluble ash
Ether extract	Crude fat (fats, oils and fatty acids)	Free fats, oils and fatty acids, chloro-phyll, sterols, antho-cyanin, carotinoids	Protein, Pıotein bound lipid	Chlorophyll, Sterol, Anatho-Cyamins, waxes etc.

Another reason the so-called proximate analysis is not adequate as it does not include many chemical factors that are important in feeding to-day. The ash gives no indication of the chemical elements in it, yet the chemical elements in the ash must be known as the deficiency of any essential mineral element will cause failure in proper animal feeding. The method also does not include vitamins. Some of the vitamins can be determined chemically, rest biologically by microbiological assay.

Because of such limitations of Weende system or proximate analysis, numerous workers over the past several years have been suggested various other procedures particularly for a logical separation of feed carbohydrates. Among them in 1938 Crampton and Maynard suggested a procedure for grouping carbohydrates of feed into cellulose, pentosans and lignin. In 1953 Ely *et al.*, proposed that the grouping of cellulose and hemicellulose as holocellulose would provide a useful parameter of digestibility. None of the above modifications were successful in predicting the total carbohydrate digestibility than the crude fibre originally suggested in Weende system.

The procedure which has recently received wide consideration as a possible substitute for the conventional crude fibre determination is that of P. J. Van Soest of Cornell in U.S.A.

2. Van Soest Method

Dr. P.J. Van Soest in 1965 developed a method which makes use of the concept that the dry matter of plant origin consists of two principal parts: *Cell wall* and *Cell contents.* Thus the method has become highly efficient to take care of the defects in the principle of estimating crude fibre and NFE by proximate analysis.

Plant cell contents consist of sugars, starch, soluble carbohydrates, pectin, non-protein nitrogen, protein, lipids and miscellaneous other water-soluble materials, including minerals and several vitamins. True digestibility is almost complete, averaging 98 per cent.

The cell walls of feeds of plant origin are not uniformly nutritious, in the sense that their principal components consist of cellulose, hemicellulose, silica, lignin, etc., singly or in such combinations as nitrogen-hemicellulose or lignocellulose and differ widely in nutrition availability depending on the kind and maturity of the plant as well as on the age and species of the animal fed. Nitrogen-hemicellulose are not at all digestible.

B. DIGESTIBILITY TRIAL

1. Conventional Type of Digestion Trial

A digestion trial involves an experiment by which the amount of nutrients actually digested and absorbed from a measured amount of feed consumed by an animal is determined.

The accurate feeding of weighed amounts of thoroughly mixed rations or individual feeds and the collection of the excreta of farm animals without any loss are important in conducting digestion trials.

Digestibility trials are conducted with animals in specially designed stalls and the series of operations may be compared roughly with the keeping of a banking account. It is obviously not possible to measure directly the amount of food that is digested, and the method adopted, therefore, is to measure the amount of food materials which the animal eats on the one hand and the excreta purged out on the other hand. The difference between the two tells us how much of the different parts of the food have been digested for further utilisation of the animal body.

The ability to utilise the nutrients of different feed varies in different species of animals because of their anatomical and physiological differences in the digestive tract. This is more pronounced in case of roughages. The ruminants have great power of utilising roughages while omnivorous and carnivorous have less of such power.

In animal nutrition when we speak of digestible nutrients, we mean the difference between the amounts of each nutrient in the feed and the faeces, that is the portion of a nutrient which is digested and taken into the body. The term is usually applied only to proteins, carbohydrates and fats. The digestion coefficient of a nutrient may then be defined as the percentage consumed in the ration which does not appear in the faeces. It is an expression of how much of each nutrient has disappeared during the passage of the feed through the digestive tract as a result of chemical reactions between feed ingredients, action of enzymes and other chemicals secreted from the animal body or by micro-organisms, and the physical action.

Digestibility of ash is not usually determined as it does not contribute to the energy content of a feed. Moreover, much of the ash in faeces is not undigested feed ash. The faeces are a pathway for the excretion of minerals from the body—minerals that have already been absorbed and which may already have served a purpose within the body. A digestion coefficient for ash, therefore, has no real meaning.

Techniques

Total Collection Method

(A) Direct Method

By this method, experimental animals are generally fed one type of feed stuff of roughage to know the amount of digestible nutrients present in it. The accurate feeding of weighed amount of thoroughly mixed individual feed and the collection of the excreta of farm animals without loss are vital for the conduction of such digestion experiments. In this regard there are eleven salient points which a beginner should know before taking up the experiment.

1. Work to do Before the Experiment. The first essential step in properly outlining an investigation is to acquire as complete a knowledge as possible of the previous research on the specific subject by a thorough study of the literature. It would be desirable after reading the literature to discuss it with others who might have got experience in this field.

After having a good background for the work to be done, one should prepare clear, accurate, comprehensive and detailed plans of the specific investigation which has been selected and may include (1) the precise descriptive name of the research project that is to be done, (2) location or locations of the work, (3) co-operating institutions or departments, (4) objective of the research, (5) names of persons participating, (6) introduction or justification for doing these experiments including a brief review of the literature, (7) the procedure: a description in simple, direct language of precisely what is proposed to be done.

2. Selection of Experimental Animals. In determining the digestibility of a feed of any class of livestock, the usual procedure is to select several animals (depending upon the species) for digestion trial. It is usually desirable that all experimental animals should be of similar breed, type, size or weight condition and age. It is preferable if they are of the same sex and that all animals used in the same experiment should have been produced in the same herd as by this they will probably have had the same pre-experimental treatment.

It is advantageous to have the animals which are castrated males except for those involving in milk production or in other female functions.

It is important that the animals for digestion experiments should be thriving, vigorous and with good appetites. So far as age is concerned, it is recommended that young adult animals or growing animals approaching maturity be used because they usually eat and perform better than those of other ages. Regarding number of experimental animals, it may be assumed that smaller the species, (sheep, goat, poultry) larger may be included for each treatment but for cattle this is not practically possible and it is said that not less than three animals should be used in each lot. If possible six animals should be used as a general convention for each treatment.

After selecting the animals, they should be clipped, dipped, drenched for internal parasites, vaccinated against such contagious diseases as may be necessary, have their feet trimmed, be ear tagged or otherwise marked, and individually weighed before they are put on experiment. It is believed that infestation with internal parasites often tends to decrease digestibility in sheep.

3. Preparation of Apparatus. The strictest attention is essential to such matters as the cleanliness of all apparatus and equipment and the sanitary conditions of the stall, surroundings and animals before and during the progress of the experiment. Scales and balances, in particular, should be checked up thoroughly. The following steps should be taken regarding balances.

1. On the day prior to weighing, remove any water that may have collected in the scale pit.
2. Clean all moving parts on the underside of the scale. Check weight marker bar and sliding indicator.
3. By placing exact weight on platform balances, check the accuracy of the balance. During the weighing operation, balance scale (set scale at zero) before each animal enters the scale box.

4. **Metabolic Stall or Crate.** A metabolism crate is actually a specially designed stall or box large enough for the experimental animal to house in controlled condition during experimental period. Here the animal enjoys freedom of movement, particularly as regards lying down and getting up. It is so designed to permit the collection of faeces and urine separately under it. In older type, the bottom is a metal grid or mesh of metal rods through which both the faeces and urine pass, the faeces being caught on a screen underneath and below the latter is a metal hopper or funnel like subfloor to catch the urine. In the type now more commonly used, the animal is confined so that he cannot turn around, and the length of the cage is adjusted to the size of the animal in such a way that the faeces fall into a properly placed container. The feed box is attached to the front, so constructed and placed as to prevent scattering. In order to avoid feed lodging at the corners of the feed trough, the bottoms of the metal boxes should be rounded at the sides; the side toward the steer (a young castrated ox) being set at a slight angle with the vertical and the edges of the box flanged to extend just beyond the wooden framework, if any. The bottom of each feed box, if of metal, should be made of one continuous piece of smooth sheet metal to eliminate joints or corners where feed may accumulate. Thus very little or no feed may be lost.

The crate may be made more portable by putting it on large castors or on 4 wheels.

In absence of any metabolic stall or crate, ordinary barn may be adapted to use for digestion experiments with minor modifications in relation to manger and faeces collection arrangement. Regarding manger, it may be mentioned that these are much larger than is common in dairy barns, made to hold large amounts of bulky feeds without spilling. The floor of the manger is sloped so that the last traces of feed remain within reach of even dwarf type of cattle. Care should be taken to prevent crevices on which feed might collect. The high cement walls between stall, 1.8 meters high in front at the mangers, prevents cows from stealing feed from their neighbours. So far as the faeces collection is concerned, it may be done either manually, whereby watchman or attendants collect the faeces behind the animals throughout the collection period. For this, at least 3 persons are to be engaged @ 8 hours per day to look after six animals for each 24 hours. Alternatively, faeces collection can also be made by using a faeces collection bag specially made for this purpose.

5. **Animal Comfort.** The comfort of the animal should be one of the factors to be considered in deciding the method to be followed for collection of faeces. One must decide which makes an animal uncomfortable: a harness strapped here and there to hold a faeces bag and then supporting the weight of the faeces bag as it fills during the day, or small stall limiting the cow's movement enough so that the faeces will fall into a pan or box placed behind it.

An essential feature of metabolism cages is that the animal must have some freedom of movement, particularly with regard to lying down and getting up. If a stanchion or a stall is so rigid as to make it difficult for cattle to lie down and get up, fatigue may result.

Good ventilation is a must for the animals. Although giving cows exercise has not been shown to influence the digestibility of feed nutrients directly by giving an opportunity to stretch the muscles during confinement at the stall will definitely lead to comfort of the animals and thereby normal metabolism will be maintained. Of course, for animals used for digestion trial if exercise is given, all care must be taken to prevent the animals from grabbing a mouthful of grass from elsewhere and no excreta should be lost. During the time of exercise, watchmen should always accompany with pails to catch any excreta.

Care should always be taken to prevent animals from the botheration of excessive flies or mosquitoes. To prevent slipping, the floors if made of concrete snould be roughened slightly during construction.

6. Feed Consumption and Residual Feed. Accurate control to obtain unvarying intake of feed from the preliminary period through the collection period is essential for the accuracy of digestion trials. When the animals refuse to eat part of the feed assigned to them, this introduces uncontrolled factors for variation in obtaining uniform results. There are various practices that may help to avoid residual feed, refused feed, weigh backs or orts, as they are called.

(i) Healthy, thrifty young animals that have good appetites are less likely to refuse feed.

(ii) Thorough mixing of moderate size, grinding and pelleting prevents animals from picking out and refusing the coarser portions of hays and other roughages.

(iii) Increasing molasses from 5-15% improves palatibility (not in chicks).

(iv) Addition of selected antibiotics have shown to influence the palatibility in some species. Similarly, certain natural and artificial flavour may increase feed intake of young pigs as much as 35 per cent.

Addition of any additives should depend on the type of technical programme.

One technique to get rid of most of the residual feed is that during the preliminary periods, feed intake should be regularised in such a way that very little or nothing is left as residual feed.

Inspite of all efforts, there remains always some residual feed in some animals during the collection period. A short guide line in respect to handling of orts is discussed below:

(i) In some investigations the waste from one feeding, either in its natural condition or after drying and grinding, are consumed by the experimental animals, if mixed with the next meal.

(ii) It has also been suggested that the waste feed that is unfit to be eaten should be added to the faeces to determine the digestible nutrients. From the strictly economic view point. this would certainly be correct, but if the purpose is to make a purely physiological study and to obtain the digestibility of the nutrients eaten, the usual method of deducting the nutrients in the feed refused from those in the feed offered to determine the amount of each nutrient actually eaten is to be preferred.

(iii) In most of the digestion experiments it is a common practice to clean out the feed through every day and any appreciable amount of orts removed before the next feed is offered. While removing the residual feed of individual animals is preserved in air dry condition for the entire collection period. At the end of this period, a representative sample from each individual collection is analysed for the nutritive value. Once it is known, the total amount of nutrients rejected by the individual animals can also be ascertained for the total quantity of the residual feed of individual animal. This is done as the residual feed mostly differs significantly from the feed offered by virtue of being more coarse or dirty. The individual nutrient content of the refused feed is deducted from the amount of the same nutrient in the feed offered. The refused feed is often higher in ash because of the dirt that the animal does not eat. Refused feed may also contain more fibre because of uneaten stems. Also, it is often lower in protein and nitrogen free-extract than the portion consumed.

7. Preliminary Periods. It is essential that the collection period of a digestion experiment be preceeded by a preliminary period of several days in which the same feed to be investigated is fed in the same weighed amounts daily as in the collection period. This is for the purpose of removing all residues of the previous feed and also of establishing as uniform a rate of passage of feed products and excretion of faeces as practicable, relative to feed intake.

Kellner stated that a preliminary period of at least five days should be allowed for ruminants. Later workers specified that the experimental animals should be subjected to a preliminary feeding of 7 to 10 days for horses and swine while for ruminants it may vary between 10–12 days. During this period feeding of the experimental feed must be of the same quantity as during the experimental period to follow.

It is known that the rumen microbial population are affected both in types and numbers by the kind of ration fed. At the time of drastic change in ration, consiberable time may be required for the kinds of micro-organisms to become stabilised to the new environment so that a more suitable microflora may develop for the efficient digestion of the experimental feed.

Maynard observed that when the amounts of hay and silage fed to dairy cows were generally identical in preliminary and collection periods as in transition periods and when the grain mixtures were little changed, short preliminary periods before collecting excreta were adequate. In experiments in which the ratio of roughage to concentrate is kept constant and only the amount of protein varies, a preliminary period of 7 days may be adequate.

Recent trend is in favour of three periods instead of the conventional two periods, one preliminary and the other for collection as follows:

1. *Period of adjustment.* This might also be termed as a preparatory, ad-libitum, adaptation, pre-experimental subperiod, change over period or period of acclimatisation. During this period the animals become accustomed to the feed, and the level at which each individual will eat is regulated. During the period the experimental animals may not be put into digestion stalls or metabolic crates, but the arrangement should be such that a careful record may be kept of the amount of feed eaten by each individual. The period may continue for 7 days or longer as needed.

2. *Preliminary period.* During this period amount of feed offered is important as it must be continued without any variation throughout this and the collection period which follows.

3. *Collection period.* The third and last period. The details in this period are discussed in the following section.

8. **Collection Periods.** After allowing the number of days that have been decided upon to continue as a preliminary period, the collection of the faeces is begun and continued throughout the collection period. The faeces obtained during the period is assumed to be from a uniform amount of feed consumed during the same number of days.

Using longer collection periods lengthens the risk period wherein accident, animal sickness, feed refusal or other disturbing circumstances may affect results significantly and might necessitate repeating the trial. Shortening the collection period, on the other hand, may also give rise to inaccuracies due to the inability to make faeces collections that are as correctly representative of the digestibility in quantity and/or chemical composition as might possibly be obtained from a longer collection period. While the brightest possible accuracy is the aim, the factors of time, labour, expense and other considerations are important in deciding the length of the collection period to obtain greater accuracy.

The length of collection periods necessary depends upon the species; longer periods being necessary in the case of herbivores, especially ruminants, than for other animals because of variability in daily faeces excretion. In general a collection period of 7–10 days for ruminants is acceptable to most.

Recently, some experts recommended that following adequate adjustment and preliminary periods, two one-week collection periods in succession, be conducted. Sample should be composited separately and chemical analysis done for each week. The data may then be calculated both by weeks and for a full 14–day collection period for the sake of comparison. Such a plan gives an excellent opportunity for checking one week against the other or the data from only the second week may be used if it appears that the first collection period should be considered as an additional preliminary period.

The days of each complete experiment may be numbered. For instance, days 1 to 14 may be designated as the adjustment period, days 15–21, the preliminary period and days 22 to 28 and 29 to 35 as collection periods.

9. Faeces Markers. With non-ruminants the time of first appearance of faeces resulting from the feeding of experimental feed can be detected if any marker is mixed-up with the feed. A good marker must have the following qualities, (1) distinctly mark the faeces resulting from the feed with which the marker was fed; (2) be insoluble and unable to be absorbed through intestine; (3) have no toxic, laxative, costive or other physiological effect on the experimental subject; (4) not contain or react with the nutrient or nutrients under investigation.

Lampblack (soot, carbon); carmine: methylene blue; ferric oxide; chromic oxide; barium sulfates; copper sulfate; bismuth subcarbonate, purple green and yellow cellophane; all of which render colour to faeces have been tried. Some have been used more extensively than others. Carmine is in use for the longest time and is favoured by some workers because of its intense red colour. In powder form, 0.25 to 1.00 gram of carmine may be mixed with the first food of an experimental period to have a distinct colour of the faeces.

With ruminants the use of markers does not result in a clear separation of the faeces because there is no marking of the beginning and end of the period. The contents of the digestive tract of ruminants do not pass through its length in the same order in which they were consumed in the feed. Markers are thus not at all satisfactory with ruminants.

10. Preparing Faeces Samples. At the end of each 24 hour collection period, faeces from individual animals are first weighed and then sampled for analysis. A 5 per cent aliquot is the amount that is most frequently kept aside as sample. With pigs, sheep or other small animals, since there is less faeces than with cattle, all or major portion of the faeces may be stored until the end of the collection period.

Usually faeces are preserved in cans, polythelene bags or in wide mouth glass jars with air tight covers. The daily samples are then labelled and if possible, stored in quick-freeze at minus 16 to 20°C until needed for making composite samples for the entire period. At the end of collection period the daily samples of faeces are brought from the refrigerator and the temperature is raised up to laboratory temperature. After that the containers, each with either one day's full amount of faeces for one animal or with a given percentage of faeces, are removed from refrigeration, weighed and finally combined to make a single composite sample for one animal for one collection period and a composite sample representing the faeces for the entire collection period is taken for analysis. From the aliquot portions two samples are taken, one larger portion for drying and the other for analysis in the fresh condition, mainly for protein estimation.

Faeces to be preserved should be free from automicrobiat (including mould) fermentation. Also care should be taken to prevent or reduce the loss of nitrogen as ammonia in drying. For these two reasons when faeces are to be dried, a mixture of HCl and alcohol should be used for preservation of faeces. H_2SO_4 at 3 per cent concentration is also a common preservator. Among other reagents, toluene, formaldehyde, thymol are all in use. Approximately 5 g of finely-ground thymol is enough for preserving daily sample of faeces under ordinary condition.

If refrigeration facilities are limited, sample should straight away be put into drier. The evidence appears to favour quick drying at 90°C to 100°C instead of low temperature for longer times whereby nutrieat losses tends to be greater. The dried samples should then be exposed to the open air (put the containers on laboratory working table covering them with net to prevent rats from stealing some of the sample) at the ordinary tempeature for 4-5 days.

After drying and equilibrating with air humidity, weigh the air dried sample. Grind them thoroughly; put the samples into tight receptacles and keep them in cold storage if possible.

It is always preferable to estimate the nitrogen content of the fresh faeces (composite sample for the entire collection period) before drying but do all other analyses on the usual air dry samples.

11. Calculation of Digestibility. In digestibility experiments, attempts are made to find out the digestibility coefficient of the food as a whole or some constituents of the food. The digestibility coefficient may be defined as the percentage of the total amount consumed which is digested and absorbed. The usual calculation of the digestion coefficient (DC) can be shown in an equation as follows,

$$\text{DC of Nutrient} = \frac{\text{kg. nutrient eaten} - \text{kg. in faeces}}{\text{kg. nutrient eaten}} \quad 100$$

The above formula is useful whenever there is no residual feed. The usual formula for the calculation of DC in which the nutrient in the residual feed is deducted from the feed offered is as follows:

$$\text{DC of nutrient} = \frac{(\text{kg. nutrient offered} - \text{kg. nutrient refused}) - \text{kg. nutrient in faeces}}{\text{kg. nutrient offered} - \text{kg. nutrient refused}} \times 100$$

Computations are made independently for each experimental animal and the average coefficient is then calculated. It has now become customary to report coefficient of the entire organic matter in the feed or ration along with usual coefficients of crude protein, crude fibre, nitrogen free extract and ether extract. Further, increasingly the digestion coefficient of the energy are being determined routinely whenever digestion experiments are conducted,

The data needed for calculating the DC are: (1) the chemical composition of feed eaten, (2) the chemical composition of the faeces, (3) the weight of the feed eaten, and (4) the weight of the faeces excreted.

Example No. 1

A bullock was fed on an average 4.0 kg of hay per day for three weeks. Over the experimental period of 7 days the animal excreted an average weight of 5.8 kg. Samples of the hay and the faeces were found to contain the percentages of composition as in Table No. 10.54 Find out the digestible coefficient of each nutrient and also the TDN per cent.

Four kg of hay actually contain 3.36 kg of dry matter while 5.8 kg of faeces contain 1.45 kg of dry matter.

The difference 1910 gram, which did not appear in the faeces, is regarded as having been digested by the bullock. This amount is 56.84 per cent of the 3360 gm of the dry matter eaten. It is said, then, that the digestion coefficient of the dry matter of the hay was 56.84. In

Table 10.54

Chemical composition of feed and faeces

(Fresh basis)

	Hay (%)	*Faeces (%)*
Moisture	16.00	75.00
Ash	6.00	2.00
Crude protein	12.57	3.22
Crude fibre	27.78	9.50
NFE	35.15	9.74
Ether extract	2.50	0.54
	100.00	100.00

the same way the percentage digestibility of each nutrient may be computed as shown in Table 10.55

Table 10.55

Digestion trial with hay

Daily average	*Dry matter (gm)*	*Crude protein (gm)*	*Crude fibre (gm)*	*Nitrogen free extract (gm)*	*Ether extract (gm)*
a. 4.00 kg hay	3360	502.80	1,111.2	1,406.00	100.00
b. In faeces	1450	186.76	551.0	564.92	31.32
c. Digested	1910	316.04	560.20	841.08	68.68
d. Digestion coefficient	56.84	62.85	50.41	59.82	68.68

Computation of Digestible Nutrients and of TDN. Digestible nutrients are also calculated on the fresh basis directly by multiplying the percentage of each nutrient by its digestion coefficient and as the result is expressed as the kilogram of digestible nutrient per 100 kg of feed, the entire equation is further divided by 100 as below:

$$\text{per cent Digestible Nutrient} = \text{per cent Nutrient} \times \frac{\text{Digestion coefficient of the Nutrient}}{100}$$

Using the data from the same digestion experiment with hay in bullocks, the digestible nutrients may be calculated as in Table .10.56

Table 10.56

	Composition % on fresh (*a*)	*Digestion coeffieient* (*b*)	*Per cent digestible nutrients* $a \times \frac{b}{100}$
Crude protein	12.57	62.85	7.90
Crude fibre	27.78	50.41	14.00
NFE	35.15	59.82	21.02
Ether extract	2.50	68.68	1.71
Dry matter	84.00	56.84	47.74

The total digestible nutrients (TDN) express the relative energy values of feeds. The calculation of TDN can now easily be made from the above Table keeping in view one more factor that 2.25 is to be multiplied with the amount of digestible ether extract because of the greater caloric value of fat which is 2.25 times more than carbohydrates or protein on unit basis

T.D.N = per cent digestible protein + per cent digestible NFE + per cent digestible crude fibre + (per cent digestible ether extract × 2 25)

$$= 7.90 + 21.02 + 14.00 + 1.71 \times 2.25$$
$$= 46.76$$

Digestibility by Difference. The method described previously is the direct method of digestion trial. In it the digestibility of most of the roughages can be found out, but with concentrates, the above method is unsuitable as concentrates fail to supply the required bulk in ruminants. The digestibility of the concentrates in such cases is found out by the method of difference. In this method digestibility of a roughage is found out first and then the concentrate mixture is added to the roughage for a second trial. The coefficient of a digestibility of the concentrate is found out by subtracting the figures obtained for the roughage alone from the figures obtained in the combined ration. The figures thus obtained may not be very accurate, as the method does not eliminate the associate action of different feeds.

Example No. 2

Find out the digestible coefficient of maize when fed to the same bullock along with same hay in the example no. 1 given in the previous section. The bullock received 4.0 kg of same hap per day along with 4.2 kg of ground maize. The average daily excretion of faeces on this mixed ration was 8.5 kg. The composition of maize ana the faeces are given in next page.

The digestible matter contained in the total ration, computed exactly like the previous example, as is shown in the first five lines (a to e) of Table 10.58. If it is assumed that the digestibility of hay (line f) was unaltered by the addition of the maize grain, it is possible to compute how much of each kind of digestible matter (protein, crude fibre, NFE and fat) in the total ration was derived from the hay, that is amount of per cent digestible nutrient in the feed. As suggested earlier, this is done by multiplying the digestion coefficient with per cent nutrient of the feed and then by dividing the entire result by 100. The remainder (line g), therefore, must have come from the maize grain (line b), and by comparison with the total amounts present in the later, the precentage digestibility (line h) or digestion coefficient of the maize is computed. The value of line f are deducted from the total digested (line e) to estimate the amount digested from the maize. The later (line g) divided by the grams of each nutrient in the maize eaten (line b), expressed as a percentage is the digestion coefficient of each nutrient. These are shown in the last line (h).

Computation of TDN of Maize

For finding out TDN, it is necessary to first calculate the value of per cent digestible nutrients of maize as below:

$$\text{Per cent Digestible nutrient} = \frac{\text{Digestible coefficient} \times \text{per cent nutrient present in maize}}{100}$$

$$\text{Per cent Digestible Crude protein} = \frac{71.76}{100} \times 9.65 = 6.924 \text{ per cent}$$

$$\text{Per cent Digestible Crude fibre} = \frac{98.12}{100} \times 1.9 = 1.864 \text{ per cent}$$

Table 10.57

Composition of Maize and Faeces (fresh basis)

	Maize grain	*Faeces*
Water	12.75	80.95
Ash	1.20	1.75
Crude protein	9.65	3.55
Crude fiber	1.90	6.50
NFE	70.85	6·75
Ether Extract	3.65	0.50
	100.00	100·00

Table 10.58

The digestibility of maize by difference

Daily average	*Dry matter (gm)*	*Crude protein (gm)*	*Crude fiber (gm)*	*N-free extract (gm)*	*Ether extract (gm)*
a. 4 kg hay	3360.0	502.80	1111.2	1406.0	100.00
b. 4.2 kg maize	3664.5	405.30	79.8	2975.7	153.30
c. Hay+Maize (a+b)	7024.5	908.10	1191.0	4381.7	253.30
d. Total faeces	1619.25	301.75	552.5	573.75	42.50
e. Total digested (c—d)	5405.25	606.35	638.5	3807.95	210.80
f. Estimated digested from hay based on % digestible nutrients*	1910.00	315.50	560.20	841.08	68.68
g. Calculated digested from maize (e—f)	3495.25	290.85	78.30	2966.87	142.12
h. Digestion coefficient of maize (g/b×100)	95.38	71.76	98.12	99.70	92.70

*The % digestible dry matter along with other digestible nutrients have already worked in example 1 under Direct Method. Those data have been utilised here since the hay used in this case is the same.

$$\text{Per cent Digestible NFE} = \frac{99.70}{100} \times 70.85 = 70.64 \text{ per cent}$$

$$\text{Per cent Digestible Ether Extract} = \frac{92.70}{100} \times 3.65 = 3.38 \text{ per cent}$$

$$\text{Per cent TDN of Maize is} = 6.924 + 1.864 + 70.64 + (3.38 \times 2.25) = 87.03$$

(B) Indicator Method

In recent years an indirect method of digestion trial has been developed. It is less time consuming and the result obtained has a clear correspondence with that obtained in the conventional method. In this method an indicator is used alone with the feed to be tested. By determining the ratio of the concentration of the indicator to that of a given nutrient in the feed and the same ratio in the faeces resulting from feed, the digestibility of the nutrient can be obtained without measuring either the feed intake or faeces output. This is done as follows:

$$\text{Faecal Dry Matter (DM)} = \frac{\text{Amount of Indicator ingested (mg/day)}}{\text{Indicator in faeces (mg/gm DM)}}$$

The digestibility of the DM in a diet can be computed as follows:

$$\textit{Indigestibility of DM (per cent)} = 100\left[\frac{\text{Indicator in diet (per cent)}}{\text{Indicator in faeces (per cent)}}\right]$$

Then, digestibility of DM (per cent) = 100 – Per cent Indigestibility of DM.

The digestibility of a specific nutrient can be computed as follows:

Digestibility per cent of a nutrient

$$= 100 - \left(100 \times \frac{\text{per cent indicator in feed}}{\text{per cent indicator in faeces}} \times \frac{\text{per cent nutrient in faeces}}{\text{per cent nutrient in feed}}\right)$$

A variety of substances have been employed as indicators such as chromic oxide (Cr_2O_3), lignin, plant pigments, indigestible nitrogen, polyethylene, glycol etc.

An ideal indicator should have the following qualities:

1. Totally indigestible
2. Pass through the tract at a uniform rate
3. Readily determined chemically.

The following criteria are expressions of digestibility:

1. Digestible DM (gm.) = DM intake (gm.) – DM in faeces (gm.)
2. $\text{Digestible DM (per cent)} = \frac{\text{DM intake} - \text{DM in faeces}}{\text{DM intake}} \times 100$
3. TDN (gm.) = (DM intake × Chem. comp.) – (DM in faeces × Chem. comp.).
4. $\text{TDN (per cent)} = \frac{(\text{DM intake} \times \text{Chem. comp.}) - (\text{DM in faeces} \times \text{Chem. comp.})}{\text{DM intake}} \times 100$
5. DE (kcal) = Energy intake (kcal) – Energy in faeces (kcal)
6. $\text{DE (per cent)} = \frac{\text{Energy intake} - \text{Energy in faeces (kcal)}}{\text{Energy intake (kcal)}} \times 100$

Abbreviation used above: DM = dry matter; TDN = total digestible nutrients; DE = digestible energy; kcal = Kilocalorie.

2 In Vivo Digestibility Methods

(i) NYLON OR DACRON BAG TECHNIQUE. The nylon bag techniques require placing of dried samples in bags made of an indigestible material such as nylon, dacron or silk which are then tightly tied. These bags are placed inside the rumen through the opening of fistulae by a veriety of techniques and after incubating for a specific time are removed. The rate and extent of digestion are measured by the loss of dry matter or nutrient content from the sample.

Because of the simplicity of the procedure and requirement of small amount of laboratory equipment (analytical balance and drying oven) and small amount of substrate to be analyzed, the technique is quite useful for evaluating the rate of forage digestion or for measuring the effect of various ration treatments, such as supplementation, on the rate and extent of digestion within the rumen.

However, the method is subject to considerable variability and is difficult to standardise. Sources of variation include: size and type of bags; cloth mesh size; sample size and fineness of grind; number of samples per trial; diet of host animal; method of suspension in the rumen; location and time in the rumen; and the method of cleaning and rinsing the bags after removal from the rumen. Attempts have been made to reduce the variability by leaving the bags in the rumen for longer periods of time; and by use of a large sample size (10 gm), a large number of samples per trial (up to 48), and by allowing the bags to move about freely with the rumen contents.

It has been further suggested that the addition of a pepsin treatment of the remaining residue in the nylon bags after removal from the rumen may improve the reliability of the method. The treatment permits more effective washing and reduces variation among triplicates, which is attributed to the elimination of microorganisms.

(ii) IN VIVO ARTIFICIAL RUMEN (VIVAR) TECHNIQUE. The Vivar technique is for studying nutrient utilisation by rumen microorganisms under controlled conditions in the rumen. The system consists of a porcelain test tube or stainless steel or glass jars fitted with bacteriological membranes to provide controlled interchange of the Vivar and rumen contents. The Vivar containers are equipped with a gas escape outlet and suspended in the rumen of a fistulated animal for the desired period of incubation. The system, though developed to stimulate conditions occurring in the living animal, appears to be of little value in its present form for the quality evaluation of forages. However, the method is useful in studying the rate phenomena in the rumen and determining the effect of changes in ration treatments on digestion and volatile fatty acid production.

C. ESTIMATION OF ENERGY CONTENT

1. CARBON-NITROGEN BALANCE TECHNIQUE. The main forms in which energy is stored by the growing and fattening animal are protein and fat since carbohydrate in the body is small in amount and fairly constant. The object of a nitrogen and carbon balance trial is to know the stored amount of protein and fat in the animal body. Once we obtain such information by estimating the amounts of these elements absorbed and living in the body and so, by difference, the amounts retained, the energy retained can then be calculated by multiplying the quantities of nutrients stored by their calorific values.

Let us take an example where a bullock was fed on an average 6,988 grams of hay and 400 grams of linseed meal. The amount of nitrogen and carbon intakes through feeding are recorded on the basis of the per cent composition of the feed ingredients and the loses of these two components through various avenues have been noted in Table 10.59. Systematic approach of calculation will ultimately lead to find out the *Net Energy gain or loss* by the bullock.

Determinations are made of the carbon and nitrogen in the food, faeces, urine, and of the carbon in the gaseous output. Thus we know the amount of carbon gained with a side by side nitrogen gain, we can easily find out the protein deposited. By subtracting the carbon of protein from the total carbon gain we can estimate the total fat stored from rest of the carbon.

Table 10.59

Calculation of energy retention of a bullock from its Nitrogen and Carbon balance

Material	*Amount*	*Nitrogen*		*Carbon*	
		Income (gm)	*Outgo (gm)*	*Income (gm)*	*Outgo (gm)*
Food:	6,988 gm hay	56.4	—	2831.7	—
	400 gm linseed (meal)	21.9	—	172.6	—
Excreta:	16,619 gm faeces	—	33.5	—	1428.7
		—	32.4	—	124.2
	4357 gm urine				
	37 gm brushings	—	1.3	—	8.0
	4730 gm CO_2	—	—	—	1290.2
	142 gm methane	—	—	—	46.6
GAIN————→		+11.1 gm		+46.6 gm	

On this ration the animal therefore, gained 11.1 gm nitrogen. Body protein contains 16.65 per cent nitrogen, hence gain of protein is:

$$11.1 \times \frac{100}{16.65} = 66.66 \text{ gm.}$$

But this protein is known to contain 52.54 per cent carbon therefore, the carbon used for this protein is:

$$66.6 \times \frac{52.54}{100} = 35.0 \text{ gm.}$$

The total gain of carbon was 46.6 gm therefore, the amount of carbon available after fulfilling the requirement of protein is:

$$46.6 - 35.0 = 11.6 \text{ gm.}$$

Fat contains 76.6 per cent carbon, therefore the fat gain is:

$$11.6 \times \frac{100}{76.5} = 15.2 \text{ gm.}$$

The final result is therefore:

A gain of 66.6 gm protein and 15.2 gm of fat energy retention.

Energy stored as protein	$(66.6 \times 4.00) = 266.6$ kcal
Energy stored as fat	$(15.2 \times 9.00) = 136.8$ kcal
NET ENERGY GAIN	$= 403.4$ kcal

Once we know the net energy retained, we can find out the heat loss by deducting the net energy from metabolisable energy:

(a) ME—Energy of heat loss = Net energy, so
(b) ME—Net energy = Energy of heat loss
(c) ME = Gross energy—Energy loss in faeces, urine, gas as methane.

Gross energy of the feedstuff, faecal energy and urinary energy can be determined by usual bomb calorimeter technique (described earlier). For methane the estimation can be done by several ways as analysing the methane of the respiratory calorimeter (described afterwords), or by adopting some formula like Axelsson's formula which is:

Methane energy in kcal $= 1083X_2^{0.638}$
Where X_2 = digested carbohydrate in kg.

For general calculation, methane production can be estimated as 8 per cent of gross energy intake.

Thus by Nitrogen Carbon technique, we can not only know the net energy (energy of retention) but also know the energy lost as heat from the animal body and thus we can compare different feedstuffs for their nutritive value.

2. BY BOMB CALORIMETER. The energy value of feeds is usually expressed in nutrition in terms of the kilocalorie and traditionally designated as large calorie. The trend, however, is slowly moving away from the use of the term calorie toward the more accurate practice of using kilocalorie by its own name.

Since Lavoisier's classic experiments on the origin of animal heat, it has been known that foods burned outside the body produce the same amount of heat as foods oxidised by the slow processes of intermediary metabolism. If, then, foods are burned and heat produced is measured, the quantity of heat expressed in kilocalories represents the *gross energy* value *of combustion* of the food. The instrument used to determine heat of combustion is known to all students of nutrition as the Bomb calorimeter. In this the food is ignited and the heat of combustion calculated from the rise in temperature of the surrounding water placed in a jacket inside the calorimeter. The data obtained regarding gross energy content of any feed stuff are precise physical measurements which represent the total energy available on oxidation. They do not represent the physiological values for the energy available to the tissues. Since the food is not completely digested and absorbed from the alimentary canal, and oxidation in the tissues is not always complete, some losses of energy are inevitable.

Thus, merely energy content of any feed does not mean the actual utilisation of that energy by the animal system. Feeds are assessed by their ability to promote energy retention in the body. To determine the energy retention, the intake of energy and losses of energy as heat in faeces, urine and as combustible gas are determined.

3. CALCULATING TDN FROM DIGESTIBILITY TRIAL AS AN INDEX OF ENERGY CONTENT OF FEED. In a number of countries including India, energy value of the feed is expressed in terms of TDN which is the abbreviation for total digestible nutrients. TDN is simply a figure which indicates the relative energy value of a feed to an animal. It is ordinarily expressed in kg or in per cent. TDN can be determined only by a digestion trial where the per cent digestible nutrients are computed on the fresh basis directly by multiplying the percentage of each nutrient, present in the feed ingredient in question (protein, fibre, N-free extract and fat) by their corresponding digestion coefficient. The value is then arrived at by adding together as below:

per cent digestible crude protein =
per cent digestible crude fibre =
per cent digestible N-free extract =
per cent digestible crude fat ×2.25 =

per cent of TDN=

To approximate the greater calorific value of fat, which contains approximately 2.25 times as much energy as carbohydrates, the percentage of digestible fat or ether extract is multiplied by 2.25. This is the result of their chemical composition. Fats contain larger ratio of carbon plus hydrogen to oxygen, i.e., fats are in a lower stage of oxidation and are, therefore, capable of yielding more energy when oxidised. It may be interesting to note that the burning of 1 gram of hydrogen produces over 4 times as much heat as does the burning of 1 gram of carbon. The formula for TDN is thus written as follows:

Per cent of TDN=Dig. Prot. %+Dig. fibre %+Dig. NFE %+(Dig. Ether Extract % × 2.25).

Total digestible nutrients is not an actual total of the digestible nutrients in a feed. In the first place, it does not include the digestible mineral matter as no direct energy is obtained from them. Secondly, the digestible fat is multiplied by 2.25 before being included in the TDN figure. The latter step is necessary to allow for the extra energy value of fats compared to carbohydrates and proteins. As a result of this step, feeds high in fat will sometimes exceed 100 in percentage TDN. (Animal fat, 175 per cent; Maize oil, 172 per cent; Dried whole milk, 110 per cent TDN content).

Since protein has a higher calorific value than carbohydrate, why has no adjustment for protein been made in the digestible protein figure? This is because losses of energy in the urine due to the excretion of nitrogen make digestible protein approximately equivalent to digestible crude fibre and digestible NFE as source of energy.

A limitation of TDN as a measure of feed energy is that it does not account for certain losses such as combustible gases and the heat increment which has been discussed before in this chapter. These losses are considerably larger for roughages than for concentrates and thus a kilogram of TDN in roughage has considerably less value for productive purposes than a kilogram of TDN in concentrates. TDN then tends to over-evaluate roughages and under-evaluate concentrates as a measure of energy for ruminants. 0.5 kg TDN in maize, better hays and poor roughages yield 1.0, 0.75 and 0.50 therm respectively.

To arrive at the quantity of energy available from a certain amount of TDN, the general accepted value is as follows:

1 kg. TDN = 4400 kcal Digestible energy
= 4.40 kcal per gram of TDN
1 kg. TDN= 3520.00 kcal Metabolisable energy.
= 3.52 kcal ME per gram of TDN.
1 kg TDN = 0.869 SE (Starch Equivalent)

It is also not very difficult to calculate the total energy value from a given value of TDN, since when the individual per cent digestible nutrients are multiplied by Atwater's physiological fuel value and on adding up, the calorific value is obtained. The Atwater's physiological fuel values although are not applicable in the case of ruminants because of low digestibility in comparison to human being, but yet the following values are still in use in calculating the calorific value of TDN.

Atwater's Physiological fuel value (ME)

Carbohydrate	4.0 kcal/gram
Fat	9.0 kcal/gram
Protein	4.0 kcal/gram

FACTORS AFFECTING THE TDN VALUE OF A FEED

A. **The Percentage of Dry Matter.** Water can in no way contribute in a positive way to the TDN value of a feed. The more water present in a feed, the less there is of other nutrients. Since the TDN value depends on the amount of carbohydrate, fat and protein, and not on water as such, any feed having less of water is expected to have more of TDN. Silage is low in TDN compared to hay mainly because of a difference in water content.

B. **The Digestibility of Dry Matter.** TDN results from the digestible portion of the nutrients present in a feed. Mineral oil has a high gross energy value, but it cannot be digested by the animal and so has no digestible energy or TDN value. Lignin would fall in similar category. Feeds high in fibre are, in general, low in digestibility and relatievly low in TDN.

C. **The Amount of Mineral Matter in the Digestible Dry Matter.** Since mineral compounds contribute no energy to the animal as such they have no TDN value. Salts like limestone and defluorinated phosphate are all digested by the animal but would have 0.0 TDN values.

D. **The Amount of Fat in the Digestible Dry Matter.** In calculating TDN, the digestible fat is multiplied by 2.25 as reasons mentioned earlier. Consequently, the more digestible fat a feed contains, other things being equal, the greater will be the TDN value. In feeds high in fats such as dried whole milk, TDN values may even exceed 100 per cent. A pure fat which has a coefficient of digestibility of 100 per cent would theoretically have a TDN value of 225 per cent $\times$ 2.25.

4. ENERGY VALUE FROM CHEMICAL COMPOSITION. Our present system of proximate analysis was developed by Henneberg and Stohmann (1868) at the Weende Experiment Station in Germany. After almost 100 years in 1965 Dr. P.J. Van Soest of U.S.A developed another method of partitioning carbohydrate portion of plant origin. At present both the systems of chemical analysis of feed are in practice in almost all the nutritional laboratories of the world.

From the gross-chemical composition of the feed sample, obtained by either of the methods, the amount of energy yielding groups of nutrients, carbohydrate, ether extract and protein are estimated. Once the amount of each component is known, estimation of the expected amount of heat of combustion can easily be made out by multiplying appropriate factors. The heats of combustion for individual carbohydrates, proteins and fats differ somewhat. The gross energy yield of sucrose, for example, was determined by Atwater to be 3.96 kcal/gram whereas starch yielded 4.23 kcal/gram. Energy yield of butterfat was found to be 9.21 kcal/gram and that of lard, 9.48 kcal/gram. For practical use, individual figures were averaged to apply to the major food stuffs (carbohydrate, fat and protein) as gross energy of food, i.e., heat of combustion.

Atwater's average Gross Energy value factors

Carbohydrate	—	4.15 kcal/gram
Fat	—	9.4 kcal/gram
Protein	—	5.65 kcal/gram

Since the gross energy value of food stuff does not represent the energy actually available to body cells, some potential energy therefore never enters the body and is excreted in the faeces. In this connection, Atwater made a large number of experiments in which he analysed the faeces of three young American men for periods lasting for 3–8 days. The following digestibility figures were obtained by him.

Carbohydrates	98 per cent digestible
Fats	95 per cent digestible
Proteins	92 per cent digestible

N.B: For digestible coefficient divide each digestible per cent value by 100.

From this the "*Atwater's factor*" for the available energy (digestible energy, DE) has been formulated. The calorific values of the three nutrients were multiplied by those corresponding digestible coefficients to get the physiological values as below:

Atwater's Digestible energy value factors

1 gram carbohydrate	$= 4.15 \times 0.98 = 4.0$ kcal
1 gram fat	$= 9.4 \times 0.95 = 9.0$ kcal
1 gram protein	$= (5.65 \times 0.92) = 5.20$ kcal

After digestion and absorption, carbohydrates and fats in human beings are completely oxidised to carbon dioxide and water in the process of cellular metabolism as in the calorimeter. Protein, on the other hand, is less efficient to be completely oxidised by the cell. In biological systems, urea, uric acid, creatinine, and other nitrogenous compounds derived from protein are excreted in the urine. Many observations of the heat of combustion of urine have shown that it contains unoxidised material equivalent to 7.9 kcal/gram of nitrogen. The value when expressed in terms of protein becomes 1.25 kcal (by dividing 7.9 with 6.25). This energy represents metabolic loss and must be subtracted from the "digestible" protein. After considering this point, Atwater has given factors for Metabolisable energy which is also known as physiological fuel value as below:

Atwater's Physiological fuel value factors

Carbohydrate	$4.15 \times 0.98 = 4.0$ kcal/gram
Fat	$9.4 \times 0.95 = 9.0$ kcal/gram
Protein	$(5.65 - 1.25 \times 0.92) = 4.0$ kcal/gram

It has already been mentioned that these values are not suitable for calculating energy values of ruminants feed as the per cent digestibility of feed components is always poor and moreover, the loss of energy in the urine is significantly higher in comparison to human beings.

Estimation of energy value of feeds obtained by multiplying the per cent composition with the appropriate Atwater's fuel value factors are thus a crude procedure for ruminants. In order to have a more precise estimate of nutritive value, the feed must be fed to the particular animal species involved (thus undergo a biological evaluation) for estimation of metabolisable energy.

D. EVALUATION OF PROTEIN QUALITY

(A) FOR NON-RUMINANTS

As discussed before, protein quality can be evaluated from the amount of digestibility, but there we do not know the efficiency with which the absorbed protein is utilised by the body. Since protein of different sources might have equal digestibility and may differ in their utilization by the body, different methods of evaluating protein have been formulated.

1. Protein Efficiency Ratio (PER). It is a measure of weight gain of a growing animal divided by protein intake.

$$\text{PER} = \frac{\text{Weight gain (gm)}}{\text{Protein intake (gm)}}$$

The PER was used as early as 1917 by Osborne and Mendal in their studies establishing differences in protein quality. It has most often been applied to studies in growing rats, but is also applicable to studies with human infants.

As carried out with rats to compare specific proteins or protein sources, a nitrogen free, otherwise adequate basal diet is used in which the protein sources to be compared are included for different groups of young animals.

It is the simplest method for evaluating protein quality since it requires only an accurate measure of dietary intake and weight gain. However, the method requires the strict adherence to certain conditions: (i) the calorie intake must be adequate; (ii) protein must be fed at an adequate but no excessive level since at high levels of dietary protein, weight gain does not increase proportionately with protein intake.

The greatest sources of error in the PER method lies in the use of weight gain as sole criterion of protein value. Weight gain cannot be assumed to represent proportional gain in body protein under all conditions.

To make a standard it has been suggested to test the protein level at 10 per cent dietary level—a level well below the level of protein ordinarily obtained in most protein rich foods.

PER is not characteristic of protein alone as it varies with different animals and condition in different laboratories.

2. Biological Value (BV). Technically, the term is defined as that proportion of the digested (and absorbed) protein that is not excreted in the urine, i.e., per cent of the absorbed nitrogen retained by the body for maintenance and/or growth. A balance trial is conducted in which nitrogen intake and urinary and faecal excretions are measured and the results are used to calculate the BV as follows:

$$BV = \frac{\text{N intake} - (\text{faecal N} + \text{urinary N})}{\text{N intake} - \text{faecal N}} \times 100$$

$$BV = \frac{\text{Retained Nitrogen}}{\text{Absorbed Nitrogen}} \times 100$$

This simplified formula measures the biological value of protein for growth purposes only. A more useful measure is one that takes account of maintenance as well. This can be accomplished by considering the metabolic and endogenous losses separately from the total faecal and urinary excretions. Biological value of dietary protein in the above sense can be expressed by the Thomas-Mitchell equation:

$$\text{per cent BV} = 100 \times \frac{\text{N intake} - (\text{faecal N} - \text{MFN}) - (\text{urinary N} - \text{EUN})}{\text{N intake} - (\text{faecal N} - \text{MFN})}$$

were MFN=*metabolic faecal nitrogen* and EUN=*endogenous urinary nitrogen.*

It will be seen that the total faecal nitrogen is corrected for the metabolic faecal nitrogen (i.e., that portion not a diet residue) and likewise the endogenous urinary nitrogn is deducted from the total urinary excretion in order to eliminate the so called wear and tear nitrogen losses that would occur even in the absence of dietary intake. If the correction is not made, i.e., MFN and EUN are not considered as in the previous case, BV obtained is designated apparent biological value.

In Thomas-Mitchell determination, it is, of course, necessary to determine the nitrogenous excretions on a nitrogen free diet or with rations containing small amounts of proteins which

Calculation of BV of a protein for maintenance and growth of the fat*

Food consumed daily (gm)	6.00
Nitrogen in food (%)	1.043
Daily nitrogen intake (mg)	62.6
Total nitrogen excreted daily in urine (mg)	32.8
Endogenous nitrogen excreted daily in urine (mg)	22.0
Total nitrogen excreted daily in faeces (mg)	20.9
Metabolic faecal nitrogen excreted daily (mg)	10.7

$$BV = \frac{62.6 - (20.9 - 10.7) - (32.8 - 22.0)}{62.6 - (20.9 - 10.7)} \times 100 = 79$$

*The example is taken from H. H. Mitchell, 1924, J. boil Chem. 58, 873.

are known to be practically 100 per cent digested in order to obtain values for metabolic faecal and endogenous urinary nitrogen. Using this procedure the metabolic nitrogen has been found to be approximately 0.1 gm for man, pigs and rats per 100 gm. dry matter consumed and 0.5 gm for ruminants.

Table 10.60

Biological values of the Protein of human food**

Animal food	*BV*	*Vegetative food*	*BV*
Whole milk	80	Potato	67
Whole egg	94	Wheat	67
Egg white	83	Oats	65

**The example is taken from H. H. Mitchell, The Protein Values of Foods in Nutrition, *J. Home Econ.*, *19*, 122, 1927.

From the Table 10.60 it is evident that animal proteins always have more BV than vegetative proteins. This is due firstly, to the fact that the animal proteins are composed of well distributed essential amino acids and secondly, they are in right amount and in proper ratio, required for animal growth. So we can reach a definite conclusion that a protein in which all the essential amino acids are present in sufficient amounts and in proper ratio will show a high biological value in non-ruminants.

3. **Net Protein Utilisation (NPU).** This is the percentage of dietary protein which is converted into body protein.

$$NPU = \frac{\text{Retained Nitrogen}}{\text{Intake of Nitrogen}} \times 100$$

Nitrogen retention may be estimated by carcass analysis. The method combines in a single index, both the digestibility and the biological value of protein.

$$NPU = BV \times \text{Digestibility}$$

The method is much less laborious but time consuming than determining BV or nitrogen balance, but is limited to those animals that are available for carcass analysis.

4. **Nitrogen Balance.** Nitrogen balance study is commonly made to evaluate protein quality in non-ruminants as well as in ruminants. The method has been described under Ruminants (B).

(B) FOR RUMINANTS

Estimation of DCP (Digestible Crude Protein). It is the most common way of expressing the protein value of feed for ruminants. As discussed previously, the term crude protein includes both the true proteins as well as non-protein nitrogenous compounds such as amides, amino acids, nitrogenous glucosides, alkaloids, ammonium salts and others present in feed stuff.

For ruminants, since the non-protein nitrogenous compounds can serve to provide the essential amino acids as a result of microbiological synthesis, distinction between true and crude protein of feeds seems no longer worthwhile.

From simple chemical analysis of the feed the amount of crude protein (true protein+non protein nitrogenous compounds) can easily be known, but the quantity present does not provide enough information on how well it is utilised in the body. Only on a digestion trial when we know the per cent absorbed, this provides some real clue about the usefulness of crude protein present in a feed stuff.

To find out the per cent digestibility of crude protein (DCP) multiply the digestibility coefficient of that protein with the crude protein content of the feed stuff.

Such trials give figures for "*apparent*" and not "*true*" digestibility owing to the presence of metabolic nitrogen in the faeces, which is not derived directly from the feed but comprises substances originating in the body, such as residues of the bile and other digestive juices, epithelial cells abraded from the alimentary tract by the feed passing through it, and bacterial residues. The apparent figures are thus lower than the true values, but since the loss of the *metabolic faecal nitrogen* is inevitable, it is better to ignore while expressing nitrogen digestibility. Usually no attempt is made to determine the true digestibility, and the values we see are all apparent values.

In general the most common practice of evaluation of food protein in ruminants is based firstly on the finding out of crude protein content. By running a digestibility trial as discussed earlier, the DCP values are then obtained. For concentrates, digestibility coefficient values are readily available in the literature, which are then used to find out the values of DCP. Roughages, due to low protein content may have sometimes negative digestible crude protein value due to greater importance of metabolic feacal nitrogen. As such a typical equation as is commonly used for both grass, hays and silages is given below:

$$\text{Per cent DCP} = (\%CP \times 0.9115) - 3.67$$

At present not only the protein values of ruminant feed stuff are tabulated as DCP but also the protein requirements of the animal are expressed as digestible crude protein requirements.

Nitrogen Balance Experiment. The method is applicable to determine the protein quality in ruminants as well as in non-ruminants. By applying the same technique the biological value (BV) of protein for non-ruminants is also estimated. The technique is equally in use to determine the protein requirements for various body functions in all classes of livestock.

The experimental technique is similar to that of a digestion trial except that in this case adequate provision for collection and analysis of urine and of any nitrogenous product such as milk should be made. When the experiment is conducted only to know the utilisation efficiency of the dietary nitrogen in terms of gaining or losing of nitrogen by the body, faeces and urine may be collected and analysed together for the sake of simplicity of the procedure. When the experimentar desires to find out simultaneously the BV of the nitrogen and digestibility separately, the collection of faeces and urine must be made separately using metabolic crate as described before.

The method actually involves an accurate account of the amount of nitrogen consumed through feed and excretion through faeces, urine and brushings (hair, feathers etc.) This must be collected and analysed under controlled conditions. Furthermore, any product for example, milk or eggs, will also need to be recorded and used as the case may be for nitrogen-content.

The method involves determination of the amount of endogenous urinary as well as that of metabolic faecal nitrogen, both of which either may by calculated from the existing formulae (See Protein Metabolism) or may be obtained by conducting actual trials which are time consuming. Feed is withheld from animals so that their bodies enter into a catabolic condition. The nitrogen excreted in the urine and faeces during this period represents the nitrogen lost through metabolic process, the values thus obtained are accordingly known as *endogenous urinary nitrogen* (EUN) and *metabolic faecal nitrogen* (MFN)

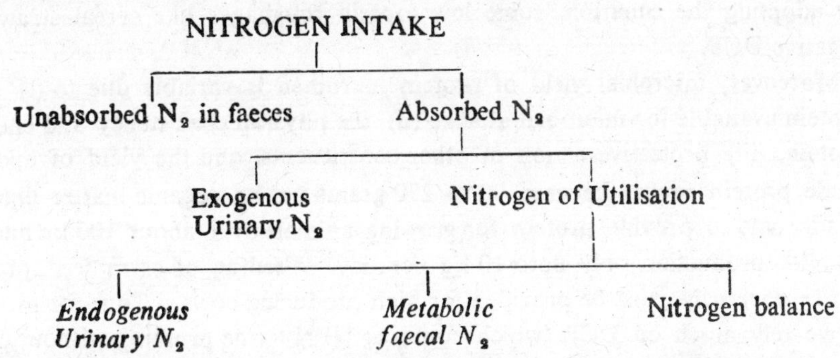

These values are then substracted from the total nitrogen values obtained in the collection of the urine and faeces during the collection period of the balance trial. Exogenous urinary nitrogen and faecal nitrogen from feed are determined by the following equations :

1. Exogenous Urinary Nitrogen = total urinary nitrogen minus endogenous urinary nitrogen
2. Faecal Nitrogen from feed = total faecal nitrogen minus metabolic faecal nitrogen

When the daily nitrogen intake is less than the total outgo from the body, the animal in that case, is in *negative nitrogen balance.* If the nitrogen intake equalled the outgo, the animal is in *nitrogen equilibrium.*

In practice, this condition can hardly be observed. An excess of intake over outgo will represent a *positive nitrogen balance,* involving a deposition and storage of protein in the body.

To measure the quality of protein of a particular feed, care must be taken that the protein is fed at an adequate amount but not at an extra high level since with a higher protein intake (than the required), there will be more of excretion. Thus it will be difficult to compare the protein quality of various feeds.

THE NEW CONCEPT TO DETERMINE REQUIREMENTS OF PROTEINS IN RUMINANTS

The method most widely used for expressing the ruminant's requirement for protein and the extent to which a certain feed could meet these requirements is one based on the measurement of *digestible crude protein* (DCP). Since this method was considered to give too much weight to non-protein nitrogen, another concept of *protein equivalent* (PE) introduced in 1925, where non-protein nitrogen fraction was assumed to be fully digestible but to have half the value of digestible true protein.

$$PE = \frac{\%\text{ Dig. Crude Protein} + \%\text{ Dig. True Protein}}{2}$$

In 1960, the method was found to underestimate the value of the non-protein nitrogen of silages etc., and the use of DCP was again proposed for feeds of ruminants.

With this conception, determination of DCP by means of digestibility trial of large number of feeds gradually become difficult particularly for roughages, which unlike concentrate feeds, have variable composition and for this regression equations for DCP on CP are used to calculate the former as below :

DCP (g/kg DM) = CP (g/kg DM) × 0.9115 − 36.7 is widely used for grasses hays and silages. By adopting the equation, some low protein roughages like cereal straws are found to have negative DCP.

Moreover, microbial yield of protein in rumen is variable due to (i) surface area of feed protein available for microbial attack, (ii) the physical consistency and chemical nature of the protein, (iii) protective action of other constituents, and the yield of microbial protein from crude protein ranges between 90 to 230 grams per kg organic matter digested. This amount is adequate to provide protein for growing animals over about 100 kg and to maintain levels of milk production only upto 10 kg per day. Feeding of extra feed protein (true proteins) per se obviously must be provided for high producing cows. Thus for providing protein needs if we rely much on DCP (which contains NPN + true protein) without caring the amount of true protein, high yielders will thus be affected.

As a result for many years there has been considerable dissatisfaction with this method.

In an attempt to overcome some of the disadvantages accociated with DCP system, protein requirements for ruminants were expressed as *Available Protein*, which is the crude protein of a define biological value that would have to be absorbed from the gastrointestinal tract to meet requirements for maintenance and production. Unfortunately the system has also number of limitations. It assumes that the faecal loss of N can be divided into a component of indigestible feed N and the other protein which represents unabsorbed secretions of N-containing compounds i.e. metabolic faecal N. In fact, faecal N consists mainly of microbial nitrogen and no such division is possible and to some extent, of biological value is in doubt. For these reasons a new conceptual approach has been made to the problems of meeting the protein requirements of ruminants particularly for high yielders.

The New Approach

In ruminants, as in other animals, the needs of the tissues are met by amino acids absorbed from the small intestine. The ideal system for calculating the nitrogen requirements of ruminants must provide, therefore, estimates of the total and individual amino acids absorbed from the small intestine. These amino acids are supplied partly by microbial protein synthesised in the rumen and partly by dietary protein which has escaped fermentation in the rumen (bypass protein). The value of dietary urea or similar NPN sources depends entirely on degradation to ammonia in the rumen by microbes and the subsequent use of this ammonia for microbial protein synthesis. The extent of the synthesis depends on the energy available to the microorganisms. Dietary protein also is degraded in the rumen by microbial attack ; the pathways of this degradation are poorly understood but the nitrogenous products include peptides, amino acids and ultimately NH_3. These products are used for the synthesis of microbial protein and there is evidence that mixed bacteria growing in the rumen incorporate considerable amounts of preformed amino acids as well as NH_3 when the diet contains protein. It is possible that this results in better microbial growth than the use of NH_3 alone but, as a net effect for the host animal, good dietary protein which is degraded in the rumen is used inefficiently.

Degradability of dietary proteins in the rumen varies among different natural protein sources and with different processing treatments.

$$\text{Degradability} = 1 - \frac{\text{Dietary protein entering duodenum}}{\text{total dietary protein intake}}$$

That part which escapes degradation (bypass protein) supplements microbial protein in providing a source of amino acids for digestion and absorption in the small intestine of the host animal.

The new system thus takes care of the amount of microbial as well as the amount of "bypass protein" requirement of ruminants i.e., proportion of degradable and undegradable amount of protein for ruminants.

Burroughs et.al in 1975 of Iowa State in U. S. A. proposed "*Metabolisable Protein*" (MP) system and Urea fermentation potential (UFP).

Metabolisable protein is defined as the quantity of protein digested or amino acid(s)

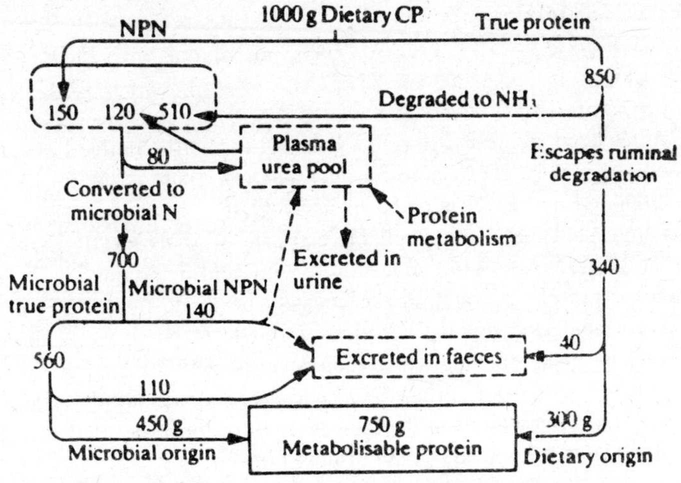

Fig. 10.30 Calculation of 'Metabilisable Protein' of diet.

absorbed in the post ruminal portion of the digestive tract of cattle and other ruminants and is available for use at tissue level. It consists partly of dietary ture protein which has escaped degradation in the rumen but which has been broken down to amino acids and are subsequently absorbed from the small intestine. Microbial protein, synthesised in the rumen, similarly contributes to metabolisable protein.

In this instance 1000 gm of dietary protein yields 750 g of MP, but this depends upon the validity of certain assumptions particularly the proportion of dietary crude protein present in non-protein form, the degradability of dietary true protein, and the efficiency of synthesis of

microbial protein, which is determined by the supply of readily available energy for micro-organisms (Fig. 10.30.)

Thus MP supplied by different diets is estimated by taking into account (i) extent of degradation of feed protein in the rumen, (ii) the amount of microbial protein synthesised in the rumen and the (iii) digestibility of these components in the small intestine. Potential microbial protein synthesis in the rumen is estimated by assessing, from the TDN content of the diet, the energy available for this purpose.

Urea fermentation potential (UFP) is a term used to indicate the amount of urea that can be utilised in a ruminant ration. **A positive UFP value of a feed represents the estimated grams of urea per kg. of feed dry matter consumed that can be used for ruminal synthesis of microbial protein.**

What is By-pass protein?

Dietary protein that escapes rumen microbial breakdown and passes to abomasum without any major biochemical changes. These are also termed as undegradable protein (UDP) or undegradable dietary nitrogen (UDN).

In the ARC protein rationing system, dietary nitrogen intake is divided as below :

$$\text{UDN} = \frac{\text{Duodenal N} - \text{microbial N}}{\text{N intake}}$$

$$\text{RDN} = 1 - \text{UDN}$$

More recently, it has been suggested that RDN should further be defined as (i) quickly degradable nitrogen (QDN) and (ii) slowly degradable nitrogen (SDN). QDN is assumed to be equal to water soluble nitrogen compound and SDN is equal to RDN–QDN.

It has also been suggested that a more reliable estimate of UDN (ADIN) which is assumed to be undegradable and indigestible even after digesting it with acid detergent.

The measurement of protein degradability can easily be made by using synthetic bags made of fine natural silk, decron material, nylon filter cloth, terylene or polyester material. The protein feed sample to be tested is kept inside the bag which then is suspended in the rumen (*in vivo*) or in artificial rumen in the laboratory (*in vitro*) for certain fixed periods, after which the portions lost is calculated as degradable amount. By subtracting the degradable amount form the total sample weight, one may get the amount of nondegradable or 'By-pass' protein portion.

Why By-pass protein?

In early lactation period of animals particularly of high yielders when substantial quantity of milk is produced and in case of growing animals where the growth rate is rapid, the microbial protein synthesized in rumen is not adequate to meet the total amino acid requirement and so it has to be supplemented with the by-pass protein.

In general a milking cow can meet her amino acid needs from the microbial protein obtained by digesting millions of dead bodies of bacteria and protozoa in her abomasum along with some amount of amino acids obtained from 40 percent by-pass protein. The total amino acid obtained is just sufficient to yield not more than 10 liters of milk per day. But for further high yielders, extra amount of by-pass protein feed is become an absolute necessity.

Why high percent of degradable protein feed in cattle ration is loss to all of us?

In rumen only bacteria utilizes nitrogen for ammonia. Protozoa mostly fed upon the bacteria for nitrogen source and convert the bacterial protein into protozoan protein. Each protozoa can engulf 60–700 bacteria in an hour at a density of 10^6/ml.

The utilization of ammonia nitrogen by bacteria also depends upon the availability of energy, carbon skeleton, S, P for preparation of all essential and non-essential amino acids to be used for bacterial body proliferation.

Thus, it has been observed that provided all components are available still the maximum ammonia nitrogen utilization by bacteria can be to the extent of 13 percent dietary crude protein (DM basis). Above this protein concentration, ruminal NH_3 increases rapidly with increasing protein or crude protein percent. *This excess NH_3-N when exceeds 5–8 mg/100 ml rumen fluid, there is an 'ammonia overflow' from the rumen.* The excess ammonia is absorbed from the reticulorumen, or passed to the lower gut, where it is absorbed and eventually a portion is converted to non-essential amino acids while the balance will form urea by the liver and excreted through urine. This is a loss to animal itself and also to owner himself.

In a cattle ration how much degradable and non-degradable protein feed should be included?

This is still under investigation of many research stations. National Dairy Development Board has already developed cattle feed having undegraded protein (UDP) also known as by-pass protein 18–22% and ruminal degraded protein 8–10% of the total protein requirement.

Table 10.61 **Composition of a by-pass protein feed as suggested by National Dairy Development Board (NDDB)**

Sl.	Material	Minimum	Maximum
1.	Moisture	8%	10%
2.	Crude protein	28%	32%
3.	Ether Extract	3%	5%
4.	Crude fibre	4%	6%
5.	R D P	8%	10%
6.	U D P	18%	22%
7.	Silica	–	2%
8.	Calcium	1.2%	1.5%
9.	Phosphorus	1.0%	1.5%
10.	Metabolisable energy (MJ/kg.)	11.5%	–
11.	Vitamin A and D_3	10,00 IU/kg.	–

Factors involved in the New Approach

The general scheme of the new approach is to calculate the amount of amino acid N of microbial origin that could be retained in the body for tissue synthesis when the maximal rate of fermentation of a particular energy input is achieved. This amount of amino acid N is compared with the total tissue needs for the particular energy input. Two alternatives present themselves :

1. **If the amount of microbial amino acid N available to the tissues is greater than the tissue needs, then the nitrogen requirement is the amount of degraded N needed by the rumen microorganisms ;**
2. **If the microbial amino acid N is less than the tissue needs, then the difference must be**

supplied by amino acids from undegraded dietary protein.

For practical calculation of N requirements simple summary equations can be derived as follows :

(a) Rumen degradable N (RDN) requirement (g/day) = 1.25 ME

(b) Amino acid N supplied to the tissues (TMN) by microbial synthesis from RDN (g/day) = 0.53 ME

(c) If total tissue N requirement, calculated by the factorial method (TN) is greater than TMN, then Undegraded dietary N (UDN) requirement (g/day) = 1.91 TN – 1.00 ME where ME is metabolisable energy requirement.

Total dietary N requirement is thus the sum of the RDN and UDN requirements.

In a proposed ration, the weights of degradable N (RDN) and undegraded N (UDN) are calculated, and these are compared with the RDN and UDN requirements of the animal.

1. If the UDN requirement of the animal is greater than the UDN content of the ration, then additional protein must be given to correct the deficiency of UDN and the weight of RDN supplied by the new ration must be calculated.

2. If the RDN requirement of the animal is greater than the RDN content of the ration, then the deficiency could be made up by urea. Alternatively, if the deficiency arises after correcting for a deficiency of UDN by supplementary protein, a source of protein of higher degradability could be used.

It is suggested that feed tables should contain values for rumen-degradable protein and undegradable protein by multiplying N with 6.25 factors rather than N as used while explaining the principles.

SOME IMPORTANT FACTS RELATED TO THE CONCEPT

1. Microbial N yield in the Rumen and Quality

For each kg of organic matter fermented, approximately 30 gm N is taken up by rumen bacteria as protein and nucleic acids.

Regarding quality of microbial protein the following points may be noted :

1. Diet does not affect the amino acid composition of individual species of bacteria or protozoa
2. Biological value of rumen bacteria & protozoa are same i.e., about 0.8 but the digestibility of bacterial protein is lower, 0.74 compared to 0.91 for protozoal protein.
3. Protozoa numbers are higher on high roughage diets than on concentrate diets.
4. Microbial protein contains 20% nucleic acid which has no value for animals.

2. Proportion of Total microbial N present as amino acid N

A value of 0.80 has been adopted for calculating N requirements. In using this factor, it must be borne in mind that the value used subsequently for efficiency of utilisation of absorbed N derived from bacteria should refer to as amino acid N and not to total N.

3. Apparent absorbability in the small intestine of amino acids derived from microbial & dietary protein

A value of 0.75 for efficiency of utilisation of apparently absorbed amino acid N from the small intestine has been adopted for both cattle and sheep.

4. Extent of degradation of dietary protein in the rumen

While the rumen contains a potent supply of proteases and deaminases, all feed proteins are not degraded to the same degree as is shown below. The figures represent degradable percent.

Urea	— 100	Soybean meal	— 60
Casein	— 90	Lucerne hay	— 60
Cotton seed meal	— 70	Maize	— 40
Groundnut meal	— 65	Fish meal	— 30.

As expected, urea is 100% degradable like soluble casein. Plants are highly variable but maize, with its high content of insoluble *zein,* is only 40% degraded. Casein a high quality protein largely converted to microbial protein, while much of fish meal, also of high quality largely passes intact into small intestine.

Proteins which are generally (but not necessarily) more soluble considered to be more degradable. The competition between passage and rumen digestion for potentially digestible substrate determines the proportion of unfermented feed passing to the omasum and abomasum. This passage (bypass protein) is important in regard to potentially digestible true protein since it will deterimine the proportion of unaltered dietary protein and amino acids reaching peptic digestion.

Moreover, when feed proteins are treated by mild heat, or chemicals such as formaldehyde or tannin, decreases rumen microbial attack by manipulating the solubility and thus increase the amount of bypass protein in the same way as described above.

Conclusions

As it stands now, the new conception to deterimine requirements of protein in ruminants makes certain questionable assumptions, and suffer the major disadvantage that no satisfactory method exist for routinely determining protein degradability The general approach although highly commendable but it should wait some more time to be introduced in regular practice after the validation under field conditions.

BALANCED RATION, ITS CHARACTERISTIC AND COMPUTATION FOR CATTLE AND BUFFALOES

Ration

A ration is the feed allowed for a given animal during a day of 24 hours. The feed may be given at a time or in portions at intervals.

Balanced ration

A balanced ration is a ration which provides the essential nutrients to the animal in such proportion and amounts that are required for the proper nourishment of the particular animal for 24 hours.

DESIRABLE CHARACTERISTIC OF A RATION

1. Liberal Feeding

Milk cows produce plenty of milk just after calving not necessarily because they are properly fed, but because they inherently do so. This inherent quality of the cow can be made use of for increasing the milk production by providing food liberally. Liberal feeding should on no account be mistaken for overfeeding. Overfeeding is doubly wasteful because it wastes food and it also injures the animal's system. By liberal feeding, one means that the animal should be provided in plenty with all the requirements which are necessary for full milk production and maintenance of her body. There should also be some allowance made for what goes as a waste in preparation and serving the food to the cow.

2. Individual Feeding

Cows of the same breed and age and receiving practically the same food and care vary widely in their productive ability. In order to obtain maximum profits, cows must be fed individually according to the individual production and requirements instead of allowing the same ration to each animal in the herd.

3. The Ration Should Be Properly Balanced

With a correct and balanced ration a cow can get the best out of all the constituents present in her food and production of milk is frequently cheaper per unit in consequence. With an improperly balanced ration much of it is wasted. What matters is not what the cow eats but what she digests; because the amount digested alone goes for milk production and maintenance of her body. A balanced ration is thus more purposeful and beneficial.

4. The Food Must Be Palatable

Digestive power and appetite are not the same in cattle at all times and under all circumstances. Much depends upon the availability of foodstuffs, force of habits and usages in a certain locality. Whatever food be given to an animal it must be to its liking. Evil smelling, mouldy, musty, spoiled and inferior foods are unpalatable and must not be given to the animals. If some excellent food is not good in taste, they should be improved by special preparations like addition of salt, or other feed additives.

5. Variety of Feed in the Ration

By combining many feeds in a ration a better and balanced mixture of proteins, vitamins and other nutrients are furnished than by depending on only a few. Variety of feeds in the ration makes it more palatable.

6. The Feeds Composing the Ration Should Be Good and Sound

It is self-evident that the addition of unsound, mouldy, musty and poor quality feeds in a ration reduces the feeding value of the mixture. Apart from this, the low quality may contain poisonous or unwholesome ingredients. Cleanliness is an important condition in quality.

7. The Ration Should Contain Enough of Mineral Matter

Every litre of milk yielded by a cow contains a little more than 0.70% of mineral matter If the amount of mineral matter in the ration is not sufficient to meet the demand in milk yield, the cow shall have to draw upon her own body supplies or fall down in milk yield. At the end of her lactation she will be left as an extremely weak animal and her milk yield in subsequent lactation will go down considerably.

8. The Ration Should Be Fairly Laxative

This is important, otherwise the food will be incompletely digested. Constipation is often the cause of most of the digestive troubles. It is, therefore, necessary to give such foods which are laxative in character.

9. The Ration Should Be Fairly Bulky

The stomach of cattles are very capacious and they do not feel satisfied unless their bellies are properly filled up. From the point of providing energy and heat generated values, indigestible fibre is not of any great importance but it pays an important role in giving a feeling of fullness to cattle. If the bulk of the ration supplied is small, however rich it might be in its nourishing constituents, cattle may fall a victim to the depraved habits of eating earth, rags, dirty refuses, etc., for filling up stomachs.

10. Allow Much of Green Fodder

Green succulent fodders are of great importance in the feeding of milch animals because of their cooling and slightly laxative action. They aid the appetite and keep the animal in good condition. Green fodders are bulky, easily digestible, laxative and contain enough of necessary vitamins. Leguminous green fodders are very rich in proteins. It should be borne in mind that at the cost of the optimum dose of concentrates, too much green fodder alone may not supply sufficient dry matter requirements.

11. Avoid Sudden Changes in the Diet

Sudden changes are often the cause of many digestive troubles, the more notable being the "*Tympanitis*", "*Impaction*", etc. These diseases reduce the milk yield and have depressing influences on the general constitution of the body of the animal. All changes of the food must be gradual and slow. An animal system receiving a certain food or a mixture of foods gets accustomed to it. It gets upset by sudden changes.

12. Maintain Regularity in Feeding

Cattle like other animals are creatures of habits and get so much used to routine that marked changes may lead to restlessness. As the feeding hour approaches, their glandular secretions become active in anticipation of the meal. Irregularity in milking and feeding tells very badly on the productive powers of an animal. The time of feeding should be evenly distributed so that the animals are not kept too long without food.

13. The Feed Must Be Properly Prepared

The feed must be well prepared. Some feeds require special preparations before administration in order to render them more digestible and palatable. Hard grains like gram, barley, wheat, maize, etc., should be grounded before feeding so that their mastication may become easy. Coarse fodders like dry jowar, bajra and green fodders of these crops should be chaffed before feeding. Some dry fodders, such as *bhusa* of cereals and legumes should be moistened. Soaking of feeds like various types of cakes and cotton seed softens them and makes them more palatable.

14. A Ration Should Not Be Too Bulky

If the ration is too bulky, the animal will fail to get all its nutrient requirements.

15. Economy in Labour and Cost

The ultimate object of rearing animals is to make profits. The cost of the feeds and the labour in feeding should be minimised to an extent that economic efficiency is not affected.

COMPUTATION OF RATION FOR CATTLE AND BUFFALOES

In the computation of ration for cattle and buffaloes, the prime consideration is to ascertain and to meet up the total requirement in terms of (i) dry matter. (ii) digestible protein, i.e., DCP and (iii) energy i.e., TDN for 24 hours.

Requirement of Dry Matter (DM)

The requirement of the quantity of dry matter depends on the body weight of the animal and also with the nature of its production. Cattle will generally eat daily 2.0 to 2.5 kg dry matter for every 100 kg of live weight. Buffaloes and crossbred animals are slightly heavy eaters and their dry matter comsumption varies from 2.5 to 3 kg daily per 100 kg body weight. This means that the animal in question should consume only so much. Naturally, all its requirements whether organic nutrients like carbohydrate, protein and fat or minerals or vitamins should come from the total dry matter that has to be allotted. Under Indian conditions, while computation of ration is made, the amount of grazing, is neglected as it is extremely poor. Since the bulk is essential, the dry matter allowance should be divided as follows:

Total dry matter (DM)—
- $\frac{2}{3}$ (as roughages)
  - $\frac{2}{3}$ dry roughages or 3/4 if sufficient legume is available
  - $\frac{1}{3}$ green roughages (If the green fodder is legume, this proportion may be only 1/4 of the total roughage ration.)
- $\frac{1}{3}$ (as concentrates)

Illustration 1

For a cross-bred cow weighing 400 kg, the dry matter requirement will be provided as indicated below·

Total DM requirement (kg) (@ 2.5 kg per 100 kg body weight)	=(4×2.5)=10
DM as concentrates (kg)	=(10×1/3)=3.33 or say 3.5
DM as roughages (kg)	=(10×2/3)=6.66 or say 6.5
DM as dry roughages (kg)	=(6.6×3/4)=4.95 or say 4.9
DM as green roughages (kg) (When legume will be available)	=(6.6×1/4)=1.65 or say 1.6

Requirement of Digestible Protein & Energy (DCP & TDN)

While calculating the total requirements of DCP and TDN one has to consider the physiological needs, or say, the purpose for which the animal has to be fed, i.e., whether the animal is just to maintain itself or in addition to carry out the advanced stage of pregnancy or whether the animal is under production. In later case it is also necessary to consider the quantity and quality of milk. The requirement of DCP and TDN requirement for all these purposes separately may be obtained from the appropriate Tables. What one has to do is to add up the additional requirements on top of maintenance requirement as per physiological condition.

Illustration 2

Find out the total requirements of DCP and TDN for a cow weighing 400 kg and yielding 10 litres of milk having 4.5 % fat.

	DCP (kg)	TDN (kg)
For maintenance	0.254	3.03
For 10 litres of milk (having 4.5% fat)	0.480	3.40
Total requirements	0.734	6.43

Computing Ration As Per Requirement

The average DCP and TDN contents of variety of feeds and fodders are already calculated by various scientists and the average values are given in appropriate Tables. From these feeds, one has to select suitable concentrates and roughages as available in the locality at a suitable rate.

Illustration 3

Compute a ration for a cow weighing 400 kg, giving 10 litres of milk having 4.5 per cent fat. The locally available feedstuff are as follows:

1. Wheat straw
2. Cowpea fodder
3. Oats (flowering) fodder
4. Maize (crushed)
5. Groundnut cake
6. Gram chuni

STEP I: Find out the requirements of DM, DCP and TDN (already worked out in previous two illustrations)

DM requirement (kg) = 10
Total DCP (kg) = 0.734
Total TDN (kg) = 6.43

STEP II: Find out the amount of DCP & TDN that are consumed through roughages:

Ingredients	*Digestible Nutrients per 100 Kg DM*		*Amount of DM (kg) to be given (Already worked out)*	*Amount of DCP & TDN given through dry matter*		*Actual amount of ingredients on fresh* basis (kg)*
	DCP (kg)	*TDN (kg)*		*DCP*	*TDN*	
(4.9 kg) Dry roughage						
Wheat straw	0	48.9	4.9	—	2.396	5.4
(1.6 kg) Green roughage						
Oats (flowering)	7.7	72.0	1.0	0.077	0.720	3.3
Cowpea	20.3	62.2	0.6	0.122	0.373	2.0
Total amount given:			6.5	1.199	3.489	

Amount of DCP and TDN given through roughages are 0.199 and 3.489 respectively. **This amount is now to be subtracted from the total requirements. The balance, i.e., (.734—.199)= 0.535 kg of DCP and (6.430—3.489)=2.941 kg of TDN to be given through concentrates.** The quantity of concentrate mixture to be given is 3.5 kg as dry matter.

STEP III: Distribute 3.5 kg dry matter among the various ingredients of the concentrate group in such a proportion that the balance 0.535 kg DCP and 2.941 kg TDN are supplied.

It is natural that while balancing the DCP and TDN requirement several trials may have to run to reach the closest figure. This might initially seem to be tiresome but little practice will make it easier.

To this amount of concentrate always add common salt and mineral mixture @ 1 percent each.

Ingredients	*Digestible Nutrients per 100 kg. dry matter*		*Amount of DM (kg) alloted now*	*Amount of DCP and TDN given through dry matter*		*Actual amount of ingredients on fresh basis**
	DCP	*TDN*		*DCP*	*TDN*	
1. Maize	7.0	87.1	1.5	0.105	1.306	1.66 kg.
2. GNC cake	49.1	77.0	0.5	0.5	0.385	0.55 "
3. Gram chuni	13.6	87.5	1.5	0.204	1.312	1.66 „
Total given			3.5	0.554	3.003	
Required			3.5	0.535	2.941	

*The dry matter per cent of all sorts of concentrates have been calculated on 90% basis.

Summary of the Calculations Made So Far:

For a cow weighing 400 kg. and yielding 10 litres of milk having 4.5% fat, the following ingredients may be given for 24 hours.

1. Wheat straw 5.4 kg.
2. Oat fodder 3.3 kg. (flowering stage)
3. Cowpea 2.0 kg.
4. Maize 1.66 kg.
5. Groundnut cake 0.55 kg.
6. Gram chuni 1.66 kg.

Salt and mineral mix each @ 1% of the concentrate mixture.

Illustration 4

Compute a ration for a cow weighing 450 kg. yielding 7.0 litres of milk having 4.5 percent fat. The cow is in advanced stage of pregnancy. The locally available feedstuffs are as follows:

1. Wheat straw
2. Oat (flowering stage)
3. Lucerne
4. Maize (crushed)
5. Sesame cake
6. Gram chuni
7. Rice bran

A. Requirement of DM

(@ 2.5 kg. per 100 kg. live wt.)	=(4.5 ×2.5)=11.25 kg.
DM as total roughages	=(11.25×2/3) = 7.5 „
DM as concentrate	=(11.25×1/3) = 3.75 „
DM as dry roughages	=(7.5 ×3/4) = 5.6 „
DM as green roughages	=(7.5 ×1/4) = 1.9 „

B. *Requirement of DCP and TDN*

	DCP (kg)	TDN (kg)
For maintenance	0.282	3.37
For 7 litres of milk having 4.5% fat	0.336	2.38
Pregnancy allowance	0.140	0.70
Total	0.758	6.45

C. *Amount of DCP and TDN that are consumed through roughages*

Ingredients	*Digestible Nutrients per 100 kg DM*		*Amount of DM (kg) to be given*	*Amount of DCP and TDN given through DM*		*Actual amount of ingredients on fresh basis (kg)*
	DCP (kg)	*TDN (kg)*		*DCP*	*TDN*	
Dry Roughages	5.6 kg					
Wheat straw	—	48.9	5.6	—	2.738	6.33
Green Roughages	1.9 kg					
Oats (flowering)	7.7	72.0	1.0	0.077	0.720	3.33
Lucerne	16.2	60.2	0.9	0.146	0.122	3.00
			7.5	0.223	3.580	

D. *Balance of DCP and TDN to be given through concentrate mixture of 3.75 kg dry matter.*

D.C.P. (0.758—0.223)=0.535 kg

T.D.N. (6 45—3.58)=2.87 kg

Ingredients	*Digestible nutrient per 100 kg DM*		*Amount of DM (kg) alloted now**	*Amount of DCP and TDN given through DM*		*Actual amount of ingredients on fresh basis (kg)*
	DCP (kg)	*TDN (kg)*		*DCP (kg)*	*TDN (kg)*	
1. Maize	7.0	87.1	0.5	0.035	0.435	0.55
2. Gram chuni	13.6	87.5	1.0	0.136	0.875	1.11
3. Rice bran	9.1	76.1	1.5	1.136	1.121	2.22
4. Sesame cake	34.0	80.0	0.75	0.255	0.600	0.28
			Given=3.75	0.582	3.033	
			Required=3.75	0.535	2.870	

N.B.: To this amount of concentrate mixture add common salt and mineral mixture @ 1% each.

*In case you find it difficult to fulfil the requirements of DCP and TDN after giving a certain proportion of ingredients, further trials should be made.

*If carotene (or green feed) is supplied, the amount of the provitamin has to be given in international units at four times the above rates (1 mg of carotene=1600 I.U.). In other words, 1 mg of carotene can replace only 400 I.U. of vitamin A.

E. Summary: For the animal in question the following ingredients may be given for 24 hours.

1. Wheat straw 6.33 kg
2. Oats (flowering) 3.33 „
3. Lucerne 3.00 „
4. Maize 0.55 kg
5. Gram chuni 1.11 „
6. Rice bran 1.66 „
7. Sesame cake 0.84 „

FEEDING STANDARDS FOR CATTLE

Modified Morrison's Standard

Table 10.62

Daily nutrient requirements of a calf growing at the rate of 0.5 kg per day during first two years and reaching adult body weight at the age of approximately 3 years

Body wt. (kg)	*DCP (kg)*	*Energy*		*Ca (g)*	*P (g)*	*Vitamin A (I.U.)*
		T.D.N. (kg)	*ME (kcal)*			
45	0.17	0.9	3290	7	6	2000
70	0.22	1.3	4680	12	10	3000
100	0.28	1.9	6900	13	10	4000
150	0.35	2.6	9360	13	12	6500
200	0.40	3.0	11500	13	12	8500
300	0.47	4.0	12600	13	12	12,500
450	0.48	5.0	13600	12	12	17,000

Table 10.63

Daily maintenance requirement of dairy stock

Body wt. (kg)	*DCP (kg)*	*Energy*		*Ca (g)*	*P (g)*	*Carotene (mg)*
		TDN (kg)	*ME (kcal)*			
250	0.168	2.02	7.27	6	6	27
300	0.197	2.36	8.50	7	7	32
350	0.277	2.70	9.72	8	8	37
400	0.254	3.03	10.91	9	9	42
450	0.282	3.37	12.13	10	10	47
500	0.296	3.64	13.28	11	11	52
550	0.336	4.00	14.40	12	12	57

Table 10.64

Requirement for production of 1 kg of milk (to be added to requirement for maintenance and also for growth if any).

Fat content of milk %	*DCP (kg)*	*Energy*		*Ca (g)*	*P (g)*
		TDN (kg)	*ME (kcal)*		
3.0	0.040	0.27	0.97	2.0	1.4
3.5	0.042	0.29	1.04	2.0	1.4
4.0	0.045	0.32	1.15	2.0	1.4
4.5	0.048	0.34	1.22	2.0	1.4
5.5	0.051	0.36	1.30	2.0	1.4
6.0	0.057	0.41	1.41	2.0	1.4
7.5	0.063	0.46	1.66	2.0	1.4

Table 10.65

Nutrients required for working bullocks per head per day

Body wt. (kg)	*Normal work*			*Heavy work*		
	DCP (kg)	*TDN (kg)*	*M.E. (Mcal)*	*DCP (kg)*	*TDN (kg)*	*M.E. (Mcal)*
300	0.33	3.1	11.2	0.42	4.0	14.4
400	0.45	4.0	14.4	0.52	4.8	17.2
500	0.56	4.9	17.6	0.71	6.4	23.1

Table 10.66

Feeding standards for a bull in service

Body wt. (kg)	*DCP (kg)*	*TDN (kg)*	*ME (kcal)*	*Ca (g)*	*P (g)*	*Vit. A (I.U.)*
500	0.43	4.5	16.2	12	12	21200
600	0.48	5.1	18.2	14	14	25400
700	0.54	5.7	20.5	15	15	29600
800	0.60	6.3	22.5	18	18	33800

Table 10.67

Additional requirement from 5th month of pregnancy (to be added with maintenance allowances)

DCP (kg): 0.14 TDN (kg): 0.70

Table 10.68 Recommended Nutrient Content of Rations for Dairy Cattle (Metric System)

Nutrients (Concentration in the Feed Dry matter)	Lactating Cow Rations: Cow Wt (kg) ≤400 / 500 / 600 / ≥700				Nonlactating Cattle Rations					Maximum Concentrations (All Classes)
	Daily Milk Yields (kg): < 8 / <11 / <14 / <18	8–13 / 11–17 / 14–21 / 18–26	13–18 / 17–23 / 21–29 / 26–35	>18 / >23 / >29 / >35	Dry Pregnant Cows	Mature Bulls	Growing Heifers and Bulls	Calf Starter Concentrate Mix	Calf Milk Replacer	
Ration No.	I	II	III	IV	V	VI	VII	VIII	IX	Max.
Crude Protein, %	13.0	14.0	15.0	16.0	11.0	8.5	12.0	16.0	22.0	–
Energy										
NE_l, Mcal/kg	1.42	1.52	1.62	1.72	1.35	–	–	–	–	–
NE_m, Mcal/kg	–	–	–	–	–	1.20	1.26	1.90	2.40	–
NE_g, Mcal/kg	–	–	–	–	–	–	0.60	1.20	1.55	–
ME, Mcal/kg	2.36	2.53	2.71	2.89	2.23	2.04	2.23	3.12	3.78	–
DE, Mcal/kg	2.78	2.95	3.13	3.31	2.65	2.47	2.65	3.53	4.19	–
TDN, %	63	67	71	75	60	56	60	80	95	–
Crude Fiber, %	17	17	17	17[a]	17	15	15	–	–	–
Acid Detergent Fiber, %	21	21	21	21	21	19	19	–	–	–
Ether Extract, %	2	2	2	2	2	2	2	2	10	–
Minerals[b]										
Calcium, %	0.43	0.48	0.54	0.60	0.37	0.24	0.40	0.60	0.70	–
Phosphorus, %	0.31	0.34	0.38	0.40	0.26	0.18	0.26	0.42	0.50	–
Magnesium, %[c]	0.20	0.20	0.20	0.20	0.16	0.16	0.16	0.07	0.07	–
Potassium, %	0.80	0.80	0.80	0.80	0.80	0.80	0.80	0.80	0.80	–
Sodium, %	0.18	0.18	0.18	0.18	0.10	0.10	0.10	0.10	0.10	–
Sodium chloride, %[d]	0.46	0.46	0.46	0.46	0.25	0.25	0.25	0.25	0.25	5
Sulfur, %[d]	0.20	0.20	0.20	0.20	0.17	0.11	0.16	0.21	0.29	0.35
Iron, ppm[d,e]	50	50	50	50	50	50	50	100	100	1,000
Cobalt, ppm	0.10	0.10	0.10	0.10	0.10	0.10	0.10	0.10	0.10	10
Copper, ppm[d,f]	10	10	10	10	10	10	10	10	10	80
Manganese, ppm[d]	40	40	40	40	40	40	40	40	40	1,000
Zinc, ppm[d,g]	40	40	40	40	40	40	40	40	40	500
Iodine, ppm[h]	0.50	0.50	0.50	0.50	0.50	0.25	0.25	0.25	0.25	50
Molybdenum, ppm[i,j]	–	–	–	–	–	–	–	–	–	6
Selenium, ppm	0.10	0.10	0.10	0.10	0.10	0.10	0.10	0.10	0.10	5
Fluorine, ppm[j]	–	–	–	–	–	–	–	–	–	30
Vitamins[k]										
Vit A, IU/kg	3,200	3,200	3,200	3,200	3,200	3,200	2,200	2,200	3,800	–
Vit D, IU/kg	300	300	300	300	300	300	300	300	600	–
Vit E, ppm	–	–	–	–	–	–	–	–	300	–

[a] It is difficult to formulate high-energy rations with a minimum of 17 percent crude fiber. However, fat percentage depression may occur when rations with less than 17 percent crude fiber or 21 percent ADF are fed to lactating cows.

[b] The mineral values presented in this table are intended as guidelines for use of professionals in ration formulation. Because of many factors affecting such values, they are not intended and should not be used as a legal or regulatory base.

[c] Under conditions conducive to grass tetany (see text), should be increased to 0.25 or higher.

[d] The maximum safe levels for many of the mineral elements are not well defined; estimates given here, especially for sulfur, sodium chloride, iron, copper, zinc, and manganese, are based on very limited data; safe levels may be substantially affected by specific feeding conditions.

[e] The maximum safe level of supplemental iron in some forms is materially lower than 1,000 ppm. As little as 400 ppm added iron as ferrous sulfate has reduced weight gains (Standish *et al.*, 1969).

[f] High copper may increase the susceptibility of milk to oxidized flavor (see text).

[g] Maximum safe level of zinc for mature dairy cattle is 1,000 ppm.

[h] If diet contains as much as 25 percent strongly goitrogenic feed on dry basis, iodine provided should be increased two times or more.

[i] If diet contains sufficient copper, dairy cattle tolerate substantially more than 6 ppm molybdenum (see text).

[j] Maximum safe level of fluorine for growing heifers and bulls is lower than for other dairy cattle. Somewhat higher levels are tolerated when the fluorine is from less-available sources as phosphates (see text). Minimum requirement for molybdenum and fluorine not yet established.

[k] The following minimum quantities of B-complex vitamins are suggested per unit of milk replacer: niacin, 2.6 ppm; pantothenic acid, 13 ppm; riboflavin, 6.5 ppm; pyridoxine, 6.5 ppm; thiamine, 6.5 ppm; folic acid, 0.5 ppm; biotin, 0.1 ppm; vitamin B_{12}, 0.07 ppm; choline, 0.26 percent. It appears that adequate amounts of these vitamins are furnished when calves have functional rumens (usually at 6 weeks of age) by a combination of rumen synthesis and natural feedstuffs.

Source: *Nutrient Requirements of Dairy Cattle,* Fifth revised edition, National Research Council, National Academy of Sciences, Washington, D.C., 1978.

FEEDING CATTLE AND BUFFALOES BY THUMB RULE METHOD

So far the conventional, or say, orthodox method of computation of ration for dairy cattle has been discussed. Although the method described is founded on scientific and rational basis, the common farmer of our country, may at times, be confounded with a labyrinth of calculation which may seem to be very simple to technical personnel. The following thumb rule may guide them to feed their livestock satisfactorily with particular reference to cases where individual attention and computation on body weight basis seem to be rather impractical.

While considering the feeding schedule of an adult dairy-cattle, proper considerations should first be made for the purpose for which the animal has to be fed. These are (1) maintenance ration, (2) gestation ration and (3) production ration. The approach here is based on practical experiences rather than scientific basis as in conventional method discussed earlier.

1. Maintenance Ration

This is the minimum amount of feed required to maintain the essential body processes at their optimum rate without gain or loss in body weight or change in body composition. The discussion on this aspect will remain limited to the concentrate part of the ration as in most parts of India, green is seldom available. In urban areas of our land, straw is considered to be the only basic roughage.

Under such circumstances, the object should be to compound concentrate mixture which will provide at least 20 per cent protein (14–16 per cent DCP) and 68–72 per cent TDN. Reasonable varieties of feed should be included so that when compounded, the mixture should be quite palatable and slightly laxative and balanced with minerals and vitamins. Variety of feed also offers other advantages, e.g., the imbalance of protein or minerals of one feed can be corrected by the other feed.

The amount of concentrate mixture and straw that will provide optimum maintenance requirement for an adult dairy cattle without any computation whatsoever are given below:

Item	*For zebu cattle*	*For cross-breed/pure breed Indian cows/buffaloes*
1. Straw	4 kg	4–6 kg
2. Concentrate mixture (with straw only or with little greens)	1–1.25 kg	2.00 kg

Let us, however, see how far in reality the above quantity satisfies the maintenance requirement of an adult dairy cattle.

Example I

As per nutrition standard it will be observed that the maintenance requirement of an adult *deshi* cow weighing 250 kg, will be DCP 0 168 kg and TDN 2.02 kg. According to thumb rule method the amount of DCP and TDN supplied as per quantities alloted will be:

Item	DCP	TDN
1. Straw 4 kg (DCP=0.0; TDN=42.0)	0.000	1.68
2. Concentrate mix. 1.25 kg (DCP=14.0 and TDN=68.0 minimum)	0.175	0.85
	0.175	2.53=Given
	0.168	2.02=Recommended

Example 2.

The nutritional requirement for an adult cow weighing 450 kg will be 0.28 kg DCP and 3.37 kg TDN (same table as for above cow). To be satisfied by thumb rule method as below:

Item	DCP	TDN
1. Straw 5 kg or more (DCP=0.0: TDN=42.0)	0.00	2.10
2. Concentrate mixture 2 kg (DCP=14.0 and TDN=68.0 minimum)	0.28	1.36
	0.28	3.46=Given
	0.28	3.37=Recommended

Now the question remains as to how to formulate the concentrate mixture that will provide 14–16% DCP and a minimum of 68% TDN without taking recourse to computation. For this the following assumptions may be made.

Oil cakes	25–35 parts	To be fortified with 1% mineral mixture, 1–2%
Millets/cereals	25–35 parts	Salt and 20–30 gm vit AD_3/100 kg, containing
Cereal by-products	10–25 parts	50,000 I.U. Vit. A and 5,000 I.U. Vit D_3 per
Pulse chuni	5–20 parts	gram

The computation of the above mixture will reveal that if quality ingredients are chosen then the above concentrate mixture will provide a minimum of 15% DCP and 70% TDN and for that a farmer need not know necessarily the computation of ration in terms of DCP and TDN. Where the principal roughage is straw, limestone powder @ 1—2% (able to pass through 150 mesh) should also be given.

Let us now take a concrete example of a type of concentrate mixture to prove that the above assumption is correct.

From the above, it will be clear that the assumption made earlier holds good and therefore a farmer need not necessarily go into details of DCP and TDN for his computation work.

A farmer desirous of producing concentrate mixture of his own should know the various types of ingredients required for making concentrate mixture ideal for livestock feeding. If he is not well conversant with the quality of raw feed ingredients and unconventional feedstuffs available in the region, he may not be able to compute an ideal concentrate mixture for his stock economically. The various types of feed ingredients generally used for computing concentrate mixture have already been discussed at the beginning of this chapter but for ready reference the names of the commonly found ingredients are mentioned here again.

1. *Protein Supplements* (Primary sources of protein)

(a) Vegetable protein supplements—oil cakes, e.g., groundnut cake, sesame cake, cotton seed cake, mustard cake, linseed cake etc.

Table 10.69

Feed stuffs (1)	DCP			TDN	
	Parts (2)	Per qnt.	As Per column 2	Per qnt.	As per column 2
Oil Cakes					
Groundnut caks	10	38	3.80	73	7.30
Sesame cake	8	32	2.56	72	5.76
Mustard cake	5	28	1.40	72	3.60
Linseed cake	5	28	1.40	72	3.60
Cereals					
Maize	20	7	1.40	80	16.00
Barley	10	8	0.80	76	7.60
Bran					
Wheat bran	15	10	1.50	65	9.75
Rice bran	10	8	0.80	66	6.60
Pulse Chuni					
Gram chuni/Arhar chuni	14	11	1.54	68	9.52
Others					
Salt	1				
Mineral Mixture	1				
Limestone Powder	1				
GIVEN			15.20		69.73
RECOMMENDED (minimum)			14.00		68.00

(b) Animal protein supplement—fish meal, skim milk powder etc. (used chiefly in compounding concentrate mixture for calves in early months).

2. *Grain supplement* (primary source of energy)—cereal grains like maize, wheat etc., millet grains like jowar, milo etc.
3. *Cereal by products* (diluents—medium energy content, and source of minerals)—wheat bran, rice bran, maize etc.
4. *Pulse chunis* (medium protein, energy source)—mung chuni, arhar chuni, massoor chuni, kalai chuni etc.
5. *Salt*
6. *Minerals*
7. *Vitamins*

In the formulation of any concentrate mixture, primary consideration is given to protein and energy content of the ration which are satisfied by selecting suitable protein supplements and grain supplements respectively. In general, cereal by-products are palatable and laxative; they furnish good amount of minerals, particularly phosphorus excepting maize and bran which are mostly used as diluents to protein and energy supplements. Pulse chunies are also palatable and supply medium energy depending on the amount of husk present in them. If a good amount of broken pulses are present then the nutritive value of these chunies is much better than brans both in protein and energy content. The addition of salt (1-2 per cent) to the concentrate mixture increases palatability and supplies sodium and chlorine to the animal. Minerals are vitally important particularly when good quality greens are not available. When straw is used as a major source of roughage, mineral and vitamin supplements are essential. Commercial mineral mixtures are available for use in cattle ration and may be used at 1-2 per cent level. Vitamin mixture (Vit. A and D_3; Vit. A—50,000 I.U., Vit. D_3 5,000 I.U., per gram) is also commercially available in suitable packs and its use @ 20-30 gm per 100 kg of concentrates will be sufficient. This amount of vitamin mixture is a must particularly when no or little greens are available to the stock. When straw is used as the sole source of roughage, the addition of 1—2 per cent limestone powder (should pass through 150 mesh) will be very beneficial.

2. Gestation Ration

In the case of pregnancy, further allowance from the fifth month of pregnancy onwards must be made for proper growth of the foetus and to keep the mother fit for optimum milk production on calving. For this, in addition to maintenance ration, a further amonut of 1.25 and 1.75 kg concentrate mixture is recommended for zebu and cross bred cow/buffaloes respectively.

Let us now examine whether in reality the above quantity satisfies the gestation requirement as recommended in the conventional method.

Example 1: The nutritional requirement for an adult cow weighing 250 kg and at an advanced stage of gestation is as follows:

Requirement:	DCP	TDN
For maintenance	0.17	2.02
For pregnancy	0.14	0.70
Total	0.31	2.72

To be satisfied by:

Items	DCP	TDN
1. Straw 4 kg or more	0.00	1.68
2. Concentrate mix 2.5 kg (1.25 for maintenance+1.25 kg for pregnancy allowance)	0.35	1.70
Given—	0.35	3.38
Recommended—	0.31	2.72

Example 2: The nutritional requirement for a cross-bred cow/Indian milch breed weighing 450 kg and at an advanced stage of pregnancy will be as follows:

Requirement:	DCP	TDN
For maintenance	0.28	3.37
For pregnancy	0.14	0.70
Total	0.42	4.07

To be satisfied by:

Items	DCP	TDN
1. Straw 5.0 kg or more	0.00	2.10
2. Concentrate mixture 3.75 kg (2.00 kg for maintenance+1.75 kg for pregnancy allowance)	0.52	2.55
Given—	0.52	4.65
Recommended—	0.42	4.07

For high yielder, it is desirable to go for liberal feeding of pregnant dams particularly cross-bred cows/buffaloes from 8th month of pregnancy of 6 weeks before calving with the object of securing full development of mammary glands for optimum milk production. For this 2.0 to 3.0 kg of concentrate for Zebu and between 4.0—5.0 kg for cross-bred/pure bred Indian cattle/buffaloes over and above maintenance requirements are recommended.

3. Production Ration

Production ration is the additional allowance of ration for milk production over and above the maintenance requirement. For Zebu 1 kg additional amount of concentrate is required for every 2.5 kg of milk over and above the maintenance requirement while the same amount of concentrate is required for every 2.0 kg of milk for cross-bred/Indian milch breed/buffaloes

As before, let us now examine whether in reality the above quantity satisfies the requirement for a milk producing cow or not by comparing the amount derived by conventional method.

Example 1; Requirement for Zebu weighing 250 kg and producing 4 kg of milk of 4.5% fat will be (by conventional method) as follows:

Requirement:	DCP	TDN
For maintenance	0.168	2.02
For production	0.192	1.36
Total	0.360	3.38

To be satisfied by:

Items	DCP	TDN
1. Straw 4 kg or more	0.00	1.68
2. Concentrate mixture 2.85 kg (1.25 kg for maintenance+1.60 kg for production)	0.40	1.94
Given—	0.40	3.62
Recommended—	0.36	3.38

Example 2: Requirement for a cow weighing 450 kg and producing 10 kg milk of 4% fat will be as follows:

Requirement	DCP	TDN
For maintenance	0.28	3.37
For production	0.45	3.16
Total requirement—	0.73	6.53

To be satisfied by:

Items	DCP	TDN
1. Straw 5 kg or more	0.00	2.10
2. Concentrate mixture 7 kg (2.0 kg for maintenance+5.0 kg for production)	0.98	4.76
Given—	0.98	6.86
Recommended—	0.73	6.53

The above two examples are sufficient to prove that the requirement of dairy cattle can be met easily by using the thumb rule method. But for buffaloes where milk is extremely rich in energy due to high fat percentage, thumb rule method does not work as efficiently as for low yielders with moderate fat percentage. An example of this situation may be studied as below:

Example 3: Requirement of a buffalo weighing 450 kg and producing 10 kg milk of 8% fat will be

	DCP	TDN
For maintenance	0.28	3.37
For production	0.69	5.06
Total requirement	0.97	8.43

To be satisfied by:

Items	*DCP*	*TDN*
1. Straw 6 kg	0.00	2.52
2. Concentrate mixture 7 kg (5 kg for production+2 kg for maintenance)	0.98	4.76
Given	0.98	7.28
Recommended	0.97	8.43

Therefore, the energy requirement of the buffalo is not satisfied.

In this example, it has been shown that by using thumb rule method, the requirement of energy (TDN) could not be fulfilled. For high yielders with high fat percentage, this kind of situation is very common. To overcome this sort of critical situation generally observed in the case of buffaloes, at least, 10 kg extra amount of green fodders like Paragrass, Maize, Guinea grass etc., should be supplied to meet the demands of energy requirement. An attempt to increase the quantum of straw to fulfill the energy requirement is likely to fail since the buffaloes will not consume 9 kg of straw for reasons of unpalatability. Therefore, in the above example, inclusion of further 10 kg of commonly found paragrass (1.4 DCP and 12.0 TDN) will add additional amount of 0.14 kg of DCP and 1.20 kg of TDN, to fulfill the energy requirement of the baffaloe ration.

If can be concluded, however, that the requirement of a crossbred cow producing more than 15 litres of milk per day or a buffaloe producing 10 litres of milk or more per day may not be met by thumb rule feeding with straw only as the roughage part of the ration unless supplemented with greens like maize, fodder, paragrass of good quality hay etc. Alternatively, TDN content of the concentrate mixture should be increased enormously (beyond 80 per cent).

So long the quantity of concentrate mixture containing 20% crude protein or 14-16 per cent DCP and 68% TDN with straw as the sole roughage are available to fulfill the energy requirements of the high yielders, there will be no problem. In rainy seasons, however, or in areas where greens are available for stock feeding, the crude protein percentage of the concentrate mixture may be reduced in line with the quantity of greens that farmer can provide to his stock, e.g., with good quality legumes like lucerne, berseem or cowpea or their hay as the roughage, the protein content of the concentrate mixture can be safely reduced to 14-16 per cent; with mixed legumes and grass or good quality paragrass, guinea grass, maize fodder, etc., as the roughage, the protein content may be reduced to 17-18 per cent protein only. Further, depending on the amount of greens/hay that a livestock owner can provide to his stock, the amount of concentrate mixture should be determined, e.g., if he can provide, say 20 kg greens like paragrass, guinea grass, dub grass etc., to his stock, this will furnish approximately 0.24—0.28 kg DCP and 2.4 kg TDN and consequently the quantum of concentrate mixture will be automatically reduced to provide the rest of the nutrients required. *Roughly speaking, for every 10 kg of good quality greens, 1 kg concentrate can be cut from the concentrate quota with the additional advantage of dry matter, TDN, minerals and vitamins in favour of greens.* A farmer feeding his cross bred cow with 7 kg concentrate with paddy straw as the roughage for production of 10 kg milk may safely reduce his feeding chart to 5 kg concentrates and 20 kg greens like paragrass/dub grass etc., plus straw. The resultant effect on milk production by

Table 10.70

Average rates of feeding of concentrates, green and dry fodder assumed for different categories of livestock and poultry

Categories of Livestock		RATES OF FEEDING PER DAY (IN Kg)		
		Concentrates	Green fodder	Dry fodder
A Cattle				
1. crossbred (milch)	....	2.75	20.00	6.00
2. females over 3 years of age :				
(i) improved cows (milch)	....	1.20	10.00	6.00
(ii) other milch cows and not calved even once	....	0.125	3.5	3.16
3. males over 3 years of age	....	0.17	4.96	5.65
4. males less than 3 years of age				
(i) crossbred (young stock)	....	1.50	10.00	2.00
(ii) other young stock	....	0.016	1.58	1.47
B. Buffaloes				
1. females over 3 years of age :				
(i) improved buggaloes	....	1.50	10.00	6.00
(ii) other milch buffaloes and those not calved even once	....	0.41	5.72	5.08
2. males over 3 years of age	....	0.109	6.51	5.43
3. less than 3 years of age	....	0.01	1.59	1.64
C. Poultry				
(i) improved layers	....	0.123	0.20	
(ii) growing stock	....	0.041	0.007	...
D. Other Livestock				
(i) improved sheep	....	0.274	...	0.40
(ii) improved pigs	....	2.50	1.00	...
(iii) hores and ponies	....	0.50	...	...

this change will be much better since it provides better nutrition by way of increased TDN minerals, vitamin etc., coupled with unidentified factor (?) present in grass juices. Further this change is also economically advantageous. At the present market rate, the cost of 2 kg concentrates having minimum 20% protein and 68% TDN will be Rs. 4.50 or more whereas the cost of 20 kg greens will be no more than Rs. 2.50 and in country side, particularly in rainy seasons, dub grass will be readily available at practically no cost. This is the reason why during the rainy season when grass grows abundantly, emaciated country cattle pick up conditions easily. It should be noted, however, that grass allowed to become over-ripe loses much of its nutritive value while it has the maximum value in the prime stage of growth.

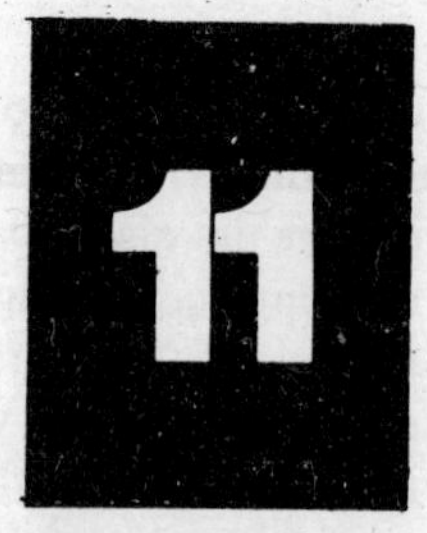

IMPORTANT CATTLE BREEDS AND THEIR CHARACTERISTICS

Zoological Classification

Cattle belong to the phylum *Chordata* (those animals having a backbone), class *Mammalia* (milk giving), order *Artiodactyla* (even-toed, hooved), suborder *Ruminatia* (cud chewing), family *Bovidae* (hollow horn), genus *Bos* (ruminant quadrupeds). Species are divided into *Bos indicus* (humped cattle), *Bos taurus* (without any hump) and *Bos bubalis* (the buffalo). Although other species were frequently mentioned by early writers, today they are mostly disregarded.

Some common terms in relation to CATTLE

Details		*Expression*	*Details*		*Expression*
Species called as	...	Bovine	Castrated male	...	Bullock or steer
Group of animals	...	Herd	Castrated female	...	Spayed
Adult male	...	Bull	Female with its offspring	...	Calf at foot
Adult female	...	Cow	Act of parturition	...	Calving
Young male	...	Bull calf	Act of mating	...	Serving
Young female	...	Heifer calf	Sound produced	...	Bellowing
New-born one	...	Calf	Pregnancy	...	Gestation

What is Breed?

A group of animals related by descent and similar in most characters like general appearance, features, size, configuration, etc., are said to be a breed. There may be considerable differences between individuals, still they have as a group many common points which distinguish them from other groups. Such a common characteristic group is termed a breed. The purity of the breed is maintained by confining the mating of animals to within the breed.

In India there are 25 well-defined breeds of cattle and 6 breeds of buffaloes in addition to a large number of non-descripts of low productivity in nature.

What is Species?

A group of individuals which have certain common characteristics that distinguish them from other groups of individuals. Within a species the individuals are fertile when mated, in different species they are not.

CATTLE BREEDS IN INDIA

According to 1988 FAO statistics on livestock population, India possesses 201.5 million cattle and 20.8 million buffaloes comprising 15.9 per cent of the world's cattle and 53.75 per cent of world's buffalo population. Thus India can feel proud of having not only the largest number of cattle and buffaloes in comparison to any country belonging to this planet, but also due to having world's best breeds of drought cattle apart from best breeds of dairy buffaloes. They are noted for their adaptability to tropical heat and resistance to most tropical diseases.

Table 11.1

COMPARISON OF TOTAL NUMBER OF RECOGNISED BREEDS OF VARIOUS SPECIES OF LIVESTOCK IN THE WORLD AND INDIA

Sl. No.	*Species*	*No. in world*		*No. in India*	
1.	Cattle	231		26	
2.	Buffaloes	16		16	(including world's best 7 milch breeds)
3.	Sheep	224		40	
4.	Goat	62		20	
5.	Pigs	54		3	
6.	Camels	?		4	
7.	Horses	20		6	
8.	Mithun	1	(Species ?)	1	(Species ?)
9.	Yak	1	(Species ?)	1	(Species ?)
10.	Poultry	?		18	

Our major handicap is that, out of 201.5 million cattle, only about 18 per cent are distributed among 26 well defined Indian breeds. Rest 82 per cent are categorised as "*Non-descript*" or the "*Local deshi cows*" characterized by their poor growth rate, late maturity and low milk production.

The family of animals that includes all types of domestic cattle are known as *Bovidae.* There are very many species belonging to the family are found throughout the world. The existing two main groups of bovidae (domestic cattle) e.g., 1. *Bos indicus* (India and Africa) and the other 2. *Bos taurus* (European), are descended from *Bos primigenius,* the original wild cattle of Europe, now no longer in existence. *Bos taurus* found in Europe and North America are all non humped cattle which were first domesticated nearly 10,000 years ago somewhere in Middle East. Our indigenous *Zebu cattle* (*Bos indicus*) or humped cattle might have been produced by selection from non-humped cattle either in South or South West Asia. The Zebu is characterised by (1) presence of prominent large hump, (2) a long face, (3) upright horns, (4) drooping ears, (5) a large dewlap and slender legs. The colour varies from white to grey and black. Zebus have relatively lower basal metabolic rate, better capacity for heat dissipation through cutaneous evaporation and thus adoptation to tropical heat, and resistance to diseases specially the tick-borne diseases than taurus cattle. In the U.S. Zebus are called *Brahman* cattle.

The domestication of zebu cattle appears to have taken place in Afganistan, Sind and Baluchistan before 4000 B.C. To-day also some zebu breeds may be located in Iraq. Zebu are believed to have been brought into India through the northern passes between 2200 and 1500 B.C., and thereafter spread along the route taken by their owners, the Vedic Aryan invaders.

For introducing some vital characteristics of zebu cattle, viz. particularly higher disease resisting power, and heat tolerating power, they have been imported from India by Southern U.S., South America and Australia for developing tropically adapted dairy/beef cattle breeds. Similarly, for last decade attempts have been made to introduce superior exotic inheritance of *Bos taurus*, into indigenous *Bos indicus* through cross-breeding. A few superior breeds/strains from such crossbred base have been evolved in cattle viz., Karan-Swiss, Karan-Fries, and Sunandini etc. Their productivity performance is superior even to those of our indigenous pure dairy breeds. Besides, they have shown reasonable adaptation to tropical heat and diseases.

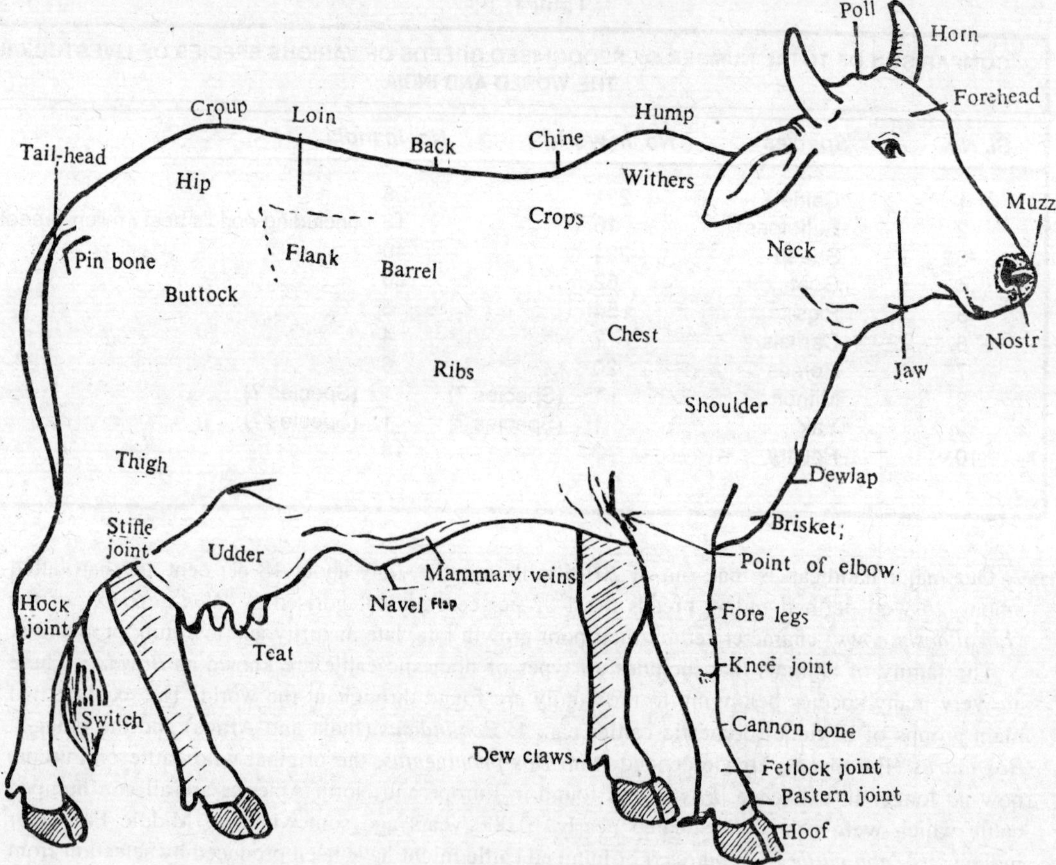

Fig.11.1 The external parts of a Cow.

CLASSIFICATION OF INDIAN BREEDS OF CATTLE

Zebu cattle are in general considered to be indigenous to the Indian sub-continent, of which India and Pakistan are considered to be their natural habitats where they have been domesticated,

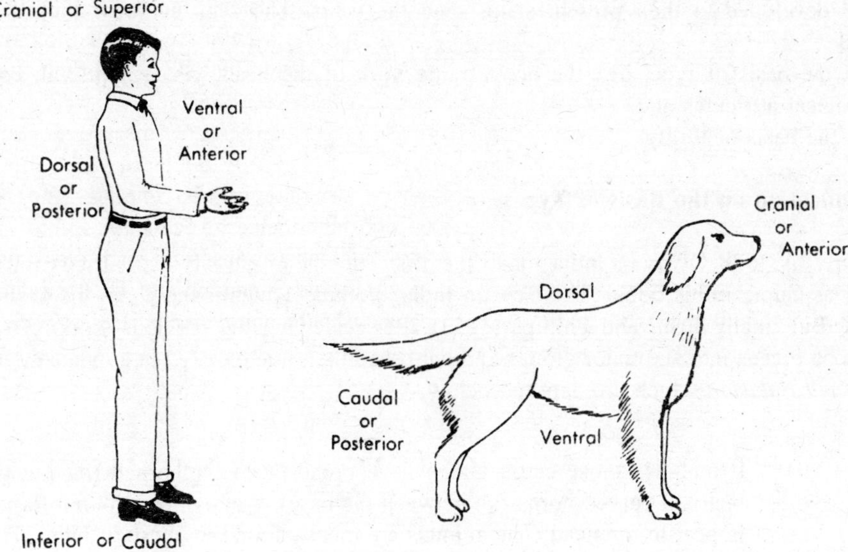

Fig.11.2 Terminology of quadruped and human compared.

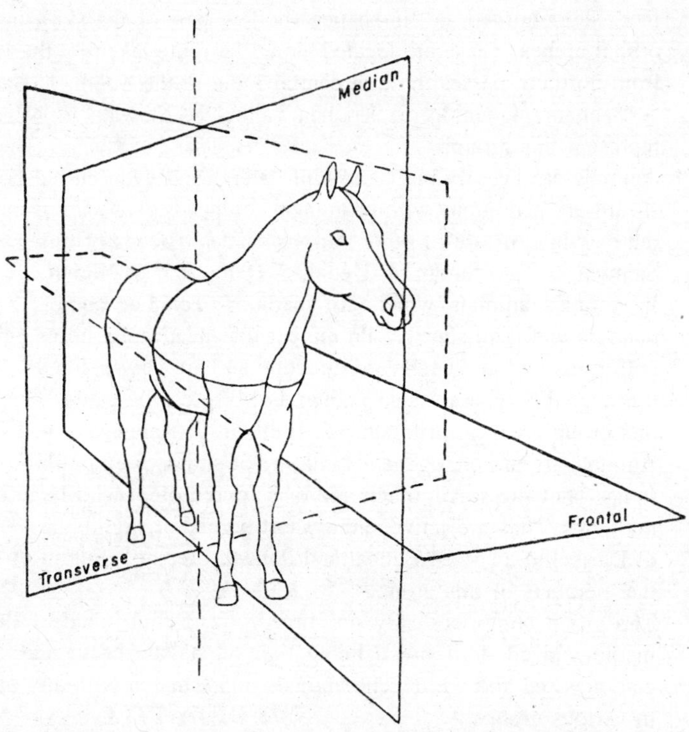

Fig.11.3 Imaginary planes of reference.

bred and developed to their present status over the years. The zebu cattle of India have been classified

A. on the basis of type, i.e., the bony frame-work of the head, visual appraisal, colour and morphological attributes and

B. on the basis of utility.

A. Classification on the Basis of Types

As early as 1938 Olver in India made the first attempt to classify the various indian cattle breeds. Das Gupta in his book "The Cow in India" volume 1 mentioned about his efforts in this direction. But finally Joshi and Phillips (1953) after reviewing the previous work, classified all Indian Zebu breeds into six major groups and published the same by FAO in a manual *Zebu Cattle of India and Pakistan* which are narrated below:

GROUP I : It includes those cattle which have broad-faced lyrehorned (having two symmetrical curved horns run between the base), grey-white coloured flat or dished in profile forehead. The animals are mostly found in Western India. The breeds under this category are 1. Kankrej, 2. Kherigarh, 3. Malvi 4. Tharparker and 5. Kankatha.

GROUP II : Cattle belonging to this group are white or light grey, narrow but slightly convex face, short horned, coffin-shaped (hollow part of the skull in front) skills and orbital arches. These are located along the route taken by the Rig Vedic Aryans from northern passes through central India to the South. 1. Hariana, 2. Ongole, 3. Bachaur, 4. Gaolo, 5. Krishna valley, 6. Mewati, 7. Nagori and 8. Rathi represent this group.

GROUP III : Animals are heavily built and with lateral and even curled horns. Dewlap and sheath are pendulous with prominent foreheads. They are usually spotted either red or white, or are of other various shades. Breeds of this group are 1. Gir, 2. Sahiwal, 3. Red Sindhi, 4. Deoni, 5. Dangi and 6. Nimari.

GROUP IV : It includes animals which are medium-sized but compact, having powerful quarters and tight sheaths. Prominent fore-head; long horns emerge from top of poll in upward and backward direction and are very pointed, grey in colour. The breed of this type are also known as Mysore type cattle. The breeds belong to this group are 1. Amritmahal, 2. Hallikar, 3. Kangayam. 4. Khillari, 5. Bargur.

Group V : Animals are of heterogeneous mixture of strains found in hilly tracts in northern India. They are small, black, red or coloured often with large patches and white markings. They are active, either short-horned or slightly large-horned. Siri breed of Darjeeling in West Bengal and Ponwar breed of Pilibhit of Uttar Pradesh are the members of this group.

Group VI : The group comprises only one breed, viz. Dhani breed of Pakistan. This is a medium sized draft breed being tight in naval sheath and dewlap. Preferred colour is red and white. The animal cannot match with any of the other breeds in various groups.

In general, the cattle from the drier regions are well built, and those from the heavy rainfall areas, coastal regions and hilly regions are smaller in built.

Table 11.2 INDIAN CATTLE BREEDS

(TOTAL 26)

Milch Breeds	Dual-purpose Breeds	Draught-purpose Breeds	
(Cows are high yielders, varies from 1,500 to 2,500 litres per lactation, bullocks are of poor quality	(Animals have characteristics intermediate between Milch and Draught breeds, milk yield varies from 1,200 to 1,500 liters per lactation	(Bullocks are excellent draft animals, while the cows are poor milkers	
1. **Gir**	1. **Hariana**	1. **Hallikar**	8. **Kenkatha**
2. **Sahiwal**	2. **Ongole**	2. **Amritmahal**	9. **Kherigarh**
3. **Red Sindhi**	3. **Kankrej**	3. **Khillari**	10. **Kangayam**
4. **Tharparkar**	4. **Deoni**	4. **Bargur**	11. **Ponwar**
	5. **Nimari**	5. **Nagori**	12. **Siri**
	6. **Dangi**	6. **Bachaur**	13. **Gaolao**
	7. **Mewati**	7. **Malvi**	14. **Krishna Valley**
	8. **Rathi**		

Out of the 26 Cattle breeds, detailed characteristics of all the 4 Milch breeds, 4 of the Dual purpose breeds and 6 of the Draught purpose breeds have been discussed in details while the breed characteristics of the remaining 12 breeds have been discussed in condensed form. However, the importance of each individual breed should be considered of equal importance.

Dual-purpose Breeds :

(Contd.)

Breed	*Home tract*	*Weight*	*Colour*	*Distinguishing Features*	*Group*	*Utility*
Nimari	Narmada Valley tract of Madhya Pradesh	M. 390.0 F. 282.0	Red with splashes of white on various parts of the body	Long and narrow face; flat forehead; moderately developed horns emerging from outer angles of poll in outward direction and carried upwards with a gentle curve to turn at points. The body is long with a straight back. Skin is fine and slightly loose. Animals are energetic and vigorous but nervous with strangers	III	Bullocks are docile and good at work. Cows are poor milkers, yielding on an average 450 to 500 kg. annually.
Dangi *(Kalkheri, Sonkheri)*	Ahmednagar, Nasik, Bansda, Sonkhed region of Maharastra & Gujarat	M 362.9 F 294.9	Broken red & white 0r black & white	Medium sized body, oily skin, small head, projecting forehead. Horns are short but thick; small ears.	III	A hardy breed. Males are excellent for work in rice field as they stand up well to heavy rainfall tracks. Females are poor milkers.
Mewati *(Kosi)*	Alwar, Bharatpur of east Rajasthan and Mathura district of U.P.	M 385.6 F 326.6	White with dark head, neck and shoulders	Long deep and powerful frames, similar to Hariana; face is also long but narrow; bulging forehead. Horns emerge from outward angles; ears pendulous. Large hump placed in front of withers. Tail is long. They are similar to Hariana breed with traces of Gir inheritance. The breed shows admixture of Gir, Rath and Naguri Cattle	II	Bullocks are powerful and docile. Cows are moderately good milkers, average milk yield is 4.55 kg. per day

Dual -purpose Breeds : (Contd.)

Breed	*Home Tract*	*Weight*	*Colour*	*Distinguishing Features*	*Group*	*Utility*
Rathi *(Rath)*	Alwar and Rajputana region of Rajasthan. Good specimens are also found in and around Bikaner district.	M 385.6 F 326.6	White or light grey	Medium sized powerfull cattle, basically similar to Hariana breed; well built and deep chest; face straight; flat forehead, eyes wide and large. Ears are short but pendulous. Well developed fore and hind quarters. Short tail with black switch	II	Bullocks are powerful and active, suitable for field and road work. Cows yield about 4.5 kg. milk per day.
Draught-purpose Breeds						
Bachaur *(Sitamarhi)*	Sitamarhi district of North Bihar.	M 385.5 F 317.5	Grey	Compact body, straight back, well rounded barrel, broad and flat forehead, prominent and large eyes. Ears are of medium size compact and firm hump. Tail is short.	II	Well known for its medium draught ability. Cows are poor milkers, yield averages about 1.35 kg per day.
Bargur	Coimbatore district of Tamil Nadu	M 340.0 F 295.0	Usually red and white. Sometimes light grey.	Body smaller than Mysore type compact; fore-head not so prominent; horns grow backwards and upwards. Hump moderately sized; dewlap fine but well mashed; tail rather short.	IV	Bullocks unsurpassable in hardiness, spiral and speed, difficult to train; cows are poor milkers.
Gaolao	Southern Madhya Pradesh, Maharastra	M 431.0 F 340.2	Females are pure white; Males grey over head, neck and humps	Body medium sized build. Very long narrow face with flat foreheads. Eyes almond shaped; ears of medium size; horns stumpy and short; voluminous dewlap. Tail comparatively short	II	Bullocks are good workers; cows are failr milkers, average milk yield is about 816.5kg. in a lactation period of 250 days.

Draught-purpose Breeds : (Contd.)

Breed	*Home Tract*	*Weight*	*Colour*	*Distinguishing Features*	*Group*	*Utility*
Kenkatha *(Kenwariya)*	Uttar Pradesh	M 344.5 F 295.0	Grey to dark grey.	Body short, deep and compact, straight back; short head and broad forehead dished. Sharp pointed ears and tail of medium length with black switch reaching below the hock. Strong horns are pointed outwards.	I	Bullocks are sturdy and fairly powerful; cows are poor milker.
Kherigarh	Lakhimpur-Kheri district of U.P.	M 476.0 F 317.5	Generally white	They have bright eyes, small active ears, short neck with well developed hump. Dwelap thin and pendulous, long tail ending in a white switch.	II	Bullocks are good for light draught and trotting purposes; cows are poor milkers; well suited for the Terai tract.
Krishna Valley	Home tract of this breed is the black cotton soil along the river Krishna and areas of Ghataprabha and Malaprabha in Karnataka.	M 499.0 F 340.0	Grey White	An admixture of Gir, Ongole and local Mysore type breeds. Long and massive body; deep and broad chest. Head comparetively small with slightly bulging forehead; small horns are curved usually emerging onwards and slightly curved up inwards.	II	Bullocks are very powerful and suitable for slow draught and heavy ploughing. Cows are fair milkers, yield about 916 kg. per lactation.
Nagori *(Nagore)*	Jodhpur and Nagore district of Rajasthan. The breed is supposed to have been evolved from Hariana and Kankrej breeds	M 408.0 F. 340.0	Generally white or grey.	Body long, deep, powerful with straight back and well developed flat forehead. Ears are large and pendulous; dewlap small and fine. Face narrow rather long. Horns moderately developed emerging from outer angles of poll in outward direction and carried upwards with gentle curve to run at points.	II	One of the most useful draught breeds of India, generally employed for road work. Cows are poor milkers, yield about 3.65 kg. of milk per day
Ponwar	Pilibhit and Lakhimpur Kheri in Uttar Pradesh	M 317.5 F 295.0	Generally black and white	Small narrow face; face small ears; big and bright eyes; hump well developed, horns long and upstanding; tail long and tapering	V	Bullocks are used for plough and load work. Cows are poor milkers.

B. Classification on the Basis of Utility

It has become customary to classify all our 26 breeds of Indian cattle on the basis of their utility. It is to be noted that these pure breeds comprises only 18 per cent of the total strength, out of which there are 4 Milch or dairy breeds, 8 Dual purpose and 14 Draught or draft breeds.

MILCH BREEDS

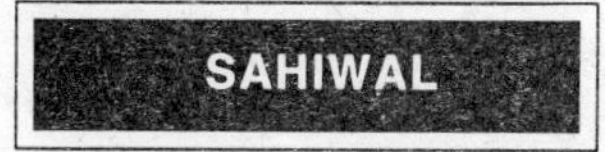

Synonym. Lola, Montgomery, Lambi-Bar, Multani.

Origin and distribution. Central and southern dry areas of the Punjab particularly in Montgomery district in Pakistan. Several pedigree herds are now being maintained in most of the large cities of Punjab, Delhi, U.P., Bihar and M.P.

• **_Distinguishing characters._ Deep body, loose skin (hence the name lola), short legs, stumpy horns, broad head and lethargic. General colours are various shades of red, pale red and dark brown splashed with white. Horns are short and thick, do not exceed 3 inches. Loose horns are common in females. Massive hump (in male), voluminous dewlap and pendulous sheath. Long whip like tail almost reaching to the ground, tapering to a good black switch. Navel flap is prominent in female. Sheath is pendulous but should not be abnormally loose or long. Males weigh about 522 kg and females 340 kg.**

Production. This is one of the best dairy breeds in India. In village the average yield is 2150 kg in 300 days lactation while at some of the farms the herd average has gone up to four to five thousand kilogrammes. Bullocks are useful for slow work.

Remarks. They are now being maintained at N.D.R.I., I.A.R.I., Government Dairy Farm (Lucknow), R.B.S. College Farm (Agra). Cattle of this breed have been exported to many parts of the tropical world. In Jamaica they have been crossed with Jersey for evolving Jamaica Hope Breed. In East Africa the breed has been utilised for upgrading the small East African Zebu cattle.

RED SINDHI

Synonyms: Red Sindhi, Scindhi, Red Karachi.

Origin and distribution. The home of this breed is round about Karachi and Hyderabad (Sindh). They are mostly imported from districts north and north-west of Karachi and Hyderabad, i.e., from the portion of Sind called Kohistan which forms the real breeding tract of this breed.

Distinguishing characters. Medium size and compact, animals having well-proportioned body, extremely docile. Thick horns emerging laterally and end in blunt points. Intelligent facial expression. Deep dark red colour varying from dun yellow in almost dark brown. Males are darker red than the cow. Heavy hump dewlap and sheath. Capacious udder with tendency to become pendulous in heavy milkers. Male weighs average 450 kg while females 295 kg.

Production. Yield as high as 5,443 kg per lactation. Average yield 1.474 kg. Bullocks suited for road and field work. They are medium paced steady workers.

Remarks. Owing to their capacity to adopt different climatic conditions the bulls are being used to grade up the local stock at N.D R.I., Naini (Allahabad), Hasur, Bangalore, Government Central Dairy (Gauhati).

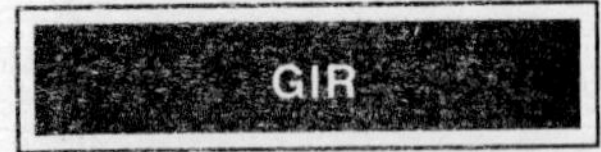

Synonyms. Kathiawarhi, Surti, Decan.

Origin and distribution. The breed probably originated in the Gir forest of South Kathiawar. They are mainly found in Junagarh State of South Kathiawar and in some other states of Western India. Herds are being maintained at N.D.R.I., (Bangalore). The breed has now migrated to the surrounding areas.

Distinguishing characters. Appearance strikingly impressive, well-proportioned body, robust constitution, proud gait and docile temperament. Ears are markedly long, pendulous resembling a tiny curled leaf. The head is moderately long but massive in appearance with prominent bony forehead, straight and levelled back are the most marking characters of the breed. Tail is long, whip-like with a black switch at the end. Skin is fine and mellow, hip bones are prominent. Colour is seldom entire varying from almost red to almost black. Spots of different colours are one of the chief characteristics of this breed. Average female weighs 386 kg while males weigh 544 kg.

Production. Cows are good milkers. Average yield 1746 kg, while some animals may go as high as 3175 kg depending on lactation when maintained properly. Bullocks are heavy and powerful, medium paced, good for draught.

Remarks. Maintained at Junagarh Farm, different goushalas of Ahmedabad, Bombay and Poona. Outside India the breed has got an excellent reputation as beef animals and large numbers have been exported to Brazil from where they have been introduced to some American countries.

THARPARKAR

Synonyms. Thari, Grey Sindhi, White Sindhi.

Origin and distribution. The home of the breed is the Tharparkar district of Hyderabad, India and cattle are now distributed in south-east Sind, Amorkot, Naukot, Dhoro Naro and Chor. The area extends up to Cutch deserts of West India; Marwar in east and Palanpur area of north Bombay.

Distinguishing characters. Medium size, deep built, short, straight and strong limbs. Strong, well-proportioned frame, broad poll and forehead is slightly convex with medium sized horns. Moderately developed dewlap with straight and moderately long back. The tail is fine with black switch. White or light grey line along the spine in young animals. Males show virility. Udder is moderately developed with 3-4 inches long teats.

Production. Cows are good yielders, bullocks suited for carting and ploughing. Average yield in village conditions is 1474 kg. However, on well maintained farms maximum yield up-

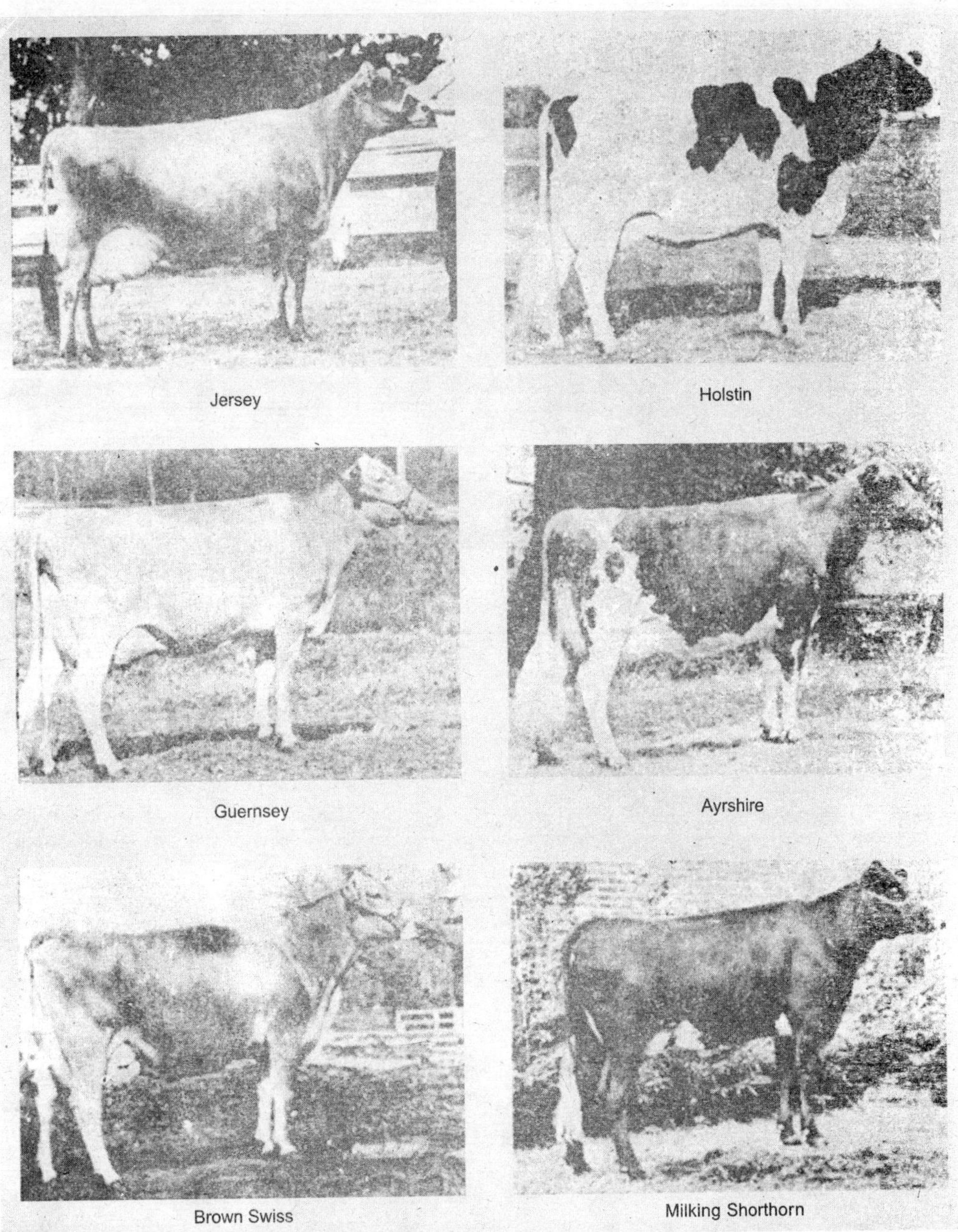

Jersey

Holstin

Guernsey

Ayrshire

Brown Swiss

Milking Shorthorn

Plate 23. (CHAPTER 11).

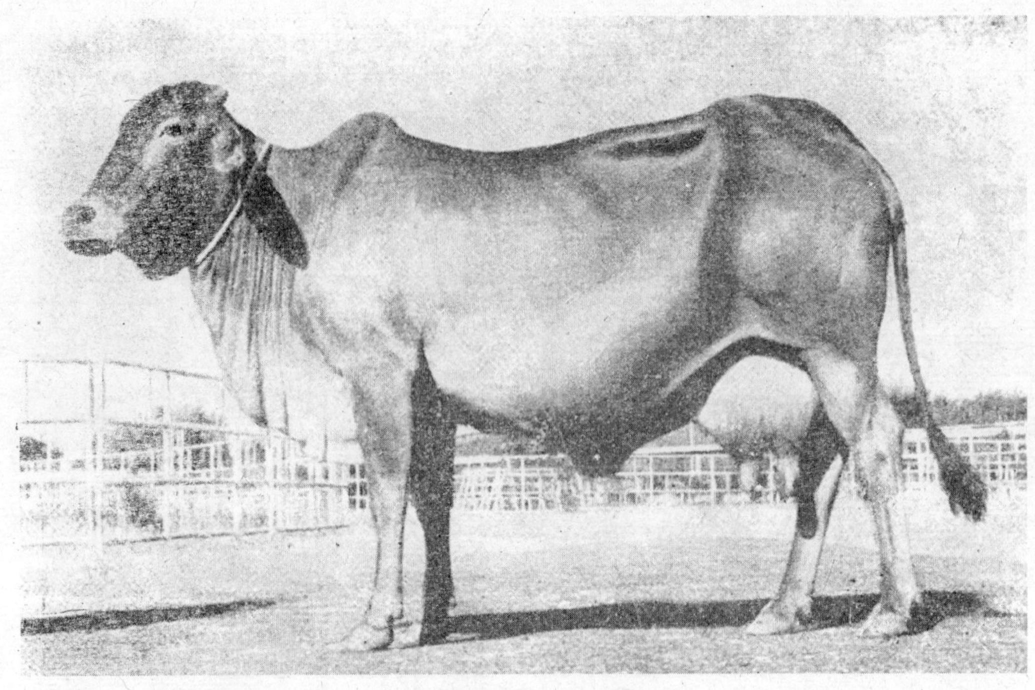

Plate 24. A Sahiwal cow.

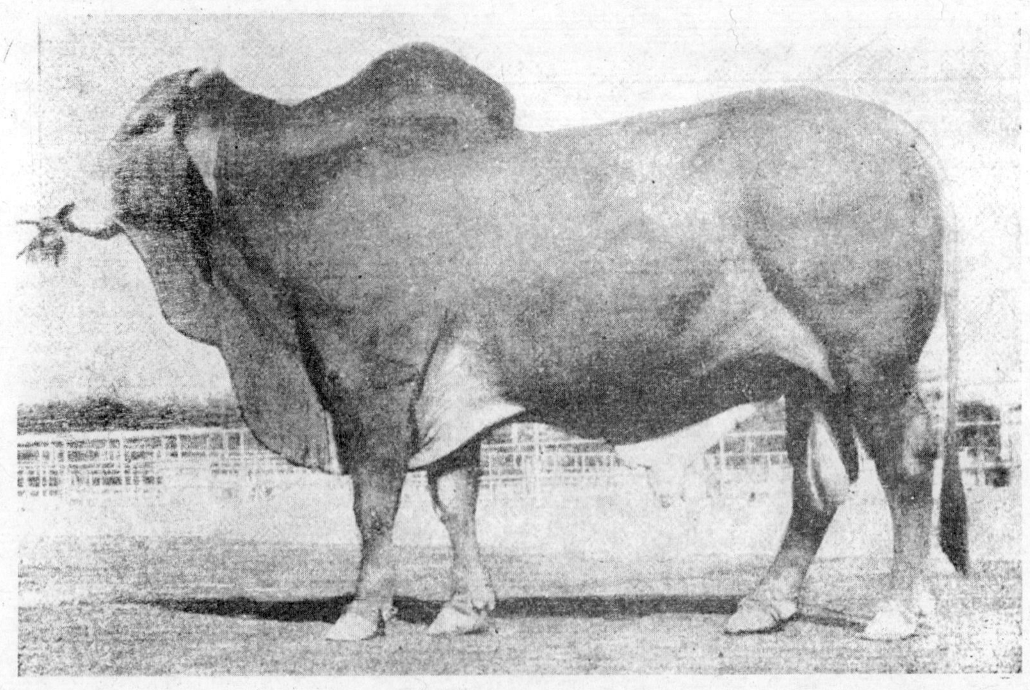

Plate 25. A Sahiwal bull.

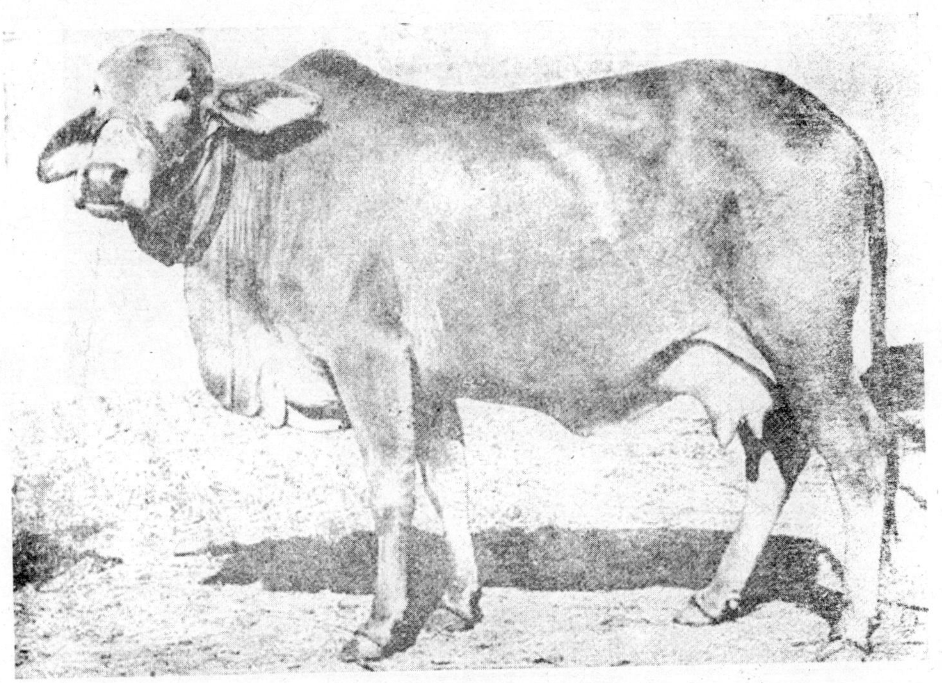

Plate 26. A Red Sindhi cow.

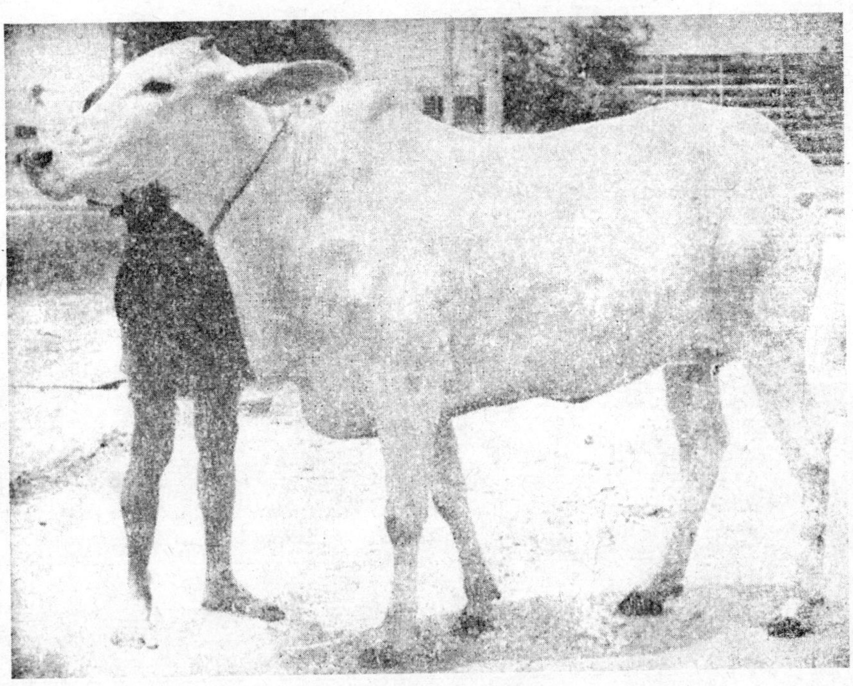

Plate 27. A Hariana heifer.

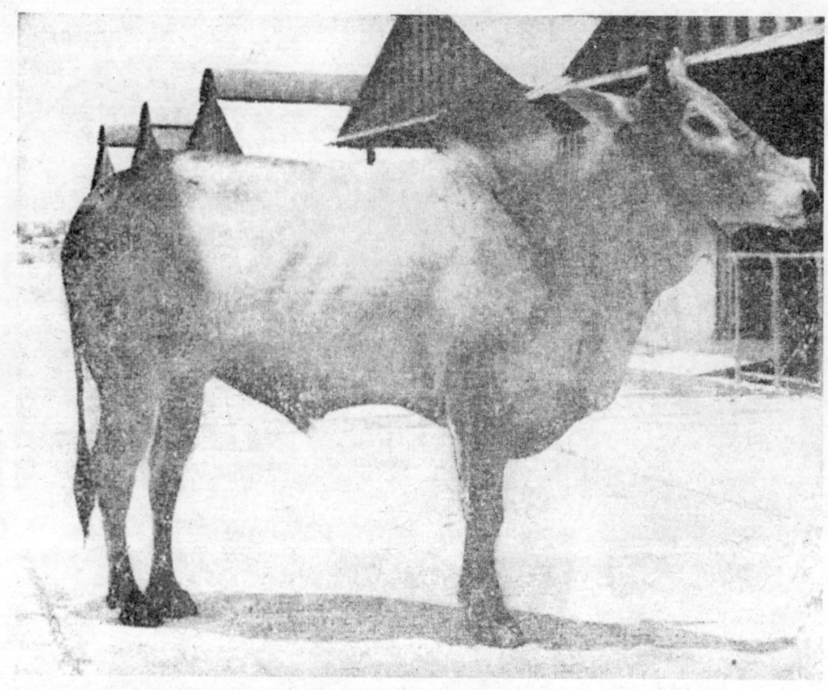

Plate 28. A Hariana bull.

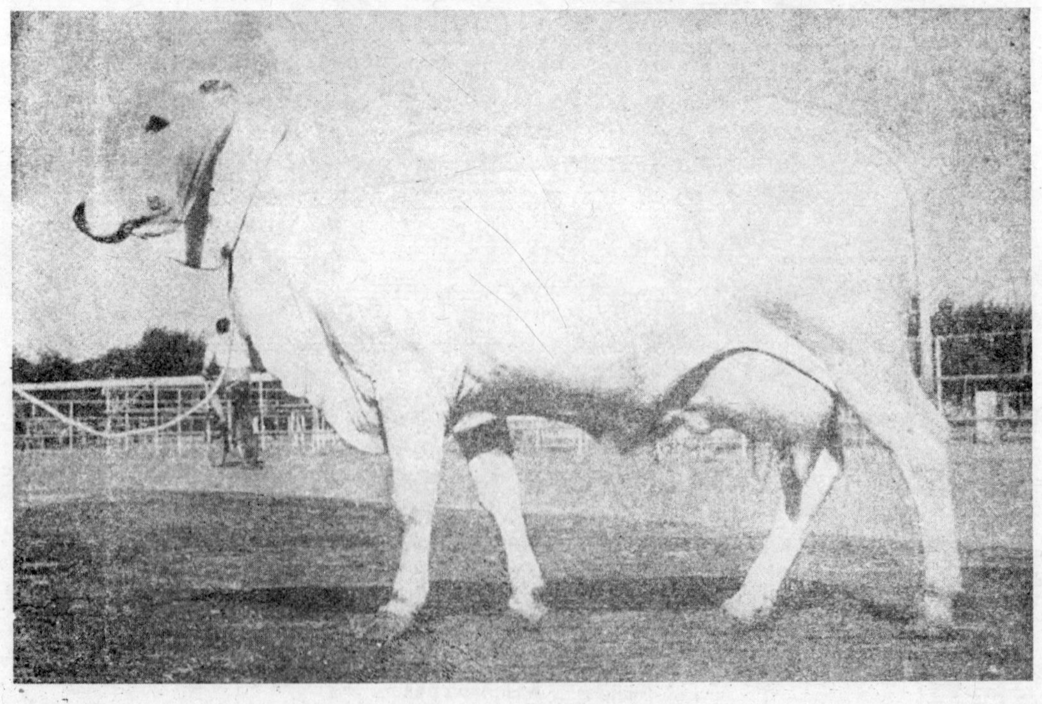

Plate 29. A Tharparkar cow.

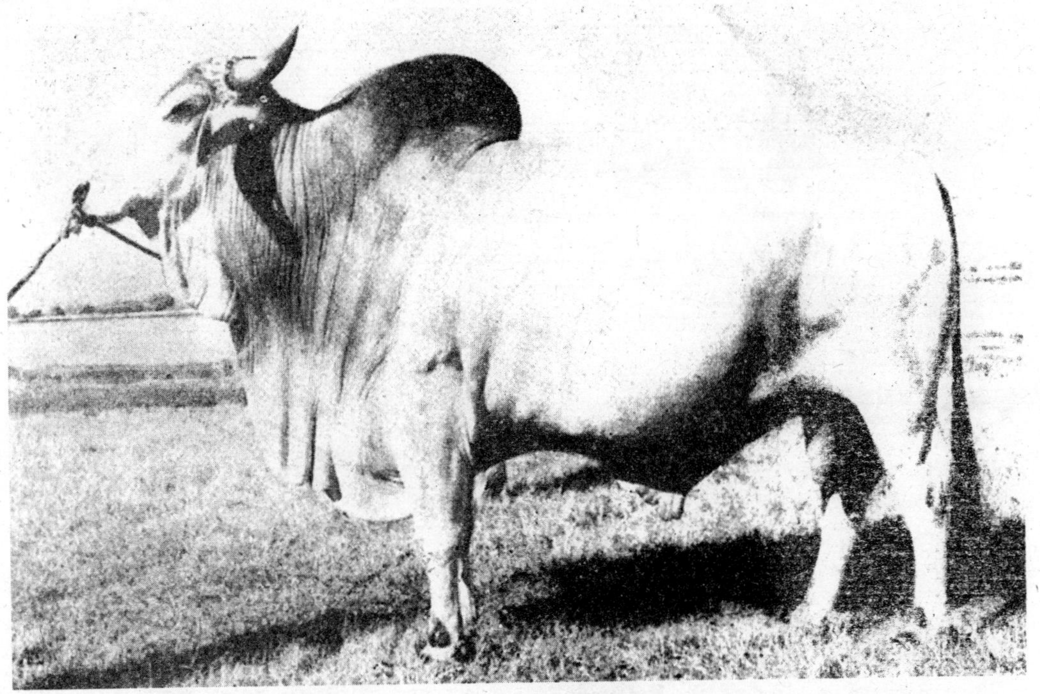

Plate 30. A male Tharparkar.

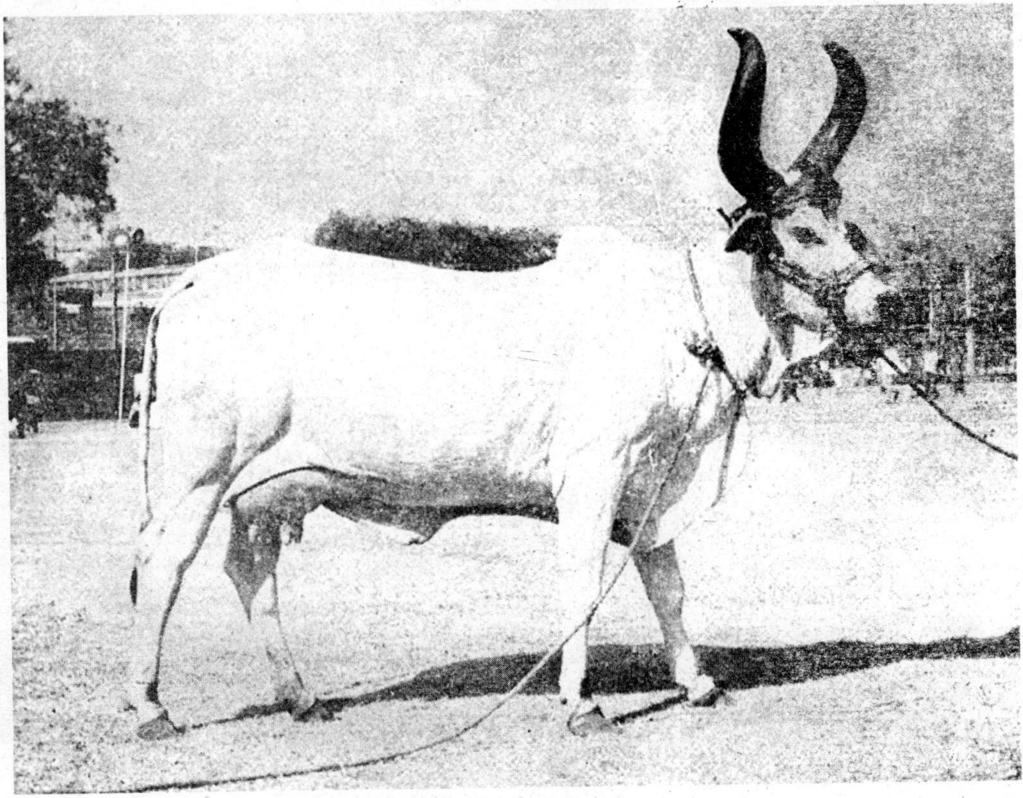

Plate 31. A Kankrej cow.

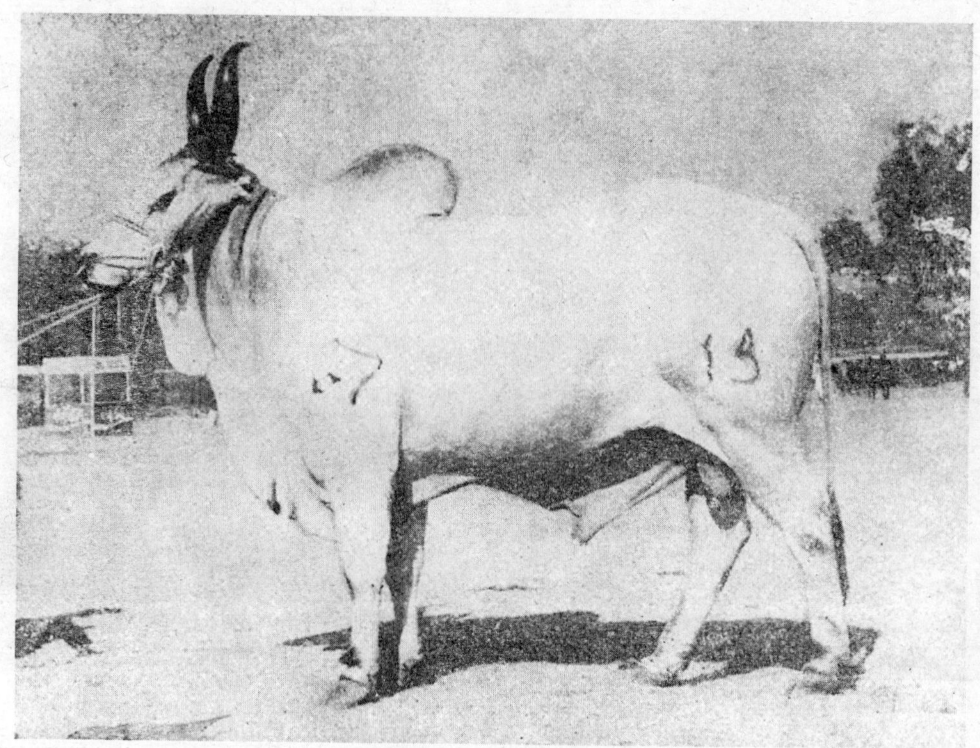

Plate 32. A Kankrej bull.

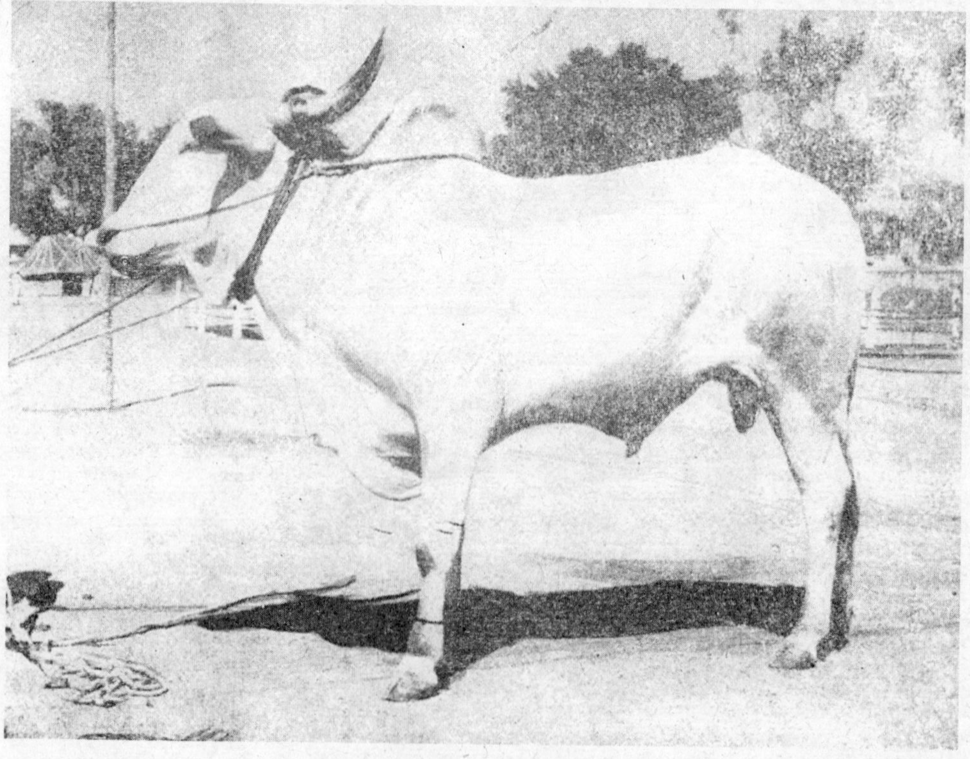

Plate 33. A Hallikar bull.

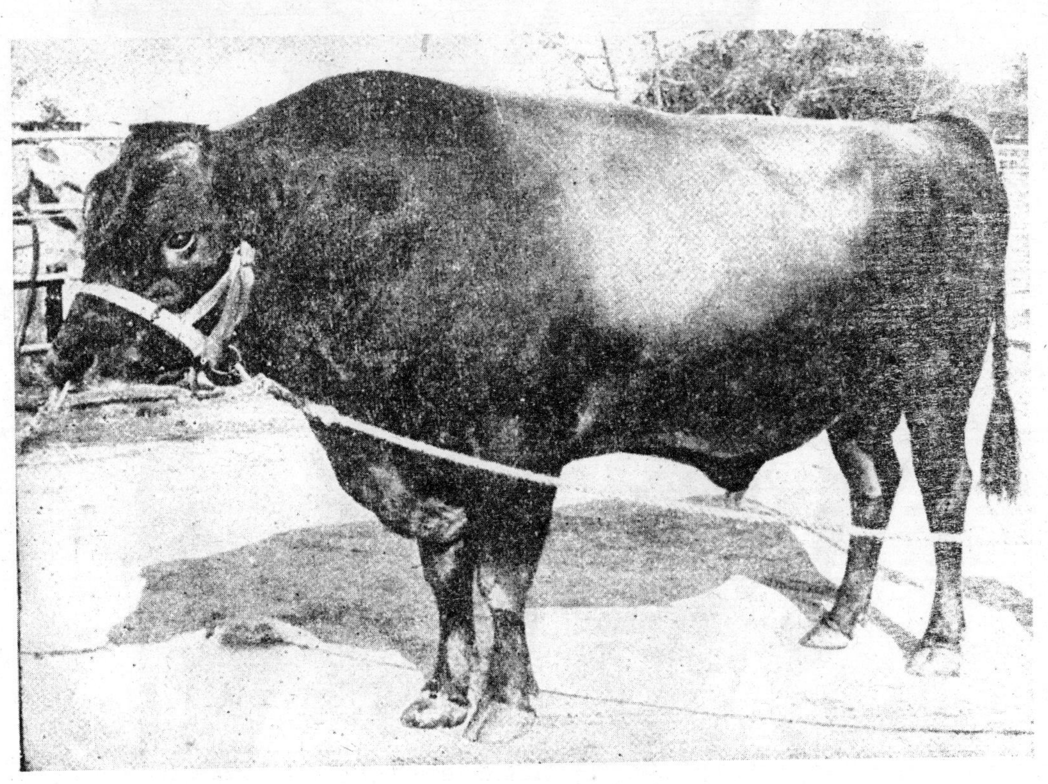

Plate 34. A Jarsey bull.

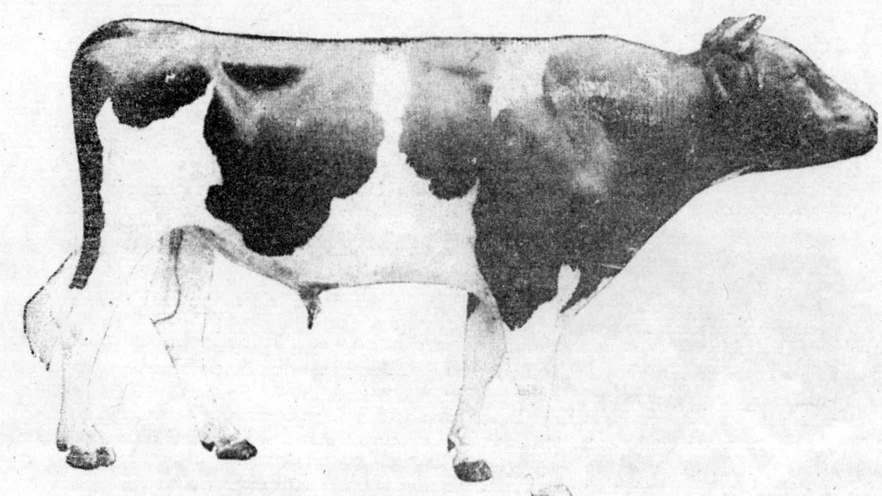

Plate 35. A Holstein bull.

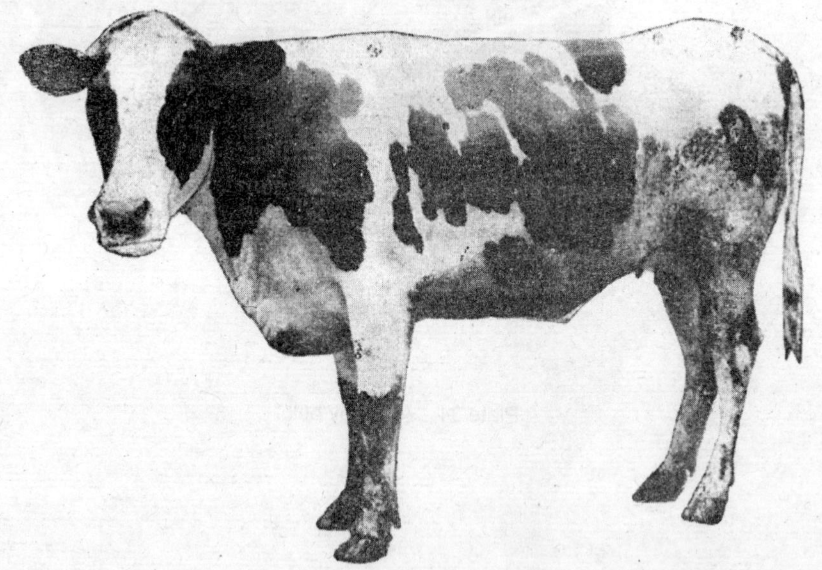

Plate 36. A Holstein x Hariana F1 heifer.

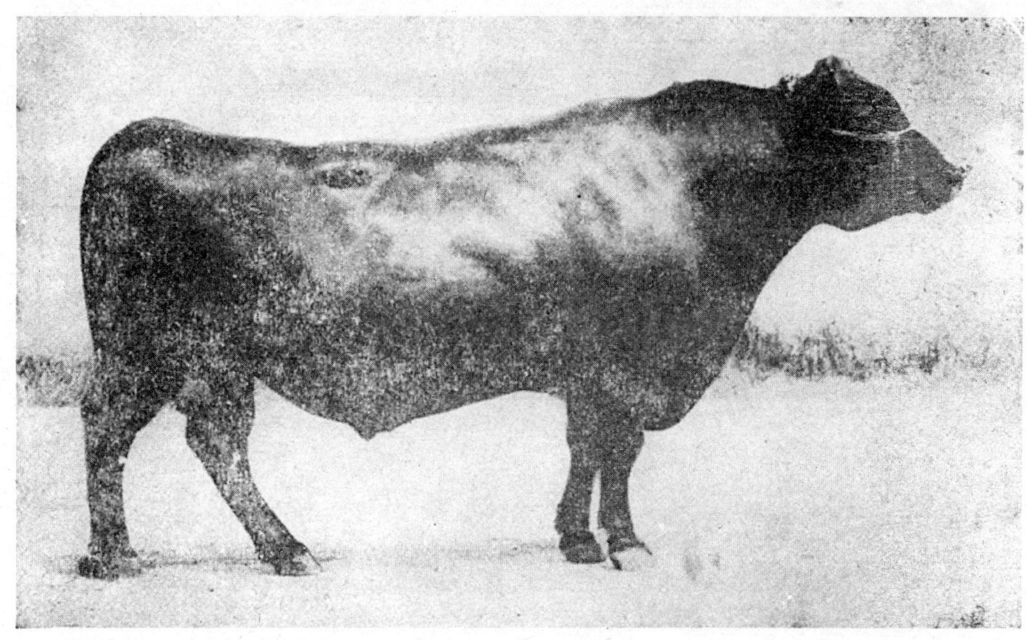

Plate 37. A Red Dane bull.

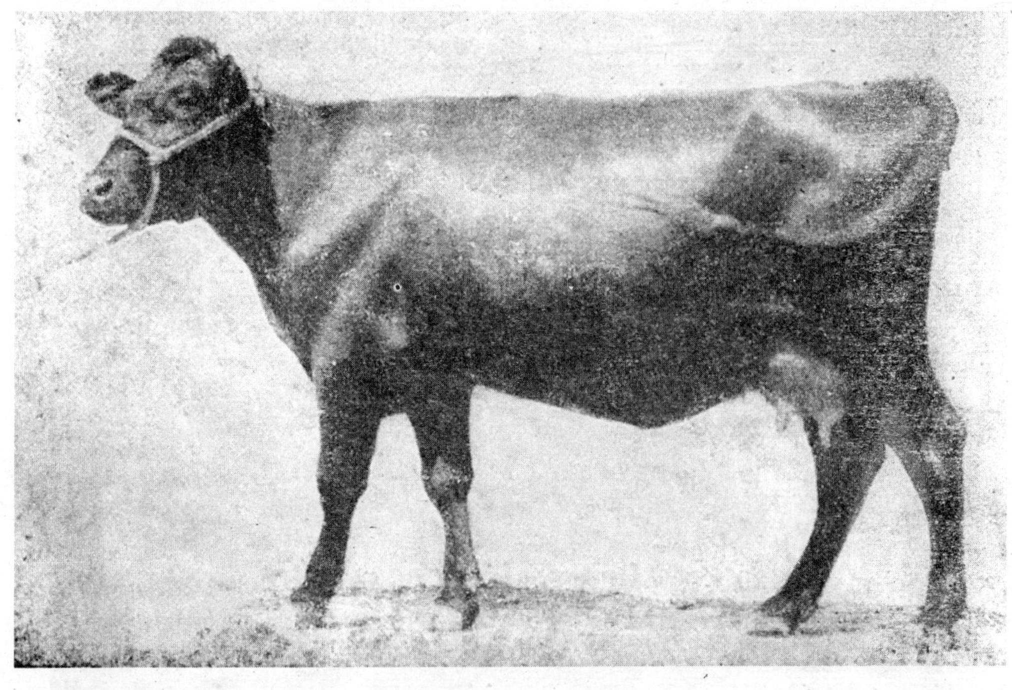

Plate 38. A Red Dane cow.

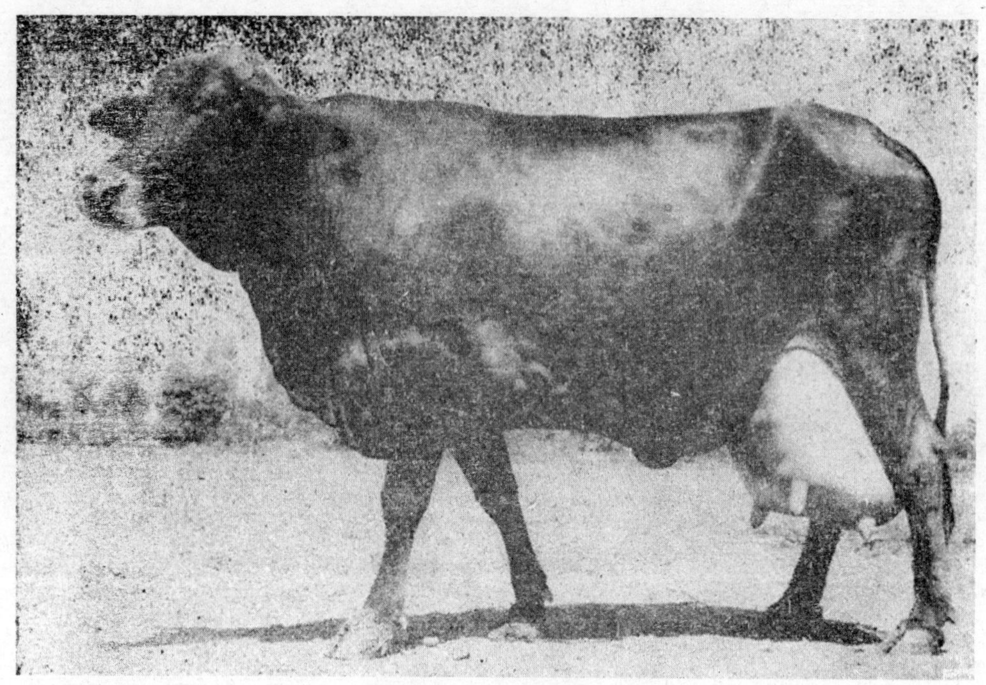

Plate 39. A Karan Swiss cow.

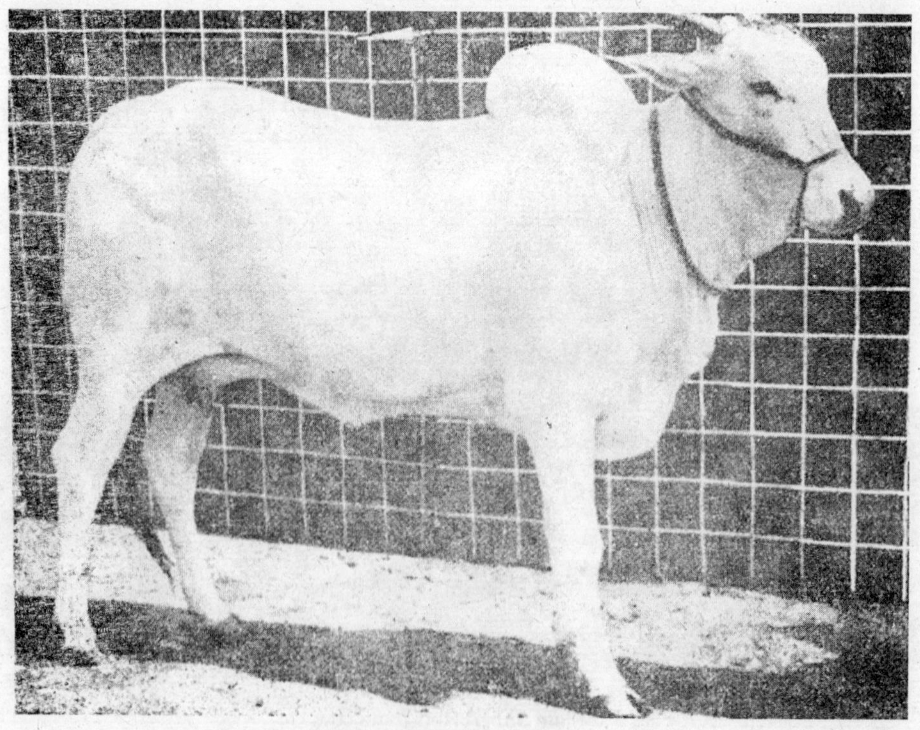

Plate 40. An Ongole cow.

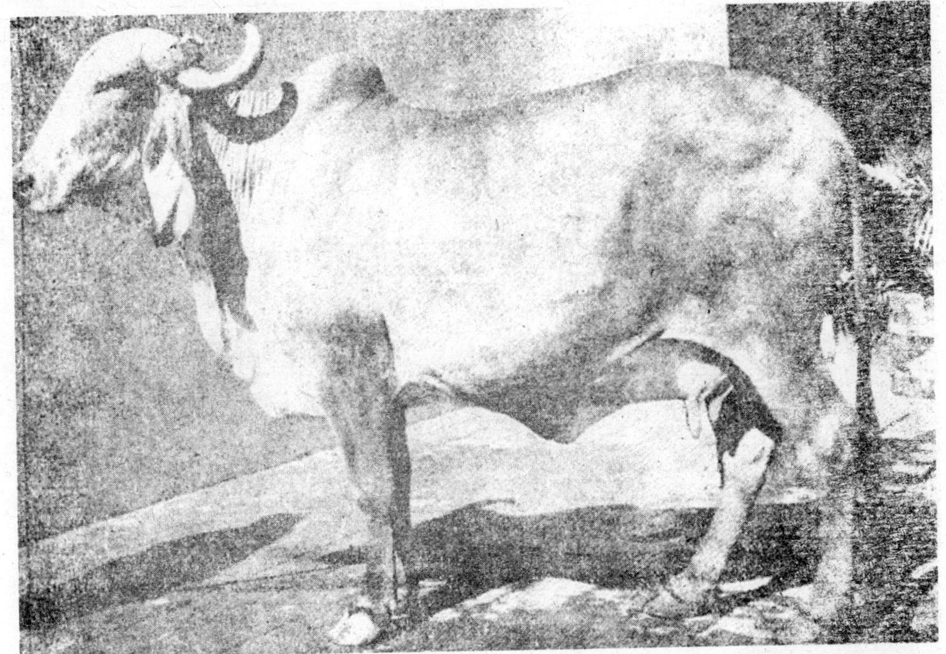

Plate 41(a). A Gir cow.

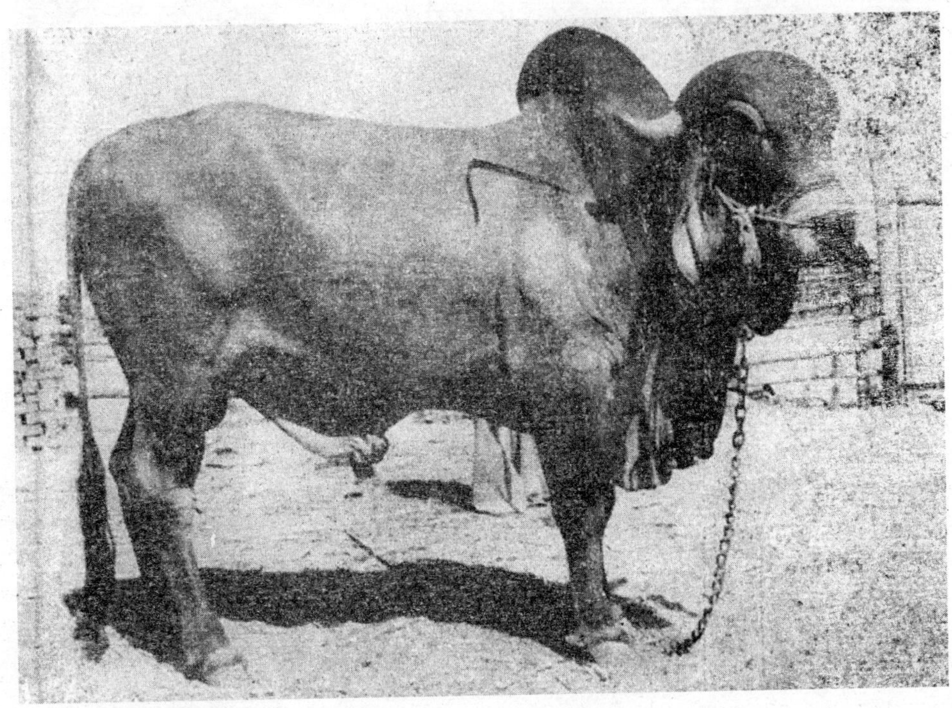

Plate 41(b). A Gir male.

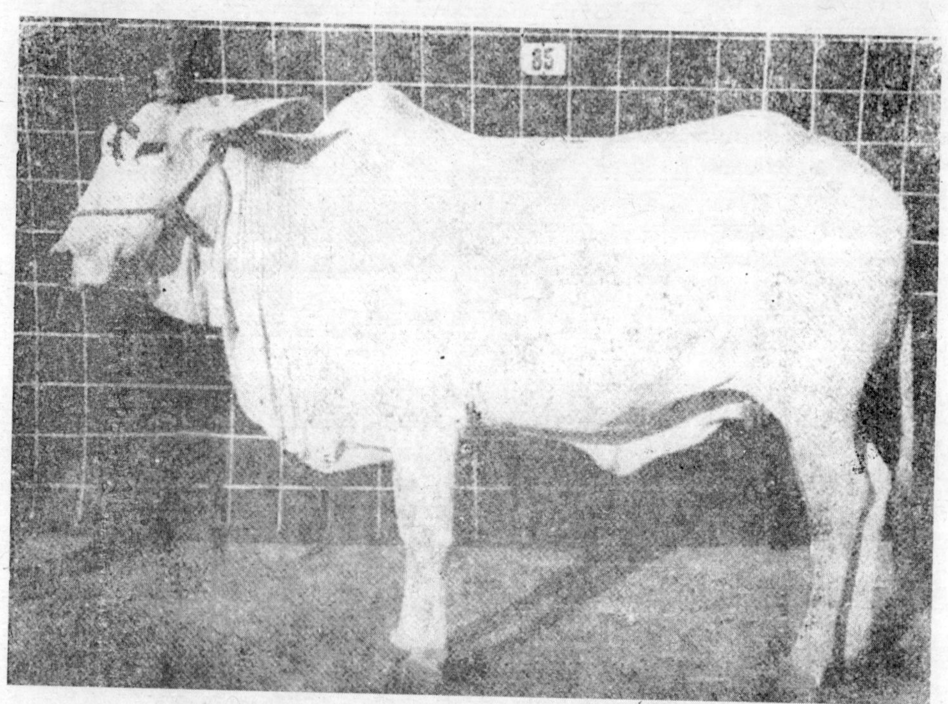

Plate 42. A Malvi cow.

to 4763 kg has been recorded.

Remarks. Tharparkar cattle are now being bred at several Government farms away from their natural home and have proved popular. Large number of these cattle have been exported particularly to Zaire, Iraq, Sri Lanka and the Philippines.

DUAL PURPOSE BREEDS

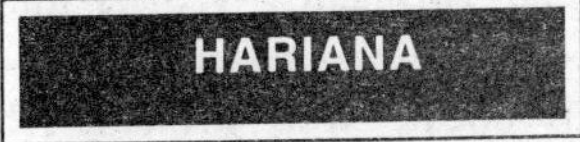

Synonym. Nil.

Origin and distribution. The breed originated in east Punjab and are now extensively found in Rohtak, Hissar, Gurgaon, Karnal and Delhi provinces. This breed also exists in more or less pure form in Jind, Nabha, Patiala, Jaipur, Jodhpur, and western U.P.

Distinguishing characters. Proportionate body, compact graceful appearance. Head is carried high, horns are short, curving upward and inward and stumpy. Popular colour is white or light grey, long and narrow face, flat forehead and a bony prominence in the centre of the poll. Small and sharp ears, skin is of fine texture and close to the body. Sheath is short, navel flap absent. Udder is capacious which extends well forward with a well developed milk vein. Legs are moderately long and lean. Pin bones are prominent and far apart in females but close in males. Tail is short, thin and tapering towards the end with a black switch reaching just below the hocks.

Production. Bullocks are good working animals for fast ploughing and road transport. Cows are average milkers with 1400 kg per lactation. Individual yield have reached upto 3266 kg.

Remarks. Animals are annually exported to all big cities of India. Pedigree herds are maintained at some Government farms.

ONGOLE

Synonym. Nellore.

Origin and distribution. Ongole tract of Andhra Pradesh, comprising Guntur, Narasaraopet, Venukonda, Kandukur taluks of Nellore and Guntur districts.

Distinguishing characters. Large, heavy and muscular. Forehead is broad with stumpy horns thick at the base and firm without cracks. Hump is well developed and erect, filled up on both sides without leaning. Animals are greatly alert and docile with good gait. Popular colour is white. Males are dark grey at extremities.

Production. Bullocks are powerful and suitable for cart and road work but are not fast. Cows are good yielders, yielding from 1255 to 2268 kg per lactation.

Remarks. Government Livestock Research Farm, Guntur has maintained this breed. In foreign countries they are considered to be good beef animals. In Brazil they are rapidly becoming a major beef breed.

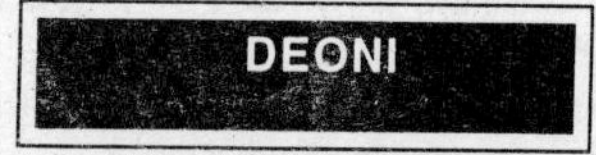

Synonym. Dongarpatti.

Origin and distribution. North-west and western portion of Hyderabad. It is allied to Dangi cattle of Bombay State.

Distinguishing characters. Resembles Gir breed, less pronounced forehead. Horns have a characteristic outward and backward curve. Lean face but not clean cut. Colour in black and white or red and white with irregular patches or spots. Deep chest, well arched ribs, straight back, strong quarters, heavy dewlap and pendulous sheath are special characters. Ears unlike Gir breed have no notch near the tip.

Production. Cows are good milkers. Average yield about 900 kg in 300 days. Milk yield goes upto 1,800 kg if well maintained. Bullocks are well suited for heavy work.

Remarks. The breed has a potentiality for future development.

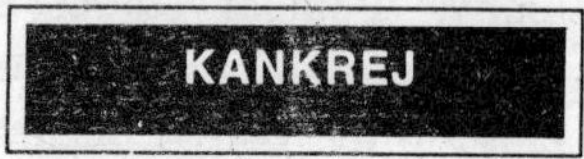

Synonyms. Bannai, Vagadia, Wadhair, Nagu, Sanehore.

Origin and distribution. The breed originated in north Gujarat in the Bombay province of India and cattle are now distributed in south-east of Rann of Kutch. Extending from north-west corner of Tharparkar district in Sind to Dholka in Ahmedabad in west.

Distinguishing characters. One of the heaviest of Indian breeds, broad chest, forehead dished in the centre, strong curved borns accompanied by skin up to some length, powerful body, straight back. Hump is well developed, tough skin, moderately developed dewlap. The colour of the male is silver grey, iron grey or black. In females colour markings are lighter. Gait is particular to breed known as 1¼ spaces (*swai chal*) with smooth movements of the body and head noticeably high. Tail is of moderate length with black switch. The animal is energetic and vigorous, excitable and nervous with strangers.

Production. Kankrej cattle are highly prized as draught cattle. Cows are fairly good milkers. Average yield is about 1,333 kg but individuals approach 3,500 kg.

Remarks. These cattle were exported in the past to North and South America for grading. in India animals are being mostly maintained at Anand.

DRAUGHT BREEDS

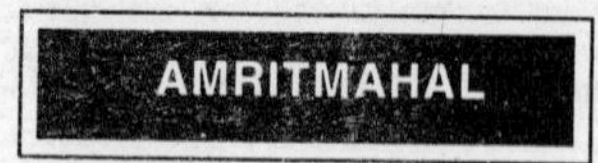

Synonyms. Nil.

Origin and distribution. The home is in Karnataka State. Government herds of selected cattle are still maintained at certain farms.

Distinguishing characters. Compact form with short straight back, well-arched ribs, powerful sloping quarters. Narrow face and prominent forehead with a furrow in the middle.

Long sweeping horns typical of Karnataka type cattle. Well developed dewlap and hump, very small sheath and close skin. Tail is of moderate length with a black switch. Grey coloured body with dark head, neck, hump and quarters.

Production. One of the best draught breeds of India. Animals are very active and famous for the power of endurance. Cows are not so good milkers.

Remarks. Nil.

KANGAYAM

Synonyms. Kanganad, Kongu.

Origin and distribution. The name is derived from the Kangayam division of Dharampuram taluk of Coimbatore district in Tamil Nadu where the breeding of this breed is a traditional affair. The breed is also found in Udamalpet, Palladam, Pollachi and in other parts of South India.

Distinguishing characters. The cattle conform largely to the Mysore type. Special points are strong horns with sharp tips. Body moderately long, straight back, short and strong neck. Moderate sized hump, wide muzzle, strong limbs, small dewlap, fine skin, very small sheath, well developed quarters and a fine tail. The colour of the bull is of grey with dark grey to black markings while the cow is white with black markings just in front of the fetlocks on all four legs and sometimes on the knees.

Production. The breed responds to good feeding and bulls are ready for service at 2.5 to 3 years of age. Heifers give birth on an average at the age of 3 years and 2 months. The cows are poor milkers yielding about 666 kg per lactation. The bulls are excellent type for hard work.

MALVI

Synonyms. Mahadeopuri, Manthani.

Origin and distribution. The breed takes its name from the Malwa tract, named after the family of kings called Malawa in Madhya Pradesh. At present the breed is mainly found in M.P. and Rajasthan. There are two types of Malvi breed which are generally recognised viz., (1) Agar type found around Shajapur district of M.P. and Jhalawar district of Rajasthan; (2) Mandsaur of Bhopal type which is comparatively smaller in size and is found in the districts of Mandsaur and Bhopal.

Distinguishing characters. Deep short and compact body. Ears are alert and short in size, short but thick horn tapering to a blunt point. Short neck, thin dewlap, short but straight and strong muscular legs. Sheath and navel flap are also short. Tail is moderately long with a black switch reaching to the fetlock. The general colour of the breed is grey to iron grey and almost black in the neck and quarters.

Production. Bullocks are good for road and field work, economical feeders and have good adaptability. Cows are poor milkers, 5-6 kg per day has been recorded by the government farms of Madhya Pradesh. The breed is essentially a good draught breed.

Remarks. Nil.

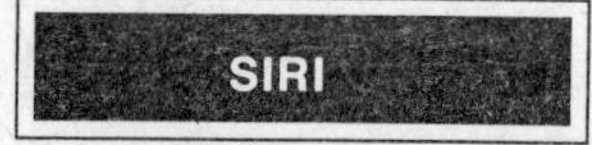

Synonym. -Nil.

Origin and distribution. These animals are found in hill tracts of Darjeeling, Sikkim and Bhutan.

Distinguishing characters. Massive body, small head, square cut, wide and flat forehead, presenting to convexity. Sharp horns, relatively small ears, well-placed hump covered with a tuft of hair at the top. Strong legs and feet, dewlap is not prominent, tight sheath, colour is black and white or red and white.

Production. Well suited for cart purposes. Bullocks are strong and of a greater size, carry 350 to 400 kg over hills. Cows are poor milkers.

Remarks. Nil.

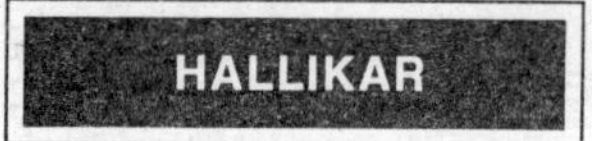

Synonyms. Nil.

Origin and distribution. The breed is mainly found in the districts of Hassan and Tumkur in Karnataka State.

Distinguishing characters. The animals are of medium size. Compact and muscular in appearance. The head is usually long with a bulging forehead, furrowed in the middle. The long horns emerge close to each other from the top and are carried backwards in a graceful sweep on each side of the neck and then gradually curving upwards to terminate in sharp points. The face is long with small ears. The coat colour is grey to dark grey with deep shadings on the fore and hind quarters. The hump is moderately developed.

Production. Bullocks are excellent draught type suitable both for road and field work while the cows are poor milkers.

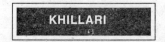

Synonym. Nil.

Origin and distribution. The breed originates from Sholapur and Satara districts and Satpura range of the former Bombay State. They are at present well distributed throughout the Maharastra State. Within this breed, the animals belong to four types, viz. (i) the Atpadi Mahal of Hanam Khillar from the former southern Mahratta State, (ii) the Mhaswad Khillar from Sholapur and Satara districts, (iii) the Thillari or Tapi Khillar from west Khandesh, and (iv) the Nakali, i.e. the imitation Khillar (Khillar means a herd of cattle).

Distinguishing characters. It has compact body with clean-cut features. The animals resemble Amritmahal breeds of cattle except that Khillari breeds look even more bigger framed. The Mhaswad Khillari is greyish males being darker over the fore-quarters and hind quarters with typical mottled markings on the face. The Tapi Khillari is white with a pink nose and pink hoofs. The Nakali Khillari is grey with tawny or brick dust colour over the fore quarters. The breed is having massive head, small eyes and ears, horns are long and pointed, emerging close to each other and follow the backward curve of the forehead. Neck is rather short and firmly set. The shoulders are tightly muscled. The barrel is long and compact with no loose skin. Legs are clean cut, straight. The hoofs are black and digits closely set. They are small in comparison with the bulk of the body.

Production. Cows are poor yielders.

Remarks. The breed is highly valued as fast paced, powerful draught animals throughout the State of Maharastra.

NEW BREEDS

KARAN SWISS

Synonyms. Nil.

Origin and distribution. The breed has been evolved at the National Dairy Research Institute, Karnal in Haryana, by breeding the Sahiwal cows with the frozen semen of Brown Swiss bulls imported from U.S.A. The breed is now distributed in many parts of Haryana.

Distinguishing characters. The mature cow attains a body weight of 400–550 kg, while a bull weighs 600–750 kg. The males are strong, sturdy and useful as draft animals. The colour of the animal varies from light grey to deep brown; sometimes a white spot is seen on the forehead. The forehead is flat to slightly dished. Ears are small. Neck is of medium size. Hump is almost non existing. Navel flap varies from light to slightly loose. Legs are proportionate in size and well set apart. Hump is long. Tail varies in length and in some cases the switch of the tail reaches the ground.

Production. The breed has excellent udder of good size, wide, deep and mostly bowl shaped. The average age at first calving is 30 months. The lactation yield is 3,355 kg in 305 days. The highest daily yield recorded is 43 kg. The fat percentage averages 4.78.

"Very recently the Government of Bangladesh has allocated over 135 crores Bangladesh taka for Second Livestock Development Project including establishment of one Livestock Research Institute at the cost of 8.5 crores taka which all will definitely bring a significant overall improvement of the Livestock Sector in Bangladesh."

SUNANDINI

Synonyms. Nil.

Origin and distribution. The breed originated in Kerala by crossing the local non-descript cattle with Jersy, Brown Swiss and Holestein-Friesian breeds followed by selection. More than two million Sunandinis now contribute to Kerala's milk production. Semen of Sunandini bulls have been exported to Tamil Nadu, West Bengal, Orissa and Karnataka.

Distinguishing characteristics. The use of number of breeds has resulted in the formation of a mosaic type of body colour and obviously the appearance vary between individuals within limits. The body otherwise is compact with well developed udder.

Production. The overall milk production per lactation is more than 2,500 litres. The cow attains the average age of first calving at 32.2 months with a calving interval of 14.15 months.

KARAN FRIES

Synonyms. Nil.

Origin and distribution. This breed has got its origin at the National Dairy Research Institute, Karnal, out of crossing between Tharparkar and Holstein-Friesian. In many parts of Haryana, the breed is now gaining popularity.

Distinguishing characters. The colour predominantly of black patches and sometimes is completely dark with white patches on the foreheads and on the switch of the poll. The udder is also dark with white patches on the teats found. The animals are extremely docile.

Production. The average age at first calving is to 30 to 32 months and the milk production is 3,700 kg with 3.8 to 4.0% fat. The intercalving period is 400–430 days.

Table 11.3

Characteristics of some foreign dairy breeds of cattle *(Bos taurus)* that are used for cross-breeding purpose in India

	Jersey	*Holstein-Friesian*	*Ayrshire*	*Brown Swiss*
Country of origin	Island of Jersey in the English channel	Holland	Scotland	Switzerland
Desirable colour markings	Fawn, with or without white markings	Blak and white	Red, mahogany, brown or combination of these with white	Distinctly brown
Av. body size (kg) female	450	675	550	625
male	675	1000	850	900
Av. gestation period(days)	280	280	278	290
Av.milk yield (lit. 305 days)	4000	6150	4840	5250
Age at first calving (months)	38	36	40	--
Distinguishing Characters	Cows have straight top lines, level rumps, sharp withers. Heads have a double dish. Animals are inclined to be nervous and sensitive. Bulls are often vicious. Capable of utilising roughages efficiently. Can withstand tropical and humid climate more than Holstein.	Animals of this breed are ruggedly built and possess large feeding capacities and udders. The head is long narrow and straight with slightly rounded withers.	Most beautiful dairy breeds. Animals have straight top lines, level rumps and good udders. They have long horns which are turned upwards. Ayrshires have shorter and thicker neck in comparison to other breeds. Animals are over-active and difficult to manage.	The breed is used for ploughing and for pulling carts as well as for milk and beef production in Switzerland. They have large heads which are usually dished and thick loose skin. Animals belonging to this breed are not as angular as those of other dairy breeds. The breed is quite, docile and easily manageable. The breed is more heat-tolerant than Jersey.
Composition of milk (percentage) :				
Fat	5.5	3.5	4.1	4.0
Protein	3.9	3.1	3.6	3.6
Lactose	4.9	4.9	4.7	5.0
Ash	0.7	0.7	0.7	0.7
Total solids	15.0	12.2	13.1	13.3

Table 11.4

Summarised data on age of first calving and the milk production, live weight, height, at withers of some Indian breeds

Breed	Age at first calving (months)	Milk production: Per lactation (kg) Normal range	Milk production: Per lactation (kg) Maximum	Milk production: Length of lactation (days)	Milk production: Fat%	Calving interval (months)	Live weight (kg): At birth Male	Live weight (kg): At birth Female	Live weight (kg): At maturity Male	Live weight (kg): At maturity Female	Height at withers at maturity (cm): Male	Height at withers at maturity (cm): Female
Hariana	32–72	635–1,497	4,536	263–320	4.0–4.8	19–21	23–25	22–24	363–544	356	132–155	127–140
Ongole	36–51	1,179–1,633	3,266	300–330	5.1	16–18	27–30	24–27	544–612	431–454	142–155	122–145
Gir	31–51	1,225–2,268	3,175	240–380	4.5-4.6	14–16	25–26	21–24	544	386	122–142	114–145
Red Sindhi	30–43	683–2,268	5,443	270–490	4.0–5.0	13–18	18–22	15–22	318–454	249–340	142–145	102–127
Sahiwal	30–43	1,134–3.175	4,536	290–490	4.0–6.0	13–18	22–24	20–22	454–590	272–408	127	117–130
Tharparkar	24–47	680–2,268	4,763	280–440	4.2–4.7	14–18	22–24	21–24	363–454	227–340	127–132	124–127
Hallikar	39–69	227–1,134	—	180	—	—	—	—	340	227	135–142	119

BUFFALO

Origin and Distribution

The domestic or water buffalo (*Bubalus bubalis*) belongs to the genus Bubalus, subfamily Bovinae, family Bovidae, is descended from the *arni* or wild Indian buffalo, and is widely dispersed throughout the southern Asia. It has been suggested that buffaloes were in the service of man as early as 2,500 to 2,100 B.C.

In recent years, the buffalo commonly known as an 'Asian Animal' has attracted global concern. The buffalo is the dairy, draught and meat animal of Asia. The Indian subcontinent is the home tract of the world's dairy buffaloes. To-day in India, the water buffalo is recognized as her milk machine. It accounts for more than half of India's total milk production, although it constitutes only one third of the total milch population. Nevertheless, its potential for milk production remains only partially tapped, as almost 80 to 85 per cent buffaloes are non-descript, yielding on an average no more than 1.5 litres of milk per day in contrast to an average of 7 to 8 litres of daily milk yield obtained from well bred milch breeds.

Some common terms in relation to BUFFALO

Details	*Expression*	*Details*	*Expression*
Species called as	... Bovine of Butaline	Castrated male	... Buffalo bullock
Group of animals	... Herd	Castrated female	... Spayed
Adult male	... Buffalo bull	Female with its offspring	... Calf at foot
Adult female	... She-buffalo or buffalo cow	Act of parturition	... Calving
Young male	... Buffalo bull calf	Act of mating	... Serving
Young female	... Buffalo heifer calf	Sound produced	... Bellowing
New -born one	... Buffalo calf	Pregnancy	... Gestation

The domesticated buffaloes may be classified into two main categories, viz., (1) the swamp buffalo (chromosomes, 2n=48) and (2) the river buffalo (chromosomes, 2n=50). They belong to the same species, *Bubalus, bubalis* but have very different habits. The former is more or less a permanent inhabitant of marsh lands, where it wallows in mud, feeds on coarse marsh grass, and is found principally in Malaya, Singapore, Philippines, Thailand, Indonesia, southern

China and other countries in the Far-East. In Philippines and some other countries it is known as the *Carabao*, and in Malaysia as the *Kerban*. The river type is the one found throughout India, Pakistan, Bangladesh, Nepal and Sri Lanka. These are primarily milch animals.

As the name implies, the water buffalo, whether of the river or the swamp type, has an inherent predilection for water and loves wallowing in water or mud pools. The river buffaloes, as a rule, shows preference for clean running water, whereas the swamp buffalo likes to wallow in mudholes, swamps and stagnant pools. Like cattle buffaloes are good swimmer.

The river and swamp buffaloes vary slightly in body structure, size and colour. A swamp buffalo is recognised by its short stocky body, short face with wide muzzle and short thin legs. These buffaloes are usually dark grey in colour, although variations from black to albinoids are found among the population. Swamp buffaloes vary in size from 300 to 600 kilograms. They are primarily used as draught animals, but they do provide small quantities of milk for a farmer's family.

In South-East Asia, the buffalo serves as the living tractor of the East. For many centuries, the swamp buffalo has been faithfully preparing the rice fields by working belly deep in liquid mud-churning. Despite its enormous size, the cud chewing, serene quadruped is so sure-footed that individual paddy fields are protected without disturbing the bunds and terraces. For decades to come, mechanization is not going to replace this trusty animal.

The meat potential of the buffalo has been amply demonstrated in Australia and Bulgaria. The suitability of buffalo as a source of good quality meat, notably more lean and having less fat compared to that from the cattle, has created a demand for it among health-conscious consumers. In India the dressing percentage has been reported to be in the range of 55.4 to 59.00 on moderate diet. In deshi male buffalo calves the dressing percentage obtained as high as 61.0, 63.0 and 64.0% maintained on high medium and low level of protein and optimum energy intake and slaughtered at about 357 kg body weight.

Another remarkable aspect of this animal is its unique ability to utilize coarse feeds, straws and crop residues, and convert them into protein and fat rich milk and lean meat. Thus buffalo fits well in poor countries having poor feed resources.

In many Asian countries, buffaloes are used in social and cultural events, e.g. buffalo racing in some South-East-Asian countries, in marriage and funeral processions in Indonesia where piebald (black and white) buffaloes have higher market price as these are prefered on such occasions, in Thailand, and as a sacrificial animal in India.

An average buffalo cow has been considered about 4 times as productive as an average indigenous cow.

Population and Production Trends

The total world buffalo population of 138.37 million is less than 10% of the total world bovine population. The annual rate of increase in buffalo population over the last 10 years was 1.7% compared to 0.7% in cattle. Largest concentration of buffaloes is in Asia and Pacific countries (133.51 million). The buffalo population has increased at a much faster rate than of cattle in India (2.0 *vs* 1.1) and Pakistan (2.5 *vs* 0.1). At present (1988), there are 75 million buffaloes are in India, followed by China (20 million), Pakistan (13 million) and Thailand (6 million).

The increase in buffalo milk production during the last 10 years was 3.7% (25.2 million tonnes in 1977 and 33.95 million tonnes in 1987) while that in cows was only 1.5%. In India buffaloes alone contribute more than 50% of the total milk produced with the increment rate of 4.1% annually.

The meat produced from buffaloes has also shown increment of 4.2% during this period (0.199 million tonnes in 1977 to 1.236 million tonnes in 1987). In India the meat production from buffalo increased 3.5% annually during last 10 years while that in China was really exciting (12.36%). Countries like Nepal, Pakistan and Indonesia have also shown increasing trend of meat production from buffaloes.

Table 12.1

Stocks and Production of Buffaloes in the world

Area	*Stocks (1000 herds)*	*Meat (1000 MT)*	*Milk (1000 MT)*
World	128102	981	31827
Africa	2410	134	—
Asia	122224	836	30413
Bangladesh	1750	7	48
Bhutan	28	—	2
China	19196	112	1560
India	64000	134	20700
Indonesia	2391	35	—
Nepal	4400	22	550
Pakistan	12777	240	7000
Thailand	6150	72	7
Europe	2664	69	55

Source: FAO Production year book 38 : 1984

Life Span

Given good management and care buffaloes are long-lived animals. It is quite common to find a reasonable milk yield or a good day's work still being achieved at upwards of 15 years of age. Buffaloes at 18 and even more may produce calves. Working buffaloes are frequently still in use at well over 20 years of their age.

Character

Perhaps the most remarkable characteristic of all breeds of buffaloes is their docility. In India it is usual to find that the care of the milking buffaloes is left to the women and girls who feed them, milk them and groom them, while the men tend the working bullocks and cows. In Thailand, and many other countries where the buffalo is the common work animal, small children tend them, riding them to the wallowing points, getting into the water with them and cleaning their ears, nostrils and eyes. There are exceptions to every rule, wild and vicious buffaloes can be encountered just as there are dangerous animals in all species, though the level of occurence is much less.

Heat Toleration

Although buffaloes are found in greatest numbers in the tropics and subtropics yet it has poor heat resistance and will suffer real distress if worked during the heat of the day, or if it is left to stand in the direct rays of the sun for long periods. Access to water or shade is essential for the well being of buffaloes. It is customary to rest working buffaloes for several hours in the middle of the day and to allow them to wallow at that time and again in the early evening when the day's work is over. Milking animals must have liberal drinking water to avoid dehydration at any time. It is thus to be noted that sudden changes of temperature and specially to the effect of cold winds and draughts may be extremely harmful to this species. In conclusions it may be remembered that heat regulating mechanism of buffaloes in comparison to cattle are less efficient. The difference may be due in part to the heavy coat of the cow preventing wetting of the skin, but more probably to the fact that the thyroid-adrenal mechanism is less efficient in the buffalo.

Wallowing

It means rolling or floundering in mud or in water. The River breeds of Indian subcontinent prefer the clear water of streams and pools bunching close together but the Swamp buffalo of China and South-east Asia likes to wallow in slime, in a mudhole accomodating one animal or very few animals only. It is seldom that buffaloes are found in areas where there is not ready access to water but wallowing is not absolutely necessary to their maintenance.

Buffaloes apparently wallow for two main reasons: 1) to regulate body temperature, and 2) to control parasites. There is no definite pattern of wallowing.

BREEDS OF INDIAN BUFFALOES

In India there are few well defined breeds with standard qualities and with specific physical characters that differentiate them unmistakably from other types as may be found in various states of the country. These are all milch breeds, but number of animals belonging to these breeds are small fraction of the total buffalo population of the country. These animals belong to a non-descript class and these vary greatly in size, weight and general features known as *deshi*. However, on the basis of regions the well defined buffalo breeds are as follows:

Table 12.2

MURRAH Group	GUJARAT Group	UTTAR PRADESH Group	CENTRAL INDIA Group	SOUTH INDIA Group
1. Murrah 2. Nili-Ravi 3. Kundi 4. Godavari **	1. Surti 2. Jaffarbadi 3. Mehsana *	1. Bhadawari 2. Tarai	1. Nagpuri 2. Pandhepuri 3. Manda 4. Jerangi 5. Kalhandi 6. Sambalpur	1. Toda 2. South Kanara

Mehsana has been developed from crosses between Murrah and Surti
Godavari is a new breed, evolved through grading up of local buffaloes of coastal Andhra Pradesh with Murrah over generations.

Out of all, six breeds viz., Murrah, Nili-Ravi, Jaffarbadi, Bhadawari, Surti and Mehsana are high quality milch breeds of the country and they all come from Northern and Western parts comprising Punjab, Rajasthan and Gujarat states. The breeds of Central and Western parts are noted as draught purpose due to the fact that they have swamp as well as river characteristics.

MURRAH GROUP

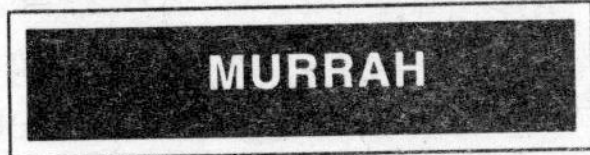

Synonym. Delhi buffalo

Origin and Distribution. The home of this breed is mainly in Punjab and Delhi, but animals are bred pure in U.P., Rajasthan and other places. Rohtak in Punjab is a well-known market from where thousands of high yielders are exported.

Distinguishing characters. Deep massive frame with short, broad back and a comparatively light neck and head. It has short, characteristic tightly curled horns, well developed udder and a long tail with a white switch reaching to the fetlock. Short massive limbs with good bone, broad hoofs and drooping quarters. Popular colour is jet black with white markings on the tail, face and extremities. The skin is soft, smooth with scanty hair. The body weight of bulls amounts on the average to 550 kg that of the she-buffaloes to 450 kg. The height

Table 12.3

Trait	I*	II**
Age at puberty	—	—
Age at first calving (months)	—	42.52
Daily lactation yield (lit.)	6.9	6.31
Lact. yield (lit.)	2076.58	1693.35
Lactation length (days)	—	299.10
Calving interval (days)	481.43	334.537
Dry period (days)	184.15	68.200
Service period (days)	172.22	144.11
Gestation period (days)	310	307-314
Fat %	6.9	—

*Data source: All India Co-ordinated Research Project on Buffalo, PAU.

**Data source: FAO Animal Production & Health Paper, 1979.

at withers on the average is 1.42 m for bulls and 1.32 m for she-buffaloes.

Production. The average milking capacity in established herds is about 1400 to 2000 kg with a butter fat content of 7 per cent of milk in a lactation of 9 to 10 months (I.C.A.R., 1966).

Remarks. The breed is the most efficient producer of milk, not only in India but probably in the world. Bulls of this breed are now used extensively for upgrading inferior stock of many countries including Thailand, Malaysia, Indonesia, the Philippines, Madagascar and Brazil. The aim is to combine the hardiness and ability of their buffaloes to convert fodder with a high degree of cellulose with the milk yield of Murrah buffalo. She-buffaloes are used in most of the important cities for the supply of milk and *ghee*.

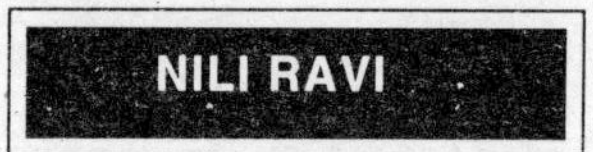

Synonym. Nil.

Origin and distribution. The Nili and Ravi are two types of buffaloes found in the valley of of Montgomery and Ferozepur. There is no essential difference between the two types although for a long time they were treated as different breeds, but closer study indicated that it was a distinction without a difference, and now they are officially treated as one breed. The best animals are found in the riverine tract along the Sutlej river, south-west of Pakpattan tehsil, Mailsi tehsil of the Multan district and Bahawalpur State.

Distinguishing characters. These animals have a medium sized, deep frame with an elongated, coarse and heavy head, bulging at the top, depressed between the eyes and ending in a fine muzzle. Horns are small with a high coil and the neck is long, thin and fine. It is the face and forehead that distinguish this breed mainly from the Murrah. The typical Nili/Ravi cow has a well developed udder. The tail is long, almost touching the ground. The colour is black but brown is not uncommon. Pink markings are sometimes seen on the udder and brisket. White markings on the forehead, face, muzzle, legs switch and around bright eyes are also seen and are much liked by the breeders.

Table 12.4

Trait	Range of value*
Age at first calving (months)	40.7—53.2
Peak daily milk yield (kg)	9.1—10.91
Lactation yield (lit.)	—
Calving interval (days)	445—525
Lactation length (days)	285—326
Dry period (days)	—
Service period (days)	—
Gestation period (days)	—
Fat %	4

*FAO Animal Production and Health Paper, 1979.

Production. Ravi breed is heavier than Nili buffalo, but their yields are hardly to be distinguished from them. Today therefore, they are not regarded to be different breeds. She-buffaloes are high milkers, average lactational yield 1600 kg in a lactation period of 250 days. Males are used for draught work.

Remarks. This is considered to be one of the best breeds of buffaloes in India, next only to the Murrah. Large numbers are exported to the big cities of the country. The name of the breed is supposedly derived from the deep blue colour (*Nili*) of the water of the sutlej river.

GUJARAT GROUP

SURTI

Synonym. Nil.

Origin and distribution. The home of this breed is in the south-western part of Gujarat state in India. The best animals of this breed are found in Anand, Nadiad and Baroda districts.

Distinguishing characters. The breed has got a fairly broad and long head with a convex shape at the top in between the horns. Horns are sickle-shaped and flat which grow in a downward and backward direction and then upwards at the tip, forming a hook. The neck is long in the female and thick and heavy in the male. The udder is well developed and finely shaped and squarely placed between the hind legs. Surti breed has got an unique straight back. They are of medium size and docile temperament.

The skin colour is black or brown and the colour of the hair varies from rusty brown to silver grey. The tail is long, thin and flexible usually with a white switch.

Production. The average lactation yield of well-bred animals is 1600 kg with a fat content of 7.5 per cent having record of yielding upto 2.500 kg.

Table 12.5

Trait	Mean ± S.E.	
	I*	II**
Age at first calving (months)	44.5 ± 20	57.83 ± 0.73
Daily lact. yield (lit.)	—	6.18 ± 0.03
Lact. yield (lit.)	1772.0 ± 10.3	1330.60 ± 11.10
Lactation length (days)	350.1 ± 54	359.42 ± 2.23
Calving interval (days)	461.1 ± 15.3	—
Dry period (days)	183.3 ± 2.00	—
Service period (days)	169.3 ± 2.54	—
Gestation period (days)	308.5 ± 0.24	—
Fat %	7.5	

*Data source: All India Co-ordinated Research Project on Buffaloes, P.A.U.
**Data source: FAO Animal Production & Health Paper, 1979.

JAFFARBADI

Synonym. Nil.

Origin and distribution. These animals are seen in their purest form in the Gir forest of Kathiawar where they are bred in large numbers, almost solely for ghee production.

Distinguishing characters. Their noticeable feature is the very prominent forehead and heavy horns which are inclined to droop on each side of the neck and then turn up at the points but not in such a tight curl as in Murrah buffaloes. Body is longer but not so compact. Dewlap and udder are well developed. Females are somewhat loose. Animals of this breed are generally black in colour. The Jaffarabadi males on the average weigh 600 kg, while females weigh 460 kg.

Remarks. Animals are heavy milkers ranging from 15 to 18 kg per day. The bulls haul heavy loads as well.

Table 12.6

Trait	Mean ± S.E.
Age at puberty (days)	1292.0 ± 36.2
Age at first calving (days)	1556.0 ± 48.9
Daily peak yield (lit.)	13.43 ± 0.8
Lactation yield (lit.)	2336.7 ± 82.50
Lactation length (days)	302.8 ± 10.2
300 days yield (lit.)	2246.0 ± 62.3
Post-partum oestrus period (days)	86.7 ± 4.2
Calving interval (days)	447.0 ± 16.25
Dry period (days)	116.4 ± 18.67
Fat %	9–10

MEHSANA

Synonym. Nil.

Origin and distribution. It derives its name from its home tract of the town Mehsana located in the north of Gujarat State. Animals of this breed are also found in Palanpur in Banaskantha district and Radhanpur and Tharad in Sabarkantha district.

Distinguishing characters. Mehsana buffaloes appear to have been derived from a mixture of Murrah and Surti blood. The breed is a medium sized animal with a low-set deep body. The skin colour is mostly jet black and occasionally brown grey with some white markings on the face, legs or tips of the tail. The breed is docile. It can stand stall feeding and can also be

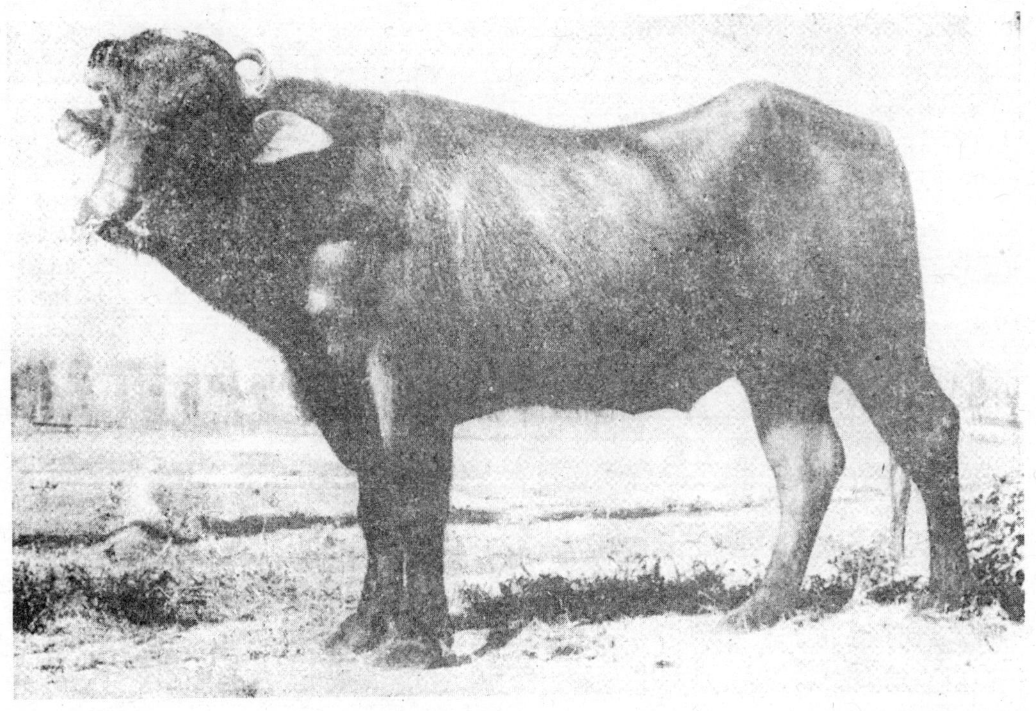

Plate 43. A Murrah male.

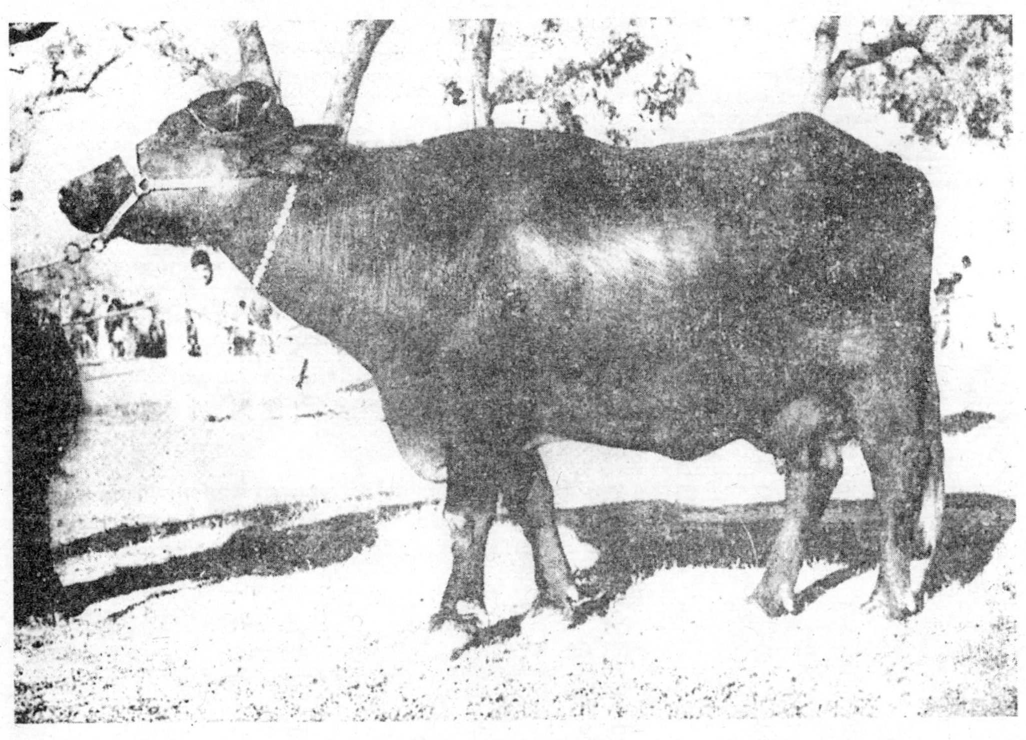

Plate 44. A Murrah female.

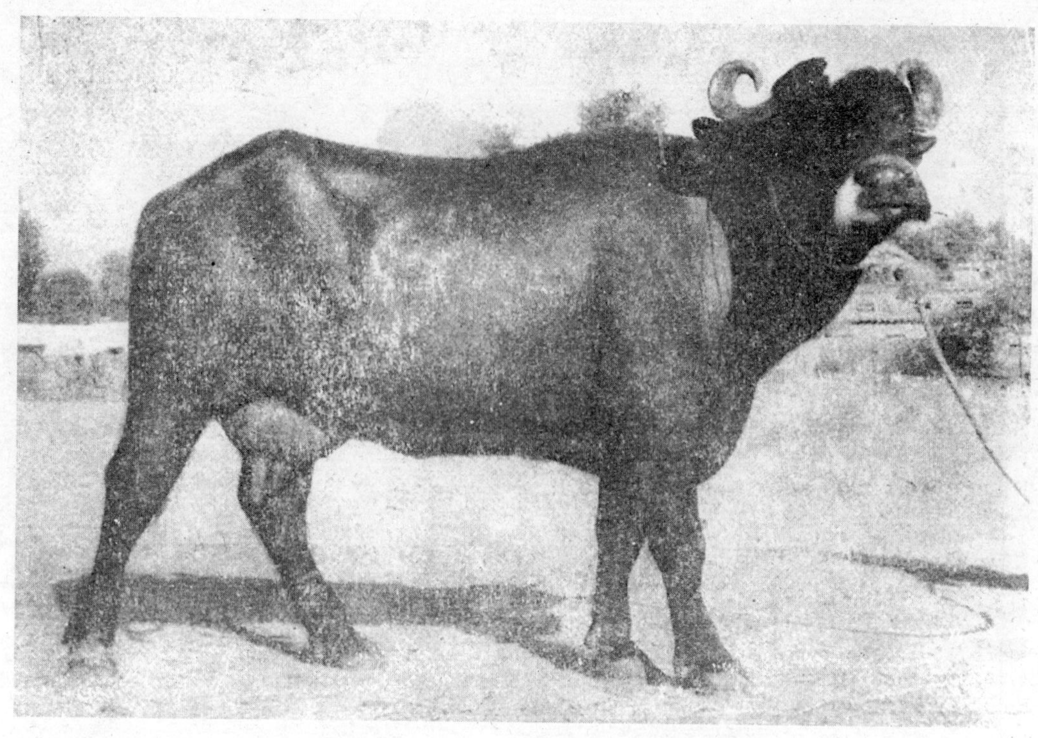

Plate 45. A Nili female buffalo.

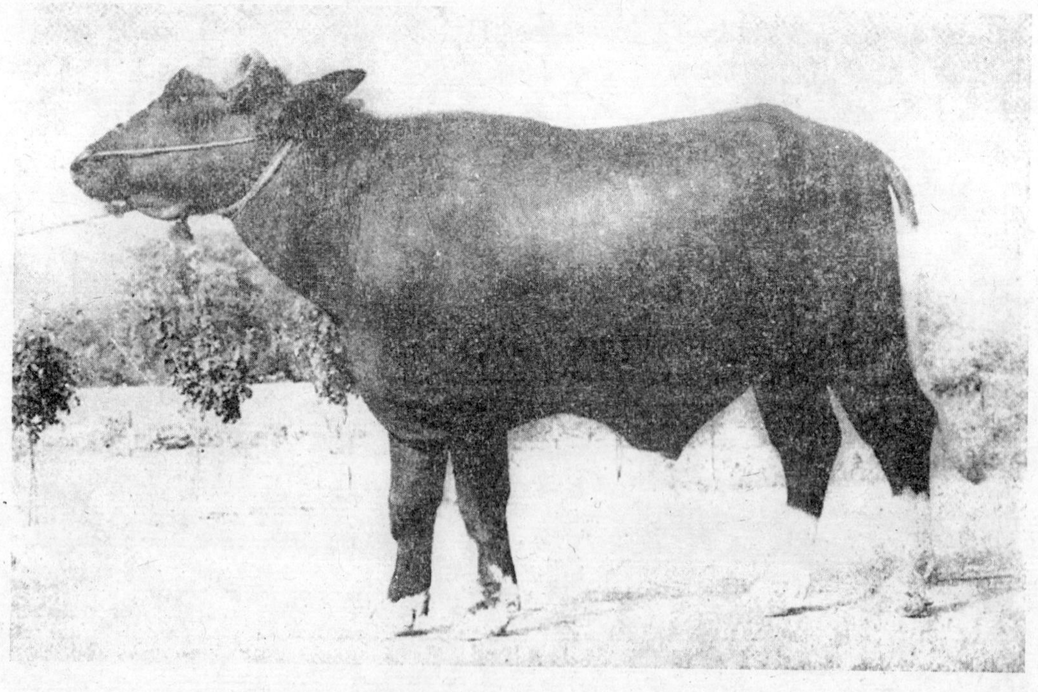

Plate 46. A Nili male.

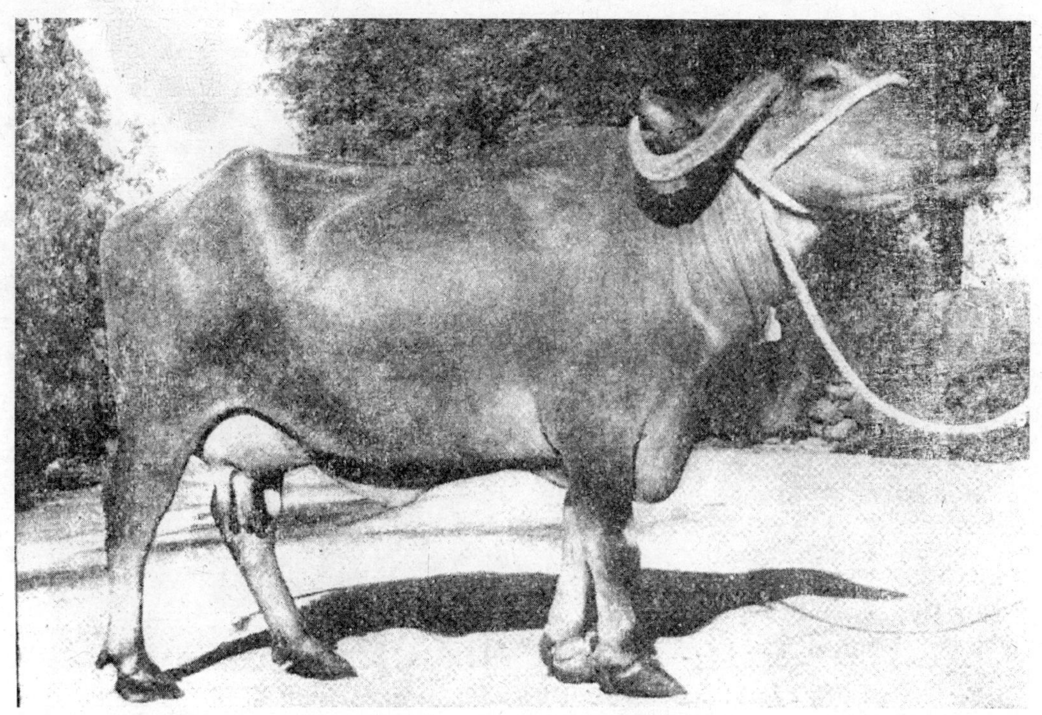

Plate 47. A Surti female.

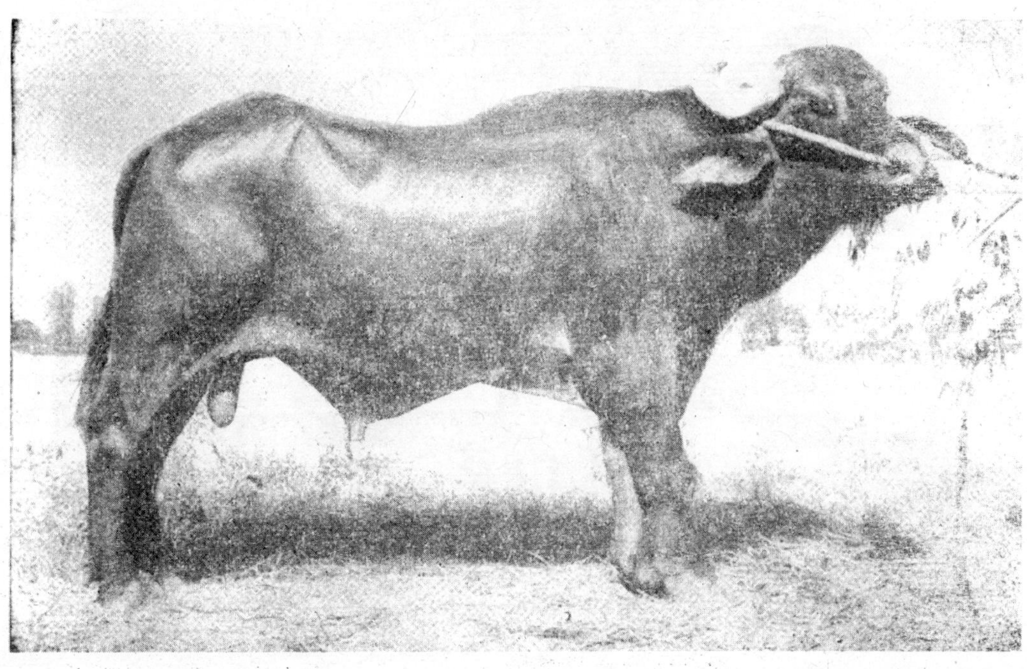

Plate 48. A Surti male.

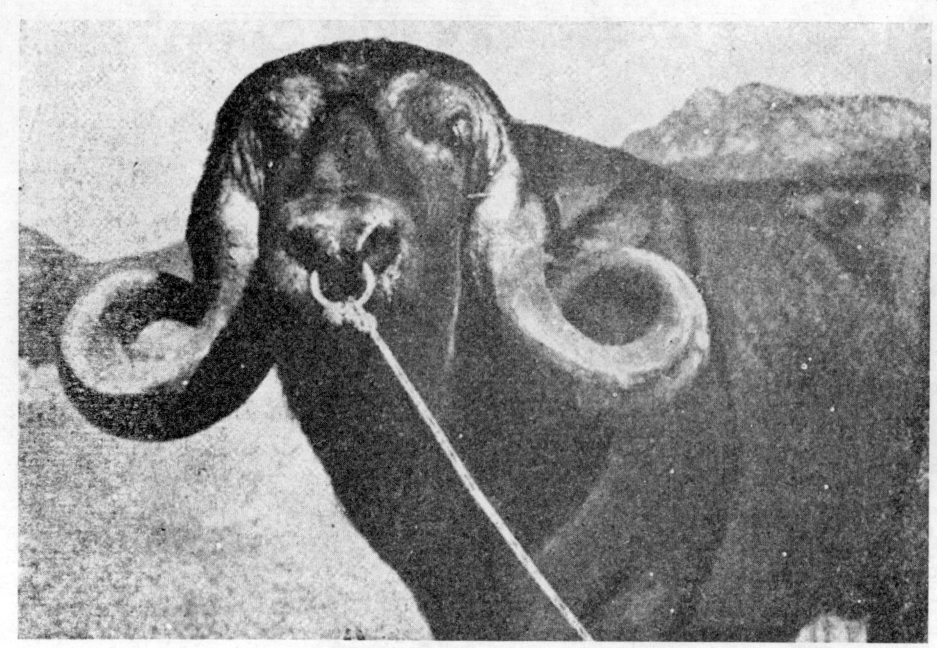

Plate 49. A Jaffarabadi buffalo.

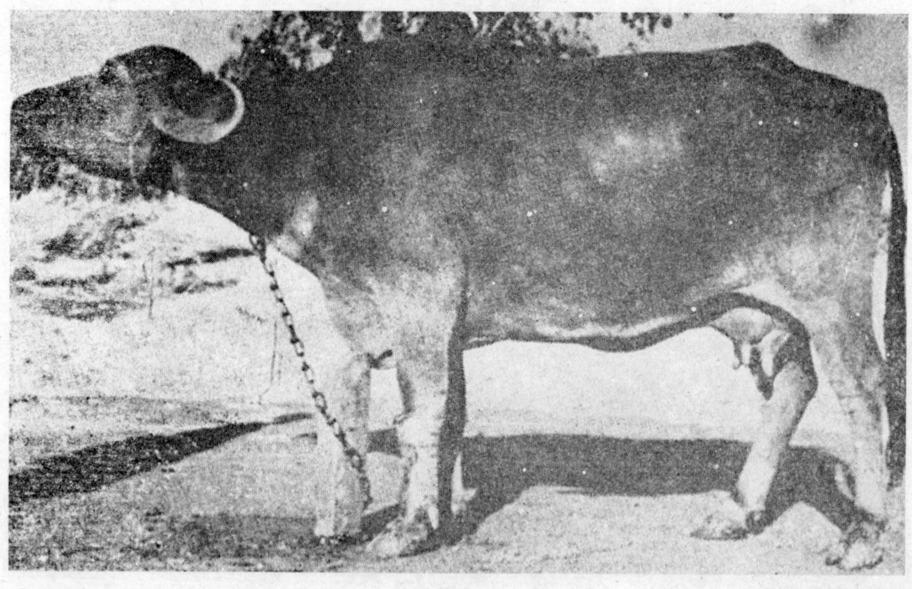

Plate 50. A Female Surti buffalo.

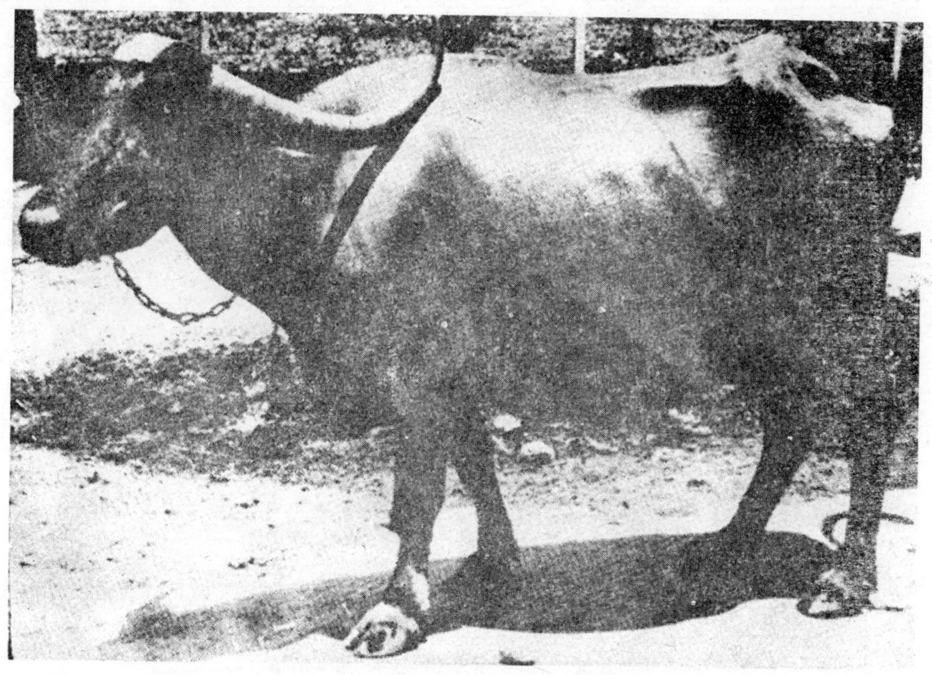

Plate 51. A Female Nagpuri buffalo.

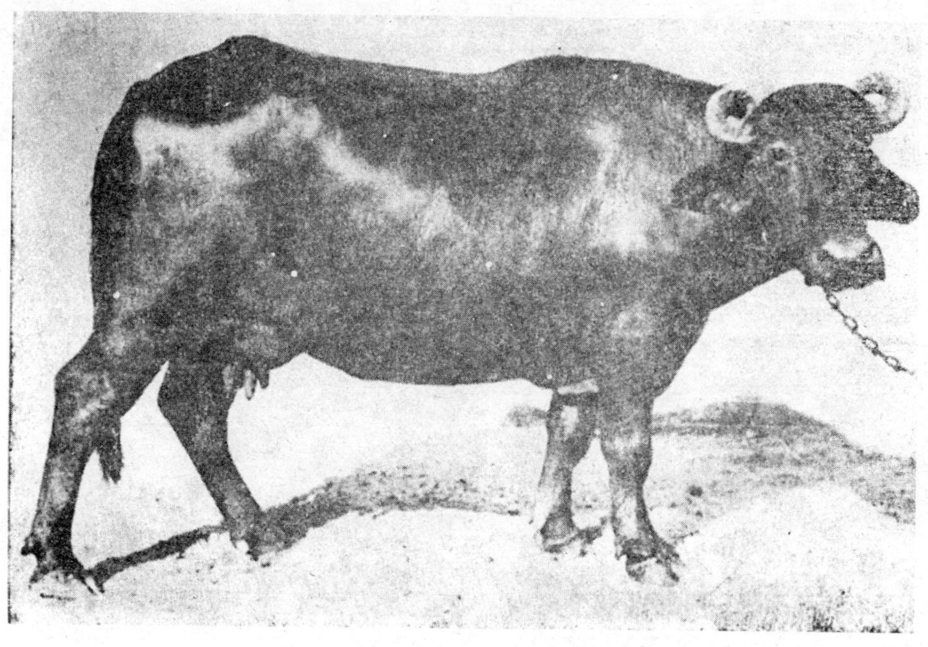

Plate 52. A Female Mehsana buffalo.

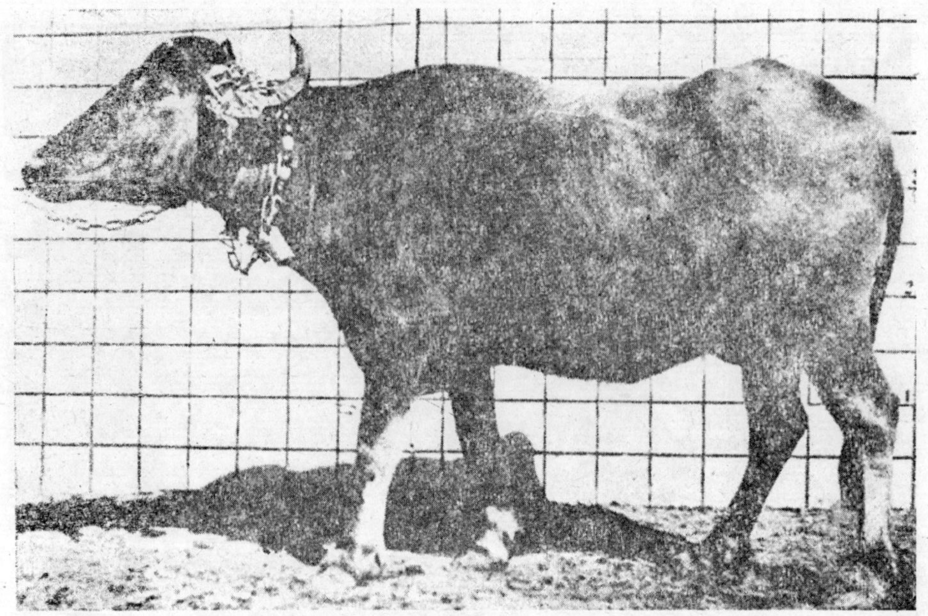

Plate 53. A Female Bhadawari buffalo.

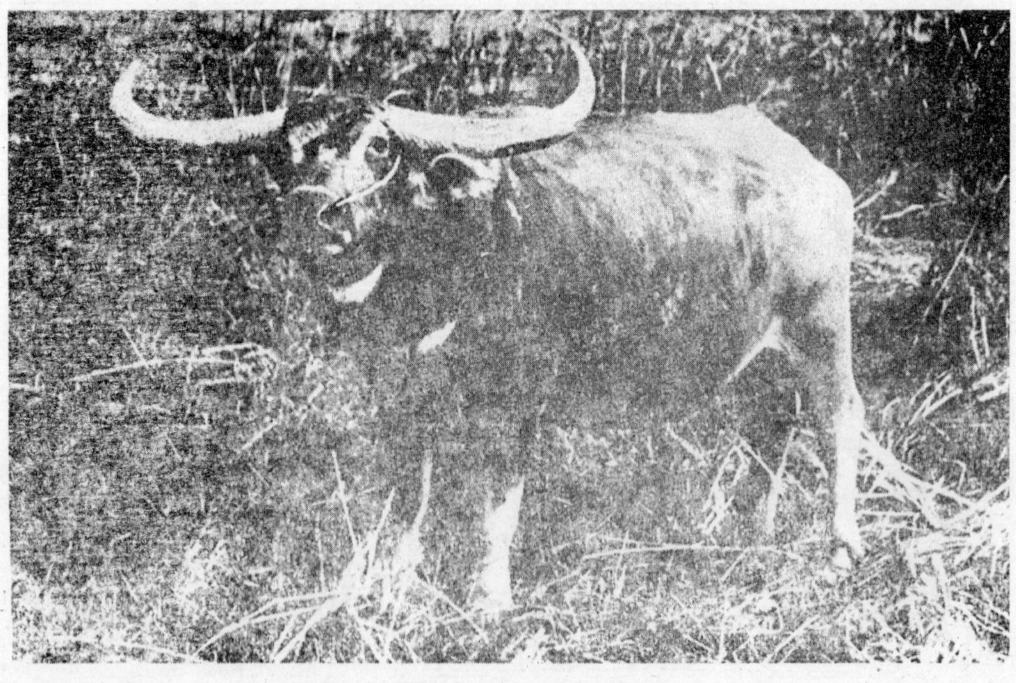

Plate 54. A Swamp buffalo.

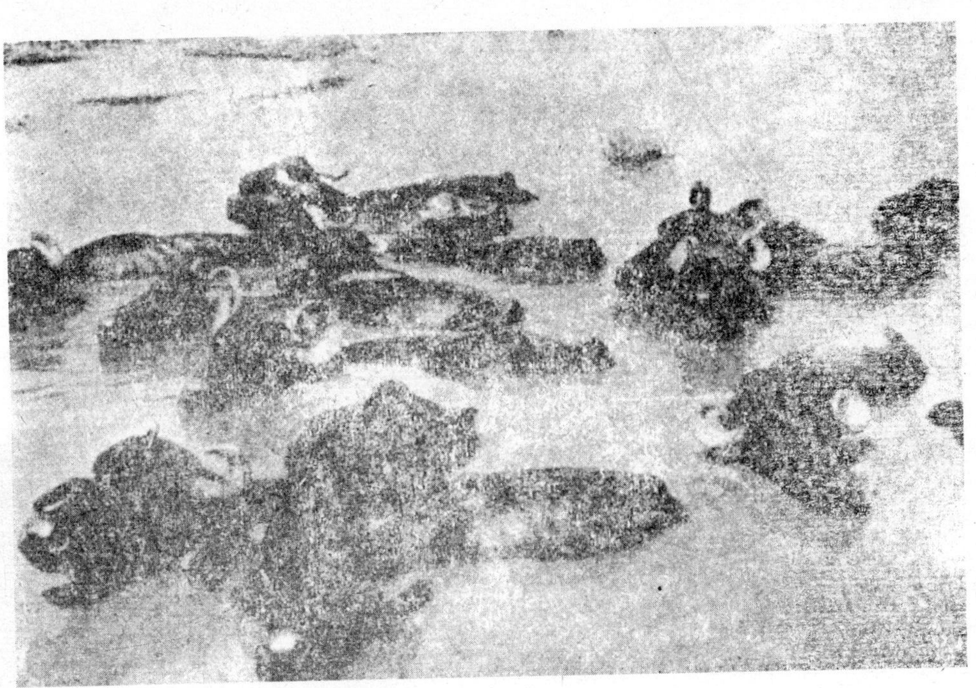

Plate 55. Buffaloes are wallowing.

reared under grazing conditions. The horns resemble the Surti or Murrah breed, *i.e.*, they may vary from long sickle type of the former to a curved knot of the latter. The neck is long and fine. As compared to Murrah breed the body is longer and tighter. It has well developed udder carried well behind, generally hind quarters are more developed than the fore-quarters with uniformly placed teats.

Table 12.7

Trait	Mean ± S.E.
Age at Puberty (months)	32.00
Age at first calving (days)	1287 ± 27.97
Calving interval (months)	16.00
Lactation yield (lit.)	1800.00
Lactation length (days)	352.00 ± 15.83

UTTAR PRADESH GROUP

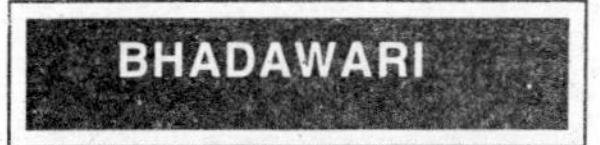

Synonym. Nil.

Origin and distribution. Bhadawari estate of Agra district and adjoining areas of Gwalior and Etawah. Animals are found scattered in the surroundings of Jamuna and Chambal rivers.

Distinguishing characters. Medium size and wedge-shaped body. Comparatively small head bulging towards horns. Legs are short but stout. Hooves of the hind quarters are more backward than fore quarters. Colour is copper, hair scanty. Barrel is short but well developed.

Table 12.8

Trait	Range of value*
Age at first calving (months)	48.3—50.78
Lactation yield (lit.)	1111—1252
Lactation length (days)	276
Calving interval (days)	453.6
Dry period	156

*FAO Animal Production and Health Paper, 1979.

Forehead is slightly broad and deep in the middle. Face is comparatively narrow with slightly marked nose. Eyes are prominent, active and bright. Udder is not so well developed but milk veins are fairly prominent. Teats are of medium size and uniform in length.

Production. Average yield ranges from 2000 to 2070 kg in a lactation period of 305 days with a high fat percentage. Males are used for draught purposes.

Remarks. Nil.

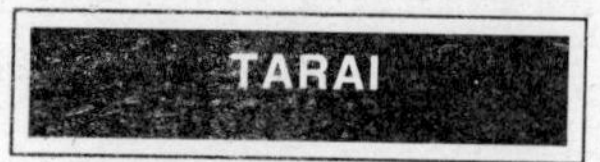

Synonym. Nil.

Origin and distribution. The breed gets the name from the *Tarai* area of U.P., where it is mostly found between Tanakpur and Ramnagar. The breed is native to hilly area. They are frequently crossed with Murrah bulls.

Distinguishing characters. It has a moderate body, slightly convex head with prominent nasal bones. Horns are long and flat with coils, bending backwards and upwards having pointed tips. The eyes are rather small but ears are long and coarse. Legs are short but strong. The tail is long, reaching below the hocks. The colour of the skin varies from black to brown. Sometimes there is a white blaze on the forehead. The switch of the tail is white.

Production. The breed is poor regarding milk production, which may be as low as 2-3 kg daily. Males are efficient draught animals used for agricultural operations as powers including transport. Tarai breed is well adapted to the difficult environmental situations and nutritional conditions of the Tarai.

CENTRAL INDIA GROUP

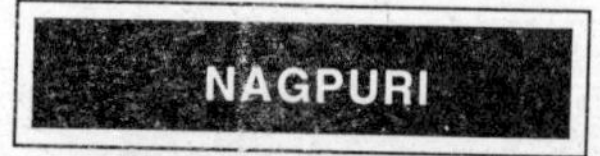

Synonym. Marathwada, Berari, Ellichpuri, Gaulani, Varad, Gauli.

Origin and distribution. As the name applies, these animals are mostly found in Nagpur including Wardha, Yeotmal, Akola, Buldana, Amrawati and Achalpur in Maharastra. The breed has got several strains differing in colour and other superficial traits.

Distinguishing characters. The colour is usually black; occasionally white markings are observed on the face, legs and switch. In general the breed is known as lighter type than those of north, not so squat and have a short tail. The face is long and thin with a straight profile. The neck is also longer with heavy brisket. It has long horns flat-curved reaches towards back over the shoulders. Naval flap is short or almost absent.

Production. Male body weight averages 525 kg while female attains about 425 kg. The average height at withers in male 142 cm and that of cows 132 cm; heart girth is 210 and 205 cm for male and female respectively.

The females are moderately good yielders, producing on an average 1,000 litres milk per lactation of 300 days with butter fat content between 7.0-8.5 per cent. The males are used for heavy draught but are slow.

PANDHEPURI

Synonym Pandharpur, Dharwari

Origin and distribution. The breed is widely distributed in south Maharastra, parts of Andhra Pradesh and Karnataka States.

Distinguishing characters. Animals are of medium size with long narrow face and very long, flat and usually twisted thin horns.

Production. Males are hardy and well suited for drought purpose.

MANDA

Synonym. Parlakimedi, Ganjam.

Origin and distribution. The animals are bred in the hills above Parlakimedi and Mandasa on the borders of Orissa and Andhra Pradesh. Basically the breed is reared in areas of thick forest usually on natural herbage and brought down to the plains for sale.

Distinguishing characters. The general colour is brown or grey with yellowish tufts of hair on the knees and fetlocks, and the switch is yellowish white. The breed is a medium sized animal. The eyes are sharp with a broad red margin around the lids. The horns are broad and semi-circular extending backward and inward. The forehead is flat with short muzzle. Neck and forelegs are also short but stout with well developed chest.

Production. Milk yield is satisfactory. Males are hardy and like a bullock can work in the hot sun. It can draw a load of about a ton but at a slow pace.

SAMBALPUR

Synonyms. Kimedi, Gowdoo.

Origin and distribution. The home tract of this breed is controversial. Originally it was known to be habitat of Sambalpur area of Orissa, later on it has been suggested that the main habitat of this breed is around Bilaspur district of Madhya Pradesh wherefrom calves are brought by 'gowdoo' (Herdman) to Sambalpur area.

Distinguishing characters. Animals are large and powerful having long, narrow barrel and prominent fore-head. Body and coat colour is generally black but it varies to brown and ash grey.

Production. Males are very active and good for drought purposes which are affected by high atmosphere temperature. Females breed regularly and produce milk satisfactorily.

KALHANDI

Synonym. Peddakimedi.

Origin and distribution. The home tract of this breed has been referred to the eastern part of Andhra Pradesh and adjoining areas of Orissa.

Distinguishing characters. A strong with broad horns and half curved running backward at the tip. Body colour is between grey and ash grey. It has well developed chest and strong fore-limbs. Eyes are prominent and large with narrow red margin around the lids. Tail is of medium length with white switch. Due to light colour it tolerates heat more than dark coloured buffaloes.

Production. Animals are docile and hardy. They are used to carry loads in hilly areas as well as for ploughing in plains. Milk yield is satisfactory.

JERANGI

Synonyms. Nil.

Origin and distribution. This breed of buffalo is widely distributed in Jerangi hills of Orissa and northern parts of Visakhapatnam and west of Ganjam in Andhra Pradesh.

Distinguishing characters. One of the dwarf breeds of buffalo and its height does not exceed four feet. Horns are conical and small, and run backward, body colour is black.

Production. Not that much good in milk production but are useful animals for ploughing in water-logged paddy fields.

SOUTH INDIA GROUP

TODA

Synonym. Nil.

Origin and distribution. The name of the breed originates from the name of *Toda* tribes of Nilgiri hills of Tamil Nadu State who rear this breed.

Distinguishing characters. These are large-sized animals having long barrel and strong build. Horns of these buffaloes are variable in shape but are usually set wide apart run outward, upward and then inward at the top. Face is short and wide. Hump and dewlap are absent, chest is broad and deep; legs are short and sturdy. Along the crest of the neck, hump area and back, there is a thick growth of hair like a mane which imparts a bison like appearance.

The animals are not always docile. All of a sudden they may become furious and dangerous particularly to unknown persons. When necessary, they fight against even tigers and other wild animals in an organised team.

Production. Females are good milkers, yields between 4.5—8.5 litres daily with an average of 7.0% fat and possesses typical well-flavoured taste.

Economic Uses of Water Buffalo

Buffalo Milk and its Quality

Dairy industry in India is mainly buffalo oriented and buffaloes have been contributing over 55% of total milk produced. The organised sector of the dairy industry mainly handles buffalo milk which constitutes nearly 95% of total milk handled by the dairy plants.

The largest number (over 80%) of buffalo cows in India and Pakistan calve during the period of July to December. Thus the buffalo dairymen in these countries are confronted with the problem of seasonal surplus milk which is usually converted into various products and short supply during the slack season. Apart from some high yielding breeds, Indian buffaloes on an average produce 500 kg of milk in a lactation in comparison to 187 kg of milk per lactation of average Indian cows. Milk yield varies widely, depending on the breed and husbandry practices. Daily yield of the lactating buffaloes in South India and Pakistan may be as low as 2–2.5 kg in a poor village animal and as high as 20.0 kg on a well managed farm. The average yield from five selected herds in India was found to be a little over 2055 kg per lactation.

In India more than 50% of the total milk production comes from the quality breeds of Indian bufaloes. The fat percentage is little less than twice as that of cow milk resulting higher profit as in India, marketing of milk is still based on the fat content.

It has about 30% more total solids, higher proportion of butyric acid, higher melting triglycerides, bigger size fat globules. The fat has less cholesterol and more vitamin E, which is a natural antioxidant. The milk is richer in calcium and phosphorus and lower in sodium and potassium. The peroxide activity in buffalo milk is 2 - 4 times higher than in cow milk.

Table 12.9

Average Composition of Cow and Buffalo Milk in India

Average percentage by weight

Constituent	Breed of Cow				Buffaloes
	Sindhi	Gir	Tharparkar	Sahiwal	
Water	86.07	86.44	86.58	86.42	83.63
Fat	4.90	4.73	4.55	4.55	6.56
Protein	3.42	3.32	3.36	3.33	3.88
Lactose	4.91	4.85	4.83	5.04	5.23
Ash (Minerals)	0.70	0.66	0.68	0.66	0.70
Solids-not-fat (SNF)	9.03	8.83	8.87	9.03	9.81
Total Solids (TS)	13.93	13.56	13.42	13.58	16.37

Source: *Annual Report 1948 of the Indian Dairy Research Institute (now known as the National Dairy Research Institute)*

Another important difference between buffalo and cow milk is that in former it is almost free from carotinoids (golden yellow in colour) due to conversion of all carotinoid materials into vitamin A (colourless) by the liver cells. That is why buffalo milk and ghee is completely white whereas ghee made from cow milk is golden yellow in colour as because of incomplete conversion of carotinoids into vitamin A inside liver cells which ultimately appears in cows milk.

The low heat capacity and high thermal conductivity of buffalo milk indicate low requirement of heat energy to achieve certain desired heat effects.

Buffalo milk is used for making mozzarella cheese in Italy. Owing to these compositional difference, buffalo milk produces better yoghurt in body and texture, allows easy separation of cream and churn of butter, provide bigger grain size in clarified butter *(ghee)*, and gives better quality desiccated milk *(Khoa)* and also acid coagulated milk *(poneer)*.

It is also a better tea/cofee whitener and make richer firm *curd* and *yoghurt*.

It is less suitable than cow's milk for making *chana* and thereby *rosogolla*. The butter made from buffalo milk is hard. Owing to lower heat stability of concentrated products, buffalo milk is unsuitable for manufacturing evaporated milk. It is also not suitable for manufacture of *cheddar, cheese*. The use of buffalo milk fat and solids not fat (SNF) in making ice-cream mix gives poor whipping quality. The high calcium and micellar casein content make buffalo milk less suitable for infant feeding; because it leads to the formation of curd with high tension.

The composition of buffalo milk like other species varies with breed. The largest use of buffalo milk in India is as such, in the liquid form, for direct consumption. It is usually standardised to about 3 percent fat by the organised diaries for marketing as liquid milk.

Table 12.10 Average percentages of constituents of milk of different breeds

Breed	Total solids	Fat	Protein	Casein	Lactose
Egyptian	16.55	7.14	3.63	3.04	4.99
Indian	17.56	7.06	4.65	—	5.07
Iraqi	17.07	7.91	—	—	—
Italian	18.90	8.50	4.50	3.60	4.60
Philippine Carabao (Swamp type)	20.36	9.65	5.26	4.24	5.29

Studies on cost of production of cow and buffalo milk, taking into consideration of number of factors such as feed, labcur, depreciation etc., showed that in rural areas good quality cows are required to be kept under better management and feeding but on the other hand buffaloes have an edge over cows due to their higher efficiency of converting coarse roughages into milk and fat.

To-day in India buffalo is the main milch animal contributing 55% of the total milk production in the country followed by 42% by cows and 3% by goats. Therefore, female buffalo calves are properly managed by the farmers so as to have a future replacement stock. Male calves are ignored and kept only for the "letting down" of milk and when become adult are used for draught or for meat.

Work

The water buffalo is the classic work animal of Asia, an integral part of the continent's traditional village farming structure. It has been estimated that buffaloes provide 20—25% of the farm power in India which is comparatively less efficient than swamp buffaloes. The farm sizes in India are small where tractor does not suit as for one tractor the farm size should be atleast 4 hectares for economic operations. Buffalo as a draft animal, has working capacity of

0.75 H.P. A sturdy single buffalo can pull a weight of 0.9 to 1 ton which is almost the same as its own weight. On a good road, a pair of buffaloes can draw a weight of upto 2 tons especially in a pneumatic cart.

As per estimates buffalo males both castrated and uncastrated are used for hauling carts and ploughing field. They plod along at about 3 km per hour. They are slow, docile and hardy workers ideally suited for agricultural operations in muddy rice fields. Their stamina and drawing power increases with body weight. In hot humid weather it is necessary to let working buffaloes cool off preferably by wallowing. Furthermore, they are less expensive than bullocks.

Buffalo Meat (Carabeef)

In Italy, Bulgaria, Czechoslovakia and Egypt buffaloes are raised mainly for meat. A

Table 12.11

Meat production (000 MT) in India

Type of meat	Year of Production				
	1975	1982	1983	1984	1985
Buffalo meat	98	130	132	134	139
Mutton and Lamb	102	132	132	133	138
Goat Meat	227	298	302	305	316
Beef and Veal	61	80	80	86	89
Chicken	88	130	137	150	158
Pig Meat	54	80	80	84	88

dressing percentage as high as 57% is obtained against 43—57% of old and unproductive buffaloes slaughtered in India and other Asian countries.

Buffalo meat production and its trade can widely expand and flourish in India as the ban on cow slaughter is not applicable to buffaloes. Buffalo meat is popular in a number of developing countries including India. As a meat animal in south Asia, India occupies the second place. Dressing percentage varies between 55—60 according to different levels of dietary protein and energy offered. In general the meat is richer in protein in comparison to meat of beef. Lysine is 44 per cent higher than even egg protein. The muscle fibres are large and fat is present in lower proportion.

Meat from much elderly animals has a poor flavour while from young ones, it is lean, tender, less fatty, palatable and considered a delicacy. The majority of buffaloes, at the present time are slaughtered when their milk production or work capacity begins to decline at the age of 9 to 12 years.

Of the total buffalo population in the country about 30% are young stock and out of this, over 50% are male calves. Buffalo calves at 1.0 to 2.0 months age can prove excellent meat producers.

Buffalo meat contains white fat as the beta carotene (the precursor of vitamin A) which is golden yellow in colour is fully converted into vitamin A which is colourless. Thus buffalo ghee is also white in colour in contrast with cow ghee which is golden yellow in colour due to presence of some amount of carotene.

Under well conducted experiments, it has been seen that the buffalo calves can attain a growth rate of 700 to 1,200 g per day from birth to 14 months of age. Buffalo broilers if reared up to 14 to 18 months of age on a well balanced ration can reach a body weight of 250 to 300 kg.

Table 12.12

Chemical Composition of Beef and Carabeef

Characteristics	*Cattle*	*Buffalo*
Moisture (%)	76.29	74.42
Crude protein (%)	19.20	20.20
Ether extract (%)	1.13	1.03
Ash (%)	1.10	1.11
Nitrogen-free extract (%)	2.28	3.24
Total pigment (mg/gm)	2.30	4.10
Myoglobin (mg/gm)	1.50	2.50
Cholesterol (mg/100gm)	54.80	64.00

Source: Arganosa, F.C. et al., 1973. *Phil. J. Nutr.* Vol. 26, No. 2, 128—143.

Other Products

Buffalo horns. When the horns are properly handled and processed they provide a variety of practical and decorative articles including buttons, toggles, combs, spoons, forks, knife handles, napkin rings, wall decorations, shoe horns etc.

Hide. The hide of the water buffalo is an important item both for export and for local industry. Pakistan is one of the world's largest producers of good quality hides and skins, and about a million water buffaloes are slaughtered annually. Leather is considered to be the most important raw material in the country's economy after jute and cotton.

Table 12.13

Value of output excluding draft power from buffaloes in 1981-82

Item	Value (Rs. million)
Milk and milk products	48800
Meat	1200
Hides	400
Dung	2600
Total	53000

Buffalo faeces. Tremendously used as fuel and organic fertiliser by the rural people.

Hair. Buffalo hairs are twice as thick as those of the bovine breeds which render suitable for brush production rather than felt.

The approximate monetary value of buffaloes in terms of its products in 1981-82 was Rs. 53,000 crores.

Breeding and Management Problems

Buffaloes are Seasonal Breeders

In tropical countries like India, she buffaloes indicate seasonal sex periodicity in respect of oestrous and conception. As much as 62.8% animals show periodicity in October to February with the peak around December and this period coincides with higher conception rate. During the period from March to September, with comparatively longer days and higher intensity of sun, ovarian activity appears to be adversely affected.

Buffalo bulls are sexually least active during hot seasons. High environmental temperature upsets the normal physiological functions affecting spermatogenesis in males and ovarian activity in the females. 82% of services take place in November. Even under A. I. conditions, 65% of the inseminations of the year are being carried out during the months of September to February. Thus 80% of buffalo calvings are recorded only in the months of July to December and minimum in hotter months.

With judicious management practices such as heat detection, protection from thermal stress, adequate and balanced ration and optimum time of insemination, the calvings in buffaloes could be evenly spread round the year to a great extent.

Silent Heat

Silent heat refers to normal follicular development and ovulations without the behavioural signs of estrus.

In summer the extreme climatic stress coupled with increased day light reduces the incidences of buffaloes coming in regular heat. During this time other reproductive problems like repeat breeding and pregnancy losses are also increased. It is generally felt that most of the buffaloes do have sub-functional ovaries causing weak or silent oestrus (in 60% cases) and such incidences are even higher than the true anestrous, especially in summer.

The research workers are trying to find out the causes of these disorders of ovarian origin and are successfully trying to correlate them with the lack of management, nutritional status of the animal and hormonal (serum gonadotrophins and steroids) profiles.

However, if due to excessive environmental stress the CL in buffaloes does not regress or partially regresses (in non-pregnant condition), it will continue to secrete progesterone and will inhibit further release of LH, thus the buffaloes will go in a state of anestrus or subestrus conditions, so long as CL does not completely regress.

Corrective Measures

1. For animals which either do not manifest oestrus or are in a state of silent oestrus or sub-oestrus firstly need managemental attention rather than therapies.

Two or three examinations with an interval of a week between each, will reveal that most of them are cases of apparent anestrus. In such cases simple utero-ovarian massage and close detection of oestrus will elleviate these conditions in most of the cases.

2. In extreme summer condition these animals should be protected from direct solar radiation by maintaining them in shaded half walled sheds. If possible animals be given showers in addition to wallowing facilities particularly at mid-day during April, May and June.

3. Parading vasectomized bulls for heat detection can be gainfully employed at organised/ large farms. Since in summer buffalo bulls soon lose libido, replacement by young high libido bulls may be thought of where it is applicable.

4. *Painting of Lugol's Iodine*: The external os is swabbed thoroughly with Lugol's solution (B. Vet. Co, Iodum 5g, pot. iodide 10g, distilled water 100 ml) with the help of a metallic swab holder (46 cm) and vaginal speculum—double application of this solution is sometimes recommended at week's interval. It is presumed that application of Lugol's Iodine on the cervix causes local irritation and bring about reflex stimulation of anterior pituitary for secretion of gonadotrophins and thus cyclicity starts.

5. Some workers have used estrogen and progesterone in anaestrus and sub-estrus cows with encouraging success. The idea behind using small doses of these hormones are to act as a positive feed back at the hypothalamus level to release gonadotrophin releasing hormone (Gn-RH) and simultaniously sensitize the gonadotrophas in the anterior pituitary so that Gn-RH may act fully to stimulate more release of gonadotrophins.

It should be noted that the method can never be considered as a substitute for good management since use of hormonal therapy might also lead to inherent weakness in the progenies.

6. Use of prostaglandin ($PGF_2\alpha$) induces luteolysis resulting in sharp fall of serum progesterone level and thus helps to bring back normal oestrus cycle. Like hormonal therapy, prostaglandin therapy also can not be recommended as a substitute of good management.

Repeat Breeding

A repeat breeding in cow or buffalo is the one which has normal oestrus, oestrus cycles as well as reproductive tract and has been bred three or more times by a fertile bull or semen yet failed to conceive.

It is possible that pathology which cannot be detected by normal clinical methods may be present which include among others, failure of fertilization, anovulation and delayed ovulation, tubal obstructions, early or latent embryonic mortalities, poor breeding and management techniques including genetic, nutritional and infectious factors. Endometritis in many cases has been found to play major factor for causing repeat-breeding. Endometritis is caused by sporadic uterine infections by a varieties of microorganisms such as *C. pyogenes*, *Coliforms*, *Pseudomonas aeruginosa*, *Streptococci* etc., viral and fungal agents along with mycoplasmal agents may also cause endometritis in cattle and buffaloes. The condition follows mainly parturition, especially abnormal ones; abortion, dystokia, retained placenta, genital prolapse, uterine inertia, traumatic lesions in the uterus, cervix and vagina. Endometritis may also occur in cows and buffaloes after coitus or after AI under unhygienic conditions.

Appropriate antibiotic treatment is advocated after conducting antibiotic sensitivity tests where repeat breeding is associated with infections of the tubular genitalia.

Daily examination of repeaters is necessary to correct the condition arising from ovarian dysfunction. Anovular heats can be detected from the absence of palpable C.L. during dioestrus. Intramascular injection of 25 mg of progesterone during early heat may help in inducing ovulation.

The golden rule, prevention is better than cure applies more appropriately to reproductive problems. The incidence can be kept under control by adopting methods such as: (1) improved feeding and management, (2) providing hygienic surroundings at the time of calving, (3) asceptic precautions at the time of inseminations, and (4) educating farmers on detection of heat and maintenance of breeding records.

Weaning

Separating calf from its mother at a very early age is a bit difficult in buffaloes due to high motherly instinct. Since the method is important to assess dam's milk production and to feed calf according to live weight a substitution technique could be followed.

A single calf is substituted for let-down of milks in a number of buffaloes and the real calves are weaned just after birth. It can be achieved by putting blinkers (materials used to shut off the side views of buffaloes) during parturition and subsequently soiling the body of substituted calf with placental secretions. The dam starts licking the substituted calf after removal of blinkers.

Calf Mortality

Buffalo calf mortality rate under one month of age averages about 10% and varies from 3—30% in individual herds. Losses upto 50% have occured in large dairy herds. A calf mortality rate of 20% can reduce net profit by 38%.

A number of factors considered responsible for this hazard, are discussed below:

1. Antibodies are not transferable from buffalo dam to her fetus through placental membranes and thus they are susceptible to various virulent diseases. In buffalo calves inspite of feeding colostrum, a low antibody titre exists. Immunoglobulin levels have been reported to be 29.73 mg/ml in day olds and the quantity increases to 35.66 mg/ml on the second day of life. On the other hand in one estimate it has been noted that colostrum which is the only source of immunoglobulin for the buffalo calf, contains 68.75 mg of immuglobulin per ml on the first day, 23.75 mg/ml on the second day and 1.01 mg/ml on the fifth day of lactation

2. Certain meteorological influences may have an effect on calf mortality rate. During the winter months, mortality may be associated with the effects of cold, wet and windy weather while during the summer it may be the hot, dry weather.

3. Most of the deaths occur during autumn and winter months before the age of 3 months. The causes of mortality in order of priority have been found (i) Pneumonia, (ii) Enteritis, (iii) Toxaemia/Septicemia, (iv) Worm infestation, (v) Bloat etc.

4. The cause of high mortality in male calves could also be due to neglecting tendency by the management particularly regarding feeding.

Some of the prescribed managemental practices including feeding practices may be followed for minimizing the mortality rate.

(a) *Housing*

In commercial herds, calves after weaning may be kept in groups in large pens where individual feeding is advocated. In small herds calves after weaning should be kept in separate pens (24 sq. ft.) upto 3 months of age to avoid suckling instinct. The methods will eliminate the possible calf scour and parasitic infestation.

(b) *Feeding colostrum*

It is the milk secreted by the udder immediately after parturition and for the following 3–5 days. It contains 20% or more protein, a little more fat, 10 to 100 times more vitamin A, three times more of vitamin D and may be tinged pink due to blood corpuscles. It acts as a natural purgative for the calf, cleaning from its intestines the accumulated faecal matter (meconium). Of much greater importance, it is through the medium of the colostrum, antibodies which protects against various bacteria and viruses are supplied to the new born calves. Colostrum coagulates at about 80° to 85° C and can not therefore be boiled.

The calves at birth after weaning should be fed colostrum within 2 hrs. and its feeding should contiue for a period of five days at the rate of 1 to 1.5 kg per day.

Table 12.14

Milk Feeding Schedule

Age (days)	*Colostrum (kg)*	*Body weight (kg)*	*Milk (litres)*
1—5	1 to 1.5	—	—
6—15		Upto 25 kg	1.0
11—15		26—30	2.0
15 and above		31—40	2.5
		41—45	3.0
		46—50	3.5
		51—55	4.0
		56—60	4.5
		60 and above	5.0

In case the dam does not give colostrum a substitute of equal nutritive value prepared from 2 eggs and an ounce of castor oil may be fed for building up resistance. It may be necessary to inject dam's serum to such a calf for augmenting antibody titre in the body. The feed efficiency ratio of buffalo calves is as high as 1 kg gain per 1.16 kg dry matter. Milk feeding schedule is given in tabular form. It is necessary to provide milk to weaned calves at body temperature preferably with supplements to make up the deficiencies of Fe, Cu, Mg, Zn and Mn. Green fodder containing upto 100 gram dry matter may be offered daily from 15 days of age onwards so that it stimulates early rumen development.

(c) *Feeding Antibiotics*

Antibiotics are necessary in calves below 3 months of age to overcome certain stress conditions developed due to clinical or sub-clinical type of scour. These drugs are usually unnecessary in calves above 3 months as by this time rumen starts functioning and antibiotics are liable to interfere in normal functioning of ruminal microbes. The details of the practices that one should follow is given in the following Table.12.16

(d) *Feeding Milk Replacer*

The objectives of feeding milk replacer to calves are primarily to reduce the cost of raising buffalo calves and also to save milk for human consumption. Milk replacer may be fed as detailed in Tabular form. It may be noted that there is a gradual decrease in milk and corresponding increase in milk replacer at the rate of 200 g milk substitute per kg milk reduction. The general principle to be followed for calculation of milk requirement is that *it should be half kg less than one tenth of the body weight*. It is also necessary to give a minimum of 1 litre of milk per day with milk replacer and the mixture should be diluted about six times with warm water to provide a drink in suspension form.

Table 12.15

Age (Days)	Colostrum Milk (lit)	Treatments 1, 2, 3,	Preventive against
1	1.5	Orally Aureomycin Nutritional formula 2 spoonful	Calf scour
1	—	Sealing navel vessels	Navel ill
2	1.5	Vitamin A concentrate (1 ml vitablend)	Night blindness
3	1.0	Piperazine adipate 1 g/4 kg live wt	Ascariasis
4	a)	Buff. serum 50 ml s/c	To raise antibody titre, against calf scour
	b)	1/2 to 1 tab. sulfadimidine	
7	1.0	As on day 3 sulfadimidine 1/2 to 1 tablet	Ascariases & dysentry
8—11		Sulment course for 4 days	Coccidiosis

1. Mineral Supplement daily
2. TM-5 or Aurofac daily
3. Rovimix in oil once a week (10,000 IU of Vitamin A)

Table 12.16

Ingredients of milk replacer

Ingredients	Quantity
Wheat	8 kg
Fish meal	12 kg
Linseed meal	40 kg
Milk (DM)	16 kg
Coconut oil	7 kg
Linseed oil	3 kg
Citric acid	1.4 kg
Molasses	8 kg
Min. Mixture[2]	3 kg
Butyric acid	0.660 litres
Antibiotic mix.	300 g
Rovimix A, B_2, D_3	15 g

1. Rate of feeding is 200 gm equivalent to one litre milk replacement.
2. The mineral mixture on 3 kg basis containing: Dicalcium phosphate 1.65 kg; chalk 0.3312 kg; sodium chloride 0.9 kg; magnesium carbonate 0.09 kg; ferrous sulphate 0.015 kg; copper sulphate 0.0021 kg; cobalt chloride 0.0015 kg; potassium iodide 0.0003 kg; sodium fluoride 0.0003 kg; zinc sulphate 0.0075 kg; manganese oxide 0.0021 kg.

Table 12.17

Schedule of feeding milk replacer diet

Age of (days)	*Live wt. (kg)*	*Milk/day (kg)*	*Milk replacer (g)*
1—5		Colostrum 1.0 to 1.5	
6—14		2	
15—18		2.0	50
19—22		minus 1/2 kg[a]	100
23—26		minus 1.0 kg	300
31—34		minus 2.0 kg	400
	40	1.0	500
	45	1.0	550
	50	1.0	600
	55	1.0	650
	60	1.0	700
	65	1.0	750
	70	1.0	800
	75	1.0	850
	80	1.0	900
	85	1.0	950
	90	1.0	1000

a) to that of half kg less than one tenth of live wt.

REPRODUCTION

Female Reproduction

Poor reproduction is a major limiting factor in buffalo production and for achieving quick genetic improvement. Buffaloes, both swamp and river, have a very high age at first calving and long calving intervals, the latter being partly due to greater lactation stress in high producing buffaloes and partly due to seasonality of breeding. Suckling of calf in both river and swamp buffaloes also results in failure of resumption of ovarian cyclicity following freshening, which adds to the lengthening of post-partum oestrous interval and calving period.

For a successful breeding to occur, a female animal must be in heat and bred at the right time after oestrous is observed. With proper nutritional management heifers could be bred successfully even as early as two years of age. Buffaloes have been reported to show less intense signs of oestrous. Teaser bull, to detect oestrus, is generally used in large herds and the kind of teaser animals usually used are vasectomized or caudectomized. Non-visual methods involve laboratory examination of vaginal mucus, determination of changes in hormonal levels in plasma and milk, monitoring body temperature and measurement of variation in physical activity.

Problems of irregular oestrous is the most important factor obstructing attainment of full reproductive and productive potential of this species. Notable reason for this is the seasonal variation and malnutrition. In such cases the ovaries become smooth/inactive or subactive. Buffaloes are reproductively more active during cooler months than hot humid months. Production from direct solar radiation and application of water to body surface effectively reduce the heat stress and increase the reproductive efficiency during hotter months.

Another system of managing anoestrous buffaloes gaining popularity among researchers is induction of oestrous. Several methods depending on the status of ovarian functions are used to induce oestrous. In the presence of corpus luteum, enucleation and/or hormone administration have been used. A safer procedure is the administration of a drug which would cause functional regression of the corpus luteum. Prostaglandin F_2 alpha and its synthetic analogues have been tried successfully to cause luteal regression. The use of drugs in the manipulation of the oestrous cycle is not only limited to heat induction in anoestrous animals but has been employed in normally cycling buffaloes also to synchronize their oestrus and thus maximize reproductive performance during the breeding season.

Anatomy of the Reproductive Organs

The structure and location of the internal reproductive organs of the buffalo are similar to those of cattle. However, the cervix is less conspicuous and the uterine horns are smaller and more coiled than in cattle. The ovaries are ovoid and measure 2–3 cm in length, 1–2 cm from surface to surface and 1–2 cm from the attached to the free border. They are located within the pelvic cavity, caudal and lateral to the uterine horns. The genital tract and ovaries, including the cyclic corpus luteum (CL) and mature follicles (> 10 mm), may be palpated per rectum.

Breeding Season

The buffalo is polyoestrous, breeding throughout the year, but rainfall, feed supply, ambient temperature and photoperiod influence the annual calving pattern. Decreasing day length and cooler ambient temperatures favour cyclicity whereas long day length and the high summer temperatures depress cyclicity. In the Indian subcontinent, most buffaloes calve between November and March.

During this breeding period, the bulls have been found to be very active sexually and the quality and quantity of semen are very high, particularly during winter (November to February). The she-buffaloes show the maximum of ovarian activity and the largest percentage of them conceive during this period.

Estrous Cycle

The estrous cycle is about 21 days which comprises four distinct phases, viz., pro-estrous, estrous, meta-estrous and dio-estrous.

During pro-estrous FSH hormone stimulates the growth of graafian follicles, which secrete oestrogen and thereby causes growth of the tubular genitalia. Vulva starts swelling and mucus secretion may start. Pro-estrous may continue for 2–3 days.

The estrous or heat period is characterised by the typical breeding behaviour of females which are then ready for mating the buffalo bull. Duration of heat usually lasts for 24–36 hours. In the later part of estrous, secretion of LH increases and that of FSH decreases and thereby causes ovulation (10–18 hours after the end of estrous) and the formation of corpus luteum (CL) in the ovary.

Following the cessation of estrous, meta-estrous lasts for 3–4 days when a sharp decline of estrogen is noted. The vulva shrinks to original form and other genitalia returns to normal size.

The last phase of estrous cycle is dio-estrous when the CL remains functional with high level of progesterone. In case of conception the CL remains active throughout the gestation period and through secretion of progesterone maintains pregnancy, stimulates mammary alveolar growth. When there is no conception, the dio-estrous lasts from 10–18 days or longer depending upon the length of estrous cycle.

Signs of Estrous

Overt signs of estrous in buffalo are not as pronounced as in cattle. Heterosexual behaviour or standing to be mounted by a male is the most reliable sign of estrous in the buffalo. Other symptoms have been narrated at the end of the chapter on Mechanisms of Reproduction.

Mating Behaviour

Mating behaviour in many respects resembles that of cattle. On contacting a female, the female sniffs her urine, then displays the 'Flehmen' reaction and proceeds to nuzzle and lick the perineum and vulva.

An oestrous female responds by standing immobile for the male to mount and ejaculate; mating lasts for 20–30 seconds. Rhythmic pelvic thursts during intromission and the forward leap at ejaculation are less marked in buffalo than cattle. The male dismounts and gradually retracts the penis into the sheath while the female remains with her back arched and tail elevated for a few minutes.

Gestation length

The gestation period varies according to breed and environment and appears to be slightly longer than cattle. It is generally quoted as being "6 weeks less than a year" (or 10 months and 10 days). The average appears to be 316 $\pm$ 5 days.

Under the usual conditions of husbandry, a female buffalo will produce its first calf at the age of $3\frac{1}{2}$ to $4\frac{1}{2}$ years and thereafter will average 2 calves in every three years upto the age of 15. Twins are extremely rare. The average time for entire process of parturition comprising (i) dilation of the cervix, (ii) expulsion of faetus, (iii) expulsion of foetal membrane is about 5 hours. Calving seldom presents any difficulty and dystocia is virtually unknown.

Placentation

The epitheliochoral placenta of the buffalo is of the cotyledonary type. The foetal membranes and fetus mostly develop in one uterine horn. Most of the 60 to 90 placentomes are distributed throughout the gravid uterine horn. As pregnancy advances the placentomes enlarge to mushroom-like structures measuring 5–7 cm in diameter.

Pregnancy Diagnosis

1. *By Rectal palpation.* Pregnancy can be accurately diagnosed per rectum from about 45 days of pregnancy. Manual slipping of the allanto-chorion is possible from about 42 to 56 days of gestation. The uterus is suspended at the level of the pelvic floor upto the fourth month of gestation, then descends to the abdominal floor. In most buffaloes placentomes and the fetus may be palpated beyond the third month of pregnancy.

2. *Hormone assays.* As in cattle, pregnancy can be diagnosed on progesterone concentrations in milk or blood plasma at 22–24 days after breeding. This test is accurate for non-pregnancy but not for pregnancy.

Table 12.18 **Calving interval (Days) in Indian buffaloes**

Breed	Range	Mean	Breed	Range	Mean
Murrah	334–537	495	Marathwada	423–430	426
Surti	461–381	461	Nili-Ravi	445–525	460
Bhadawari	453.6	453	Non-descript	—	480

Calving Interval or Intercalving Period

The interval between the subsequent calvings is known as calving interval or inter-calving period, which is a significant trait for the assessment of the life time production potential of buffaloes.

Parturition

(a) *Signs of Approaching Parturition*

About 1–2 weeks before parturition, the female exhibits marked abdominal enlargement, udder development, hypertrophy and oedema of the vulval lips. As parturition approaches, the animal isolates herself from the rest of the herd. The relaxation of the pelvic ligaments leads to an elevation of the tail head while liquefaction of the cervical seal of pregnancy results in a string of clear mucus hanging from the vulva, particularly when the animal lies down.

(b) *Initiation of Parturition*

About 15 days before parturition, plasma levels of both oestrone and $PGF_{2\alpha}$ metabolite increase and reach peak values. At parturition there is a sharp decline of plasma concentration of progesterone with a significant increase of cortisol.

(c) *Stages of Labour*

About 12–24 hours before parturition, uterine contractions increase both in frequency and amplitudes causing the animal some abdominal discomfort. It takes about 1 to 2 hours to dilate the cervix along with rhythmic contractions of longitudinal and circular muscle fibre of the uterus (Stage I labour).

As the fetus enters the birth canal, the dam lies down and starts straining (Stage II labour). The allantochorion ruptures before it reaches the vulva. Next, the fetus, within the amnion, appears at the vulva. Strong abdominal contractions lead to the rupture of the amniotic sac and the delivery of the fetus, usually in anterior presentation and dorsal position, with extended limbs. This stage of labour lasts 30 to 60 minutes but may extend upto six hours, particularly in primipara. After delivery, abdominal straining ceases and the fetal membranes are expelled within 4–5 hours (stage III labour). Twinning is rare in buffalo and the incidence is less than 1 per 1000 births.

(i) *Feed in Relation to Reproduction*

Inadequate feeding and improper management of growing buffalo calves prevents full expression of their potential for growth. This causes delay in attaining sexual maturity both in males and females. Well-fed and well-managed buffalo heifers usually attain sexual maturity a year or more earlier than the poorly fed animals. Similarly, the poor level of nutrition during the later part of pregnancy, the problem of rebreeding after calving before the summer sets in and difficulties in detection of animals in oestrous during summer, result in long intercalving periods. Feeding calcium and phosphorus as per the requirement in lactating buffaloes helps to ensure early post-partum breeding.

(ii) *Heat Stress and Reproduction*

Reproduction in buffaloes is adversely affected by heat stress. Buffaloes protected from high ambient temperature and direct solar radiation along with adequate nutrition show improvement in their reproductive performance. Heat detection in buffaloes through behaviour symptoms is not possible. Non-availability of male to detect heat when the animals are confined and stallfed or tethered for stable grazing, adds to the problems of poor calf crop in both the river and swamp buffaloes. Bull parading during the cooler hours of the day or night even during summer would help to detect the animals in heat. This could be taken advantage of by shortening the calving interval and breeding the animals throughout the year, and thus reduce the peak and trough pattern of milk production in the Indian subcontinent. In case of farmers maintaining one or two buffaloes essentially under confinement and stall feeding, frequent urination can be used as best criterion for oestrous detection.

(iii) ***Endocrinology of female reproduction***

Not much work has been done on basic endocrinology of buffaloes. Some of the animals, even on attaining 5 years of age, do not exhibit oestrous in spite of the endocrine rhythm. Ovaries in such animals lack responsiveness to gonadotrophins and show poor folliculogenic activity. The FSH and LH levels, both in pituitary gland and in circulation, are also normal in such animals. There is therefore a need for investigating causes of gonadal insensitivity to gonadotrophic hormones in buffaloes. FSH concentration is the highest and LH the lowest at the peak breeding period. FSH : LH ratio remains narrow in summer. There is a need for investigating the specific receptor concentration for individual hormones at cellular level in the target organs. Elaborate experiments need to be designed by using hormonal agonist and anti-agonist, and active and passive immunization methods for bringing about extrinsic alternations in the hormones and receptor complexes.

The endocrinological parameters responsible for poor oestrous expressivity also need to be studied. Higher levels of plasma progesterone in anoestrous buffaloes and differences in plasma progesterone levels in buffaloes with phasic and non-phasic endocrine profiles have been reported. The animals with phasic profiles though anoestrous could be brought into oestrous by administering prostaglandins. Higher levels of circulating prolactin also appears to be most important interfering hormone in the secretion of ovarian hormones. Further studies involving prolactin and gonadotrophin receptors at ovarian level would be required.

(iv) ***Other Aspects of Female Reproduction***

Weaning is not normally practised because of the fear of problems in letting down of milk. Weaning of buffalo calves at birth or after utilizing colostrum especially in first calvers and raising them on commercial replacers is feasible, practical and economical. It will substantially reduce incidence of delayed post-partum oestrous.

Male Reproduction

Anatomy

The reproductive organs are like those of the bull but the testes and scrotum are smaller and the penile sheath is less pendulous. As in cattle, the testis and epididymis can be palpated through the scrotal wall whereas the prostate, seminal vesicles and ampullae can be felt per rectum.

Over the last two decades considerable attention has been given to understand environmental and biological constraints in sexual behaviour and semen production, elucidate the basic structure and functional characteristics of buffalo spermatozoa in relation to fertility. Endocrinological basis of male fertility, in vitro processing and short and long term preservation of semen, and fertility of chilled and frozen buffalo semen have been studied.

Endocrinology of Male Reproduction

The endocrinological studies showed that in river type buffaloes the plasma concentration of testosterone is low at 1 month of age (0.14 ng/ml) and increases gradually by 5 months. Thereafter the testosterone level fluctuates around this level until about 14 months of age and reaches 1 ng/ml at the age of 24 months. The level of androstenedione is highest at 2 months and declines gradually to reach very low level by 8 months indicating feedback mechanism which switches on the sequences of event leading to initiation of spermatogenesis. In indigenous buffaloes of Sri Lanka the lowest testosterone levels are found at 1–4 months of age with two prepuberal elevations at 5–6 months and 12 months of age. The swamp buffaloes are reported to have 3 elevations at 7, 10 and 16 months of age, followed by sustained rise after 20 months while in the Malaysian swamp buffaloes the testosterone level remains very low up to 2 years of age. In adult animals LH and testosterone have shown typical episodic and pulsatile pattern of secretion. Differences in hormonal profile between different seasons have been reported.

Further researches on histochemical and endocrinological profiles are needed to understand the reason for long leg period between completion of spermatogenesis and ability to ejaculate adequate number of sperms. Effect of draught work on hormonal profiles, libido and spermatogensis also needs further investigation. Such studies may reveal other possible methods for decreasing the age at puberty and maintaining optimum sexual activity for prolonged period.

(i) ***Factors Affecting Libido and Semen Quality***

The size and weight of testes are significantly lower in buffaloes than in cattle, and are reflected in relatively poor libido and semen production and quality. The scrotal circumference and testicular volume have large and positive correlation with body weight and age. The age at first ejaculation in buffalo males is rather very late. The time lag between testosterone secretion (12 months) to support spermatogenesis and onset of spermatogenesis (16 months) and the achievement of puberty (21/2–4 years) is considerably long. The possibility of reducing this age through better feeding and possible administration of exogenous gonadotrophic hormones needs to be examined. It may be possible to obtain usable semen at 21/2 years of age.

High ambient temperature and direct solar radiation adversely affect libido and semen production. Administration of exogenous gonadotrophins has produced variable results. Intramuscular injections of prostaglandins (PGF2) 1 hour before semen collection reduced the reaction time and resulted in increased ejaculate volume without affecting the total and live sperm concentration.

The major problems of male fertility are poor libido, quantitative and qualitative reduction in buffalo semen during summer, and wide range of variability in libido, semen production, and quality and freezability among bulls. The spermatogenic efficiency of the buffalo is only 43%. Although these problems are mostly related to nutrition and physical environment, specially heat stress, there are large genetic differences which could possibly be exploited in improving performance of males.

Water buffaloes provide 20–30% of farm power in China, Thailand, Indonesia, Malaysia and the Philippines. In India 60% of the total farm power is derived from draught animals, out of which about 10 per cent is from buffaloes. In spite of the large contribution of buffaloes towards farm power, little work has been done to improve and make maximum use of the draughtability of swamp buffaloes kept primarily for draught. Buffaloes can pull loads greater than six times their body weights but their usual load carrying capacity is 1.5 to 2.0 tonnes, i.e. 3 to 4 times of their body weights. These loads can be pulled for 2–3 hours continuously and for 6–8 hours in a day during winter and 5–6 hours during summer with rest pauses in between. Working of buffaloes increases heart rate, respiratory activity, body temperature and plasma volume and develops a mild alkalosis. During hot summer, they exhibit distress symptoms. Studies in Pakistan showed that milk production could be maintained when the buffalo cows were fed adequately and used for work under favourable environmental conditions.

Artificial Insemination (AI) in Buffalo

In India AI has been practised in buffaloes for over 30 years but has lagged behind cattle largely because of the difficulty of detecting oestrous. Chilled semen (5°C), diluted in a variety of extenders is still widely used in buffalo AI.

Buffalo semen can be frozen in extenders used for bovine semen. One such extender is a tris-buffer containing 7% glycerol and 20% egg yolk. Extended semen is packed in 0.25 or 0.5 ml French straws to contain 30 million motile spermatozoa per dose. Straws are exposed to nitrogen vapour at α –120° to –140°C for 7 to 10 minutes before being stored in liquid nitrogen. Semen should be thawed at 37 to 40°C. The post-thaw progressive motility of buffalo semen varies from 35 to 60%.

The optimum time of insemination in relation to oestrous and ovulation has not been determined for the buffalo. Most inseminations are usually performed between 12 and 24 hours from the onset of oestrous. At this time, the cervix is sufficiently dilated for the deposition of semen in the uterine body by the recto-vaginal technique of AI.

Nutrition

Buffaloes are mostly found in countries where feeds, fodders and pastures are limited and are of poor quality. In spite of this situation, the buffaloes have thrived reasonably well and relatively better than cattle.

The findings on the comparative functional rumen developments as well as the rumen fermentation activities have, in general, led to the belief that *buffaloes are more efficient converters of low-grade roughages* for different body functions.

(A) ***Nutritional Requirements***

Energy and protein requirements have been worked out for maintenance and milk production. The metabolizable enery requirement:

(a) for maintenance ranges from 97.8 to 188.8 Kcal/$W^{0.75}$ kg in dry and lactating buffaloes,

(b) for milk production ranges from 1,171 to 1,863 Kcal/Kg 4% FCM.

The DCP requirement (a) for maintenance in dry and lactating animals ranges from 1.28 to 3.48 g/kg $W^{0.75}$ kg, (b) for milk production ranges from 126.6 to 166.34 g/100 g of protein secreted in milk.

The dry-matter intake (per unit body weight) of buffaloes is lesser than that of cattle.

(B) ***Superiority of Buffaloes to Cows in Feed Utilization***

Buffaloes have high efficiency of feed utilization when fed on high roughage (fibrous) diets. The digestibility of dry matter and crude fibre/neutral detergent fibre in most of the situations is also comparatively higher in buffaloes than in cattle. Possible reasons for better utilization of nutrients in buffaloes are:

(i) large rumen volume,
(ii) high rate of salivation (associated with pH control, recycling of nitrogen and sulphur),
(iii) slower rate of passage of digesta through the reticulorumen,
(iv) slow rumen motility,
(v) higher cellulolytic activity of microbial population, and
(vi) lesser dry-matter intake per unit body weight.

Buffaloes fed on low-grade roughages can maintain a positive nitrogen balance, when supplemented with higher NPN-based rations. The concentrations for total nitrogen and ammonia nitrogen is higher in the rumen of buffaloes than of cattle. This may be due to better activity of intra-cellular deaminases of microbes. This is also substantiated by the high proteolytic activity in rumen of buffaloes.

(C) *Rumen Environment in Buffaloes*

The microbial population (protozoa, total viable bacteria, amylolytic and proteolytic bacteria) is higher in rumen of buffalo than of cattle. The number of oscillospira is 10–25 times higher in buffalo rumen liquor than in cattle. This may be responsible for greater protein synthesis in buffalo rumen. The higher numbers of iodophylic organisms in the rumen of buffaloes than of cattle also help in better utilization of nitrogen from simpler sources (NPN) for synthesis of microbial protein for the host. The rumen concentration of total VFA is higher in buffaloes than in cattle. The proportions of propionic acid and butyric acids as compared to acetic acid also are higher in buffalo rumen fluid.

(D) *Improving Utilization of Poor-quality Roughages and Crop Residues*

Chemical treatment of poor-quality roughages which are common feed for buffaloes helps in improving intake and digestibility. Such forage supplement to the tune of 30–50% of dry matter of feed or 0.9 to 1.5% of live weight will be optimum for production and much cheaper than providing supplemental nutrients through costly concentrate feeds. Examples of such feeds include supplementation of urea molasses with green forage, viz., cultivated leguminous fodder, leaves of cassava, gliricidia, leucaena, water hyacinth, groundnut and sweet potato vines.

Health

Almost all the diseases recorded in cattle occur in buffaloes but may differ in the degree of incidence and pathogenicity.

Buffaloes show higher degree of resistance to a number of diseases, e.g. brucellosis and foot-and-mouth disease (FMD). However, with regard to FMD this statement is disputed by some workers. They are however more susceptible to pasteurellosis, bovine maligant cattarrh and rinderpest. Buffaloes also suffer from bovine viral diarrhoea (BVD), mucosal comples, buffalo pox, infectious bovine rhinotracheitis (IBR) and buffalo lymphosarcoma.

Buffaloes have high incidence of parasitic diseases because of their wallowing nature. They have high risk of helminthic infestation and sarcoptic mange during periods of draught. Buffaloes suffer from nutritional haemoglobinurea, acidosis and alkalosis. They are exceptionally more susceptible to degnala disease which occurs in traditionally non-paddy growing areas when buffaloes are fed on paddy straw. This disease results in gangrene of extremities ultimately resulting in death. Degnala disease is possibly due to mycotoxicosis and/or selenium toxicity.

Buffaloes also have high incidence of anoestrous and torsion of uterus. Genital mycoplasma an important cause of infertility both in male and female buffaloes.

Calf mortality in buffaloes is very high. Ascariasis and *Toxocara vitulorum* are the major causes of calf mortality in addition to neonatal diarrhoea and pneumonia. Rota and corona viruses along with virulent strains of *E. coli* are associated with diarrhoea. PI3 chlamydial agents and other micro-organisms are responsible for pneumonia. Lack of full immunological competence and depressed cellular immune responses would require colostrum feeding to provide immunoglobulins to protect the neonates from these infections. These infections appear to be more severe, and could possibly be due to inadequate availability of maternal antibodies because of the limitations of their absorption from colostrum.

The buffalo calves are also more prone to adverse effects of inclement weather conditions. Early suckling after birth, hygienic conditions of quarters where calves are maintained, regular deworming and protection against ectoparasites and administration of pro-biotic (e.g. lactobacillus bacteria) may help in reducing calf mortality.

Prepartum reproductive disorders in buffaloes include dystocia, antepartum prolapse and abortion. The management of post-partum disorders will depend largely on the extent and nature of the problem. Most of the puerperal metritis cases are due to retained placenta and abortion. The relatively high prevalence of metritis and other genital tract infections in buffaloes is, in part, due to practices of inserting the tail, a stick, hand or the wrist into the vagina to assist milk let down and to tranquilize viscious buffaloes prior to milking in Iraq, and the practice of inflating the vagina by mouth or through a tube in Iraq and India. The isolates most commonly found in infectious endometritis are *Corynebacterium pyogenes*, *Streptococcus* sp. and *Staphylococcus aureus*. Since these isolates are usually sensitive to the more common antibiotics, treatment of infections of the genital tract involves uterine infusion and/or systemic antibiotic administration. Brucellosis is one of the infectious diseases of buffaloes which is better prevented than treated because it is not readily amenable to antibiotic treatment and it is of public health importance. Leptospirosis is another zoonotic disease affecting buffalo reproductive tract. However, its role in causing abortions and infertility is not explained. Genital tuberculosis involving ovary, oviduct and uterus are rare though reported.

Relevant Information about Buffalo

1. Most of the female buffaloes show sign of heat at night and it has been observed to be maximum at midnight.
2. The oestrus symptoms is also weaker in buffaloes when compared to cows which become still weaker during the hot dry months (April to June) and is known as silent heat.
3. High buffalo calf mortality is one of the serious problems among farmers. Exposure to draft and damp, wet bedding specially in rainy season and in winter leads to high incidence of Pneumonia. Gastro-enteritis is the second highest cause of buffalo calf mortality. The disease may be due to viral, bacterial or parasitic infections. All care must be taken to offer good quality feeds at optimum quantity.
4. Services are given before feeding, as bulls seem to perform more quickly if this procedure is followed. If the interval between two successive services is long (7–10 days or more), the bull is allowed to serve a second time, since the first ejaculate may contain a number of dead spermatozoa.

5. Buffaloes are less discriminating in foraging and therefore consume a larger quantity of coarse fodder that is not readily eaten by cattle. This might be one of the reasons why buffaloes thrive better than do cattle on coarse fodder.
6. Buffalo bull attains sexual maturity later than ox bull.
7. Because of lower heat tolerance, the shelter requirements of the buffalo are different from those of the cattle. During hot summer months, buffaloes need special comfort for which they love to have wallowing.
8. Buffalo bulls are more apt to develop strong autoganism among themselves than dairy or beef bulls and thus requires extra attention for keeping them apart. Fights between buffalo bulls are dangerous and frequently end in fatality.
9. Buffaloes are comparatively more susceptible to some diseases like Rinderpest, Haemorrhagic septicaemia (pasteurellosis) than the indigenous cattle managed under comparable conditions.
10. India possesses the largest number of buffaloes (64.48 million in 1985), the figure is about half of the world's total buffalo population (128.7 million). India is followed by China, Pakistan, Thailand, the Philippines, Nepal, Indonesia, Vietnam, Burma, Turkey, Sri Lanka, Iraq, Iran, Bangladesh and other countries.
11. Management of buffaloes shall include adequate attention for their exercise, supply of adequate clean feed, allowing bath and wallowing, sanitary management, regular vaccination programme and other regular care and attention as are practised in dairy cattle.
12. Buffaloes have a low cost of milk production per litre which is a net outcome of physiological superiority of buffaloes over cows.

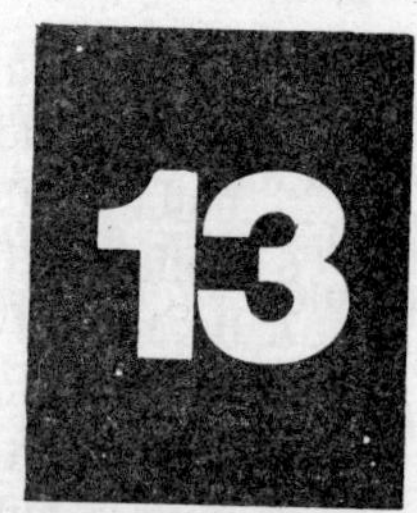

DAIRY FARM MANAGEMENT

What is Management?

It is said that management is the art and science of combining ideas, facilities, processes, materials and labour to produce and market a worthwhile product or service successfully.

Thus, a manager is an organiser and a converter—he converts resources into products. This is just as true for our dairy farm as for our biggest industries. The managers of motor company convert labour, steel, rubber, plastics into falcons. We convert labour, soil, fertility, hay, silage, and other inputs into milk. These transformations do not occur by happenstance. They are the result of a purposeful and premeditated force called management, a process we shall examine more closely.

Functions of Management

From a gerneral point of view, a manager must perform five major functions; he must plan, organise, co-ordinate, direct and control.

Another way of expressing these managerial functions is to consider the manager's role as a "decision maker", i.e., who must decide what to do, how to do it and when. This decision-making responsibility distinguishes the manager from the hired worker who awaits to be told. Thus, the functions of management may be outlined as *steps* in decision-making, sometimes called the "management process". For successful performance of these processes, the manager must:

(1) OBSERVE. Gather information about all resources available, new technologies which may apply, alternative market outlets, sources of capital credit needed and other items affecting successful operation;

(2) ESTABLISH GOALS. Clearly set out the objectives he wants to achieve;

(3) IDENTIFY PROBLEMS. Find the obstacles, or "stumbling blocks," which hinder progress towards goals;

(4) ANALYSE. Compare alternative methods of reaching goals, considering for each plan the income potential, the capital needed, the labour required, etc.;

(5) DECIDE. Choose a plan of action and set out a clearcut procedure for getting under way;

(6) ACT. Put his chosen plan into operation;

(7) BE RESPONSIBLE. Assume responsiblity for the consequences of actions taken;

(8) EVALUATE. Measure results and compare accomplishments with goals and standards of performance;

(9) CONTROL. Keep a careful check on production level, labour efficiency, cost, investments, etc.;

(10) ADJUST. Keep the operating system flexible to take advantage of new developments which are applicable.

One will not take time, of course, to work through these processes formally for every decision made. With some practice, however, it may become a way of reasoning and planning which may be applied to any problem to be solved. For major decisions, such as buying a farm, closing a long-range plan of operation or making a major adjustment in operations, it should be followed carefully, using the appropriate tools outlined below.

Tools of Management

One of our first jobs as a farm manager is to be well-informed about many kinds of information affecting our business. Should decisions cannot be made consistently on the basis of erroneous information, some of the tools which are helpful in acquiring accurate information about our business and in guiding our management decisions are as follows:

(1) FARM RECORDS. No business of any consequence can be operated successfully without a good system of accounting. For a dairy farm, these accounts should include the following as a minimum:

(a) *Complete inventories* at the beginning and end of each year—including a summary of all assets, debts and net worth;
(b) *Production records* (including main animal products and their by-products);
(c) *Current expenditures and receipts* (including quantities sold);
(d) An annual *production* and *financial summary*; and
(e) An *analysis* of the year's records to determine strong and weak points of the business and to serve as a guide to wiser adjustments.

(2) COMPARATIVE (BLOCK) BUDGETING. This is a quick and effective way to compare alternative system of organizing our overall farm business from the standpoint of capital, labour requirements, and the net income potential. These budgets are based upon long-run expectations of yields, prices and costs.

(3) ANNUAL BUDGETING. This is a "must" to guide year to year adjustments in an operating system. Annual budgets are based on the current outlook for yields, prices and costs. They give a preview of the coming year's business and often allow one to correct mistakes in judgment *before* they happen.

(4) PARTIAL BUDGETING. This is a shorter process of comparing the costs and returns from alternative adjustments in some part of our business, such as the "pros and cons" of some new technology.

It is worthwhile repeating that all kinds of budgets used in planning for the future—one of our major responsibilities as a planner—must be based upon reliable information. Careful analysis of our own records, a study of analysis from similar farming operations and an up-to-date knowledge of the results of new research will provide the data needed.

CARE OF THE COW AND CALF DURING AND AFTER PARTURITION

Success in dairying depends largely on the proper care and efficient management of the herd. All dairy operations must be planned with due regard to the comfort of the animals. Care of pregnant cows during and after calving, therefore, should receive the personal attention of the dairy farmer, otherwise he is likely to make many costly mistakes. Few hints are given here for his guidance.

A. Caring for the Cow

1. Usually a dairy cow will carry her calf a period of 282 days (gestation period). However, they may range from 270 to 290 days after conception. If accurate breeding records have been kept, which every farmer should do, the date can be calculated to within one to ten days. Knowing expected date of calving is a "*must*" for taking all future care of the pregnant cows.
2. In handling advanced pregnant cows, care should be taken to prevent them from being injured by slipping on stable floors or by crowding through doorways, or by mounting cows or bulls that are in heat. Separate the pregnant cows from rest and allow them to live in a little isolated way.
3. Symptoms that an animal is about to calve include swelling of the udder, swelling of the vulva and dropping away ligaments around the tail head. At this stage she should be housed in calving pen. Birth usually takes place in one or two hours. The room should be clear, well ventilated, well bedded and finally, disinfected. Alternatively a small well grassed pasture free from trash or manure and close to the framstead (to get some observation) make a good calving place except during monsoon and cold months.
4. The majority of domesticated animals require little or no assistance in the actual act of parturition, provided they are in a reasonably healthy and vigorous state. At the same time, it is advisable that someone shall be at hand to give any help if some emergency arises. At the first sign of calving, the front feet of the calf should appear first, then the nose. Any abnormality in presentation requires immediate attention by a veterinarian. Remember that if the labour prolongs for more than 4 hours, abnormal presentation is probable (dystokia), immediately provide veterinary aid.
5. After parturition the exterior of the genitalia, the flanks and tail should be washed with warm clear water containing some crystals of potassium permanganate or *Neem* leaves boiled in water. This will give a good antiseptic wash.
6. Keep the cow warm to prevent her from chill and it is desirable to give her warm water or warm *Gur sarbat* to drink just after parturition.
7. It is normal for the udder to become large and swollen just before calving. Controversy exists as to whether or not the udder should be milked out before calving. Special precautions should be exercised to see that old nails, loose glass pieces, etc., do not cut and injure the swollen udder. Milk the cow partially to avoid milk fever after parturition.
8. The placenta will normally leave the cow within 2-4 hours. If it is not expelled between 8-12 hours, administer *Ergot* mixture. Beyond 12 hours, apply manual help by a veterinarian.

   When the afterbirth (placenta) has been discharged, it should immediately be buried deeply. All care should be taken to avoid licking or ingestion of placenta by the cow as the practice adversely reduce milk yield due to excessive protein intake.
9. There are always dangers that high producing cows will develop milk fever and mastitis. The dairyman should remain alert for any symptoms of the diseases. To avoid milk fever, it is best not to draw all the milk from the udder for a day or two after calving. To avoid mastitis, regular tests should be made by a veterinarian.
10. Feed the cow at first only bran mash moistened with lukewarm water to provide laxative effect. Some green grass may also be given. After 2 days a mixture of oats, bran and linseed mash can be used to replace the bran mash. If the cow is in good

condition at the time of calving the amount of feed during these two days does not matter. The amount of concentrates should then be gradually increased with the aim of reaching full dosages in two weeks.

B. Caring for the Newborn Calf

1. Immediately after the calf is born, make sure that all mucus is removed from the nose and mouth. If the calf does not start to breathe, artificial respiration should be used by alternately compressing and relaxing the chest walls with the hands after laying the calf on its side.
2. Apply tincture of iodine to the navel at birth, and dust with boric acid power. If a long cord is attached to the navel, swip it off about 2" from the body before applying iodine. The navel cord should not be tied but allowed to drain.
3. Under most conditions the calf will be on its feet and ready for suckling within an hour. Some assistance at this stage is useful. Much infection can be prevented if an attendant cleans the udder before the calf nurses.
4. Be sure the calf gets first milk (colostrum) at least for 48 hours. The antibodies present in colostrum protects the calf against diseases and has a laxative effect. The rate of milk feeding should be about 10% of the calf's weight per day, upto a maximum of 5-6 litres per day. If scouring occurs, the milk allowance should be reduced to 1/2 or less until the calf recovers.
5. If possible, follow weaning system (to remove the calf from the dam). Usually the calf is separated permanently from its mother after the first feeding because it simplifies management and reduces the food and labour costs for rearing. At present, there is a great variation in practice regarding the best time to remove the calf from the dam. Some dairymen allow the calf to remain with its dam for 2 or 3 days or until the milk is suitable to put in the regular supply. It probably makes little difference as to when the calf is removed from its dam.
6. The calf is best maintained in an individual pen or stall for the first few weeks. This allows more careful attention to individuals. After about 8 weeks of age, it may be handled with a group.
7. Take body weight of the cow if possible and identify the calf by tatooing.
8. At the age of 15 days, 30–40 .cc. of H.S. serum should be inoculated into the calf.
9. Dehorn the calf at an early age preferably within 15 days.
10. Teats of the udders of heifer in excess of four are usually best removed. Frequently limited amounts of milk may be secreted by extra teats creating difficulty at milking time.
11. At the age of 3 months, the calf should be vaccinated against anthrax and 15 days, thereafter it should be vaccinated against B.Q.
12. Details of calf rearing may be learnt under the heading "Raising the dairy calf" discussed elsewhere in this chapter.

HOUSING FOR DAIRY CATTLE

An efficient management of cattle will be incomplete without a well planned and adequate housing of cattle. Improper planning in the arrangement of animal housing may result in additional labour charges and thus curtail the profit of the owner. During erection of a house for dairy cattle, care should be taken to provide comfortable accommodation for an individual cattle. No less important is the (1) proper sanitation, (1) durability, (3) arrangements for the production of clean milk under convenient and economic conditions, etc.

Location of Dairy Buildings

The points which should be considered before the erection of dairy buildings are as follows:

1. **Topography and drainage.** A dairy building should be at a higher elevation than the surrounding ground to offer a good slope for rainfall and drainage for the wastes of the dairy to avoid stagnation within. A levelled area requires less site preparation and thus lesser cost of building. Low lands and depressions and proximity to places of bad odour should be avoided.

2. **Soil type.** Fertile soil should be spared for cultivation. Foundation soil as far as possible should not be too dehydrated or desiccated. Such a soil is susceptible to considerable swelling during rainy season and exhibit numerous cracks and fissures.

3. **Exposure to the sun and protection from wind.** A dairy building should be located to a maximum exposure to the sun in the north and minimum exposure to the sun in the south and protection from prevailing strong wind currents whether hot or cold. Buildings should be placed so that direct sunlight can reach the platforms, gutters and mangers in the cattle shed. As far as possible, the long axis of the dairy barns should be set in the north-south direction to have the maximum benefit of the sun.

4. **Accessibility.** Easy accessibility to the buildings is always desirable. Situation of a cattle shed by the side of the main road preferably at a distance of about 100 meters should be aimed at.

5. **Durability and attractiveness.** It is always attractive when the buildings open up to a scenic view and add to the grandeur of the scenery. Along with this, durability of the structure is obviously an important criteria in building a dairy.

6. **Water supply.** Abundant supply of fresh, clean and soft water should be available at a cheap rate.

7. **Surroundings.** Areas infested with wild animals and dacoits should be avoided. Narrow gates, high manger curbs, loose hinges, protruding nails, smooth finished floor in the areas where the cows move and other such hazards should be eleminated.

8. **Labour.** Honest, economic and regular supply of labour be available.

9. **Marketing.** Dairy buildings should only be in those areas from where the owner can sell his products profitably and regularly. He should be in a position to satisfy the needs of the farm within no time and at a reasonable price.

10. **Electricity.** Electricity is the most important sanitary method of lighting a dairy. Since a modern dairy always handles electric equipments which are also economical, it is desirable to have an adequate supply of electricity.

11. **Facilities, labour, food.** Cattle yards should be so constructed and situated in relation to feed storages, hay stacks, silo and manure pits as to effect the most efficient utilisation of labour. Sufficient space per cow and well arranged feeding mangers and resting areas contribute not only to greater milk yield of cows and make the work of the operator easier but also minimises feed expenses. The relative position of the feed stores should be quite adjacent to the cattle barn. Noteworthy features of feed stores are given:

(a) Feed storages should be located at hand near the centre of the cow barn.
(b) Milk-house should be located almost at the centre of the barn.
(c) Centre cross-alley should be well designed with reference to feed storage, the stall area and the milk house.

Types of Housing

The most widely prevalent practice in this country is to tie the cows with rope on a *Katcha* floor except some organised dairy farms belonging to government, co-operatives or military where proper housing facilities exist. It is quite easy to understand that unless cattle are provided with good housing facilities, the animals will move too far in or out of the standing space, defecating all round and even causing trampling and wasting of feed by stepping into the mangers. The animals will be exposed to extreme weather conditions all leading to bad health and lower production.

Dairy cattle may be successfully housed under a wide variety of conditions, ranging from close confinement to little restrictions except at milking time. However, two types of dairy barns are in general use at the present time.

1. The loose housing barn in combination with some type of milking barn or parlour.
2. The conventional dairy barn.

LOOSE HOUSING SYSTEM

Loose housing may be defined as a system where animals are kept loose except milking and at the time of treatment. The system is most economical. Some features of loose housing system are as follows:

1. Cost of construction is significantly lower than conventional type.
2. It is possible to make further expansion without much changes.
3. Facilitate easy detection of animals in heat.
4. Animals feel free and therefore, proves more profitable with even minimum grazing.
5. Animals get optimum exercise which is extremely important for better health and production.
6. Overall better management can be rendered.

The floor and manger space requirement of dairy cows are give in Table 13.1

Other Provisions

The animal sheds should have proper facilities for milking barns, calf pens, calving pens and arrangement for store rooms etc. In each shed, there should be arrangement for feeding, manger, drinking area and loafing area.

The shed may be cemented or brick paved, but in any case it should be easy to clean. The floor should be rough, so that animals will not slip. The drains in the shed should be shallow and preferably covered with removable tiles. The drain should have a gradient of 1" for every 10' length. The roof may be of corrugated cement sheet, asbestos or brick and rafters. Cement concrete roofing are too expensive.

Inside the open unpaved area it is always desirable to plant some good shady trees for excellent protection against direct cold winds in winter and to keep cool in summer.

Table 13.1

Types of Animals	Floor space per animal (Sq. feet)		Manger length per animal (inches)
	Covered area	Open area	
Cows	20-30	80-100	20-24
Buffaloes	25-35	80-100	24-30
Young stock	15-20	50-60	15-20
Pregnant Cows	100-120	180-200	24-30
Bulls Pen	120-140	200-250	24-30

Cattle Shed. The entire shed should be surrounded by a boundary wall of 5′ height from three sides and manger etc., on one side. The feeding area should be provided with 2 to 2½ feet of manger space per cow. All along the manger, there shall be 10″ wide water trough to provide clean, even, available drinking water. The water trough thus constructed will also minimise the loss of fodders during feeding. Near the manger, under the roofed house 5′ wide floor should be paved with bricks having a little slope. Beyond that, there should be open unpaved area (40′ × 35′) surrounded by 5′ walls with one gate. A plan for such a house along with the plan for calves shed and their sections are shown in Fig. 13.1. It is preferable that animals face north when they are eating fodder under the shade. During cold wind in winter the animals will automatically lie down to have the protection from the walls.

Shed for calves. On one side of the main cattle shed there shall be fully covered shed 10′ × 15′ to accommodate young calves. Such sheds with suitable partitioning, may also serve as calving pen under adverse climatic conditions. Beyond this covered area there should be a 20′ × 10′ open area having boundary wall so that calves may move there freely.

In this way both cattle and calve sheds will need in all 50′ × 50′ area for 20 adult cows and followers. If one has limited resources, he can build ordinary, *katcha/semi katcha* boundary walls but feeding and water trough should be cemented ones. The estimated cost of brick boundary wall, cement sheets, roofing on pipes and angle irons are give as per 1981 market price.

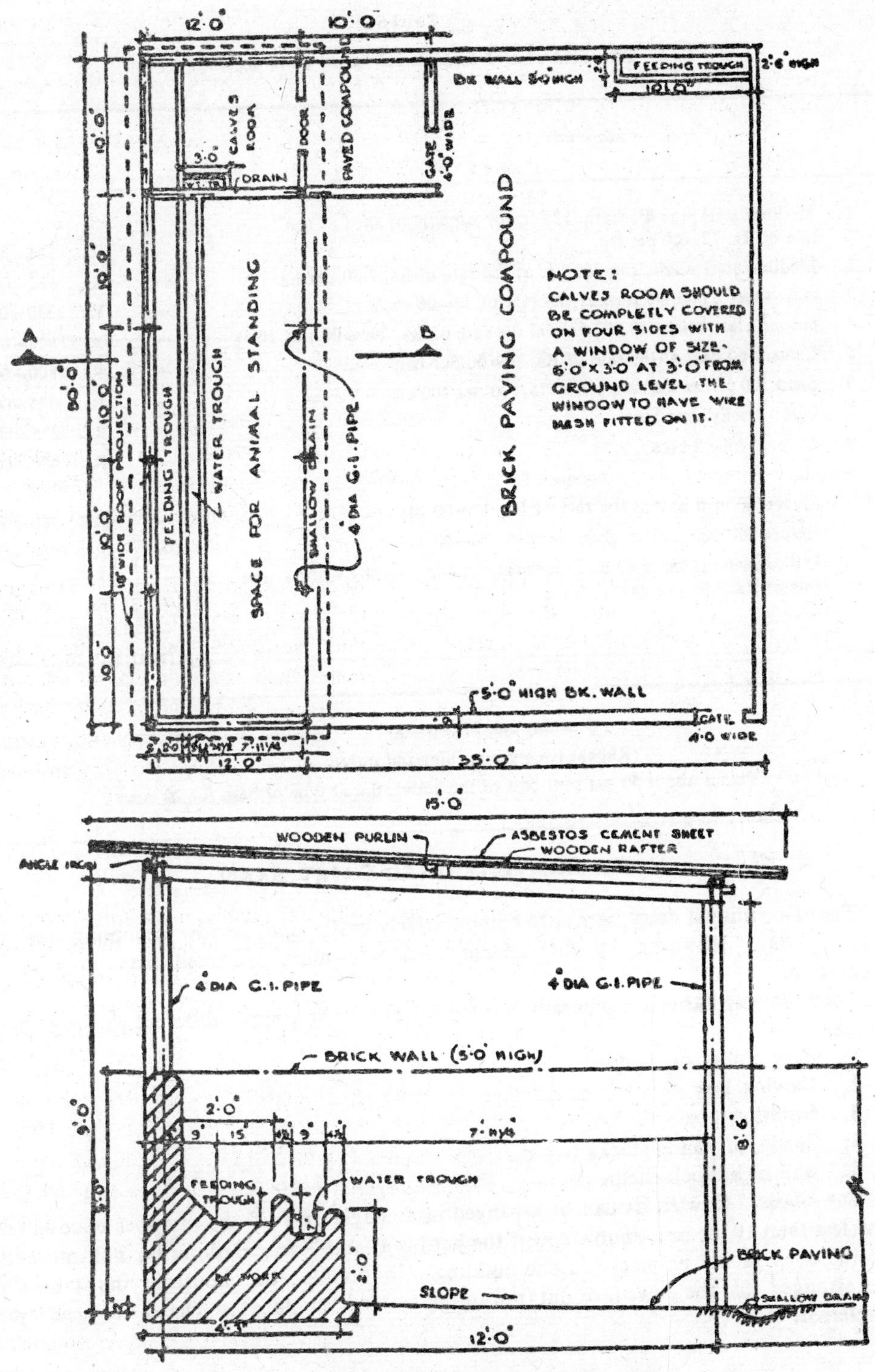

Fig. 13.1. Plan for Loose Housing to accomodate 25 cows with followers.

Table 13.2

Estimated cost of loose house for 20 cows and followers

	Materials		*Cost*
1.	Medium steel pipe 4" width, 127 ft. for support of shed at the rate of Rs. 12—00 per ft.	—	Rs. 1524—00
2.	Medium steel angle iron 240 kg. at the rate of Rs. 2.80 per kg.	—	Rs. 672=00
3.	A.C. sheet 2 met. 45 nos. at the rate of 30=00 each	—	Rs. 1350=00
4.	Second class bricks 40,000 nos. at the rate of Rs. 290=00 per 1000	—	Rs. 11600=00
5.	Cement 60 bags at the rate of Rs. 30=00 per bag	—	Rs. 1800—00
6.	Sand 500 cft. at the rate of Rs. 75=00 per 100 cft	—	Rs. 375—00
7.	Door 4'×6½' one No.	—	Rs. 275—00
8.	Gate 4' wide 2 Nos.	—	Rs. 450=00
	Labour		
	Mason 60 men unit at the rate of Rs. 15=00 day	—	Rs. 900=00
	Helper 200 men unit at the rate of Rs. 8=00 day	—	Rs. 1600—00
	Skilled man mazdoor 40 units for erection and sheeting work at the rate of Rs. 8.50 per day	—	Rs. 320—00
			Total Rs. 20,866—00

or Say Rs. 21,000—00

(Rupees twenty-one thousand only).

Note: This is about 50 per cent cost of the conventional type of barn for 20 cows.

CONVENTIONAL DAIRY BARN

The conventional dairy barns are comparatively costly and is now becoming less propular day by day. However, by this system cattle are more protected from adverse climatic condition.

The following barns are generally needed for proper housing of different classes of dairystock on the farm.

1. Cow houses or sheds
2. Calving box
3. Isolation box
4. Sheds for young stocks
5. Bull or bullock sheds.

Cow Sheds. Cow sheds can be arranged in a single row if the number of cows are small, say less than 10, or in a double row if the herd is a large one. Ordinarily, not more than 80 to 100 cows should be placed in one building. In double row housing, the stable should be so arranged that the cows face out (tail to tail system) or face in (head to head system) as preferred.

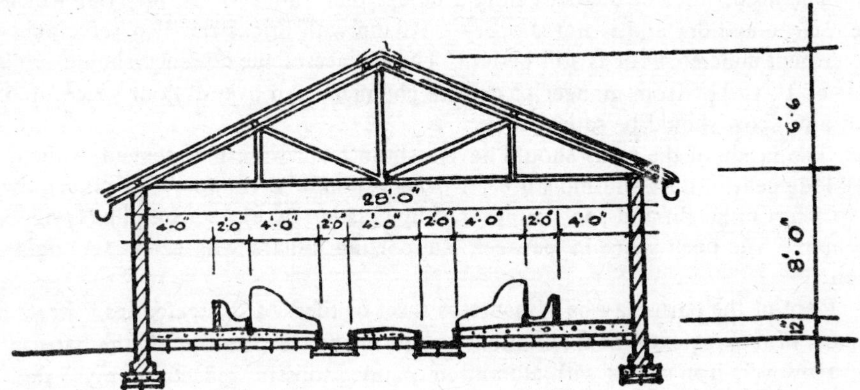

Fig. 13.2. Tail to tail arrangement.

Advantages of tail to tail system

1. Under the average conditions, 125 to 150 man hours of labour are required per cow per year. *Study of time:* Time motion studies in dairies showed that 15% of the expended time is spent in front of the cow, and 25% in other parts of the barn and the milk house, and 60% of the time is spent behind the cows. Time spent at the back of the cows is 4 times more than the time spent in front of them.
2. In cleaning and milking the cows, the wide middle alley is of great advantage.
3. Lesser danger of spread of diseases from animal to animal.
4. Cows can always get more fresh air from outside.
5. The head *gowala* can inspect a greater number of milkmen while milking. This is possible because milkmen will be milking on both sides of the head *gowala.*
6. Any sort of minor disease or any change in the hind quarters of the animals can be detected quickly and even automatically.

Advantages of face to face system

1. Cows make a better showing for visitors when heads are together.
2. The cows feel easier to get into their stalls.
3. Sun rays shine in the gutter where they are needed most.
4. Feeding of cows is easier, both rows can be fed without back tracking.
5. It is better for narrow barns.

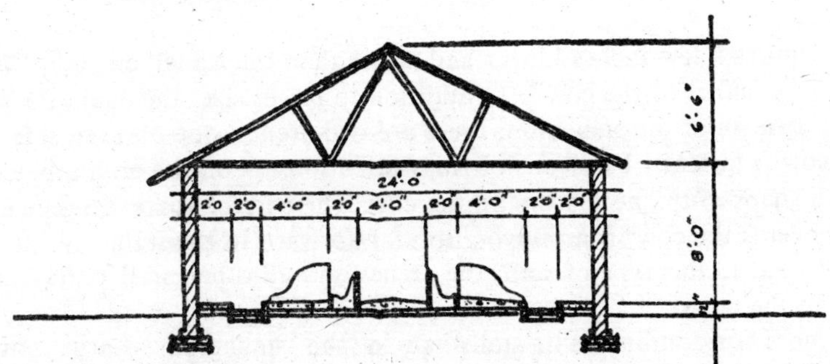

Fig. 13.3. Face to face arrangement.

Floor. The inside floor of the barn should be of some impervious material which can be easily kept clean and dry and is not slippery. Paving with bricks can also serve ones purpose. Grooved cement concrete floor is still better. The surface of the cowshed should be laid with a gradient of 1″ to $1\frac{1}{2}$″ from manger to excreta channel. An overall floor space of 65 to 70 sq. ft. per adult cow should be satisfactory.

Walls. The inside of the walls should have a smooth hard finish of cement, which will not allow any lodgment of dust and moisture. Corners should be round. For plains, dwarf walls about 4 to 5 feet in height and roofs supported by masonry work or iron pillars will be best or more suitable. The open space in between supporting pillars will serve for light and air circulation.

Roof. Roof of the barn may be of asbestos sheet or tiles. Corrugated iron sheets have the disadvantage of making extreme fluctuations in the inside temperature of the barn in different seasons. However, iron sheets with aluminium painted tops to reflect sunrays and bottoms provided with wooden insulated ceilings can also achieve the objective. A height of 8 feet at the sides and 15 feet at the ridge will be sufficient to give the necessary air space to the cows. An adult cow requires at least about 800 cubic feet of air space under tropical conditions. To make ventilation more effective a continuous ridge ventilation is considered most desirable.

Stall design. The two main types of dairy barn stalls are the stanchion stall and tie stall.

1. *The Stanchion Stall*

It is one of the standard dairy cow stalls. It is equipped with a stanchion for fastening a cow in place. Usually there is a stall partition in the form of a curved pipe between the stalls to keep the cows in place and to protect their udders and teats from being stepped on by other cows.

The stanchion should be so constructed and arranged as to allow the cows the greatest possible freedom. There should be several links of chain at the top and bottom of the stanchions and sufficient room on each side of it to permit the animal to move its head from side to side. It is important to provide for the comfort of the cows and to line them up so that most of the droppings and urine go to the gutter. Practically, it is not possible to fit every cow to her stall properly. To compensate this, many stanchions have adjustments so that they can be set forward if the cow is too large for the stall or backwards if the cow is too small. The cow can be fastened easily and quickly with the stanchions and is held more closely in place than other types of ties. However, she is held more rigidly and therefore, the stanchion is less comfortable than other types of fasteners.

2. *The Tie Stall*

The tie stall requires a few inches longer and wider than the stanchion stall. It is designed to provide greater comfort to the cow. In addition to larger size, the chain tie gives the cow more freedom. Instead of the stanchion, there are two arches, one on each side of the neck of the cow. The cow is fastened by means of rings fitted loosely on the arch pipes and connected to a chain which snaps to the neck strap on the cow. The correct space between arches is 10–12 inches. This prevents the cow from moving too far forward in the stall.

It is important that in this type of stall, the arches and all other stall parts are kept lower than the height of the cows.

The cow has more freedom in the tie stall than in the stanchion. Large cows and those

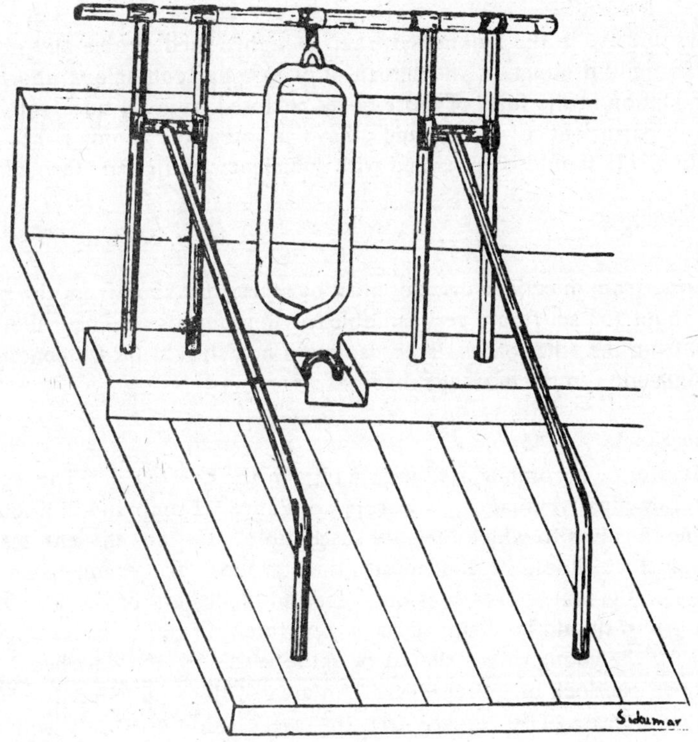

Fig. 13.4. A stanchion for Cattle.

with large udders get along better in them because of freedom they enjoy. It is not desirable to have a tie chain in a small stall.

Manger. Cement concrete continuous manger with removable partitions is the best from the point of view of durability and cleanliness. A height of 1′-4″ for a high front manger and 6″ to 9″ for a low front manger is considered sufficient. Low front mangers are more comfortable for cattle but high front mangers prevent feed wastage. The height at the back of the manger should be kept at 2′-6″ to 3′. An overall width of 2′ to 2½′ is sufficient for a good manger.

Alleys. The central walk should have a width of 5′-6′ exclusive of gutters when cows face out, and 4′-5′ when they face in. The feed alleys in case of a face out system should be 4′ wide, and the central walk should show a slope of 1″ from the centre towards the two gutters running parallel to each other, thus forming a crown at the centre.

Manure gutter. The manure gutter should be wide enough to hold all dung without getting blocked, and be easy to clean. Suitable dimensions are 2′ width with a cross-fall of 1″ away from standing. The gutter should have a gradient of 1″ for every 10′ length. This will premit a free flow of liquid,excreta.

Doors. The doors of a single range cowshed should be 5′ wide with a height of 7′, and for double row shed the width should not be less than 8′ to 9′. All doors of the barn should lie flat against the external wall when fully open.

Calving Boxes

Allowing cows to calve in the milking cowshed is highly undesirable and objectionable. It leads to insanitary milk production and spread of disease like contagious abortion in the herd. Special accommodation in the form of loose-boxes enclosed from all sides with a door should be furnished to all parturient cows. It should have an area of about 100 to 150 sq. ft. with ample soft bedding. It should be provided with sufficient ventilation through windows and ridge vent.

Isolation Boxes

Animals suffering from infectious diseases must be segregated soon from the rest of the herd. Loose boxes of about 150 sq. ft. are very suitable for this purpose. They should be situated at some distance from the other barns. Every isolation box should be self contained and should have separate connection to the drainage disposal system.

Sheds for Young Stocks

Calves should never be accommodated with adults in the cow shed. The calf house must have provision for daylight ventilation and proper drainage. Damp and ill-drained floors cause respiratory trouble in calves to which they are susceptible. For an efficient management and housing, the young stock should be divided into three groups, viz., young calves aged up to one year, bull calves, i.e., the male calves over one year and the heifers or the female calves above one year. Each group should be sheltered in a separate calfhouse or calfshed. As far as possible the shed for the young calves should be quite close to the cowshed. Each calfshed should have an open paddock or exercise yard. An area of 100 square feet per head for a stock of 10 calves and an increase of 50 square feet for every additional calf will make a good *paddock*.

It is useful to classify the calves below one year into three age groups, viz., calves below the age of 3 months, 3-6 months old calves and those over 6 months for a better allocation of the resting area. An overall covered space of:

(a) 20-25 square feet per calf below the age of 3 months,
(b) 25-30 square feet per calf from the age of 3-6 months,
(c) 30-40 square feet per calf from the age of 6-12 months and over, and
(d) 40-50 square feet for every calf above one year, should be made available for sheltering such calves. An air space of 400 to 500 cubic feet per calf is a good provision under our climatic conditions. A suitable interior lay-out of a calf shed will be to arrange the standing space along each side of a 4-feet wide central passage having a shallow gutter along its length on both sides. Provision of water troughs inside each calf shed and exercise yard should never be neglected.

Bull or Bullock Shed

Safety and ease in handling a comfortable shed for protection from weather and a provision for exercise are the key points while planning accommodation for bulls or bullocks. A bull should never be kept in confinement particularly on hard floors. Such a confinement without adequate exercise leads to overgrowth of the hoofs creating difficulty in mounting and loss in the breeding power of the bull.

A loose box with rough cement concrete floor about 15′ by 10′ in dimensions having an adequate arrangement of light and ventilation and an entrance 4′ in width and7′ in height will make a comfortable housing for a bull. The shed should have a manger and a water trough. If possible, the arrangement should be such that water and feed can be served without actually entering the bull house. The bull should have a free access to an exercise yard provided with a strong fence or a boundary wall of about 2′ in height, i.e., too high for the bull to jump over. From the bull yard, the bull should be able to view the other animals of the herd so that it does not feel isolated. The exercise yard should also communicate with a service crate *via* a swing gate which saves the use of an attendant to bring the bull to the service crate.

IDENTIFICATION OF FARM ANIMALS

The identity of an animal has to be established soon after its birth. Many dairymen name their cows but do not have any marks for their identification except as they know them. For a small herd the naming of animals may serve the purpose to some extent, but for large farms and moreover with pure breed animals, it is always necessary to put some sort of identification marks on each animal.

Cattle can be marked by ear-tag, tattoo, number tags attached around the neck or horn chain, branding numbers on horns or hips, ear notches, photograph or by colour sketches.

Ear-tagging. Ear-tags are metal pieces with number or letters engraved on them. There are two types of ear-tags, self-piercing tags and tags that require a hole in the ear made with a ear punch. Generally the tags are inserted within one-third of the way out from the base of the ear, generally on the upper edge of the ear with the number on top.

Tattooing of cattle. Tattooing the ears is another method of marking cattle belonging to light coloured ears. The method is to punch several small holes with a die (meant for this purpose) in the form of numbers or letters through the skin on the inside of the ear and then

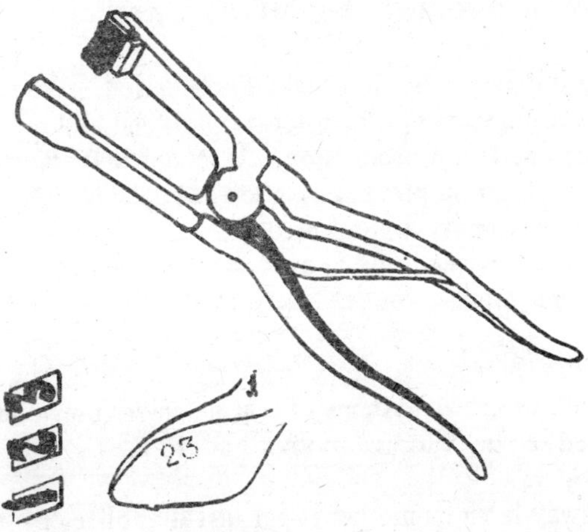

Fig. 13.5. A tool for Tattooing.

fill them with tattoo ink. If done correctly, this is a permanent mark. The usual practice is to start the marking with '001' and continue the same up to '999'. Its disadvantage is that animals must be caught and the inside of the ear cleaned to be able to read the indentifying marks.

Number Tags. Some cattle owners prefer metal tags, large enough to be read at a distance in place of tattooing or ear tagging their cattle. The metal tags are fastened to neck chains. The objection of this method is that, their is a chance that they may be lost.

Branding. The most common method of marking and identifying dairy cattle is by branding. Branding should be done at an early age of the animal, preferably before the calf is weaned. A heated number of symbol is gently pressed on the body of the animal. It causes partial burning of the tissue and produces a permanent scar of the identical shape.

Branding is also done by a cold stamping iron. In this type of branding, a branding liquid is used and the stamp is dipped in that liquid and then applied in the same way as with hot iron. In this type of branding the wound takes considerable time to heal.

The greatest disadvantage of this method is that a permanent damage is caused to the skin of the branded animal which reduces the values of its hide. The best place for branding is the lower part of the thigh which comes at the marginal end of the hide and is of lesser value.

Ear Notching. Notches cut in the ears make a rather easy method to identify animals. A notch represents a number depending on its location, whether in the top, bottom or end of ear, and also, which ear it is in. Few dairymen are not willing to disfigure the ears of their cattle in this way and they adopt some other methods. The method is common in swine and sheep.

Putting Identification Marks on Poultry and Sheep

Poultry birds are generally marked with light aluminium wing tags carrying either individual or group numbers. It is generally done after the first day of hatching and a separate coloured or numbered leg band may be used when the birds are mature.

In case of sheep, tattooes and ear-tags are used for marking. Flock marks may also be put by a special mark on wool by means of marking fluid.

RAISING THE DAIRY CALF

The future of any herd depends on how calves are raised. Whatever a calf may be, the outcome of a scientific breeding system, if it is not properly fed and managed, it will not attain the large size necessary for maximum production. It is said that "good animals are raised, not purchased". Nobody can go on purchasing good animals of high pedigree endlessly. One has to raise one's own calves to make a good herd.

Due to the high mortality of calves in India because of mismanagement, calf rearing should be taken up on scientific lines and economically achieved.

System of Calf Rearing

There are mainly the following two systems of rearing calves prevailing in this country.

1. The calf is allowed to stay with its mother and to suckle only a little before and after the cows are milked.

2. The calf is taken away from its mother either just after birth or after 2 or 3 days of birth. Some calf raisers prefer to allow the calf to be with its mother till the colostrum period. After that, feeding and management of the calf will be entirely in the hands of the dairyman. This is called the "*Weaning system*".

Advantages of Weaning

(1) If the calf accidently dies, there is no difficulty in regular milking of the cow.

(2) With calves suckling the dams under ordinary conditions of stall feeding, there is no way of controlling the right amount of milk to be taken by the calf. By following a weaning system the calves can be fed economically and just as much as may be necessary for them.

(3) In this way the calf can be saved from some diseases like diarrhoea, scours etc., which are results of uncontrolled feeding.

(4) The actual yield of milk of the cow—the essential item of dairy farming—can be entered in the milk record.

(5) Total yield increases—If the owner wants milk in quantity he must practise "weaning system".

(6) The calf can be culled out at any early age.

(7) Milking without a calf is more hygienic and sanitary.

Because of the multifarious advantage, the weaning system is getting more popular in India. A number of military dairy farms, government and improved private dairy farms have already adopted this method.

Raising calves on scientific lines is discussed below.

1. Feeding and Management of the Calf before Birth

The raising of a dairy calf begins even before it is born. Cows which are not fed properly will give birth to under-nourished calves. Since the unborn calf makes most of its growth during the last 3 or 5 months before birth, special care must be taken to feed the cows liberally at that time. The additional food will not only enter in the growth tissues of the calf but will also help the mother to stand the strain of parturition normally. She should have free access to grazing fields. If she is in a low condition, she should get 2-3 kg. of grain in addition to grazing for maintenance, and one kg of grain for each 2½ kg of milk in addition to all the good quality roughages she eats. Every effort must be made to keep a cow from being constipated as this increases the possibility of dystokia (difficult in parturition).

2. Care of the Calf after Birth

(A) Treatment of the calf. It varies with the system of rearing. If the calf is removed from its mother after 3 days, one should allow the cow to lick her calf just after calving so as to make it dry and for calf's comfortable breathing. In case of weaning just after calving, one should clean all the slimy mucus by rubbing with a clean and soft towel or smooth dry paddy straw just as an imitation of the way the cow licks. The sooner the calf is dry the less chance there is of its being chilled specially in winter months.

(B) Treatment of the navel cord. By means of sterilised scissors, the navel cord is detached to ½″ from the body. Generally, a 30 per cent solution of tincture iodine is painted on the exposed part of the navel cord for disinfection.

3. Feeding Calves

Feeding colostrum. It will vary with the system followed, but whatever system may be practised, the calf must receive the first milk which the cow gives after calving and is called colostrum. Be sure to feed the calf enough of colostrum between 2 to 2.5 litres daily for the first 3 days following its birth. Any excess colostrum may be fed to other calves in the herd in amounts equal to the amount of whole milk normally fed. If possible where a cow is milked before calving, freeze some of the colostrum for later feeding to the calf. None of it should be wasted. The digestibility of colostrum increases when it is given at a temperature between 99°F and 102°F. The importance of colostrum can be felt more from the following virtues.

(a) The protein of colostrum consists of a much higher proportion of globulin than does normal milk. The globulins are presumed to be the source of antibodies which aid in protecting the animal from many infections liable to affect it after birth.
Gamma-globulin level in blood serum of neonatal calves is only 0.97 mg/ml at birth. It increases to 16.55 mg/ml level after first colostrum feeding at 12 hr and subsequently on the second day shows a peak of 28.18 mg/ml. This level more or less persists till the reticuloendothelial system of the calf starts functioning to produce antibodies.

(b) The protein content of colostrum is 3 to 5 times as that of normal milk. It is also rich in some of the materials, of which copper. iron, magnesium and manganese are important.

(c) Colostrum contains 5–15 times the amount of vitamin-A found in normal milk, depending upon the character of the ration given to the mother during the rest period.

(d) Colostrum is also superior to milk in having a considerably greater amount of several other vitamins which have been found essential in the growth of dairy calves, including riboflavin, choline, thiamine and pantothenic acid.

(e) Colostrum acts as a laxative to free the digestive tract of faecal material.

Teaching the calf to drink. When the calf is allowed to stay with its mother, its natural instinct automatically leads the calf nearer the udder of its mother within half-an-hour to one hour of its birth. However, calves who are weak may need a little assistance to search out the teats.

In case of weaning system, teaching the calf to drink becomes necessary. This is an operation that requires considerable patience, as some calves are slow in learning to take milk from a pail. One should pour about a quart of the mother cow's milk into a clean pail used for feeding calves and bring the nose of the calf in contact with milk. This is best accomplished by allowing the calf to suck the finger of the feeder so that its head may be guided into the pail and then the hand of the feeder can be gradually lowered into the bucket and submerged in the milk sufficiently deep to allow a little milk to be taken by the calf. By continuous feeding it will learn to drink.

In some farms it is thought preferable to feed the young calf during the first 3 or 4 weeks of life from a nipple pail, that is, a pail equipped with a rubber nipple which the calf sucks. The nipple pail has the advantage in that the calf takes the milk more slowly, and is thus less likely to have digestive upsets.

When nipple pails are used, one should rinse them thoroughly after each feeding.

Feeding whole milk. In feeding whole milk, calves may be fed as per feeding schedule. While feeding whole milk the following points should be remembered.

(a) As far as possible provide milk from the calf's mother.

(b) Feed milk immediately after it is drawn.

(c) At other times, warm milk to body temperature.

(d) The total amount of milk may be fed at 3 or 4 equal intervals up to the age of 7 days and then twice daily.

Feeding skim milk. On many farms, large quantities of separated milk are available for feeding to calves and other livestock. Excellent dairy calves can be raised by changing them from whole milk gradually after two weeks of their age. Here again the feeding schedule should be followed.

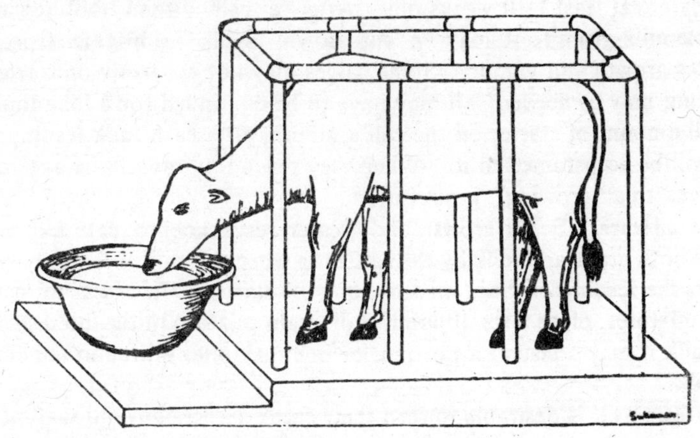

Fig.13.6. Drinking milk from pail.

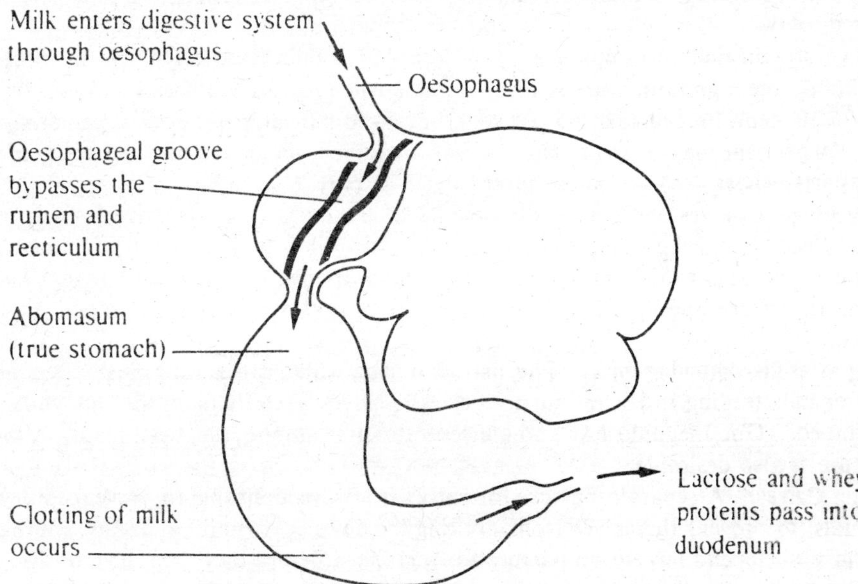
Milk enters digestive system through oesophagus
Oesophagus
Oesophageal groove bypasses the rumen and recticulum
Abomasum (true stomach)
Lactose and whey proteins pass into duodenum
Clotting of milk occurs

Fig.13.7. Diagrammatic representation of the digestive system of the very young calf.

Feeding dried skim milk, whey or buttermilk. In case these products are avilable at a reasonable rate, they can be fed to calves. The above dried products are mixed with water at the rate of 1 kg to 9 kg of water and then it is fed as skim milk. To avoid digestive troubles the mix should always be fed to calves after warming it upto 100°F.

Feeding calf starters. The expense and labour involved in raising calves when either liquid whole milk of skim milk is used have caused many dairy farmers to turn the calf to "Calf starter" method. Calf starter is a mixture consisting of ground farm grains, protein feeds and minerals, vitamins and antibiotics. One continues to feed whole milk to calves receiving starter until they are at least 1-10 weeks old. After a calf attains the age of 2 weeks the amount of whole milk given to it may be cut down. Milk feeding is especially helpful in promoting better growth and vigour. Some calves may not eat freely on starter and in such cases milk feeding may be needed. It may have to be continued for a long time. One should then rub a small amount of starter on the calf's mouth, after each milk feeding for a few days when the calf will be accustomed to it. When they reach four months of age, one should then transfer the calves to a "growing" grain ration.

Feeding grain mixture. Better growth and greater resistance to calf ailments result from consumption of both grain and milk by the calf than when the calf is fed only on milk. At the age of 7–15 days the feeding of grain mixtures may be started. In order to get calves accustomed to grain mixtures, place a small handful of grain mixture in the used pail. As the calf is finishing its milk it may consume a portion, or one may offer a little in the hand immediately after feeding milk.

For educated farmers it is desirable to feed their cattle as per conventional method, i.e., based on the requirement to DCP and TDN which are backed by scientific experiments. A table of requirements of calf growing @ 0.5 kg. per day during first two years and reaching adult body weight at the age of approximately 3 years is already given. Average thumb rule requirement is discussed below.

Excessive protein rich grain mixture is not desirable as milk is already rich in proteins. A medium high protein grain mixture is most suitable when milk is fed freely. A grain mixture of oats—35 per cent, linseed cake—5 per cent, bran—30 per cent, barley—10 per cent, groundnut cake—20 per cent may be fed to the calves. Another good mixture consists of ground maize—2 parts, wheat bran—2 parts, linseed meal—1 part.

Feeding silage. Calves at their ages between 3 to 6 months may be given small amounts of silage. Feed 1 to 2 kg daily to calves aged up to 3 to 4 months and then increase these amounts by about 500 gm. per day for each month of the calf's age. Use every precaution to ensure the quality of the silage fed. Mouldy or damaged silage may lead to indigestion.

Feeding after discontinuing milk. The period during which calves are most often neglected is soon after milk feeding is discontinued. Feed the calves liberally from the time milk feeding is discontinued. Good legume hay and concentrates are among the best feeds, although a good pasture is also desirable.

Pasturing Calves. A separate pasture for calves is always desirable to prevent injury by the older animals, to prevent the calves from exciting the cows by running about among them. If calves have to depend largely on pasture for their feed before they are 12 months of age, they will not grow normally, as they are unable to obtain adequate feed from pasture alone.

Allow the calves' access to a constant supply of fresh water and common salt. If the pasture consists of non-legume grass growing on an acid soil, it is better to give the calves some mineral supplement, such as steamed bone meal of feeding grade.

Providing minerals. Milk is one of the best sources of calcium and phosphorus, and as a rule, calves suffer no deficiencies in these mineral during the milk feeding period. High quality legumes are excellent sources of calcium, grain mixtures are, on the other hand, good for phosphorus. Unless these feeds are freely consumed after the milk feeding period is passed, one should supply a mineral mixture or starter at the rate of 2 per cent. If calves are located in a region where goitre (big neck) in calves has been found, use iodised salt instead of ordinary salt.

Supplying antibiotics. Recent experiments indicate that aureomycin and terramycin will increase the growth rate of dairy heifers without any apparent effect upon reproduction or milk production. Aureomycin fed in the milk at the rate of 80 miligrams of auremycin hydrochloride per calf per day from 4 to 116 days of age produced the following results:

1. Increased the gain in growth from 10 to 30 per cent.
2. Improved the appetite.
3. Decreased the number of cases of calf scours.
4. Produced smoother hair coats.

4. Housing the Calf

The object of housing is to provide shelter to the calves against sun, rain and other inclemencies of weather.

In rearing of young calves, it is desirable that an open exercise paddock directly communicating with their shelter and feeding house should be provided. The exercise yard should not be of a lesser area than 3 square yards for each calf and the calf shelters should provide 10 square feet of floor area for each animal. Calf pens should be located close to the cow sheds, and clean drinking water should always be accessible to them. If possible, calves of different ages, viz., under three months, three to six months and over six months till they are weaned, should be housed separately for better management and care. Details about construction measurements are discussed under housing.

5. Dehorning the Calf

This is a process by which the horns of an animal are removed after birth by treating the tender horn roots with a chemical, mechanical or electrical dehorner. Dehorning of yearlings and older animals is painful and results in considerable bleeding. The practice is, therefore, to dehorn the calf before it is 10 days old. Up to this age the horn button does not become attached to the skull.

Advantages of dehorning:

(a) Dehorned animal will need less space in the sheds.
(b) Horned animals are a danger to the operator.
(c) Cattle with horns inflict bruises on each other that may result in heavy economic losses.
(d) Dehorned animals can be handled more easily.

Disadvantages of dehorning:

(a) Animals with a nice horn have a style. This sometimes is an advantage in exhibition and cattle shows.

(b) Some breeds have got an important identification marks for horn e.g., Kankrej, Kangayam, etc.

(c) Animals with horn can defend themselves.

Methods of Dehorning

(A) **Chemical**. The chemicals commonly used are caustic soda. They come in a white stick about the size of a blackboard chalk or in a commercially prepared dehorning paste. The procedure to dehorn a calf by caustic potash is as follows:

(i) Clip the hair around the base of the horn button in order to expose the base of it for application of the dehorning preparation. Apply a ring of petroleum jelly near the base of the horn button.

(ii) In using a caustic potash stick, hold it carefully by the help of a caustic potash holder and then rub it over the button several times using a circular motion, until the skin at the baes of the button begins to soften and the button bleeds slightly.

(iii) Treat the second button similarly. Check the first button treated to see if it and its base have been well covered. The skin at the base will crack easily if enough caustic has been applied.

(iv) Confine the caustic to the very base of the button. Any excess caustic may run, removing the hair from the skin and injuring the eyes as well.

(B) **Mechanical**. (i) *Clippers and Saws:* When older cattle are to be dehorned, especially designed clippers or saws are used. A considerable amount of bleeding may follow operation. To prevent bleeding, the main horn artery should be tied off with a cotton or silk thread. This may be done by sliding a sewing needle under the artery to pull thread in place before tying. It is necessary when sawing or clipping the horns, to take about one-half inch of skin in order to get at the horn roots.

(ii) *Rubber Bands:* Some farmers have reported successful dehorning of older cattle by using the rubber band method. The chief advantage is that no open wound results such as happens when clippers or saws are used to dehorn. The dehorning is accomplished by first making a groove around the base of the horn in about the same place it would be cut with a saw or clipper, and then using the elastrator to slip a rubber band over the horn and into the groove. The rubber band shuts off the circulation and the horn gradually comes off.

(C) **Electrical**. Electrical dehorners are seldom used in India. The rod is heated with electricity and has an automatic control that maintains temperature at about 1,000°F. Applying the electric dehorner to the horn button for 10 seconds is sufficient to destroy the horn cells.

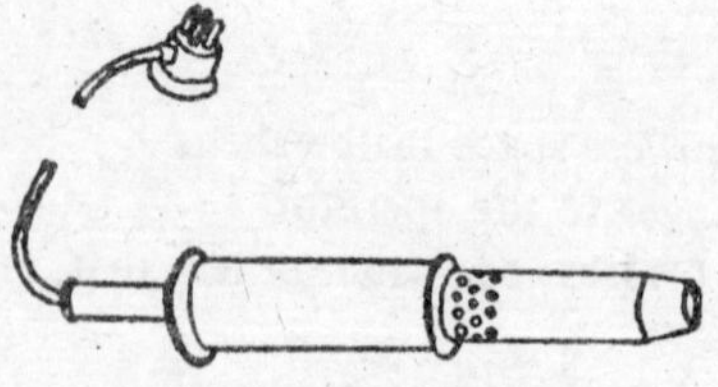

Fig. 13.8. An electric Dehorner.

6. Marking the Calf

Marking of calves for identification is an important managerial operation. For registration of pure breeds, calves must be identified. The different methods of marking an animal has been discussed previously.

7. Removing Extra Teats

Extra teats beyond the normal four are unsightly and should be removed when the calf is between one and two months' old. The best method for removing an extra teat is to disinfect the area around the teat and clip it off with a pair of sterilised scissors. Usually there is no bleeding, if at all bleeding is considerable, holding a cotton pack over the wound for a few minutes will stop it.

8. Castrating the Bull Calf

Castration is the unsexing of the male or female and consists in the removal of both testicles or ovaries respectively. It is probably the most common and oldest of all surgical operations. Its objects are to prevent reproduction, to increase faster gains, to produce a more desirable type of meat and to make the animal docile and easier to handle.

Calves, lambs and pigs should be castrated while they are young; the best time is between 8–10 weeks for calves, about 2 weeks for lambs and about 1 week for pigs.

There are three methods of castrating a bull calf which are as follows:

1. By making an operation in the scrotum where the vas deferens are disconnected from the scrotum. Thus the spermatozoa will not be able to flow out of the penis.
2. Castration with the help of a Burdizzo's castrator. The method is also known as

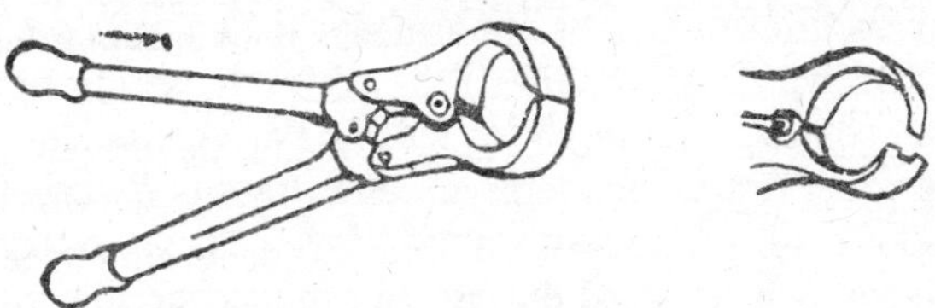

Fig.13.9. Burdizzo's Castrator.

   "bloodless castration". The castrator crushes each cord separately an inch or two above the testicles. While performing castration by this method, the following precautions should be taken:
   (a) The cord does not slip away at the time of operation.
   (b) Castrator should not press on any folds of the skin.
   (c) The Burdizzo is not placed too low to crush the testicles.
3. Recently a new method has been developed in western countries where they use a strong and tight rubber ring around the cord at the very early age of the calf. This creates a constant pressure. When the testicles have been absorbed, the ring drops down.

9. Preventing and Controlling Diseases in Calves

One of the most difficult problems in raising dairy calves is that of preventing and controlling diseases. In recent years, much has been learned about disease control, and now many of the causes of previous losses can be controlled. Diseases like white scours, common scours, pneumonia, ringworm and different internal parasitic attack are most prevalent in calves.

Adequate precautions must be taken to prevent all such types of diseases. Details of health control measures are discussed under "Other essentials in dairy cattle management" of this chapter.

MANAGEMENT OF CROSS-BRED COWS

The foreign breeds used for cross-breeding purposes in India are Holstein Fresian, Brown Swiss, Red Dane and Jersey. Among these, Holstein is the highest milk yielder (over 6,000 litre per lactation) although the fat percentage of its milk is somewhat low (3.5 per cent). Jersey is the breed of small sized animals, with relatively high fat content in its milk (4.5–5.0 per cent) and can suit the hill areas. The milk production potentiality of Jersey is estimated at 4,000 litre per lactation. The other two foreign breeds, i.e., Brown Swiss and Red Dane are in between Holstein Fresian and Jersey regarding their milk production and fat content.

At present it is advisable to maintain 50 per cent exotic blood in the cross-bred animals in plains of India whereas 62.5 per cent in the hilly areas. This level may be achieved by using inter-mating or forward crossing of F_2 generations respectively.

All over the country cross-breds are gaining popularity for their higher milk yields as compared to buffaloes and other cows. Although no unusual care is needed for this category of livestock but still there are certain fundamental points which should always be kept in mind while rearing a cross-bred cow.

Dairy cattle are homothermous (maintain constant body temperature) and therefore, when the environmental temperature rise or falls abnormally, the animals are in stress. In general, for cross-breds (such as Brown Swiss × Sahiwal) the critical temperature leading to a decline in milk yield at higher level comes at about 90° to 95°F. For comparison, this critical temperature is 70°-80°F for Holstein Fresian and Jerseys. For Brown Swiss it is between 85°-90F. The comfort zone for all cross-breds is between 65°-75°F. These findings show that milk yield of cross-bred cows is likely to be affected during the summer months of April to August. In case of male, extremely high temperatures, coupled with high humidity lead to degeneration of testicular epithelium, thereby causing inferior quality of semen production. This situation may be partly avoided by providing ample shady trees during summer months. It has also been observed that exposure of cross-breds to high environmental temperature in summer reduces the feed intake.

Second point of importance in the management of cross-bred animals is disease control. In general, cross-breds are having less disease resisting character in comparison to any Indian pure breeds. It has been observed that cross-bred animals are prone to foot and mouth disease. To check the spread of this disease, breeders are advised to get their cross-bred stock vaccinated against foot and mouth and all other contagious fatal diseases. Mastitis is the next important disease which may very often be found in cross-bred animals. An occasional check up for mastitis is a must for cross-bred owners.

Cross-bred animals are also very much suceptible to all kinds of parasitic infections. As such, rigorous preventive measures should be taken right from the early age. Deworming with piperazine compounds should be practiced once during 1-2 months followed by 3-4 months and

5-6 months. For adult cattle follow direction of the veterinarians. Remember, calf mortality in cross-bred is high due to parasitic infection in comparison to Indian pure breeds.

The next important consideration is about the nutritional aspect of cross-breds. By virtue of being high yielders, their nutritional requirements have to be higher. It has been calculated that the energy need for such high yielders can never be met with only succulent fodders, supplementation of concentrate mixture (having high energy content) is a must. As a thumb rule, for the sake of economy, feed the cross-breds 1/10th of its body weight of green fodders along with concentrate mixture as discussed in the nutrition chapter of this book.

For better physiological efficiency of work production in cross-bred bullocks, it is observed that during the cooler months of the year and also during the early morning and evening parts of the summer months ploughing or any other types of hard work was almost the same in both Indian and cross-bred bullocks. Care must be taken to prevent cross-bred bullocks from doing any hard work during the hottest part (noon and aftenoon) of the summer months. The following observations may be noted in support of this statement.

Research was carried out at the National Dairy Research Institute to determine the physiological efficiency of work production in cross-bred bullocks. The cross-bred bullocks were compared with pure-bred Hariana bullocks with regard to pulse rate, respiration rate, and capacity to cart and plough during different seasons of the year. The data are recorded in Table 13.3.

The time taken for ploughing a given area was almost the same in both the breeds of bullocks during cooler months of the year. Even though cross-bred bullocks showed rise in pulse rate and respiration, they did not show distress symptoms even after continuous work without any break for 4 hours.

Table 13.3

Breed	*Season*	*Pulse/mt. (4 hr. continuous work)*			*Respiration rate per mt. (4 hr. continuous work)*			*Area ploughed in 6 hr. (m^2)*
		Initial	*Final*	*Difference*	*Initial*	*Final*	*Difference*	
Cross-bred	(Winter)	63	79	16	24	35	11	2,970
Hariana		49	60	11	23	35	12	3,320
Cross-bred	(Summer)	60	78	18	34	60	26	2,860
Hariana		51	70	19	25	42	17	3,070
Cross-bred	(Hot-humid)	59	78	19	45	69	24	2,440
Hariana		51	66	15	35	52	17	2,903

KEEPING RECORDS IN THE DAIRY FARM

It is impossible to run any kind of business profitably without proper records. A dairyman who does not have a fairly accurate record of the amount of feed given to the cows in his herd, and of the amount of milk and butterfat which they produce is certainly not conducting his business efficiently. Unless accurate records are kept, the best cow in a herd is likely to have equal rank with the poorest, at least in the mind of the owner.

Preservation of Permanent Records

There are three general methods of preserving records, individual conditions will determine which one is best suited to each case. Records may be kept in any of the following ways:

1. In books with permanent leave
2. In loose leaf books or files
3. Envelopes

There are advantages in using books with permanent leaves for some records, whereas the loose leaf books or files and envelopes are better for others. For breeding records, the permanent leaf book has the advantages of being safer, as the separate pages cannot get loose. However, it is cumbersome, as old records which must be handled frequently are exposed to the danger of being lost if the whole book is lost. The loose leaf records, however may be divided and only those records that are in use at a particular need be kept at hand while other old leaf records may be put away for safe keeping. The loose leaf records also have the advantage that all the data relating to an individual animal may be kept together so that when it is desired to get any information upon a certain cow, all such information will be together in one book.

Kinds of Records

Several kinds of records may be kept in a dairy farm. Some of them are more important to the breeder of pure bred grade animals. Records of production should be kept by all dairymen. The important records which should be kept are discussed below:

Milk Record Register

1. Economic feeding. Milk record is a guide to correct feeding. It enables feeding to be regulated according to the quantity of milk produced by the cows. The yields of heavy milker may be pushed up by generous feeding and feed given to the low producers reduced to the extent necessary. Feeds account for over 60% of the total cost of producing milk. Correct feeding avoids wasteful expenditures and increases the profits of a dairyman.

2. Realising proper prices. The performance of the cows and their immediate parents are taken into consideration by purchasers, and people are willing to pay more for animals whose performances are known. When the cows without any milk records are purchased, their capacity for production has to be judged by external characters at the purchaser's risk.

3. Keeping in touch with cows. Milk and feed records keep the dairyman in touch with the individual animals. Fall in milk yield of any individual cow is noted and thereby the owner can readily note the early stages of any ill-health or improper management of the animals concerned.

4. Registration in the central herd book. Persons interested in registering their cattle under the Central Herd Book can fulfil their wishes only when they have got such milk records.

5. Pedigree can be maintained. Pedigree is an important register for dairy cattle. To complete this register it is a compulsory task to enter individual milk yield regularly.

6. Selection of bulls. Milk recording enables breeders to select suitable bulls, whose dams are known to be good milkers. By the help of this record, progeny testing of the bull is done.

Cattle Feed Register

To know how much profit a cow is making, it is necessary to find out not only the production of cow but also the amount of feed that she has consumed. It is also necessary, especially

Service Register of Cows

Name of the dairy farm ....

Address ....

Breed ....

Serial No.	No. of cows	Date of last calving	Date of service	Time of service	No. of bull	Expected date to calve	Date to be dried off	Date of calving	Weight of the calf	Sex of the calf	Time taken for the expulsion of placenta	Remarks

Officer-in-charge

Feed Indent Sheet

To

The Store Keeper. ....

Please issue the following rations for...

....

Particulars of animals | Rate of feeding

Serial No.	Ingredients	For animals in milk and young calves		For dry stock and adult calves		Total
		Percentage	Quantity	Percentage	Quantity	
1.	Groundnut Cake					
2.	Rice Bran					
3.	Arahar Chuni					
4.	Gram ..					
5.	Wheat Bran ..					
6.	Pea ..					
	Total ..					
7.	Mineral Mixture..					
8.	Salt ..					

For special animals

Signature of Receiving Officer

Signature and designation of Indenting Officer

Calf Register

Name of the farm...

Address..For the month of..............19.....

Serial No.	Date of numbering	Ear No.	Sex of the calf	Sire	Dam	Disposal		Remarks
						How the calf was disposed	Date	

Officer-in-charge.

Feed Register

Name of the farm..Address..............................
For the month of...19.....

Number of Cows	Date / Grain Ration No....		Hay		Silage		Other feed	
	A.M.	P.M.	A.M.	P.M.	A.M.	P.M.	A.M.	P.M.

Officer-in-charge

Milk Record Sheet

Name of the farm..Address..............................
For the month of...19.....
Owner of the herd..........................Post Office.......................District.................

Date	Time	Name and number of cows	Name and number of cows	Name and number of cows	Name and number of cows	Name and number of cows
1	A.M.					
	P.M.					
2	A.M.					
	P.M.					
3	A.M.					
	P.M.					
19	A.M.					
	P.M.					
30	A.M.					
	P.M.					
31	A.M.					
	P.M.					

Officer-in-charge

Health Record of the Individual Cow

Name of the farm.......................................Address...

Sex.........................Age...............No............Herd No...........Breed...............

Tuberculosis Tests		General Health				
Date	Results					

Brucellosis Tests						
Date	Results					

Officer-in-charge.

Lactation Record

Name of the farm.................. Address........................

For the Year........................

Animal's particular number	Months of the year										Yield in lit. during lactation period	Average fat %	No. in days in a lactation	Date and days dry off	Re-marks
	Jan.	Feb.	Mar.	April	May	...	...	Oct.	Nov.	Dec.					

Officer-in-charge.

Stock Register of Cattle

Name of the farm........................ Address..................

For the Year.........................

Serial no. and name of the animal	Tattoo No.	When purchased	Date of birth	Value	Approximate age when purchased	Pedigree		How disposed off	Page of Herd Register	Remarks
						Dam	Sire			

Officer-in-charge.

in large herds, to have some form on which to put down the amount of feed that each cow should receive. It is almost impossible for any individual to remember the amount of feed that should be given to each individual cow. Usually such a record should be changed after every week or fortnight. This should be filled out according to the production of the individual cow and should be fastened near the feed bin. The amount of grain mentioned on the sheet should be carefully weighed at each feeding. The roughages need not be weighed at each feeding but should be weighed at least once a month so that some idea of the amount given is known.

In large farms, it is an usual practice to number different grain mixtures that has been fed to the herd.

Calf feeding requires a somewhat different form since calves are fed whole milk, skim milk, grain and hay. These can easily be made to conform to the conditions.

Breeding Record

The servicings are recorded in two ways—bull wise and cow wise. In the former, all cows mated to a particular bull are recorded while in the latter all bulls that have serviced any particular cow are noted down. The combination of both is essential as it gives a cross check.

Cattle History and Pedigree Sheet Register

Cattle history deals only about the life of a particular animal, viz., the name, brand number, performances, diseases suffered and the cause of disposal, or the reason of death. Cattle pedigree sheet deals only about the history of ancestors of a particular animal.

Health Record

It is desirable to have a record of the health of the cows in a herd. This includes a place for the tuberculosis test, abortion test, and the general health, etc. Sometimes by a study of the health record of an animal, the reason for an unexpected result may be found.

Calf Register

When a calf is born, it is entered in this register. The register contains the calf's tatoo or notch number, its date of birth and sex, the weight at birth, etc. The calf register also furnishes the information whether a particular calf was reared or culled out.

Financial Record

Of all records maintained in a farm, the financial records such as cash book, stock book are the most valuable registers from the standpoint of profit and loss of any type of commercial dairy herd.

HANDLING THE BULL

Ringing

The ring is a safeguard in handling, and every bull should have one in his nose, even if he is regarded as gentle and easy to handle.

When the bull is between 8 months and a year old, a ring should be put in his nose. A copper ring 2 to 2½ inches in diameter is satisfactory at this time, but it should be replaced by a larger and stronger gun-metal ring when he reaches 2 years of age. Rings are likely to wear and develop sharp edges, which may cut through the septum. Such rings should be replaced.

It is well to place two rings in the nose of an especially unruly bull.

The ringing operation is not difficult and can be done with but little trouble if it is gone about in the right way. Tie the bull's head fast so that he cannot jerk. Grasp his nose firmly, with the fingers. (Pl. 56) (A). Push a trocar, with cannula (B) through the cartilage that separates the nostrils. Then pull the trocar, but leave the cannula (C). Put one end of the opened ring in the cannula (D), then withdraw the cannula, leaving the ring in the nose (E). Close the ring and replace the screw in it (F). File or sandpaper the joint until it is smooth. Do not tie the bull or lead him by the ring until the nose is healed and soreness gone, which will be from a week to 10 days.

Instead of a trocar and cannula, some breeders use a sharp pocket knife with good results. Some rings are provided with a sharp point which when opened can be used to pierce the cartilage in the nose. There are also special nose punches on the market.

Occasionally a bull pulls the ring out, tearing out the septum of his nose. This is usually caused by sudden jerking on a tight rope, being tied too short, or getting the ring caught on something. An accident of this kind is rather serious, as there is no entirely satisfactory way to remedy the condition. In some cases, the ring is placed higher up, or the cartilage is pierced the opposite way and the ring placed in a vertical position. If this is done, it is not advisible to tie the bull by the ring, as it may be torn out again. Smaller rings may be placed on either side of the torn place, with a larger ring through them. Then this may work all right in some cases, but is not always successful, as the three rings may give the animal considerable trouble in eating and may get caught on objects.

If the nose is torn out, the bull should be confined in a stall and the pen so arranged that it will not be necessary to handle him a great deal. If handling is necessary, it should be done only with a strong chain or leather halter which tightens across the nose when the lead rope is pulled. There are special halters in the market designed for cases of this kind.

Sometimes a veterinarian can make a surgical repair of the torn nose, joinining the torn ends again so that a ring can be worn.

Throwing or Casting

It may be necessary at times to throw and tie a bull for certain minor operations. This can be done with an inch rope preferably of cotton, which is softer and more pliable than hemp. The rope should be 40 to 50 feet long, depending on the size of the animal. One end is looped around the neck and tied with a rigid knot that will not slip. A half hitch is then

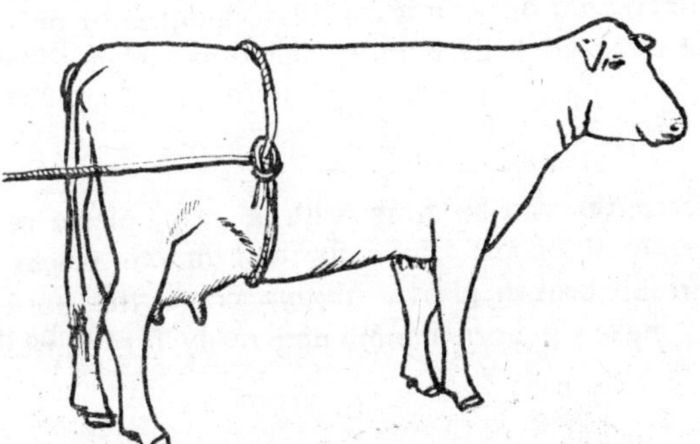

Fig. 13.10. The application of an udder kinch to control forward movement of the hind-limb of a Cow.

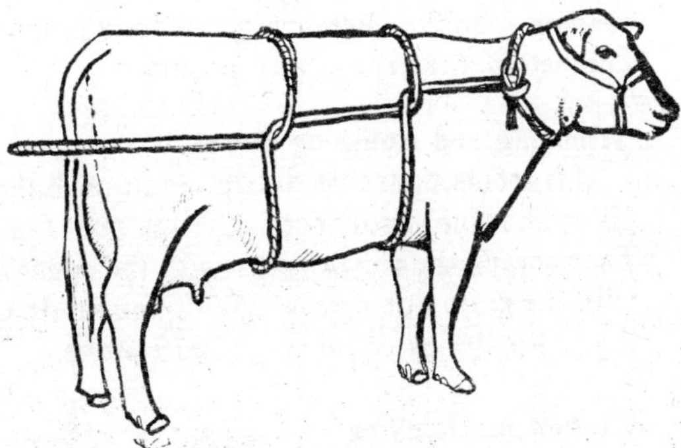

Fig. 13.11. Reuff's method of Casting.

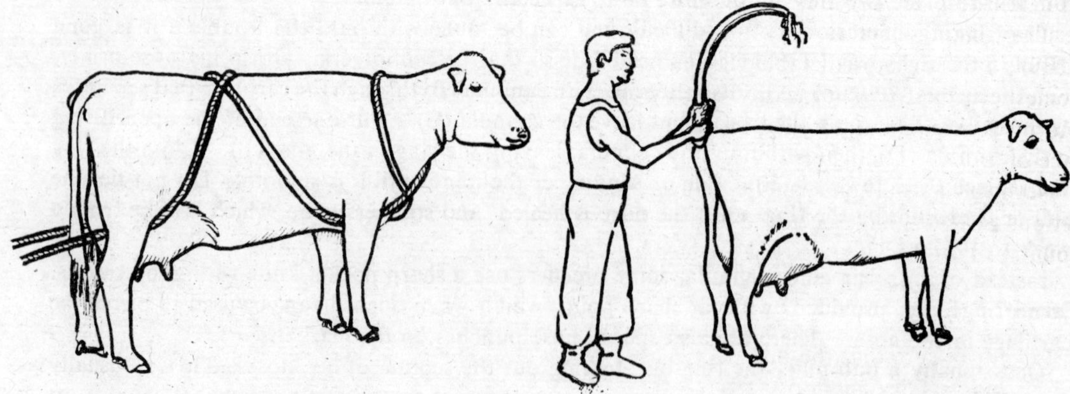

Fig.13.12. An alternative method of adjusting the rope for castrating Cattle.

Fig.13.13. Restraint of hind-limb movement in a stalled cow by uprooting tail.

taken around the chest and one also around the flank. The hitch must be well down on the side of the body. By pulling steadily on the free end of the rope, the animal falls to the ground, usually on the opposite side from the way the head is turned. The animal should always be casted (heavily pregnant animal should never be cast) on a large well strawed yard or grassed area. Have plenty of help at hand.

Trimming the feet

Bulls kept in close quarters with little exercise frequently develop longer hoofs. This condition is not only unsightly, but may become so painful that the bull cannot stand or walk squarely. Then, too. it brings on various other troubles, such as sore feet. The hoofs should be trimmed, or they will break off or disfigure the animal's feet. Hoofs of young animals often can be trimmed with a long handled chisel, pincers or hoof knife while the animal is standing on a hard dirt or plank floor. The sole and the cleft between the claws cannot be got at in this way, in that event it may be necessary to throw and tie the animal.

Care must be taken not to cut too far back or too deep as there is danger of cutting into the quick, which may result in lameness and foot infection. Considerable practice is required to become a proficient hoof trimmer. It is unlikely that one can learn all techniques by only reading a book. Better ways include practicing on small heifers under the supervision of a competent and experienced person,

Trimming and Polishing Horns

If it seems desirable to trim and polish the horns, this can be done with a rasp, pieces of glass, and fine sandpaper. Use the rasp first to smooth off the dead tissue and uneven places. Then scrape the rough spots with the edges of freshly broken glass. Always scrape the horn with the grain not across. With fine sandpaper, make the horn smooth and ready for polishing. Apply linseed oil and pumice stone.

Caution in Handling

Always handle a bull in a firm manner and never trust him. Many accidents have resulted from trusting the so-called gentle bull. It often happens that a man is injured or killed as a result of taking chances.

Bulls have an unpredictable viciousness of disposition probably unequalled by any of our domestic animals. They easily qualify as the most dangerous beast on the farm. Their enormous strength and killing instinct when aroused should never be discounted, even in the face of a docile life history.

Never take a bull on a public highway unless he can be kept under absolute control. Many serious accidents have occurred as a result of allowing so-called gentle bulls to graze along country roads or when driving them to and from pasture with cows on public highways.

Care of Breeding Bull

1. Make sure that the bull is typical of the breed and comes from parents with high index of production.

2. Do not use the bull for breeding purpose unless it attains proper maturity, i.e., 3 to 3½ years.

3. It should be free from communicable diseases.

4. Allow the bull to move about and have regular exercises, otherwise they are likely to put on fat and become slow at service.

(The trend of today is to avoid natural mating and to follow artifical insemination for better cross-breds).

DETERMINATION OF AGE OF CATTLE

The teeth serve animals as organs of prehension, mastication, and are used as weapons of offense and defence. According to their form and location in the mouth, the teeth are classified as *incisors*, *canines* and *molars* ("cheek teeth"). The incisors (central, laterals and corners) are situated in the front. The incisors are prehensive organs in all animals. They are absent from the upper jaw of the ruminating animals (cattle, sheep, goat etc). In lower jaw there are eight incisors, in the non-ruminants canines are behind the incisors and are typical of carnivorous and omnivorous animals and are used mainly for fighting purposes. In ruminants the upper jaw has no canines, and in the lower jaw they have moved forward, assuming the function and shape of the incisors. Cheek teeth (premolars and molars) are 24 in number, 6 on each side of each jaw (right upper, lower and left upper, lower). The anterior 3 of these 6 teeth are premolars and the posterior three are molar.

In most mammals and in all the domestic mammals—two set of teeth develop. The first set, consisting of fewer teeth than the second, appears early in life and is called the *deciduous* (D) or temporary or milk teeth. It is gradually replaced by the permanent dentition during the animals growth period. The deciduous dentition provides the young mammal with a fully functional, though smaller set of teeth that can be accomodated by its small jaws. As the jaws grow longer, new *permanent* (p) teeth are added and the deciduous teeth are gradually replaced by permanent teeth. Incisors (I), Canines (C) and Premolars (P), with the exception of the first premolar, are replaced. The molars (M), which erupt caudal to the premolars, are not present in the deciduous dentition. Replacement is gradual and follows a definite sequence, so that some deciduous and some permanent teeth are in use at the same time. As the developing permanent tooth pushes to the surface, it presses on the roots of the worn-out deciduous tooth and gradually cuts off its nutrition. The deciduous tooth becomes loose, eventually dies and is displaced.

The eruption and wearing out of the incisors of the cattle are related to their age and it is due to this fact that within certain limits it is possible to estimate the age of domesticated animals.

Teeth of the Cattle

The incisors are absent from the upper jaws of all ruminants including cattle, their place being taken up by the "dental pad". The incisors in the lower jaw are slightly movable in a direction.

The eight incisors are chisel-shaped and do not have flat tables and infundibulum. The incisors are described as centrals, first intermediate, second intermediate and corner incisors. *The canines are absent in all ruminants.*

The premolars and molars are also more or less chisel shaped and progressively increase in size from first to last. The premolars and molars have well-formed grinding surface.

The dental formulae of all ruminants including cattle, buffalo, sheep and goat are as follows:

Deciduous (Temporary) or milk teeth

$2\ (DI\frac{0}{4}Dc\frac{0}{0}Dp\frac{3}{3}) = 20$ total teeth where D=deciduous, C=canine, P=premolar & M = molar teeth

Permanent

$2\ (I\frac{0}{4}C\frac{0}{0}P\frac{3}{3}M\frac{3}{3}) = 32$ total teeth

The age estimation of our dairy cattle can also be done by examining the incisors teeth, which may be mentioned as follows.

The calf is born with two central incisors and the other incisors start coming out as the calf advances in age. When the calf is five to six months old, eruption of all the eight temporary incisors are complete, which are again replaced by permanent teeth in due course; the permanent teeth are smaller but broader with distinct neck between the root and crown and paler in appearance.

With the advancement of the animals age, the teeth start wearing off and the changes in the teeth at different periods of life span serve as the indicator of the animals' age. At the age of ten months the two dental temporary incisors show signs of wearing; when the animal is about months, the two lateral incisors start wearing off. At the age of about 1½ years, the whole set of milk teeth are flattened by the action of time.

At the age of about two years, the two central temporary incisors are replaced by the permanent ones; at the age of three years, the two intermediate incisors also get replaced; and at four years of age the corner incisors are also replaced.

At 5½—6 years, the entire set of eight teeth is completely replaced by the permanent teeth set.

Table 13.4.—Formulas and Eruption of Deciduous Teeth

	Horse	Cow	Sheep	Pig	Dog
	Deciduous Formulas				
	3 0 3 2(DI–DC–DP–) 3 0 3	0 0 3 2(DI–DC–DP–) 4 0 3	0 0 3 2(DI–DC–DP–) 4 0 3	3 1 4 2(DI–DC–DP–) 3 1 4	3 1 4 2(DI–DC–DP–) 3 1 4
	Deciduous Eruption				
Incisors					
DI 1	Birth to 1 wk	Birth to 2 wk	Birth to 1 wk	2–4 wk	4–5 wk
DI 2	4–6 wk	" " "	1–2 "	1½–3 mo	4–5 wk
DI 3	6–9 mo	" " "	2–3 "	Birth or before	4 "
DI 4	———	" " "	3–4 "	———	———
Canines					
DC1	———	———	———	Before birth	3–4 wk
Premolars					
DP1	———	Birth to few da	2–6 "	5 mo	4–5 mo
DP2	Birth to 2 wk	" " "	2–6 "	5–7 wk	4–5 wk
DP3	" " "	" " "	2–6 "	U–4–8 da	3–4 wk
DP4	" " "	———	———	U–4–8 da L–2–4 wk	3–4 wk

Deciduous Incisors	DI	Day	da	Upper	U
Deciduous Canines	DC	Week	wk	Lower	L
Deciduous Premolars	DP	Month	mo		
		Year	yr		

Table 13.5.—Formulas and Erutpion of Permanent Teeth

	Horse	Cow	Sheep	Pig	Dog
	Permanent Formulas				
	3 1 3–4 3 2(I–C–P—M–) 3 1 3 3	0 0 3 3 2(I–C–P–M–) 4 0 3 3	0 0 3 3 2(I–C–P–M–) 4 0 3 3	3 1 4 3 2(I–C–P–M–) 3 1 4 3	3 1 4 2 2(I–C–P–M–) 3 1 3 3
	Permanent Eruption				
Incisors					
I1	2½ yr	1½–2 yr	1–1½ yr	1 yr	4–5 mo
I2	3½ yr	2–2½ yr	1½–2 yr	16–20 mo	4–5 mo
I3	4½ yr	3 yr	2½–3 yr	8–10 mo	4–5 mo
I4	———	3½–4 yr	3½–4 yr	———	———
Canines					
C	4–5 yr	———	———	9–10 mo	4–5 mo
Premolars					
P1	5–6 mo	2–2½ yr	1½–2 yr	12–15 mo	5–6 mo
P2	2½ yr	1½–2½ yr	1½–2 yr	12–15 mo	5–6 mo
P3	3 yr	2½–3 yr	1½–2 yr	12–15 mo	5–6 mo
P4	4 yr	———	———	12–15 mo	5–6 mo
Molars					
M1	9–12 mo	5–6 mo	3–5 mo	4–6 mo	4 mo
M2	2 yr	1–1½ yr	9–12 mo	8–12 mo	U5–6 mo
M3	3½–4 yr	2–2½ yr	1½–2 yr	18–20 mo	6–7 mo

Incisors, I; Canines, C; Premolars, P; Molars, M; Day, da; Week, wk; Month, mo; Year, yr.

After the age of six years, changes occur in the level of these permanent incisors. At 6-7 years the central incisor, at 7-8 years the 1st intermediate incisor, at 8-9½ years the 2nd intermediate incisors and by 11th year the corner incisors get worn out; by the age of 11 years the incisor teeth become smaller due to wear and tear.

By the 12th year of age, the dental tables become square instead of oval and the teeth stand apart leaving space between them.

After the age of 12 years, age estimation by examining the teeth becomes practically difficult, and after this age, the productive life of our dairy cattle also become lost.

OTHER ESSENTIALS IN DAIRY CATTLE MANAGEMENT

1. Daily Inspection

An ideal dairy farm manager should make a regular routine to visit the herd every morning. His first duty will be to look for any diseased animal. In the morning when the animals are let out, he can spot those which have come into heat. When the animals return from grazing, it will be possible for him to observe any injuries, amount of forages taken by individual animal (from the flanks of the animal), any other indisposition can also be detected from the appearance or behaviour of any animal. When attending a cattle farm with a large herd, the dairy manager has to rely considerably on the help of the attendants as the manager also supervises other works like purchase of feeds and stores, and marketing of produce. Still he should formulate a plan of giving collective attention to those important items as a daily routine.

2. Regularity of Care

The dairy cow is a creature of habit. Everyday the same routine of feeding, milking and caring for her should be followed.

A major change in her daily programme may have effects upon her production and health. Most cows can, however, come accustomed to slight amount of change.

3. Kindness in Handling

A cow should always be treated with kindness if she is to maintain production. The beating of a cow should never be allowed under any circumstances. We must not treat our cows as wild beasts, on the other hand we should treat our animals with full affection.

4. Grooming Dairy Cows

Grooming should form a part of daily routine in a well-kept herd. Grooming or brushing is essential as it removes dirt and loose hairs from the body. Regular grooming and removing manure or litter from their bodies not only help to keep the hide pliable but also make possible the production of clean milk. The clipping of the long hair from the udder and hind legs and the rear flanks will have to prevent accumulation of filth . Further it improves blood circulation.

The equipment needed for grooming are a blunt type-comb for removing the coarse material or manure from the cow and a heavy bristle brush for the main grooming job. If no brush is available, coarse rope (made of paddy straw, coconut straw, or dried grass) turned into a pad will be a good substitute. The movements of the brush should be along the direction of the body hairs.

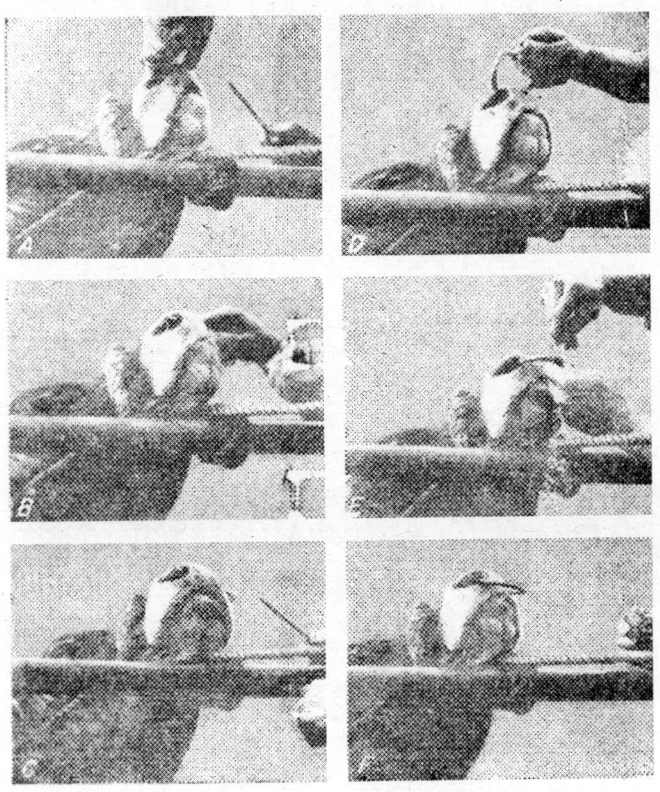

Plate 56. Ringing the bull (Chapter 13).

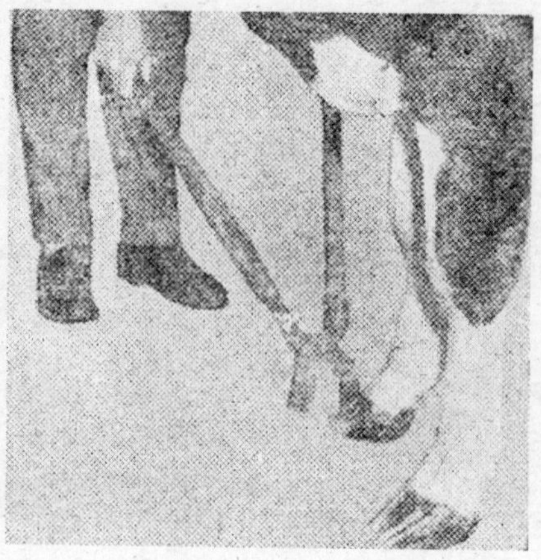

Plate 57(a). Trimming feet, clipping off the toe of the hoof with pincers (Chapter 13).

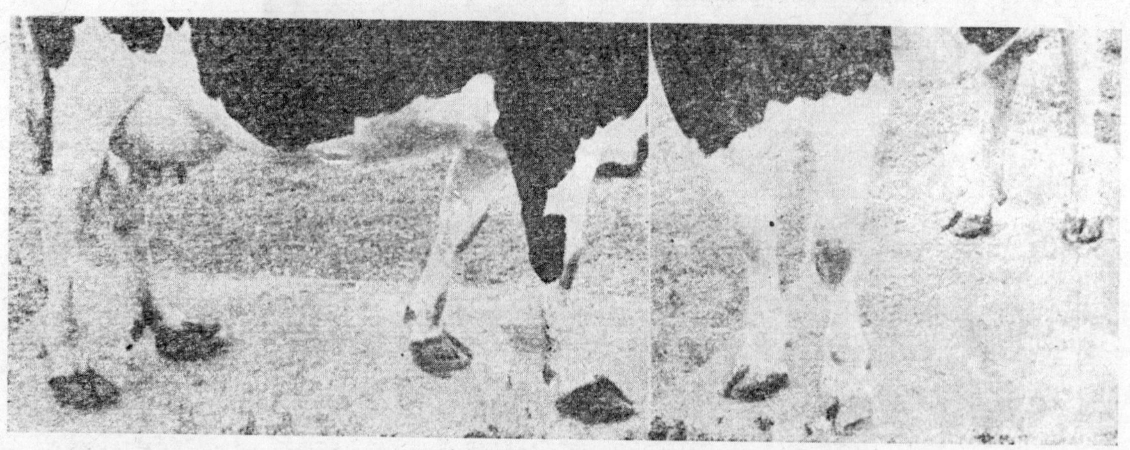

Plate 57(b). Cow on the left needs trimming of all her four feet. The same cow, on right after, trimming and she can stand squarely on all four feet (Chapter 13).

5. Drying off Cows

It is generally considered that a cow should remaln dry for a period before calving, for four principal reasons:

(1) To rest the organs of milk secretion
(2) To permit the nutrients in the feed to be used in developing the foetus instead of producing milk
(3) To enable the cow to replenish in her body the stores of minerals which have become depleted through milk production
(4) To permit her to build up a reserve of body flesh before calving.

Practical experience has shown that cows denied of a dry period will give less milk in the following lactation than those allowed a period of rest.

Methods of drying. Three methods of drying off a cow are in use: (1) incomplete milking, (2) intermittent milking, and (3) complete cessation.

Incomplete milking. Dairymen who follow this system do not extract all the milk from the udder at milking time for the first few days after the drying-off period has begun. Later they milk intermittently but never completely. After the production decreases to only a few litres daily, milking is stopped.

Intermittent milking. Under the procedure, the cow which is to be dried off will be milked once a day for a while, then once in every next day, and finally milking will be stopped altogether.

Complete cessation. From practical observations it has been found that complete cessation of milking can be recommended safely with cows producing as much as 10 litres of milk per day. In drying a cow by this method, the udder fills until pressure increases enough to stop secretion inside the udder. After the cessation of secretion, the milk is gradually re-absorbed from the gland until it becomes completely dry. The cow should not be milked during the stage of re-absorption as this releases the pressure within the gland and secretion is again initiated, resulting in a prolonged period of drying off.

Length of dry period. Cows should always be in at least a medium state of flesh at time of calving. For this reason, thin cows should have longer dry periods than those carrying more flesh. For cows which are well fed and are in good condition at the time of drying off, it is suggested that the dry period should be 40 to 80 days, the shorter period being for low producers. Thin cows should remain dry for longer periods.

6. Detecting Heat

Detection of heat followed by artificial insemination or natural mating is one of the prime essentials in dairy cattle management. It has been observed in many developed countries that due to lack of this timely act (which again may be due to negligency or ignorance of the dairymen) dairy farms suffer from proper detection of heat and that is why so much emphasis have been placed on correct timing in artificial insemination work. For this the dairymen should have careful observation and some experiences in detecting heat at proper time.

7. Pregnancy Diagnosis

Pregnancy diagnosis is directly related to the economy of dairy management. As early as 1½ to 2 months of pregnancy the status can easily be detected by any experienced veterinarian. In many instances, the dairyman becomes overconfident about the success of his artificial insemination, without proper check up as because his cows are not repeating heat for a second time and may even waits up to about 5 to 6 months; lately dairyman realizes that there are many factors other than normal pregnancy which are responsible for non-return of heat. Early detection of pregnancy of an animal thus becomes an indispensible job of any herd owner.

8. Milking

1. Observe regular milking hours and as far as possible equal milking intervals should be followed.
2. After washing the animal, practice only dry hand milking. Use the full hand method followed by strippings. Do the milking quickly, gently and completely.

9. Health Control Measures

These include (1) vaccination against various viral and bacterial diseases, (2) testing programme and (3) deworming programme.

Vaccination

The human endeavour to fight disease has been a problem since time immemorial. The initial scientific application of biological products was established by Jenner's work on the effectiveness of cowpox in immunization of human beings against small-pox. Jenner's (1798) observation forms the starting point of the evolution of biological products.

The science of immunology and evolution of biological products then remained dormant for about a century, but thereafter the microbiologists started probing into various microbes fatal to man and animals. The last decade of the 19th century proved to be the golden era of bacteriology and immunology. During this period appeared the classic works of Pasteur on anthrax, fowl cholera and rabies; Salmon and Smith (1885) on swine paratyphoid; Koch (1890) (1891) on tuberculosis; Behring and Kitasato (1890) on diphtheria antitoxins; Ehrlich's (1892) exposition of the principles of immunity; and of Metchnikoffs (1901) on immunological studies. These studies opened up a new lease of life to the suffering humanity and animals.

The research work on development of biological products in India was taken up at the imperial Bacteriological Laboratory, established at Poona (now Pune) in 1890 by the Government of India.

After two years it was found that the climatic conditions at Pune were not altogether suitable for carrying on the finer operations of biological research and it was decided to shift the Laboratory to Mukteswar, in the foot-hills of Himalayas, in 1893. In 1901 a branch laboratory was built on a site at 'Kurgaina' about 4 km from Bareilly, wherefrom it was moved in 1913 to its present commodious site at Izatnagar and was called Imperial Veterinary Serum Institute, Izatnagar, in U.P. which eventually became the Biological products Division of the Indian Veterinary Research Institute, and the main biological products unit of the country.

How to Make a Vaccination Programme Successful?

To-day it is well established that vaccination is one of the most effective ways of preventing specific diseases by inducing immunity in animals. Unfortunately not all types of vaccination are capable of imparting life long immunity. Thus it is essential to know the period of effectiveness of a particular vaccine, the dosage and route of vaccination and the storage conditions for stocking vaccines. The following aspects may be helpful for making the vaccination programme successful.

1. Perform vaccination only in healthy stock.
2. Cows in advanced pregnancies should never be vaccinated.
3. Calves between 4–6 months should be vaccinated.
4. During any outbreak of disease, vaccination programme should never be carried out.
5. Keep all vaccines under refrigeration until ready for use. At the time of vaccination, the reconstituted vaccines, particularly the live viral vaccine, should be kept on ice.
6. Follow strictly the manufacturers directions.
7. Destroy all unused vaccines which could not be used within validity period.
8. Clean up and disinfect all equipment and clothing after the vaccination performed by trained and qualified personnel.
9. Keep a record of the brand, kind and batch number of vaccines used for various animal species with dates.

I. VACCINATION PROGRAMME

1. Rinderpest (A viral disease). The advent of tissue cultural rinderpest vaccine (TCRPV) has revolutionised the control programme. This is the single vaccine which has been found to be safe and immunogenic in indigenous, pure exotic and cross-bred cattle of various blood levels. The vaccine has also been found to be effective in calves and animal having advanced stages of pregnancy.

The duration of immunity with this vaccine have been shown to be about 3 years in India. Cattle are vaccinated as early as 6–8 months of their age followed by annual vaccination where the disease is more prevalent.

2. Foot and Mouth Disease (A viral disease). The vaccine used for the disease is known as polyvalent tissue culture vaccine. Calves below one month of age are given 20 ml (1/2 adult dose) of vaccine followed by a second dose of similar strength within next 21 days. At the age of 5–6 months, the calves are again vaccinated, using 40 ml at this stage. Hereafter annual vaccination is recommended. In case of highly susceptible costly exotic animals six-monthly vaccination may be done against yearly vaccination. (The quantity of vaccine given depends upon dilution). The vaccine is given subcutaneously on the dewlap region.

3. Haemorrhagic Septicaemia (A bacterial disease). The vaccine used is H.S. oil adjuvant vaccine. First vaccination at 6–8 months of age followed by regular annual vaccination is the recommendation. The vaccine may be subcutaneously injected preferably a month or two before the onset of rainy season.

4. Anthrax (A bacterial disease). As early as 6–8 months calves are vaccinated with Anthrax Spore Vaccine (living). Hereafter annual vaccination is recommended preferably before the onset of rainy season.

5. Black Quarter (A bacterial disease). The vaccination programme against this disease always commences after 3 weeks from the time of vaccinating the animal with H.S. Adjuvant vaccine. Annual vaccination is recommended. About 5 ml of B.Q. Polyvalent vaccine is given as subcutaneous injection.

6. Brucellosis (A bacterial disease). Brucella abortus (strain 19) living vaccine is used for immunisation of female calves of 6-9 months of age @ 5 ml per animal administered subcutaneously. Males are not vaccinated. Immunity once developed after the vaccination will remain active and gradually declining in succeeding pregnancies.

II. TESTING PROGRAMMES. Animals should be tested for tuberculosis, brucellosis and Johne's disease once every six months in the initial stages and later on, depending upon the health status of the herd, the test can be carried out annually. Positive reactors should be eliminated. Besides these, strict hygienic measures should be adopted. The breeding bulls should be completely free from infection.

III. DEWORMING PROGRAMMES. Deworming against the infestation of internal parasites (endoparasites) should be undertaken bi-annually, i.e., at the onset of monsoon and again after the end of monsoon.

1. **Ascariasis amongst calves.** Calves of about 6 weeks of age should be dosed with piperazine salts @ 1 gm/4 kg. body weight. Among other medicines, vermicides or vermax may be used as per direction of the veterinarian.

2. **Gastroenteritis.** Cattle above 3 months of age should be dosed with Thiabendazole @ 100 mg per kg body weight while Phenothiazine may be dozed @ 10 gm per 50 kg body weight.

3. **Liver flukes/Amphistomes.** In areas where fluke worm infestation is prevalent, use of hexachloroethane (Avlothane) @ 10 gm per 50 kg body weight is given. The total amount of the medicine is generally splitted into 2 doses spaced at 24 hours.

What precautions should be taken against contagious diseases ?

1. Vaccination programme as stated should strictly be followed.
2. The affected animals should be segregated from the healthy ones so as to prevent the spread of the disease.
3. The carcasses of the animal should be burnt or buried 6 feet deep in lime under ground.
4. Disinfect the shed in which any diseased animal is kept.
5. Spraying of cattle and shed should be done once a quarter. In the case of severe tick or lice infestation, spraying may be done at weekly intervals.

10. Culling of Dairy Animals

On a well organised dairy farm number of animals goes on increasing which provides a basis of selection by culling the undesirable ones. The following categories of the animals ought to be culled from the herd.

1. Animals which are suffering from contagious disease,
2. Animals having stunted growth,
3. Problem breeders,
4. Low yielders,
5. Long intercalving interval, short lactation and longer dry period.

11. Control of Bad Habits

Certain bad habits are prevalent among the cattle such as suckling another cow or herself, kicking during milking, fence and rope breaking etc. Unless they are properly treated from the first observation, it becomes a difficult problem to get rid of such practices in later stages. Some of the common bad habits are discussed below:

Suckling. Every dairyman has had experience with cows that suck themselves or other cows, thus causing losses of milk, contamination of the udder and sometimes indigestion of the animal concerned. There seems to be no satisfactory explanation of why they do so. To prevent this perversion, the cow should be separated from the rest of the herd. A cradle or a bull ring is put in the cow's nose and then two or three other rings are attached to it. A special ring that has some sharp progs soldered on to it, is very effective. This system does not interfere with the animals' normal eating.

Licking Some animals, specially calves, get into the habit of licking other calves during the milk-feeding period. This ultimately leads to the indigestion of hair which get entangled with the curdled milk in the stomach and forms hair balls. On further accumulation of such hairs, balls continue to grow in size and lead to serious disorders which may be transmitted to other calves. One of the precautionary methods is to rub a pinch of salt or mineral mixture on the tongue of the calf after each feeding. Repetition of this system will enable the calf to forget this habit. Some use rope-net or wire gauze muzzles to control this vice. Young calves of this nature can best be kept in individual pens or tied so that they cannot reach others.

Kicking. Many heifers or cows kick when the are milked. It may be mainly because of handling by an unskilled milker or may be by nature vicious.

Before applying any remedial measure, it will be wise to search for the reasons of such habit. It may be possible that the cow is suffering from some disease of the udder or teats. Sometimes bad milking method may compel the animal to do so. In such cases proper treatment will bring the cow in order. But when the cow by nature is vicious, in that case one method is to tie the head high. Another is to tie a rope around the body of the cow just in front of the udder. In severe cases, anti-linking chains can be used. A clamp fits over each hock and a chain fastens them together. Sometimes a piece of rope is used to tie the hocks by making a loop like the figure '8'. Unless crossed between the two hocks. the strap will slip down when the cow struggles.

Fence breaking. Some animals have the habit of breaking their fence of the enclosure in which they are grazed on jumping over the fences. The habit is formed due to the feeling that on the other side of the fence the grasses are more green or plenty. There is little that will stop a rougish cow except proper hitching arrangements and good fences.

Table 13.6

Vaccination Programme for Cattle and Buffalo

Disease	*Nature of vaccine*	*Age and Season at vaccination*	*Immunity*	*Remarks*	*Dose*
Anthrax	A suspension of living spores of a non-encapsulated avirulent strain of *Bacillus anthracis* in 50 per cent glycerine saline	All ages, 4-6 months onwards, in endemic areas Feb to May	The immunity is established in 10 days after vaccination and lasts about one year	The vaccinated animals may have a mild febrile reaction for 2-3 days after vaccination; annual repetition of vaccination necessary	2 ml S/c
Haemorrhagic septicaemia	A suspension of formalinized agar-washed culture of *Pasteurella multocida* in liquid paraffin and lanolin	All ages, 4-6 months onwards May to June	The immunity is established in about 21 days and lasts about one year	In some animals a slight swelling may develop at the site of vaccination, this and a mild fever may persist for 2-3 days; annual repetition of vaccination necessary	5 ml S/c
Black-quarter	A mixture of broth cultures of *Clostridium chauvoei* and *Cl. septicum* rendered sterile by formalinization	All ages, 4-6 months onwards All season	The immunity is established in about a fortnight and lasts about one year	A slight swelling at the site of inoculation may develop and persist for 2-3 days; annual repetition of vaccination necessary	5 ml S/c
Brucellosis	A suspension of the living culture of *Brucella abortus* (strain 19)	Although older animals may be vaccinated, the usual procedure is to vaccinate claves of 6-9 months	Durable immunity which persists satisfactorily over the first or second pregnancies; boosted by natural inapparent infections	A mild rise of temperature may be seen 1 to 2 days after vaccination. The temperature comes down very soon. A hard and painful swelling develops at the site of inoculation and persists for about a week	5 ml S/c
Rinderpest	A freeze-dried preparation of spleen pulp of goats artificially infected with the 'Mukteswar' strain of rinderpest virus (GTV)	All ages, 4-6 months onwards Winter months	Durable immunity lasting several years	The vaccine is used for imunizing plains cattle; vaccination may be repeated every 3 years	1 ml S/c

(Contd.)

Disease	Nature of vaccine	Age and Season at vaccination	Immunity	Remarks	Dose
	A freeze-dried preparation of blood, spleen and mesenteric lymph glands of rabbits artificially infected with the lapinized strain of the rinderpest virus	All ages, 4-6 months onwards Winter months	Durable immunity lasting several years	A mild rise of temperature may be observed after vaccination. The vaccine is used for crossbred and other cattle susceptible to G.T.V. and animals in advanced pregnancy. Vaccination may be repeated every 3 years	5 ml S/c
	A freeze-dried bovine kidney-cell-culture rinderpest virus vaccine	All ages, 4-6 months onwards Winter months	Durable immunity lasting several years	The vaccine is used for exotic and other highly susceptible cattle and animals in advanced pregnancy. Vaccination may be repeated every 3 years	
Foot-and-mouth disease	Formalin-inactivated, aluminium hydroxide gel absorbed polyvalent goat kidney-cell-culture virus vaccine, incorporating types 'O', 'A', 'C' and 'Asia 1'	All ages, 4-6 months onwards, although animals younger than 4 months may also be vaccinated Nov to December	Immunity is established after about a fortnight of vaccination and persists for 6-8 months. The immunity is conferred upon the animals for a longer duration with repeated vaccinations	The vaccine is used for protecting exotic and other highly susceptible cattle against the foot-and-mouth disease. There is no systemic reaction seen after vaccination, although a somewhat painful local swelling may develop at the site of vaccination. The swelling either disappears completely in course of time or gets reduced appreciably	10 ml S/c

S/c - Sub-cntaneous

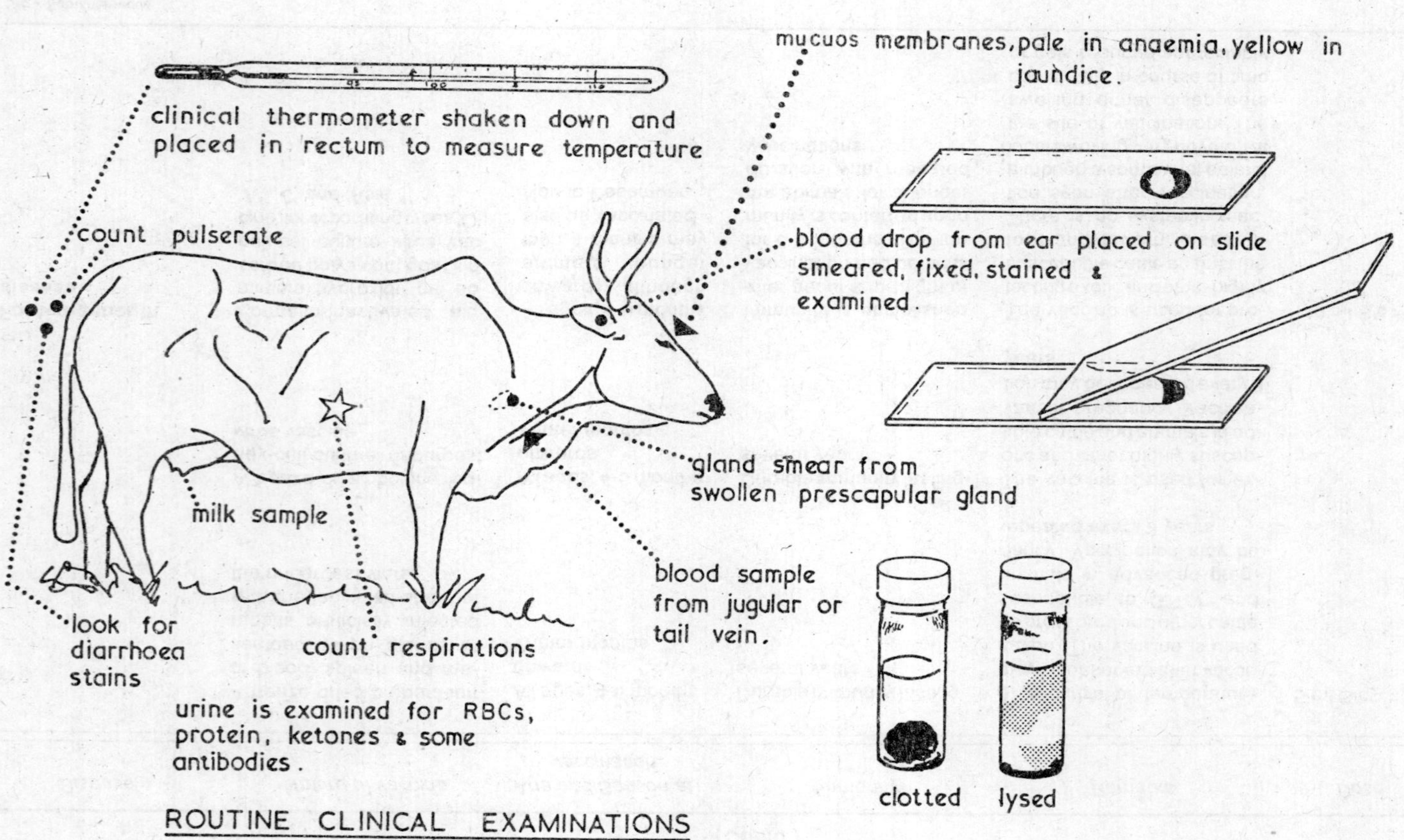
clinical thermometer shaken down and placed in rectum to measure temperature
count pulserate
mucuos membranes, pale in anaemia, yellow in jaundice.
blood drop from ear placed on slide smeared, fixed, stained & examined.
gland smear from swollen prescapular gland
blood sample from jugular or tail vein.
milk sample
look for diarrhoea stains
count respirations
urine is examined for RBCs, protein, ketones & some antibodies.
clotted
lysed
ROUTINE CLINICAL EXAMINATIONS

Fig. 13.14

Table 13.7

Probable dates of parturition in different species bred on various dates

Date of Services	AVERAGE DATES OF PARTURITION					
	Dairy Cow (282 days)	*Water Buffalo* (316 days)	*Doe* (150 days)	*Ewe* (148 days)	*Sow* (114 days)	*Mare* (336 days)
Jan. 1	Oct. 11	Nov. 13	May 31	May 25	Apr. 24	Dec. 3
Jan. 16	Oct. 26	Nov. 28	June 15	June 10	May 9	Dec. 18
Feb 1	Nov. 11	Dec. 14	July 1	June 28	May 26	Jan. 3
Feb. 16	Nov. 26	Dec. 29	July 16	July 13	June 10	Jan. 18
Mar. 1	Dec. 9	Jan. 11	July 29	July 26	June 22	Jan. 31
Mar. 16	Dec. 24	Jan. 26	Aug. 13	Aug. 9	July 7	Feb. 15
Apr. 1	Jan. 9	Feb. 11	Aug. 29	Aug. 27	July 23	Mar. 3
Apr. 16	Jan. 24	Feb. 26	Sept. 13	Sept. 11	Aug. 7	Mar. 18
May 1	Feb. 8	Mar. 13	Sept. 28	Sept. 25	Aug. 22	Apr. 2
May 16	Feb. 23	Mar. 28	Oct. 13	Oct. 10	Sept. 6	Apr. 17
Jun. 1	Mar. 11	Apr. 13	Oct. 29	Oct. 26	Sept. 22	May 3
Jun. 16	Mar. 26	Apr. 28	Nov. 13	Nov. 10	Oct. 7	May 18
Jul. 1	Apr. 10	May 13	Nov. 28	Nov. 25	Oct. 22	June 2
July 16	Apr. 25	May 28	Dec. 13	Dec. 13	Nov. 6	June 17
Aug. 1	May 11	Jun. 13	Dec. 29	Dec. 29	Nov. 22	July 3
Aug. 16	May 26	Jun. 28	Jan. 13	Jan. 10	Dec. 7	July 18
Sept. 1	Jun. 11	Jul. 14	Jan. 29	Jan. 26	Dec. 23	Aug. 3
Sept. 16	Jun. 26	Jul. 29	Feb. 13	Feb. 10	Jan. 7	Aug. 18
Oct. 1	Jul. 11	Aug. 13	Feb. 28	Feb. 15	Jan. 22	Sept. 2
Oct. 16	Jul. 26	Aug. 28	Mar. 15	Mar. 12	Feb. 6	Sept. 17
Nov. 1	Aug. 11	Sept. 13	Mar. 31	Mar. 28	Feb. 22	Oct. 3
Nov. 16	Aug. 26	Sept. 28	Apr. 15	Apr. 12	Mar. 10	Oct. 18
Dec. 1	Sept. 10	Oct. 13	Apr. 30	Apr. 27	Mar. 2	Nov. 2
Dec. 16	Sept. 25	Oct. 28	May 15	May 12	Apr. 9	Nov. 17

Table 13.8

Normal pulse rate, respiration rate and body temperature of common livestock

Animal	*Pulse rate/mnt*	*Respiration rate/mnt*	*Body temperature (F°)*
Horse	30–40	8–12	100.4–100.8*
Cattle	45–55	12–16	101.8–102.4**
Sheep	70–80	12–20	101.3–105.8***
Pig	70–80	10–16	100.9–104.9
Goat	70–80	12–20	101.3–105.8
Dog	90–100	15–30	100.9–101.7
Cat	100–120	16–32	101.0–102.0
Fowl	300	15–30	105.0–107.0

***In youth higher; **In milk cows higher; ***In full fleece heifer and in oldder age lower.**

Table 13.9

Incubation Period

The time that elapses between infection and appearance of systems of a disease is known as incubation period.

The average incubation periods for the commoner infectious diseases are :

Anthrax	12 to 24 hours or more
Black-quarter	1 to 5 days
Braxy	12 to 48 hours
Distemper	3 days to 3 weeks
Dounne	15 to 40 days
East Coast fever	10 to 20 days
Erysipelas (swine)	2 to 3 days
Foot-and -mouth disease	2 to 12 days
Heart-water	11 to 18 days
Influenza	3 to 10 days
Lymphangitis. epizootic	8 days to 9 months
Piroplasmosis. British bovine	14 days at earliest
Piroplasmosis. other forms	Up to 3 weeks
Pleuro-pneumonia. contagious bovine	3 weeks to 3 months
Pleuro-pneumonia. contagious equine	3 to 10 days
Rabies	10 days to 5 months
Rinderpest	4 to 5 days
African horse-sickness	6 to 8 days
Strangles	3 to 8 days
Surra	5 to 30 days
Swine fever	5 to 15 days
Tetanus. horse	4 days to 3 weeks
Tetanus. Ox	5 to 8 days
Texas fever	6 weeks
Tuberculosis	2 weeks to 6 months

14

PIGS

Zoological Classification

Swine belong to the phylum *Chordata* (vertebrates) class *Mammalia* (milk giving), order *Artiodactyla* (even-toed, hoofed animal), family *Suidae* (non ruminants), genus *Sus* Linn. The European breeds of domestic swine were derived from the local wild pig, *Sus scrofa,* whereas the breeds in the Far Eastern parts of the globe were derived from another wild pig, *Sus vittatus.* The two types inbred readily. The modern breeds of pig evolved from different crossings between the two original types and the present day domestic pig, *Sus domesticus* is the result of thousands of years of evolution through gradual domestication.

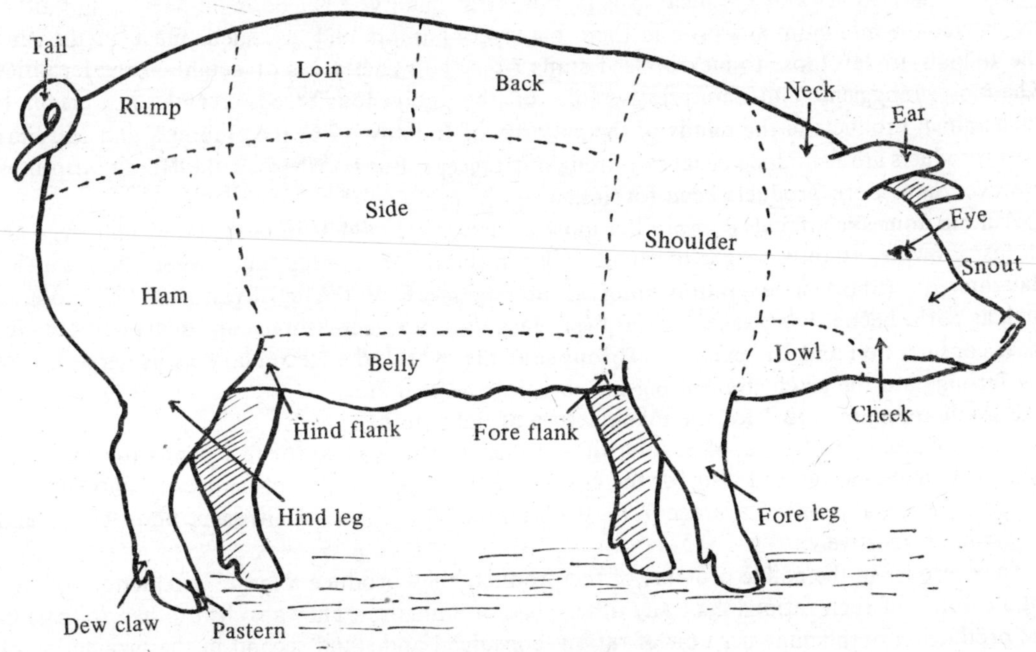

Fig. 14.1. The salient points of Pig.

Population and Production Trend

China ranks first in the world as a pig rearing country where the number is around 300 million which counts more than 1/3 of the world pig population followed by U.S.S.R., USA,

Brazil and West Germany. In India according to estimated population of 1982 the country had 10 million pigs. Of these Uttar Pradesh has got the highest contribution followed by Bihar, Andhra Pradesh and Tamilnadu.

Table 14.1

Pig population in India

Year	1951	1956	1961	1966	1972	1977	1982
Population (Million)	4.4	4.9	5.2	5.0	6.5	7.6	10.0

At present there are no Indian breeds of pigs, however, the type of pigs which are found throughout the country may be divided into four kinds, viz., wild pigs (*Sus scrofa cristatus*), domesticated or indigenous pigs, exotic breeds of pigs and upgraded stock of pigs such as Large-White Yorkshire, Middle-White Yorkshire, Landrace, etc.

In India pig raising and prok industry are in the hands of traditional pig keepers belonging to the lowest socio-economic stratum with no means to undertake intensive pig farming with good foundation stock, proper housing, feeding and management. They are compelled to follow old and primitive methods with common village hogs which could properly be designated as scrub animals. The small sized animals do not have any definite characteristics, grow slowly, produce small litters and the meat type is of inferior quality. The poor farmers cannot afford to provide the minimum attention in their managerial affairs and as such most of the time the animals are left loose to pick up feed stuffs from the waste areas of neighbouring localities. The most unhygienic and unimpressive life of the indigenous breeds creates an aversion to such animal products in the minds of the majority of Indians. For the Hebrews and Muslims, pork products are forbidden because of religious precept. But no where in the Hindu scriptures, however, have pork products been forbidden.

Among domestic animals pigs are the most prolific, 6–12 piglets in every litter, and they are all fast growing, attain a weight of about 68 kg in about 6–8 months time, when they can be slaughtered. (Shortest generation interval among meat producing livestock) Pig products such as pork, bacon, ham, sausages, lard (pig fat), etc., are increasingly in demand both for local consumption and for export. Throughout the world the secondary considerations of pig farming are the production of pigskin, bristles and manure.

Pigskin are mainly used for the manufacture of light leather goods.

Pigs manure is widely used as a fertiliser either for the soil or for fish ponds for the production of methane gas and also for the culture of the algae which can be used as animal feed. Pig manure contains on an average 0.70, 0.60 and 0.70 per cent of nitrogen, phosphorus and potassium respectively.

They recover in the edible proteins of the product, they produce a large production of the total calories of their rations than any other class of animals. They also lead other animals in the production of thiamine per unit of ration consumed and stand second in the production of niacin, and are third as producers of riboflavin and iron. However, swine store little calcium in the edible portion of their carcasses and no vitamin A or D.

PIGGERY DEVELOPMENT WORK IN INDIA

Before the introduction of five-year plans, except for some sporadic import of a few superior quality pigs of exotic breeds by a few missionary organisations, no concerted or organised measures were taken to improve pig production in the country. The organisation of pig production in rural areas has now been concentrated around the bacon factories. During the second and third plan periods establishment of the following eight bacon factories was the beginning of an attempt made for piggery development in the country. The details regarding the location and installed capacities of these are given in Table 14.2

Table 14.2

Bacon factories and their installed capacities (1972–73)

Name of the factory	*Capacity per day (pigs)*
Bacon Factory, Gannavaram, Krishna Dist. (A.P.)	100
Bacon Factory, Borivili, Bombay, Maharashtra	100
Bacon Factory, Haringhata, Mohanpur, W.B.	10–20
Bacon Factory, Central Dairy Farm, Aligarh, U.P.	100
Bacon Factory, Kuthattukulam, Ernakulam, Kerala	50
Bacon Factory, Kanke, Ranchi, Bihar	50
Pork Processing Plant, Kharar, Punjab	10–20
Bacon Factory, Alwar, Rajasthan	50

Unfortunately at present, none of the bacon factories are working even at fifty per cent of their installed capacity. Necessary steps are now being taken up to remove constraints for appropriate breeding programmes in the Regional Pig Breeding Stations attached to bacon factories to ensure steady supply of quality pigs.

Inspite of pig development programmes and establishment of bacon factories, pig farming has not yet become popular to any considerable extent. A trend is, however, observable that apart from poor and a section of sophisticated urban population the middle class people are also gradually developing taste for pork and pork products. On the basis of available indicators of demand the requirements of pork and pork products have been estimated by the National Commission on Agriculture (1976) for the years 1985 to 2000 A.D. are given below along with the number of pigs to be slaughtered to meet the desired demand.

Table 14.3

Year	*Type of demand*	*Quantity of pork and pork products (million tonnes)*	*Number of pigs to be slaughtered (million)*
1985	High	0.11	2.4
	Low	0.08	1.8
2000 A.D.	High	0.17	3.1
	Low	0.12	2.2

There are 82 state pig breeding farms where pure-*exotic* breeds of pig as well as their crosses are being maintained. With a view to encourage scientific pig breeding in these farms, exotic pigs are also imported.

Characteristics of Swine and Their Production

1. *Superior feed conversion power.* The capacity of swine to transform large amounts of vegetable concentrated feeds into valuable animal feed as pork, bacon, etc., has brought them to their present pre-eminence in animal science. They produce more live-weight gain from a given weight of feed than any other class of meat animals except carefully managed broilers. On an average pigs now produce 100 kg gain from 300 to 350 kg feed, i.e., a kilogram of pork can be produced on as little as 3.0 to 3.5 kilograms of feed.

This capacity to digest and assimilate food is measured by dividing the liveweight increase of the pig into the weight of food eaten by the pig. The numerical result of this simple division is known as the feed conversion ratio or factor, and is defined as the weight of feed required to put on one unit of liveweight, e.g.,

Liveweight increase of pig = 90 kg
Feed consumed by pig = 270 kg

Feed conversion ratio $\frac{270}{90} = 3$ kg feed per kg live weight gain

Factors affecting this ratio

(*i*) *Age of the pig.* The ratio increases with age. For a 6 weeks old piglet only 2 kg of kreep feed are normally required to produce 1 kg liveweight gain. For a bacon pig approaching slaughter weight it could take over 6 kg of meal.

(*ii*) *Quality of feed and feeding system.* Feed nutritionally unbalanced will not give good conversion rates. Wasteful feeding also leads to poor results.

(*iii*) *Exposure to extreme weathers.* Extreme cold or hot weather do not provide the ideal conditions for efficient feed conversion.

(*iv*) *Genetic variation.* Marked genetic variation exists within breeds and improvement can be realised by selection of breeding stock with low food conversion factors.

(*v*) *Healthy condition.* This is the topmost prerequisite for obtaining maximum feed efficiency ratio. Intestinal parasites might be one of the significant causes for wide ratio.

2. *Swine store fat rapidly.* No other animal produces per unit of live weight, so much fat in so short a time or at the expense of so little feed. They have more separable fat than separable lean in their carcass. The waste fat problem in swine is very important. Feed efficiency will not be improved until excess fat is eliminated.

3. *Swine are prolific and bring quick return.* Swine grow rapidly, mature quickly and are prolific as judged either by the number of piglets (6-12) they produce at one birth or by the fact that the same sow may be managed to raise two litters of pigs a year. A unit of 10 sows and 1 boar will produce about 160 piglets during the first year.

Gilts may be bred between the age of about 8-9 months farrow when approximately 13 months old, and their pigs, if kept healthy and fed well, will weigh more than 80 kg each by the time they are about 6 months old. Thus the economic returns come quickly.

4. *Enterprise requires moderate investment.* The initial investment in getting into the business is small since swine require a small investment for buildings and equipments and are

well-adapted to the practice of self feeding, labour is kept to a minimum.

5. Swine excel in dressing percentage, yielding 65-80 per cent of their live weight when dressed in packer style with head, leaf fat, kidneys and ham facings removed. On the other hand, cattle dress only 50-60 per cent, and lambs and sheep 45-55 per cent. Moreover, because of the small production of bone, the percentage of edible meat in the carcass of the hogs is greater.

6. Pork is most nutritious. Because of the higher content of fat and the slightly lower content of water, the energy value of pork is usually higher than that of leaf of lamb.

7. Because of the nature of the digestive tract, the growing fattening pig must be fed a maximum of concentrates and a minimum of roughages. Where or when grains are scarce and high in price, this may result in high production cost.

8. Because of the nature of their diet and their extra-ordinarily rapid growth rate, they are extremely sensitive to unfavourable rations and to careless management.

9. Swine are very susceptible to numerous diseases and parasites.

10. One of the major disadvantages of raising hogs has been the expense of hog-tight fences. The cost of such a fence is considerably higher than the cost of a fence that will turn cattle or sheep.

11. Sows should have skilled attendants at the time of furrowing.

12. Because of their rooting and close grazing habits, hogs are hard on pasture.

BREEDS OF SWINE

At present there are about 60 recognised breeds of domestic pigs in the world. All have 38 somatic chromosomes. Out of these the Large White Yorkshire, Middle White Yorkshire, Landrace, Berkshire, Tamworth, Chester white, Duroc and Hereford are noteworthy. The most common breeds used in India are described below.

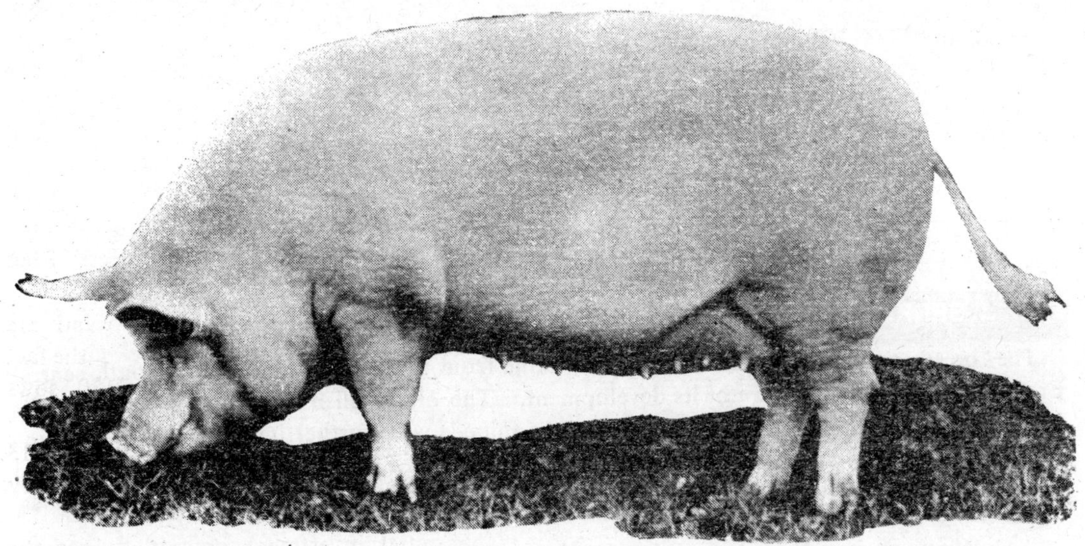

Fig. 14.2. A Large White Yorkshire Sow They Are Prolific Breeders

LARGE WHITE YORKSHIRE

The Large White Yorkshire is a popular English Bacon breed which had its origin nearly a century ago in Yorkshire and neighbouring countries in northern England. Yorkshire sows are noted as good mothers. They not only farrow and raise large litters, but they are great milkers.

Colour:	Entirely white in colour. Black pigment spots, called "freckles" do not constitute a defect, though they are frowned upon by breeders.
Head:	Moderately long, face slightly dished, snout broad, wide between the ears.
Neck:	Long, fine and proportionately full to shoulders with wide and deep chest.
Back:	Long, level and wide from neck to rump.
Legs:	Straight and well-set, level with the outside of the body, with flat bone.
Skin:	Fine, white, free from wrinkles.
Live weight:	Mature boars weight from about 300 to 450 kilograms, while average sow weights from 250 to 350 kg.
Carcass quality:	Possess necessary length, gives a first grade bacon, good ham and a comparatively light forequarter.

MIDDLE WHITE YORKSHIRE

This breed was evolved in Yorkshire of Northern England by crossing the Large White with smaller breed of Yorkshire extraction. The breed is accepted as an excellent pork pig, reaching slaughter weight early and with a high percentage of lean meat to bone. The breed is hardy, grows rapidly, but is not so prolific as the Large White. In India the breed has been extensively used for improving the indigenous stock in rural areas.

Colour:	White in colour.
Head:	Moderately short, straight jaw, short snout.
Neck:	Fairly light, medium length, proportionately and evenly set on shoulders.
Back:	Long and level to root of the tail with well sprung ribs.
Legs:	Straight and fairly short, well set apart, fine and flat bone, standing well up on toes and a good walker.
Skin:	Free from coarseness, wrinkles or any spots.
Live weight:	Mature boars generally weigh 270 to 360 kilograms.

BERKSHIRE

The breed originated in and takes its name from Berkshire, a country in south-central England which was the centre of its development. The old English hog, a descendant of the boar, served as foundation stock and these early animals were further improved by introducing Chinese, Siamese and Neopolitan blood. The breed is now highly valued as producer of good quality pork. In India specially in the South the breed is popular for upgrading programmes.

Colour:	It is black with "six white points", that is white on feet, nose and tail, but more than 10 per cent white of an animal disqualifies it.

Head:	It has a short head with dished face and its ears are erect.
Back:	Long, level arched narrow back.
Legs:	Straight and well set long legs.
Live weight:	Full grown boars weigh between 275 to 375 kg. Sows weigh from 200 to 290 kg.
Carcass quality:	Its reputation throughout the world has been for meaty, well balanced carcass with a high cut-out value.

Other Important Breeds

LANDRACE

The origin of this breed is in Denmark, where it has been bred and fed to produce the highest quality bacon in the world. The breed is white in colour, although black skin spots 'freckles' are rather common. The breed is characterised by its long, deep side; square ham; relatively short legs; trim jowl; heavy lop ears. The carcass is more lean than that of the meat. There is less back fat and lard. The breed is noted for prolificacy and for efficiency of feed utilisation. In U.S.A. the breed has been extensively used for developing crossbred foundation. In India the Landrace stock have been imported with the same objective.

TAMWORTH

The breed originates from central England. The breed derives its name from the town of Tamworth, which is located on the river Thames. Golden red colour, varies from light to dark. Extremely good bacon type. The individuals are long-legged with long, smooth sides and strong backs. The head is strikingly long and narrow with a long snout and fairly large ears that are carried somewhat erect. The carcass produces bacon on the finest quality. The sows are prolific and careful mothers, and the pigs are excellent foragers. Mature boars weigh upto 350 kg and the mature sows from 250 to 300 kg. The breed has been widely used for cross-breeding purposes in the tropics, particularly in Southeast Asia. They thrive under close confinement feeding, but they must be well-managed and fed. Landrace is susceptible to sunburn.

DUROC

North-eastern United States gave rise to one of the most popular U.S. breeds—the Duroc which is the outcome of blending of two breeds, Jersey Reds and Durocs of New York.

The breed is moderately red coloured with shades varying from a golden to cherry red colour. The Duroc is noted for excellent rate of gain and feed efficiency. Maturing early, the Duroc sow has large litter and is a good mother. The carcass is considered as a good meat type. The weight of mature boar is about 400 kg and of sow it is normally 350 kg. The breed is now popular both in South east Asia and in the American tropics mostly due to its colour, hardiness and fast growth.

CHESTER WHITE

The breed had its origin in the south-eastern Pennsylvania, principally in Chester and Dela counties of U.S.A. The foundation stock included important pigs of English Yorkshire, Lincolnshire and Cheshire breeds. As the name indicates, the breed is white in colour with some bluish spots sometimes found on the skin. Chester White sows are very prolific. The pigs are good feeders; they mature early and make good gains.

HEREFORD

It is one of the newer breeds of swine. The breed was originated in Missouri in the U.S.A. The most distinctive characteristic of the Hereford breed is their colour marking, which is similar to that of Hereford cattle. It is two-thirds red in colour, either light or dark with constant white face. The white colour must appear on at least two feet and extend upto an inch or more above the hoof. In size, the Hereford is smaller than the other breeds of swine and in general are of compact type.

Some common terms in relation to PIG

Details		*Expression*	*Details*		*Expression*
Species called as	...	Swine or Sus	Castrated male	...	Hog or stag or barrow
Group of animals	...	Drove or stock or herd	Castrated female	...	Spayed
Adult male	...	Boar	Female with its offspring		Suckling
Adult female	...	Sow	Act of parturition	...	Farrowing
Young male	...	Boarling	Act of mating	...	Coupling
Young female	...	Gilt	Sound produced	...	Grunting
New-born one	...	Piglet or pigling	Pregnancy	...	Gestation

SELECTION

Selection of a Gilt or Sow

In selecting a gilt or sow, the primary aim is to secure a female that will produce large litters of fast growing pigs capable of being fattened to marketable weights at an age of six months or less. (In the practical swine enterprise, 'growing-fatting' generally refers to that period from weaning to market weight of almost 100 kg. Because hogs are fattened at an early age, the process really refers to both growing and fattening).

Appearance or type. Before selecting a gilt or sow by its appearance, have a clear mental picture of the desirable type. In selecting a gilt or sow on the basis of appearance, consider the following main points; (1) general form or types; (2) size or weight for age; (3) development in the regions of high-priced cuts of pork; (4) quality.

As for form or type, a desirable gilt or sow presents a well-balanced appearance. From the side view, the top line appears as a strong uniform arch; the underline is straight; the legs are medium in length; the sides are deep and long. As viewed from the front or rear, the shoulders, back, loin and rump are fairly wide, and the width is carried uniformly from front to rear.

Gilts do not show as much depth of body as sows and consequently appear more "leggy" at the younger age. A desirable animal has a large heart girth, as indicated by the distance around the body just behind the shoulders. The head is trim in appearance with good width at the snout and between the eyes. The face is medium in length, varying somewhat with the breed. The various characteristics of the head and ears and the colour should conform to those desired for the particular breed to which the animals belong. In size or weight, a good gilt or sow in average condition is large for her age.

A good gilt or sow shows a reasonable amount of development in the regions of the high priced cuts of pork chops, which come from the back and loin; ham which comes from the rear quarters and bacon, which comes from the sides. Therefore, select animals having wide, full hams. Give preference to a body that is wide over the back and loin and long and deep. Do not expect gilts to show development in these regions as do mature sows.

Pedigree. A pedigree is the statement of an animal's ancestry. In addition to the names and herd-book numbers of the animals in each of several generations, usually it includes also the date of birth of each animal and the name of the breeder. It may extend back to the beginning of a breed's record history, or only for two or three generations.

In a real sense, a pedigree is good or bad, according as the individuals in it are good or bad. The better the individuals, the more uniform they are in the type of performance desired, the more prepotent and uniform the breeding qualities of the individual may be expected to be.

Performance or productive ability. While appearance and pedigree are important, it is even more desirable to consider actual performance, or productive ability, of an animal. In the case of a gilt or a sow, one measures efficiency of rate of gain as shown by its weight for its age. In the case of a sow, secure information on the number of pigs in each litter that she has farrowed, number of piglets raised per litter and the weight of the litter at 56 days usual weaning time or a later age.

Prepotency or transmitting ability. Prepotency is the ability to transmit characteristics to the offspring to a marked degree. It refers to either male or female. From a genetic standpoint, there are two requisites that an animal must possess in order to be prepotent: (1) dominance and (2) homozygosity. If a given sire or dam possess a great number of genes that are completely dominant for desirable type and performance and if the animal is relatively homozygous, the offspring will closely resemble the parent and resemble each other, or be uniform, in that case we will say that the animal is a prepotent. One should be careful to note whether this prepotency stands for desirable or undesirable qualities before arriving at any conclusion. Since gilts are purchased before they have pigs, it is not possible to determine their prepotency, transmitting ability, as can be done with a sow.

Selecting a Boar

Often we hear the saying this boar is one-half the herd which is literally true since he passes on one-half of the genes to the pigs he sires. While selecting a boar, take into account most of the considerations mentioned for selecting a gilt. As for type secure a boar that answers the general description given for a desirable type of gilt or sow. A desirable boar is larger for his age and heavier of bone than a gilt, and he shows masculinity and ruggedness, rather than feminity.

As with a gilt, a bear should be 4 to 6 months of age at the time of selection since serious defects in type are not so likely to develop after this age is reached.

Female Reproductive Organs

The genital organs of the sow resemble in general those of the cow, but a few special features may be noted.

The ovaries of the sow are concealed in an ovarian bursa. They are rounded and the surface is lobulated with follicles and corpora lutea. Mature follicles may have a diameter of about a third of an inch (7 to 8 mm), while that of corpora lutea it is about half an inch or more (12 to 15 mm). There is no sharp demarcation between the fallopian tubes and the horns of the uterus. The uterus present several sticking features. The body of the uterus is about 2 inches long. The horns are extremely long and flexible, and can be moved about freely. They are arranged in numerous coils and appear very much like loops of intestine. In the non-pregnant animal they may be 4 ro 5 feet long. The extremities of the horns taper to about the uterine tubes. The neck is remarkably small (about 10 cm). The cervix is

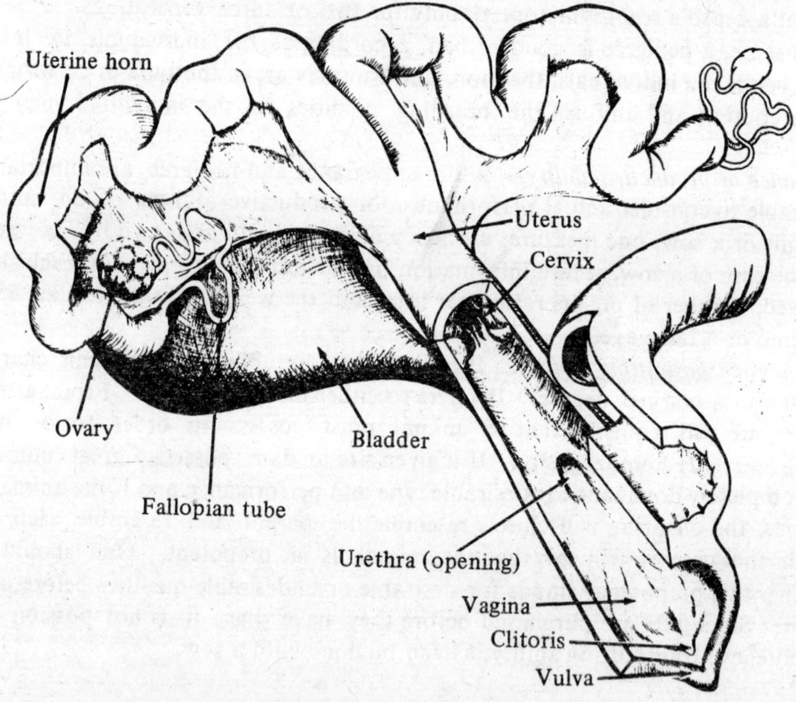

Fig. 14.3. Reproductive organs of Sow.

closed by numerous rounded prominances which dovetail together and protects the uterus from contamination. During service the penis of the boar may enter the cervix for passageway of sperms. Again during parturition, the cervix becomes relaxed before piglets can be expelled. The cervix is thus capable of several modifications in structure, depending on the physiological need of the female. The vagina is about 4 to 5 inches long and small in diameter. The

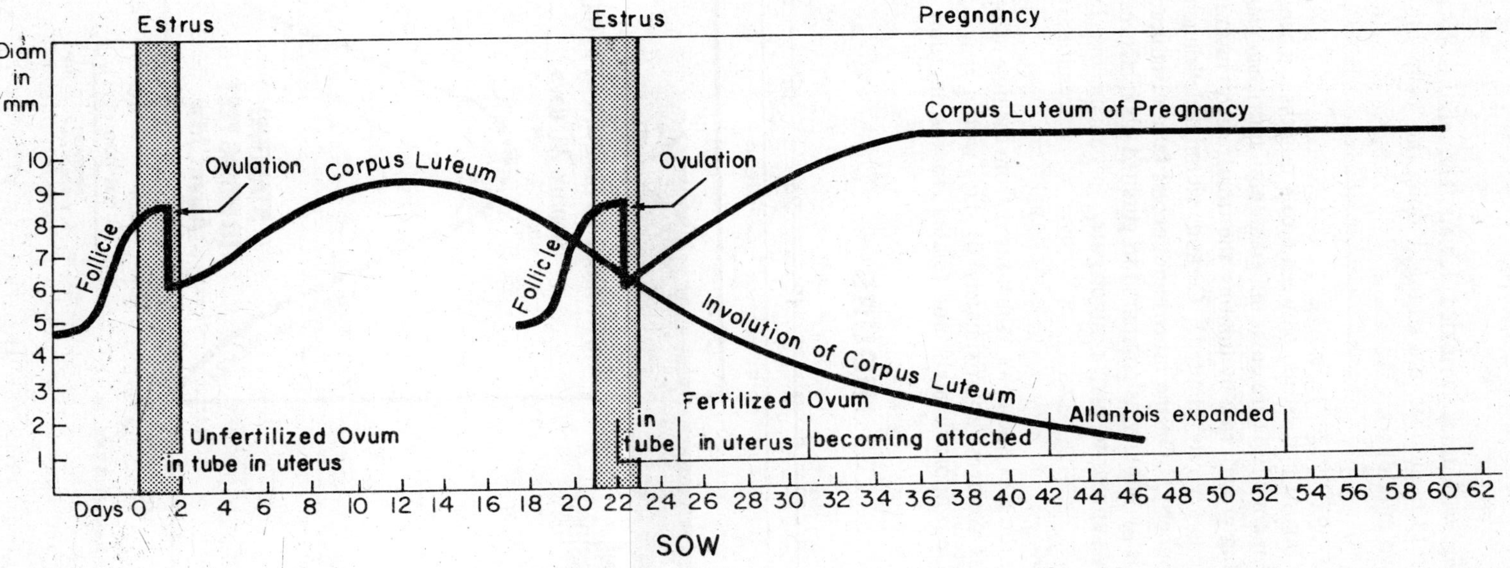

Fig. 14.4 The estrous cycle of the sow. (Slightly modified from Corner.) (Dukes, The Physiology of Domestic Animals, courtesy of Comstock Publishing Co.)

vulva is about 3 inches long, with thick wrinkled labia. The clitoris is long and flexible. The mammary glands, 10 to 12 in number, are arranged along the belly in the rows. Each gland have one teat with two milk ducts.

Sexual Maturity

Most gilts reach puberty (age at first estrus) between 6 to 8 months. There is some effect of genetics on puberty but the main effects are environmental, e.g., nutrition plays a great role in age at puberty. Retarding growth rate by limiting the total feed intake delays puberty specially if the energy intake is severely limited. Certain vitamin deficiencies (Vitamin B_{12}) have been shown to delay puberty. On the other hand, excess fatness induced by self feeding of gilts has been shown to delay puberty as compared to gilts fed a slightly restricted amount of feed. Variation among breeds appear to play a minor part.

Estrus Cycle and Heat Period

The length of the cycle in the gilts and sows as measured from the time of onset of one estrus to the onset of the next estrus averages approximately 21 days with a range of about 18 to 24 days. The length of the cycle is approximately not related to the duration of the estrus but

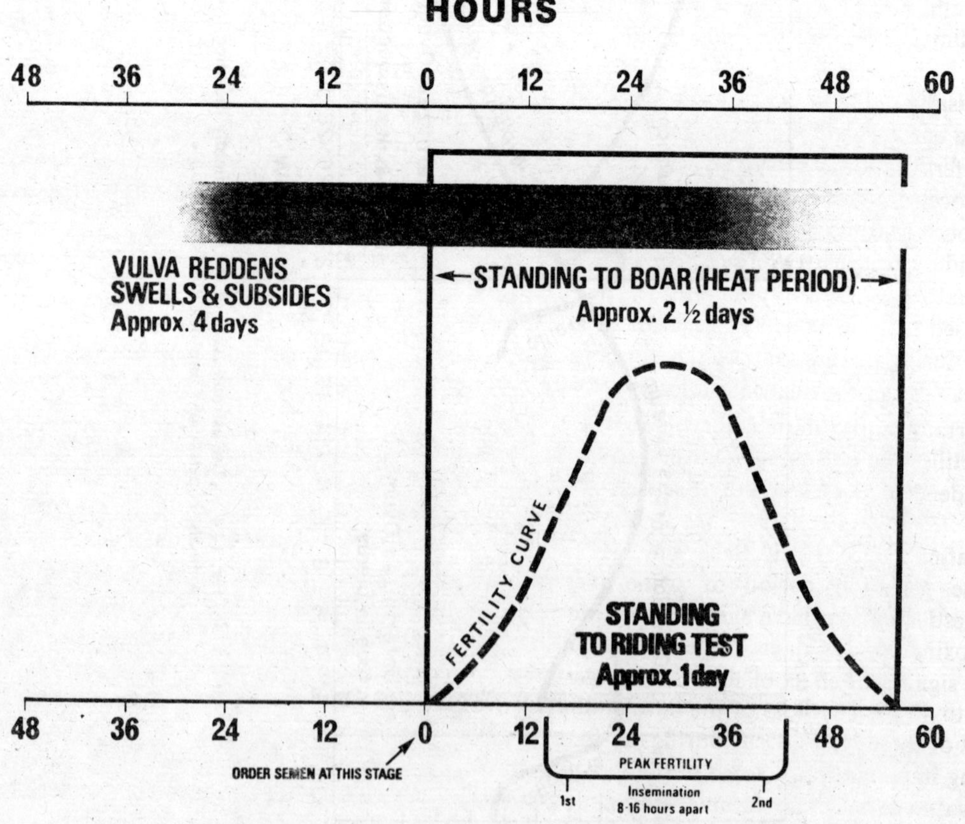

Fig. 14.5. Optimum time for the insemination of the Sow.

there are breed differences in the average cycle length. Ovulation with external manifestation of estrus is rare in swine. The external sign of estrus include: (i) enlargemet of the vulva 2 to 8 days before the onset of heat, (ii) reddended and swollen vulva sometimes associated with mucus discharge, and (iii) behavioural changes including restless activity, mounting other animals, both male and female and allowing mounting by other swine. On more careful examination the experienced observer detects.a characteristic immobility response when pressure is applied to the back region. Attempts have been made to relate vaginal smear, to stage of estrus in an attempt to utilise more effectively artificial insemination.

Estrus itself lasts for 2 to 2½ days and recurs every 19–23 days throughout the years. Gilts however, tend to remain on heat for only about one day.

Ovulation

In sow ovulation occurs late in the estrus. There are apparently breed differences not only in the length of the estrus period but in the time in which ovulation occurs. On the average ovulation occurs approximately 48 hours after the onset of estrus. The interval from the first to last ovulation, at a given estrus varies from 1 hour in length to perhaps as long as 7 hours. Sows are prolific (giving birth to several offspring at one time) animals and the rate of ovulation varies considerably with 10 to 20 ova being the usual range. Parity, age, nutritional level and breed influence ovulation rate. Gilt have a lower ovulation rate than sows and the number of ova produced by gilts increases with successive estrus.

Fertilisation

The entrance of the sperm into the ovum and the subsequent formation of pronuclei constitutes fertilisation. Normally, a single sperm enters the ovum but occasionally polyspermy does occur. This is generally associated with aging of the egg and may exceed 10 per cent incidence in some cases. In the sow fertilisation occurs only 6 to 10 hours after mating. This coincides with the travel of the ova down the oviduct and their union at that point with spermatozoa. By 14 hours after natural mating, essentially 100 per cent of all ova will be fertilised. It has been suggested that mating or artificial insemination would be accomplished only during the first-half of the estrus period and never after 36th hour following onset of estrus. Recent evidence indicates that age of sperm at the time of insemination is also important in maximum embryo survival. The first division occurs very shortly after the time of fertilisation and in eggs flushed from the fallopian tube 2 to 3 days following mating there is evidence of 3 or 4 cell divisions having already taking place.

Gestation and Maternal Behaviour

The gestation period of swine averages about 114 days (3 months 3 weeks 3 days). Domesticated pigs have shorter gestation period than that of wild pigs, the latter averaging approximately 124 days. There are small breeds and size differences have been noted. There is no significant effect of litter size on gestation length in swine. It is not uncommon to have a 30 to 40 per cent loss of the developing fetus between the first and 114th day of gestation. Most of these losses occur during the first 25 days which would correspond to the period preceding implantation. Some of the deaths are probably due to genetic defects within the sperm or ova; and an unfavourable uterine environment is conditioned in part by the ovarian hormones, estrogen and progesterone; and hormone imbalances may be involved. The high correlation between uterine length and embryo survival suggests that uterine crowding is a cause of embryonic death. While full-feeding prior to ovulation does increase ovulation rate, it is also a cause of embryonic mortality after conception has occurred.

The litter size tends to increase slightly with each succeeding litter upto a maximum over the fifth to seventh litters and it then generally declines. The average increase between the first and sixth litter is about two.

Females become increasingly docile during pregnancy and reduction of physical activity is influenced by the increased body weight associated with advanced pregnancy. Occasionally they show sign of excitement and often bite walls and fences seeking an outlet. In confinement they tend to cover any available holes, and in doing so will pack their water container with straw. The pitch of the voice is lower and when such sows are either startled or crowded into small areas, their attitude becomes more aggressive, suggesting maternal protection. The female selects a site and begins to prepare a nest for her litter 1 to 3 days before farrowing. If shelters are not available, she establishes a definite area for nest building, and attempts to keep it clear and dry. In concrete pen, her nesting tendencies are frustrated by the surroundings, but she still selects a nest site.

Farrowing appears to follow a diurnal pattern: parturition is rare in the morning and early afternoon, more frequent in late after noon and most frequent at night.

A few nursing sows show a potentially fertile heat period 2-3 days after furrowing, while others may exhibit estrus in the later stages of lactation. In both cases a higher plane of nutrition is supposed to assist these developments. All sows are potentially most fertile during post-weaning heat. If weaning is carried out before the piglets are 3 weeks of age the average time lag before estrus is about 10 days, with some variation. When weaning occurs during fourth week onwards then the delay is only 3–5 days and there is less variation. It may be possible to induce the sow to come on heat by a technique of partial weaning which entails the daily separation, at 3 weeks of age, of sow from litter for 12 hours each day, for 5 or 6 consecutive days; she is then mated and the piglets are allowed to resume normal access to her milk supply for the next 4 or 5 weeks.

The advantage of early weaning, from the reproductive point of view, is the potential increase in piglets produced per sow per year. *Flushing* of the sows (the increasing of the energy content of sow's ration for 6 days or so before the expected time of estrus and for a few days after mating) may increase the number of young born. The number of piglets may vary from 4–5 upto 20.

Male Reproductive Organs

In the male the essential organ the gonad corresponding to the ovary of the female is the testicle or *testis*, and two testes are normally present. They are carried in the external body cavity in the scrotum, where they become located after migration out of the body cavity through the inguinal canal by approximately the 100th day of prenatal life. In between the scrotum and the testis there is a tough capsule covering the testis known as *tunica albuginea.* The testis are carried in a near vertical position with the head of the *epididymis* on the ventral end and its body on the anterior surface. The greater part of each testis is composed of the *seminiferous tubules* in which, following a number of cell divisions, there are formed the male sperm cells known as the *sperms* (singular spermatozoa). The *spermatozoa* passes from the tubules into the coiled tube attached to the rear of the testis, known as *epididymis.* Each sperm represents a single free moving cell, and consists of an egg-shaped head in which is the nucleus, a short cylindrical body and long, thin, whip-like tail by which it drives itself along. The sperm is only about 1/500 of an inch in length and very large numbers are produced. In the tissue between the seminiferous tubules are the interstitial cells which produce testicular hormone responsible for developing the secondary sexual characters of the male, induction of libido, etc. As it is produced regularly and not at recurrent intervals, there is no sexual cycle in the male as there is in the sow. The *interstitial tissue* in boars is somewhat more plentiful than in other animals. The seminiferous tubules form a network of irregular epithelium lined spaces, the *rete testis.* From this there is usually one large duct emerging on the dorsal surface of the testis to join the head of the epididymis. The epididymis consist of a long, highly convoluted tube which increases in diameter as it reaches the point of transition into the

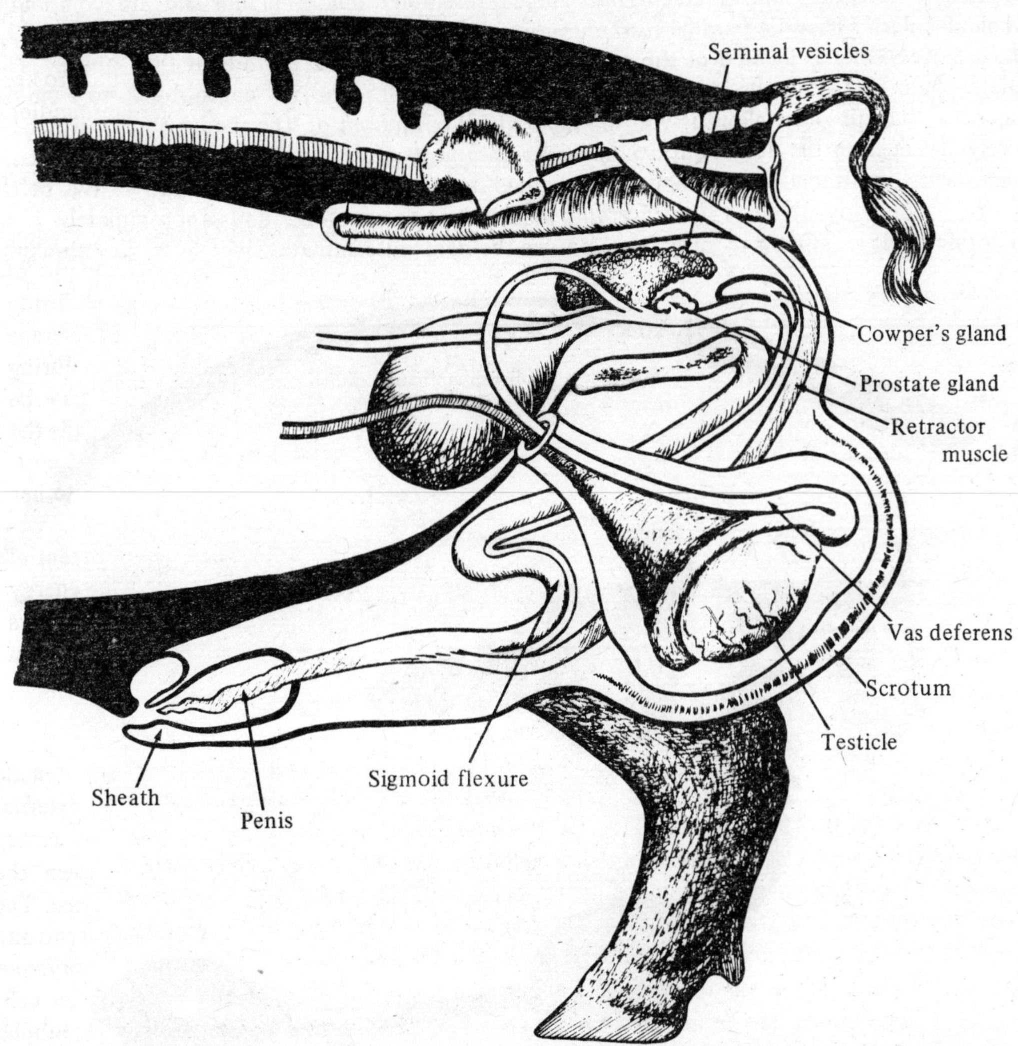

Fig. 14.6. Reproductive organs of Boar.

vas deferens. The total length of the epididymal tube is several metres. The vas deferens is approximately 25 to 30 centimetres long with an outside diameter of approximately 2 mm and an inside diameter of approximately ¼ of this. On each side of the pelvic urethra lie the *seminal vesicles.* The vesicular seminales are exceedingly large and extend into the abdominal cavity. The bulbourethral glands are very large and dense than other animals. They cover the neck of the bladder, the Cowper's, the prostate and the vas deferens. They are elongated, hollow, branched, tortuous tubes. There is no main central duct but rather a series of large ducts which branched and anastoms and finally converge to form one single duct which enters the urethra just ventrolateral to the vas deferens opening. Thus the openings from the vas deferens and the seminal vesicles into the urethra represent four seperate openings located in close proximity to each other. The Cowper's glands (*bulbourethral* glands) resembles mucous glands and are compound tubuloalveolar. They lie parallel to the urethra and are attached to it on the ventral sides. The excretory duct is located at the posterior end and enters the urethra at that point. The general shape of the glands is cylindrical, approximately 15 cm in length by 3 to 5 cm in diameter. The prostate gland is multilobular gland composed of the body (bulb) which is closely attached on the dorsal surface of the urethra at its anterior end and of the *pars disseminata* which is attached to the body of the gland itself but imbedded in the wall of the pelvic urethra. The body weighs 15 to 25 grams and is 4 or 5 cm long and approximately 1 to 2 cm thick. It is difficult to surgically remove the pars disseminata, since it is so intimately

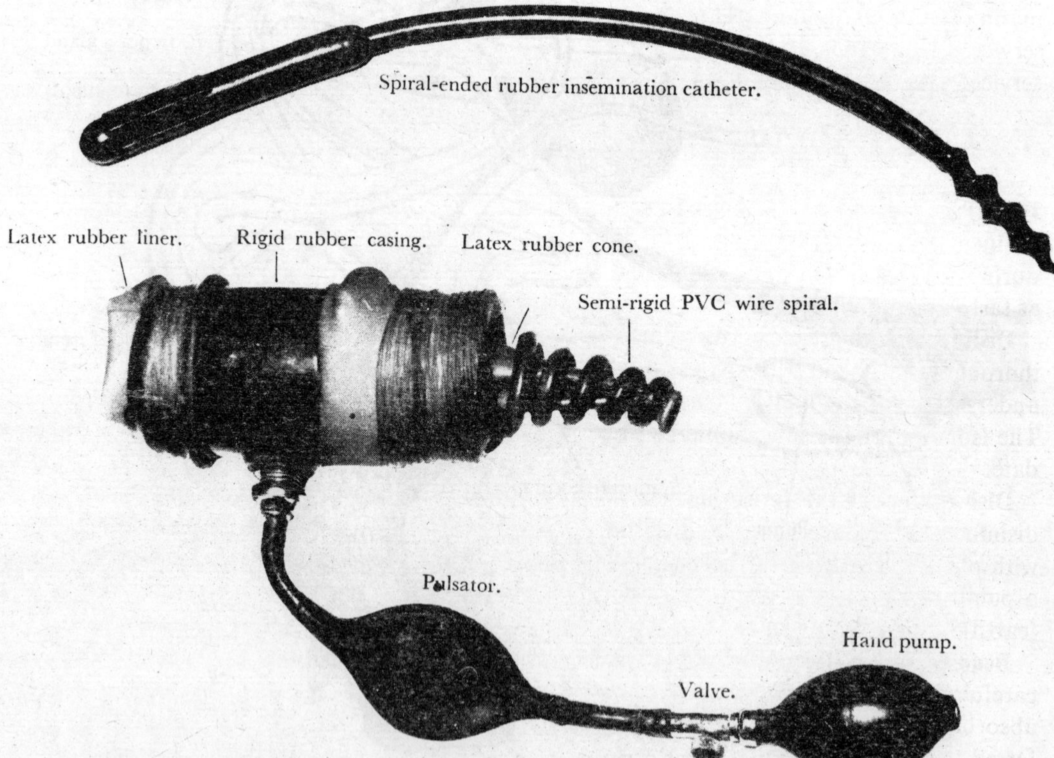

Fig.14.7. An artificial vagina for semen collection from the boar and a cathetor for artificial insemination of the Sow.

embedded in the urethral wall. The prostate contains large branching cavities and irregularly shaped ducts and alveoli There is abundant connective tissue capsule about the outside of the gland. The pelvic urethra is about 20 to 25 cm long from its origin at the neck of the bladder to the entrance of the excretory ducts at the posterior end and consists of approximately equal proportions of glandular and muscular tissue. The pars disseminata of the prostate is conspicuous at its anterior end because of its yellow colour. The penis in the sexually mature boar measures from 50 to 75 cm in length and 1 to $1\frac{1}{2}$ cm in diameter. The end has a corkscrew twist to the left. The penis arises at the *bulbo cavernosus*. Two retractor muscles are attached to the ventral surface anterior to the regions of the sigmoid flexture.

Puberty of Boar

The boar generally reaches puberty at the age of 8 months. The age of physiological maturity (i.e., presence of spermatozoa capable of fertilisation) may differ from the time when the essential elements of mating behaviour appear. Spermatozoa are present in the testis as early as 4 to 5 months of age but there is some delay before gametes are capable of fertilising ova. Level of feed intake during the growing period has an influence on age at puberty, a full-feeding programme being associated with early puberty. Mature size is not reached until approximately 1 year of age. The number of services allowed will vary with the age, development, temperament, health, breeding condition, distribution of services and system of mating (hand mating and pasture mating). In general young boars should be limited to one service per day and not more than twice a week while older boars may be used from two services a week upto twice a day at the maximum.

MANAGEMENT OF SWINE

1. Caring for the Sow and Litter at Farrowing Time

Since the sow produces several offsprings when she farrows and the pigs are easily injured during the first few days of their lives, an individual pen is needed for each sow and her litter at farrowing time and for at least 3 to 5 days following farrowing.

Disinfection of pregnant sow. Before moved into the farrowing quarters, the sow should be thoroughly scrubbed with soap and warm water, specially in the regions of the sides, and undersurface of the body. This will remove adhering parasite eggs and other disease germs. The isolation of the sow should be practised about 3 or 4 days prior to expected farrowing date.

Disinfection of the farrowing pen. The farrowing pen should be thoroughtly cleaned and disinfected to reduce possible infection. This may be done by scrubbing the walls and floors with phenyl water. A further precaution is to apply a 4 per cent standard disinfectant, using a pump spray to force it into all the crevices and angles. In case the floor is "*Katcha*" (earth), 2 or 3 inches of the top layer should be removed, then replaced with fresh earth.

Bedding of the farrowing pen. When the pens are thoroughly dry, they should be bedded carefully. The kind and amount of bedding to use is a matter of personal liking. Any good absorbant that is dry and will lie close to the floor is satisfactory. Rye or wheat straw is preferred to oat straw. Cut straw, any fine stemmed hay, saw dust or shavings are good as these interfere little with the efforts of the new born pig to reach the mother's teat.

Good housing. Hogs are sensitive to extreme heat and cold and require more protection than any other class of animals. This is specially true at the time of parturition. The type of farrowing pen which seems best adapted to the weather and other conditions should be used. The main requirements for satisfactory housing are that the quarters be dry, sanitary, and well ventilated and that they provide good protection from heat, cold and winds.

The guard rail. A guard rail around the farrowed pen is an effective means of preventing sows from crushing their pigs. The importance of this simple protective measure may be best emphasised by pointing out that approximately one-half of the young pig losses are accounted for by those pigs that are laid on by their mothers. The rail should be raised 8 to 10 inches from the floor and should be 8 to 12 inches from the wall.

Artificial heat helps to save young pigs. With early spring or winter pigs, especially in Northen India, a supply of artificial heat is necessary if chilling of the new born-pigs is to be avoided. An old stove or heater fixed up at one end of the central house is often the means of preventing chill. It must be remembered, however, that there is considerable fire hazard from this practice. The electric pig brooder is a much safer heating unit. The principles involved are identical to those of electrical chick brooder except for the canopy.

2. Care of the Litters during the First Eight Weeks

The first time when the sow goes to the trough after farrowing, some of the bedding should be renewed removing the soiled straw only; the main bed should be left undisturbed for a few days. Proper attention should be given to the new-born piglets which require a special treatment during the first eight weeks.

Needle teeth. An examination of the mouth of pigs at birth will show that they have eight small tusk-like teeth, two on each side of both upper and lower jaws. These teeth are normal, inclined to flatness, have sharp edges and generally are brown in tinge, at the tip. Needle teeth often are the cause of irritation and pain to the sow when the pigs nurse, specially at first when the udders are tender. Moreover, the pigs may bite or scratch each other and infection may start and cause serious trouble.

Pig growers who give their pigs most attention, as a rule, remove these immediately after birth. The operation may be done with a small pair of pliers or with strong forceps made specially for the purpose (tooth nipper) very close to the gum.

Creep feeding. Creep feed is that normal feed, given to suckling pigs behind a barrier (or creep) which allows them access to the feed but excludes the sow.

It has always been said that "young gains are cheap gains". This is due to (1) the higher water and lower fat content of the young animal in comparison with older animal, and (2) the higher feed consumption and coversion unit of weight of young animals. These factors have encouraged more and more creep feeding of pigs and other animals. The practice of self feeding of concentrates to young animals in a separate enclosure away from their dams is known as creep feeding.

Weaning

Fifty years ago pigs were weaned 8-12 weeks of age and sometimes even later. This has started to decrease and now some producers are weaning at 3-5 weeks of age due to latest technical know how. Fifty years from now pigs may be weaned very shortly after birth and the sow will serve primarily as an incubator for them. Baby pigs will be raised in cage and fed milk replacers. This will decrease baby pig losses to just a few per cent as compared to the 20–25% death loss which occurs between birth and weaning now.

Indian farmers most often allow single furrowing once in a year. Under such non-intensive conditions the piglets are allowed a long suckling period and weaning takes as late as on 12 weeks of age.

However, the traditional eight week weaning as was in developed countries is also now uncommon. The more usual ages are:

5–6 weeks; (widely followed by average farmers)
3–4 weeks; (followed by educated farmers).

Ther is some development in weaning below three weeks. The earlier the swine producer weans pigs, sows will rebred earlier and for this know-how, facilities and well trained personnel will be needed to operate successfully.

In weaning system it is best to remove the sow from the piglets rather than the other way round, so that at least they remain in the same environment, thus avoiding the double stress of weaning and a change of surroundings.

Advantages & Disadvantages of Early Weaning (3–6 weeks of age)

Advantages

1. The earlier it takes place the greater the potential annual production of piglets per sow. Usually sows come on heat within a week of weaning and thereby by reducing weaning age to 3–4 weeks, 4–5 weeks and 5–6 weeks, the litters per sow per year will be 2.35, 2.0 and 1.8 respectively as the average gestation period is only of 114 days. Thus sows are rebred earlier.

2. The piglets will be heavier and more uniform in size due to the fact that sow reaches maximum milk flow about 3 weeks after furrowing and the trend is downward by the fourth

Table 14.4

Guidelines to successful early weaning

Guideline	Age in weeks				
	1	2	3	4	5
Minimum pig weight (kg)	2.3	4.0	5.5	6.8	9.5
Furrowing house temp. (C)	24.0	21.0	21·0	19.3	15.5
Minimum floor space per pig (sq. ft)	4.0	4.0	4.0	5.0	6.0
Minimum number of pigs per linear foot of feeding space	5	5	4	4	4
Maximum number of pigs per linear foot of water space	12	12	12	10	10
Maximum number of pigs per group	10	10	10	20	25

week. Early weaning will mean the baby pig can obtain more to eat than if it continues to nurse the sow to 8 weeks of age. Of course, the prestarter and starter feed used must be of high nutritive value.

3. Better disease control. Earlier weaned pigs have fewer diseases and parasites which are transmitted from the sow to her piglets.

4. Savings on the sow's feed. Against this savings, however, one must figure the cost of the prestarter and starter feeds the young pigs eat.

5. Less weight loss of the sow. This means the sow may be sold after furrowing if she is no longer needed or if the market price is favourable.

Disadvantages

1. Requires fortified, well balanced and highly palatable prestarter and starter feeds.
2. Requires excellent management and technical know-how.
3. Requires excellent sanitation practices.

Castration. It is essential that boar pigs to be fattened for market be castrated when young. It is usual to castrate boar pigs at 4 to 6 weeks old.

In preparation for the operation, the pigs should be kept off feed 10 to 12 hours. An assistant should hold the pig by grasping the front and hind legs of either side with the pig's back resting on the ground. Before starting the castration, the hands should be thoroughly washed with soap and water and rinsed in a good disinfectant. The knife also should be disinfected both before and after making the incision. The testicle on one side is held firmly between the thumb and fingers of the left hand, while an incision is made by a single stroke of a sharp knife, parallel to the middle line of the body and then draw the testicle out. Draw the cord attaching to the testicle out an inch or two, and if it does not break scrape it off with the knife blade.

Remove the other testicle similarly. Wash the wound with a mild disinfectant solution.

Marking of pigs. As with other kinds of livestock, it is an essential item to mark individual animals as early as they are born. For pigs ear notching, ear tattooing, body tattooing, metal ear clips and branding are in use. Out of the methods listed, ear notching at farrowing time is a universal practice. The ear notches are usually made with special ear marker or an ordinary harness punch. No universal system is employed; each individual producer has his own ideas upon the subject.

3. Caring for the Herd Boar

Many hog raisers follow the plan of keeping or buying a young boar each year, keeping him as a boar only until the breeding season is over, then castrating him and sending him to market. By following this plan no special care need be given to him.

The more efficient raisers of market hogs and breeders of pure breeds prefer to retain boars to older ages, especially if their first crop of pigs indicates that they are highly successful sires.

Separation of the mature boars. It is usually advisable to keep mature boars separated in different boar pens. Boar pens should be so constructed as to accommodate one or at the most two mature boars of equal size.

Unequal size pairing may cause damage to the smaller boar from fighting and there might be a situation where the stronger one will have a tendency to deceive the weaker one from its

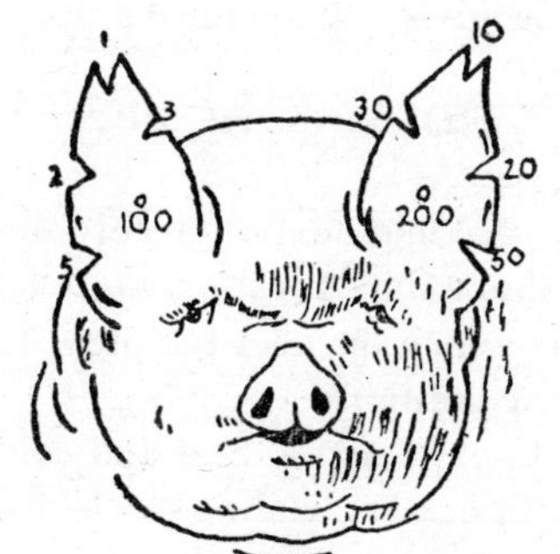

For 274 mark 200 + 50 + 20 + 3 + 1

Fig. 14.8

normal share of feed. It is a good practice to study the behaviour of the boars before selecting the pair for a single pen.

Range allowance. A serious mistake is made when a boar is confined to a very small filthy lot. An area of 30 feet wide and 100 feet long would give ample range for a boar. A lot that is quite high, dry, and well drained is preferred.

Rations for boar. A commonly suggested mixture of feeds for herd boars may be as follows; maize 40 per cent, oat 40 per cent, and a high protein supplemental mixture having 15 to 16 per cent protein. This composition may be modified to suit local conditions, considering the availability and economy of various feeds. Barley, wheat, sorghum grain may substitute maize. Oats may be replaced by grains of somewhat similar composition as wheat or barley. In the absence of good pasture, lucerne or berseem should be included in the ration either as such or as hay. A mineral mixture should be self fed.

Boars should not be allowed to become fat. Limit the feed to the needs of the boar. If the boar is young, make the allowance great enough to permit normal growth—about 1.5 kilogram of feed daily per 45 kg. of live weight. Mature boars usually need about one-half of this amount or about 750 grams of feed per 45 kg of body weight. Plenty of water is needed daily as a part of the ration.

Exercise. Outdoor exercise throughout the year is one of the first essentials in keeping the boar in a thrifty condition. When there is a lack of pasture, arrangement of properly fenced range is a must. Older boars may refuse to take sufficient exercise voluntarily, in which case the keeper should resort to driving the boar daily or provide some other means of exercise.

Ranting. Some boars pace back and forth along the fence, often "chopping their jaws and slobbering". Such action is called ranting. Young boars that take to excessive ranting may go off feed, become "shieldy" and fail to develop properly. Isolation from other boars or from the sow herd is an effective means of quieting such boars.

Clipping the tusk. As boars reach the age of two years or more, certain teeth called tusks appear on the sides of the jaws; they grow long and sharp and are dangerous to the caretaker as well to other animals. As soon as they become long enough to be dangerous, cut them back. It is wise to take the help of a veterinary surgeon. A boar treated properly, given plenty of company and handled sympathetically everyday will usually be reasonably docile even with the tusk. Even then it is advisable to clip the tusk.

HOUSING OF PIGS

Good housing with adequate accommodation incorporating all essential requirements of pigs must be provided so that the animals can grow quickly and efficiently. This is only possible through scientific housing which includes the provision for fresh air, exercise, sunlight protection from inclement weather conditions.

Pigs are very much susceptible to extremes of heat and cold and wide variations in temperature. Pigs are poorly provided with heat regulating mechanism and sweating only takes place from the snout. So it is difficult to keep them cool in hot weather. Temperature in a pig house is, therefore, one of the most important factors to be taken into consideration while erecting a pig house particularly in tropical countries.

Systems of Housing Pigs

Pigs are kept under two systems—open air system and indoor system. A combination of the two is, however, followed in most places in this country. Both these systems have advantages and disadvantages. The size of the enterprise, the type of pigs to be produced, the availability of land and the climatic conditions are the guiding factors for choosing the housing system. In case of farms with small holdings no special purpose pig house is necessary but in a specialised farm accommodating a large number of animals, there may be the necessity of constructing special purpose houses for different categories of stocks e.g., breeding stock and store pigs. The housing system will also vary depending on whether the pigs are kept under pasture or indoor, or a combination of the two.

Location

The farm should be located near the city where there is a heavy demand of pork products. This is particularly necessary to avoid the cost of transport of feed and other stuff as also for disposal of animals. Where pedigree pigs are sold in large numbers it is advantageous to locate the house near a railway station. Proximity to public utilities like electricity, gas and water supply will be an added help to the farm. At the same time the farm should not be situated in the municipal areas where there might be objection in future from health authorities as also for future possibilities of expansion.

Layout of building has a marked influence on efficient working. The most important item to be considered is the facility for proper sanitation with a good drainage system. The building should be situated in such a way that doors and windows will receive maximum sunlight and the pigs will get shelter from prevailing direction of the wind.

Enclosures

Permanent enclosures are necessary for permanent buildings and portable enclosures are necessary for rotational system where usually portable type of buildings are used. Permanent enclosures are usually provided by fences. Woven wire and chain linked wire-netting of 2″-3″ mesh of number 8 or 10 SWG are quite suitable. Pig fences should be 3′ to 5′ high and closely

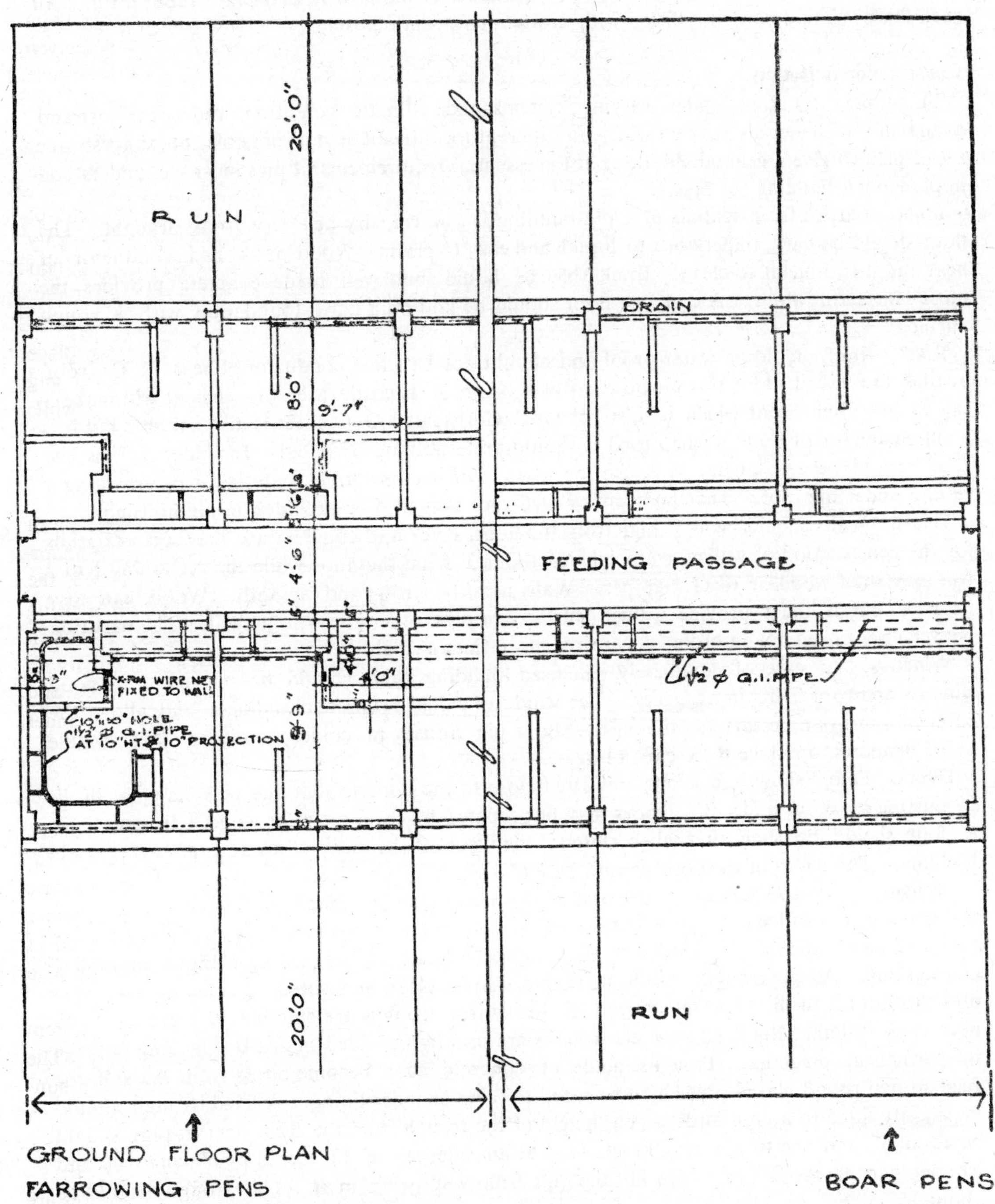

Fig. 14.9 Ground floor plan of farrowing and of Boar pens.

fitted to the ground with a single strand of barbed wire under it so that pigs cannot lift it. All such fences should be tightly fitted with strong intermediate posts.

Constructional Details

Since pigs are kept under varying systems and climatic conditions and as the cost and availability of materials vary so widely in different localities it is not possible to suggest one set of plan to give a generalised idea but the essential requirements of pigs must be understood in planning a building for pigs.

Floor. One of the essentials of a pig building is a warm, dry bed free from draught. The floor should be hard, impervious to liquid and easy to clean. Wood is a bad conductor of heat and it is difficult to clean. Brick absorbs liquid but well made concrete provides the most satisfactory floor. A concrete floor should be laid on a hard foundation with a rough surface.

Roof. Roof should be water proof and should not be a bad conductor of heat. R.C. roof or tiles are excellent for this purpose. But R.C. roof is costly, asbestos cement will make a satisfactory light roof which is also cheap. Corrugated G.I. sheet is also suitable but it is good conductor of heat so when used it should preferably be insulated. In colder regions the roof should be insulated. This can be done with an insulating material or by providing a ceiling under the roof. Thatched roof or tiled roof may also be provided in pig housing.

Walls. Walls should be 4′-5′ high from the floor. Brick and concrete are the best materials for the construction of walls for a height of about 3′ from the floor while the remaining 1 or 2 feet may be of wood or 1″ G.I. pipes. Walls must be strong and smooth. Wood can also be used but it must provide a flush surface to pigs, otherwise will gnaw it. The partition between pens need not in ordinary cases be more than 4′ high.

Windows. In case of completely enclosed building there should be provision of good window and roof lights in a piggery. The windows would promote cleanliness and allow the entry of sunrays necessary for the pigs. Many pig houses in colder countries have double gazed windows to reduce the escape of heat.

Doors. Doors should be strong and fitted close to the floor so that the pigs may not lift it by putting its snout under it. Doors may be prepared by sheet metal or wood. In any case a door should be such that when closed it may cut off the entry of air and rain water in the building. The width of the door should be 2′6″ to 3′.

Troughs. About 72 per cent of the cost of pig production is debited to food. So the position and construction of feed trough is considered to be an important factor. A trough space of about 12 inches should be provided to each pig to facilitate proper feeding without scrambling and fighting. All pig troughs should be strong, easy to clean and fitted in such a way that pigs can not tilt them. Portable galvanised heavy iron troughs are suitable in piggeries with deep litter system. But fixed concrete troughs are usually provided beside the feeding passage in permanent piggeries. Troughs made of concrete soon become pitted from acids in the feed so half round glazed pipes may be fitted to form an inner lining. A fixed trough should be slightly tilted to a plug outlet. The height of the trough from the floor next to pigs should be about 6″ and the trough may be divided at an interval of 12 inches by placing iron and wooden bars across trough to prevent the pigs from wallowing in it. The trough should be about 15″ wide.

Water supply. Water is required for cleaning and drinking purposes. Fresh drinking water should always be available to the pigs all the year round. Automatic drinking bowls

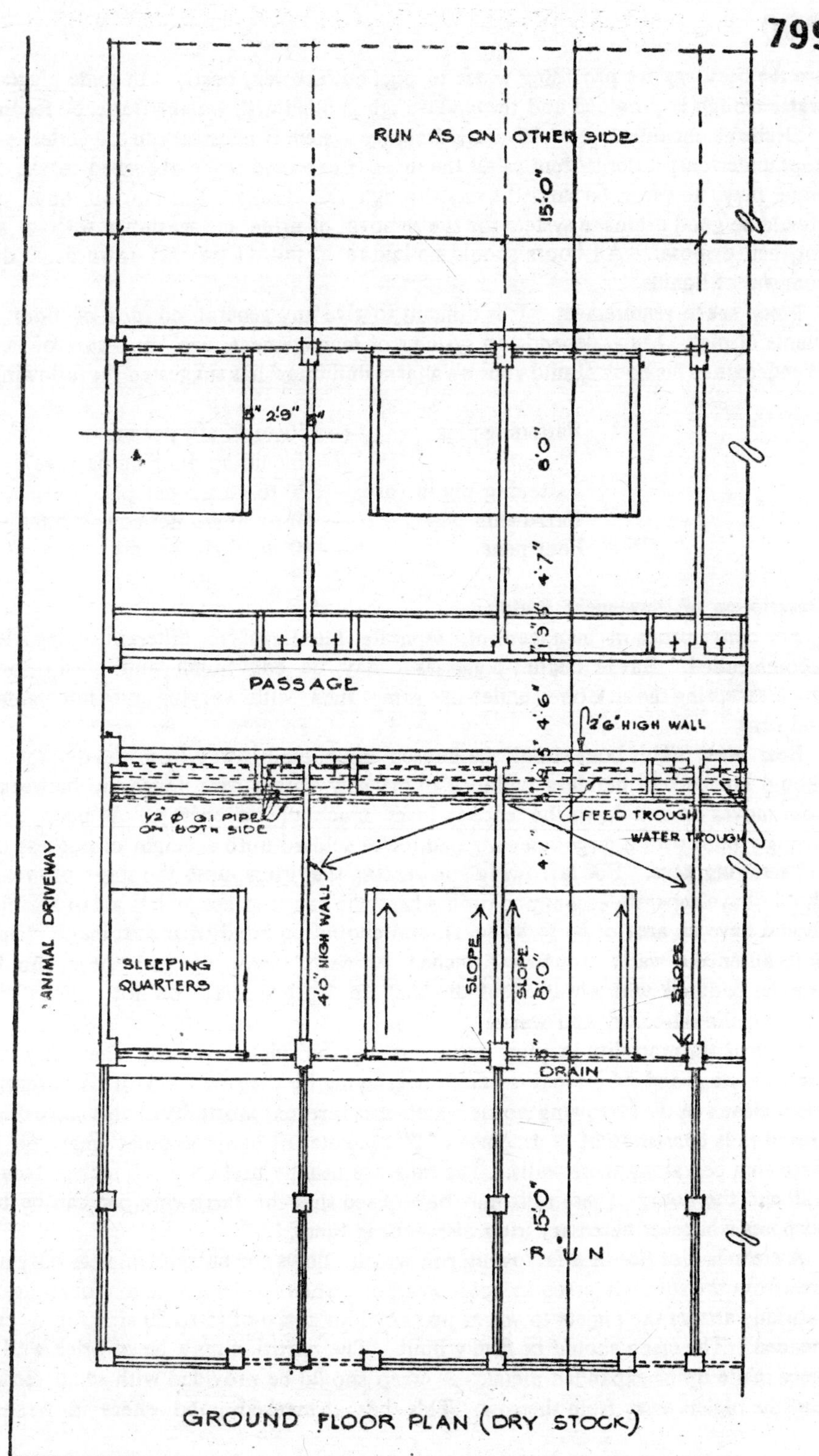
RUN AS ON OTHER SIDE
15'0"
5" 2'9" 5"
8'0"
4'7"
1'3"
PASSAGE
4'6"
2'6" HIGH WALL
½" Ø GI PIPE ON BOTH SIDE
FEED TROUGH
WATER TROUGH
4'1"
ANIMAL DRIVEWAY
SLEEPING QUARTERS
4'0" HIGH WALL
SLOPE
SLOPE
8'0"
SLOPE
DRAIN
15'0"
RUN
GROUND FLOOR PLAN (DRY STOCK)

Fig. 14.10

are the best way for providing water to pigs but are very costly. In some piggeries no separate water trough is provided and the feed trough is filled with water after each feeding.

Drainage facilities. No elaborate drainage system is necessary in piggeries where pigs are kept under deep litter system as all the urine is expected to be absorbed in the litter. Surplus water may, however, be carried away through the drains. But in all other piggeries there should be good drainage system for the removal of urine and washings with a suitable system for their disposal. All floors should be laid to a fall (1 in 72) towards a drain for rapid removal of liquid.

Floor space requirement. It is difficult to give any generalised idea of floor space requirements of pigs. Much depends on systems of management, age and size of animals. Frank Wenderson in his book 'Build your own farm buildings' has suggested the following requirements:

Fattening pigs	—	10 to 16 sft. per pig (including dunging passage)
Fattening pig in yards	—	30 to 40 sft. per pig
Farrowing pigs	—	60 to 80 sft. per sow & litter
Boar pens	—	40 to 50 sft. per pig.

Description of Permanent Buildings

For convenience in management, separate buildings for different categories of stock is recommended. But in smaller piggeries it may be convenient and cheap to house all the stock excepting the sick ones under the same shed with varying measurements of paddocks and pens.

Boar pens. This boar should be housed individually away from the dry sow unit. A boar should not be kept beside a paddock of dry sow with a wire fence in between as when the boar moves up and down the fence it loses much of its energy. A boar house should be strongly built with a large open air paddock enclosed upto a height of not less than 4½ feet.

Farrowing pens. For farrowing and rearing the litters, upto the stage of weaning, the sow should have separate accommodation where she can find her piglets all to herself. A farrowing should have an area of 60 to 80 sq. ft. and should be fitted with automatic drinking bowl or in its absence a water trough. Attached to each farrowing pen there should be a small exercise paddock with a wallow of about 8" in depth specially on hot regions of our country. The pen should be dry and warm.

Most of the mortality in pigs occur among the piglets during the early period of their suckling stage and major loss is due to overlaying by the sow. So it is essential to provide some means in the farrowing house which may prevent mortality at this stage due to trampling. Guard rails consisting of G.I. pipes of 2" diameter or bamboo poles may be placed in the farrowing pen along these walls. The rails are usually fitted 8 to 10 inches from and off the wall and the floor. These rails may be so fixed that the farrowing pen can be used for other purposes whenever necessary after dismantling them.

A creep is a device in a farrowing pen which allows the entry of piglets only as a protected area from the sow. A creep in cold weather, when provided with some heating unit, will naturally attract the piglets to warm up. A floor space of 15 to 20 sft. for a creep is recommended. The creep should be firmly built. The partition may be of brick wall 4' high or a fence made up of expanded metal. A creep should be provided with small feeding trough to feed the piglets away from the sow. This has a marked good effect in weaning weight of piglets. The floor of a farrowing pen may be kept warm and dry by spraying saw dust or similar material.

Dry sow and gilts. Dry sows and gilts do not require any special purpose buildings. They should be housed away from the breeding boars. Fully or partially covered yards or loose boxes may be used for dry sows and gilts.

Weaners and fatteners. A layout for convenient working may be a single or double row of pens with a feeding passage in front of or in between them. There should be an enclosed run attached to each pen so that the pigs can get enough fresh air, sunlight, exercise and have dunging space. The pen may be of rectangular shape with the feeding passage on its length and there should not be any door along the feeding passage so that all the frontage may be available for a continuous feed trough. In warm areas it will always be advantageous to have a wallowing tank 8″ deep in every run for the health and comfort of the pigs.

Segregation shed. Under the intensive system it is very difficult to control any outbreak of infectious disease. So a separate segregation shed away from the main units is necessary. Care should be taken to see that the wash water from the segregation shed does not pass through the drains beside the main units.

Other buildings. Food godown, store for miscellaneous equipment and office buildings should be located as near to the main piggery buildings as possible for facilities of work. Construction of these buildings will depend on the size of the herd and the capital available. A weighing yard with a few holding pens should be constructed centrally for periodical weighing of stock.

DIGESTION IN PIGS

From the diagram of the gastro-intestinal tract of the pig (Fig. 14.11) it may be seen that the pig has a large caecum and colon indicating that the pig is more related to the herbivore than to the carnivore. In fact that pig, like human beings, is considered an omnivorus animal as its feed is both of animal and vegetable origin.

Uptake and Mastication of Feed

Whenever ground concentrates mixed up with any liquid like water or skim milk is offered to the pig, it dips its snout to the bottom of the trough and sucks the mixed feed with the help of the tongue. Longer particles like grass or beets are chewed by the molar teeth. Since the angles of the mouth are situated far back, part of the mouth will always remain above the surface of the trough. The portion which remains above the surface sucks air together with the mixed feed. The suction of air into the mouth and rapid chewing movements with open lips cause the characteristic smacking and surping sounds. After the uptake of feed in the mouth, it is thoroughly mixed up with saliva. The amount of saliva depends upon the type of feed. Less the moisture content of the feed, more will be the secretion of saliva.

There are three salivary glands (a) parotid glands, lying in the space below the ear and behind the border of the lower jaw; (b) the submaxillary glands, lying just within the angle of the lower jaw and (c) the sublingual glands, which lies at the side of the root of the tongue. Each of these glands are paired, so that actually there are six glands. The parotid glands produce serus, an alkaline fluid, which normally contains small amounts of the enzyme *amylase*, aids in hydrolysing the carbohydrates. The activity is many times less than that found in human saliva. The secretion from the other salivary glands contains no enzyme. The carbohydrate portion of the diet is thus subjected to amylase action in the mouth which is continued for some time in the stomach until the acid in gastric juice has inactivated the enzyme.

Digestion in the Stomach

The wall of the stomach is full of glands. The ducts of these gastric glands open into the stomach cavity, so that as the gastric juice is produced it pours directly into the stomach cavity. Three types of cells have been described in the gastric glands. They are (1) parietal cells which secrete HCl, (2) neck cells which secrete mucin, a mucus substance; (3) chief cells which produce enzyme pepsinogen which later on changes into pepsin. Thus the gastric juice is composed of water, mucin, pepsin and HCl.

Even though food does not remain long enough in the mouth for amylase to complete the carbohydrate digestion, the action of the enzyme continues long after the food has entered the stomach. The pH optimum for amylase is about 7, however, it will continue to act until the pH has fallen to 4.5. The first phase of gastric secretion is called the amylolytic phase. Bacterial carbohydrases and carbohydrases of the feed will also show activity during the amylolytic phase of gastric digestion. Through the action of these enzymes starch and other polysaccharides are broken down to soluble carbohydrates such as, erythrodextrin and, to some extent, to maltose.

As stomach juice penetrates the swallowed feed the pepsin starts to break down the feed proteins. There will then be the phase with both amylolytic and proteolytic activity, the amyloproteolytic phase of gastric digestion. Through the action of pepsin and HCl the feed protein are broken down to peptides. The pH optimum for pepsin is about 2.

When the pH fall below 4 the amylase activity is completely inhibited and the only enzyme acting is pepsin. It is to be noted that the various phase of digestion in the stomach go on concomitantly.

No lipases are secreted from the stomach glands. Gastric juice may show weak lypolytic activity due to lipases reflexed from the small intestine into the stomach. These lipases may liberate some free fatty acids from ingested lipids. However, the main change of feed lipids in the stomach is a result of gastric motility which by churning and kneading turn the lipids into a coarse emulsion.

Digestion in the Small Intestine

The liver and pancreas are the two large glands connected to the first part of the small intestine. By peristaltic movement of the small intestine the content is mixed and transferred through three parts, viz., duodenum, the jejunum and the ilium. In the small intestine the digestion is continued through the action of the enzymes from the intestinal glands and from pancreatic secretion.

There is a continuous formation and secretion of bile in the liver. Part of this bile is stored in the gall bladder and part of it flows directly through the duct to the small intestine. In liver bile the percentage of dry matter is about 3 whereas bladder bile has about 16 per cent dry matter. The higher dry matter content in the bladder is due to absorption of water from the gall bladder. The major organic components of bile are the bile pigments and the bile salts with significant amounts of lipids as phospholipids (mainly lacithin and lyso-lecithin) and some cholesterol are present. Bile salts are sodium and potassium salts of glycocholic or taurocholic acid. The reaction is usually weak alkaline with a pH of about 7 to 8.

Pancreas is both an endocrine and exocrine gland. The endocrine secretions, insulin and glucagon are not considered here. There are three proteolytic zymogens in pancreatic juice namely, trypsinogen, chymotrypsinogen and a procarboxypeptidase. All three zymogens are then rapidly converted into active enzymes such as trypsin, chymotrypsin and carboxypeptidase respectively. Apart from proteolytic enzymes the pancreatic juice, which is clear and distinctly alkaline contains several other lypolytic and amylolytic enzymes. The pig secretes from 7 to 15 litres of pancreatic juice per day.

The duodenal mucosa contains branched coiled tubular glands called *Brunner glands*, that give an abundant secretion. It is viscous, sticky fluid with an alkaline reaction. The pH of duodenal juice from pigs ranges from 8.4 to 8.9. The alkali and mucin or mucin like substances in the secretion protect the intestinal mucosa from injury by the acid chyme coming from the stomach. There might be some digestive enzymes in the duodenal secretion.

When the acid chyme from the stomach is mixed with the alkaline secretion from the liver, the pancreas and the intestinal gland, the acid is partly neutralised and the pH of the intestinal content rises slowly as the content is passed down through the tract.

The lipolytic activity of pancreatic juice is due to a specific enzyme, pancreatic lipase which removes only fatty acid residues linked to primary hydroxyl groups (α groups) of triglycerides. The rate of lipase action is increased by emulsifying agents such as bile salts, lecithin and lysolecithin.

The digestion of starch initiated by salivary amylase is continued by the action of pancreatic amylase, resulting starch into maltose and isomaltose. Ingested carbohydrates with different glucosidic linkages are attacked by other carbohydrases present in the intestinal secretions. The products of the action of these carbohydrases are different disaccharides. The epithelial cells of the small intestine contain four enzymes, lactase, sucrase, maltase and isomaltase, which are capable of splitting the disaccharides lactose, sucrose, maltose and isomaltose respectively, into their constituent monosaccharides. There is much reason to believe that these enzymes are located in the brush border of the cell linning the lumen of the intestine and that the disaccharides are digested as they come in contact with this border. The digested products are then immediately absorbed into the portal blood.

However, it is important to note that raw potato starch and cellulose are not digested by the the intestinal enzymes in the pig. Part of these substances are digested by bacterial fermentation in the large intestine including caecum.

Digestion in Caecum and Colon

It has been known for a long time that the pig can digest crude fibre to some extent and that this digestion is entirely dependent upon bacterial fermentation in the caecum and colon. The digestible coefficient of crude fibre of normal swine varies from 10 to 90 per cent. The variations are probably due to (1) changes in the intestinal flora which again varies with the type of diet. In normal pigs there are 10^8 to 10^9 micro-organisms per gram of caecal contents, The predominating species are lactobacilli and streptococci, and (2) to the amount of cellulose in the ration. It has been estimated that the optimum level of crude fibre in swine ration should be about 6 to 7 per cent.

The products of bacterial fermentation of cellulose are volatile fatty acids (VFA) with acetic acid as the predominant acid. The average composition of mixed VFA from the caecum of pigs is as follows: 62 per cent acetic acid, 28 per cent propionic acid and 10 per cent butyric acid.

Cuthbertson and Philipson in a review stated "If the products of bacterial decomposition

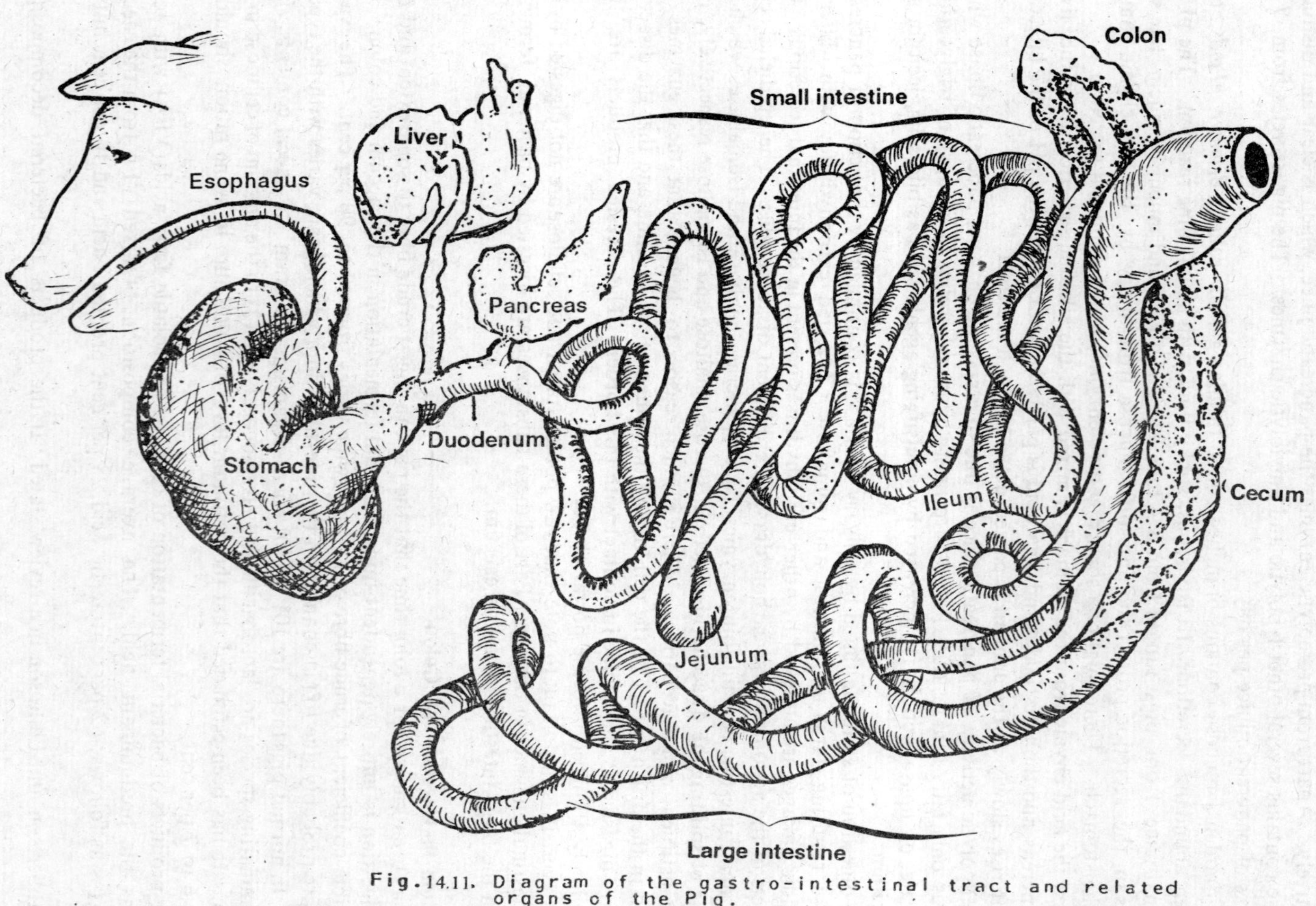

Fig. 14.11. Diagram of the gastro-intestinal tract and related organs of the Pig.

of cellulose in the large intestine of omnivorus can be utilised as productively by pigs as by ruminants then fodder cellulose should have a value for fattening pigs not much inferior to that of oats".

VFA produced in the caecum and colon of pigs are rapidly absorbed in the blood system and are readily utilised by the animal.

Regarding proteins, substantial amount of digestible proteins are absorbed after hydrolysis in the small intestine. Some amount of amides and non essential amino acids are catabolised and due to deamination results in the formation of ammonia which is readily absorbed through caecum and colon. Since ammonia is a toxic substance, it is converted into urea and excreted again. This process results in loss of energy. The extent to which it normally occurs in pigs is unknown.

Micro-organisms are capable of synthesising several water soluble vitamins and thus plays a role in the normal supply of these elements. The beneficial effect which is sometimes observed by the addition of antibiotics may be due to a depression of pathological micro-organisms. The advantage of a general and continuous addition of antibiotics to swine ration is, for many reasons, doubtful.

NUTRITION OF PIG

Problems in Supplying Feed Nutrients to Pigs

Successful swine production requires a carefully planned and efficient feeding programme. Diets that would suffice a few years ago are not adequate now because of more specialisation and intensification of the swine farming.

Through proper breeding and selection, rapid growing strains of swine have been developed. Owners of the farms now plan to market their hogs at 5 months of age instead of 7–8 months that was in practice a few years ago. Apart from this planning for larger litters (piglets at a time) and breeding to farrow twice a year forces the swine producers to adopt refined methods of scientific feeding programmes.

1. **Need for balancing the diets.** To have the profitable and efficient production, pigs must be provided with sufficient protein, minerals, vitamins, fats and carbohydrates in their daily ration. For this, swine producers must know the nutrient requirements of the pig, the characteristics of a good diet and the nutritive value of the feeds used in pig diets. They also need to learn how to put all the information together into a well balanced and economical feeding programme.

2. **Avoiding small pig losses.** About one-third of the pigs farrowed die before they reach market. This results in a huge loss to swine producers each year, the blame although cannot be solely entrusted to faulty nutrition, but nutritional deficiencies account for a good part of them. Thus the losses can significantly be lowered down by adopting a sound feeding programme for the newly born pigs.

3. **What makes a good ration?** While thinking of a good pig ration, most nutritionists think in terms of 'nutrients' which can be of any food constituent that aids in the support of animal life. These now consist of 10 essential amino acids, 18 vitamins, about 15 essential mineral elements, some essential fatty acids, carbohydrates and some unidentified factors.

These nutrients are required to be furnished in such correct proportion, level and form as will meet the full demand of the pigs at their particular age and physiological conditions.

While selecting the nutrients it should be considered that a good diet should also be palatable. Certain feed ingredients when added to the ration increase palatability and others decrease it. Thus a knowledge of feeds; specially of unconventional agro-industrial by-product is extremely necessary with regard to their overall effect on palatability.

Table 14.5

Essential data required for the calculation of rations for pigs and for assessment of their performance

Class and liveweight of pigs (kg)	*Nutritive ratio required in the ration*	*Average daily feed intake (kg)*	*Expected average daily liveweight gain (kg)*
Piglets (Birth to 14)			
Creep feed for weaners	1.0:4.0-4.5	0.14-0.7	0.32
Weaners (14-23)			
Starter rations	1.0:4.5	0.7-1.4	0.29
Growers (23–54)	1.0:4.5-5.5		0.64
25		1.4	
32		1.8	
41		2.0	
Fatteners (45–91)	1.0:5.5-7.0		0.84
45		2.3	
59		2.5	
68		2.5-2.7	
Pregnant gilts and sows	1.0:5.0	2.3	
Suckling gilts and sows	1.0:5.0	5.4 or 0.9 plus 0.5 for each suckling pig	
Boars	1.0:5.0		
<15 months of age		2.7	
>15 months of age		2.3	

Source: Durrance, K.L. (1971), *Basic Information for Swine Production*, University of Florida: Gainsville.

An ideal ration usually contain a variety of feeds and supplements, which tend to improve the balance of the diet and thus prevent certain nutritional deficiencies.

All care must be taken to avoid toxic substances which might be incorporated due to the addition of some high percentage of unconventional feed stuffs in the ration.

Similarly feed ingredients specially of oil cakes which are apt to become rancid must be guarded against. Rancid diets are not only low in palatability but also destroys certain nutrients including some vitamins.

4. **Nutrient requirements of the pig.** The recommended nutrient levels given in Table 14.6 are to be used as a guide. In most cases, they do not contain a margin of safety. Some of the important factors which affect nutrient needs and thus alters the recommended levels are summarised in Table 14.5

Table 14.6

Nutrient requirements of growing swine fed *ad-libitum*: percentage or amount per kilogram of air-dry diet

Nutrients	*Requirements*				
Liveweight (kg)	*5–10*	*10–20*	*20–50*	*35–60*	*60–100*
Daily gain (kg)	*0.30*	*0.50*	*0.60*	*0.75*	*0.90*
(1)	*(2)*	*(3)*	*(4)*	*(5)*	*(6)*
Energy and Protein					
TDN (%)	70.4	79.4	74.8	74.8	74.8
Digestible energy[a] (kcal)	3,500	3,500	3,300	3,300	3,300
Metabolisable energy[a] (kcal)	3,360	3,360	3,170	3,170	3,170
Crude protein[b] (%)	22	18	16	14	13
Inorganic Nutrients (%)					
Calcium	0.80	0.65	0.65	0.50	0.50
Phosphorus	0.60	0.50	0.50	0.40	0.40
Sodium	—	0.10	0.10	—	—
Chlorine	—	0.13	0.13	—	—
Vitamins					
Beta-carotene (mg)	4.4	3.5	2.5	2.6	2.6
Vitamin A (IU)	2,200	1,750	1,300	1,300	1,300
Vitamin D (IU)	200	200	200	125	125
Vitamin E (mg)	11	11	11	11	11
Thiamine (mg)	1.3	1.1	1.1	1.1	1.1
Riboflavin (mg)	3.0	3.0	2.6	2.2	2.2
Niacin[c] (mg)	22.0	18.0	14.0	10.0	10.0
Pantothenic acid (mg)	13.0	11.0	11.0	11.0	11.0
Vitamin B_6 (mg)	1.5	1.5	1.1	—	—
Choline (mg)	1,100	900	—	—	—
Vitamin B_{12} (μg)	22	15	11	11	11

Table 14.6 (*Contd.*)

(1)	(2)	(3)	(4)	(5)	(6)
Amino acids (%)					
Arginine	0.28	0.23	0.20	0.18	0.16
Histidine	0.25	0.20	0.18	0.16	0.15
Isoleucine	0.69	0.56	0.50	0.44	0.41
Leucine	0.83	0.68	0.60	0.52	0.48
Lysine	0.96	0.79	0.70	0.61	0.57
Methionine + Cystine[d]	0.69	0.56	0.50	0.44	0.41
Phenylalanine + tyrosine[e]	0.69	0.56	0.50	0.44	0.41
Threonine	0.62	0.51	0.45	0.39	0.37
Tryptophan	0.18	0.15	0.13	0.11	0.11
Valine	0.69	0.56	0.50	0.44	0.41

[a] These suggested energy levels are derived from maize-based diets. When barley or medium or low-energy grains are fed, these energy levels will not be met. Formulations based on barley or similar grains are satisfactory for pigs weighing 20–100 kg, but feed conversion will normally be reduced with the lower-energy diets.

[b] Approximate protein levels required to meet the essential amino acid needs. If cereal grains other than maize are used, an increase of 1 or 2 per cent of protein may be required.

[c] It is assumed that all the niacin in the cereal grains and their by-products is in a bound form and thus is largely unavailable.

[d] Methionine can fulfill the total requirement; cystine can meet at least 50 per cent of the total requirement.

[e] Phenylalanine can fulfill the total requirement; tyrosine can fulfill 30 per cent of the total requirement.

SOURCE: *Nutrient Requirement of Swine*, Seventh Revised Edition, National Research Council, Washington, D C. 1973.

5. Variation in individual requirements. Nutritive requirements of animals are achieved on the basis of the performance of a group of animals. The average of the group is used to determine rate of gain and feed efficiency. Thus chances will always remain when the recommendation which is applicable for a group may be deficient for some individual animals who have a higher requirement or for some reason do not utilise it efficiently.

6. Variation in availability of nutrients in feeds. Availability of any nutrients present in the feed stuff varies due to various reasons depending on their form. A swine feeding trial should be the best criterion for determining whether a certain combination of feeds supplied by manufacturer is adequate in certain nutrients.

7. Variation in results with natural versus purified diets. Almost all the nutrient requirements that have been determined for pigs are based on purified diet experiment. It is most likely that as compared to purified diets, there is some difference in the availability of nutrients in practical type of ration. Many of the nutrients, such as minerals and vitamins, are added to purified diets in relatively pure forms. This is not the state of affairs in natural diet where vitamin and minerals are present in various forms. Moreover, the two different diets will have as different effect on the intestinal synthesis of certain nutrients which subsequently

Table 14.7

Daily nutrient requirements of growing swine

Nutrients	*Requirements*				
Liveweight (kg)	*7.5*	*15*	*27.5*	*47.5*	*80*
Feed intake (Air-dry (kg)	*0.600*	*1.250*	*1.700*	*2.500*	*3.500*
Dry matter (kg)	0.54	1.12	1.53	2.25	3.15
Energy and protein.[a,b]					
TDN (kg)	0.48	0.99	1.27	1.87	2.62
Digestible energy (kcal)	2.100	4.370	5.670	8.250	11.552
Metabolisable energy (kcal)	2.020	4.200	5.390	7.920	11.090
Crude protein (kg)	0.132	0.225	0.272	0.350	0.455
Inorganic Nutrients					
Calcium (kg)	0.0048	0.0081	0.0110	0.0125	0.0175
Phosphorus (kg)	0.0036	0.0063	0.0085	0.0100	0.0140
Sodium (kg)	—	0.0013	0.0017	—	—
Chlorine (kg)	—	0.0016	0.0022	—	—
Vitamins					
Beta-carotene[c] (mg)	2.6	4.4	4.4	6.5	9.1
Vitamin A (IU)	1,300	2,200	2,200	3,2500	4,550
Vitamin D (IU)	132	250	340	312	437
Vitamin E (mg)	6.6	13.8	18.7	27.5	38.5
Thiamine (mg)	0.8	1.4	1.9	2.8	3.9
Riboflavin (mg)	1.8	3.8	4.4	5.5	7.7
Niacin[d] (mg)	13.2	22.5	23.8	25.0	35.0
Panthothenic acid (mg)	7.8	13.8	18.7	27.5	38.5
Vitamin B_6 (mg)	0.9	1.9	1.9	—	—
Choline (mg)	660	1.125	—	—	—
Vitamin B_{12} (μg)	13.2	18.8	18.7	27.5	38.5
Amino Acids (g)					
Arginine	1.6	2.8	3.4	4.4	5.7
Histidine	1.5	2.5	3.1	3.9	5.1
Isoleucine	4.1	7.0	8.5	10.9	14.2
Leucine	5.0	8.4	10.2	13.1	17.1
Lysine	5.8	9.8	11.9	15.3	19.9
Methionine+cystine[e]	4.1	7.0	8.5	10.9	14.2
Phenylalanine+tyrosine[f]	4.1	7.0	8.5	10.9	14.2
Threonine	3.7	6.3	7.6	9.8	12.2
Tryptophan	1.1	1.8	2.2	2.8	3.7
Valine	4.1	7.0	8.5	10.9	14.2

[a]These suggested energy levels are derived from maize-based diets. When barley or medium or low-energy grains are fed, these energy levels will not be met. Formulations based on barley or similar grains are satisfactory for pigs weighing 20–100 kg, but feed conversion will normally be reduced with the lower-energy diets.

[b]Approximate protein levels required to meet the essential amino acid needs. If cereal grains other than corn are used, an increase of 1 or 2 per cent of protein may be required.

[c]Carotene and vitamin A Values are based on 1 mg of beta-carotene equalling 500 IU of biologically active Vitamin A. Vitamin A requirements can be met by carotene or vitamin A or both.

[d]It is assumed that all the niacin in the cereal grains and their by-products is in a bound form and thus is largely unavailable.

[e]Methionine can fulfill the total requirement; cystine can meet at least 50 per cent of the total requirement.

[f]Phenylalanine can fulfill the total requirement; tyrosine can fulfill 32 per cent of the requirement.

Source: *Nutrient Requirement of Swine*, Seventh Revised Edition, National Research Council, Washington, D.C. 1973.

Table 14.8

Nutrient requirements of breeding swine: percentage or amount per kilogram of air-dry diet

Nutrients	*Requirements*		
Liveweight (kg)	*110–250*	*140–250*	*110–250*
Energy and Protein			
TDN (%)	74.8	74.8	74.8
Digestible energy (kcal)	3,300	3,300	3,300
Metabolisable energy (kcal)	3,170	3,170	3,170
Crude protein (%)	14	15	14
Inorganic Nutrients (%)			
Calcium	0.75	0.75	0.75
Phosphorus	0.50	0.50	0.50
NaCl (salt)	0.5	0.5	0.5
Vitamins			
Beta-carotene (mg)	8.2	6.6	8.2
Vitamin A (IU)	4,100	3,300	4,100
Vitamin D (IU)	275	220	275
Vitamin E (mg)	11.0	11.0	11.0
Thiamine (mg)	1.5	1.0	1.5
Riboflavin (mg)	4.0	3.5	4.0
Niacin (mg)	22.0	17.5	22.0
Pantothenic acid (mg)	16.5	13.0	16.5
Vitamin B_{12} (μg)	14.0	11.0	14.0
Amino Acids (%)			
Arginine	—	0.34[b]	c
Isoleucine	0.37	0.67[b]	c
Histidine	0.20[a]	0.26[b]	c
Lucine	0.66[a]	0.99[b]	c
Lysine	0.42	0.60[b]	c
Methionine + cystine	0.28	0.36[b]	c
Phenylalanine + tyrosine	0.52[a]	1.00[b]	c
Threonine	0.34	0.51[b]	c
Tryptophan	0.07	0.13[b]	c
Valine	0.46	0.68[b]	c

[a]This level is adequate; the minimum requirement has not been established.

[b]All suggested requirements for lactation are based on the requirement for maintenance + amino acids produced in milk by sows fed 5–5.5 kg of feed per day from which amino acids are 80 per cent available.

[c]No data available, it is suggested that the requirement will not exceed that of bred gilts and sows.

Table 14.9

Daily nutrient requirements of breeding swine

Nutrients	*Requirements*					
	Breed Gilts	*Breed Sows*	*Lact Gilts*	*Lact sows*	*Young Boars*	*Adult Boars*
Liveweight (kg)	*110–160*	*160–250*	*140–200*	*200–250*	*110–180*	*180–250*
Feed intake (air-dry) (kg)	*2,000*	*2,000*	*5,000*	*5,500*	*2,500*	*2,000*
Dry matter (kg)	1.8	1.8	4.5	5.0	2.3	1.8
Energy and Protein						
TDN (kg)	1.5	1.5	3.7	4.1	1.9	1.5
Digestible energy (kcal)	6.600	6.600	16.500	18.150	8.250	6.600
Metabolisable energy (kcal)	6.340	6.340	15.840	17.420	7.920	6.340
Crude protein (kg)	0.280	0.280	0.750	0.825	0.350	0.280
Inorganic Nutrients						
Calcium (kg)	0.0150	0.0150	0.0375	0.0412	0.0188	0.0150
Phosphorus (kg)	0.0100	0 0100	0.0250	0.0275	0.0125	0.0100
NaCl (salt) (kg)	0.0100	0.0100	0.0250	0.0275	0.0125	0.0100
Vitamins						
Beta-carotene (mg)	16.4	16.4	33.0	36.3	20.5	16.4
Vitamin A (IU)	8,200	8,200	16,500	18,150	10,250	8,200
Vitamin D (IU)	550	550	1.100	1.210	690	550
Vitamin E (mg)	22.0	22.0	55.0	60.5	27.5	22.0
Thiamin (mg)	3.0	3.0	5.0	5.5	3.8	3.0
Riboflavin (mg)	8.0	8.0	17.5	19.3	10.0	8.0
Niacin (mg)	44.0	44.0	87.5	96.3	55.0	44.0
Pantothenic acid (mg)	33.0	33.0	65.0	71.5	41.3	33.0
Vitamin B_{12} (μg)	28.0	28.0	55.0	60.5	35.0	28.0
Amino Acids (g)						
Arginine			17.0	18.7	NA	c
Histidine	4.0	4.0	13.0	14.3	NA	c
Isoleucine	7.4	7.4	33.5	36.9	NA	c
Leucine	13.2	13.2	46.4	51.0	NA	c
Lysine	8.4	8.4	30.0	33.0	NA	c
Metionine+cystine	5.6	5.6	18.0	19.8	NA	c
Phenylalanine+tyrosine	10.4	10.4	46.9	51.6	NA	c
Threonine	6.8	6.8	25.5	28.1	NA	c
Tryptophan	1.4	1.4	6.5	7.2	NA	c
Valine	9.2	9.2	34.0	37.4	NA	c

[a]Expected daily gain for bred gilts is 0.35–0.45 kg; for bred sows, 0.15–0.30 kg and for young boars, 0.25–0.45 kg.

NA=Not available, intakes 25 per cent greater than those of bred gilts are suggesed to adequate.

[c]Data unavailable, intakes equal to those of bred sows are suggested to adequate.

affect their need in the diet. Thus there is some difference in the requirement of nutrients under two sets of conditions.

8. **Stress condition may cause variation.** Stress condition such as temperature, moisture, humidity, improper and irregular feeding, poor housing, etc., can alter the need for certain nutrients. In such cases specially prepared stress feeds are used containing higher levels of nutrients with added additives. Thus pig producer needs to apply good judgment when increasing nutrient levels above standard requirement like NRC requirements.

9. **Variation due to Nutrient inter-relationships.** It is extremely difficult to suggest the requirement of certain nutrients until their inter-relationships with other nutrients are known. Examples of few such inter-relationships are choline and methionine; methionine and cystine; phenylalanine and tyrosine; niacin and tryptophan; calcium-manganese and copper; zinc-copper and protein; copper-zinc and iron; vitamin-D-calcium and phosphorus; iron and phosphorus; moybdenum-copper and sulfur; sodium and potassium; biotin and pantothenic acid; B_{12} and methionine; vitamin E and selenium. All these inter-relationships explain why there is some variation in the nutrient requirements.

10. **Variation due to peroxidising of lipids in the ration.** The very presence of peroxidising lipid can destroy certain nutrients. Unless some antioxidants are previously added, the requirement for the nutrients which are affected will be higher.

11. **Variation due to faster growth.** Nutrient requirements as suggested quite a few years ago may not be adequate for the modern day pig having faster growth rate, high feed efficiency ratio and a lean carcass.

12. **Variation due to subclinical disease level.** This refers to a condition when an animal suffers from some disease but nothing seems to be wrong externally. However, it causes the pig to perform below the normality and thereby requires special attention for increasing selective nutrients in the diet.

13. **Variation due to other factors.** Factors other than already discussed are: (a) environmental temperature, (b) destruction of nutrients by light or irradiation, (c) antibiotics, hormones and other feed additives in the diet, (d) absorption of nutrients on colloids in the feed and in the intestinal tract, (e) toxins from aflatoxins or other deleterious compounds present in the feed, (f) enzymes, such as thiaminase, in feeds which destroy nutrients.

Thus the recommended nutrient levels given in Tables 14.6 to 14.9 are to be used as a guide. Some margin of safety needs to be used with certain nutrients. The safety factors will vary with the different situations encountered. The only best way to know whether a diet lack certain nutrients is to run a feeding trial and to ascertain whether the addition of the nutrients are sufficient and beneficial.

PROTEIN REQUIREMENTS OF THE PIG

Swine must have good quality protein in the diet. Protein levels are important but not merely as important as proper amino acid balance. If proteins are fed that do not contain adequate amounts of the dietary essential amino acids, then these amino acids must be added in the form of higher quality protein or as the specific amino acids.

The growing pig needs a dietary source of each of the 10 essential amino acids and in addition, needs some of the non-essential ones as an additional source of nitrogen. Tryptophan, lysine and methionine are the amino acids most likely to be deficient in swine rations consists mostly of grains and their by-products.

The main functions of protein in animal body have already been described in Chapter 10. Thus swine require a regular intake of protein without which pigs suffer from reduction in growth or loss of weight. Ultimately, for maintenance of body functions protein will be withdrawn from certain tissues. Since the antibodies are composed of protein, any sort of deficiency will lower down the resisting power of the animals against any disease. Adequate protein in the diet not only maintain vigour but also prevents from becoming ill.

I. Essential Amino Acids

Being monogastric, pigs require a constant supply of eight out of 22 amino acids naturally found in animal body of pig. All these 8 amino acids are known as "essential amino acids" since either the body cannot synthesize them or if synthesized these are not in sufficient quantities as required by the animal.

The eight essential amino acids, which must be included in swine diets, are given below as % of total diet.

Isoleucine	0.63	Phenylalanine	0.88
Leucine	0.75	Threonine	0.56
Lysine	0.95	Tryptophan	0.15
Methionine	0.56	Valine	0.63

At least one-half of the methionine requirement can be met by cystine, and one-half of the phenylalanine requirement can be met by tyrosine. Lysine is the first limiting amino acid in swine growth and is often considered critically when balancing rations. As long as the amino acid requirements are met, some variation in the total protein level of the diet will not adversely affect rate of gain.

II. Quality of Dietary Protein

A good quality dietary protein is that which can supply the various essential amino acids at proper amount and ratio. If one essential amino acid is deficient then the other essential amino acids can only be utilised upto the level of the deficient one. This means that deficiency of even a single essential amino acid will cause the entire diet to be inadequate. For this reason it is a must that feeds low in one or more of the essential amino acids should be fed in combination with other protein sources, otherwise swine will make inefficient use of the protein supplied by that feed leading poor growth.

Proper combinations of vegetable, animal and fish proteins can be made to supply all the essential amino acids.

III. Time factor in Protein Feeding

Since amino acids are not stored in the system to any appreciable extent, animals do better if they are fed all the required, essential amino acids at the same time. It has already pointed out earlier that lack of any one essential amino acid in the diet will decrease the use of all the others. Many pig producers prefer to feed maize or other cereal grains at any time of the day followed by supplying or protein supplement in the morning and only cereal grains in the evening with good results. But when the interval of supplemental protein feeding was increased to 36 or 48 hours (two and three feeding of cereal grains than one feeding of protein supplement) there is a decrease in rate of gain, efficiency of feed utilisation and nitrogen retention resulted.

Table 14.10

Limiting amino acids for pigs

Feedstuffs	*First order*	*Second order*	*Comments*
Soybean meal (dehulled)	Methionine	Threonine	The meal must be properly heated to destroy inhibitory factors.
Meat and Bone	Tryptophan	Methionine	Good source of calcium and phosphorus
Barley	Lysine	Threonine	Lysine is about 0.5%
Wheat	Lysine	Threonine	Lysine is about 0.5%
Milo bran	Lysine	Threonine	Lysine is about 0.2%
Maize	Lysine	Tryptophan	Lysine is about 0.2%
Linseed meal			
Cotton seed meal	Lysine	Methionine	Lysine is about 1.5%. Contains gossypol
Sunflower-seed meal	Lysine	Methionine	—

IV. Excess Protein

Excess protein in the diet is equally bad as feeding diet deficient in protein. First of all excess protein in the feed cannot be stored except in limited quantity thus the unwanted amount is thrown out of body through urine as ammonia or urea. This is a direct way of taxing kidney. The remainder of the protein molecule serves as a source of energy or is stored as fat. Thus excess protein is not entirely wasted but definitely uneconomic since energy from carbohydrate source is comparatively cheaper.

V. Effect of Amino Acid Deficiencies

The effect of feeding diets having deficiency of individual essential amino acid is discussed as below:

1. LYSINE. Swine diet mostly comprises cereal grains and their by-products, all are more or less deficient in lysine. A deficiency of lysine causes reduced appetite, loss of weight, poor feed efficiency, rough, dry hair coat and a general emaciated condition. The lysine requirements of the pig are shown in Tables 14.7 to 14.9.

2. TRYPTOPHAN. Tryptophan is another essential amino acid which is present in most of the cereal grain at low levels. The bulk of the tryptophan which is metabolised by an enzyme 2, 3-dioxygenase ultimately turns into nicotinic acid. Tryptophan is thus to be regarded as a provitamin for nicotinamide. But the reverse reaction does not occur. Deficiency in the diet causes a loss in weight, poor feed consumption, depraved appetite, rough hair coat and symptoms of inanition in the pig.

3. METHIONINE. This is an essential amino acid which in the normal course of its metabolism provides sulphur for the synthesis of cysteine and cystine but the reverse reaction does not

occur. When the diet is adequate in cystine, methionine is no longer needed for cystine synthesis instead, it is used as methionine to form new tissues and carry out the functions for which methionine is required.

Deficiency of this amino acid results in reduced rate of gain and efficiency of feed utilisation.

Methionine has got another inter-relationship with choline. The acid can furnish methyl groups for choline synthesis. Diet which is mildly deficient in both, adding either one will improve growth.

Methionine also has a key role in transmethylation, the process by which methyl groups are transferred to appropriate acceptors to give physiological important compounds such as creatine and adrenaline.

4. THREONINE. Like that of lysine and methionine, synthesis of threonine depends on the formation of aspartic acid semialdehyde, which cannot be made in most higher animals. Consequently, threonine is also regarded as an essential amino acid. During catabolism it is finally converted into succinyl coenzyme A.

Occasionally threonine is found to be a limiting amino acid in the monogastric diet. Deficiency will lead lowered feed consumption, slow growth rate and poor feed utilisation.

5. ISOLEUCINE. A branched chain essential amino acid is transaminated to 2-keto acid, oxidatively decarboxylated and subjected to several further reactions, resulting the formation of equimolar proportions of acetyl coenzyme A and propionyl coenzyme A.

Cornell workers observed that a lack of isoleucine in the diet decreased rate of gain, feed efficiency ratio and nitrogen retention.

6. VALINE. The acid may be the third or fourth limiting amino acid in some swine feeds like soybean meal, wheat, etc. Deficiency causes lowered feed consumption, poor growth rate and feed efficiency.

7. HISTIDINE. It may be the fifth limiting amino acid in bone and meat meal. A deficiency in diet leads to poor growth and feed efficiency ratio. The pharmacologically important substance histamine is formed from histidine by decarboxylation of histidine.

8. PHENYLALANINE. Phenylalanine is another essential amino acid. The normal catabolism of the acid proceeds by hydroxylation to tyrosine. This means that if the diet contains enough of tyrosine, phenylalanine which is a dietary essential acid, will not be used up for the synthesis of tyrosine rather it will then perform the reaction for which phenylalanine is exclusively required. A deficiency of the amino acid in the diet resulted in decreased growth and efficiency of feed utilisation.

9. ARGININE. The compound is of immense importance in urea synthesis. In general, it is prevalent in all common pig diets. Like other essential amino acids, arginine deficiency also causes slower growth and poor efficiency of feed utilisation. The compound can be synthesised at a rate sufficient to allow 65-70 per cent of normal growth but a small amount of arginine in daily ration of pig must be ensured to fulfill the total requirement.

10. LEUCINE. The compound is moderately distributed in all feed ingredients used for pig and hardly one can expect deficiency symptoms arise out of scarcity of the compound in daily diet.

VI. Urea as Protein Substitute

Urea, the compound which is used in dairy cattle ration as substitute of natural protein, is not at all beneficial to pigs. Thus the use of urea in swine ration is completely banned.

VII. Balance of Amino Acids

A diet should not only contain all the desired type of essential amino acids, but those acids should be present at right proportion. In one study it was observed that pigs benefited from receiving 0.1 per cent level of DL-Lysine with a maize-cottonseed meal diet. Level of lysine greater than 0.1 per cent appeared to depress growth, whereas levels lower than 0.1 per cent failed to support maximum growth. Evidently, amino acids need to be fed at the right amount and also in the right proportion with other essential amino acids for maximum benefit.

VIII. Protein Requirements of the Pig

Advanced scientific knowledge about vitamins and mineral nutrition have made it possible to feed less protein in swine ration. In the past protein requirements were high as the protein supplement used to supply some factor other than amino acids (minerals and vitamins).

Due to the fact that now we have more information about the amino acid content, their availability, variations in feed, requirement of the animal at various stages of their growth, the proper balance of the essential amino acids, effect of processing on the nutritive value of protein, the protein requirement has been found to be lowered at present-day feeding standard and it is expected that future knowledge may further reduce the requirement. Again, it must be remembered that grains will vary in protein and amino acid content depending upon the area of the country in which they are grown and a safety factor must be provided to take care of this variation.

Table 14.11

Protein requirements of swine

Class of animals	*Live weight range (kg)*	*Total feed intake (kg)*	*Crude protein content of diet (%)*	*Crude protein needed daily (kg)*
Growing-finishing	5–10	0.60	22	0.132
	10–20	1.22	18	0.219
	20–35	1.66	16	0.265
	35–58.5	2.45	14	0.343
	58.5–100	3.42	13	0.444
Breed gilts	105–155	2.00	14	0.280
Breed sows	155–245	2.00	14	0.280
Lactating gilts	130–200	5.00	15	0.750
Lactating sows	200–245	5.40	15	0.810
Young boars	105–175	2.45	14	0.343
Adult boars	175–245	2.00	14	0.280

SOURCE: Cunha, T.J., J.P. Bowland, J.H. Conrad, V.W. Hays, R.J. Meade, and H.S. Teague, N.A.S.—N.R.C. Publication (1973).

While discussing the protein requirement of pig, it must be considered very important that young pigs require more protein in the diet than older animals which are storing less protein and more fat in their bodies.

IX. Effect of Processing on Amino Acids

An excellent review by R.J. Meade [*Jr. Animal Sci.*, Vol. 35, 713 (1972)] gives the following information on the effect of processing on amino acids in feeds.

1. Too much overheating of protein supplemented feeds affects the availability of all amino acids of which lysine seems to be the most heat sensitive and destroys earlier.
2. Processing has got little effect on the availability of amino acids present in soybean meal, and groundnut meal.
3. Amino acids of fish meal are on the other hand subjected to vary in their availability when fish meals are overheated or scorched.
4. Similarly the amino acids of meat and bone meal will have reduced availability if the meals are overheated in processing.

CARBOHYDRATE AND FIBRE

Swine diets compose chiefly of carbohydrates which make up about 75 per cent of the dry matter in most plants.

Of all types of carbohydrates, sugars and starches are readily digested whereas cellulose which, along with lignin forms bulk portion of the plant materials, has low digestibility for the pig. This is due to the fact that the digestive tract of the pig consists mainly of a simple stomach of relatively small capacity in contrast to the compound stomachs of cattle, buffalo, sheep and goat and the large caecum of horses. In all these species ruminal microbes play an important role in converting complex carbohydrates into simpler forms.

During the first two weeks of life, piglets can not effectively digest starch. Carbohydrate in the diet during this time should come from glucose and lactose during the first week and from fructose and sucrose during the second week. After pigs reach two weeks of age, they have the necessary enzymes in the digestive tract to digest starch. Pig pre-starters and starters fed during the first two weeks after birth of the pig should provide carbohydrate in a form that the pig can utilize.

Fibre Utilisation by the Pig

As has already stated, the pig is less able to utilise crude fibre in comparison of other ruminants and horses. The digestive system of the pig lacks cellulolytic enzymes and it is due to microbial secretion of cellulase at pigs caecum and colon that a small amount of fibre is digested. The end products of microbial digestion of the cellulose in the alimentary tract of the pig are mainly the steam volatile fatty acids which are produced in and absorbed from the caecum and the colon.

There is no agreement as to what level of fibre pigs can utilise. This lack of information may be due to differences in source of fibre feed, level of fibre in the experimental diets, level of other nutrients in the diet, plane of nutrition, age and weight of the pigs, etc. It has been observed that heavier the pig the more the fibre it can use. The stage in which a forage is harvested also makes a great difference as crude fibre of plants harvested at an early age are more digestible than that cut at late. The explanation that may be cited for this behaviour is that as the plants gets matured, the deposition of lignin in the cell wall will also increase and will render the feed less digestible.

Many scientific reports favour the inclusion of 5 to 6 per cent fibre as the maximum to include in the diet, but some think a figure of 6–8 per cent crude fibre for inclusion. However, for sow it has been agreed that diets may contain 10–12 per cent fibre.

FATTY ACIDS, FAT AND ENERGY

The practical swine diets consisting of grain and protein supplements should supply enough fat required for normal physiological functions of pig. But when diets consist of cassava, starch or other carbohydrate sources (lacking in fat) as the main sources of energy plus a solvent-extracted oil cakes as protein source, there may be a possibility of fatty acid deficiency. Such deficiency could also occur in animals weaned at an early age and when fed milk substitute diets. It is thus important that these diets contain a source of fat and that it be protected against rancidity.

Need for Essential Fatty Acids (EFA)

In the daily diet of pigs the presence of essential fatty acid is a must. All the three unsaturated fatty acids viz., linoleic (C-18 with two double bonds), linolenic (C-18 with three double bonds) and arachidonic (C-20 with four double bonds) are designated as essential fatty acids since body cannot synthesize these fatty acids from any other sources. The top priority has been given to linoleic acid since it alone if present in sufficient amount in animal body (through feed) will either be converted into two other acids or will serve the metabolic roles played by both linolenic and arachidonic acids.

They function as (i) integral part of the lipid-protein structure of cell membranes, (ii) as lipoprotein enzymes, (iii) precursor of prostaglandin by virtue of the fact that linoleic acid is converted into arachidonic acid from which the prostaglandins of various types are synthesized, (iv) source materials for thromboxanes.

A deficiency of EFA in the young growing pig results in (a) scaly skin necrosis particularly in tail region, (b) dullness, (c) dry hair coat. In later stages, (d) a brownish gummy exudate and necrotic areas appear about the ears and under the flanks, (e) retarded sexual maturity and (f) an abnormally small gall bladder.

Practical swine rations contain various grain and grain by-products will supply adequate amounts of EFA. The excess amount will be used for energy. Rations for adult ruminant animal should not contain more than 3-5 per cent fat, the non-ruminants require about 15-20 per cent. Too much fat in the ration will reduce feed intake and increase the chances of digestive upset and may cause diarrhoea. High level of unsaturated fat in swine diets can result in soft pork.

In terms of EFA, 2 per cent level of linoleic acid for growing pigs upto 11-14 weeks of age and later on 1 per cent of the total digestible energy as linoleic acid for pigs from 15 weeks to slaughtering time have been reported to optimize growth and efficiency of energy utilisation. However, Agricultural Research Council (ARC, 1981) has advocated higher amounts of EFA for pigs, viz., pigs upto 30.0 kg should get 3.0 per cent linoleic acid in their diets while for body weights above this upto slaughtering time the amount should be 1.5 per cent of total dietary energy.

Table 14.12

Fat content of some feedstuffs

Feedstuff	Composition		
	Fat (%)	Linoleic (%)	% of DE from Linoleic
Cereal grains			
Maize	3.9	1.8	4.7
Oats	4.0	1.5	4.9
Wheat	1.7	0.6	1.6
Barley	1.9	0.2	0.6
Protein sources			
Soybean	0.8	0.3	0.7
Whey, dried	0.8	—	—

Adding Fat to Diet

There are certain special advantages in adding fat to the diet which are as follows: (1) minimise dustiness of feeds, (2) improves feed efficiency, (3) increases acceptability and palatibility, (4) improves physical appearance, (5) increases ease of pelleting, (6) reduces feed wastage in feeding, (7) decreases carotene loss.

But, there are some disadvantages in adding fats to the diet which are as follows: (1) feeds difficult to handle while adding of fat goes on, (2) feed need be stabilised with a suitable antioxidant to prevent rancidity.

With growing-finishing pigs, higher levels of fat (10-20 per cent) in the diets are in practice.

Energy Values of Feeds

At present most of the information available on energy values for feeds used by swine are expressed in terms of TDN where assumptions and approximations are used in the calculation. But, it is always preferred to express the values in terms of calories, measured directly by calorimeter and expressed either as digestible energy (DE) or as metabolisable energy (ME). The energy content of feed can easily be compared with that of excreta or of energy level of urine. Thus this an additional advantage obtained when energy values are expressed in terms of either DE or ME.

To change to the caloric system, it is necessary to convert TDN values to DE or ME. For this when DE values are computed from TDN, *1 kg of TDN has an average DE value of 4,500 kcal. With mixed feeds for pigs, ME values approximate 96 per cent of DE values.* Value for methane gas production in swine has been accepted as 1.1 per cent of DE which is negligible.

ANTIBIOTICS AND OTHER ANTIMICROBIAL COMPOUNDS

Antibiotics are chemical substances, produced by micro-organisms, which in small concentration have the capacity of inhibiting the growth of or destroying other micro-organisms. Hundreds of antibiotics exist, but only a few are beneficial for animal feeding.

The subject has been discussed at length in Chapter 10: Judicious use of effective antibiotics will not only bring fast rate of gain and high feed efficiency but also increase conception rate, favouring rate and litter size. Dr. Krider of Purdue University in U.S.A. estimated that the proper use of antibiotics for sows and in creep diets could save one more pig per litter and that each dollar spent for antibiotics for animal feed use returned 5-8 dollars in increased returns to the producer. The degree of antibiotic response has been summarised by him as presented in Table 14.13

Table 14.13

Effect of adding antibiotics to swine diets

	Per cent increase in	
	Rate of gain	*Feed efficiency*
Early weaned at 15-20 lb to about 40-50 lb	20–40	7–15
30 + to 100-125	9	1.4
100 lb to market	10.6	6.1
Weaning to market	10.7	5.1

Recommendation on Antibiotic Use

It is very difficult to recommend exact antibiotic levels which will suit all farm conditions situated throughout the world. This is because the farms vary in sanitation and other stress conditions. The following two Tables give the recommended antibiotic levels made by the National Research Council (NRC) and Kentucky research workers for pigs at their various ages.

Table 14.14

NRC recommended antibiotic levels

Item	*Pig weight (kg)*	*Antibiotic per ton of feed (gm)*[a]
Baby pigs	4.5-11	40
Growing pigs	12–30	10–20
Finishing pigs	30–98	10
Therapeutic level for pigs doing poorly	—	50–100[a]
Supplement to be fed free-choice with gain	—	50–100

[a]If pigs are in very poor condition and will not eat, the antibiotic can be given in the drinking water.

Table 14.15

Kentucky recommended antibiotic levels

Stage of production	*Relative level*	*Suggested range (gm/ton)*[a]
Prebreeding and breeding	Moderate to higher levels	100-200
Gestation	None unless disease and environmental stress exists	0-20
Farrowing	High levels	100-200
Lactation	Moderate levels	0-40
Pre-starter (early weaned pigs)	High levels	100-250
Starter (12-25 lb in weight)	High levels	100-250
Grower	Moderate levels	50-100
Finisher	Low levels	20-50

[a]Gram per ton needed varies with type of antibiotic and the health problem involved.

MINERAL REQUIREMENTS OF THE PIG

There are 104 elements in the periodic system. With the exception of the organically bound elements having molecular weight of 16 or less (i.e., hydrogen, oxygen, carbon and nitrogen), all other elements are considered inorganic elements or more commonly termed as minerals. Of the 104 minus 4 (organically bound elements), i.e., 100 elements, only a few (about 40) occur in measurable amounts in the body. All are not essential for body processes and these are constituents of animal food and thus occur in animal body. In fact the essentiality of any mineral is known from its metabolic role in the body.

Vital Functions of Minerals and Effect of Deficiency

Each of the essential mineral elements serves the body in one or more of the following four different ways: (a) as a constituent of skeletal structures, (b) in maintaining the colloidal state of body matter and regulating some of the physical properties of colloidal system (viscosity, diffusion, osmotic pressure), (c) in regulating acid-base equilibrium, (d) as a component or activator of enzymes and/or other biological units or systems. Thus, it may be said that nearly every process of the animal body depends on one or more of the mineral elements for proper functioning.

A lack of minerals in the diet may cause any of the following deficiency symptoms: (a) reduced or poor appetite; (b) poor growth, (c) rickets, (d) soft of brittle bones, (e) beading of the ribs, (f) stiffness or malformed joints, (g) posterior paralysis, (h) goitre, (i) pigs born hairless, (j) failure to come in heat regularly, (k) poor milk production, (l) weak or dead young.

Table 14.16

Elemental composition of the body of most animals

Elements	*Percentage of body weight*		*Approx. no. of grams in a 70 kg man*
A. Organically bound elements			
Oxygen	65.0	96%	45,500
Carbon	18.0		12,600
Hydrogen	10.0		7,000
Nitrogen	3.0		2,100
B. Inorganic elements			
Calcium	1.5	3.45%	1,050
Phosphorus	1.0		700
Potassium	0.35		245
Sulphur	0.25		175
Sodium	0.15		105
Chlorine	0.15		105
Magnesium	0.05		35
Iron	0.004		3
Manganese	0.003		0.2
Copper	0.002		0.1
Iodine	0.00004		0.03
Others	Present in trace amounts only		

SOURCE: Hawk, P.B., B.L. Oser and W.H. Summerson, *Practical Physical Chemistry* (13th edition), The Blakiston Co., New York (1947).

Mineral Content of the Animal Body

At the present time only 20 elements (21 in ruminants where it includes cobalt) are considered essential for pigs. They are calcium, phosphorus, magnesium, sodium, potassium, choline, sulphur, manganese, irŏn, copper, iodine, zinc, fluorine, vanadium, molybdenum, selenium, chromium, tin, nickel and silicon. The following five elements are considered probably essential, arsenic, barium, bromine, cadmium and strontium.

The details about the metabolism, sources, functions, deficiency symptoms of individual minerals have already been described in Chapter 10. The exact requirements of minerals for pigs have been given in Tables 14.6 to 14.9

VITAMIN REQUIREMENTS OF THE PIG

Vitamins are organic compounds required for normal growth and the maintenance of animal life and are needed only in very small amounts. They are not related to each other as are proteins, carbohydrates and fats. All are different in structure and functions.

Although pigs synthesise some of the vitamins in large enough quantities to supply their daily needs such as vitamin C, most other vitamins must be supplied in pigs diet. The following 15 vitamins are required daily by the pigs.

Fat soluble vitamins	*Water soluble vitamins*
Vitamin A	Thiamin, Riboflavin
Vitamin D	Niacin, Pantothenic acid,
Vitamin E	Pyridoxine, Choline,
Vitamin K	Biotin, p-amino benzoic acid
	Folic acid, B_{12}, Inositol

A detailed discussion about the nature and physiological properties of all these vitamins have been described in Chapter 10. The recommended levels for pigs at their various stages of growth have been given in Tables 14.6 to 14.9.

The following factors are listed below which have had an effect on the increased need for vitamins in swine diets.

1. Selection for meat type and faster growing pigs.
2. Genetic differences in animals which can alter vitamin needs.
3. Trend toward complete confinement and slotted floors which lessens opportunity for coprophagy (eating of faeces). Faeces contain many vitamins.
4. The depletion of certain nutrients in soil which contributes lower concentration of some pro-vitamins in feed ingredients.
5. Modern methods of handling and processing feeds and their effect on nutrient level and availability.
6. Inter-relationships among various nutrients can affect vitamin need.
7. Tendency to adopt earlier weaning which increases need for vitamins in these diets.
8. Increased stress and subclinical disease level conditions because of closer contact among animals in confinement.
9. Presence of antimetabolites in feeds can increase certain vitamin needs.
10. Molds in feed significantly increase the need for more vitamins in the diet.

Considering the above factors it may be concluded that the recommended level, as suggested by nutritionists from time to time are simply a guide line, the livestock producer must consider various other factors while adding vitamins in the diet of pigs. Deficiency of a single vitamin may result a tremendous economic loss to the owner. Many farmers are reluctant to buy the necessary vitamins to balance their diets. But doing this is being *"penny-wise and pound foolish"*. Is is always profitable to buy necessary vitamins that are necessary for pig ration.

Guidelines in Formulating Swine Ration

In all commereial farms pigs are maintained as intensive animals and fed a diet based on concentrates. These are either purchased as balanced diet or made up from home produced cereals mixed with protein-rich feed ingredients, minerals, vitamins and feed additives to correct the deficiencies. Dependable protein, mineral and vitamin premixes are available as supplements in open market. For purposes of convenience and facilitating ration formulation for pig at their various ages and stages of production some guidelines are narrated below.

Table 14.17
Types of Rations and Feeding Programme for Swine

Ration	Source	Age or size of Pig	Level of protein (%)
Milk replacer (pre-starter or creep ration)	Commercial	7-10 days after birth to all piglets including orphan piglets under 3 weeks of age or until the piglets weaned and weight from 3.5 to 6.5 kg body wt.	20
Starter	Commercial	From the day of weaning 3-5 weeks of age to about 20 kg body weight	18
Growing-Finishing	Commercial or farm mixed	20 kg onward upto 35 kg body wt.	16
Growing-Finishing	Commercial or farm mixed	35 kg onward upto 70-90 kg body wt.	13
Pre-gestation	About 10—14 days prior to expected breeding, the female should be fed a ration that will make for gains of 0.5-1.0 kg per day.		14-16
Gestation	Limited feeding is a must for gestating gilts and sows. Two to three weeks prior to farrowing, feeding level should be increased to about 500 grams per day.		12
Furrowing	Reduce feed intake slightly 4-5 days before and after furrowing. Laxative and bulky rations (wheat bran and oats can be substituted for about half of the regular diet) should be fed starting 10 days before furrowing and during the first week of lactation. Small amount of linseed meal may also be included. On the day the sow furrows, she should be given no feed for 10-12 hrs except water.		14-16
Lactation	Feed requirements are greater than gestation. The nutrients required by the sow for milk production is greater than for producing young.		16
Boars	Young boars upto 57 kg need a ration containing 18% protein which may be reduced to 16% as the boars grow from 57 to 90 kg.		16-18

Some of the pointers in formulating rations and feeding of swine in general are discussed below:

1. Presently most of the Indian pig farmers experience difficulties in computing their own pig ration at home due to lack of experiences and thus purchase commercial feeds from open market. However, some knowledge of the nutritional needs of pigs and of the composition of the feeds may be useful to individuals for efficient feeding as per requirement with minimum cost.

2. Feeding standards for pigs now evaluate the pig's energy requirement in *Megajoules* of digestible energy (DE) per day. Protein evaluation is based although on *Crude protein* (CP), but it actually means about the requirement of specific amino acids in feed, e.g. lysine, methionine, cystine, threonine, tryptophan etc., with lysine being the most important.

3. Based on cost, feed ingredients of similar nutritive values may be interchanged while formulating ration.

4. Maintaining overall protein content of the ration is not the final aim in feed formulation but the quality of amino acids and their ratio should be taken into consideration.

5. When proteins of animal origin predominate, required mineral balance may be obtained by allowing hogs free access to a 2-compartment box or self-feeder with (a) trace mineralised salt in one side, and (b) a mixture of 1/3 salt (for purposes of palatability) and 2/3 monosodium phosphate or other phosphorus supplement, in the other side. In case when dietary proteins constitutes most of the sources of vegetable protein, add a third compartment to the mineral box and place in it a mixture of 1/3 rd salt (trace mineralised) and 2/3 ground limestone or oystershell flour.

6. Except for gestating sows and boars of breeding age, hogs are generally self fed. All of the ingredients may be mixed together and placed in the self-feeder. In case the cereal grains and protein supplements are hand-fed, the grain and supplement should be fed separately.

7. All grains in mixed feed should be ground (maize-medium; wheat-medium to coarse; barley-fine; sorghum-fine to medium; oats-fine). Generally slop feeding (feeding of wet mesh) is not superior to dry feeding as the former method require more time and excessive labour. Palleting of feed is recommended when feed contains more of fiber.

8. The most convenient way to feed animals on a farm is to prepare the complete ration as per recommended levels for different classes and offer the pigs the recommended amount distributing it in two or three times a day which they will eat without waste.

9. Antibiotic and other chemotherapeutic agents are carefully added to swine diets to secure an even distribution. Use only those materials specifically authorised for swine.

FEEDING OF PIGS

Proper feeding is an extremely important item of management since feed represents a very high percentage of the total cost of production of a pig, sometimes as high as 80 per cent. Pig grows at a very faster rate and thus the demand for feed are very high. A baby pig may weigh 1.4 kg when it is born and 163 kg by the time it reaches 18 months of age. Thus in 18 months it multiplies its weight by 120 times. This is about 12 times faster than a calf which weighs 41 kg at birth and will weigh 408 kg after 18 months. When pigs are fed over generous rations, pigs fatten very rapidly and also uneconomic.

Pig is omnivorous, i.e., it can eat all types of feed. Although it likes to graze or chew forages but due to its nature of single stomach it cannot live entirely on roughages. The typical mouth and teeth of the pig which is different from ruminants, enable it to pick up feed from the surface of the soil or to root it out from the ground. Incidentally pigs thrive best on feeds which are commonly used by human. To avoid the competition for the feed by human and pigs, it should be the pig farmer's aim to use the cheaper agro-industrial by-products and to supplement them by the more expensive nutritious feeds to the point that true economy dictates.

Pigs require different rations at different stages of life. As the pig grows older, protein, mineral and vitamin requirements in proportion to body weight significantly decrease. Animal protein in particular, is more indispensable for young than for the older animal, and the ability of the pig to deal with roughages increases with age. The younger the pig the more critical the period becomes. Consequently higher quality and more fortified diets are needed.

Due to varying physiological needs of the pig during its life, the pig is fed different diets at different ages as per following:

1. *Pre-Starter ration* (Creep Feeding)

The dry pre-starter feeds also known as creep ration or milk replacer are usually offered to the piglets when they are about of 2 kg body weight or 7–10 days old. This should be

Table 14.18

Composition of creep feed as suggested by University of Kentucky, U.S.A.[a]

Ingredient	Diet[b]			
	1	*2*	*3*	*4*
Ground yellow corn	533	561	327	355
Dried skim milk	800	800	400	400
Solvent soybean meal (50%)	282	302	484	504
Fish solubles	50	50	50	50
Dried whey (high lactose)	—	—	400	400
Sugar (cane or beet)	200	200	200	200
Distilers' dried solubles	50	—	50	—
Stabilised fat	50	50	50	50
Calcium carbonate	8	8	10	10
Dicalcium phosphate	—	2	2	4
Iodised salt	5	5	5	5
Trace mineral mix	2	2	2	2
Vitamin premix	20	20	20	20
Antibiotic mix[c]	+	+	+	+
	2000	2000	2000	2000
Calculated analysis				
Protein (%)	24.0	24.0	24.0	23.0
Calcium (%)	0.69	0.71	0.70	0.72
Phosphorus (%)	0.60	0.60	0.60	0.60

[a]For pigs weaned earlier than 3 weeks of age

[b]Values in pounds per ton

[c]Antibiotics should be added to provide 100–250 gm/ton.

continued till piglets are weaned and weigh from 6.5 to 8.5 kg body weight. Piglets are used to encourage dry feed consumption as a means of supplementing the sow's milk.

Creep feed should contain about 20% protein a major portion of which should be of animal origin. Moreover, the feed should have more of minerals and vitamins with low fibre content and finally it should be highly palatable.

A few examples of computed rations are given below. As already pointed out the cost, chemical composition and availability should be considered first before computing a ration.

Dr. S.K. Ranjhan an eminent scientist in the discipline of Animal Nutrition and his co-workers in India have suggested the following composition for creep mixture.

Table 14.19

Creep mixture

Ground yellow maize	40 kg
Skimmed milk	10 kg
Groundnut cake	10 kg
Til cake	10 kg
Wheat bran	10 kg
Molasses	10 kg
Fish meal	6 kg
Brewars yeast	2 kg
Mineral mixture	2 kg
Add. Vitamin (A, B_2, D_3 (Rovimix))	10 g
	100.00 kg

Composition of complex mineral mixture	
Sterilised bone meal (Finely powdered)	45.0 kg
Ground chalk	10.0 kg
Di-Calcium phosphate	12.0 kg
Common salt	30.0 kg
Yellow oxide of iron (Ferrous sulphate)	0.5 kg
Potassium iodide	0.25 kg
Starch	0.75 kg
Sodium carbonate	0.75 kg
Sodium Thiosulphate	0.75 kg
Add for 100 kg.	
1. Cobalt chloride	55.0 g
2. Copper sulphate	265.0 g
3. Manganese sulphate	330.0 g
4. Zinc sulphate	750.0 g

As a general guide creep feed may be prepared as below:

1. Maize 65 per cent	It can be replaced by sorghum, broken wheat, broken rice, tapioca

2.	Groundnut cake 14 per cent	This also can be replaced by other oil cakes such as soybean oilmeal, sesame oil cake, linseed cake, coconut cake
3.	Molasses 5 per cent	
4.	Wheat bran 10 per cent	This may be replaced by rice bran
5.	Fish meal 5 per cent	This may be replaced by meat meal, meat scrappings, skim milk powder, butter milk
6.	Mineral mixture 1 per cent	
7.	Antibiotics —	
	100	

Table 14.20

[1]Composition of a starter's diet as suggested by the University of Kentucky, U.S.A.

Ingredient	*Diet*[2]			
	1	*2*	*3*	*4*
Ground yellow maize	873	948	981	1035
Solvent soybean meal (50%)	516	490	556	504
Dried skim milk	—	100	—	100
Fish solubles	50	50	—	—
Distillers' dried solubles	50	—	—	—
Dried whey (high lactose)	300	200	300	200
Stabilised fat	50	50	—	—
Sugar (cane or beet)	100	100	100	100
Calcium carbonate	15	14	15	14
Dicalcium phosphate	19	21	21	20
Iodised salt	5	5	5	5
Trace mineral premix	2	2	2	2
Vitamin premix	20	20	20	20
Antibiotics[3]	+	+	+	+
	2000	2000	2000	2000
Calculated analysis				
Protein (%)	20.0	20.0	20.0	20.0
Calcium (%)	0.70	0.70	0.70	0.69
Phosphorus (%)	0.60	0.60	0.60	0.60

[1]For creep diets and for weaned pigs weighing 12–30 lb
[2]Values in pounds per ton.
[3]Antibotics should be added to provide 100–250 gm/ton.

2. *Starter ration*

The ration offered to piglets from the day of weaning to about 20 kg body weight. It is almost similar to the prestarter ration except that the skim milk powder is replaced by either fish meal or meat meal. At some places where skim milk powder is available at cheaper rate, the pre-starter ration is continued.

3. *Growing—Finishing ration*

After the pigs have a good start and weigh about 20 kg, they should be switched from starter to grower diet as by attaining this body weight it has almost passed a nutritional critical period and after that they will do well on relatively simple ration. For some swine, producers use a mixture of starter and grower diet until the pig looks thrifty in appearance. The ration contains about 16 per cent protein, having some percentages of animal protein and fibre.

When piglets grow about 35 kg body weight they are offered lighter, bulkier finishing ration for production of lean (bacon) carcasses. These rations contain lower level of animal proteins and energy and during the phase, it is possible to replace larger proportion of cereal grains with grain processing by-products bringing the protein per cent upto 13. The replacement of cereal grains results in proportionate fall in the energy contents of the rations bringing in lower growth response of pigs. Some energy demand is met through the increased intake of low energy feeds. The ration in general continued from 35 kg till the animals grow up to a body weight of 70 kg when they are economical for slaughter in India. In U.S.A slaughtering is economical at their 90 kg body weight.

The following are some of the formulated composition of grower's ration suggested by Dr. S.K. Ranjhan, Professor of Eminence in Animal Nutrition. Rations are grouped on the basis of the inclusion of cereals and non-cereal grains.

Grower's ration

I. Cereal Rations

1.	Maize	30.00 kg	2.	Maize	20 kg
	Groundnut cake	20.00 ,,		Milo	10 ,,
	Wheat bran	40.00 ,,		Groundnut cake	10 ,,
	Fish meal	7.5 ,,		Wheat bran	40 ,,
	Mineral mixture	2.5 ,,		Til cake	10 ,,
	Vitamin mixture			Fish meal	7.5 ,,
	(Rovimix A, B_2, D_3)	10.0 g		Mineral Vit. supplement	2.50 ,,
3.	Maize	60.0 kg	4.	Maize	20.0 kg
	Wheat bran	10.0 ,,		Milo	15.0 ,,
	G.N. cake	10.0 ,,		Any other grain	15.0 ,,
	Til cake	10.0 ,,		Wheat bran	10.0 ,,
	Fish meal	7.5 ,,		Rice polishing	10.0 ,,
	Mineral and Vit.-mix	2.5 ,,		G.N. cake	40.0 ,,
				Til cake	10.0 ,,
				Fish meal	7.5 ,,
				Mineral and Vit. supplement	2.5 ,,

II. Non Cereal Rations

1.	Wheat bran	70.0 kg	2.	Rice polishing	70.0 kg
	G.N. cake	20.0 ,,		G.N. cake	20.0 ,,
	Fish meal	6.5 ,,		Fish meal	6.5 ,,
	Mineral mixture	3.0 ,,		Mineral mixture	3.9 ,,
	Common salt	0.5 ,,		Common salt	0.5 ,,
	Rovimix (A, B_2, D_3)	10 g		Rovimix (A, B_2, D_3)	10 g
	(Growth rate 0.7 lbs/day/head)			(Growth rate 0.65 per day per head)	
3.	Wheat bran	60.0 kg	4.	Rice polishings	60.0 kg
	Yellow maize	10.0 ,,		Yellow maize	10.0 ,,
	G.N. cake	20.0 ,,		G.N. cake	20.0 ,,
	Fish meal	6.5 ,,		Fish meal	6.5 ,,
	Mineral mixture	3.0 ,,		Mineral mixture	3.0 ,,
	Common salt	0.5 ,,		Common salt	0.5 ,,
	Rovimix (A, B_2, D_3)	10 g		Rovimix (A, B_2, D_3)	10 g
	(Growth rate 0.8 lbs/day per head)			(Growth rate 0.7 lbs/day per head)	
5.	Wheat bran	35.0 kg	6.	Wheat bran	30.0 kg
	Rice polishings	35.0 ,,		Rice polishings	30.0 ,,
	G.N. cake	10.0 ,,		Yellow maize	10.0 ,,
	Til cake	10.0 ,,		G.N. cake	10.0 ,,
	Fish meal	6.5 ,,		Til cake	10.0 ,,
	Mineral mixture	3.0 ,,		Fish meal	6.5 ,,
	Common salt	0.5 ,,		Mineral mixture	3.0 ,,
	Rovimix (A, B_2, D_3)	20 g		Common salt	0.5 ,,
				Rovimix (A, B_2, D_3)	10 g

Note: Expected growth rate with the above rations (about 0.5 kg) per head per day with a feed efficiency of 4 kg of meal to one kg live weight gain.

Composition of some finisher rations as suggested by Prof. S.K. Ranjhan, the pioneer worker in Animal Nutrition are given below:

I. Cereal ration

1.	Maize	40.0 kg	2.	Maize	20.0 kg	3.	Maize	25.0 kg
	Wheat bran	30.0 ,,		Milo	20.0 ,,		Any other grain	15.0 ,,
	G.N. cake	12.0 ,,		Wheat bran	20.0 ,,		Rice polishings	33.0 ,,
	Til cake	10.0 ,,		Rice polishings	10.0 ,,		G.N. cake	12.0 ,,
	Fish meal	5.5 ,,		G.N. cake	12.0 ,,		Til cake	10.0 ,,
	Mineral mixture	2.5 ,,		Til cake	10.0 ,,		Fish meal	5.5 ,,
	Rovimix (A, B_2, D_3)	10 g		Mineral mixture	5.5 ,,		Mineral mixture	2.5 ,,
				Rovimix (A, B_2, D_3)	10 g		Rovimix (A, B_2, D_3)	10 g

II. Non Cereal Rations

1.	1. Wheat bran	75.0 kg	2.	Wheat bran	70.0 kg	3.	Wheat bran	40.0 kg
	2. G.N. cake	17.0 ,,		G.N. cake	12.0 ,,		Rice polishings	30.0 ,,
	3. Fish meal	5.0 ,,		Til cake	10.0 ,,		G.N. cake	10.0 ,,
	4. Mineral mixture	2.5 ,,		Fish meal	5.5 ,,		Til cake	10.0 ,,
	5. Common salt	0.5 ,,		Mineral mixture	2.5 ,,		Fish meal	5.5 ,,
	6. Rovimix (A, B_2, D_3)	10 g		Rovimix (A, B_2, D_3)	10 g		Mineral mixture	2.5 ,,
							Rovimix (A, B_2, D_3)	10 g

The pig farmers may also compute the finisher ration out of the ingredients available in their locality if they followed the following composition.

		For alternate substitutes see page 581
Maize	45 per cent	
Groundnut cake	20 ,,	,,
Molasses	5 ,,	—
Wheat bran	25 ,,	,,
Fish meal	3 ,,	,,
Mineral mixture	1.5 ,,	—
Salt	0.5 ,,	—

Table 14.21

[a]Composition of a finisher diet as suggested by the University of Kentucky, U.S.A.

Ingredient	*Diet*[b]		
	1	2	*3*
Ground yellow maize	1691	1712	1684
Solvent soybean meal (44%)	168	196	256
Meat and bone meal	50	50	—
Distiller's dried solubles	50	—	—
Calcium carbonate	11	10	16
Dicalcium phosphate	9	11	23
Iodised salt	10	10	10
Trace mineral premix	1	1	1
Vitamin premix	10	10	10
Antibiotics[c]	+	+	+
	2000	2000	2000
Calculated analysis			
Protein (%)	13.1	13.1	13.0
Calcium (%)	0.60	0.59	0.60
Phosphorus (%)	0.50	0.50	0.50

[a]For pigs weighing 125 lb to market weight.
[b]Values in pounds per ton.
[c]Add antibiotics to provide 20–50 gm/ton.

4. *Gestation ration*

An excellent, well-balanced diet is very important during gestation. Gilts have greater requirements than mature sows because their diet will have to take care of their growth as well as that of the developing foetus. Thus gilts need more feed per 100 kg of body weight.

Approximately, two-thirds of the growth of the foetus is made during the last month of the gestation period when demands for nutrients are at a maximum point. Again the increased needs are primarily, for proteins, vitamins, and minerals. During gestation, it is also necessary that body reserves be stored for subsequent use during lactation.

Most swine producers will feed 2.0 to 2.5 kg mixed feed during the breeding period, and then decrease to about 1.5 kg during the major part of gestation. Then they increase feed intake to 2.5 kg during the 3 or 4 week period prior to furrowing. If this level of feeding results in the animals becoming "over-fat", it should be decreased. If, conversely, this level of feeding results in the gilts and sows becoming too thin, it should be increased accordingly. The gilts and sows should be kept in a thrifty condition, not too fat nor too thin, but somewhere in between.

In addition to the above limited feeding system, the use of pasture should be considered for valuable quality protein, minerals, vitamins and exercise. On the basis of quality and quantity (not more than 10–12 per cent) of fiber consumed, the corresponding amount of dry matter of mixed concentrate feed may be reduced.

A ration for gestating females may be of relatively coarse in structure. The ration for gilt should contain 16 per cent CP, while that for sows it may be 14 per cent during the first two thirds of gestation followed by 16 per cent for the rest period.

The following composition may be followed:

Maize	**50 per cent**	**For substitutes see page 713**
Groundnut cake	**20 ,,**	**,,**
Molasses	**5 ,,**	**—**
Wheat bran	**18 ,,**	**,,**
Fish meal	**5 ,,**	**,,**
Mineral mixture	**1.5 ,,**	**—**
Salt	**0.5 ,,**	**—**

5. *Furrowing ration*

It is considered good practice to feed highly and with bulky feeds from 4-5 days before and after furrowing by substituting wheat bran, oats, ground legume hay or dehydrated lucerne meal. At furrowing, about one-third of the ration may be made up of these bulky feeds.

Adding bulk to the ration at furrowing may help prevent constipation and reduce problems with mastitis-metritis-agalactia (MMA). Make sure that there is a good supply of fresh water at furrowing time.

6. *Lactation ration*

The feed requirements of the sow during lactation are considerably greater than during gestation. This is because the increase of nutrients required by the sow for milk production is greater than for producing young. There is considerable variation in the amount of milk produce by sows. This is dependent on the diet fed, the inherent ability to produce milk, the number of pigs in the litter etc. On an average feed a ration containing 16 per cent total protein at the rate of 4.5 to 6.0 kg per day to gilts and 5.5 to 6.5 kg per day to sows. A full feed of high energy, low fiber diet is necessary for maximum milk production during lactation.

AMOUNT TO FEED

The most convenient way to feed animals on a farm is to prepare the complete ration recommended for different classes and provide the pigs with a free choice to eat liberally without any waste. Two to three times feeding daily is the common practice. Animals learn to anticipate their feed. Accordingly, they should be fed with great regularity. The following is the approximate amount of dry feed they will consume.

Table 14.22

Average feed consumption and efficiency of gains in body weights of pigs at various ages

Age months	*Probable live wt. (kg)*	*Amount of feed consumption per head/day (kg)*	*Cumulative feed consumption/pig (kg)*
1–2	15	0.50	15.0
2–3	27	1.00	45.0
3–4	40	1.25	82.5
4–5	50	1.50	127.5
5–6	60	2.00	187.5

Table 14.23

Approximate water requirements of pigs

Class of pig	*Water requirements (in litre)*
Growing pigs (weeks of age)	
8–12	3.5
13–18	6.0
19–24	7.5
25	8.0
Pregnant gilts and sows	
First 3 months	10–15
Last 3 months	16–20
Lactating sows with	
5–7 piglets	20–25
8–10 piglets	22–27
11–14 piglets	28–35
Boars	20–25

Note: If water is used for cleaning and washing, requirements may be considered double the figure given here.

Feeding Systems and their Effect on Performance

The way in which a pig will utilize a ration will depend upon many factors. Important among these are:

1. The rationing system used, e.g. *ad lib.*, restricted, appetite.
2. The form in which the food is presented, e.g. dry foods, wet foods.
3. The way in which it is presented, e.g. in troughs, in self-feeders, on floor.

1. Rationing System

Ad lib feeding. This system, which can employ meal, cube and liquid forms, in labour saving in operation and allows the pigs to fulfil their full quicker growth potential. There is rather a lot of food wastage and comparatively lower efficiency of food conversion. The finished carcases tend to be rather fat. Over-eating sometimes occurs and may give rise to digestive disorders. Meal rations have to be evenly ground, otherwise pigs fed *ad lib.* may select and eat the less coarse elements in a meal and reject relatively fibrous portion. Cubes do not have this disadvantage. Generally speaking, young animals are fed *ad lib.* up to 45 kg live weight by which time they will be consuming 1.8 kg of meal per day. Potential prokers and heavy hogs may be kept on *ad lib.* feeding, but baconers will be put on to restricted feeding at this stage.

Restricted Feeding

The animals are given a measured amount of food once, twice or thrice a day, the total daily ration being usually about 0.45 kg less than they would consume if fed *ad lib.* In general the growth (relative to the *ad lib* fed animal) is restricted, but the efficiency of food conversion (EFC) is improved. The carcases grade well as there is generally a satisfactory lean: fat ratio compared to animals fed *ad lib.*

Appetite Feeding

This is compromise between *ad lib.* and restricted feeding. The pigs are given as much food as it is thought they can clear up in 15-20 minutes, and if some is left over, the next feed is made smaller. If all is cleared well before the end of 20 minutes, extra food is provided next time. This system is supposed to give excellent growth rates without the laying down of too much fat in the carcass.

2. Form in which the feed is presented

Dry foods

These can be either meals or cubes which may be fed either *ad lib* or restricted. The advantages of complete pelleted cubes over meals are:

1. Slightly less waste—specially on floor feeding

2. Less dust in the house, therefore, less coughing and less possibility of respiratory disease.
3. Slightly better food conversion rate (5-10 per cent) which may be due to heat in the cubing process altering digestibility. Hogs will increase in average daily gain by 2-5 per cent.

The disadvantage in feeding dry cubes is its higher cost.

Wet foods: (Dry meals mixed with water)

The method involves mixing predetermined amounts of feed and water prior to or at the time of feeding. When properly used, this method can practically eliminate feed dust and minimise respiratory diseases. The method requires extra time and thus involves extra labour. Research has shown no difference in rate of gain, dressing percentage, carcass measurement or in carcass quality in pigs fed on wet or dry feeds.

3. Ways of presentation of feed

Trough Feeding

Trough can be used for restricted feeding of liquid, meal or pelleted feeds. All the pigs fed at one time and hence there should be sufficient trough space, e.g. a 90 kg baconer will need about 30 cm of trough length and a heavy hog about 40 cm.

Floor Feeding

The food material in the form of meal or cubes, is scattered on the floor once or twice a day. The method is recommended for pigs weighing more than 30 kg live-weight. Feeding in the sleeping area encourages cleanliness, since pigs are less inclined to dung where they eat. The method is a useful system where trough space is limited.

Self-Feeders

These are usually constructed in the form of a non-spill trough with cross partitions so that only one pig can be fed in each subdivision. Ground cereals and protein supplements may be fed separately and at free choice. Generally pigs fed free choice rations in separate feeders or compartments will not make as uniform or as fast gains as pigs fed a complete mixed ration.

Essential Factors influencing welfare of PIGS

GENERAL :

1. Always buy your stock from a pedigree and disease-free herd.
2. Feed adequate balanced ration to the growing pigs, finishers and breeding stock.
3. Deworm the herd every quarter.
4. Vaccinate the pigs every year against diseases for which vaccines are available.
5. Provide adequate shade and shelter and ample water especially during the summer season.
6. Do not breed gilts weighing less than 70 kg. Do not breed gilts on the first day of heat, mate the gilt on secor and third day of onset of heat.

HOUSING :

1. The building must be well lit to ensure good management, hygiene and disease control.
2. There must be space for essential behavioural needs of the pigs, freedom to stand up, lie down, stretch t.eir limbs and groom themselves.
3. Competition for feeding, watering, resting should be avoided.
4. The main requirements for satisfactory housing are that the quarters be dry, sanitary and well ventilated and that they provide good protection from heat, cold and winds. Remember that all body functions depend on fresh air and oxygen.
5. Separation of various age groups is a great advantage in feeding and management which all help in growth rate and in reduction of diseases.

CARE OF SOWS :

1. Deworm sows three weeks before farrowing.
2. Transfer the pregnant gilt to farrowing pen one week before farrowing.
3. Give laxative feed to pregnant gilts three days prior to farrowing.
4. Avoid over feeding three days prior to farrowing and 12 hours after farrowing, Provide guard rails and bedding to the farrowing house.
5. Keep close watch on sows during farrowing without disturbing them.
6. Feed adequate balanced ration to the suckling mothers along with sufficient clean drinking water.
7. Breed sows at first heat after weaning with outstanding boars.
8. Wash the sow's udder with soapy disinfectant before she enters the farrowing pen so that the piglets do not get infected while nursing. The farrowing pen should be clean and disinfected.
9. Proper lighting in a farrowing pen is important.

CARE OF PIGLETS :

1. Clean the mouths and nostrils of the piglets immediately after their birth and induce them to suck milk from the dams. Prevent the piglets from being overlayed by dam.
2. Protect newborn piglets from cold by providing comfortable and warm housing (70-75°F).
3. To protect piglets from pernicious anaemia, give them iron injections during the first week of age or paint the teats of mother with a mixture of ferrous sulphate and molasses.
4. Provide palatable feed to the piglets when 15 days old. Ensure equal quantity of ration to each piglet.
5. Feeders should be placed always under shelter.
6. Wean the piglets at eight weeks of age and castrate all the males not required for breeding at weaning. Weigh the growing pigs at regular intervals, weekly up to weaning and monthly thereafter.
7. Always keep in touch with the local veterinarian.

15

POULTRY

WHAT IS POULTRY ?

The term 'poultry' applies to a rather wide variety of birds of several species and it refers to them whether they are alive or dressed (slaughtered and prepared for market). The term applies to chickens, turkeys, ducks, geese, swans, guinea fowl, pigeons, pea fowl, ostriches, pheasants, quail and other game birds.

The study of birds which are not classed as poultry is known as *ornithology*.

Nomenclature and Breeds of Fowl

The fowl has been domesticated since 2000 B.C. Zoologically the fowl belongs to the genus *Gallus* of the family *Phasianiae*. The domestic fowl is called simply *Gallus domesticus*. The ancestors of the domestic chicken originated in Southeast Asia: and has been subjected to extensive breeding for size, colour patterns, conformation and egg laying ability during long domesticated history. Like other birds, it has a coating of feathers, no teeth, soc-like appearance and legs with spurs. The very presense of comb distinguishes it from other birds. Fowls are having a relatively high breathing and pulse rate, and body temperature ranges from 105° F to 109° F which is higher than that of other domestic animals.

There are 8 types of combs ; of these only the single, rose and pea are common.

Regarding colour patterns there are about 13 common colours observed in poultry birds, these are (1) White, (2) Buff (light yellow), (3) Blue, (4) Black, (5) Barred, (6) Red, (7) Span-

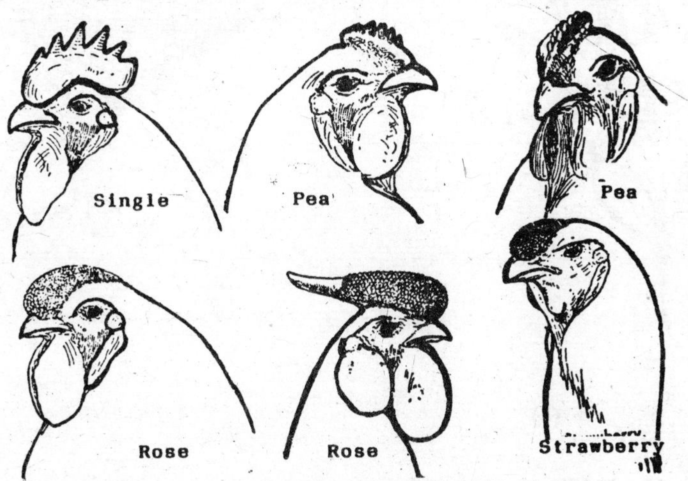

Fig. 15.1. Types of standard male combs.

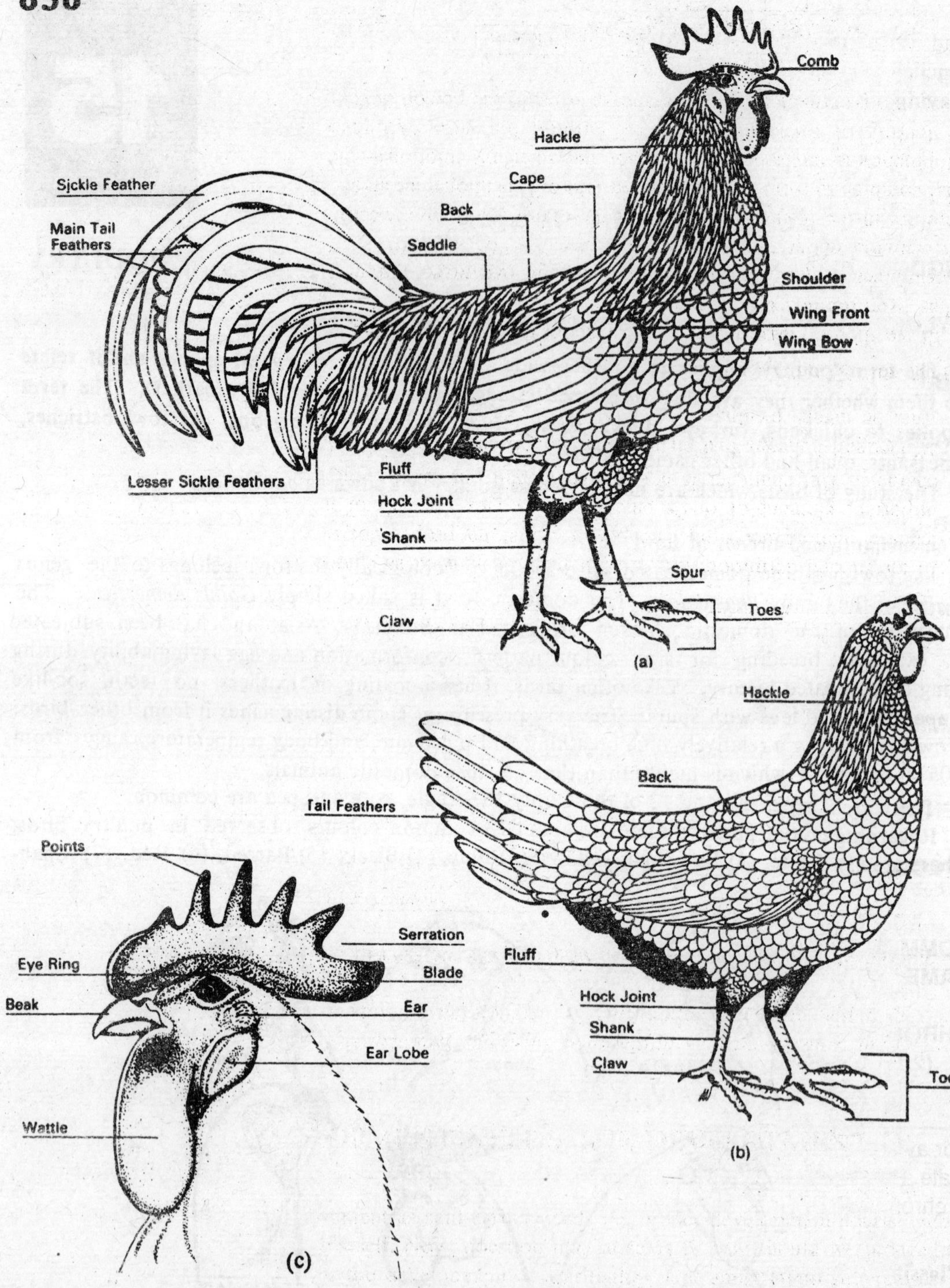

Fig. 15.2 External parts of fowl. (a) male, (b) female, (c) the head of the chicken

glad (glittering spot), (8) Mottled (two colours folded together), (9) Laced, (10) Crecentic penciled, (11) Parallel penciled, (12) Stippled (painted in dots or separated touches), (13) Striped (having stripes of different colours).

ZOOLOGICAL CLASSIFICATION

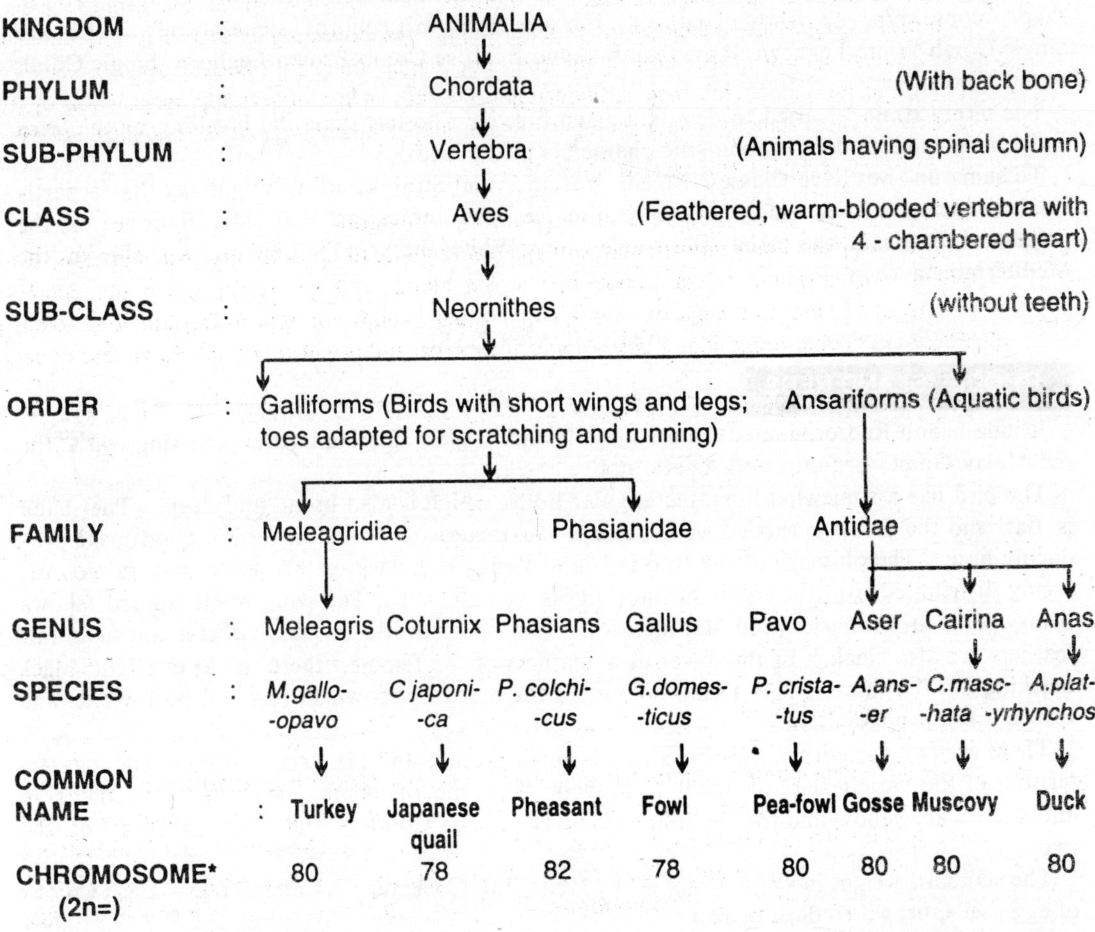

For avian it was once thought that the femaleswere XO, having one fewer chromosome than the male. Recent studies, however show that the female has a very small sex chromosome, called the w chromosome. Thus the female is Xw (sometimes called Zw).

Classification of Fowls

Fowl may be classified on the basis of utility, economic value or fancy purpose and these include (1) Meat type, (2) Egg type, (3) Dual purpose, (4) Game, (5) Ornamental, (6) Bantam

Birds of distinct type and colour patterns admitted to the standard are termed as standard breed.. They are further classified as (1) Class, (2) Breed, (3) Variety, and (4) Strain.

The term "Class" is used to designate groups of breeds which have been developed in certain regions or geographical areas; thus the class name—Asiatic, Mediterranean, English, Polish, American, French, etc.

The term "breed" denotes an established group of bird having the same general bony shape, weight and some common characteristics.

"Varieties" represent a sub-division of a breed, distinguished either by colour pattern, shape, comb type or feather pattern. For example in Leghorns, some of the varieties are Single Comb White Leghorn, Rose Comb Leghorn, Rose Comb Brown Leghorn, Single Comb Buff Leghorn, etc.

The term "strain" is used to denote a given breeder who has done the breeding on the bird and has introduced certain economic characters in the bird.

To sum up we have Classes, Breeds, Varieties and Strains and we might say that a particular bird is a Banerjee Single Comb White Leghorn indicating that Mr. Banerjee is the breeder of the strain, the variety is a single Comb White, the breed is Leghorn and it is in the Mediterranean class.

AMERICAN CLASS

RHODE ISLAND REDS

Rhode Island Red originated from Rhode Island in New England after crossing with the red Malay Game, Leghorn and Asiatic native stock.

The bird has a somewhat long, rectangular body, which is also broad and deep. The back is flat and the breast is carried well forward—characteristics which make it a good meat producing bird. The plumage of the Rhode Island Red is rich dark or brownish red in colour, evenly distributed over the entire surface, and is well glossed. The wing when spread shows black both in primaries and secondaries. The tail coverts, sickle feathers, and main tail feathers are also black. In the lower neck feathers of the female, there is also slight black marking at the base. The usual colour of the breed is, brownish red, but buff, white and brown are not uncommon.

There are two varieties of this breed: (1) Single Comb, and (2) Rose Comb. The characteristics of the varieties are identical aside from the type of comb. In both cases the skin and shanks are yellow and the ear lobes red. The Single Comb is the more popular of the two.

The standard weight in kg is: Cock—3.8; Hen—3.0; Cockerel—3.4 and Pullet—2.5. Colour of egg shells, brown to dark brown.

PLYMOUTH ROCK

The Plymouth Rock is one of the most popular breeds in America, largely because it is a bird good size, with excellent fleshing properties and good egg laying abilities. Birds of this breed have long bodies and have good depth of body. They have single combs. Mature birds weigh from 3.5 to 4.5 kg. There are seven varieties of Plymouth Rocks, each distinguished by its plumage. They are: (1) Barred, (2) White, (3) Buff, (4) Silver pencilled, (5) Blue, (6) Partridge, and (7) Columbian.

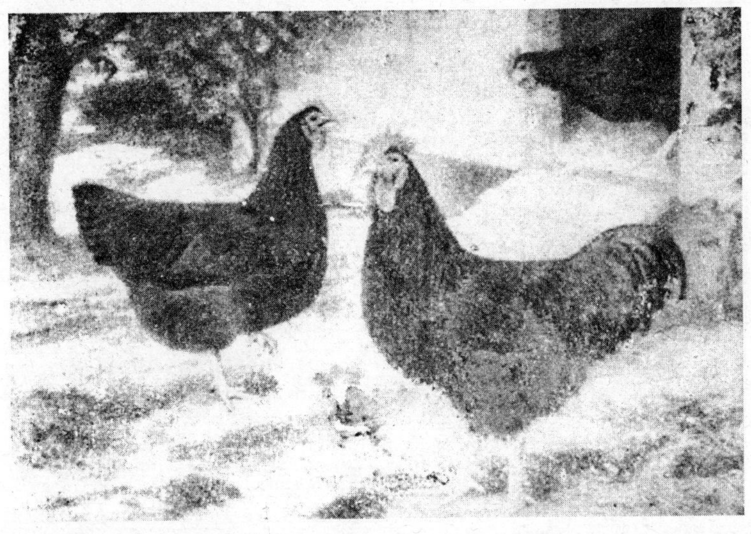

Plate 58. S.C. Rhode Island Red (Chapter 15).

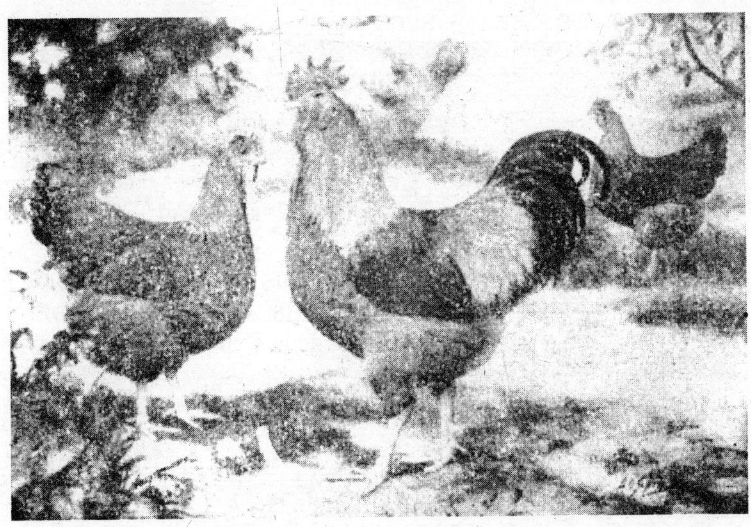

Plate 59. New Hampshires (Chapter 15).

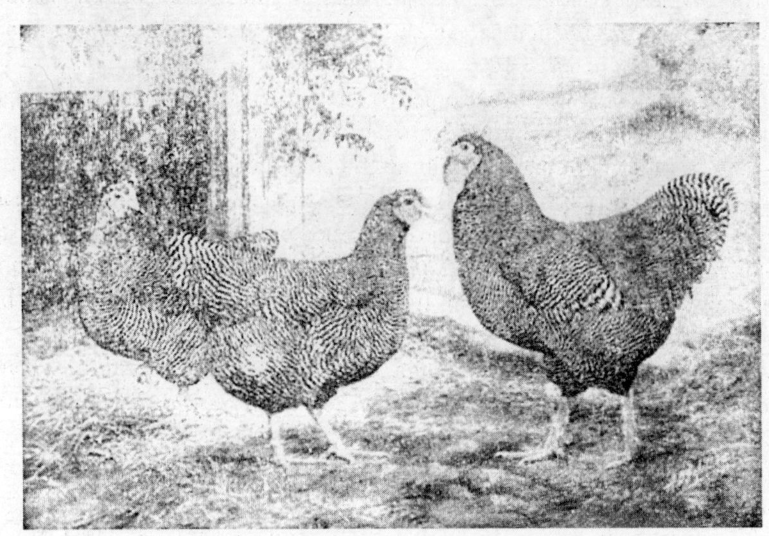

Plate 60. Barred Plymouth Rocks (Chapter 15).

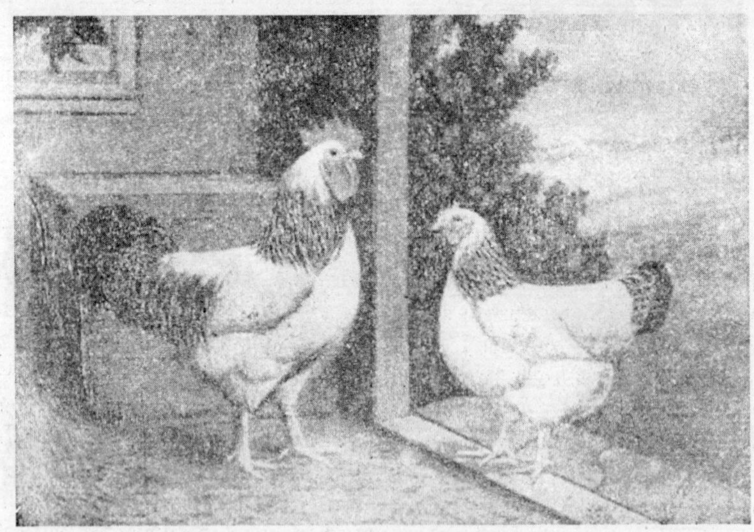

Plate 61. Light Sussex (Chapter 15).

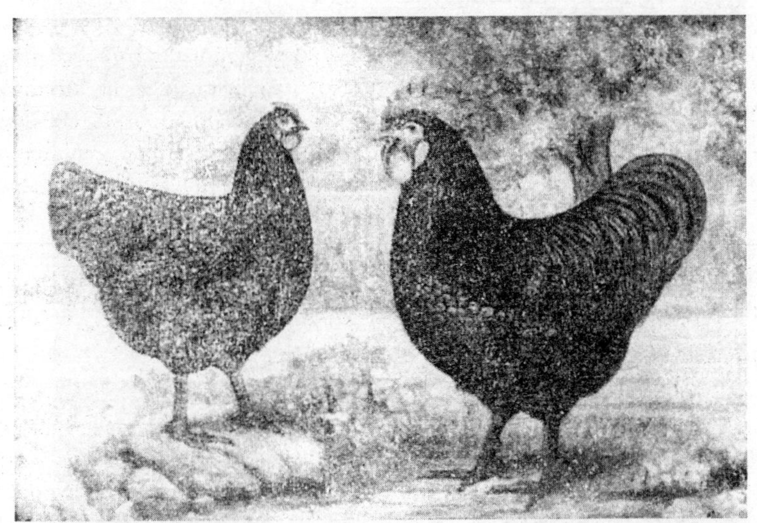

Plate 62. Australorps (Chapter 15).

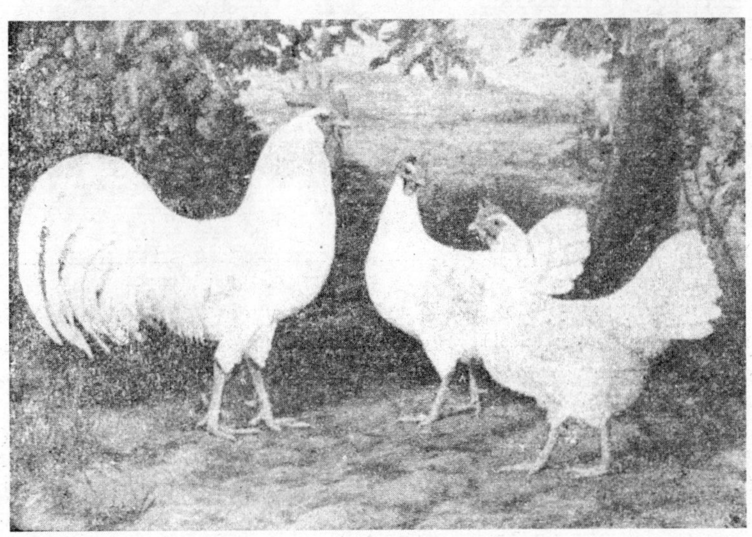

Plate 63. S.C. White Leghorns (Chapter 15).

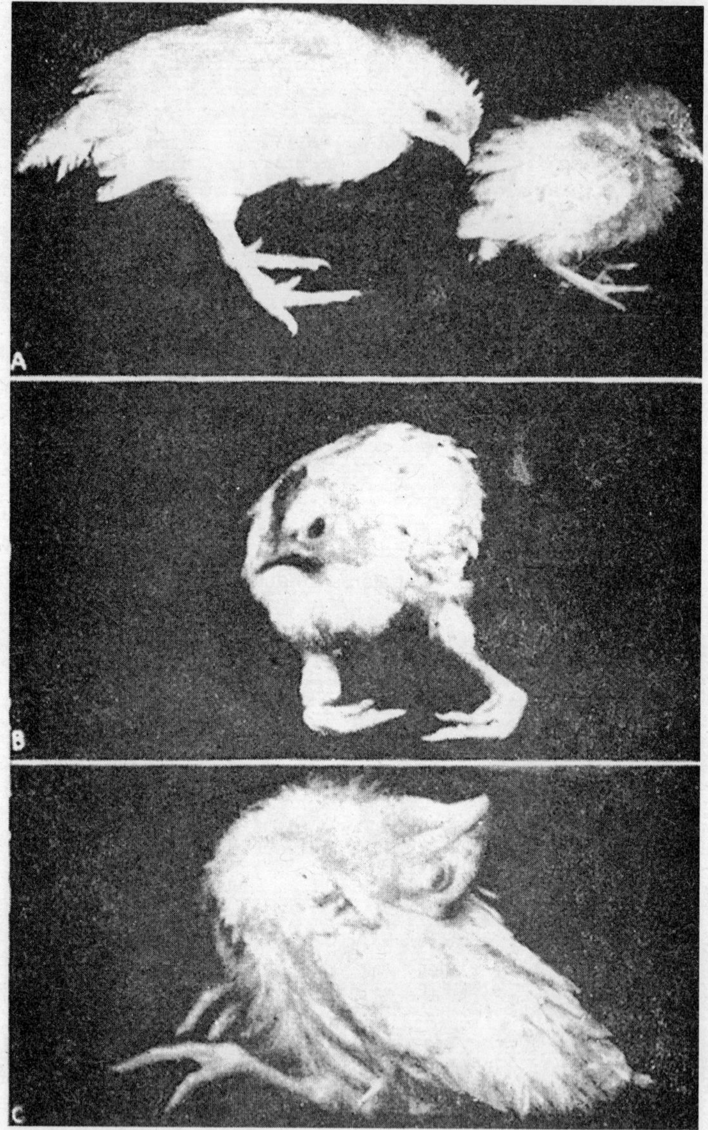

Plate 64. Effects of vitamin deficiencies. A. Effect off nicotinic acid deficiency on chick growth. B. Riboflavin deficiency in a young chick. Note the curled toes and the tendency to squat on the hocks. C. Head retraction caused by a deficiency of thiamin (Chapter 15).

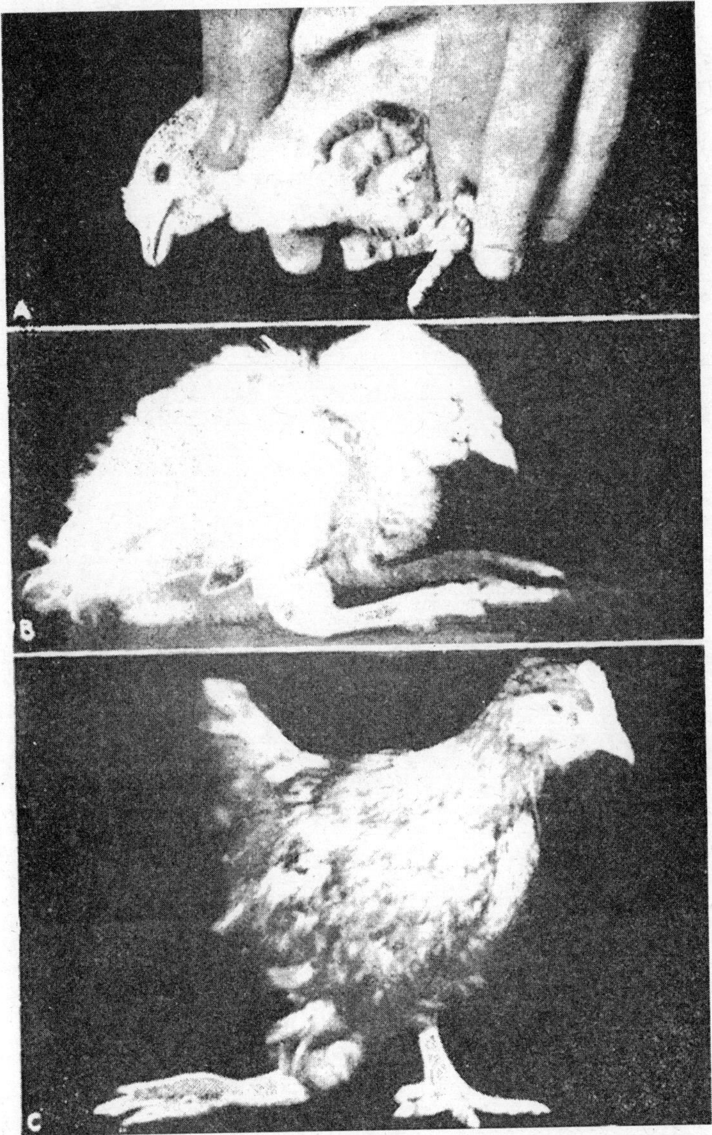

Plate 65. Effect of vitamin deficiencies. A. Biotin deficiency. Note the severe lesions on the bottom of the feet, and the lesions at the corner of the mouth. B. An advanced stage of pantothenic acid deficiency. Note the lesions at the corner of the mouth, and on the eyelids and feet. C. Perosis or slipped tendon resulting from a deficiency of managanese. This condition may also be caused by a deficiency of choline, biotin, nicotinic acid or folic acid (Chapter 15).

Table 15.1 Important characteristics of Some Representative Breeds of Chickens

Breed	Standard Weight, Kg.		Type of Comb	Colour of Earlobe	Colour of Skin	Colour of Shank	Shanks Feathered	Colour of Egg
	Cock	Hen						
American Breeds:								
Plymouth Rock	4.3	3.4	Single	Red	Yellow	Yellow	No	Brown
Wyandotte	3.8	2.8	Rose	Red	Yellow	Yellow	No	Brown
Rhode Island red	3.8	2.8	Single and rose	Red	Yellow	Yellow	No	Brown
Jersey black giant	5.9	4.5	Single	Red	Yellow	Black	No	Brown
New Hampshire	3.8	2.8	Single	Red	Yellow	Yellow	No	Brown
Asiatic Breeds:								
Brahma (light)	5.4	4.3	Pea	Red	Yellow	Yellow	Yes	Brown
Cochin	5.0	3.8	Single	Red	Yellow	Yellow	Yes	Brown
Langshan (black)	4.3	3.4	Single	Red	White	Bluish-black	Yes	Brown
English Breeds:								
Australorp	3.8	2.8	Single	Red	White	Dark slate	No	Brown
Cornish (dark)	4.5	3.4	Pea	Red	Yellow	Yellow	No	Brown
Dorking (silver-gray)	4.0	3.1	Single	Red	White	White	No	White
Orpington (buff and white)	4.5	3.6	Single	Red	White	White	No	Brown
Sussex	4.0	3.1	Single	Red	White	White	No	Brown
Mediterranean Breeds:								
Leghorn	2.7	2.0	Single and rose	White	Yellow	yellow	No	White
Minorca (S.C. black)	4.0	3.4	Single	White	White	Dark slate	No	White
Ancona	2.7	2.0	Single and rose	White	Yellow	Yellow	No	White
Andalusian (blue)	3.1	2.5	Single	White	White	Slaty blue	No	White

In general the plumage is greyish white, each feather crossed by almost black bars which should be even in width, straight and should extend down to the skin. Each feather should end with a narrow, dark tip which, with the alternate dark and light bars, give a bluish cast or shade to the surface colour.

Solid black or partly black feathers may occur in some birds of practically all strains in this variety. Black spots on the shanks are also common, particularly in females. All these strains indicate purity of breeds.

Barred Plymouth Rock. In this variety, the male birds have black and white bars of equal width, whereas in female the white bars should be as wide as the black bars.

White Plymouth Rock. White Plymouth Rocks have been used extensively in broiler production. The plumage is white throughout and usually free from black ticking, brassiness and creaminess. The variety was developed from a sport of the Barred variety.

NEW HAMPSHIRE

The shape of the body of the bird is less rectangular than that of the Rhode Island Red. The plumage is chestnut red, but is not so well established as in the Rhode Island Red. It has a single comb. In females the lower neck feathers are distinctly tipped with black. The main tail feathers are black, edge with medium chestnut red. In both sexes the under colour is light salmon.

The breed is a good-producer of large brown shelled eggs. The standard weight in kg Cock 3.8; Hen 2.7; Cockerel 3.4; Pullet 2.5.

ASIATIC CLASS

BRAHMA

The breed was developed in India and exported to America and England about one hundred years ago. The original birds were light in colour. Brahmas are massive in appearance, well feathered and well proportioned. They have pea combs. Mature birds weight from 4 to 5 kg. Three varieties of Brahmas have been produced: (1) Light, (2) Dark, and (3) Buff.

Light Brahma. The light Brahma is most popular because of its colour and its size. Mature birds weigh about 500 gm more than birds of the other two varieties.

The colour pattern of the light Brahma is similar to that of the Columbian Plymouth Rock and the Columbian White, the hackle feathers are black with white edging, and the main tail feathers are black, with the exception of top feathers of the female, which are laced with white. The shanks, toes and beak are yellow.

Dark Brahma, In the male the hackle is greenish black with an edging of white. Plumage in front of the neck is black. The wing bow is white and the primary wing feathers and tail feathers are black.

In the female, the head and the upper neck are silver grey, the wing bows are steel-grey with black pencilling and the primary wing feathers are black with a narrow edge of steel-grey. The back is steel-grey, with the same black pencilling as on the breast, body and fluff. The tail is black except for the top two feathers, which are grey underneath. The shanks, toes and beak are yellow.

ENGLISH CLASS

SUSSEX

The breed developed in England about 200 years ago primarily as table birds. It has a long body, shoulders are broad with a good depth from front to rear and the bird in general has excellent fleshing qualities. Males of this breed have a single comb and coloured beaks, shanks and toes. The standard weights in kg are Cock 4.0; Hen 3.1; Cockerel 3.4; Pullet 2.7. The varieties are described below:

Light Sussex. The plumage is quite similar to that of the Columbian Plymouth Rock and Columbian Wyandote. This variety appears to lay well during summer months in India.

Red Sussex. The plumage is deep rich red in both sexes. The only exception to the Red are found principally in the primaries where the lower webs are black with a narrow edging of red, and in the secondaries, where the upper webs are black like that of the tail colour. The under colour of all sections in both sexes is red with a slight bar of slate.

AUSTRALORP

The breed was developed in Australia where for many years it has been bred principally for egg production rather than meat. It is also very fleshy which makes it a good dual purpose breed.

The back is somewhat long, and the body slopes gradually towards the tail. It has a good depth of body, and more closely feathered than the Orpington. The comb is single, the body is black, plumage is lustrous greenish black in all the sections, the under colouring is dull black.

The "Austro White" a hybrid cross between the Australorp male and the White Leghorn female, has proved to be an excellent layer with good vigour and is maintained in large flocks in commercial egg farms of India. The standard weight of Australorp in kg is: Cock 3.8; Hen 3.0; Cockerel 3.4; Pullet 2.5.

ORPINGTON

Orpingtons were developed in Kent in England. They are long, deep and broad and well rounded, with a full breast and a broad back. They are little more loosely feathered than breeds of American class. Orpingtons have single combs. Mature birds weigh from 4.5 kg.

There are four varieties: (1) Buff; (2) Black; (3) White; (4) Blue. Only the Buff Orpington has made much popularity in America.

Buff orpington. It was evolved from Buff Cochin, Dark Dorkings, and Golden spangled Hamburgs. The plumage is the same as in other Buff breeds, such as the Buff Plymouth Rock. The shanks and toes are white.

MEDITERRANEAN CLASS

LEGHORN

Out of the important breeds classified as Mediterranean breeds, the Leghorn is by far the most popular. It is the word's number one egg producer. The breed originated in Itlay and so far there are 12 varieties. Only three varieties, however, have become popular. They are:

(1) Single Comb White; (2) Single Comb Buff; and (3) Single Comb Light Brown.

The breed is small, active, and reputed for the harmony of its various parts. In appearance the Leghorn is the neatest of all birds. It is small and very compact in form, carries the tail rather low and has a small head with well set comb and wattles. It has a relatively long back, prominent breast, and comparatively long shanks.

The shape of comb is quite important to Leghorn fanciers. The single comb of the male should be of medium size and should stand erect, with five uniform, deeply serrated points. The front point of the female should stand erect, but the remainder of the comb should gradually slope to one side.

The White, Buff and Brown varieties are subdivided further on the basis of the character of the comb. i.e., whether it is rose or single comb. All the varieties have yellow beaks, skin, shanks (legs) and toes.

In India about 50 years ago White Leghorn fowls were introduced by Christian missionaries and fanciers in U.P., Travancore-Cochin and few other States; the indigenous non-descript fowls in the villages were graded up with the White Leghorns. Today, White Leghorns are one of the most popular breeds throughout the plains of India.

Leghorns are known for their stylish carriage. Mature birds weigh from 2.0 to 2.7 kg.

MINORCA

Minorcas, originally called Red-Faced Black Spanish, are the largest and heaviest of Mediterranean breeds of poultry. Long strong bodies, large combs, long wattles, large white ear lobes, large and full tail moderately elevated, with firm muscular legs set squarely under the powerful looking body, are the distinct characteristics of this breed. The beak, shanks and toes are black.

An excellent producer of large white eggs. Colour of skin white; the egg shell is chalk white in colour. This breed was at one time even more popular than the Leghorn because of the superior size of its white eggs, but is now dropping out of favour probably because of the decline in production. The standard weight in kg. : Cock 4.1 ; Cockerel 3.4 ; Hen 3.0 ; Pullet 2.8.

Blood-The Circulatory System

In contrast to their reptilian ancestors, fowl have four-chambered hearts, which allow efficient circulation to the lungs to provide sufficient exchange of O_2 and CO_2 to support a high rate of metabolism. The blood of a chicken makes up about 8% of the body weight in chicks one to two weeks of age and about 7% of the weight of a mature hen. This is similar to the blood volume of turkeys, which was reported to be 7% in breeder hens.

The heart rate of a mature small fowl, such as a white leghorn, is about 350 beats per minute. Larger breeds such as the Rhode island red have lower heart rates averaging about 250 beats per minute. A typical heart rate of resting turkeys is 200 beats per minute, but rates as low as 160 and as high as 275 beats per minute are not unusual. Dropping a day-old chick has been shown to increase the heart rate from 300 beats per minute to 560. The deep body temperatures of mature chickens and turkeys are about 41.9° C (107.4°F) and 41.5°C (106.7°F), respectively.

Table 15.2 **Heart rate in Birds**

Type of Bird	Heart Rate Beats/Minute
Quail	500-600
Chicken	250-475
Turkey	200-275
Pigeon	220
Goose	200

Blood pressure – Blood pressure of chickens of all ages is measured as mm Hg. Even the pressure of the developing embryo may be recorded. As with human beings, there are two measures : (1) systolic pressure (arterial), and (2) diastolic pressure (as the blood returns to the heart).

Following are the recognized blood pressures of adult chickens :

Table 15.3

	Systolic Pressure	Diastolic Pressure
	(mmHg)	(mmHg)
Adult female chicken	140–160	130–134
Adult Male chicken	180–195	145–150

Genetic factors exert a strong influence on blood pressure in turkeys. The broad breasted bronze turkey, a variety of turkey which became known for its tendency to have a high incidence of mortality due to aortic rupture, has among the highest values of blood pressure known for birds or mammals. Hypertensive and hypotensive turkeys which have been developed by genetic selection are potentially valuable models for research on the control of blood pressure.

The blood functions in transport of oxygen and carbon dioxide, transport of nutrients to body cells, in temperature regulation, and in transport of important metabolites, hormones, and waste products to appropriate places in the body. Chicken blood contains from about 2.5 to 3.5 million red blood cells per cubic millimeter depending on age and sex. The blood of adult males contains about 500,000 more red blood cells per cubic millimeter than are found in the blood of a hen. Turkey blood contains about 2.5 million red blood cells per cu mm. As in chickens, this value will vary with age and sex. Avian red blood cells contain a nucleus, in contrast to the red blood cell of a mammal. The red blood cells contain the hemoglobin, the oxygen-carrying pigment of blood. About 30% of the volume of whole blood of a young chick, poult or laying hen and approximately 40% in adult male chickens and turkeys in made up of cells. The life span of erythrocytes of chickens averages from 28-35 days, about one- half that of humanus.

The spleen is an organ associated with the circulatory system, found near the gizard in the abdominal cavity, in which red and white blood cells may be formed, and which may act as a reservoir for red blood cells.

Nervous system

The nervous system regulates all organs and consists of many parts. The brain represents highly concentrated nerve cells, the basis for all nerve stimuli. Hearing and sight are well developed, with the chicken being able to distinguish colours; but the ability to smell is of low magnitude. The sensitive taste buds enable the bird to develop a liking for certain feed flavours that in part determines the type of food the bird eats.

Chickens have an ability to learn; they learn to recognize large numbers of pen mates at a young age, and their ability increases with age.

Respiratory system

The respiratory system of chickens consists of

Nasal cavaties	Bronchi
Larynx	Lungs
Trachea (windpipe)	Air sacs
Syrinx (voice box)	Air–containing bones

Lungs of the chicken are small compared with those of mammals. They expand or contract only slightly, and there is no true *diaphragm*. The lungs are supplemented by nine air sacs and the air–containing bones. They have four pairs of air sacs dvided equally into *thoracic* and *abdominal air sacs*, plus one singular *interclavicular sac.*

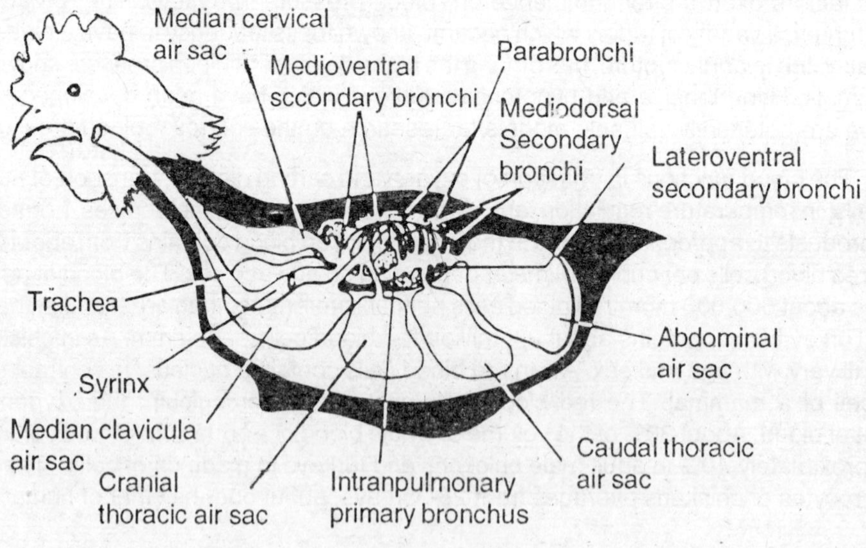

Fig. 15.3 Respiratory system of the chicken.

Air freely moves in and out of the air sacs, but the lungs are responsible for most of the respiration. Both the lungs and air sacs function as a cooling mechanism for the body when moisture is exhaled in the form of water vapour.

The respiratory rate is governed by the carbon dioxide content of the blood; increased levels increase the rate, which varies between 15 and 25 cycles/min in the resting bird.

THE DIGESTIVE SYSTEM AND ITS FUNCTION

A bird cannot be classed as a simple stomach animal, and yet its digestive system is somewhat similar. Very little digestion takes place in poultry through bacterial action, and moreover poultry can digest smaller amounts of fibre than any other class of farm livestock.

The structure of the alimentary canal of the bird suggests that the digestive process is rapid and that it resembles both the carnivora and herbivora in certain particulars. The relative shortness in length is a carnivorous characteristic, while the thorough pulverising of the feed in the gizzard corresponds to mastication in the herbivora.

Following is a brief description of the digestive organs in poultry and its function.

Mouth Parts

The distinctive character of the mouth of the bird is the absence of lips and teeth. These parts are replaced by a horny mandible on each jaw, forming the beak.

The tongue is shaped like the barbed head of an arrow with the point directed forward. The barb-like projections at the back of the tongue serve the purpose of forcing the grain toward the entrance to the gullet when the tongue is moved from front to back. The amount of saliva is very small.

Esophagus

The esophagus or gullet is distinguished by its enormous expansibility. Food passes from the mouth through the esophagus to the crop and onwards.

Crop

The crop is an enlargement of the esophagus, and is used for storing and softening the food. Food is gradually sent to the stomach as needed by contraction of the walls of the crop.

Proventriculus

Two or three inches beyond the crop, an enlarged muscular portion of the esophagus will be seen, about ½ to ¾ inch in diameter and from 1¼ to 2 inches long. This is the proventriculus, a small organ which receives the food from the crop. On the inner surface are the openings of various glands, which secrete gastric juice and some acids. These liquids are mixed with the food and assist in further softening it. This glandular stomach does not appreciably detain the food.

Gizzard

The gizzard is heavily muscled, reddish-green colour, and located just back of the proventriculus. Probably some gastric digestion takes place in the gizzard, but this organ functions chiefly in crushing and grinding food. It is the largest single organ of the body. The gizzard is composed of two pairs of thick, powerful muscles covered internally with a thick, horny epithelium.

In fact the gizzard functions as a filter, in such a way that fine material enters the duodenum in about one minute after ingestion by a fowl, while coarse material is retained much longer to be ground by the contractions of the gizzard.

Duodenum

Placed in the section of the small intestine which forms a fold immediately after the

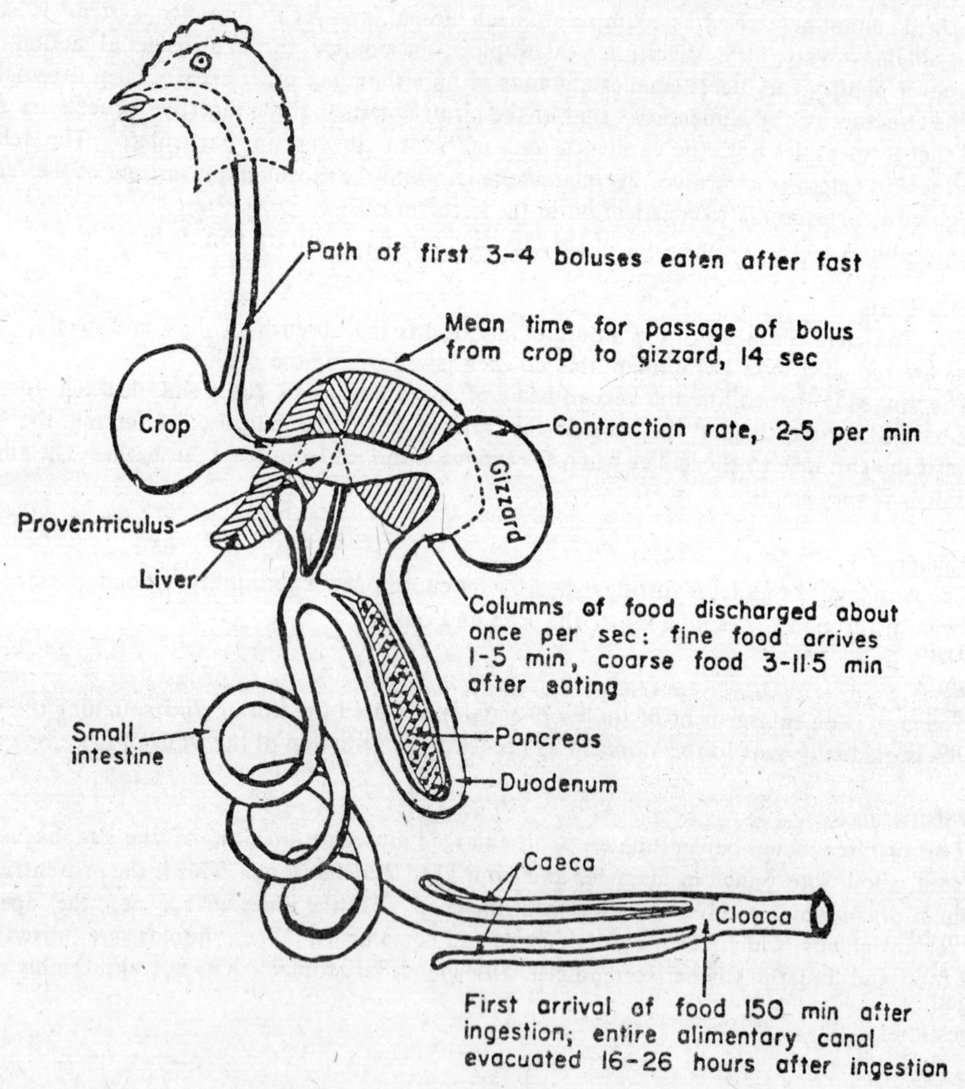

Fig. 15.4. The digestive system in a Chicken.

digestive canal leaves the gizzard, this loop,. or fold of the intestine is the duodenum, which supports the pancreas.

Gastric digestion, together with some pancreatic digestion, takes place in the duodenum.

Table 15.4

The Digestive Enzymes of the chicken

Where Found	*Substrate*	*End Product*
Mouth		
Amylase	Starch	Glucose, maltose, dextrins
Proventriculus		
Pepsin	Protein	Peptides
Small instestine		
Produced by pancreas		
Amylase	Starch	Glucose, maltose, dextrins
Lipase	Fat	Fatty acids, monoglycerides
Trypsin, Chymotrypsin, Elastase	Protenins	Amine acids small peptides
Carboxypeptidase		
Produced by intestinal mucosa		
Oligo-1,6-glucosidase	Dextrins	Glucose
Maltase	Maltose	Glucose
Sucrase	Sucrose	Glucose and fructose
Amino peptidase, dipeptidases	Peptides	Amino acids

Pancreas

Lying between the folds of the duodenum, this organ is relatively longer in birds than in mammals. It secretes a fluid known as the pancreatic juice, that contains proteolytic, amylolytic and lipolytic enzymes which vigorously hydrolyse proteoses, peptones, starches and fats. The pancreatic juice empties into the duodenum.

Liver

This is a large, several lobed, dark red organ. It is more or less flat, even more so at the extremities. It is the largest gland in the body. The liver secretes the bile.

Two ducts convey the bile from the liver to the terminal part of the duodenum. The one from the right lobe of the liver is enlarged to form the gall bladder in which the bile is temporarily stored. The one from the left lobe has no such enlargement. They enter the duodenum together. The gall bladder can be easily identified by its dark green colour. Bile aids in the digestion of fat.

Spleen

This round reddish body is found near the liver. It is usually from $\frac{1}{4}$ to $\frac{1}{2}$ inch in diameter.

Its function is little known. Some authorities believe that the white corpuscles of the blood accumulated in the spleen are rebuilt or cast from the body.

Small Intestine

It makes up the digestive tract from the gizzard to the caeca. It is about 2½ feet long in mature bird. The inner surface is lined with mature villi, which may be seen washing under water.

Besides its digestive function, the small intestine also acts as an organ of absorption of the feed ingredients in simpler form.

Caeca

At the junction of the small and large intestines are two blind sacs, 5–7 inches in length. These open into the intestine as one end, but have no outlet at the other. They appear to serve as temporary storage organs for faecal material, and some absorption may take place in them. They also aid in the digestion of fibre.

Large Intestine

It lies between the junction of the caeca and extends for a short distance up to the exterior opening of the cloaca. Short villi project into the lumen of the tract for further absorption of the digested materials (in mammals villi are absent in the large intestine).

Cloaca

The faecal material from the rectum and urine from the kidneys pass into this organ. The materials are mixed and excreted through the vent.

Urinary System

From each kidney, the urine, in the form of a white pasty material, passes through the ureter to the cloaca, where it is subsequently voided with the faecal matter from the cloaca.

MALE REPRODUCTIVE SYSTEM

The male reproductive system produces male reproductive cells (spermatozoa), meant for introducing them into the oviduct of the female for fertilisation of the egg and secondly for producing a hormone which influences sex characters.

The male reproductive system consists of the testes, vas deferenes, and papillae or rudimentary copulatory organs.

Testes

The testes are two small ovoid organs situated at the anterior end of the kidneys in the dorsal body wall. The left testis is usually larger than the right one. Each testis consists of a larger number of slender tubes, called seminiferous tubules, from the linings of which the reproductive cells are given off. The spermatozoa are then carried out of the testes by the seminal fluid, which is also produced in the testes. Millions of these are produced and expelled in the seminal fluid.

Vas Deferens

The vas deferens are the two tubes pursuing a wavy course from the testes to the cloaca. They convey the spermatozoa and seminal fluid from the testis to the cloaca.

Papillae

The rudimentary copulatory organ of the male is located on the median ventral portion of one of the transverse folds of the cloaca. At the time of mating sperms are introduced by the papillae into the oviduct in the cloacal wall of the female.

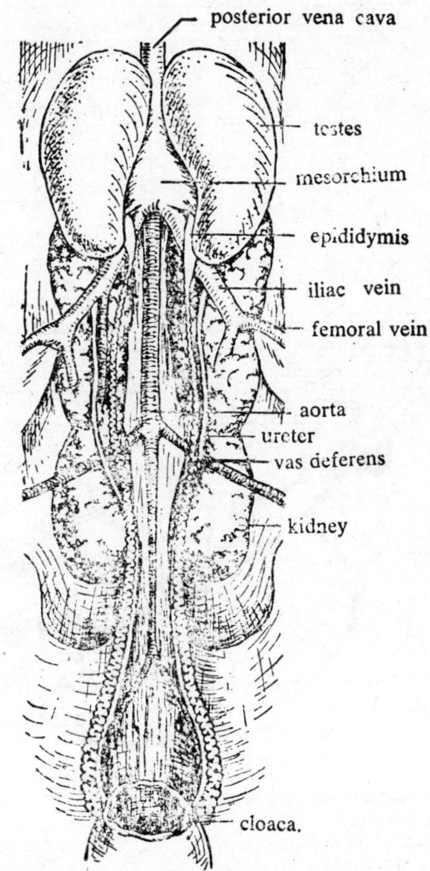

Fig. 15.5 Male urinary and reproductive organs.

Cloaca

The enlarged section of the alimentary canal that connects the large intestine and vent is called the cloaca. The vent is the external opening of the cloaca. Sperms from the testes, faecal material from the large intestine and urine from the kidneys all pass through the cloaca and are eliminated through the vent.

FEMALE REPRODUCTIVE SYSTEM

The female reproductive system differs greatly from that of mammals. The reproductive cell, also known as a gamete, ovum or egg, is an article of food. It is large and enclosed with a food supply for embryo development.

The reproductive system of the female consists of primary and accessory sexual organs, the ovary and the oviduct with its five parts: infundibulum, magnum, isthmus, uterus, and vagina.

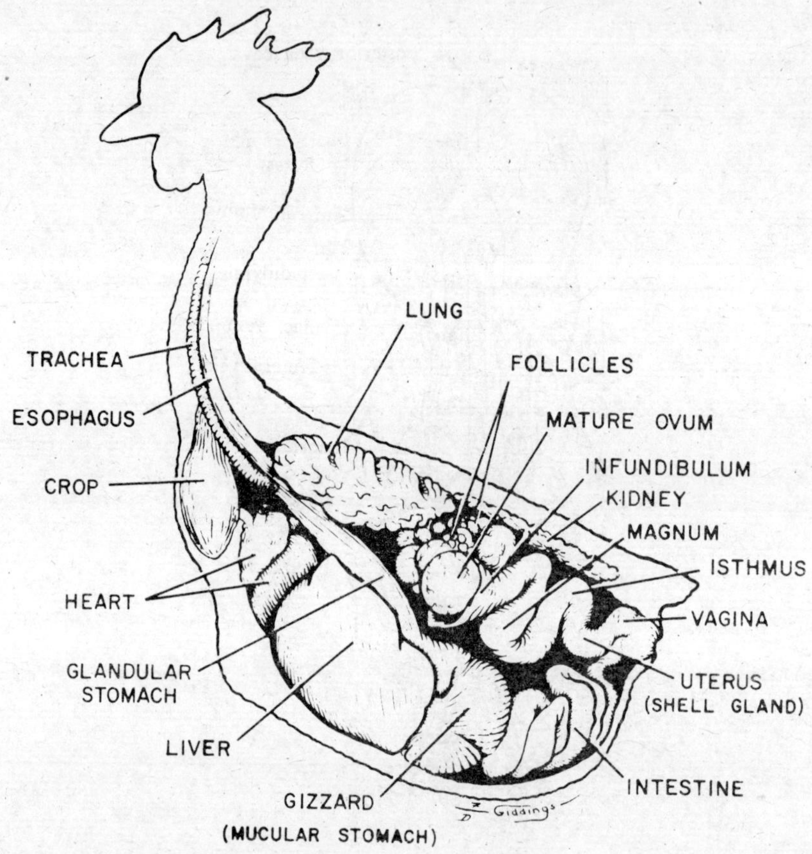

Fig.15.6 Reproductive organs of the hen in relation to other body organs. The single ovary and oviduct are on the hen's left side; an underdeveloped ovary and oviduct are sometimes found on the right side, having degenerated in the developing embryo.

Ovary

At hatching time the female chick has two ovaries and two oviducts. Normally, only the left one develops, the right persisting if at all, only as a functionless rudiment. A few cases have been reported, however, in which both right and left ovary and oviduct were present and functioning in a mature pullet. This is very rare.

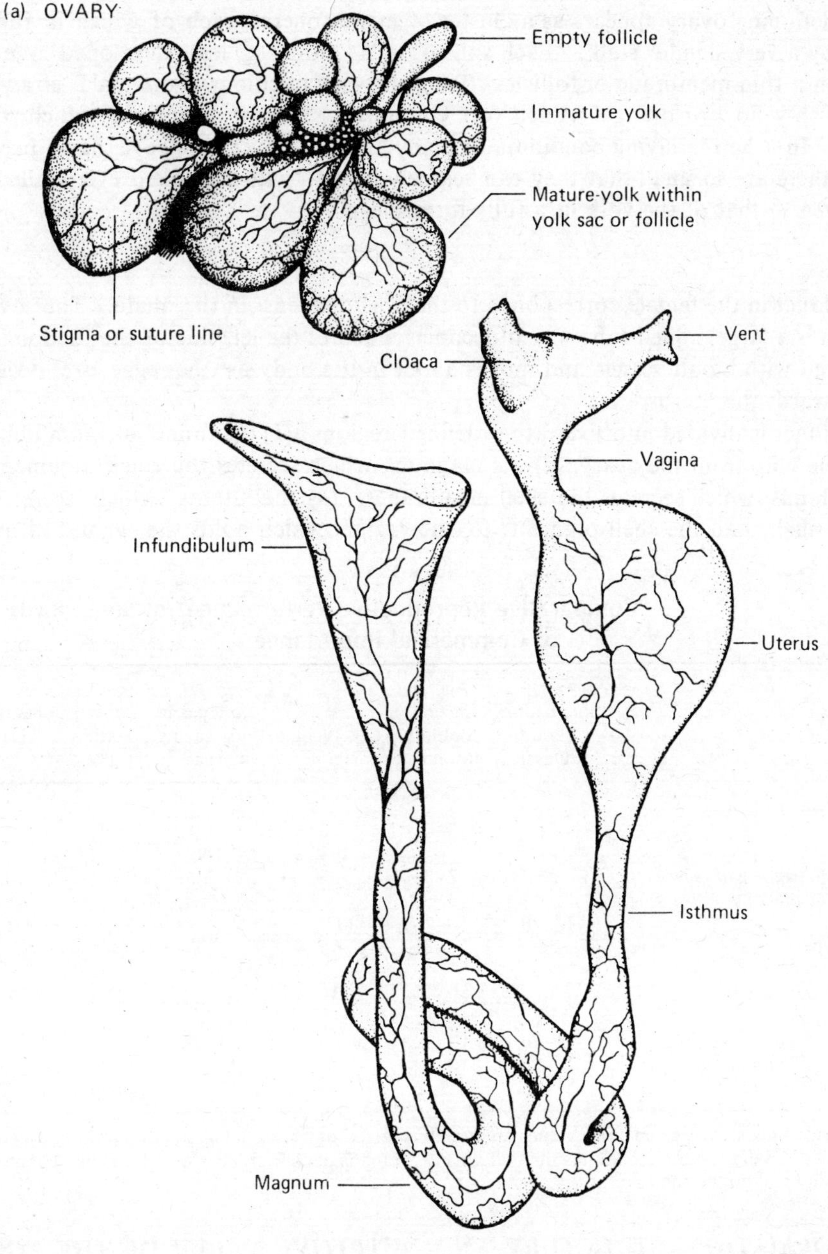

Fig. 15.7 Ovary and oviduct of the chicken. (From the *Egg Grading Manual*, USDA Ag Handbook #75.)

The functioning ovary appears as a cluster of many spheres, each of which is independently attached by a very slender stalk. Each sphere is a more or less developed ovum or yolk enclosed in a thin membrane or follicle. The yolk vary in colour from pale straw colour to deep reddish-yellow or orange. Each yolk contains a germinal disc, from which the embryo develops. In a hen in laying condition, as many as 900 to over 3,600 ova have been counted. Many of them are so small that they can scarcely be seen with the naked eye, while others vary in size even to that of the yolk in a fully formed egg.

Oviduct

The oviduct in the female corresponds to the vas deferens in the male. The oviduct in a laying hen is a large, coiled tube which occupies much of the left side of the abdominal cavity. It is covered with blood vessels and moves about in the body as the eggs are developed and moved towards the uterus.

The oviduct is divided into five rather defined regions: (1) the funnel or infundibulum, which receives the yolk from the ovary; (2) the magnum, which secretes the thick albumen or white; (3) the isthmus, which secretes the shell membranes; (4) the uterus, which secretes the thin white, the shell, and the shell pigment; (5) the vagina, which holds the egg until it is laid.

Table 15.5

Comparative Reproductive Performance* of Some Birds of Commercial Importance

Species	Incubation Period (Days)	Age at Sexual Maturity (Months)	Egg Weight (gm)	No. Eggs in First Laying Year	Fertility (%)	Hatchability of Fertile Eggs (%)
Chicken *(Gallus gallus)*						
Layer	21	5–6	58	300	97	90
Broiler	21	6	65	180	92	90
Turkey *(Meleagris gallopavo)*	28	7–8	85	90	83	84
Duck *(Anas platyrhynchos)*						
Layer	27–28	6–7	60	300	95	75–80
Meat type	28	6–7	65			
Goose *(Anser anser)*						
Small type	30	9–10	135	30–70	70	70
Large type	33	10–12	215			
Pheasant *(Phasianus colchicus)*	24–26	10–12	30	50–75	95	85
Guinea fowl *(Numida meleagris)*	27–28	10–12	40	80–200	90	95
Quail *(Coturnix coturnix)*	15–16	1.5–2	10	300	90	75–85

*Only general figures are given since values are greatly affected by breed, location and nutrition. In particular the values given in the last three columns depend greatly on management practices, and it is likely that fertility and hatchability will be the same for all species.

FORMATION, STRUCTURE AND NUTRITIVE VALUE OF THE EGGS

The knowledge of the formation and structure of the egg is essential for an understanding of fertility, embryo development, egg quality, any disease of the female reproductive organs.

Yolk Formation

The ovarian tisssue appears as a cluster of tiny ova or yolks. During the early stages of

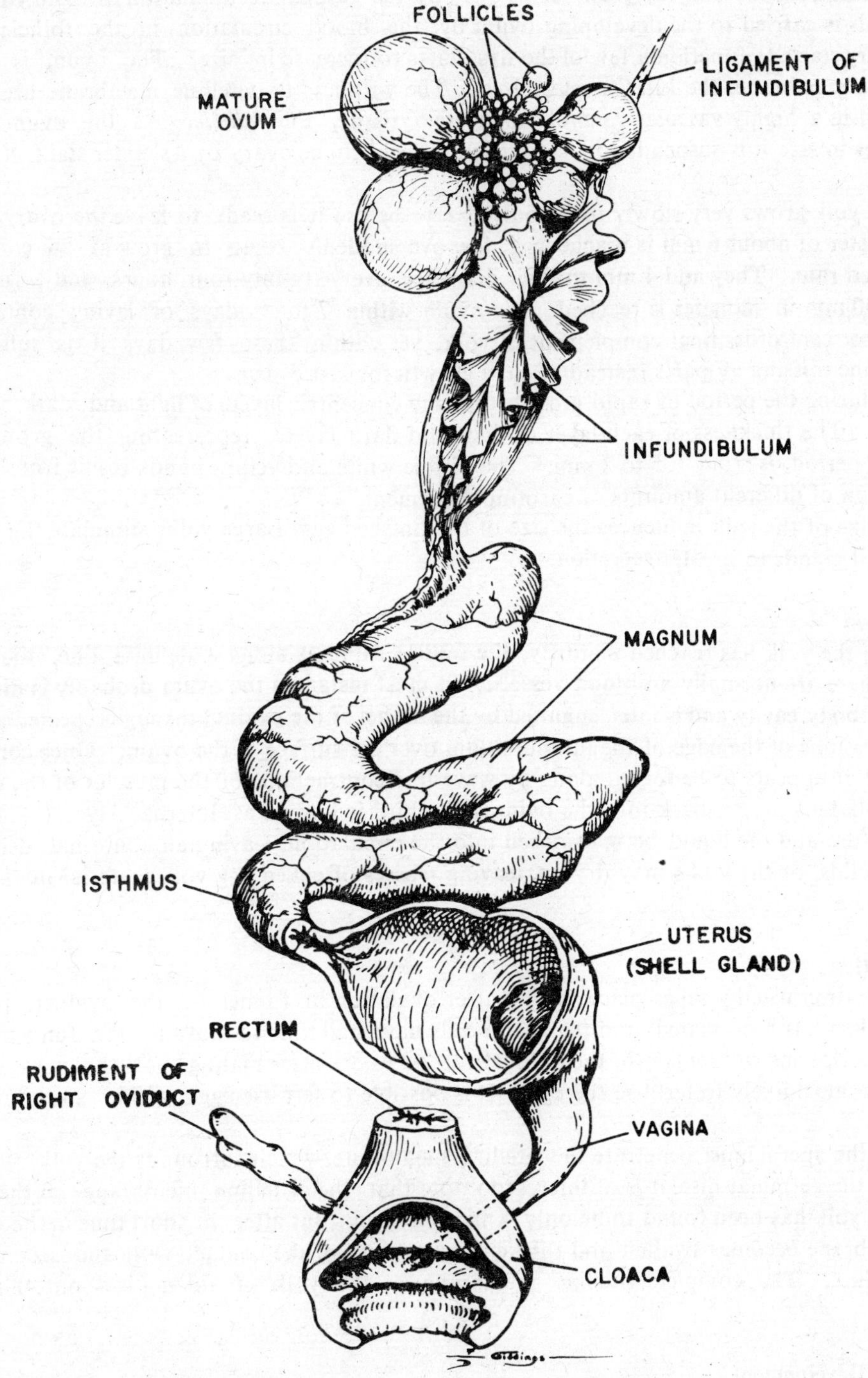

Fig. 15.8 Reproductive organs of the hen.

yolk formation, the oocytes grow very slowly by the gradual accumulation of light yolk. Food materials is carried to the developing ovum by the blood circulation in the follicle. When the ovary starts to function a few of the ova starts to increase in size. The ovum is enclosed in a thin membrane, the *Vitelline membrane.* The yolk and its vitelline membrane are in turn enclosed in a highly vascular coat of connective tissue, the *follicle.* As the ovum or yolk increases in size it is suspended in its follicle and held to the ovary by a slender stalk, the follicle *stalk.*

Each yolk grows very slowly for about 10 days before it is ready to leave the ovary. When a diameter of about 6 mm is reached, a few ova suddenly begin to grow at an enormously increased rate. They add 4 mm to their diameter every twenty-four hours, until full size of about 40 mm in diameter is reached. An ovum within 7 to 9 days of laying contains less than 1 per cent of its final complement of yolk, yet within these few days it is sufficient to supply the missing 99 parts instead of slow growth for last 3 days.

It is during the period of rapid growth that the concentric layers of light and dark yolk are formed. The thickness of each layer of light and dark layers, representing the growth in a 24-hour period, is from 1.5 to 2 mm. The visible white and yellow bands result from periodic deposition of different amounts of carotinoid pigment.

The size of the yolk influences the size of the finished egg. Large yolks stimulate the albumen and shell glands to greater secretion.

Ovulation

When the yolk has reached maturity, the follicle ruptures along a definite line, the stigma, where there are normally no blood vessels. In most instances the ovum probably is discharged into the body cavity and is later engulfed by the funnel of the oviduct through repeated advances and recessions of the edge of the infundibulum over the surface of the ovum. Once completely enclosed, it appears to be forced along by wave-like contractions of the muscles of the oviduct. If the yolk fails to get back into the oviduct the bird is known as internal layer. The yolks may rupture and the liquid be reabsorbed into the circulation, leaving an abnormal deposit of yellow solids, or the yolks may dry up, leaving masses of caked egg yolk material in the body cavity.

Fertilisation

Fertilisation usually takes place shortly after ovulation in funnel of the oviduct, provided that the hen has been mated, and the sperm cells have had time to move to the funnel of the oviduct. Sperms will remain in the oviduct for 2-3 weeks after mating, but the newest sperm is the one most likely to fertilise the egg. It is possible to fertilise eggs within 24 hours after mating.

Since the sperm must penetrate the vitelline membrane, which surrounds the yolk, in order to reach the germinal disc, it is of interest to note that the vitelline membrane on the freshly ovulated yolk has been found to be only 4 microns thick. But after the short time in the oviduct, the membrane becomes swollen and thickens, as a result of the contact with the secretions of the oviduct. The complete vitelline membrane of the yolk of laid egg is about 48 microns thick.

Embryo Development

The fertilised ovum starts cell division and embryo development soon after fertilisation. It continues during the period approximately by 24 hours when the egg remains in the oviduct. The germ spot or blastoderm increases in size and there is some change in the consistency of the white and yolk. Unless the fertile egg is held below 82°F after it is laid, there will be further germ development. It is, therefore, desirable to produce infertile eggs at all times except when they are not needed for hatching.

Secretion of Thick White

Immediately upon being grasped by the mouth of the oviduct the ovum or yolk is forced through the oviduct by ciliary action or by peristaltic movements of the walls of the oviduct to the magnum region. It requires about 3 hours to pass through this region. The inner surface of the magnum section of the oviduct is lined with goblet cells that secrete albumen. At this region the yolk acquires the mass of firm white albumen, which makes up about one-half of the total white, by volume. Hens that lay eggs containing a relatively high percentage of thick white have more goblet cells. The thick white percentage tends to decrease from about April to July in most flocks.

Formation of the Shell Membranes

The yolk, surrounded with its thick white, passes from the magnum through a short section of the oviduct known as the isthmus. Here the two shell membranes are added and the shape of the egg is determined. An isthmus of large diameter tends to result in thick round eggs, while on of small diameter tends to result in long slender eggs.

It is an interesting fact that these membranes are so formed as to enclose the yolk and thick white rather loosely. They do not plump out until the egg receives its final quota of white in the uterus.

Addition of Thin White and Shell

The developing egg passes from the isthmus into the uterus, where it remains for about 24 hours. The inner layer, between the inner and outer layers of thick white, becomes apparent

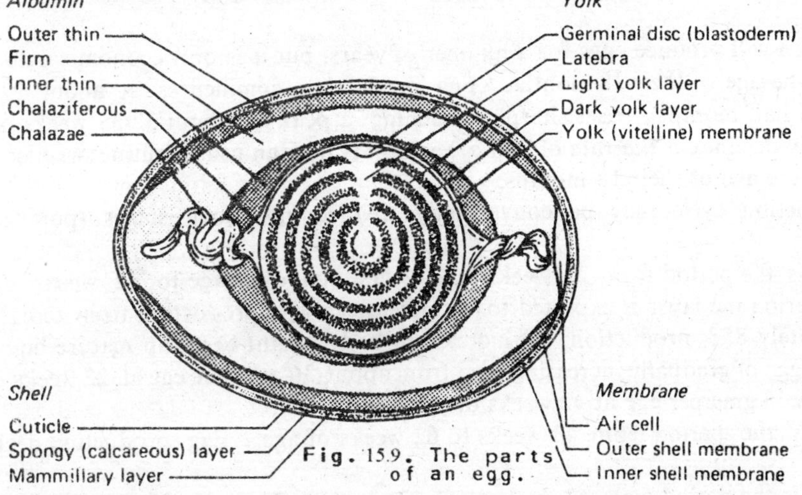

Fig. 15.9. The parts of an egg.

while the egg is in the uterus as a result of the albumen rotating around the yolk. The thin white, composed of water and a mineral solution consists largely of sodium, calcium and potassium. The inner and outer layers of thin white each comprise about 20-25 per cent of the total white.

In addition to the formation of the inner and outer layers of thin white, the uterine glands also secrete material for the shell, consisting largely of calcium carbonate. It is carried to the uterus by the blood circulation. It is interesting to note that the calcium of blood is nearly double at the laying stage. High temperature always tends to reduce shell thickness.

Table 15.6. **Agmark standards for market table eggs**

Grade	Weight (g)	Shell	Aircell	White	Yolk
A-Extra large A-Large A-Medium A-Small	60 and above 53-59 45-52 38-44	Clean, unbroken and sound, shape normal	Up to 4 mm indepth practicaly regular or botter	Clear, reasonably firm	Fairly wellcentred, practically free from defects, outline indistinct.
B-Extra large B-Large B-Medium B-Small	60and above 53-59 45-52 38-44	Clean to moderately stained, sound and slightly abnormal	8 mm in depth, may be free and slightly bubbly	Clear, may be slightly weak	May be slightly off centered, outline slightly visible.

EGG PRODUCING CARRIER OF A LAYING HEN

A laying hen will produce eggs for a number of years, but it is only economical to keep the layers up to the age of their 18 months. Egg production commences at about 22 weeks of age (five and half months), rises sharply, reaching a peak at about 32-35 weeks of age, and then gradually declines at the rate of half a week. It is thus an usual routine practice to replace the layers at the age of their 18 months.

The production cycle may be conveniently divided into three stages (popularly called phases).

Phase I is the period from 22 weeks (age of first laying) of age to 42 weeks of age and during this period the layer is expected to (1) increase in egg production from zero to a peak of approximately 85% production; (2) increase in body weight to attain mature body weights; (3) produce eggs of gradually increasing size from about 36 gms per egg at 22 weeks of age to approximately 58 gms per egg at 42 weeks of age.

Phase II is the period from 43 weeks to 62 weeks of age. Egg production declines upto 65 per cent.

Phase III is the period from 63 weeks upto 72 weeks. The egg production is less than 65 per cent.

A typical production, body weight and feed consumption curve for a laying flock is shown.

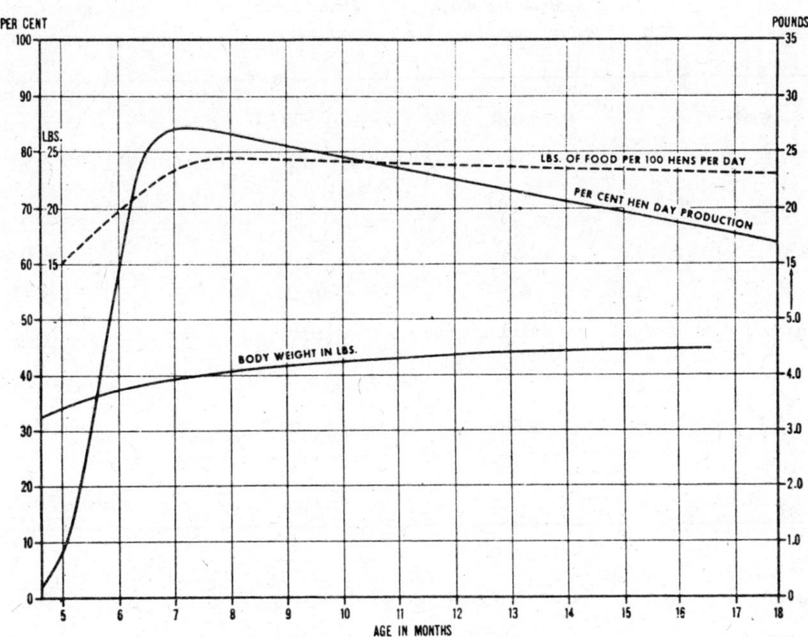

Note the changes in egg production, body weight and feed consumption of Single Comb White Leghorn hens during their production period.

TEN FACTORS AFFECTING EGG SIZE

Breeding. Most breeders develop strains which will produce egg sizes required by the market. Random sample test results are a very good guide for comparing the egg size of different strains in the market.

Feeds. Most rations in the market are well balanced. However, if an unbalanced stale, or badly mixed feed is given, smaller eggs may result.

Feed restriction. All birds should be able to get food when they want it. Any restriction on feed, whether due to lack of enough feeder space, forgetting to feed the birds or from using stale food, will lower feed consumption and reduce egg size.

Lack of water. Water that is too hot, too cold or dirty will be unpalatable to the birds—they will not drink enough, food consumption will fall and egg size will suffer. Keep the water fresh and clean and look out for any faulty drinkers supply.

Protein level. Rations containing less than 15 per cent protein are liable to give smaller egg size. Although this is not likely to be a problem with commercially compounded rations, home mixers should keep a careful check on the point.

Table 15.7

Nutritive value of eggs

	Recommended daily allowance for moderately active man	*Quantity in 1 egg*	*Quantity in 1/2 pint milk (approx. 280 ml.)*
Energy (kilo calories)	3,000	90	205
Proteins (g)	70	6.6	9.6
Fat (g)	50	5.5	10.3
Carbohydrate (g)	570	...	14.0
Calcium (g)	0.8	0.03	0.37
Phosphorus (g)	0.9	0.12	0.28
Iron (mg)	12	1.6	0.10
Vitamin A (I.U.)	5,000	600	600
Vitamin D (I.U.)	400	50	...
Vitamin B_1 (mg)	1.5	0.095	0.10
Vitamin C (mg)	75	2.0	6
Riboflavin (mg)	2.0	0.19	0.25
Nicotinic acid (mg)	18	0.04	0.08

Laying-house temperature. Experiments have shown that egg size can be at least 1 oz. per dozen less at temperatures over 70°F than at 55°. It is important, therefore, to keep house as cool as possible during hot weather.

Disease. Most disease will upset the birds, giving decreased feed consumption. This can only lead to lower production and egg size. Good hygiene and management will reduce this risk.

Age of maturity. Birds which mature early, such as those reared during increasing daylength, will lay smaller eggs than birds reared on a constant daylength or a decreasing daylength.

Age of birds. Birds at 20 to 26 weeks of age will lay smaller eggs than at 40 to 50 weeks. Maximum egg size can be expected when the birds reach about one year old. Egg size tends to get smaller just before birds stop laying.

Egg cooling and storage. It is important to cool eggs as quickly as possible after they are laid and to store them at a temperature of 50 to 55°F, otherwise they will lose weight by evaporation. This may result in poorer grading results, and so a poorer economic return.

ABNORMAL EGGS

Double-yolked eggs. Such types are due probably from two ova ripening at the same time, or one ovum being pushed back into the oviduct at the same time when another ovulation takes place. The type is more common in pullets than older birds. Probably newly functioning ovary and oviduct takes time to work normally.

Meat spots. Sometimes found either on the yolk or in the white of egg. Spots are generally degenerated blood clots resulting from haemorrhages in the ovary or oviduct.

Blood spots. May be found as a result of haemorrhages of small blood vessel in the ovary or oviduct. The follicle probably does not rupture along the stigma, where there are normally no blood vessels, or else the rupture occurs before ovulation. If the spots are found in the white of the egg, it indicates a haemorrhage in the wall of the oviduct.

Soft shelled eggs. The conditions generally result from the failure of the shell glands to secrete normal composition (may be due to calcium deficiency) or from the peristaltic constrictions becoming so violent as to hurry the egg through the uterus.

Small yolkless eggs. This type of egg is due to the stimulus produced by some foreign substance, such as a blood clot or piece of membrane, gaining entrance into the oviduct and passing along in the same manner as the yolk. The passage of the particle will stimulate the albumen, shell membrane and shell glands to secrete their particular products.

An egg within an egg. After an egg has been formed it may be forced back up to the funnel region by reverse peristaltic action. As it again passes the oviduct, albumen, shell membranes and shell are added.

Foreign-matter in eggs. Feather, and other foreign-matter, sometimes find their way into the oviduct and become included in the albumen; they pass through the egg formation stages and thus become embodied in the egg.

Pale yolks. These may be caused by constitutional anaemia, but are more likely due to lack of carotene and other colouring substances. Pale yolks usually occur during the winter months, and by increasing the amount of maize or maize meal in the ration, this defect may be rectified.

Rotten new-laid eggs. These are laid by an over-fat hen, a bird with oviduct disease, or one with vent gleet, which has affected the oviduct. The egg, when completely formed, has been unable to pass out of the oviduct on account of one of these reasons and has, therefore, remained bad.

SELECTION AND IMPROVEMENT

Selection, as used in connection with breeding, refers to the choosing of parents for the next generation. Its skilled performance is the foundation of constructive breeding practice. Success in poultry production is just as dependent upon the use of good breeding stock as it is in crop production. A farmer who plants seed with poor yielding ability gets a poor yield, likewise a poultry breeder who selects poor males and hens for the breeding flock to start poultry farm will definitely run at a loss, no matter, whether good feed, management and disease control practices are adopted.

Therefore, before selecting birds for starting a poultry farm a hasty or hurried decision should be avoided or selection should not be made for sentimental reasons or because of someone having purchased a particular pair of birds from a definite farm running profitably.

Careful selection of birds pays a poultryman in different ways and to get a really good foundation stock, a few basic points noted below may be followed.

1. Number of necessary removals during the laying year is reduced.

2. Culls are eliminated.
3. Average egg production is higher.
4. Profit is greater.
5. Segregation of best birds for breeding purposes is made possible.
6. Appearance of improved flock from the standardisation view-point.
7. Late maturing individuals can be excluded.
8. Production of subsequent generation of higher quality individuals is aided.
9. The spread of disease is retarded through the elimination of diseased individuals.

Selection of individual males and females for breeding may be based on:

1. The past in which the pedigree of the individual examined for several preceding generations.
2. The present in which the appearance or performance of the individual and its sibs (sisters and brothers) is used in making final judgement.
3. The future in which the breeding worth of the individuals is judged by the appearance or performance of its descendants, usually only its sons and daughters.

Two or more of these bases may sometimes be used in combination, especially the second and third. The constructive breeder attempts by selecting individuals which are pure for certain desirable genes and through intelligent mating, to assemble in new individuals still more desirable combination of genes.

Pedigree Selection

A good individual with a good ancestry is preferable to an equally good individual with a poor ancestry, but it should be emphasised that a good ancestry only improves the chances for better breeding performance and is no guarantee for such performance.

Since genes and chromosomes occur in pairs and are halved for any individual in each generation, it is immediately apparent that a particular remote ancestor can have very little influence on the genetic make-up of an individual which is considered in selection.

Pedigree selection is of value in a broad sense in that one would certainly choose a breeding cockerel whose dam had laid 250 eggs in preference to one whose record was only 150. But one should also remember that two cockerels from the 250 eggs hen may give widely differing performance as measured by the egg production of their daughters. Furthermore, a difference between 250 eggs and 150 eggs in a dam's record may be important in selection, whereas a difference between 275 and 250, or even between 300 and 250 would seem negligible.

Appearance and Performance

Vigour. Good health or vigour is the first prerequisite qualification in a bird to be used for breeding purposes. This is evident by its behaviour and body characteristics.

Birds with good vigour are active and take an interest in things going on around them. They walk, run, fly, scratch, sing, cackle or crow, and show sex interest.

They have a broad, long, deep body, with a good capacity for handling feed and producing eggs.

The head gives a good indication of the health of the bird. Rice said,—"The bird carries its health certificate on top of its head". This refers to the comb. A large bright red comb indicates good vigour, while a small, pale or dark comb indicates low vitality or disease condition.

Breed type. Birds to be maintained as breeders should be representative of the breed and variety to which they belong. A variety is a sub-division of a breed used to distinguish groups of the same breed as fowls differing in colour of plumage, shape of comb, and other characteristics.

Head. The appearance of the head is variable because of differences in size, shape and expression. Hens with coarse, phlegmatic, masculine, or "beefy" heads are not likely to lay many eggs. Those with clear-cut rugged, alert heads that are at the same time fine in quality, are likely to be among the best layers in the flock.

Eye. A good individual should have bright, prominent, well-placed eyes. They should not be depressed nor show evidence of physical debility. The so-called "pearly" eye and the retraced pupil are commonly associated with fowl paralysis.

Beak. The beak should be relatively short, strong, well-curved and in proportion to the head of the bird. The mandibles should meet properly and not overlap each other nor be deformed in any other manner. Such deformities are likely to interfere with the food consumption of the bird and consequently with the production.

Face. The face of the individual should be clean-cut and lean, yet should not present a pinched-in appearance. If (in facing the front of the bird's head) the face of the fowl is narrow and the eyes appear to be closed, it is undesirable and is usually an indication of low vitality.

The comb and wattles should be of reasonable size, well placed and fine in texture. A smooth, velvety feel indicates good texture.

Condition of comb, vent and abdomen. With some simple practice it has become a minor matter to distinguish a layer from a non-layer. This can be done by closely examining the following parts of the bird.

(*a*) *Comb*: The comb is a secondary sexual character. It tells us what is going on in the ovary. If the comb is dry, hard and scaly, the hen may still be laying but she will soon stop.

If the hen has been out of laying but the ovaries are expanded and she is coming back into production, the comb indicates the fact. It begins to swell; the blood rushes to the tips of the points, and they become hot, soft, waxy, brighter in colour and fall.

The comb is reddest and hottest just before laying commences. As soon as laying starts, the comb gradually cools and becomes somewhat lighter in colour.

(*b*) *Pubic bones:* When a bird is laying, the pubic bones—the two small bones extending along the sides of the body towards the vent are spread apart to such an extent that 2 or 3 fingers can be placed between them. During non-laying period the pubic bones become thin and pliable. In a poor-layer, the pubic bones are close together and can barely accommodate one finger space between them.

(*c*) *Vent:* When a hen is laying heavily the vent is greatly stretched during the exclusion of egg. It is, therefore, much larger than when she is not laying. During laying period it is oval in shape, pliable and moist.

(*d*) *Abdomen:* When the bird is laying heavily the abdomen is much larger than at other times. The intestines and oviduct are expanded in the laying hen because they are distended and stretched by larger quantities of food and by egg. It has also been found that the heart, gizzard, crop, etc., are much larger than in a poor layer. The skin covering the abdomen is soft and pliable. Usually 3 or 4 fingers are accommodated between the end of the keel and the ends of the pubic bones. The abdomen is constricted, the skin becomes thick and the space between the end of the pubic bones and of the keel shortens in case of non-layers.

Body conformation. To lay a large number of eggs a bird should have a good body with the following characteristics:

1. A flat, broad back that carries well but towards the pubic bones.
2. A wide heart girth.
3. Good depth of body that increases towards the abdomen in a bird in laying condition.
4. Good span between the pubic bones and keel bones.
5. Thin, straight pubic bones set well apart.
6. Good quality of skin.
7. Body wedge-shaped from back to keel bone.
8. Legs set well apart.
9. Good fleshing in all parts of the body.
10. Reasonably long keel bone.
11. A widespread of lateral processes.

Proportionate Measurements

Body measurements should be considered from the standpoint of their relationship to the size of the individual. A bird of the Asiatic or American class, for instance, may actually have large body measurements than one of the Mediterranean class, but in proportion to the size of the individuals, the former may have a much smaller proportionate capacity and consequently be a poorer producer. Each breed should be judged on the basis of the characteristic breed size. A bird should be well proportioned and have skeletal development consistent with its size.

Quality. Quality is devoted by the character of the bird, as evidenced by the examination of the shanks, keel and pubic bones. The bone formation should be sufficiently rugged for the size of the individual but should not tend towards coarseness. The shanks should appear wedge-shaped. Rounded shanks are not good. The pubic bones should be pliable, pointed and thin when bird is in production. The keel should be sufficiently long to support the abdomen and should be refined nature.

The skin should be loose, pliable and of velvety quality.

Plumage is sometimes used as an index in selection. This is particularly possible when the hen is nearing the end of her laying year, as this time the feathers of a high producer are usually brittle, rough, broken and soiled, whereas normally in such birds, due to the pliability of the skin the feathering is generally loose.

Pigmentation

This also gives some information regarding a bird's past production, in case of hens having yellow skin and shanks. During the period of production, the yellow xanthophyl pigment in the feed eaten is used for colouring the yolks and the body gradually loses its reserve supply of yellow pigment. The order of disappearance of pigment from the body and the approximate period of egg production required to bleach the body structures are follows:

Vent	... 1–2 weeks
Eye rings and Ear lobes	... 2–4 weeks
Beak	... 6–8 weeks
Shanks	... 12–20 weeks

The pigment first leaves those structures having the best blood cii :ulation. When a bird stops production, the pigment return in the same order it left and approximately twice as fast.

Moulting

Moulting is the act or process of shedding and renewing feathers. The shedding and renewal of feathers normally occurs once a year, though it may occur in certain individuals twice in a year and more rarely, only once in a period of two years. Hens usually moult in the following order: (1) head, (2) neck, (3) body (including breast, back and abdomen), wing and tail. Not only this, but there is a high degree of regularity about the order of moult within the several sections. The wing primaries, for example, begin to drop before the secondaries. The

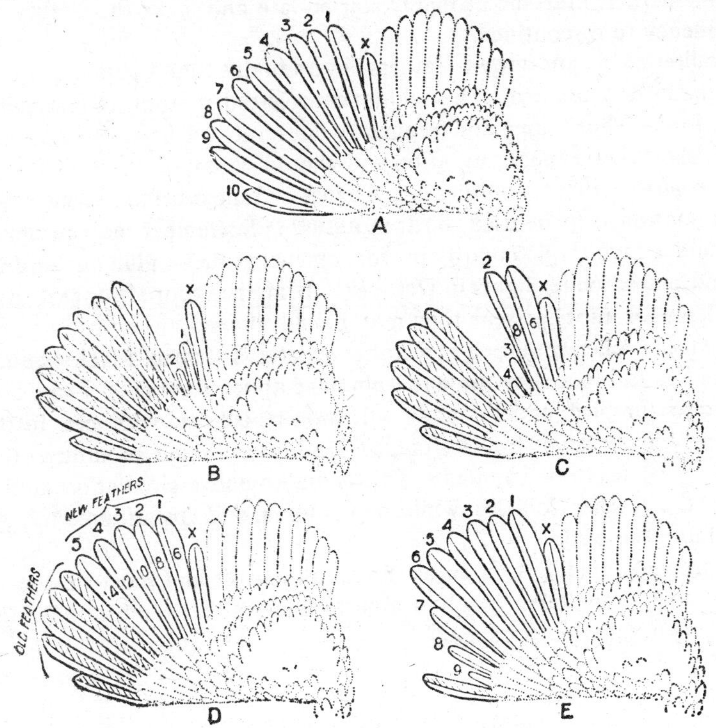

Fig. 15.10 A. A normal wing showing the primary feathers, 1 to 10. They are separated from the secondaries (shown in dotted line) by the short axial feather, X. B. The beginning of a wing moult. 1 and 2 are new feathers growing in. C. An eight week moult. D. An unusual instance in which only five primaries are moulted. E. A wing as it appears near the completion of normal moult.

first primary to be shed is the inside one, next to the axial feather, and the remainder are shed in succession until the last one to be dropped is the outermost primary near the tip of the wing.

Birds inherit the tendency to shed their plumage annually. An early moulter, under normal conditions, is a poor layer. A late moulter, under normal conditions, is a good layer. The nature of moulting both at the starting time and its duration should be considered while judgeing a bird's laying ability.

Hens seldom lay and shed feathers at the same time. A high producing bird may, for a short time, moult and lay simultaneously; but usually she sheds more rapidly, and is declining in production when moulting begins. When her wing feathers commence to drop, it is a sign that she is nearly or quite through laying. The fact that a hen sheds rapidly though early, stamps her as being better than the common early moulter that sheds slowly. Presumably, a hen does not stop laying because she moults, but rather moults or stops laying because her physical condition is such that she cannot support egg production and continue nourishment of the feathers.

In general it may be said that there are three kinds of moulters in the birds hatched during the usual spring season: early, medium and late.

1. *Early moulter.* The bird ceasing to lay in June, July or early August, shows that she has a short laying period, that she probably started late and lacks the vitality, laying capacity, or inherited tendency to discontinue.

The early moulter sheds and grows feathers so gradually that a person may not observe the process unless the bird is handled. She seldom completes her moult in less than 3 or 4 months. She then rests for a short time and frequently does not get back into production for some time. In brief, she takes a longer vacation and should be culled.

2. *Medium moulter.* Birds moulting late August or September are termed medium moulters. If artificial illumination is to be used, birds moulting in September may be segregated, allowed to recuperate under favourable conditions for renewing their plumage and recovering their body weight, and placed under lights in October. If after about 4 weeks of non-laying the birds are to be kept for another year they may be culled.

3. *Late moulter.* A hen moulting in October or later is termed a late moulter. The feathers are dropped rapidly, and in a short time the plumage appears rough. There may be a few old feathers clinging to the bird, and her body will soon be covered with pin feathers. Hens are rarely seen during July or August in this ragged condition. While moulting, the late moulter is quite timid and dislikes to be handled. This is due to active circulation and sensitive nerve development in the feather follicles while new plumage is being grown. At this time the slightest touch hurts the bird.

The feathers grow in rapidly, as soon as the moult is over and most of the birds are back in production as early moulters. Such a moult indicates that the bird has high vitality and therefore usually is a superior producer.

Temperament

A good layer is more active, more alert, and yet at the same time more easily handled than a poor layer. She is among the first off the perch in the morning among the last on it at night. When not on the nest she is busy and business-like, scratching or ranging in an eager search for food. The appetite of a great layer is seldom satisfied.

Broodiness

If a bird is to lay well, it must not be broody much of the time. Broodiness is the external evidence of the maternal instinct and is a dominant sex-linked character. Unless breeders are selected for non-broodiness, the offspring will show more broodiness each year with a decline in egg production.

Light breeds, such as Leghorns, are less broody than general purpose breeds, such as Plymouth

Rocks. Within a given breed or variety there are strains with much less broodiness than is found in others.

Precosity or Sexual Maturity

By sexual maturity is meant the number of days between the date a pullet is hatched and the date she lays her first egg. Early sexual maturity is determined by at least two dominant genes; one is autosomal and the other is sex linked, although probably other genes are involved.

Pullets hatched during February, March and April are of two types regarding sexual maturity. Those hatched early, i.e., in February and the beginning of March are definitely better than those hatched in the latter part of this period. It has been suggested that this difference is associated with the relative length of daylight.

Females for breeding purposes should be selected on the basis of their earliness of sexual maturity as that of their dams and their sisters.

Persistency

Implies that a bird continues to lay well toward the close of her first laying year. Length of laying during a year is influenced not only at the beginning of the first egg laid, but also at the end of the period the last egg is laid. The tendency to continue laying eggs up to a longer time say up to the next winter is known as persistency and it has much the same effect at the end of the year as early maturity does at the beginning.

Lack of persistency is easily determined, as a rule, by the beginning of an early moult. Some hens moult as early as June and others as late as December, so that it is easily possible to have a difference of one hundred and eighty days of a laying year on account of this one factor.

The common practice of culling laying flocks in late summer is based on the fact that persistency is highly correlated with total annual egg production. Culling out the early moulters automatically removes many of the low producers from the flock.

Trapnest Records

From all considerations trapnesting is the only means of obtaining a definite check on the productivity of an individual. It also provides the opportunity to study egg size, colour, texture and shape and production intensity and persistency. Naturally it gives a material index for use in the selection of birds. Many poultrymen have a tendency to pay considerable attention to "trapnesting records" and not enough to physical make-up. A wise procedure is to first select the birds according to handling qualities and then resort to the trapnest for conformation of the selection. Neither method of selection is as efficient as the combination of both.

Progeny Test

Family and progeny records are essential in breeding for improvement in characters of low heritability such as egg production, hatchability and viability. The final and most valuable test for a breeder is the kind of progeny that it produces. It is not, how many eggs a hen lays that counts, but the number her daughters will lay. If a bird is to be valued as a breeder, it must be able to transmit desirable characters to its offspring. The progeny test is also used for the purpose of distinguishing between individuals which are homozygous and those which are heterozygous for some simple character such as rose comb and white skin colour.

It is highly important to select sires of superior breeding value because the average sire has about ten times as many chicks as the average dam.

The breeding programme should be bared on the selection of outstanding families.

HATCHING THE EGGS

The process of hatching, by which, in the span of 21 days, a microscopic germ is changed into a downy chick, capable of walking, eating and experessing its needs by its voice and actions seems nearly magical. With such rapid development and change within the egg, great care must be exercised to provide correct conditions if a good percentage of strong chicks is to be hatched. No detail should be overlooked in giving the eggs every chance to hatch, and each chick a chance to live, since upon their ability to do this may rest the success or failure

Table 15.8

Guide for selection and culling layers

Character	*Good layer: keep*	*Poor layer: cull*
I. Vigour	Strong	Weak, unthrifty
II. Breed type	Wedge shape body	Shallow and tendency towards rocker keel
III. Head	Neat, refined	Beefy, crow head
1. Comb and Wattles	Full, red, waxy, warm and velvety	Very long, thin and sharp pointed
2. Eyes	Full bright, alert	Dull, sleepy
3. Beak	Stocky, well curved	Very long, thin and sharp pointed
4. Ear lobes	Full waxy and velvety	Shrunked and coarse
IV. Neck	Stocky, rather short	Long and thin
V. Body	Capacious	Limited capacity
1. Back	Broad and straight	Narrow and crooked
2. Sides	Deep, straight	Shallow, barrel-shaped
3. Keel bone	Long and properly curved	Short and crooked
4. Pelvic bones	Wide apart, thin	Close together, thick
5. Skin	Thin, soft, oily	Thick, dry, rough
6. Abdomen	Large, soft, free from fat	Small, hard, with thick fat
7. Vent	Full, larger and moist	Small, dry
8. Feathers	Warm and soiled	Clean and perfect
VI. Legs	Wide apart, well-set	Close together, knock-kneed
1. Shanks	Thin and soft in back	Full, hard and round in the back
2. Toe nails	Stocky, well curved	Long, thin
VII. Temperament	Alert, active, friendly	Shy, nervous, quacky
VIII. Moult	Late and rapid	Early and slow

of the poultry enterprise. Let us first take this problem starting from the selection of hatching eggs.

Selection and Care of Hatching Eggs

1. **Egg size.** The size of the eggs used for hatching is important because there is a high correlation between the size of eggs used and the size of the chicks hatched. Neither small sized egg nor very big sized egg should be selected. It is always desirable to select eggs approximately 58 gm each. Eggs in which the proportion of white to yolk is about 2:1 usually hatch better than eggs having wider or narrow ratios. The yolk portion is rich in carotene, hence a growth promoting substance is always desirable. Abnormal shaped egg should always be discarded.

2. **Shell colour.** In case of varieties of chickens that lay white shelled eggs, all eggs used for incubation should be free from tints, except for the first few tinted eggs laid at sexual maturity.

For brown coloured eggs medium and dark brown eggs hatch better than light brown eggs.

3. **Shell texture.** When shell texture is poor due to deficiency of calcium or vitamin D the result, of course, is associated with low hatchability, otherwise the mottled appearance of the egg shell as observed by candling does not appear to be related to hatching results.

4. **Cracked shells.** All eggs should be tested for cracked shells, and this can be done quite readily by tapping two eggs together. If there is a resonant sound, both eggs are sound in shell; but if there is dull sound, one of the eggs is cracked and should not be used for incubation.

5. **Tremulous air cells.** Care should be taken in shipping or delivering eggs to a hatchery to avoid excessive shaking which sometimes results in a condition known as "tremulous air cells", a condition that tends to lower hatchability.

6. **Soiled egg.** Soiled eggs should not be washed in water before setting, as washing with water opens up the pores and this interferes with the hatching results. If the dirt is not excessive, it should be removed with a knife. Highly soiled eggs should not be set.

7. **Age of egg.** In hot weather, eggs should not be kept for more than 3 days but in winter they may be kept for 7 to 10 days.

8. **Turning.** Turning eggs is not necessary if they are not held longer than one week during the storage period.

Always collect the hatching eggs from the best birds where good, strong and healthy males are used for mating.

The Best Time to Start Hatching

The best time to raise chickens altogether depends upon the climate in which the chickens are to be raised.

July, August and September are the most favourable months for raising chickens in Punjab, U.P. and Madhya Pradesh because of (1) low rainfall, (2) suitable room temperature. Before July the heat is very great and after September the winter is too much. Both the conditions are unfavourable for chickens.

In places like Simla, Nainital, Mussoorie, Darjeeling, Assam and where ever the cold is severe during the cold season and moisty air during the rain, March, April, May and June are the favourable months for raising chickens.

In West Bengal and all other places of India where there are no westerly hot winds, chickens can be raised most successfully from October to end of March.

Natural Hatching

Natural hatching or hatching of eggs by hen is a primitive but most effective method to get a high percentage of success. It is particularly claimed that the hen is more to be trusted and consequently some breeders trust special sittings of egg which are to produce future stock cockerels.

Selection of the hatching hen. Pullets are not recommended for this purpose. The ordinary *deshi* hen is ideal for hatching chickens as she is a close sitter, and owing to her light weight, there is little possibility of eggs being broken.

The hen should be thoroughly broody. A broody hen can be recognised by her constant determination to sit in her nest. The hen must be in perfect health, and have all her feathers on her. Hens in moult should always be rejected.

The hen should be thoroughly dusted with a good insecticide, such as gammaxane or sodium fluoride. A further dusting ten days later will ensure its complete freedom from lice and ticks.

Sometimes hens will lay several eggs during natural hatching. Every egg placed under a hen should be marked distinctly so that if any eggs are laid in the nest may be detected and removed.

Best time to set hen. The best time to set a hen is at night, as at this time she is more likely to settle down to her job. Besides, when eggs are put under the hen at night, the chickens are more likely to appear on the night of the 21st day, and will have the whole night to rest and gain strength.

The nest. The nest on which the hen is placed must be made in a quiet corner where she will not be disturbed. An earthen pot, about 15 inches in diameter and 8 inches deep, is filled three-quarters with earth or ashes. Over the earth a fine, soft hay, straw or leaves are placed, and the latter pressed down to make a hollow. A quantity of flowers of sulphur or an insecticide powder is sprinkled over the nest, and after the eggs have been placed on the hollow, the hen is gently seated on them and left undisturbed.

Apart from an earthen pot any other vessels of wood or tin, etc., of any specification can be made use of on the same principles. Great care should be taken to provide a nest just large enough for the hen to properly sit in. The nest must not be too large, or else the eggs will roll away from under the hen and become chilled and spoiled.

A sitting hen must not be kept in a damp, dirty, draughty or badly ventilated place.

Care of sitting hens. Before putting the hen on the eggs she must be placed under a basket and fed and watered; a plentiful supply of good grain must be given. It is a good plan to set a hen on half a dozen dummy eggs, and allow her to sit and settle down for 2 or 3 days. By this way the hen will acquire all the qualities of broodiness and then the dummy eggs should be removed and the good eggs are placed under her.

The sitting birds should receive clean water twice daily and adequate amount of whole grains and limestone grit. Sloppy foods of all description should be avoided as they tend to produce loose droppings and consequent soiling of the eggs.

Hens ought to come off their eggs at least once every day. The temporary change from the cramped position is good for the hen and the exposure to the fresh air gently benefits the eggs. If the hen does not come off her nest, she may have to be lifted off the eggs.

It becomes important to see that she gets her food and a little exercise at the same time of the day. She should be allowed to go back to her nest after about 20 minutes.

Care of the hatching eggs. Some breeders insist that the eggs should be laid on their sides which aids the foster mother to turn the eggs regularly every day. Eggs should be placed about $1\frac{1}{4}''$ apart.

After the eggs have been placed under the hen, all that needs to be done is to inspect them every day to see that they are all right.

When the weather is very hot and dry it may be necessary to sprinkle warm water of 102°F over the eggs in order to give moisture. In West Bengal it is generally not necessary due to normal humidity.

It is a sound practice to sprinkle flowers of sulphur over the nests and eggs just a day or two before the chickens appear.

Rats often are a nuisance as they steel eggs from under the hens. The only remedy is to keep the hen with her eggs in a box with a good strong bottom and $\frac{1}{2}''$ mesh wire-netting sides.

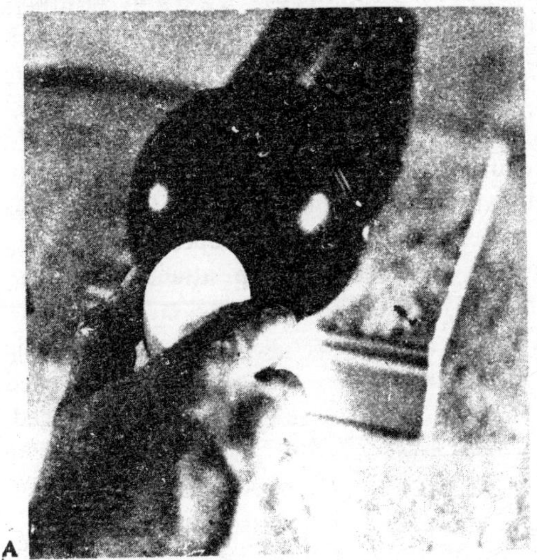
A

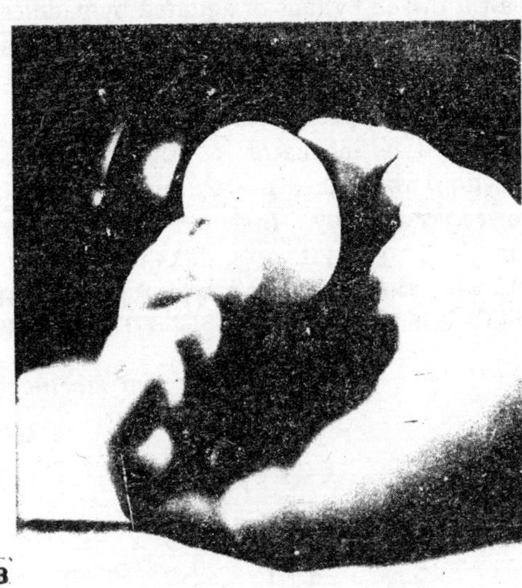
B

Fig. 15.11 Hand candling of eggs : (a) Egg placed at candling light with palm of hand down, (b) Hand turned with a snap of the wrist to cause egg contents to move within the shell.

Infertile and addled eggs are generally examined from the nest after the 7th or 10th day of sitting. For this purpose there are different methods of testing, of which candling of eggs is the most common. If the egg is perfectly transparent, like a new-laid egg, it is infertile; but if a small dark body is seen floating about the centre of the egg, it contains a chicken. After 21 days, if the egg has a partly-formed chicken in it, or is rotten, then it is addled. If the chicken is fully formed and is dead in the shell, it is spoiled. If the germ has formed in the egg and not hatched, it is fertile, but has been addled or spoiled by some cause, for which the eggs may be to blame.

The other method of testing fertile good eggs is as follows:

On the 19th or 20th day of hatching fill a large bowl with hot water (exactly at 102°F), place the testing eggs in the water. After a minute the fertile eggs containing live chickens will wriggle in the water; this is caused by the chickens endeavouring to make escape from the shells. The infertile and addled eggs will float about, but will not wriggle.

The eggs must be allowed to remain only one minute in the water, and then taken out, properly dried and put back under the hen.

Number of eggs under a hen. The size of the hen and the state of the weather must decide the number of eggs to be placed under her. It is better to place a few. Small country hens should have only 6 eggs in the warm weather and 4 in the cold weather. Under no condition should the number of hatching eggs exceed 7 or 8 under a country hen.

Artificial Incubation

Improvement in the design and construction of incubators, have made artificial incubation so reliable that machines have largely, and on most farms completely, replaced broody hens. Incubators can be roughly classified as: (a) hot water radiation from pipes in the egg chamber; (b) hot air infusion, or warm air pouring directly into the egg chamber; (c) forced-draft, where the air is driven by fans or agitated by paddles. Out of these hot air flat type and hot air mammoths are very common and are discussed below:

Hot Air Flat Type Incubators

The flat type incubator is usually of small capacity, ranging from 50–500 eggs. Full instructions about their use are supplied with the machines, and these instructions are to be followed very strictly. In general fresh air enters get warmed by the hot air tubes at the side of the machine, and as it cools, sinks towards the floor and escapes by the vent or openings at lower levels. Fig.15.12 illustrates a typical flat type of incubator, heated by oil lamp attached to the side of the incubator. The eggs rest on wire bottomed trays fitted some 6–8 inches below the

HOT AIR INCUBATOR

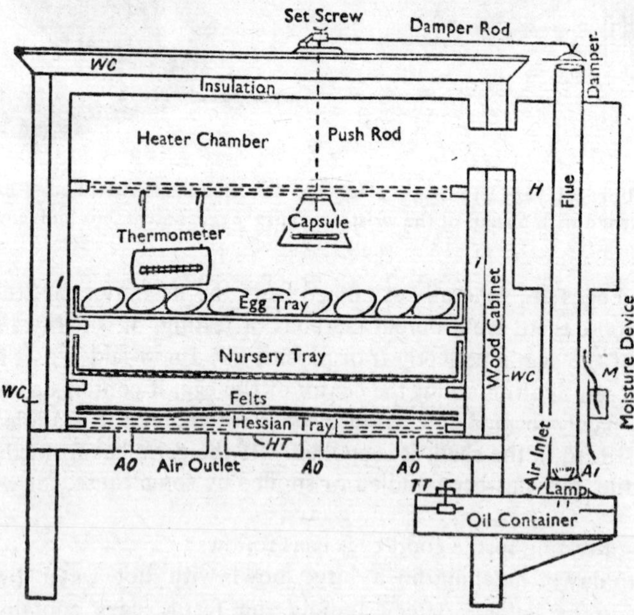

Fig. 15.12 WC = wood cabinet; H = hot air; AO = air outlet.

hessian of the heating chambers. Under this tray is another tray, this having a floor of hessian, and is known as the nursery tray. Most of the machines of this type have a glass window fitted to the front of the hatching egg tray. The tray itself is especially made short, so that when pushed fully back there is a space of two inches between its front edge and the front of the machine, the idea being that the dried chicks, being attracted by the light, come forward to the window and fall through to the cooler and less crowded nursery tray below. The heat regulating principle in these incubators is simple. When the temperature of the incubator rises above the level to which it is previously adjusted, the capsule (made up of two thin metal sheets welded together containing small amount of ether) expands and forces the push rod upwards, and this in turn lifts the damper off the exhaust flue, but as soon as the inside temperature falls below the required point, the damper closes down and all the heat goes into the incubator. In this incubator only one thermometer is necessary. To provide the necessary moisture, one type of machine has a trough fitted with a wick which enters the double wall of the lamp flue, and in evaporation charges the heating and rising air with extra moisture. Some have two small troughs which slide into fitments attached to the two inner side walls of the egg compartment and are filled with warmed water about hatching time. Others fit a small type of water tray with sponge or hessian over or in it and rests under the eggs in place of the nursery tray. In most flat type incubators the eggs are turned by hand. It is important that the eggs should be turned in opposite directions each time.

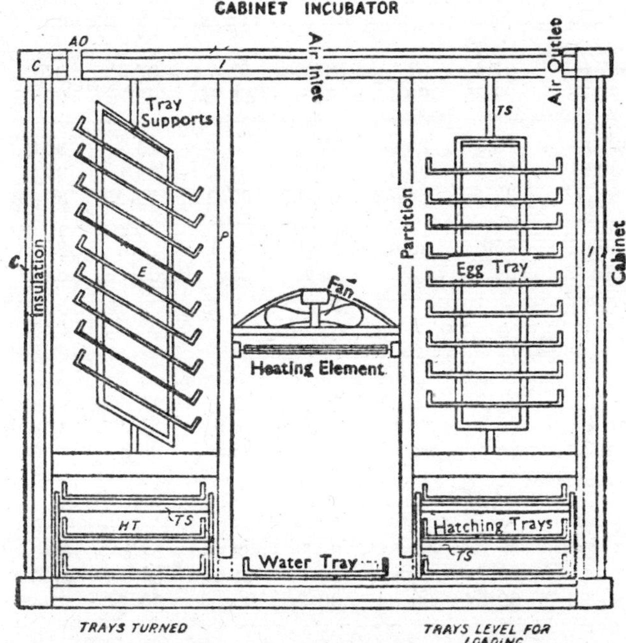

Fig. 15.13 AO = air outlet; HT = hatching tray; E = egg tray; C = cabinet.

Hot Air Mammoths

The chief difference between these machines and the flat type are: (1) the eggs are placed in the upright position with the broad end upper-most, (2) the eggs are turned by tilting the trays through 40–45° each side of the horizontal, and (3) the ventilation and internal air circulation are mechanically controlled by some arrangement of fans. In this case the heat is controlled by a thermostat, which either cuts in or out with the heater unit, and is set at a quarter degree each way. Should the machine rise a quarter degree above the setting, then the heat is turned off, and when it drops to a quarter degree the setting, then it cuts in again, thus the incubator steadily runs to a half degree. The methods of turning the eggs vary with the make of machines some by a wheel attachment at the side and some by a lever, but they all result in the egg tray, which during the period of incubation is tilted at an angle.

MANAGEMENT OF INCUBATORS DURING INCUBATION

1. Levelling of the incubator. Levelling may be accomplished by the use of a spirit-level and if the level is not even, the damper rod will not function normally thus will affect the temperature regulation of the incubator.

Table 15.9

Forced-air Incubator Requirements *	*Chicken*	*Turkey*	*Duck*	*Muscovy Duck*	*Goose*	*Guinea*	*Pheasant*	*Peafowl*	*Coturnix Quail*
Incubation period (days)	21	28	28	35–37	28–34	28	23–28	28–30	17
Temperature* (degrees C/F., dry bulb)	37.6 99.75	37.4 99.25	37.5 99.5	37.5 99.5	37.4 99.25	37.6 99.75	37.6 99.75	37.4 99.25	37.4 99.25
Humidity (degrees C/F., wet bulb)	29.4–30.6 85–87	28.3–29.4 83–85	28.9–30.0 84–86	28.9–30.0 84–86	30.0–31.1 86–88	28.3–29.4 83–85	30.0–31.1 86–88	28.3–29.4 83–85	28.9–30.0 84–86
Do not turn eggs after	19th day	25th day	25th day	31st day	25th day	25th day	21st day	25th day	15th day
Temperature during last 3 days of incubation (degrees C/F., dry bulb)	37.2 99.0	36.9 98.5	37.1 98.75	37.1 98.75	36.9 98.5	37.2 99.0	37.2 99.0	36.9 98.5	37.2 99.0
Humidity during last 3 days of incubation (degrees C/F., wet bulb)	32.2–34.4 90–94	32.2–34.4 90–94	32.2–34.4 90–94	32.2–34.4 90–94	32.2–34.4 90–94	32.2–34.4 90–94	33.3–35.0 92–95	32.2–34.4 90–94	32.2–34.4 90–94

*For still-air incubators add 1–2°C. (2–3°F) to the recommended operating temperatures.

2. Sanitation and fumigation. (1) Sweep the compartment and brush out all fluff and debris. Also clean out the incubator room and when all clearing up has been completed spray the floor with disinfectant. (2) Scrub the egg trays, carrier-rack and the water trays with disinfectant. Reassemble them and leave them outside the machine for a short time to air. (3) Replace the rack and trays in the compartment. (4) For routine fumigation add about 50 cc of 40% formaldehyde to 25–30 grams of potassium permanganate crystals into an enamel basin near the fan to ensure even distribution. The above quantities are required for 100 cubic feet of incubator capacity.

3. Regulating incubator. A trial run of the incubator at the beginning of each hatching season, regardless of the incubator new or old is a must. The thermometer should be checked comparing with a standard thermometer. The wick of the lamp should be new, of sufficient length to last during the incubation period. The thermostat should be regulated according to the manufacturer's instructions, and the machine operated at a temperature of 103°F for at least 24 hours to make sure that the machine is alright.

4. Placing eggs. Arrange the eggs in egg tray in rows either on their sides in the case of flat type incubators or upright, with the broad end up in cabinet-type machines.

5. Regulating temperature. For flat type incubators the temperature will depend upon the design of the incubator and the height of the thermometer bulb above the eggs. Most satisfactory results are secured with a temperature of 101°F during the first week followed by 102°F during the second week and 103°F during the 3rd week of incubation.

6. Sufficient ventilation. When the amount of CO_2 in the air exceeds 2 per cent, the hatchability of eggs decreased rapidly. On the 21st day of incubation about 140 to 150 times as much air is required as on the first day. This emphasises the need for good ventilation and particularly the necessity of keeping the ventilation outlets well opened during the later stages of incubation.

7. Turning of eggs. Best hatching results are obtained when the large ends of the egg is kept uppermost. Eggs should be turned daily, starting with the third day of incubation. The number of turning during the early stages of incubation should be 4 to 6 times daily. After about a week the number of turnings may be regulated at 8 hours equal interval. Cease turning after 18th day. The object of turning the egg is to prevent the embryo sticking to the shell membrane.

8. Testing eggs. Incubated eggs should be tested (candled) on the 7th and 14th day as explained under 'natural hatching'. The infertile eggs may be sorted, hard boiled and later ground up as part of chicken ration.

9. Care during hatching. Care of the hatching eggs (sprinkling flowers of sulphur, egg testing, etc.) from the day of setting upto 18th day may be taken as same with that as described under natural hatching. On the 19th day the nursery tray should be placed. A good hatch is that when the chicks are out of their shells before the end of 21st day. As activity increased with the pipping of the shells, the temperature is likely to run very high, and the moisture too low. It is of no use to assist a chick to come out of its shell as usually in such cases the chick becomes weak or crippled. The chicks which have hatched should remain in the incubator without any feed for at least 18 to 24 hours. After drying off and fluffed out, the temperature should be gradually reduced to 93° to 95°F for "hardening off" the chicks before transferring them to the brooder.

Causes of Poor Hatches and "Dead in the Shell"

Poor hatches may be the result of unhealthy stock, incorrect mating, or breeders fed on a deficient ration. Inefficient operation is a major cause of poor hatches, and points to watch are as follows:

1. Preparation. Before eggs are set the machine should be run for a few days to check for temperature variations and general performance. Have on hand spare capsules, the thermometers, mercury tubes, micro switch and an element. Organise these matters in the off season.

2. Age of eggs. It has been observed that preserved eggs at 55°F to 60°F give better results only for one week, after this the percentage of hatchability will decrease if eggs are stored beyond 7 days to the extent of 10% for each subsequent day.

3. Turning of eggs. The eggs should not be roughly shaken, particularly in the delicate early stages. Turning should be 2 to 3 times during 24 hours up to about 17th day. On 18th day onwards there should not be any turning.

4. Time of turning. Turning should take place night and morning, at the same time each day.

5. Infertile eggs. Causes of infertile eggs are as follows:

(a) Insufficient or too many hens per male bird
(b) Underfed males
(c) Lice-infested males
(d) Eggs held too long
(e) Over fat hens
(f) Cross-mating of a light and heavy breed
(g) Cold conditions early in the season
(h) Very inbred lines

6. Moisture Control. A thick wick in the wet-bulb thermometer will give a lower temperature than required, and a thin wick that becomes hard will give too high a reading. Inefficient wicks can be a major cause of poor hatches.

7. Control of ventilators. Ventilators should be neither closed right up to hold humidity nor opened too much to reduce it. Instead the control should be carried out by reducing or increasing the surface area of water in the trays. Insufficient ventilation can cause many "dead in the shell".

8. Air circulation speed. Too slow a circulation will result in hot and cold places in the machine, and too high a speed will mean excessive drying out of the eggs. Check the recommendations for the type of machine. If pulleys are replaced on the incubator see that they are of the correct size.

9. Malformed or crippled chickens. Excessive low or high temperatures are the principal cause of these, and another cause is incorrect turning of eggs wrong way up in the trays.

10. Thermometers. Thermometers should be tested before each hatch. A rough check is to take one's own temperature in the mouth if the reading is 98.4° F the thermometer will be a good one. A thermometer reading with a 2° inaccuracy, particularly if it is 2° under the correct temperature, could cause almost a complete failure in electric forced draught machines.

11. Dead in shell. If death in shell comes in early stage (3 to 5 days), insufficient turning, incorrect fumigation, or incorrect temperature could be the cause. If death in shell has occurred between 12 and 14 days, suspect excess moisture in the early stages, general condition of the breeding stock, or incorrect feeding such as insufficient riboflavin in the feed. If death in shell has occurred in the last stage (18-21 days), temperature, humdity or ventilation have not been right. Other causes could be rough handling in transfer or chilling through a delay in the process of transfer or due to failure of electric supply.

12. Weak and small chickens. Weak chickens can result from over heating, small chickens from small eggs or insufficient moisture. Chickens breathing heavily may be affected by disease or by too much moisture. Musty chickens often result from low temperatures or insufficient ventilation.

Table 15.10

Nutritional Deficiencies of the Breeders that Affect hatchability

Deficient Items	Embryonic Description
Vitamin A	Failure to develop normal blood system. Embryonic malpositions.
Vitamin D_3	Rickets. Lack of phosphorus. Stunted chicks and soft bones resulting from improper calcification of eggshells.
Vitamin E	Reduced fertility. Bulging eyes. Inadequate embryonic vascular system. Exudative diathesis (edema). Embryonic mortality 1 to 3 days.
Vitamin K	Prolonged embryonic blood clotting time. Hemorrhages and blood clots in embryo and extraembryonic blood vessels. Hemorrhagic syndrome of embryos and newly hatched chicks.
Riboflavin	High mortality 9 to 14 days, edema, atrophied leg muscles, clubbed down, curled toes, enlargement of the sciatic nerve sheaths, and dwarfing are indicative of too little riboflavin. Reduced hatchability 2 weeks after breeder rations become deficient.
Pantothenic Acid	Abnormal feathering. Subcutaneous hemorrhages in embryo. Chicks hatch in a weak condition and most fail to survive.
Biotin	Perosis. Short long bones (micromelia). Shortened and twisted bones of the feet, wings, and skull. Webbing between third and fourth toes. Parrot beak. Excessive mortality between 1 to 7 days.
Vitamin B_{12}	Embryonic malposition with head between legs. Edema. Short beak. Poor muscle development. High embryonic mortality 8 to14 days.
Folacin	Similar to biotin deficiency. Chicks die shortly after pipping the shell.
Vitamin B_6	Reduced hatchability.
Calcium	Rickets. Reduced hatchability. Short and thick legs, wings, and lower mandible. Pilable beak, legs, and neck. Edema.
Phosphorus	Rickets. Soft legs and beak. High embryonic mortality between 14 and 16 days.
Manganese	Skeletal abnormalities. Chondrodystrophy (short wings and legs, abnormal head and parrot beak). Imperfect development of inner ear. Retarded growth. Edema. Abnormal down.
Zinc	Micromelia. Skeletal deformities (absence of rump, wings, legs, and toes). Underdeveloped eyes. Tufted down. Newly hatched chicks are weak and cannot stand, eat, or drink. Chick mortality increased soon after hatching.
Selenium	Subcutaneous fluid. Exudative diathesis (edema). Degeneration of the pancreas. Reduced hatchability. Selenium deficiencies are enhanced when the breeder diet is low in Vitamin E.

(Contd.)

Excessive Items	
Selenium	Selenium is very toxic at high levels. Edema. Crooked toes. High embryonic mortality.
DDT	Affects chick growth, egg production, and livability, but not hatchability.
PCBs (polychlorinated biphenols)	Toxic to developing embryos. Hatchability drastically reduced, but egg production and fertility not affected.
Nicarbazin	Brown eggshells lose their pigment. Hatchability decreases up to 32 %.

Analysing Poor Hatchability

Observation and Possible Causes

Eggs exploding

Bacterial contamination of eggs
Dirty eggs.
Improperly washed eggs
Incubator infection

Clear eggs

Infertile
Eggs held improperly
Too much egg fumigation
Very early embryonic mortality.

Bloodring (embryonic death, 2-4 days)

Hereditary
Diseased breeding flock
Old eggs
Rough handling of hatching eggs
Incubating temperature to high
Incubating temperature too low

Dead embryos second week of incubation

Inadequate breeder ration
Disease in breeder flock
Eggs not cooled prior to incubation
Temperature to high in incubator
Temperature too low in incubator
Electric power failure
Eggs not turned

Observation and Possible Causes

Air cell too small

Inadequate breeder ration
Large eggs
Humidity too high, 1 to19 days

Air cell too large

Small eggs
Humidity too low, 1 to 19 days

Chicks hatch early

Small eggs
Leghorn eggs versus meat type eggs
Incorrect thermometer
Temperature too high, 1 to 19 days
Humidity too low, 1 to 19 days

Chicks hatch late

Variable room temperature
Large eggs
Old eggs
Incorrect thermometer
Temperature too low, 1 to 19 days
Humidity too high, 1 to 19 days
Temperature too low in hatcher

Fully developed embryo with beak not in air cell

Inadequate breeder ration
Temperature too high, 1 to 10 days

Fully developed embryo with break in air cell

Inadequate breeder ration
Incubator air circulation poor
Temperature too high, 20 to 21 days
Humidity too high, 20 to 21 days

Chicks Pipping early

Temperature too high, 1 to 19 days
Humidity too low, 1 to 19 days

Chicks dead after pipping shell

Inadequate breeder ration
Lethal genes
Disease in breeder floock
Eggs incubated small end up
Thin-shelled eggs
Eggs not turned first 2 weeks
Eggs transferred too late
Inadequate air circulation, 20 to 21 days
CO_2 content of air too high, 20 to 21 days
Incorrect temperature, 1 to 19 days
Temperature too high, 20 to 21 days
Humidity too low, 20 to 21 days

Malpositions

Inadequate breeder ration
Eggs set small end up
Odd-shaped eggs set
Inadequate turning

Sticky chicks (albumen sticking to chicks)

Eggs transferred too late
Temperature to high 20 to 21 days
Humidity too low, 20 to 21days
Down collectors not adequate

Sticky chicks (albumen sticking to down)

Old eggs
Air speed too slow, 20 to 21 days
Inadequate air in incubator
Temperature too high, 20 to 21 day

Chicks too small

Eggs produced in hot weather
Small eggs
Thin, porous eggshells
Humidity too low, 1 to 19 days

Chicks too large

Large eggs
Humidity too high, 1 to 19 days

Trays not uniform in hatch or chick quality

Eggs from different breeds
Eggs of different sizes
Eggs of different ages when set
Disease or stress in some breeder flocks
Inadequate incubator air circulation

Soft chicks

Unsanitary incubator conditions
Temperature too low, 1 to 19 days
Humidity too high, 20 to 21 days

Chicks dehydrated

Eggs set too early
Humidity too low 20 to 21 days
Chicks left in hatcher too long after hatching completed

Mushy chicks

Unsanitary incubator conditions

Unhealed navel, dry

Inadequate breeder ration
Temperature too low, 20 to 21 days
Wide temperature variations in incubator
Humidity too high, 20 to 21 days
Humidity not lowered after hatching completed

Unhealed navel, wet and odorous

Omphalitis
Unsanitary hatchery and incubators

Chicks cannot stand

Breeder ration inadequate
Improper temperature, 1 to 21 days
Humidity too high, 1 to 19 days
Inadequate ventilation, 1 to 21 days

Crippled chicks

Inadequate breeder ration
Variation in temperature, 1 to 21 days
Malpositions

Crooked toes

Inadequate breeder ration
Improper temperature, 1 to 19 days

Spraddle legs

Hatchery trays too smooth

Closed eyes

Temperature too high, 20 to 21 days
Humidity to low, 20 to 21 days
Loose down in hatcher
Down collectors not adequate

DISEASE AND HATCHABILITY

Several poultry diseases that affect the parent breeder flock have an effect on the developing embryo, hatchability, and chick quality, other disease organisms establish themselves in the hatchery and incubators to infect future hatches. Many of the pathogenic organisms produce similar conditions, high embryonic mortality, weak chicks, and whitish diarrhoea. Therefore, it is almost impossible to differentiate the source of infection by observations of the dead embryos or the newly hatched chicks. Only a laboratory examination will determine the organism involved.

The important ones involving incubation and chick quality are as follows :

pullorum disease
Arizona disease
fowl typhoid
paratyphoid
aspergillosis
omphalitis
Escherichia coli infection
infectious bronchitis
Newcastle disease
avian encephalomyelitis
Mycoplasma gallisepticum infection
Mycoplasma synoviae infection
aflatoxosis (toxin poisoning)
laryngotracheitis

BROODING AND REARING

Systems of Brooding

Brooding units are designed to house chicks from one-day old until they no longer need supplementary heat (0-8 weeks). *Growing pens* are used from the end of the brooding period until the broilers are sold or the pullets moved into permanent laying houses (upto 20 weeks).

Laying pens or cages are used for pullets and hens from the time they start to lay until they are culled and sold at the end of the laying period (upto 78-80 weeks).

There are two general systems of brooding: (1) natural method, and (2) artificial method.

In deciding on the method of brooding to use, it must be remembered that if artificial methods of incubation have been practised, then artificial methods or brooding should follow.

Natural Brooding

Natural brooding, once the only method used in brooding chicks, has been quite largely replaced by artificial methods. The natural method is used on farms where only few chickens are raised each year. *Deshi* hens as a class are ideal mothers as they possess a strongly developed maternal instinct, moreover, because of their small structure they seldom injure the young chicks by trampling on them. Depending upon her size, a hen will brood 15-20 chickens. The broody hen will provide all the warmth required by the chicks. Before placing the chicks with the hen she should be examined for her good health and free from lice, etc.

Rearing coop. A rearing coop is made up of packing box material which is about 2 feet square, sloping down from front to back, say about 2 feet height in front and 18 inches at the back. The essential requirements of such a coop are dryness, durability, ventilation, cheapness, roominess and safety. Wire enclosed runways are a desirable attachment for brooding coops.

Food for chicks and mother. For the first week, it is, advisable to give small quantities of feed frequently, perhaps every two hours; this should consist of a chick mash, mixed with water or milk to a crumbly consistency, and this at first may be given on a board, in or close to the coop.

The hen must not be neglected and she should have a suitable wet or dry balanced growers mash. Care must be taken to see that the feed for the hen is so arranged that the chicks do not get access to it. Clean water must always be available for hen and chicks.

Other managerial practices. The cage should be cleaned and sprayed regularly to hold mites and similar pests under control. Wire netting of suitable mesh should cover the top of the run and the floor of the coop to prevent damage from rats, cats, owls and other predatory animals. During the first week vaccination against Marek's and Ranikhet disease should be provided. Debeaking during the first week is desirable. At the age of 6-8 weeks vaccinate to prevent fowl pox and Ranikhet diseases.

Movement of coop and run. Frequent moving of the coop along with its run to a fresh site will prevent out-break of disease and parasitic infestation. It is also desirable to let the chicks and broody hen in the sun for a short time once or twice a day.

Artificial Brooding

Artificial brooding is the handling of newly born chicks without the aid of hen. It is accomplished by means of a temperature controlled brooder (rearer or foster mother). Artificial brooding has several advantages over the natural method, namely: (1) chicks may be reared at any time of the seasons ; (2) thousands of chicks may be brooded by a single person; (3) sanitary condition may be controlled; (4) temperature may be regulated; and (5) feeding may be undertaken according to plan.

There are many types, styles and sizes of brooder units on the market that employ a variety of fuels. The equipment usually is rated by the manufacturer according to the number of chicks that may be started under each unit. The essentials of a good brooder are: a dependable mechanism for controlling temperature and regular supply of fresh air, dryness, adequate light, space, easy disinfection, protection against chick enemies, safety from fire, and economy in construction. For heating such brooders, use of coal, kerosine oil, gas, electricity are used depending upon the availability of such materials and the capacity of the poultrymen. From the point of temperature regulation, electricity is the best. Basket brooders and brooders from packing cases are very popular where small number of chicks are raised. For

Table 15.11

Floor space, temperature and water space for chicks in Artificial Brooder

Age	*Floor space*	*Brooder temperature*	*Water space*
First week	100 to 120 sq. cms. per chick	95°F	Start on shallow pans to avoid crowding, use 4 waterers per brooder.
2-4 weeks	250 to 300 sq. cms. per chick	90°F...2nd wk. 85°F...3rd wk. 80°F...4th wk.	Provide 4-6 waterers of 3 litre capacity per brooder. Fill waterer at least twice daily.
5-8 weeks	700-800 sq. cms. per chick	80°F	Use water trough with adjustable stands. Keep waterers at chicks' shoulder level, 2 cm. space per chick.

large number of chicks, battery brooders of multiple tiers having adjustable feeding and water trough with thermostatically heat regulating mechanism are very common now-a-days.

MANAGEMENT OF CHICKS IN THE BROODER

1. Adjust the temperature as per requirement of the chicks. In case of oil heating, see that there is no defect in the stove or lamp. Chicks should not get access in heated parts of the lamp at any cost.
2. Avoid a damp poultry house; in case of dampness, however, a deep litter can solve the problem.
3. Discourage litter eating by the chicks, scatter mash over egg case flats when the chicks are first taken out of their boxes. Keep chick hoppers filled. Provide balanced standard mash.
4. Keep provision for the entrance of fresh air.
5. Chicks may be taught to roost when they are from 4-6 weeks old. Early roosting will help to reduce over crowding and prevent litter borne infections.
6. Provide clean, fresh water in front of the birds at least twice daily.
7. Chicks, after 3 weeks old may be provided chopped green grasses.
8. Clean the brooders including feed hoppers daily.
9. Follow a regular vaccination programme.
10. Avoid overcrowding as this will lead slow growth and mortality.
11. Keep the brooder in such a place that cold wind and rain does not get in.
12. Daily inspect the condition of birds and their faces for any sort of abnormality. Keep in touch with any veterinarian for the help at the time of need.
13. It is always advisable to check the fittings, temperature control, feed and water trough arrangement before shifting the chicks in the brooder.

HOUSING AND EQUIPMENT

Need for Poultry Housing

The chicken as a wild jungle fowl, sought safety and rest on the high limbs of a tree or in the thick underbush. The jungle served for protection against the hot sunlight. Nature's object, with poultry is to cause the hen to reproduce herself and to maintain the race to which she belongs on the basis of survival of the fittest. On such natural conditions of wild state they lay very few eggs, and these only in the spring of the year.

But under modern conditions the hen is required to lay many eggs throughout the year, and this object can best be achieved if a comfortable shed is provided for them. So, in conclusion we can say that poultry is housed for comfort, protection, efficient production and convenience of the poultry man.

Essential of Good Housing

Comfort. The best egg production is secured from birds that are comfortable and happy. To be comfortable a house must provide adequate accommodation; be reasonably cool in summer, free from drafts and sufficiently warm during the winter; provide adequate supply of fresh air and sunshine; and remain always dry. Given these the hen responds excellently.

Protection. Includes safeguards against theft and attack from natural enemies of the birds such as the fox, dog, cat, kite, crow, snake, etc. The birds also should be protected against external parasites like ticks, lice and mites.

Convenience. The house should be located at a convenient place, and the equipment so arranged as to allow cleaning and other necessary operations as required.

Location of Poultry House

In planning a poultry house, the location should be taken into consideration. In selecting site for poultry houses the following factors should be considered.

1. **Relation to other building.** The poultry house should not be close to the home as to create unsanitary conditions. On the other hand it should not be too far away either because this will require more time in going to and for in caring for the birds. In general at least three trips should be made daily to the poultry house in feeding, watering, gathering the eggs, etc.

2. **Exposure.** The poultry house should face south or east in moist localities. A southern exposure permits more sunlight in the house than any of the other possible exposures. An eastern exposure is almost as good as a southern one. Birds prefer morning sunlight to that of the afternoon. The birds are more active in the morning and will spend more time in the sunlight.

3. **Soil and drainage.** If possible the poultry house should be placed on a sloping hillside rather than a hilltop or in the bottom of a valley. A sloping hillside provides good drainage and affords some protection.

The type of soil is important if the birds are to be given a range. A fertile well drained soil is desired. This will be a sandy loam rather than a heavy clay soil. A fertile soil will grow good vegetation which is one of the main reasons for providing range.

If the poultry house is located on flat poorly drained soil, the yards should be tiled, othere wise, the birds should be kept in total confinement.

4. **Shade and protection.** Shade and protection of the poultry house are just as desirable as for the home. Trees serve as a windbreak in the winter and for shade in the summer. They

should be tall, with no low limbs. Low shrubbery is no good as in their presence the soil becomes contaminated under the shrubbery, remains damp, and sunlight cannot reach it to destroy the disease germs. One thing we should remember that plenty of sun shine should be available at the site.

Housing Requirements

Floor space. The smaller the house the more square feet are required for each hen. Bigger pens have more actual usable floor space per bird than smaller pens. The recommendations as suggested might be useful regarding floor, feeders and watering space.

For economic production of laying hens it is always better to keep them in small units of

Table 15.12

Floor space requirement per bird

S. No.	*(Age weeks)*	*Floor space per bird (cm²)*	
		Light breeds	*Heavy breeds*
1	0 to 8	700 minimum	700 minimum
2	9 to 12	950 minimum	950 minimum
3	13 to 20	1900 minimum	2350 minimum
4	21 and above	2300 to 2800	2800 to 3700

Table 15.13

Feeder space requirement per bird

S. No.	*Age (weeks)*	*Feeder space per bird (linear cm.) Minimum*
1	0 to 2	2.5
2	3 to 6	4.0
3	7 to 12	7.5
4	13 and above	10.0

Table 15.14

Amount of water required and watering space for chicken

Age (weeks)	Water space per chick in linear inches	Amount of water per 100 birds (litres)
0-4	1/4 (0.6 cm)	2.8- 4
5-8	½ (1.2 cm)	12-14
9-12	4 (10 cm)	20-25
13-16	5 (12.5 cm)	35-40
16 and above	6 (15 cm)	45-48

15 to 25 birds. This number can go up to a maximum limit of 250 birds. In commercial poultry farms, units of 125 or so are advisable. Where there is a long house, partitioning at every 20 feet should be made to eliminate drafts, etc.

Ventilation. Ventilation in the poultry house is necessary to provide the birds with fresh air and to carry off moisture. Since the fowl is a small animal with a rapid metabolism, its air requirements per unit of body is high in comparison with that of other animals. A hen weighing 2 kg and on full feed, produces about 52 litres of CO_2 every 24 hours. Since CO_2 content of expired air is about 3.5 per cent, total air breathed amounts to 0.5 litre per kg live weight per minute.

A house that is a tall enough for the attendant to move around comfortably will supply far more air space than will be required by the birds that can be accommodated in the given floor space.

Temperature. Hens need a moderate temperature of 50°F to 70°F. Birds need a warmer temperature at night, when they are inactive, than during the day. The use of insulation with straw pack or other materials not only keeps the house warmer during the winter months but cooler during the summer months. Cross ventilation also aids in keeping the house comfortable during hot weather.

Dryness. Absolute dry conditions inside a poultry house is always an ideal condition. Dampness causes discomfort to the birds and also gives rise to diseases like colds, pneumonia, etc. Dampness in poultry house is caused by: (1) moisture rising through the floor; (2) leaky roofs or walls; (3) rain or snow entering through the windows; (4) leaky water containers; (5) exhalation of birds.

Light. Daylight in the house is desirable for the comfort of the birds. They seem more contended on bright sunny days than in dark, cloudy weather. Sunlight in the poultry house is desirable not only because of the destruction of disease germs and for supplying vitamin-D but also because it brightens the house and makes the birds happy. Birds do fairly well when kept under artificial lights.

Sanitations. The worst enemies of the birds, i.e., lice, ticks, fleas and mites are abundant in poultry houses. They not only transmit diseases but also retard growth and laying capacity. The design of the house should be such which admits easy cleaning and spraying. There should

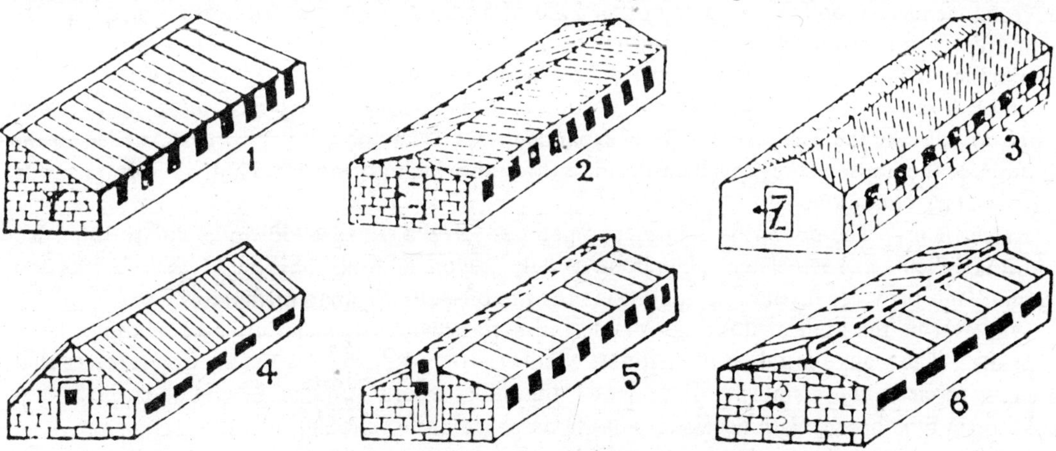

Fig. 15.14 Types of roofs for poultry houses.

be minimum cracks and crevices. Angle irons for the frame and cement asbestos or metal sheets for the roof and walls are ideal construction materials, as they permit effective disinfection of the house. When wood is to be used, every piece should be treated with coaltar, creosote, or similar strong insecticides before being fitted.

Styles of Poultry Houses

The style of the poultry house makes little difference as long as the birds are provided. There are several styles of poultry houses with reference to types of roofs.

Shed types. They are the simplest of poultry house and by far the most useful and practical type of house that can be used under different climatic conditions and for different systems of poultry keeping. The slope of the roof needs only be slight in the plains, while in the hills where snowfall is heavy or in heavy rainfall, it ought to be sufficiently steep. The shed-roof types of houses may be either portable or stationary. The portable house is generally a small one, not exceeding $8' \times 6'$ while the stationary types can be made of any dimensions.

Gable type. This type requires more material and labour for construction. Some poultry-men put a ceiling floor in gable roof houses and use the space in the gable for storage. The type is more suitable in rainfall areas. Here, again gable type may be stationary or portable.

Combination type. Such houses have double pitch roofs in which the ridge between the two slopes is not midway from front to back. Most of the houses have the long slope to the rear. Like the gable type, the combination roof requires more material and labour than the shed roof.

House Construction

Roofs. In India the cement-asbestos sheeting, corrugated iron and zinc sheets are commonly used as roofing material. Cement-asbestos sheeting although very satisfactory and durable is expensive. Corrugated iron and zinc sheets are equally satisfactory and the cost is lower than cement-asbestos.

Floors. The floor of a laying house should be free from dampness, with a smooth surface without cracks, easy to clean and disinfect, rat proof and durable.

Concrete floor. A well laid concrete floor is the safest way to meet these requirements and is recommended in preference to any other kind of a floor. Concrete floors laid on the ground conserve warmth from the earth in winter.

Wire mesh floor. Wire mesh floor or preferably mesh of expanded metal is the best for portable houses. The expanded metal although more expensive is stronger, more durable and does not sag like the wire mesh. The expanded metal having $\frac{1}{2}'' \times \frac{1}{2}''$ mesh, nailed to the bottom of the house makes excellent flooring through which all the excreta drop out ensuring best sanitary condition.

Katcha floor. The poor village farmer sometimes prefer this sort of floor due to low cost, but it is difficult to keep clean. The floor usually becomes foul, harbours disease germs and vermin, and provides favourable conditions for the onset and spread of diseases.

Whatever be the kind of flooring, it is desirable to provide dry clean litter as bedding.

Walls. The walls should be water-tight, wind-proof, and finished with interior surfaces that are easy to clean and disinfect. Except for the hills where summer is cool and winter very cold, open type houses with necessary adaptions prove quite suitable.

In plains where safeguarding is assured from enemies, the walls may be of expanded metal wire mesh on all the sides and the roof will be on some special iron frame. In winter it will be necessary to cover those mesh with gunny bags, etc.

Ventilation. If built of brick, the south side of the house ought to be enclosed with half-inch mesh wire netting; on the north, east and west, high up near the roof, there should be some openings, 12″ × 6″, covered with the same kind of wire netting. This will afford perfect ventilation at all seasons, and the house will not be too warm in the summer or too cold in the winter.

Door. The door of the house must be on the south, and made of an angle iron frame covered with ½″ mesh wire netting. The size of the room should be always large enough to allow a man to conveniently get through.

Windows. At least 1½ square feet openings for each 10 square feet of floor space is recommended for the plain areas of India. In the hill regions where it becomes cold in winter and not too warm in summer, this size may be reduced to half. All openings should be covered with 1″ wire netting. Equal openings on opposite sides of the house or even on all four walls are desirable. Be sure to make the roof overhang at least 18″, preferably 36″ out from the wall to cut down radiation through the window opening.

POULTRY HOUSE EQUIPMENT

The poultry house should be equipped with roosts, nests, feed hoppers, water containers and other items which are essential for satisfactory production. It should be simple in construction, cheap, movable, easily cleaned and disinfected whenever necessary.

Perches or roosts. Chickens start roosting when they are eight weeks old. Apart from catering to the natural instinct or desire of the chickens to get above the ground at night, perches help materially to keep the bird's feet and plumage clean.

Make perches from long wooden bars of two square inches rounded at the top and flat at the bottom. Fix these perches about 16 inches above the ground and near about the walls in such a way that they can be removed for disinfection. Give at least a 12-inch space between two perches. Each bird will need about 8 inches of the perch to roost.

The rear perches should rest a little higher than those at the front, if they are arranged to be horizontal with the length of the house. This will encourage some of the birds that like to roost high to go to the back perches. Paint the perches occasionally with creosote to prevent insects.

Nest boxes. Each pen of laying birds should be provided with nest boxes for laying eggs. It should be roomy, movable, cool and well ventilated, dark and conveniently located. Nests are usually constructed 14 inches square, 6 inches deep and with about 15 inches head room. All metal nests are preferred to wood nests because of easy cleaning and less chance of becoming infested with mites. Empty kerosene tins make excellent boxes. One nest should be provided for every 5 or 6 hens. Dark nest are desirable because they result in less scratching in the nest, less egg breakage and less egg eating. A wooden packing case 18 inches square or a wide mouthed earthen pot can be a suitable nest. Place some sand or soft hay or straw inside.

Nests sometimes are also placed inside a run but in that case care should be taken to prevent crows, etc., by covering the top of the run with wire netting.

Trapnests. Each nest is provided with a trap door so that when the poultryman releases the hen from the nest he can identify her and mark her leg-band number on the egg. There should be one nest for every 3 or 4 birds. Trapnests differ from regular nests in that they are provided with trap doors by which birds shut themselves in when they enter.

For convenience of the caretaker, the nests should be placed 18 to 20 inches above the floor.

Feed hoppers. The essential features of satisfactory feed hoppers are that they (1) avoid wastage of feed, (2) prevent the birds from getting their feet into the feed and from roosting on

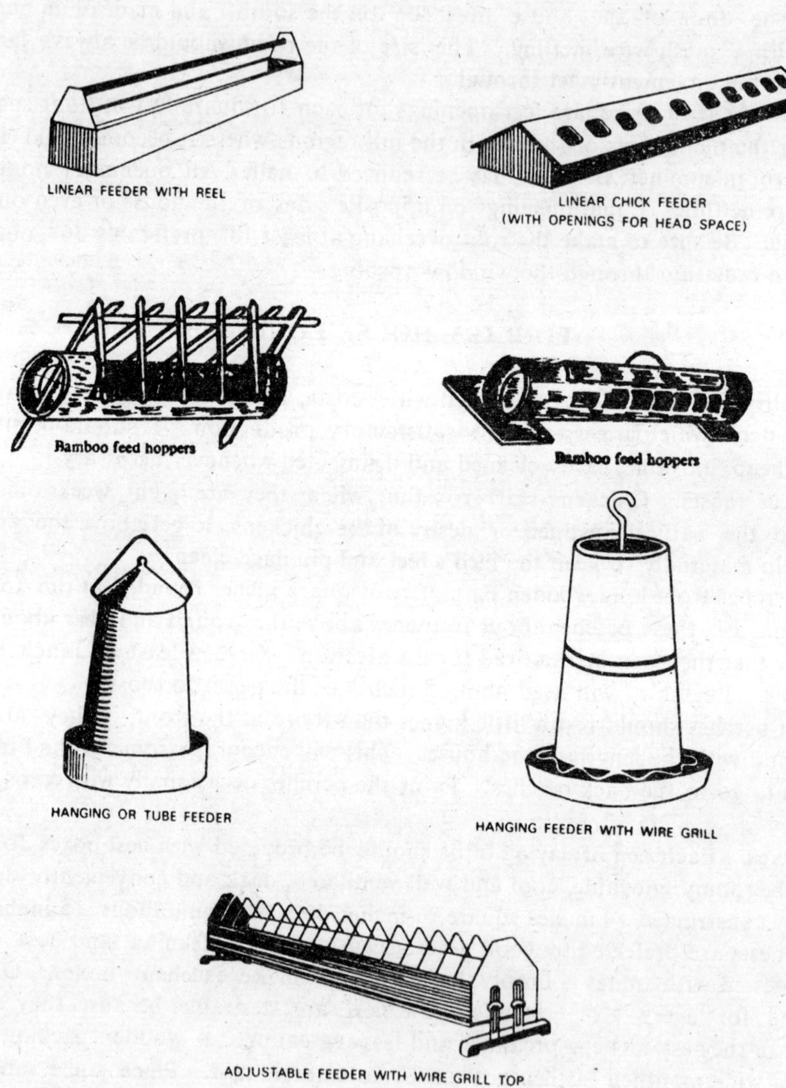

Fig.15.15. Types of Feeders.

the hopper, (3) are easy to clean, and (4) make it easy for the birds to eat from the bottom of the hopper.

Troughs, pots and pans used for feeding should be of suitable size depending on the age and size of the birds. Some of the designs are shown in the diagram (Fig.15.15).

Watering devices. An ample supply of water should be made available at all times, or egg

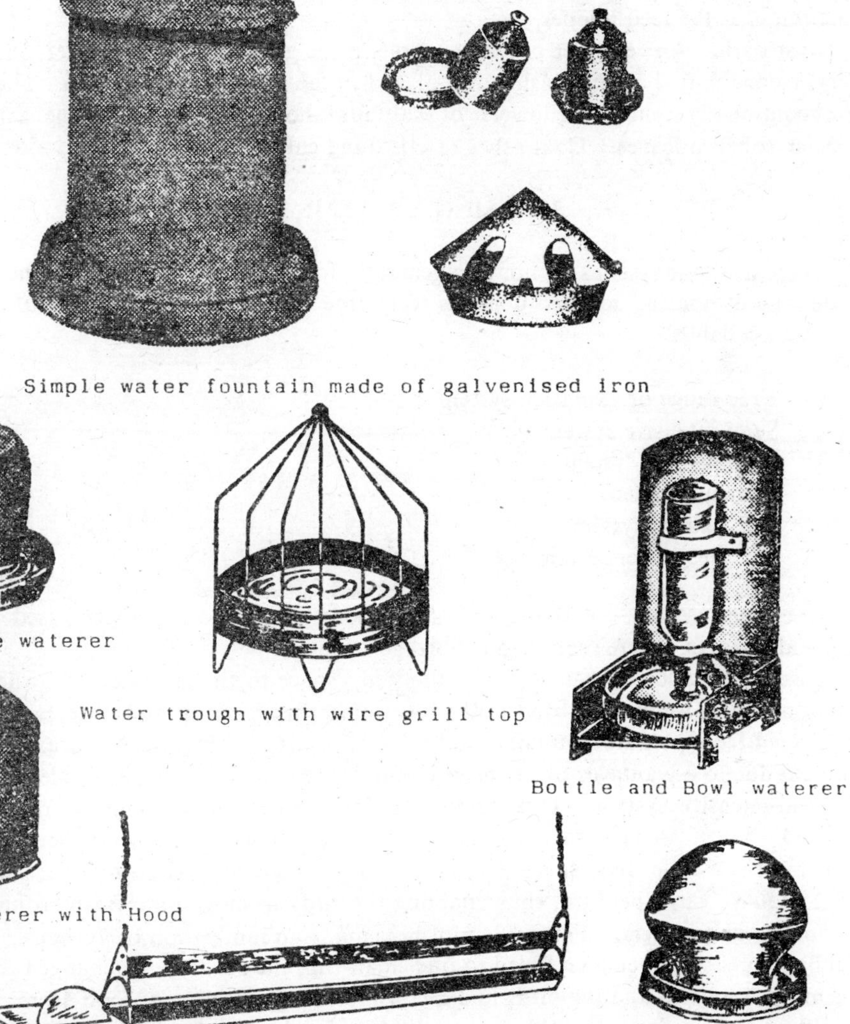

Fig.15.16. Types of Waterers.

production is liable to be affected. The water container should contain clean water, kept cool in summer, and be easily cleaned because contaminated water tends to spread certain diseases from bird to bird.

A wide variety of watering utensils satisfying the above needs can be had. Some of the designs are shown in the diagram (Fig.15.16).

Grit and shell container. Ordinary hoppers made either of wood or metal can be used for oyster shells or other grit. It is advantageous to have the source of calcium for egg shell formation near the feed hopper.

Dust bath. An earthen pot or a whole in the ground, 2′ in diameter, should be filled with dry, clean, shifted earth or ashes and placed in the shed on the east side. The container should be continually refilled. Flowers of sulphur should be added to the ashes, also some dry coarse tobacco leaves. Coal ashes or cowdung cake ashes may be used alternatively.

HOUSING SYSTEMS OF POULTRY

There are four systems of housing generally found to follow among the poultry keepers. The type of housing adopted depends to a large extent on the amount of ground and the capital available.

1. Free-range or extensive system
2. Semi-intensive system
3. Folding unit system
4. Intensive system
   A. Battery system
   B. Deep litter system

Free-range system. This method is the oldest of all and has been used for centuries by general farmers, where there is no shortage of land.

This system allows great but not unlimited, space to the birds on land where they can find an appreciable amount of food in the form of herbage, seeds and insects, provided they are protected from predatory animals and infectious diseases including parasitic infestation. At present due to advantages of intensive methods the system is almost obsolete.

Semi-intensive system. This system is adopted where the amount of free space available is limited, but it is necessary to allow the birds 20-30 square yards per bird of outside run. Wherever possible this space should be divided giving a run on either side of the house of 10-15 square yards per bird, thus enabling the birds to move onto fresh ground.

Folding-unit system. This system of housing is an innovation of recent years. In portable folding units birds being confined to one small run, the position is changed each day, giving them fresh ground and the birds find a considerable proportion of food from the herbage are healthier and harder. For the farmer the beneficial effects of scratching and manuring on the land is another side effect.

The disadvantages are that food and water must be carried out to the birds and eggs brought back and there is some extra labour involved in the regular moving of the fold units.

The most convenient folding unit to handle is that which is made for 25 hens. A floor space of 1 square foot should be allowed for each bird in the house, and 3 square feet in the run, so that a total floor space to the whole unit is 4 square feet per bird, as with the intensive system.

A suitable measurement for a folding house to take 25 birds is 5 feet wide and 20 feet long, the house being 5′ × 5′, one-third of the run The part nearest the house is covered in and the remaining 10′ open with wire netting sides and top.

Intensive System

In this system the birds are confined to the house entirely, with no access to land outside, and it is usually adopted where land is limited and :xpensive.

This has only been made possible by admitting the direct rays of the sun on to the floor of the house so that part of the windows are removable, or either fold or slide down like windows of railway train to permit the ultraviolet rays to reach the birds. Under the intensive system, Battery (cage system) and Deep litter methods are most common.

A. Battery system. This appliance is the inventor's latest contribution to the commercial egg farmer. This is the most intensive type of poultry production and is useful to those with only a small quantity of floor space at their disposal. Nowadays in large cities hardly a poultry lover can spare open lands for rearing birds. For all such people this system will prove worthy of keeping birds at minimum space.

In the battery system each hen is confined to a cage just large enough to permit very limited movement and allow her to stand and sit comfortably. The usual floor space is 14 × 16 inches and the height, 17 inches. The floor is of standard strong galvanised wire set at a slope from back to the front, so that the eggs as they are laid, roll out of the cage to a receiving gutter. Underneath is a tray for droppings. Both food and water receptacles are outside the cage. Many small cages can be assembled together, if necessary it may be multistoried. The whole structure should be of metal so that no parasities will be harboured and thorough disinfection can be carried out as often as required. Provided the batteries of cages are set up in a place which is well ventilated, and lighted, is not too hot and is vermin proof and that the food meets all nutritional needs, this system has proved to be remarkably successful in the tropical countries. It may be that as it requires a minimum expenditure of energy from the bird, which spends all its time in the shade, it lessens the load of excess body heat. The performance of

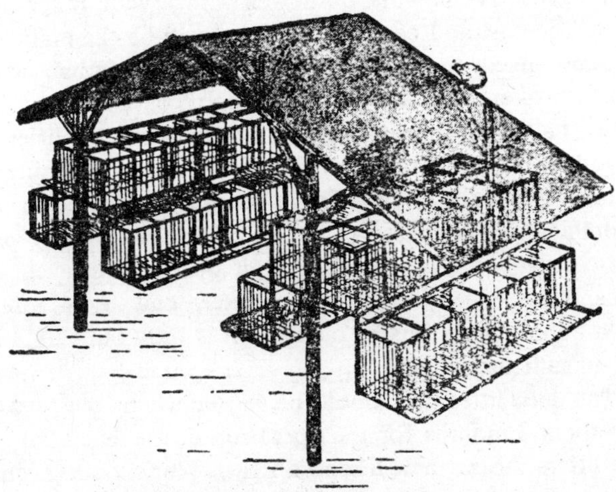

Fig. 15.17 Battery system.

each bird can be noted and culling easily carried out. Pullets, which are more often used than birds of over one year, should be placed in the cages at least one month before they are expected to lay.

The feeding of birds in cages has to be carefully considered, as the birds are entirely dependent on the mash for maintenance and production. To supply vitamins A and D, cod-liver oil, yeast, dried milk powder are useful, and fish meal or other animal protein, and balanced minerals and some form of grit must be made available.

As in each cage there will be only pullets so one can never expect fertilised eggs, hence the vegetative eggs will be there, which can be preserved for a longer time than fertilised eggs at ordinary room temperature but can never be used for hatching purposes.

B. Deep litter system. In this system the poultry birds are kept in large pens up to 250 birds each, on floor covered with litters like straw, saw dust or leaves up to depth of 8–12 inches. Deep litter resembles to dry compost. In other words we can define deep litter, as the accumulation of the material used for litter with poultry manure until it reaches a depth of 8 to 12 inches. The build-up has to be carried out correctly to give desired results which takes very little attention.

Basic Rules Needed

1. Do not have too many birds in the pen—one bird for every 3½ to 4 and preferably 5 square feet of floor space.
2. Provide sufficient ventilation to enable the litter to keep in correct condition.
3. Keep the litter dry. This is probably the master work in a deep litter system. If the litter gets soaked by leaking from roofs or from water vessels, it upsets the whole process and would have to start over again. All probable precautions should be taken to maintain the litters completely dry.
4. Stir the litter regularly. Turning the litter (just like digging in a garden) at least once weekly is very important in maintaining a correct build-up of deep litter.

How deep litter is started? For deep litter we can use many materials as a medium for starting the build-up in a pen. It can work quite well with a wide range but organic materials should always be used. The cost and ease of obtaining will be the main guide. Suitable dry organic materials like straw (needs to be cut into 2 or 3 inch lengths), saw dust, leaves, dry grasses, groundnut shells, broken up maize stalks and cobs, bark of trees in sufficient quantity to give a depth of about 6 inches in the pen should be used. When the litter has built up it would be very difficult for anyone to say what material was initially used. Nothing else has to be added. The droppings of the birds gradually combine with the materials used to build up the litter (the bacterial action commences as a result). When a pen is not overcrowded, these can be regularly absorbed and correct condition maintained, if stirring and even distribution is kept up. In about 2 months, it has usually become deep litter, and by 6 months it has become built-up deep litter. At about 12 months of old stage it is fully built up. Extra litter materials can be added to maintain sufficient depth.

When to start it? The deep litter pen should be started when the weather is dry, and is likely to remain so for about 2 months for the operation of the bacterial action which alters the composition of the litters. Start new litter with each year's pullets and continue with it for their laying period.

Deep litter in wet areas. Laying birds can be kept quite successfully in a shed built off the ground—in fact birds can be kept in houses with 2 or 3 floors one above the other. Sometimes the litters may get damp in spite of all precautions, at that time about 0.5 kg of superphosphate may be thoroughly mixed up with litters spreading in 15 square feet of floor space. When this is not available hydrated lime (but never quicklime) can be used at the same level.

Advantages of Deep Litter System

1. Safety of birds. Birds on range or even in a netted yard can be taken by wild animals, flying birds, etc. When enclosed in deep litter intensive pen which has strong wire netting or expanded metal, the birds and eggs are safe.

2. Litter as a source of food supply. It may come as surprise to learn that built-up deep litter also supplies some of the food requirements of the birds. They obtain "Animal Protein Factor" from deep litter and some work indicates that this could mean that birds obtain sufficient of this to enable a suitable feed ration to be prepared with only a vegetable protein such as groundnut meal included in the feed. The level of vitamins such as riboflavin increases up to nearly three-fold, according to experiments conducted. The combination of this and the Animal Protein Factor is necessary to good hatchability of eggs and early growth of chickens.

3. Disease control. Well managed deep litter kept in dry condition with no wet spots around waterer has a sterilising action. The level of coccidiosis and worm infestation is much lower with poultry kept on good deep litter than with birds (or chickens) in bare yards and bare floor sheds particularly where water spillage is allowed.

4. Labour saving. This is one of the really big features of deep litter usage. Cleaning out poultry pens daily or weekly means quite a lot of work. With correct conditions observed with well managed litter there is no need to clean a pen out for a whole year; the only attention is the regular stirring and adding of some material as needed.

5. The valuable fertiliser. This is a valuable economic factor with deep litter. According to McArdle and Panda, 35 laying birds can produce in one year about 1 tonne of deep litter fertiliser. The level of nitrogen in fresh manure is about 1%, but on well built-up deep litter it may be around 3 per cent nitrogen (nearly 20% protein). It also contains about 2 per cent phosphorus and 2 per cent potash. Its value is about 3 times that of cattle manure.

6. Hot weather safeguard. This is an important feature in a hot climate. The litter maintains its own constant temperature, so birds burrow into it when the air temperature is high and thereby cool themselves. Conversely, they can warm themselves in the same way when the weather is very cool. Accordingly, it is a valuable insulating agent.

BREEDING SYSTEMS

A large number of mating systems are being used in poultry breeding. There is no evidence, however, to indicate that any one system is best for all purposes. Following is a brief discussion of the procedures, advantages, disadvantages of each system.

Out-crossing. The mating of birds of the same variety but of different strains is called outbreeding. The object is to hold the good traits already in one family line and to capture the good ones from the other one. Or, it may be an attempt to get rid of the undesirable traits in one line and obtain only the good ones from another line.

Grading. This system involves the mating of superior males with successive generations of breeding hens of the same breed or variety. The system is followed until the progenies produced approach the quality of the males used. To avoid disadvantages of inbreeding one particular cock should not be used for a number of times, but different cocks of the same breed should be selected.

This method is, therefore, of great importance for improving indigenous poultry existing in our villages.

Cross breeding. The mating of pure-bred males of one breed with pure bred females of another breed is known as cross breeding. This method has been popular in livestock breeding. Cross breeding in chickens has resulted in higher hatchability, more efficient and faster gains, and lower chick mortality. Hybrid vigour resulting from cross breed utilised extensively in broiler production.

Line breeding. Line breeding is similar to inbreeding but involves the breeding of birds less closely related. The mating of cousins or grand-sire and grand-daughters are examples of line breeding. It is done to conserve and perpetuate the good traits of certain outstanding birds. It tends to produce a homozygous genetic condition.

Inbreeding. It is the mating of such closely related birds as (1) brother to sister, (2) son to dam, (3) sire to daughter. It is done primarily to intensify the degree or homozygosity. The practice has not proved satisfactory with poultry.

Bad as well as good characteristic become mixed in inbreeding.

Top crossing. This system of breeding has been used successfully in swine production and is finding its place in poultry breeding. It involves the mating of inbred males with females which are not inbred.

Tests must be made to determine the inbred lines which cross with the flock involved. The 'nicking' ability of each line must be determined.

A single inbred line in top crossing is much cheaper than a four inbred top cross. Only line has to be determined.

Single cross top crossing. This system involves the mating of single cross males to pure-bred females. Two proven inbred lines are maintained to produce the single cross males. This system has also proved desirable in swine production.

Single cross males normally demonstrate a reproductive performance far superior to that of the inbred, and equal or superior to that of pure-breds.

Methods of Mating

The methods of mating used will have a marked influence on fertility and consequently on the number of offsprings used. Most common methods of mating are flock and pen mating. Stud mating and artificial insemination are sometimes used in experimental work.

Flock mating. It is also known as mass mating.

Other things being equal, better fertility is obtained from flock matings than from pen matings, probably due to the competition among males in flock mating which results in more matings and better fertility. One male is sufficient for 15 to 20 hens, but number varies with the size and age of the hens. In flock matings the percentage of chicks hatched is unknown.

Pen mating. In pen mating a pen of hens is mated to a single male. If the birds are trap-nested and the hen's leg-band number recorded on the egg, it is possible to know the parents of every chick hatched from a pen mating. About the same number of hens are mated with a male as in the case of flock mating. Fertility is not so good in pen mating as in flock mating. This is because, certain hens may not like the cock or vice-versa.

Stud mating. In stud mating the females are mated individually with a male kept by the owner in a coop or pen. Thus this system involves more labour than flock mating. The birds should be mated at least once each week in order to maintain good fertility.

Stud mating may be used where hens are kept in laying batteries. It is also used when a very valuable male is being used as a breeder.

Artificial insemination. This system is not practical in poultry breeding work although it is possible to follow the system. It is used in experimental work and may be used in turkey breeding where poor fertility is encountered.

POULTRY NUTRITION

Nutrition is the process of furnishing the cells inside the animal with that portion of the external chemical environment needed for optimum functioning of the many metabolic chemical reactions involved in growth, maintenance work, production and reproduction.

Nutrition encompasses the procurement, ingestion, digestion and absorption of the chemical elements which serve as food. In addition it includes the transport of these chemical elements to all cells within the animal organism in the physical and chemical forms most suitable for assimilation and use by the cells.

Principles of Poultry Feeding

Poultry feeding is one of the important branches of poultry science, since feed-cost alone accounts for 60-65 per cent of the total farm expenses. It is in the interest of every poultryman to be able to get as much chicken meat or as many eggs for every rupee that he spends on the feed as possible.

The problems involved in the feeding of fowls in recent times are multifarious because of modern farming conditions such as: (i) increased cost of poultry feed; (ii) confinement rearing of poultry; (iii) inclusion of agro-industrial by-products in poultry; and (iv) increase in flock size and high flock density.

While computing ration for poultry birds, the following facts should be considered:

(i) Poultry birds have no lips or teeth, hence require a more concentrated ration.

(ii) Their digestive tract having a simple stomach is comparatively short, digestion is quite rapid. It takes about 2½ hours for feed to go from mouth to cloaca in the laying hen, and 10 hours in a non-laying hen. Therefore, the nutritive requirements of poultry are more precise.

(iii) Unlike ruminants, where micro-organisms synthesise a sizeable portion of essential amino acid, vitamin B complex, vitamin K in the stomach, the poultry completely depend upon the dietary source for all such nutrients (all essential amino acids, vitamin B complex, etc.).

(iv) Poultry birds are fed collectively rather than individually.

(v) Due to higher rate of metabolism poultry require a more exact ration.

Nutrients—Their Nature and Functions

The term nutrient means any single class of food, or group of like feeds. that aids in the support of life and makes it possible for birds to produce meat or eggs. They are classified according to physical, chemical and biological properties into following groups:

1. Water
2. Proteins
3. Carbohydrates
4. Fats and oils
5. Minerals
6. Vitamins
7. Feed additives (not a nutrient, but added to enhance the quality of the nutrients)

1. Water. The internal environment of an animal is basically a water medium in which transport of nutrient occurs, metabolic erections take place, and from which wastes can be eliminated. Water makes up 85 per cent of the body of day old chicks gradually decreases as chickens grow older, reaching a level of about 55 per cent in mature chickens at 42 weeks of age. The water content of whole egg is about 65 per cent.

Ordinarily, chickens consume about 2 to 2.5 gms of water for each gram of feed consumed during the starting and growing period and from 1.5-2.0 gms of water per gm of feed as laying hens. Since an average poultry ration contains no more than 10 per cent water, a good supply of clean drinking water is essential for poultry and egg productions.

2. Proteins. In poultry, the products produced consists mainly of protein. On a dry weight basis the carcass of an 8 weeks old broiler is more than 65 per cent protein and the egg contents are about 50 per cent protein. Typical broiler rations will contain from 22 to 24 per cent protein and in layers ration the amount varies between 16-17 per cent.

From the standpoint of nutrition, the amino acids that make up the protein are really the essential nutrients rather than the protein molecule itself.

Table 15.15

Twelve Essential Amino Acids Required by the Growing Chick,

Essential	Nonessential
Arginine	Alanine
Cystine	Aspartic acid
Histidine	Glutamic acid
Isoleucine	Glycine
Leucine	Hydroxyproline
Lysine	Proline
Methionine	Serine
Phenylalanine	
Threonine	
Trytptophan	
Tyrosine	
Valine	

Tyrosine is synthesised from Phenylalaine, cystine from methionine, hydroxylysine from lysine. Under some conditions glycine or serine synthesis may not be sufficient for most rapid growth; either serine or glycine may need to be supplied in the diet.

The amino acid needs of the growing chickens and laying hens are met in practice by proteins of plant and animal sources. Generally, it is necessary to choose more than one source of dietary protein, (i.e., animal and vegetable sources) to meet the amino acid requirement of the chicken.

Of the essential amino acids, listed above, lysine, methionine, arginine, glycine and tryptophan are referred as "critical" amino acids, since these are usually deficient in ordinary practical poultry ration. This is because cereal grains are usually low in critical amino acids which make up a large proportion of a usual poultry ration. It is thus a must to include a good proportion of animal protein like fish meal, etc., in poultry ration to ensure the inclusion of all critical amino acids

3. Carbohydrates. The main function of carbohydrates in the diet is to provide energy to the animal. The polysaccharides of major importance are starch, cellulose, pentosans and several other complex carbohydrates. Although cellulose and starch are composed of glucose units, chickens possess enzymes that can hydrolyse only starch. Cellulose, therefore, is completely indigestible. Cereal grains and their by-products are excellent source of starch and thus constitutes a bulk of poultry ration.

4. Fats. Fats make up over 40 per cent of the dry egg and about 17 per cent of the dry weight of a broiler. Although fats supply concentrated form of energy (2.25 times more energy than carbohydrate and protein) their inclusion as true fats or oils in the ration is seldom practised because of high cost and the risk of rancidity which develops on prolong exposure to air, heat, sunlight, etc. Most feed ingredients (maize, barley, safflower, milo, wheat, rice bran, etc.) contain 2-5 per cent fat and that is enough for the inclusion of one essential fatty acid (Linoleic acid), which must be present in the young growing chicks or they will grow poorly, have an accumulation of liver fat and be more susceptible for respiratory infection. Laying hens with diets deficient in linoleic acid will lay very small eggs that will not hatch well.

5. Minerals. The body of the chicken and the egg excluding shell contain nearly 4 and 1 per cent mineral matter respectively. The elements known to be required in the diet of poultry are calcium, phosphorus, sodium, potassium, magnesium, chlorine, iodine, iron, manganese, copper, molybdenum, zinc and selenium. The importance of each element may be learnt from chapter 10 of this book. Usually the grains and vegetable protein ingredients are relatively poor in mineral contents when compared with those of animal protein feed stuffs. The common mineral supplements in poultry feed are as follows:

(i) Limestone
(ii) Bone meal
(iii) Oyster shell
(iv) Sodium chloride
(v) Dicalcium phosphate
(vi) Manganese sulphate
(vii) Potassium iodide
(viii) Superphosphate.

6. Vitamins. Vitamins most commonly function as coenzymes and regulators of metabolism. The 13 vitamins required by poultry have been summarised in tabular form (Table 15.16). Apart from natural sources, commercial vitamin mixture suitable for poultry are also available. One point to remember, of course, is that the natural vitamins are likely to have other factors associated with them. These may be other recognised nutrients or they may be unidentified factors. Diets continuously deficient in any one of the required vitamins will seriously tell initially upon the egg production and then the life of the chickens.

7. Feed additives. A full discussion including importance of various feed additives has been made separately as below.

MODERN FEED ADDITIVES FOR POULTRY

Efforts to produce human feeds from animal sources more efficiently and at lower cost have stimulated continued research for new additives. Considerable information has accumulated about the multifarious utility of various feed additives.

Additives are never nutrients. They either singly or in combinations are added to a basic feed, usually in small qualities for the purpose of fortifying these with certain nutrients or stimulants or medicines. Often they are called "non-nutrient" feed additives. The inclusion of most of these materials in poultry ration are controlled by law in most of the countries. Some of the useful effects of such non-nutritive feed additives are discussed below:

A. Additives that promote Feed Intake or Selection

Like people, most of the animals have taste and aroma preferences, some feed are more liked by them than others.

1. Antioxidants

All feeds are susceptible to spoilage, but those which are high in fat content are specially prone to antioxidation followed by rancidity. Most animals will refuse to eat spoiled feed. But when feed is limited, they may consume it with digestive disturbances resulting in many cases. To curb the oxidation of feeds antioxidants are routinely added to many livestock feeds.

Antioxidants are compounds that prevent oxidative rancidity of polyunsaturated fats. In absence of these there may rancidity also cause destruction of Vitamins A, D, and E, and several of the B complex vitamins. In some cases the breakdown products of rancidity may react with the epsilon amino groups of lysine and thereby decrease the protein and energy values of the diet. Some common antioxidants are: BHT (Butylated hydroxytoluene); Santoquin; Ethoxyquin; BHA (Butylated hydroxyanisode); DPPD (Diphenyl paraphenyl diamine). All are added at 0.01% level in poultry feed.

2. Flavouring Agents

These are feed additives that are supposed to increase palatability and feed intake. There is need for flavouring agents particularly (1) when highly unpalatable medicants are being administered, (2) during attacks of diseases, (3) when animals are under stress, and (4) when a less palatable feed stuff is being incorporated in the ration.

"Poultry Nector", a flavouring agent has been studied initially at Misissippi University (U.S.A.) and proven to give consistant improvement in performance when added at 0.05% to poultry diets particularly when less palatable ingredients are used.

3. Pellet binders and Additives that alter Feed texture

Pellet binders are products that enhance the firmness of pellets; among them, (1) sodium bentonite (clay), (2) liquid or solid by-products of the wood pulp industry, consisting mainly of hemicelluloses, or combinations of hemicellulose and lignins, (3) molasses or fat are sometimes added to feed as an aid in pelleting, as well as a concentrated source of energy, (4) guar meal is another example. All are added @ 2.5% of the diet.

B. Additives that Enhance the Colour or Quality of the Marketed Product.

Many marketing concerns have 'brain washed' consumers into believing that broilers having a deep yellow coloured shank are of top quality. A similar situation exists relative to eggs, in which deep yellow yolks are considered to be highly desirable. Consequently, Xanthophylls are routinely incorporated into broiler feeds. Another synthetic carotinoid, Canthaxanthin when added @ 2-10 grams per tonne of feed along with yellow maize and lucerne helps to produce orange-yellow colour in the shanks and skin of broilers along with yolks.

C. Additives that Facilitate Digestion and Absorption

1. Grit

Since poultry do not have teeth to facilitate grinding of feed, most grinding takes place in the thick muscled gizzard. Grit is added to supply additional surface area of the feed by grinding those inside the gizzard. Oester shell, limestones are common grits. Gravel and pebbles have been used successfully as long lasting sources of grit.

2. Chelates

Chelating agents, such as EDTA, are sometimes used to increase the availability and absorption of certain minerals. In chicks zink absorption is enhanced through addition of EDTA.

3. Enzymes

These are complex protein compounds produced in living cells which cause changes in other substances without being changed themselves. They are organic catalysts.

For common poultry diets, the enzymes of the digestive system cause normal hydrolysis of the dietory proteins, carbohydrates and fats. Thus no benefit may be expected from the use of enzyme preparation as feed additives unless feed composed of higher amounts of barley, wheat, sunflower, rye, ricebran or oat grains are fed to chickens. Barley to a large extent than wheat contain compounds named beta-glucans which give viscocity to the contents of the digestive tract. Such viscous material interferes with the activity of all digestive enzymes. Very small concentration of beta-glucans, 0.75 to 1.0% can produce this effect. The beta-glucanase in the enzyme products, by breaking down the beta-glucans, reduces the viscocity of the feed in the digestive tract and thus facilitates the action of natural digestive enzymes. The cellulases in the enzyme products would act on the cellulose present in the cell walls of grain by-products like rice bran, rice polish, wheat bran and other crude fibres present in other feed ingredients in the feed and would improve availability of nutrients from these products. The enzyme preparations which are being marketed are Agrozyme, Diazyme, Zymo-pabst, Porzyme and Avizyme etc.

4. Probiotics

Probiotics are live cultures of useful bacteria along with medicine in which they were grown. The organisms used are beneficial strains of lactobacillus and streptococcus. The reasoning behind the use of probiotic is that ingestion of these organisms would lend an increase in their number in the digestive tract. Their dominance would reduce the population of undesirable organisms like *E. Coli* and thus save the birds from the toxins that these undesirable organisms produce in the digestive tract.

5. Antibiotics

These are substances which are produced by living organisms (molds, bacteria, or green plants) and which have bacteriostatic or bactericidal properties.

As early as 1949, it was observed that chickens fed with vegetable protein gain in more weight when they were fed antibiotics 5-10 mg. per kg. of feed.

The probable modes of action of antibiotics follow:

1. They may spare certain nutrients. Studies in some cases indicated that antibiotics can replace inadequate intakes of certain vitamins and amino acids.
2. They may selectively inhibit growth of nutrient-destroying organisms while promoting growth of nutrient producing organisms.
3. They increase feed and/or water intake.
4. They may inhibit growth of organisms which produce toxic waste products or toxins.
5. They may kill or inhibit pathogenic organisms (a) within the gastrointestinal tract, or (b) systemically.
6. They may improve the digestion and subsequent absorption of certain nutrients.

The normal levels of incuusion are 4 grams per tonne of feed for the narrow spectrum, viz., penicillin, streptomycin etc., and 10 grams per tonne for the broad spectrum types, viz., tetracyclines, aureomycin etc. Higher levels of antibiotics (50 to 100 grams per tonne) may be used only after the careful consideration of disease level.

D. Additives that alter Metabolism

1. Hormone:

Hormones are chemicals released by a specific area of the body that the transported to another region within the animal where they elicit a physiological response.

Hormonal preparations are added in the diet of chickens with a view to bring about desirable metabolic changes so that increased egg production or carcass fat deposition in birds could be achieved. These fall into about following four categories:

a) Anabolic compounds are chiefly progesterone and related steroids which may stimulate protein metabolism. The objectives are clear, but to-date results have not been promising.

b) Oestrogens in the form of Diethylstilbesterol (DES) were used for several years largely as a subcutenious implant in broiler chicken. It resulted carcass quality having more tender and tastier. However, since hormone residues remain present in carcass, its use in chicken feed is now prohibited in U.S.A.

Dienestrol diacetate is the only feed additive of this type that is currently approved at a level of 0.0023 to 0.0035 percent in the feed for the last 4-10 weeks to improve the carcass quality of broilers and roasters. The practice must be discontinued at least 48 hours before slaughter. It must not be fed to laying hens or breeding stock.

c) Thyroxine and related compounds are reported to stimulate growth and to improve egg production during the later part of the laying year. They are usually given in the form of iodinated casein at levels of 100 to 200 grams per ton (110 to 220 mg./kg.) of feed. Results from the use of iodinated casein have been variable may be due to the differing needs of individual birds. A slight excess dose may bring about moulting and drop in egg production.

E. Additives that affect Health Status

1. Antifungal additives are agents that destroy fungi. Fungi can affect feed intake and subsequent production through contamination at one or more of four stages in the feeding chain: (1) in the field before harvesting, (2) during storage, (3) at mixing, and (4) within the animal itself. Once contaminated, fungi can pose problems through the production of toxins, alterations of the chemical composition of the diet, or alterations of the metabolic functioning of the animal ingesting or harboring the fungus. Production of aflatoxin by *Aspergillus flavus* is a classical example which is carcinogenic (tumor producing).

The best method of controlling fungal infestation is to dry all feeds below 12 percent moisture. Additionally, mold inhibitors should be added to high moisture feed that are exposed to air during storage. Sodium propionate, sodium benzoate, quaternary ammonium compounds, acetic acid and certain antifungal antibiotics as nystatin or copper sulfate etc. are added to concentrate feeds to prevent further growth by molds. The toxicity of aflatoxin-contaminated feed can also be reduced by irradication of ultraviolet light or exposed to anhydrous ammonia under pressure.

2. Anticoccidial drugs are used to control coccidial infections which is a parasitic disease caused by microscopic protozoan organisms known as coccidia, which live in the cells of the intestinal lining of livestock. At least eight species of coccidia affect chicken: *Eimeria tenella, E. necatrix, E. maxima, E. acervulina, E. brunetti, E. hagani, E. praecox* and *E. mites.*

There are over two dozen coccidiostats combinations commercially available. Bifuran supplement, Amprol-25%, Embazin, Zonamix, Nitrofurazone, Furazolidone etc. etc. are very common coccidiostats. Most of these inhibit further proliferation of parasites during their sexual cycles. Coccidia tend to develop resistance to a coccidiostat to which they are exposed over a long period of time. When resistant forms appear, a change to another coccidiostat will usually restore control of the disease.

3. Antihelmintic Drugs. Chickens are subject to infestation with a wide variety of parasites, external and internal. External parasites can be eliminated by use of available insecticides. Likewise intestinal worms can also be killed or expelled by feeding suitable vermifuges (wormers).

The four most common intestinal parasites are large roundworms (*Ascaris*), cecal works (*Heterakis*), capillary worms (*Capillaria*), and tape worms (*Taenia*). Of these, the large round worms are more easily expelled; cecal worms, capillary worms and tape worms, in the order given, are less easily expelled.

Antihelminties generally require more than one administration. The first administration kills those worms which are present in the body; and subsequent wormings kill those worms which hatched from eggs after the initial dose.

Table 15.16

Vitamin deficiency symptoms in poultry and the principal natural sources of these vitamins

Vitamin	*Deficiency symptoms*	*Principal natural sources*
Vitamin A	Retarded growth, general weakness, emaciation, staggering gait, ruffled feathers, mortality, watery or sticky eyelids, xerophthalmia, creamy white pustules on roof of mouth and along esophagus, ureates in kidney tabules and ureters. In young and adult birds a cheesy exudate from eye and sticky discharge from nostrils is often observed. Egg production and hatchability are markedly reduced.	Cod-liver and other fish oils, animal liver meals, green grasses, yellow corn, lucerne green or dried, maize gluten meal, leaf meals from tropical legumes.
Vitamin D	Rickets—leg weakness, stiff legged gait, crooked keels, beaded ribs, swollen hocks, soft bones, ungainly manner of balancing body, appear unthrifty, depigmentation of feathers, and mortality; in adults, fragile bones, thin-shelled eggs, reduced egg production and hatchability.	Cod-liver oils and certain other fish oils or concentrates. Deactivated animal sterol. Sunshine by irradiation of sterols under the skin, ultraviolet ray lights by similar irradiation.
Vitamin E (α-tocopherol)	Encephalomacia ("Crazy chick" discase) incoordination of movement, frequently unable to stand, turns in circle, edema beneath skin and hemorrhage in cerebellum. In turkeys, enlarged hock disorder and dystrophy of smooth muscle of gizzard lining reported. In ducks, dystrophy of skeletal muscle. In adults, reduced hatchability in chickens and turkeys.	Green forage, vegetable oils, whole and sprouted grains, lucerne meal.
Vitamin K	Prolonged blood clotting time. Hemorrhages develop internally and subcutaneously on the legs, breast, abdomen, neck, under the wings, and in the intestinal tract.	Lucerne, kale, green leafy vegetabies, meat scraps, fish meal.
Vitamin B_1 (thiamine)	Polyneuritis—retracted head, retarded growth, reduced appetite, extreme weakness, ataxia, emaciation, impairment of digestion, convulsions, and death.	Whole grain, wheat by-products, yeast, liver meal, groundnut meal, molasses, grasses, lucerne, rice by-products.
Vitamin B_2 (riboflavin)	"Curled toe" paralysis (toes curl inward) and paralysis of legs, retarded growth, diarrhea, tendency to walk on hocks, hypertrophy and softening of brachial and sciatic nerves and dry scaly skin, severe dermatitis in poults at corners of mouth, vent, eyelids and footpads. In adults, reduction in egg production and hatchability, dwarfed embroys showing edema, degeneration of Wolffian bodies, and 'clnbbed down" condition. Embryo motality peak at about th eleventh day of incubation.	Liver meal, yeast, milk by-products. Concentrates made from fermentation residues, lucerne leaf meal, young grasses, kidney, some fish meals, distillers' solubles.

(Contd.)

Vitamin	*Deficiency symptoms*	*Principal natural sources*
Vitamin B_6 (pyridoxine)	Retarded growth, hyper-excitability, tend to run aimlessly, flapping their wings with head down, repeated convulsions with distended or twisted neck, complete exhaustion and death. In adults, loss of appetite, reduced egg production and hatchability, loss of weight and death.	Liver meal, yeast, rice bran, meat (muscle tissue and glands), cane molasses, fish, wheat and rice by-products, lucerne.
Vitamin B_{12} (cyanocobalamine)	Reduced growth, poor feathering and mortality in young chicks. In adult hens, poor hatchability of fertile eggs. Chicks that do hatch have low "carryover" and show high early mortality unless injected with or fed, high levels of vitamin B_{12}	Fish meal, liver, whey, soybean oil meal, cow manure, egg yolk, egg white, various fermentation products.
Pantothenic acid	Retarded growth, ragged feather development, dermatitis lesions on eyelids, at corners of mouth, around vent and sometimes on top of the feet, liver damage and changes in spinal cord may develop. In adult fowls, lowered hatchability and impaired egg production result.	Liver meal, yeast, cane molasses, groundnut meal, milk by-products, wheat bran, rice bran, soybean meal, lucerne leaf meal, kale cabbage, broccoli, cauliflower, cucumbers, fermentation residues, maize, distillers solubles grasses.
Nicotinic acid (niacine)	Poor growth, poor feathering inflammation of the mouth and tongue ("black tongue"), perosis, reduced feed consumption and occasionally dermatitis on skin and feet of young chicks and poults. In poults, enlarged hock disorder; in ducks and goslings, bowed legs occur. In adults, poor egg production and reduced hatchability.	Yeast, liver meal, rice bran, wheat feeds, groundnuts, greens, meat (muscle tissue), maize distillers' solubles.
Folic acid (Folacin)	Retarded growth, poor feathering depigmentation of feathers in coloured chicks and poults, reduction in red blood cell numbers and hemoglobin (anemia), reduction in white blood cells, occasionally perosis, and high mortality. In poults, cervical paralysis (paralysis of neck) also observed. In adults, anemia, weight loss, reduced egg production and lowered hatchability.	Green leafy plants, grass, spinach, lucerne, etc. Yeast, liver, kidneys. Whole grain supplies enough in poultry rations.
Biotin	Poor growth, perosis and severe dermatosis. Bottoms of feet become roughened and crack open, then dermatitic lesions also appear, at	Liver, yeast, potatoes, kidneys and other glands, milk, cane molasses, lucerne leaf meal, grasses. Whole

(Contd.)

Vitamin	*Deficiency symptoms*	*Principal natural sources*
	corners of mouth and on eyelids as described for pantothenic acid deficiency. In adults, impaired hatchability with embryos showing skeletal deformities including parrot beak and short legs.	grain supplies enough in the poultry ration.
Choline	Poor growth, perosis (slipped tendon), poor feed utilisation, unthrifty appearance and slight increase in liver fat. Practical rations for adult fowl appear to contain adequate levels of choline.	Liver meal, meat, fish, whole grain, wheat by-products, milk by-products, groundnut meal, soy-bean oil meal.

SOURCE: *Poultry Feeding in Tropical and Subtropical Countries*, FAO Rome, 1964.

REQUIREMENTS FOR POULTRY FEEDS

Chickens of different ages require different levels of nutrients. The Indian Standards Institution (ISI) has prescribed the standard specifications for starting, growing and laying chicken feeds to serve as a guide for the feed manufacturers and poultry keepers in the country in their publication number ISI: 1974 – 1977. The nutrient requirement of chicken feeds are detailed in Table 15.17.

Poultry feeds are of the following three types:

1. *Starting poultry feed:* An all mash ration to be fed to chicks upto the age of 8 weeks.
2. *Growing poultry feed:* A ration to be fed to growing chickens after 8 to 20 weeks or until laying commences.
3. *Laying poultry feed:* A ration to be fed to laying birds after 20 weeks onwards or after laying commences.

Feeding Broilers

A broiler, also known as fryer is a young chicken, which grow very fast and can be marketed during the ages between 8 to 12 weeks old. By this time it attains about 1.5 kg live weight. It may be of either sex, tender-meated with soft, pliable, smooth, textured skin and flexible breast bone cartilage.

Broiler rations are especially formulated in such a way that they promote an early rapid growth. Usually broiler rations are prepared in such a way so that the feed contains relatively high energy and high protein when compared with the feed of chickens other than broilers. A protein per cent between 22 and 24 are fed to broilers for the first 5–6 weeks to obtain rapid early growth. These rations are called broiler starter rations. After this period, broilers are

fed with a different type of ration having relatively less protein and more energy for fattening. Such a feed is known as broiler finisher ration. The ideal composition of broiler feed is given in Table 15.17.

Table 15.17

ISI requirements for chicken feeds

	Broiler starter (0-6 weeks)	Broiler finisher (6-9 weeks)	Chick (0-8 weeks)	Grower (8-20 weeks)	Layer (20-80 weeks)	Breeder (20-80 weeks)
Metabolizable energy (kcal/kg)**	2900	3000	2700	2700	2700	2800
Crude protein** (%)	22	19	22	16	18	18
Crude fibre* (%)	6	6	7	8	8	8
Acid insoluble ash* (%)	3	3	4	4	4	4
Total sulphur amino acid* (%)	0.75	0.75	0.75	0.5	0.5	0.5
Lysine* (%)	0.9	0.9	1.0	0.7	0.5	0.5
Methionine** (%)	0.35	035	035	0.25	0.25	0.25
Vitamin A (IU/kg)	6000	6000	4000	4000	8000	8000
Vitamin D_3 (ICU/kg)	600	600	600	600	1200	1200
Thiamine (mg/kg)	2	2	6	6	6	6
Riboflavin (mg/kg)	5	5	5	5	5	8
Pantothenic acid (mg/kg)	12	12	10	10	15	15
Nicotinic acid (mg/kg)	40	40	30	20	20	20
Biotin (mg/kg)	0.1	0.1	0.1	0.1	0.15	0.15
Vitamin B_{12} (mg/kg)	8	8	15	15	15	30
Alpha tocopherol (mg/kg)	20	20	10	10	10	20
Choline chloride (mg/kg)	1400	1400	1300	—	—	1300
Linoleic acid** (%)	1	1	1	1	1	1
Salt (NaCl)* (%)	0.6	0.6	0.6	0.6	0.6	0.6
Calcium* (%)	1	1	1	1	2.75	2.75
Available phosphorus* (%)	0.5	0.5	0.5	0.5	0.5	0.5
Manganese (mg/kg)	60	60	55	55	55	55
Iodine (mg/kg)	1	1	1	1	1	1
Iron (mg/kg)	40	40	20	20	20	20
Copper (mg/kg)	4	4	2	2	2	2
Zinc (mg/Kg)	50	50	—	—	—	—
Moisture* (%)	10	10	10	10	10	10

* Maximum.
** Minimum. ISI 1974-1977 (Third revision).

Table 15.18

Inter-relations between nutrients in poultry rations

	BROILERS		***REPLACEMENT PULLETS (EGG OR MEAT TYPE)***			***Laying and breeding hens (egg and meat type)***
	0-6 weeks	***6-9 weeks***	***0-6 weeks***	***6-14 weeks***	***14-20 weeks***	
Calorie : protein (C/P)	139 : 1	160 : 1	145 : 1	180 : 1	241 : 1	190 : 1
Calcium : phosphrous	1.4 : 1	1.4 : 1	1.4 : 1	2 : 1	2 : 1	4.5 : 1
Vitamin D_3 (ICU/kg)	200	200	200	200	200	200
Arginine : lysine	1.12 : 1	1.09 : 1	1.09 : 1	1.05 : 1	1.03 : 1	1.6 : 1
*Methionine : cystine	1.15 : 1	1.14 : 1	1.14 : 1	1.14 : 1	1.14 : 1	1.12 : 1
Phenylalanine : tyrosine	1.14 : 1	1.16 : 1	1.16 : 1	1.1 : 1	1.16 : 1	?
Tryptophan (%) at	0.2	0.2	0.2	0.16	0.12	0.11
Niacin (mg/kg)	27	27	27	11	10	10

* Methionine content in ration should not be less than 0.46 for 0 t0 6 weeks old chicks.

Table 15.19

Essential amino acid requirement of poultry

(Expressed as % of protein)

Amino acid	*Starting chicks*	*Broilers and capons*	*Laying hens*
	(1)	*(2)*	*(3)*
Arginine	6.0	5.0	6.0
Lysine	5.5	6.0	5.0
Methionine	3.8	4.5	3.6
Or			
Methionine and	2.0	2.5	2.0
Cystine	1.8	2.0	1.6
Tryptohan	1.0	1.3	1.0
Glycine	5.0	6.0	–
Histidine	2.0	2.0	1.9
Leucine	7.0	7.5	7.5
Isoleucine	3.8	4.0	5.0
Phenylalanine	6.5	8.0	6.4
Or			
Phenylalanine and	3.5	4.0	4.4
Tyrosine	3.0	4.0	2.0
Threonine	3.5	4.0	3.5
Valine	4.3	4.5	5.0

NOTE: Values based on

1. N.R.C of U.S.A.
2. Lewis D. (1963), Based upon Maximum N_2 retention in 2–3 week broiler chicks.
3. Card and Nesheim (1966).

Table 15.20

Classification and composition table for poultry feeds*

Feed ingredient	ME (kcal/kg)	D.M.	C.P.	C.F.	E.E.	N.F.E.	Total ash	Acid Insol. Ash	Ca	P.	Lys.	Met.	Tryp.
Energy feeds:													
Bajra grain	2642	89.6	12.7	2.2	4.9	78.2	2.0	1.50	0.13	0.72	0.42	0.24	0.18
Cashew bran	—	94.4	16.9	6.9	27.1	45.4	3.7	0.10	0.45	0.40	—	—	—
Cashew kurna	—	95.7	18.4	9.5	52.9	15.6	3.6	0.40	0.50	0.60	—	—	—
Jower	2645	87.3	10.3	3.6	4.6	78.1	3.4	—	0.18	0.32	0.32	0.28	0.08
Lentils dehusked	—	94.2	24.6	0.7	1.0	71.1	2.6	0.36	0.20	0.83	0.97	0.32	0.26
Maize bran	—	93.7	8.5	14.9	1.4	73.8	1.4	—	0.07	0.13	—	0.03	0.06
Maize damage	—	89.7	10.1	2.8	3.9	80.1	1.7	0.39	0.25	0.40	0.21	0.18	0.16
Maize grit	2742	90.8	13.6	5.3	2.1	76.1	2.9	1.23	0.22	0.35	1.01	1.20	1.35
Maize opaque-2	—	—	9.9	—	—	—	—	—	—	—	0.34	—	—
Metha	—	92.1	20.6	8.6	6.1	60.9	3.8	0.45	0.35	0.80	—	—	—
Molasses	2400	73.6	2.8	—	—	86.3	10.9	0.44	1.51	0.66	—	—	—
Mowha flour	—	80.0	6.0	8.7	0.3	78.7	6.3	—	—	—	—	—	—
Oak kernels	—	—	5.4	2.1	10.2	79.4	2.9	—	0.13	0.15	—	—	—
Oats	—	91.7	14.7	13.5	4.6	60.8	6.4	—	0.11	0.41	0.38	0.23	0.10
Rice deoiled	2235	92.3	14.1	13.8	1.7	53.4	17.0	8.37	0.37	1.80	0.45	0.44	0.15
Rice kani	2345	90.7	7.9	1.4	1.7	87.1	1.9	0.66	0.11	0.48	0.06	—	—
Rice polis	2937	91.8	12.7	11.2	13.9	48.6	13.6	6.77	0.27	1.37	0.40	0.38	0.25
Salseed cake	3096	90.4	10.4	3.4	2.9	79.6	3.7	2.16	0.24	0.16	0.60	0.38	0.41
Starch	3938	89.4	10.6	0.03	0.09	99.4	0.28	0.04	—	—	—	—	—
Tapioca flour	3000	—	2.9	10.9	0.7	77.0	8.5	—	0.58	0.12	0.06	0.006	0.005

(Contd.)

Feed ingredient	ME (kcal/kg)	D.M.	C.P.	C.F.	E.E.	N.F.E.	Total Ash	Acid Insol. Ash	Ca	P	Lys.	Met.	Tryp.
Tapioca waste	—	90.4	4.1	15.9	1.5	72.5	6.0	—	0.58	0.19	—	—	—
Wheat bran	1069	88.9	14.7	11.3	3.8	62.3	7.9	—	0.19	1.12	0.50	0.16	0.18
Wheat damaged	—	89.9	9.5	2.3	2.3	81.9	4.0	1.66	0.08	0.41	—	—	—
Wheat dust	—	92.1	12.3	18.3	2.3	57.3	9.6	—	0.52	0.33	0.37	—	—
Protein Supplements:													
Blood meal	1420	88.8	73.4	0.7	—	—	6.0	3.0	0.32	0.31	4.79	0.66	0.88
Liver residue meal	—	90.9	65.4	1.3	15.8	11.9	5.6	—	—	—	3.85	0.89	0.50
Meat meal	2319	92.5	56.2	2.2	11.9	8.7	21.0	9.17	2.68	2.06	3.73	0.80	0.60
Poultry by-product meal	—	93.0	56.4	0.9	17.8	7.6	17.3	2.20	3.95	1.73	—	—	—
Casein	—	95.6	80.2	—	—	—	—	—	—	—	—	—	—
Coconut cake	1190	91.0	22.6	12.5	8.7	49.4	6.8	—	—	—	0.70	0.32	0.32
Cotton seed cake	1556	92.3	25.9	25.4	8.6	33.7	6.4	0.79	0.52	0.86	0.76	0.45	0.35
Dhaincha	—	91.2	28.3	11.0	5.8	50.7	4.2	0.10	0.30	0.55	2.30	0.60	0.67
Fish meal	1834	93.8	43.1	3.6	4.3	11.5	37.5	22.85	7.16	1.67	3.01	1.19	0.80
Frog meal	—	97.4	68.2	0.4	4.9	2.4	24.1	—	11.75	5.38	—	—	—
Gram baked dry	—	94.5	38.8	10.7	6.6	38.1	5.8	—	—	—	—	—	—
Bengal gram	2496	65.1	14.0	6.5	5.7	68.2	5.6	—	0.20	0.28	0.31	0.29	0.20
Black gram	2614	92.4	20.8	6.1	6.4	60.8	5.9	0.19	0.34	0.51	0.29	—	—
Gram chuni	2320	87.6	29.2	12.1	7.0	45.7	6.0	—	1.30	1.30	0.94	0.23	0.18
Gram red dehusked (Arhar)	—	93.1	21.7	0.9	1.9	71.0	4.5	0.08	0.19	0.92	0.69	0.74	0.14
Gram green (Mung)	—	93.5	19.7	5.2	1.3	70.1	3.7	0.32	0.25	0.84	—	0.41	0.13

(Contd.)

Gram horse (Kulthi)	2614	93.6	20.1	8.3	5.7	63.1	2.8	0.12	0.35	0.53	—	—	—
Groundnut cake (expeller)	2596	91.5	40.9	8.9	7.9	36.4	5.9	0.86	0.23	0.59	1.50	0.42	0.53
Groundnut cake (deoiled)	2328	93.3	57.9	11.2	2.2	27.2	10.8	2.24	0.31	0.67	1.51	0.43	0.71
Guar dal	—	89.7	48.0	5.3	7.4	23.7	5.1	—	0.26	0.79	—	—	—
Guar meal	—	91.0	42.6	10.9	6.2	35.1	5.8	0.59	0.54	0.70	2.94	—	0.59
Meat scrap with shell	—	89.7	55.2	1.0	14.5	11.9	17.4	—	—	—	—	—	—
Linseed oil cake	—	94.0	29.6	11.1	10.4	42.6	6.3	—	—	—	0.94	0.51	0.44
Maize gluten feed	2315	92.3	26.9	5.1	4.8	59.6	2.3	—	—	—	—	—	—
Maize grit	2742	90.8	13.6	5.3	2.1	76.1	2.9	0.21	0.31	0.15	0.33	0.26	0.07
Mustard oil cake	2373	91.3	35.1	8.2	14.1	33.4	9.2	1.20	0.89	1.78	0.99	0.72	0.68
Mustard cake (deoiled)	—	—	41.96	11.68	1.43	35.91	9.02	—	1.01	1.11	2.25	0.79	0.18
Neem seed cake	—	—	34.0	27.4	2.8	29.2	6.6	5.60	0.74	0.57	—	—	—
Ramtil cake	2817	96.6	36.0	18.6	8.9	28.3	8.2	1.85	0.62	0.96	1.37	—	—
Rape seed cake	—	87.6	36.0	10.4	12.8	31.4	9.4	—	1.12	1.05	—	—	—
Rubber seed cake	—	85.9	25.4	25.0	9.7	50.3	9.6	—	0.37	0.33	—	—	—
Safflower oil cake (decorticated)	—	92.8	42.2	8.5	8.2	32.2	8.9	—	0.40	0.51	—	—	—
Safflower oil cake (undecorticated)	—	95.0	23.1	29.9	5.5	36.9	4.6	—	—	—	—	—	—
Sesame cake	1882	90.7	39.1	4.7	9.3	34.3	12.6	1.50	2.46	1.42	1.04	0.84	0.72
Spent coffee cake powder	—	90.8	19.4	17.7	1.2	56.2	5.5	—	—	—	—	—	—
Sunflower cake	2230	89.1	37.2	11.6	10.9	32.6	7.7	0.62	0.43	1.14	—	—	—
Sunhemp meal	—	91.1	40.0	9.3	5.4	40.3	5.0	0.36	0.47	0.68	2.1	0.52	0.57
Taramira cake	—	96.9	40.5	8.0	9.5	35.9	6.1	1.04	0.57	0.71	0.97	—	0.55
Yeast sludge	—	91.8	32.1	1.8	1.3	46.3	18.5	—	6.05	0.41	—	—	—
Mineral supplements:													
Egg shell meal	—	98.2	5.8	—	0.3	1.4	92.5	—	33.63	—	—	—	—
Limestone	—	99.9	—	—	—	—	99.6	—	34.42	3.02	—	—	—
Feed additives:													
Penicillin mycelium residue	—	—	17.9	5.6	5.5	35.8	35.2	—	3.80	0.17	—	—	—
Penicillium mycelium waste	—	91.8	31.9	8.4	6.7	34.5	18.5	—	3.97	1.12	1.24	0.46	0.37

(Contd.)

Feed ingredient	ME (kcal/kg)	D.M.	C.P.	C.F.	E.E.	N.F.E.	Total ash	Acid Insol. Ash	Ca	P.	Lys.	Met.	Tryp.
Terramycin waste	—	96.6	31.7	7.2	4.1	15.4	41.6	—	—	—	0.73	0.84	1.05
Dry Roughage:													
Agathi leaf meal	—	—	32.3	6.7	6.1	45.1	9.5	—	3.26	0.22	—	—	—
Berseem leaf meal (dehydrated)	—	89.7	15.3	23.5	3.7	42.8	14.7	—	—	—	0.66	0.30	0.29
Cowpea leaf meal	—	21.2	21.1	17.7	9.4	36.1	15.7	3.53	4.45	0.46	—	—	—
Guar leaf meal	—	14.2	22.5	9.7	3.5	49.9	14.4	2.36	3.98	0.33	0.52	—	—
Groundnut plant meal	1812	92.1	14.4	32.5	3.1	37.4	12.6	—	1.69	0.34	—	—	—
Lucerne leaf meal	—	95.6	20.3	16.0	4.0	51.1	9.6	0.23	2.25	0.35	—	—	—
Lucerne dehydrated	—	91.0	19.1	21.6	2.8	42.1	14.4	—	1.83	0.45	—	—	—
Maize husk	1512	92.3	9.7	13.7	2.0	70.5	4.1	3.17	0.63	0.12	0.43	0.26	0.13
Mowha residue	—	—	14.5	30.9	5.4	31.0	1.3	—	—	—	0.76	—	0.55
Sugarcane bagasse	—	—	2.5	33.1	3.7	46.4	14.3	—	0.74	0.07	—	—	—
Sunhemp leaves	—	—	34.7	13.6	10.2	30.4	11.1	—	2.17	0.36	—	—	—
Tapioca leaf meal	—	90.9	15.4	22.8	12.2	41.1	8.5	—	1.43	0.25	—	—	—
Miscellaneous:													
Linseed	—	97.9	28.9	6.3	40.5	21.4	2.9	0.03	0.44	0.53	—	—	—
Potato peelings	—	16.9	10.0	2.4	2.1	81.5	4.0	—	0.21	0.32	—	—	—
Salseed	2827	92.0	8.1	3.2	16.4	69.0	3.3	0.96	0.19	0.17	9.48	0.33	0.36
Soybean meal	—	89.9	41.7	6.3	21.2	26.0	4.8	—	0.36	0.90	2.31	0.51	0.72

Abbreviations
M.E.=Metabolisable energy, *D.M.*=Dry matter, *C.P.*=Crude protein, *C.F.*=Crude fibre, *E.E.*=Ether extact, *N.F.E.*=Nitrogen free extract, *Ca*=Calcium, *P*=Phosphorus, *Lys*=Lysine, *Met*=Methionine, *Tryp*=Tryptophan.

**Compiled by*—The Division of Poultry Research, Indian Veterinary Research Institute, Izatnagar, Bareilly, U.P.

METHODS OF FEEDING

A well balanced ration improperly fed will not give the most satisfactory results unless a satisfactory method is followed. Some of the popular methods of feeding are as follows:

1. **Whole grain feeding system.** By this method birds are allowed to have their required ingredients kept before them in separate containers. The system though permit birds to balance their ration according to individual needs, however, it appears doubtful. This old and abandoned system offers no particular advantage. While it entails the use of several feed hoppers and a considerable amount of time to keep them filled.

2. **Grain and mash method.** This method is slightly better than the previous one. It involves feeding of grain mixture along with balanced mash. By this, one can increase or decrease the protein level as desired. Unless the poultryman is exceptionally skilled, the method will lead to bad performances.

3. **All mash method.** In this method of feeding, all the feed ingredients are ground, mixed in required proportion and fed as a single balanced mixture. This method is desirable for all types of poultry grown under litter and cage system. By this, birds, cannot have the opportunity to have selective eating and moreover the quality of eggs produced are of uniform quality.

Table 15.21

Formulae of some economic poultry ration

I. *Starter Ration (0-8 weeks)*

Ingredients ↓ *Ration* →	*1*	*2*	*3*	*4*	*5*	*6*	*7*	*8*	*9*
					Per cent				
Yellow maize	—	—	—	—	—	16	17	16	10
Rice polish (10% oil)	31	46	61	60	40	40	40	40	40
Deoiled rice polish	—	—	—	—	20	—	—	—	—
Wheat bran	10	—	—	—	—	10	10	10	10
Maize grit	20	15	—	—	—	—	—	—	10
Maize gluten feed	15	15	10	—	—	—	—	—	—
Maize gluten meal	—	—	10	1	—	—	—	—	—
Groundnut cake	10	10	15	16	16	20	20	10	10
Maize steep fluid (on dry basis)	—	—	—	—	—	—	—	10	10
Fish meal (or) meat meal	10	10	10	5	5	10	5	10	5
Silk worm pupae meal	—	—	—	5	5	—	4	—	4
Limestone	1.5	1.5	1.5	1.5	1.5	1.5	1.5	1.5	1.5
Steamed bone meal	1.0	1.0	1.0	1.0	1.0	1.0	1.0	1.0	1.0
Common salt	0.5	0.5	0.5	0.5	0.5	0.5	0.5	0.5	0.5
Vitamin and mineral mixture*	1.0	1.0	1.0	1.0	1.0	1.0	1.0	1.0	1.0
Antibiotic	+	+	+	+	+	+	+	+	+

*Contains 22 grams $MnSO_4$, 1000,000 IU. Vitamin A, 500 mg Riboflavin & 75000 I.U. Vitamin D_3.

II. Growth Ration (9 weeks to 20 weeks)

Ingredients ↓ *Ration*→	*1*	*2*	*3*	*4*	*5*	*6*	*7*	*8*
				Per cent				
Yellow maize	20	20	—	—	—	20	20	—
Rice polish	40	40	51	61	61	40	40	56
Wheat bran	10	10	10	10	10	6	6	10
Maize grit	—	—	10	—	—	—	—	10
Maize gluten meal	6	6	5	5	5	—	—	—
Maize steep fluid	—	—	—	—	—	10	10	10
Groundnut cake	10	10	10	10	15	10	10	10
Fish meal (or) meat meal	10	5	10	10	5	10	5	5
Silk worm pupae meal	—	5	5	—	—	—	5	5
Limestone	1.5	1.5	1.5	1.5	1.5	1.5	1.5	1.5
Steamed bone meal	1.0	1.0	1.0	1.0	1.0	1.0	1.0	1.0
Common salt	0.5	0.5	0.5	0.5	0.5	0.5	0.5	0.5
Vitamin and mineral mixture*	1.0	1.0	1.0	1.0	1.0	1.0	1.0	1.0

*Containing 22 gms $MnSO_4$, 1000.00 I.U. Vitamin A, 500 mg Riboflavin and 75000 I.U. of Vitamin D_3.

III. Layer Ration (Parts Per 100)

Ingredients ↓ *Ration*→	*1*	*2*	*3*	*4*	*5*	*6*	*7*
				Per cent			
Maize	—	—	20	20	—	10	20
Rice polish	30	30	40	50	55	50	30
Deoiled rice polish	—	—	—	—	—	—	20
Wheat bran	10	10	—	—	10	5	—
Maize grit	25	—	—	—	—	—	—
Maize gluten meal	5	—	10	—	10	5	—
Maize gluten feed	—	20	—	—	—	—	—
Groundnut cake	10	10	5	20	15	15	20
Fish meal or meat meal	—	—	—	5	5	5	5
Silk worm pupae meal	5	5	5	—	—	—	—
Molasses	10	15	15	—	—	—	—
Pencillin mycelia	—	5	—	—	—	—	—
Limestone	3	3	3	3	8	3	3
Bone meal	1	1	1	1	1	1	1
Salt	0.5	0.5	4.5	0.5	0.5	0.5	0.5
Vitamin and mirreral mixture*	0.5	0.5	0.5	0.5	0.5	0.5	0.5

*Contains 25 gms $MnSO_4$, 5000 I.U. Vitamin A, 500 mg Riboflavin and 50000 I.U. Vitamin D_3.

However, ground feeds are not so palatable and do not retain their nutritive value so well as unground feeds.

4. Pellet method. Pellets are made of dry-mash under high pressure. These are quite hard and cylindrical shape and is being extensively used in Western countries. The greatest advantage in using pellets is that there is little waste in feeding. The disadvantage is that pellets are expensive—about 10 per cent more expensive than that of feeds not pelleted.

5. Restricted or controlled feeding. The method involves restrictions of feeding pullets during 6-20 weeks of age instead of *ad libitum* feeding as is practiced at present in most poultry farm. Reduction in feed cost, delayed sexual maturity but improved egg production curve, along with a reduction in the number of small eggs laid are some of the advantages of this system.

Feed restrictions to birds can be made by a number of ways, viz., (1) Skip a-day programme; (2) alternate day feeding, (3) restriction of feeding time, etc. Before adopting this practice, the readers should gather further information in this aspect to suit his particular condition as none of the methods are suitable for all conditions.

Ten Principal Points for Consideration of Poultry Feed Formulation

(1) Feeds must contain all essential nutrients in right amount and proportion required for the purpose for which it is fed.

(2) Chickens of different ages require different level of nutrients, hence only the accepted standards as per age should be followed accordingly.

(3) Ingredients chosen for preparation of poultry mashes must be palatable.

(4) While selecting ingredients for preparation of poultry mashes, nutritional value of each ingredient should be evaluated *vis-a-vis* cost.

(5) Chickens have no teeth to grind grains or oil cakes, hence these ingredients should be crushed into proper sizes in keeping with age of the chicken.

(6) Micro-nutrients and non-nutrient feed additives should be carefully chosen and mixed up meticuously for effective results.

(7) Include agro-industrial by-products to minimise cost and select a variety of ingredients to make good deficiency of one by the other.

(8) While selecting an ingredient care should be exercised to judge its optimum level of inclusion as many of the ingredients are likely to be deleterious at higher level.

(9) Fungal infested ingredients should always be avoided.

(10) Care should be taken to select optimum C/P ratio for the purpose for which feeds are compounded.

$$C : P \text{ ratio} = \frac{\text{Metabolisable energy in Kcal/kg diet}}{\text{\% Protein in the diet}}$$

The recommended C : P ratio for the diet of various classes of chickens are as under :

Starter chicken (0-8 weeks)	135 : 1
Grower chicken (8 - 20 weeks)	140 : 1
Layer chicken (20 weeks onward)	170-180 : 1
Starter broiler chicken (0-6 weeks)	135 : 1
Finisher brolier chicken (6 week onward)	155 : 1

Table 15.22

Rates of inclusion of some common poultry feed ingredients.

Ingredients	*Range of inclusion for* *Chicks*	*Growers & Layers*
Energy Sources	0-50	0-50
Maize	0-3	0-5
Rice polish (deoiled)	0-30	0-30
Rice polish	0-50	0-50
Salseed cake	0-3	0-5
Tapioca meal	0-10	0-10
Triticale	0-30	0-30
Wheat bran	0-10	0-15
Vegetable Protein sources		
Groundnut cake (Expeller/deoiled).	0-50	0-40
Cotton seed cake	0-5	0-5
Linseed cake	0-5	0-10
Maize gluten meal	0-10	0-10
Maize oil cake	0-10	0-10
Mustard Cake	0-5	0-10
Niger cake	0-15	0-15
Safflower cake	0-15	0-15
Sesame seed meal	0-10	0-10
Soyabean meal (heat-treated)	0-30	0-30
Sunflower cake	0-10	0-20
Guar meal	0-6	0-6
Animal protein Sources		
Fish meal	3-15	3-10
Blood meal	0-3	0-3
Feather meal (hydrolysed)	0-5	0-5
Meat meal	0-7	0-8
Silk worm pupae meal	0-5	0-5
Miscellaneous		
Lucerne meal	0-3	0-5
Bone meal	0-2	0-2
Lime stone	0-2	2-6
Pencillin mycelium	0-2	0-2
Salt	0-0.5	0-0.5

Source : Department of Agriculture & Cooperation, Ministry of Agriculture, Government of India, New Delhi.

HOW TO COMPUTE A RATION FOR CHICKEN?

A farmer interested in compounding poultry mashes should have the basic knowledge of various types of raw ingredients as to their efficacy and nutrient composition *vis-a-vis* cost to make any mash effective for his flock. A short description has already been made in regard to various feed ingredients. However, they may be broadly classified as follows:

(i) *Protein supplement:* (Primary source of protein)

(a) Vegetable protein supplement—e.g., groundnut, soybean cake, mustard cake, maize gluten, etc.

(b) Animal protein supplement—Fish meal, skim milk powder, liver meal, etc.

(ii) *Energy supplement:*

(a) Primary source of energy—Cereal grains like maize, wheat, millet grains like jowar, milo, rice polish etc.

(b) Cereal by products (Diluents—medium energy content and sources of minerals) e.g., wheat bran, rice bran, maize grit, etc.

(iii) *Salt,* (iv) *Mineral,* (v) *Vitamins*

(vi) *'Non-nutrient feed additives—e.g., antibiotic, antioxidants, etc.*

In the formulation of poultry ration, the farmer has to consider first protein and energy and their ratio to each other what is known as C/P ratio. Protein again should be provided that it satisfies the requirement in terms of amino acids with particular reference to Lysine, Methionine and Cystine. Then the ration should also fulfil the requirement of mineral with particular reference to calcium and available phosphorus. It should also satisfy the requirement of both fat soluble and water soluble vitamins.

Having various points as above in mind, a poultryman desirous of compounding a poultry mash, e.g., layers mash should first find out from the Table the requirement of various nutrients of layers mash and then proceed to satisfy these requirements by selecting proper protein and energy rich ingredients supplemented with minerals, vitamins, etc. Experience suggests that if formulation is made as per following assumption, then a lay farmer can manage to prepare his own layers mash without going for meticulous calculation.

Protein rich supplement:	Vegetable port. suppl.	: 18–22
	Animal port. suppl.	: 5–8
Energy rich supplement:	Cereals, millets	: 60–65
Mineral supplement :	Calcite	5
	Standard mineral mixture	2–3
Vitamin supplement :	Standard Vit. AB_2D_3 complex.	

Example 1

To cite a concrete example in terms with above assumption a model pattern of formula for layers mash is given below which will satisfy in terms of protein (with particular reference to amino acid make up), energy, mineral and vitamin, etc.

Maize	46 parts
Wheat	20 ,,
Fish meal	6 ,,
Groundnut cake	15 ,,
Til cake (black)	5 ,,
Calcite	5 ,,

Any standard mineral mix.	2.5
Dicalcium phoshate/bone meal	0.5
	100

Add to this Rovimix (Vit. AB_2D_3) @250 gm/qtl and if possible also add **Rovibe** (**B complex**) @20 gm/qtl.

Example 2

For the sake of economy, however, the above formula may be modified in the following pattern which will be almost equal in production value as the original one:

Maize	19
Wheat	7
Tapioca chips	10
Rice polish	17
Rice bran (deoiled)	5
Molasses	5
Salseed cake	4
Groundnut cake (deoiled)	8
Maize gluten/til cake	7
Mustard cake (deoiled)	5
Fish meal/silk worm pupae meal or liver meals	5
Calcite	5
Standard mineral mixture	2.5
Dicalcium phosphate/bone meal	0.5
	100

Table 15.23

Average growth rate and feed requirements for egg–type chickens.

Age in weeks	*Average weight of bird (gms.)*	*Cumulative feed in kgs. per 1,000 birds*
4	275	650
8	590	1,900
12	850	3,400
16	1,100	5,000
20	1,300	7,000
24	1,550	10,000
30	1,600	14,500
40	1,700	22,000
60	1,700	37.000
80	1,700	52,000

Add to this Rovimix (Vit. AB_2D_3) @ 250 gm/qtl [and where possible Rovibe (B complex vitamin) @ 20 gm/qtl for better hatchability, if required].

By this way various economic rations can be formulated using agro-industrial by-products intelligently.

RAISING OF BROILERS

What is Broiler ?

A broiler or fryer is a young chicken of either sex below 8 to 10 weeks of age weighing 1.5 to 2.0 kgs body weight, with a tender meated soft, pliable smooth textured and flexible breast. *Roaster* on the other hand is also a young chicken but are much older (12 to 16 weeks) and heavier than broilers. It may be of either sex but tender meated, with soft, pliable, smooth-textured skin and breastbone cartilage which are somewhat less flexible than that of a broiler or fryer.

Breeds and Breeding for Broiler

Parental broiler flocks consists of a female line and a male line are selected at their eight weeks of age. Those which weigh the most in each brood are the ones chosen for breeding purposes. The female lines usually have been developed from birds of White Rock background and the male lines from birds of Cornish ancestry.

Hybrid vigour in next generation is obtained by systematic matings that may involve crossing of different breeds as stated, may be among different strains of the same breed or inbred lines. The male lines for producing broilers usually have dominant white feathers and are selected for rapid growth ; meat characteristics, such as breast width, body depth, live market grade, dressing yield and rapid feathering. Female lines used producing broilers must also have outstanding growth rate, high hatchability and good but not outstanding, production of eggs of desirable size and texture.

Progeny test and family selection have been effective in the development of broiler lines.

The end product of all well planned selected crosses should be to produce a chick which will be modern white in colour, yellow shanked, grows faster than either of the parents (hybrid vigour) with a tender meated and flexible breast cartilage. All these characters of broilers depend on the genetic make up of their parents which themselves are not broilers.

A coordinated project for the evaluation of suitable strains of White Cornish, White Plymouth Rock, New Hampshire and Rhode Island Red fowls for the production of commercial hybrid broiler chicken in the country has been taken up by the Indian Council of Agricultural Research.

Demand and Supply of broilers

The National Commission on Agriculture in its report estimated the demand for poultry meat during 1985 to touch 1,50,000 tonnes and in 2000 A.D. 3,00,000 tonnes. In case of broilers, the number has been estimated at 17.2 millions for 1985 and 71.8 millions for 2000 A.D.

The development of our own superior strain of meat type chicken would help to minimise the present day importation of parent stocks and thus help in conserving foreign exchange.

Facts pertinent to an understanding of broiler performance

1. At any given age, males are heavier than females.
2. Weekly increases in weight are not uniform ; gains increase each week until reaching a maximum at about the eight week for straight-run (both sexes together).
3. Weekly feed consumption increases as weight increases.
4. Generally the more feed consumed, the better the feed conversion at a given age.
5. Fast gains are efficient gains ; as weekly gains increase, feed efficiency increases.
6. Healthy birds consume more feed and have better feed conversion than sick birds.
7. The greater the activity, the lower the feed efficiency.
8. Cannibalism results in lowered feed consumption, growth and feed conversion.
9. Changes in temperature cause changes in feed consumption ; broilers eat about 1% more feed for each 1°F decrease in temperature, and they eat about 1% less feed for each 1°F rise in temperature. Very high temperatures drastically reduce feed consumption and cause poor feed conversion.
10. Flock are not uniform, with the result that all birds are not of the same weight at market time. The males are heavier than the females. But neither sex is uniform ; there are large, medium, and small cockerels and pullets.
11. Broiler growing efficiency is usually measured in the following three ways :
    (a) Mature live body weight
    (b) Feed conversion over the life of the bird
    (c) Age to reach a desired weight, or growth rate.

Broiler Housing

In modern commercial broiler production, the bird spends its entire life in one house ; that is, it is not brooded in a special brooder house, then moved to another house for growing for broiler raising is basically a brooding operation.

The broiler house should be located in such a way, (i) to take advantage of prevailing wind for ventilation and sun for light, (ii) ground elevation should be higher than surrounding ground level to permit good water drainage away from building, (iii) should be readily accesible to power, water supply and sewage.

There are of course many different styles and designs of houses, and even more variations in equipment. The important thing is that broiler houses and equipment provide comfortable conditions, including adequate feed and water, so that the birds can perform at the highest level of which they are genetically capable. A satisfactory broiler house must protect against heat and cold, high winds, and inclement weather.

Management Practices for Broilers

1. Poultry house temperature

Temperature is important. On the first week 95°F is quite comfortable. This may be reduced at the rate of 5°F weekly until 70°F is reached on the sixth week. When chicks circle wide, it is too hot. If they tend to crowd, under the hover it is too cool. In either case, adjustment is needed immediately.

2. Ventilation of Broiler house

The main functions of ventilation are to maintain Oxygen, keep CO_2 at low level, remove dust or moisture and ammonia from the house and maintain required temperature. Air movement requirements are best determined by observing bird comfort, litter condition, and odour build up. If necessary exhaust fan may be used.

3. Lighting for Broilers

Many operators prefer to use all-night lights, about 15 watts to each 200 square feet of floor area during early growing period. Growing chicks in semi-darkeness by using red bulb keeps the chicks quiet, prevents cannibalism, and may have a slight effect on feed efficiency. Most broiler growers provide light in the brooder house 24 hours a day throughout the entire growing period. One 60 watt bulb for each 200 square feet of floor space.

4. Floor space requirement

Broilers will require from 0.8 to 1.0 square feet of floor space per bird.

5. Debeaking

In addition to preventing cannibalism, debeaking usually lessens mash feed wastage. Electric debeakers are now available and chicks are debeaked when only one day old.

6. Sexing

In view of high feed prices, formulation of rations according to sex has certain economic advantages. They may be sexed by vent, colour, or rate of feathering. If the two sexes are

Table 15.24

ESTIMATED GROWTH AND FEED CONSUMPTION RATES OF BROILERS[1]

	Feed consupmtion					
Age	Per week	Cumulative	Average Gain in Body Weight per week	Average Weight per Bird	(kg.) Meat per 100 (kg) Feed	(kg.) Feed per (kg) Meat
(wk)	(kg)	(kg)	(kg)	(kg)		
1	0.11	0.11	0.09	0.13	–	–
2	0.18	0.30	0.10	0.24	–	–
3	0.32	0.61	0.17	0.41	–	–
4	0.43	1.04	0.20	0.61	–	–
5	0.50	1.54	0.25	0.86	–	–
6	0.60	2.15	0.27	1.14	53.0	1.89
7	0.70	2.85	0.27	1.41	49.5	2.02
8	0.78	3.63	0.30	1.70	47.5	2.13
9	0.92	4.55	0.30	2.00	44.0	2.27

[1]Lankford, L.T. and T.L. Barton, Guide to Broiler Production, Leaflet 180, University of Arkansas, April 1974.

separated, the males may be marketed first and the females may be given the extra floor space and retained longer for heavier weights. Other differences between the sexes are :

(i) Males are about 1% heavier than females at hatching time.

(ii) Males grow faster than females and weigh more at a given age. At normal market age, males attain the same weight as females about 9 days earlier.

(iii) At 6-10 weeks of age male birds lay down progressively less fat and show a higher incidence of breast blisters.

(iv) Females need less protein than males, as they grow more slowly.

(v) Females show less response to chemical growth promoters than males.

(vi) Males convert feed to meet more efficiently than females.

7. **Broiler feeds**

Since feed constitutes about 70% of the cost of producing broilers, it is important to give special attention to it. Broilers are usually fed with two types of ration, broiler starter and broiler finisher (Table 15.25). The former ration is fed upto 5 weeks of age and the latter is continued till the age of marketting. From the Table ,it may be noted that starter ration is having more protein (21-22%) and less metabolisable energy, 2,900 kcal than the finisher ration, 19-20% protein & 3000 kcal per kilogram of feed. The finisher diet, containing

Table 15.25

Recommended rations (per quintal of feed) for broilers.

Composition	*Unit*	*Broiler Starter (0-6 Weeks of age)*	*Broiler finisher (6–9 Weeks of age)*
Yellow Maize	kg	45.0	48.00
Rice Polish	kg	10.7	17.7
Groundnut Cake	kg	30.0	22.0
Lucerne meal	kg	1.0	1.0
Fish Meal	kg	11.0	9.0
DL-methionine	gm	40	-
Mineral Mixture	kg	2.0	2.0
Vitamin A+B_2+D_3+K	gm	30	30
Vitamin B_{12}	gm	20	20
Vitamin K	mg	100	100
Potassium Iodide	mg	20	20
Manganese Sulphate	gm	10	8
Zinc Carbonate	gm	10	8
Antibiotic feed supplement	gm	50	50
Zinc Bacitracin	gm	100	100
Coccidiostat	gm	50	50

Source : Department of Agriculture & Cooperation, Ministry of Agriculture, Government of India, New Delhi.

Table 15.26

Body weight and feed consumption of broiler*

(M=Male & F=Female)

Weeks	Body weight gm		Feed consumption weekly gm		Feed consumption cumulative gm	
	M	F	M	F	M	F
1	107	105	82.5	81.5	82.5	81.5
2	250	230	182	161	264.5	242.5
3	460	410	329	280	593.5	522.5
4	700	600	434	357	1,027.5	879.5
5	960	810	539	227	1,566.5	1,306.5
6	1,300	1,060	700	560	2,266.5	1,866.5
7	1,670	1,340	805	679	3,071.5	2,545.5
8	2.060	1,630	945	770	4,016.5	3,315.5

*Feed conversion after 8 weeks: 1.95 and 2.03 by M and F chicks respectively.

Source: *Nutrition of the Chicken* by Scott, Milton F., Nesheim, Malden C. and Young, Robert J., Pub. M.L. Scott and Associates, Ithaca, New York, 1969, p. 76.

Table 15.27

Average feed consumption of starter and grower birds (per bird per day)

Age (weeks)	White Leghorn (light breeds; g)	White Rock/ Rhode Island Red (heavy breeds; g)	Age (weeks)	White Leghorn (light breeds; g)	White Rock/ Rhode Island Red (heavy breeds; g)
1	6.5	6.5	13	60.0	65.0
2	13.0	14.0	14	62.0	65.0
3	17.0	17.0	15	62.0	65.0
4	24.0	26.0	16	55.0	70.0
5	32.0	36.0	17	70.0	75.0
6	37.0	42.0	18	75.0	80.0
7	40.0	45.0	19	75.0	80.0
8	49.0	54.0	20	80.0	87.0
9	53.0	60.0	21	85.0	90.0
10	58.0	60.0	22	88.0	100.0
11	60.0	65.0	23	90.0	100.0
12	60.0	65.0	24	97.0	110.0

Table 15.28. Feed consumption of laying birds

Egg production (%)	Feed consumption (g/day)
0	84
10	88
20	93
30	98
40	103
50	107
60	110
70	120
80	125

increased levels of fat and xanthophyll pigments, aids in the development of the uniform yellow skin colour.

8. Broiler Health Programme

A health programme is fundamental to successful broiler production. A suggested disease prevention and control programme follows :

(i) Start with disease-free chicks.

(ii) Vaccine chicks against Ranikhet and Marek's disease at the hatchery.

(iii) Use effective drugs in the feed, or a vaccination programme to prevent coccidiosis.

(iv) Keep feed free from aflatoxin.

(v) Do not allow visitors or attendants inside the broiler house unless they wear disinfected boots and clean clothing.

(vi) When there are several age groups on the farm, always care for the youngest birds first while performing daily routine works.

(vii) Rework built-up litter. When built-up litter is used, all caked and wet litter should be removed and replaced with fresh, clean litter before chicks arrive.

(viii) Cover floor with clean litter at least 3 in. deep after each clean out, Wood shavings, rice hulls, straws cut into small pieces are suitable litter materials.

9. Marketing Broilers

Most broilers are marketed when they are between 7 and 8 weekof age. For the most part, marketing involves moving the birds from the house in which they are produced to the consumers house. Improper handling of broilers immediately prior to and during shipment will result in excess bruises, and lowered quality. Such losses may be minimised as follows :

(i) Discontinue grit feeding at least 2 weeks prior to marketing (usually grit is not fed after 5 weeks of age)

(ii) Let the feeders became empty about 2 hours before catching and remove the waterer to prevent bruises during catching.

(iii) Catch and load properly by : (a) using an experienced attendant, (b) working under a dim blue light at night, (c) corraling them in small groups, (d) grasping them by shanks with no more than 4 or 5 being carried at a time.

(iv) Protect the in-transit birds from extremes in weather. In hot weather, protect against overheating in shipment by using open crates and avoiding lengthy stops in route.

USE OF AGRO-INDUSTRIAL BY-PRODUCTS IN POULTRY RATIONS

In India, the cereal grains which form the major source of energy for poultry are in short supply. They are costly and are required by people who are mostly vegetarians. Animal proteins are also in short supply and costly. Most of the Indian work on poultry nutrition has been concentrated upon investigations to utilise farm and industrial by-products as substitutes for maize, fish meal and even conventional oil cakes. With a view to compute balanced and economical rations a brief review of some of the important ingredients is discussed.

A. Protein Supplements

1. *Mustard cake.* Complete replacement of groundnut cake with mustard cake is not possible. Work done at I.V.R.I. and other places showed that mustard cake (expeller variety) could be included in chick starter or broiler diets upto 10% level. Work done at Bidhan Chandra Krishi Viswavidyalaya, West Bengal, showed that the deoiled variety of mustard cake could safely be included in chicken ration replacing groundnut cake upto the tune of 100 per cent.

2. *Mahua cake.* Trend of research work indicates that mahua residue may be included upto 10 per cent replacing groundnut cake.

3. *Meat meal.* Meat meal has been shown to replace 50 per cent of fish meal in chick rations. Variation in the nutritional value of meat meal is largely found to be determined by calcium and essential available amino acid content of the meal.

4. *Blood meal.* Reports indicate that upto 3 to 5 per cent blood meal replacing fish meal, can be satisfactorily used in chick ration.

5. *Liver meal.* Results indicate that upto 10% liver meal (liver dry residue) replacing fish meal can be used in chick ration.

6. *Silk worm pupae meal.* Satisfactory growth and egg production have been obtained replacing some part of maize and the whole of fish meal with silk worm pupae meal. However, some workers found that silk worm pupae meal could only replace 50% of fish meal in chick starting ration.

7. *Guar meal.* A by-product from guar gum industry. Results indicate that raw guar meal proved detrimental to chick growth above 6.5 per cent inclusion in the rations but toasting or autoclaving or supplementation with 0.1 per cent hemicellulose enzyme, significantly improve its nutritive value.

8. *Ram til cake.* The cake is extensively found in Maharashtra, M.P., Andhra Pradesh, Mysore and Orissa. It has been found to replace satisfactorily upto 50 per cent and 10 per cent of groundnut cake in the chick and layer rations respectively.

9. *Cotton seed cake.* It can replace groundnut cake upto 15 per cent. However, in layers continued use of this cake is known to cause yolk mottling on storage of eggs.

10. *Safflower oil meal.* It can replace groundnut cake upto 25 per cent.

11. *Soybean meal.* The product can easily replace groundnut.

12. *Hatchery by-product meal.* The meal is prepared from infertile eggs and dead germs, etc., and can be fed replacing 33 per cent of fish meal in the ration.

13. *Karanja cake.* The cake is one of the newer additions to the list of substitute oilseed cakes. Work conducted at Bidhan Chandra Krishi Viswavidyalaya, West Bengal showed that Karanja cake (*Pongamia glabra*) in its deoiled form can be included in chicken ration upto 8 per cent replacing other conventional oil cakes. The cake other than deoiled form is highly toxic for the chickens.

B. Energy Supplements

1. *Rice polish (bran).* The product is an excellent substitute for maize and can easily substitute maize upto 40–50 per cent in chick starter or layer ration. The deoiled form is also extensively used upto 20–35 per cent replacing ordinary rice polish.

2. *Salseed and deoiled salseed meal.* The results indicate that salseed and sal cake could be used in chick ration upto 5 per cent and in layer ration upto 10 per cent replacing an equal quantity of maize.

3. *Millets (Kodo, Sawan, Kanjui, etc.).* The work on Economic poultry rations scheme in U.P. showed that 10–14 per cent saving in feeding cost could be achieved by replacing maize with 24 per cent Kodo and sawan.

4. *Damaged grain.* Results obtained so far have indicated that upto 30 per cent damaged maize and 60 per cent damaged wheat could be used to replace good quality grain for chicks. However the extent of damage is to be considered first before inclusion in the chicken ration.

Table 15.29. Meat production in India (1000 MT)

Species	1975	1980	1985	% increase over 1975
Beef and veal	71	74	89	23.35
Buffalo meat	117	120	135	15.38
Mutton and lamb	117	120	135	15.38
Goat meat	269	270	315	17.10
Pork	56	70	85	51.78
Poultry meat	101	113	180	78.22
Total	821*	870*	1036*	

*Includes meat from other sources.

BIOTECHONOLOGY IN POULTRY FEED INDUSTRY*

Though the term "Bio-technology" has come into common usage in recent times, we have been using "Bio-technology" as such for a long time. In its broadest sense the word "Biotechnology" would cover all those techniques in which processes going on in living organisms are utilized for purposes other than those intended by nature. Curd making is "Bio-technology", since in this "technique" the property of the organism lactobacillus to produce lactic acid is utilized by us in curd making. Silage preparation is just another "Bio-technology".

In animal feeding we have been using brewer's, dried grains, liver meal, fish meal, antibiotic, synthetic, aminoacids—all products of bio-technology—for quite sometime. There are however, some products that are being introduced in the animal feeds in the past few years and when one talks about Bio-technology in feed industry, it is these products that one has in mind. Thus in the present paper we would restrict ourselves to these products only. These products mainly include, enzymes, yeast cultures, bacterial cultures and their metabolites, diet acidifiers and mold inhibitors.

Enzymes

The enzymes used are mostly harvested from microbial or fungal cultures. They are generally a combination of proteinases—those that breakdown proteins, of amylases—those that digest starches—betaglucanases those that act on betaglucan and cellulases which split up cellulose. These enzyme products are recommended as feed additives and are claimed to improve the availability of nutrients to the birds. Under normal circumstances, high energy diet which is composed of maize and soyabean extractions is efficiently digested by the poultry. The inclusion of the enzyme products in such diets, therefore, would not cause much improvement. But, the diets based on barley, wheat, sunflower, ricebran, wheatbran, rice polish etc., would stand to benefit by the addition of suitable enzyme products. Barley and wheat contain compounds named betaglucans. Barley contains higher amount of these compounds than wheat. In the digestive tract betaglucans give viscocity to the contents of the digestive tract. Such viscous material interferes with the activity of digestive enzymes. Very small concentration of betaglucans, 0.75% to 1.0% can produce this effect. The betaglucanase in the enzyme products, by breaking down the betaglucans, reduces the viscocity of the feed in the

Table 15.30

Effect of incorporation of enzyme products on broiler performance

Type of diet	Enzymes added	Final Weight	Feed consumption ratio
High Energy	0	1.79 kg	2.0
High Energy	500 mg/kg	1.90 kg	1.89
Low Ènergy	0	1.62 kg	2.36
Low Energy	1000 mg/kg	1.80 kg	1.98

* The material is taken from "Pashudhan, Vol. 5, (January 1990) written by Dr. S.P. Netke, an eminent animal nutritionist.

Table 15.31

Beneficial effects of probiotics in broilers

	Feed without probiotic	Feed with probiotic
Gains in weight	460 grams	491 grams
Feed consumption	993 grams	991 grams
Live weight index	100	107
Feed conversion index	100	93.5

digestive tract and thus facilitates the action of natural digestive enzymes. The cellulases in the enzyme products would act on the cellulose present in the cell walls of grain by products like, ricebran, rice polish, wheat bran and crude fibre present in other feed ingredients in the feed and would improve availability of nutrients from these products. The proteinases and amylases supplement the activity of natural digestive enzymes. The results of a study presented in Table 15.30 illustrates the ad vantages. derived from the use of enzyme products in poultry feeding.

Table 15.32

Effect of dietary acidifiers on mortality of chicks

	Acidifier not added	Acidifier added
Mortality	3.1	2.9
Feed Conversion	1.96	1.9

These results show that the improvement in the performance of the broiler fed with low energy diets was much higher than that of broilers fed with high energy diets. The birds fed with low energy diets performed as well as those fed with high energy diet when the former was supplemented with enzymes. The enzyme products that one intends to use should however satisfy some conditions. First of all the enzymes present in the products must be active. They must be able to withstand the action of other proteolytic enzymes in the digestive tract and should not be inactivated by the pH levels in the digestive tract. It must also be kept in mind that if the diet is pelleted the enzymes added would be inactivated. If these conditions are not satisfied by the enzyme products, their addtion in the diet would not be advantageous.

Probiotics

These are another class of products made available by Bio-technology. The name indicates that they are just opposite of ''antibiotic'' in the sense that ''antibiotics'' are ''against life'', and ''probiotics'' are ''for life''. The term however, is misleading. The correct name should have been ''amibiotics'', i.e., ''friendly organism''. What are supplied as probiotics are live cultures of useful bacteria along with medicine in which they were grown. The organisms used are beneficial strains of lactobacillus and streptococcus. The reasoning behind the use of probiotic is that ingestion of these organisms would lend an increase in their number in the digestive tract. Their dominance in the digestive tract would reduce the population of undesirable organisms like, E. Coli and thus save the birds from the toxins that these organisms produce in the digestive tract. A typical example of the beneficial effects of the use of probiotics is presented. in Table 15.31.

It is also claimed that addition of probiotics improves the performance of layers and that it is particularly useful under stress conditions when E. Coli proliferates in the digestive tract to the disadvantage of the bird. In other words, ''probiotics'' is the biotechnical tool to manipulate the microbial population in the digestive tract. Here again, to derive the benefits from its addition to the diets the probiotics should contain those types of bacteria that inhibit the multiplication of E. Coli. These bacteria when ingested must be resistant to the action of gastric juice and bile salts. They must be able to attach themselves firmly to the intestinal wall and should be able to multiply in the surroundings present in the intestines. All the products ''available as probiotics'' may not satisfy these conditions and to that extent would be incapable of conferring the desired benefits.

Many producers use the process of microencapsulation to protect the bacteria till they are released in the intestines. Such products would be more promising than the others. As is the case with enzyme, additions the organisms present in probiotics would be destroyed by the high temperatures developed in pelleting.

Yeast Culture

These are dried products containing yeast *(Saccharemyces cervisiae)* along with the medium on which they were grown. Their incorporation in the feed is claimed to improve the feed intake, feed efficiency and egg quality. How, exactly they produce the beneficial results is not fully understood. Some studies indicate that the yeast additions have been useful with diets that contain readily fermentable carbohydrates.

It is argued that products of fermentation of these carbohydrates inactivate the intestinal toxins that reduce the appetite of the birds or they may directly stimulate the feed consumption. It is also felt by some that the presence of glutamic acid in the yeast culture used increases the palatability of the feeds. The yeasts are known to concentrate zinc in their cells. When the cells rupture the zinc which is in the chealted form and is therefore, highly available is released in the intestinal tract. The yeast has been shown to improve the microbial digestion in the hind gut. The yeast also facilitates the growth of *Lactobacillus* and *Streptococcus.* Their use along with probiotic in the diet thus can be beneficial. Many probiotics, therefore, contain yeast in addition to *Lactobacillus* and *Streptococcus.* Though there are extensive studies on the use of yeast culture in ruminants very few studies have been reported on the use of yeast culture in poultry. In these studies too it has been used in combination with Lactobacillus.

Diet Acidifiers

These are a combination of organic acids obtained as metabolites of micro-organisms. It is claimed that the use of such acidifiers provides proper pH for the growth of Lactic acid bacteria in crop and thereby influences the composition of microbial population in the intestine, in favour of *Lactobacillus.* In young calves the acidifiers facilitate early clotting of milk and thereby improve its digestibility. It is felt that acidifiers by providing proper pH in the stomach would facilitate the digestion of protein in poultry too. Under normal conditions ingestion of diet raises the pH of the stomach content. It comes down to preingestion value in a few hours in claves. The use of acidifiers in claves had been shown to shorten this time and thereby improve the digestibility of milk proteins. It is, however, difficult to extrapolate these findings to the poultry because the food stays in the stomach only for a short time. The few studies published have shown reduction in mortality of chicks when acidifiers were used.

It would be seen that the three products, probiotics, yeast culture and diet acidifiers probably act by favourable manipulation of microbial population and there are some manufacturers who have drawn up detailed feeding programmes using all these three products.

Mold Inhibition

Another important tool of Biotechnology is mold inhibitors. These are the mixtures of organic acids which when added to water or diet reduce the fungal contamination. Since *Aspergillas flavus*—the aflatoxin producing fungus—is also controlled by the mold inhibitor it is finding wide acceptance by the consumers. Sime feed manufacturers in this country are routinely adding this to the feed to improve the keeping quality of the diet and control fungal contamination of the feed right from the time it is prepared till it is consumed by the birds.

It might be mentioned here that fungal contamination of the feed can take place in the feed mill, in transport, during storage at the farm and in the feeders themselves. Use of mold inhibitor would keep such contamination under check.

The information about the products discussed would, however, indicate that these products are very sensitive and need utmost care in their production and in ensuring their stability during storage. One should critically evaluate the products offered as regards the credibility of their claims.

Use of right type of products can certainly help the economics of poultry keeping.

MANAGEMENT - EGG PRODUCTION STOCK

Regardless of the size of the poultry enterprise, the basic unit is the individual bird. The single organism is the only part of the operation that actually produces monetary worth. This is most apparent when an entire flock dies before producing an egg or before it is sent to the processing plant.

Even the most sophisticated record system and financial backing are of minor consequence in comparison to the basic needs of the bird. The needs are feed, water, protection from the elements (disease, rain, wind, rough handlers, etc.) and fresh air.

The poultry producer will always be making decisions based upon immediate pressures, but decisions and concerns should be taken care of in a sequence of priorities.The number one priority is to satisfy the needs of the birds discussed above. Refinements are than possible, and the process of refinement is then a steadily rewarding process.

COMMON DEFICIENCIES

Here is a list of the most common management faults found in poultry houses :

1) Dirty water troughs.
2) Insufficient water space.
3) Insufficient feeder space.
4) Insufficient litter in nests —— dirty eggs.
5) Improper ventilation —— houses too tight, usually. This is a very common deficiency in developing industries.
6) Feeders too full or improperly adjusted so that feed is wasted.
7) Tendency to give too much medication.Constant medication is an indication that the manager is using drugs as a substitute for basic management.
8) Wrong medication, due to failure to obtain competent diagnosis.
9) Allowing weeds or tall crops to block air flow from the poultry building.
10) Allowing lice and mites to build up enough to cause production drops —— due to lack of parasite inspections.
11) Failure to follow a vaccination program. Many flock owners have problems with flocks that have not been vaccinated properly with even the most common vaccines.

12) Caked or damp litter in the poultry house.

13) Cannibalism caused by crowding, lack of feed or water space, or improper ventilation.

14) Insufficient grit and shell hoppers when self-feeding of calcium is used.

15) Floor eggs due to housing birds after production has begun or failure to install nests early.

16) Insufficient or improperly hung nests — too high.

17) Failure to gather often enough.

18) Failure to keep feed consumption, mortality and production records.

19) Improper egg storage.

20) Failure to close nests at night which allows the layers to roost in the nests.

21) Failure to allow adequate lighting — not enough light receptacles and dirty light bulbs.

22) Failure to follow advice of one good service person.

If the above items are taken into consideration and eliminated as deficiencies, the manager has provided to the birds the necessary needs and is capable of refining the management of the operation.

Table 15.33

Schedule of vaccination against prevalent diseases in chick's age

Chick's age	*Disease*	*Name of Vaccine*	*Storage*	*Immunity*	*Route*	*Dose*
1 day	Infectious Bronchitis (IB)	Egg-adapted IB Vaccine	6 months at refrigerator temperature	Not worked out	Intra-nasal	Two drops
1 day	Marek's Disease (MD)	Cell-free or Cell-associated turkey herpes Virus	As indicated by the manufacturer	Not worked out	Intra-muscular or intrapenitoneal	As per manufacturer's instruction
4-5 days	Ranikhet Disease (Newcastle Disease) (RD)	Ranikhet Disease Vaccine Strain F	3 months in a refrigerator and 10 days at room temperature	15 weeks	Intra-nasal or intra-ocular	Two drops
4-5 days	Fowl pox	Pigeon pox	2 months in refrigerator	6-8 weeks	Feather follicles	Swab
6-8 weeks	Fowl pox	Chick embryo-adapted fowl pox	2 months in refrigerator	Lifelong	Wing-web	Two pricks
9-12 weeks	Ranikhet Disease (Newcastle Disease)	Ranikhet Disease Vaccine R_2B (Mukteswar strain)	3 months in refrigerator, 7 days in summer, 10 days in other seasons	Lifelong	Intra-muscular	0.5 ml

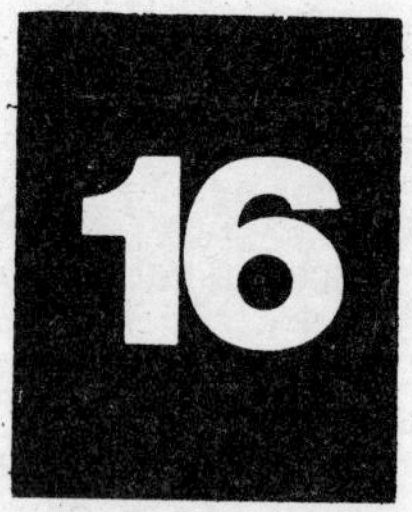

GOAT

The goat was the earliest ruminant domesticated around 9000 to 7000 B.C. References are made to goat in early biblical literature when it provided milk, meat, hides, fibre and manure. The Harappa toys contain representation of goat. Two seals from Mohenjo-daro show a wild Bezoar, of Western Asian goat with enormous curled and side spreading horns. On the basis of the archaeological evidence, the centre of goat domestication extends over Iraq, Iran, Jordan, Turkey and Palestine around 7000 B.C.

Some common terms in relation to GOATS

Details		*Expression*	*Details*		*Expression*
Species called as	...	Caprine	Castrated male	...	Castrated or wether
Group of animals	...	Flock or band	Castrated female	...	Spayed
Adult male	...	Buck	Female with its offspring	...	Suckling
Adult female	...	Doe	Act of parturition	...	Kidding
Young male	...	Buckling	Act of mating	...	Serving
Young female	...	Goatling	Sound produced	...	Bleat
New -born one	...	Kid	Pregnancy	...	Gestation

From these centres of domestication people migrated during pre-historic times with their goats and other animals. Two main routes of dispersion of goats from Western Asia are thought to have been used from as early as 2000 B.C., 1) The 'silk road' from Persia and Afghanistan through Turkestan to Mongolia or to North China, and 2) The route to the Indian sub-continent through the Khyber Pass followed by Indo-Aryan people.

The goat is a hollow-horned ruminant belonging to the mammalian order Artiodactyla, sub-order Ruminantia, family Bovidae and either of the genera *Capra* or *Hemitragus*. The distinction between the two genera was first based on horn-form but it has since been confirmed genetically about distinguished characteristics.

Goat which belongs to the genus *Capra* has possibly been developed from the following 5 wild species: (i) *Capra hircus*, the true goat including the Bezoar; (ii) *Capra ibex*, the ibexes; (iii) *Capra caucasica*, the Caucasian tur; (iv) *Capra pyrenaica*, the Spanish ibex; and (v) *Capra falconeri*, the Markhor.

It appears that the Markhor and the Bezoar gave rise to the majority of the Indian and central Asian breeds.

Perhaps the first successful attempt of standardization of a breed was Angora goat, originated in Central Asia, and was brought to Anatolia in Turkey during 5th century B.C. The breed is exceptionally valued for mohair (soft white wool). Another creation of a breed "Cashmere" has also originated in Central Asia for its production of pashmina (undercoat of this breed, which is very fine soft wool) now found in India at high altitude areas. Pashmina is used to produce high quality clothing and when blended with wool, it is known as felt. The first modern milk goat breed developed in Switzerland by the end of last century.

It is estimated that in the world there are about 102 descript breeds and types of goats, 95% of them are in developing countries, India having 20, Pakistan 25 and China 25 breeds of goats respectively.

To-day India ranks first for its genetic resources and numerical superiority of goats in the world (115.52 million in 1990).

A goat produces per year around 130 kg of dry manure which improves the soil fertility through its nutrients (more than cow or buffalo manure) and also by its residual effect on reducing soil pH. Annual production of goat's manure, casings and offals recorded in 1984 to the extent of 40,000 kg. The word manure refers to mixture of animal excrements consisting of undigested feeds plus certain body wastes and bedding.

Goats are less prone to toxic effects of toxic shrubs like lantana, tithonia and acanthus as judged by clinical symptoms. They have high dry matter and fibre digestibility, and thus can subsist on poor woody vegetation which no other species will consume.

In Asia and Africa, the major contribution of goats is towards meat and skins. The goat skins are highly valued and have large export market, both in the processed form and as products. Perhaps, the value addition in goat skin processing is much larger than any other product including fibre.

There is much less risk in goat farming especially in drought prone areas where large mortality occurs due to frequent droughts because of their higher prolificacy and capacity to recover flock size. There are much less housing requirements and management problems with goats. Woman and children essentially look after herding, feeding and health care of goats. The involvement of woman increases as the farm size decreases, and the men are forced to seek off-farm employment.

Most goats are maintained in small holder situation, integrated with crop farming; however, there are large flocks maintained under nomadic system. Except in Europe and America, where large dairy goat herds are maintained under intensive management for commercial milk production, and the milk is primarily utilized for making cheese and yogurt. Goats are essentially raised under extensive system of management.

In spite of the neglect of goat by development planners, primarily due to misconception of the role in ecological degradation, their number has increased relatively more than other species, specially in Asia. India has the largest population of goats and 35% of the total meat consumed comes from this species.

Goats contribute to the subsistence of small holders and landless rural poor. They also produce meat, milk, fibre, skins and manure and transport power, especially in high altitudes as in Himalayas. A Gaddi goat can carry up to 10 kg of load on much steep slopes than could be negotiated by mule, the most versatile drought animal. Goats along with sheep have an important role in income generation, capital storage, employment generation and improving household nutrition. Being small in size, the meat can be consumed by the family and would not need refrigeration. Goats are also utilized as biological control for brush and undesirable forbs. The browsing, if controlled, accelerates vegetative growth of trees, shrubs and surface vegetation. The role of goat in causing ecological degradation and desertification is highly exaggerated and is more due to misconception. The goat in fact acts as seeding machine of trees, especially hard-coated seeds which would not germinate unless acid treated; such seeds while passing through the animal get their hard coats softened and get pelleted. These pelleted seeds have greater germination capacity.

Goat milk is easily digestible because of smaller sized fat globules making softer curd. It also has much less allergic problems than milk of other species of livestock. It has medicinal qualities. Goats can be milked as often as required preventing milk storage problem. The total annual production of 959,000 MT of goat's milk corresponds to 2.9% of the total milk produced in India including cow and buffalo. Its nutritive value does not differ appreciably from that of cows milk. The mineral content is slightly higher than cow due to presence of relatively higher amount of calcium, phosphorus and chlorine content. However, it has lower iron value.

Table 16.1 Means with their standard errors for lactational parameters in Indian goat breeds

Breed	Lactation yield (kg)	Lactation length (days)	Av. daily yield (kg)	Peak yield (kg)	Dry period days	References
Jamunapari	158.06±4.49	187.80±4.29	0.996±0.05	3.205	115.0±3.00	23, 9, 25
Beetal	173.95±1.27	181.70±1.94	1.278±0.02	—	125.5±6.84	23, 15, 7, 26
Barbari	95.58±2.78	152.3±4.80	0.760±0.18	2.100	155.3±0.60	23, 9, 10, 8
Sirohi	73.80±1.21	158.7±1.35	0.468	0.696±0.01		3, 10
Malabari	66.33±8.37	172.5±12.4	0.457	—	145.2±11.8	6, 8, 21
Jhakrana	121.80±8.82	114.60±18.47	0.988	—		8

Goat meat is commonly called *Chevon* and is usually low in fat. It contributes about 35% to the total meat production of the country from livestock (except poultry), through sacrifice of 33.94 million goats annually. Best quality meat is obtained from 6–12 months old goats. Dressing percentage is between 43 to 53 per cent. Export of goat's meat started in seventies and by now India is exporting to as many as 20 countries. At present the internal demand is 20 times higher than the present production. The contribution of goat's milk and meat production is minimal. It is thus apparent that an increase in individual production of the indigenous is essential to boost the natural production.

There is a large genetic variability in goats. There are 102 descript breeds and a large number of less descript or less known breeds. Of these, half are in Asia, India having 20, Pakistan 25 and China 25. India has contributed superior goat 'germplasm' for improvement of goats in South Asia and South-East Asia. Unfortunately some of these are fast declining in numbers.

Considering the economic importance of goat in national economy, the Government of India has set up Central Institute for research on Goats at Makhdoom near Mathura in U.P.

Table 16.2

Contribution of goats to the Indian economy

Products	Quantity (metric tonnes)	Estimated value (million rupees)	% Contribution
Meat[1]	0.7	32862.6	79.3
Milk[2]	1500.0	9.0	-
Skins[3]	76.3	5341.0	12.9
Pashmina[4]	48.0	24.0	-
Hair (raw)[5]	15300.0	122.1	0.3
Offals[6]	0.15	3052.0	7.3
Blood[7]	20700.0	61.0	0.2
Dung[8]	0.03	1.5	-
Urine[8]	0.01	0.5	-

1 Based on a goat population of 109 million in 1990, 70% offtake, an average slaughter weight of 20kg and a dressing percentage of 48%. The average price of goat meat is Rs. 45/kg.
2 In tonnes, based on a value of Rs. 5/-kg.
3 Refer to million pieces and valued at Rs. 70/- piece.
4 In tonnes. Based on a population of 400000 animals, yield, of 20 g/head and a price of Rs. 500/ kg.
5 In tonnes. Estimated at 200 g hair/skin form the number of skins produced valued at Rs. 8/kg.
6 Estimated at 8.0% of live weight (legs, rumen and intestine) and valued at Rs. 34/ offals/head.
7 Estimated at 3.4% of live weight, 40% consumption, valued at Rs. 2/- per animal.
8. Expressed as N equivalent in urea. Dung and urine production are 300 g and 150 ml/ head a day in an animal with average live weight of 20 kg. The average N contents were 1.3 g/100g DM in faeces and 0.9 g/100 ml urine respectively. Estimated as N equivalent in urea costing Rs. 2.25/- per kg.

Source: Fifth International Conference on Goats, 2-8 March, 1992, New Delhi, India

In mountainous regions as in Jammu and Kashmir and Himachal Pradesh flocks of 100 to 500 animals are raised in high valleys during summer while in winter flocks are raised in lower valleys. In the plains, goats are raised by the socio-economically weaker sections of population at lower cost since raising are limited through grazing on the waste land, agricultural by-products, garden and kitchen wastes. The flocks mostly comprise of 2 to 5 goats. In urban areas goats, are however, raised without much grazing, i.e., mostly under stall-fed conditions.

BREEDS OF INDIAN GOATS

At present there are 20 breeds of goat in India although majority of them do not have specified defined characters. A population in a given locality, with characters distinct from other population in the vicinity and with a distinct local name, has usually been considered as a breed. The breeds are now classified on the basis of four agro-climatic conditions of the country, e.g., (1) the north western and central arid and semi-arid region; (2) the southern peninsular region; (3) the eastern region; (4) northern temperate region.

Majority of the breeds (60% of the total) are found in the North-western region. The breeds of this region are also larger in body size and more productive than the breeds of other regions. Jamunapari, Beetal, Jhakrana, Surti and Barbari are the prize breeds of this region. Black Bengal is the only breed of eastern region which is highly priced for its flesh and skin and has very wide distribution. The breeds of southern peninsular region are tall and leggy in general and their level of production is low.

I. The North-Western Arid and Semi-arid Region

The region comprises the States of Punjab, Haryana, Rajasthan and Gujarat including plains of U.P. and M.P. The region has the largest number (29 million) of goats comprising 43% of the total goat population of the country. The characteristics of some important breeds are discussed below:

JAMUNAPARI

Distribution. It is the biggest and most majestic breed of goats in India. The breed has been extensively utilised to upgrade indigenous breeds for milk and meat (dual-purpose) and has been exported to neighbouring countries for the same purposes. Its home is between Jamuna, Ganges and Chambal rivers.

Pure stocks are found in Etawah districts of U.P. The breed is distributed at Agra and Mathura apart from Morena districts of Madhya Pradesh.

Breed characteristic.

i) *Size* (Average)

	Adult male	*Adult female*
Body weight (kg)	50–60	40–50
Body length (cm)	77.0	75.0
Chest girth (cm)	79.0	76.1

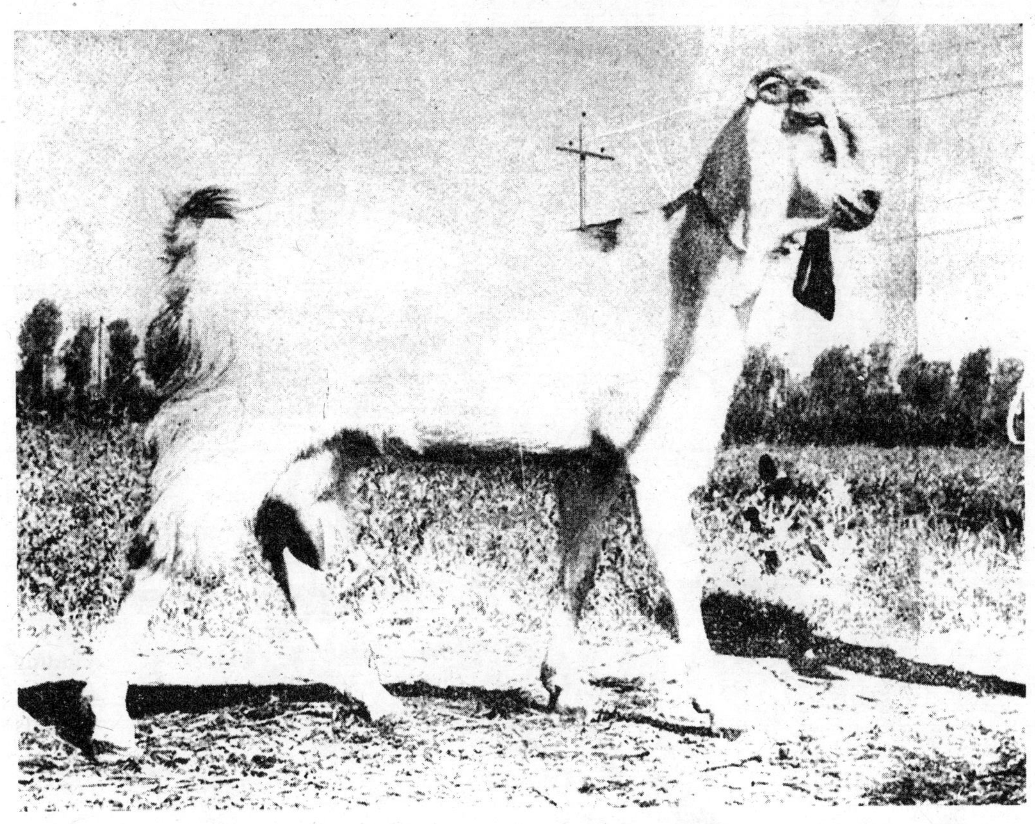

Plate 66. A female Jamunapari goat.

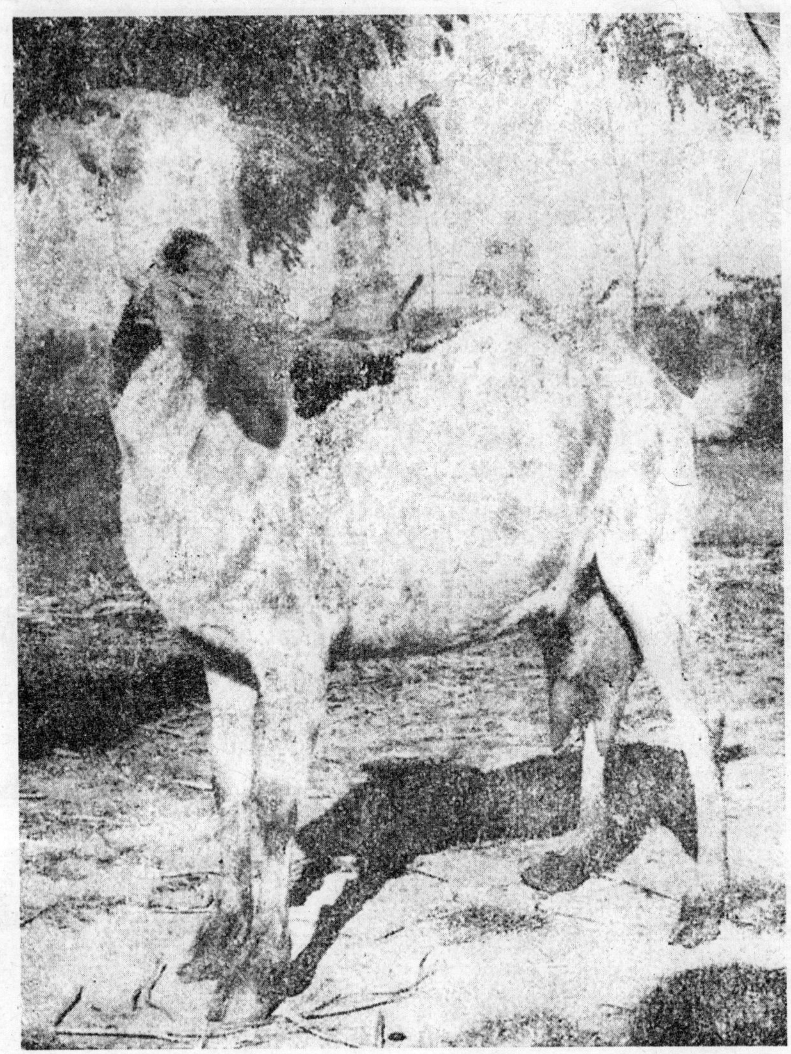

Plate 67. Barbari female.

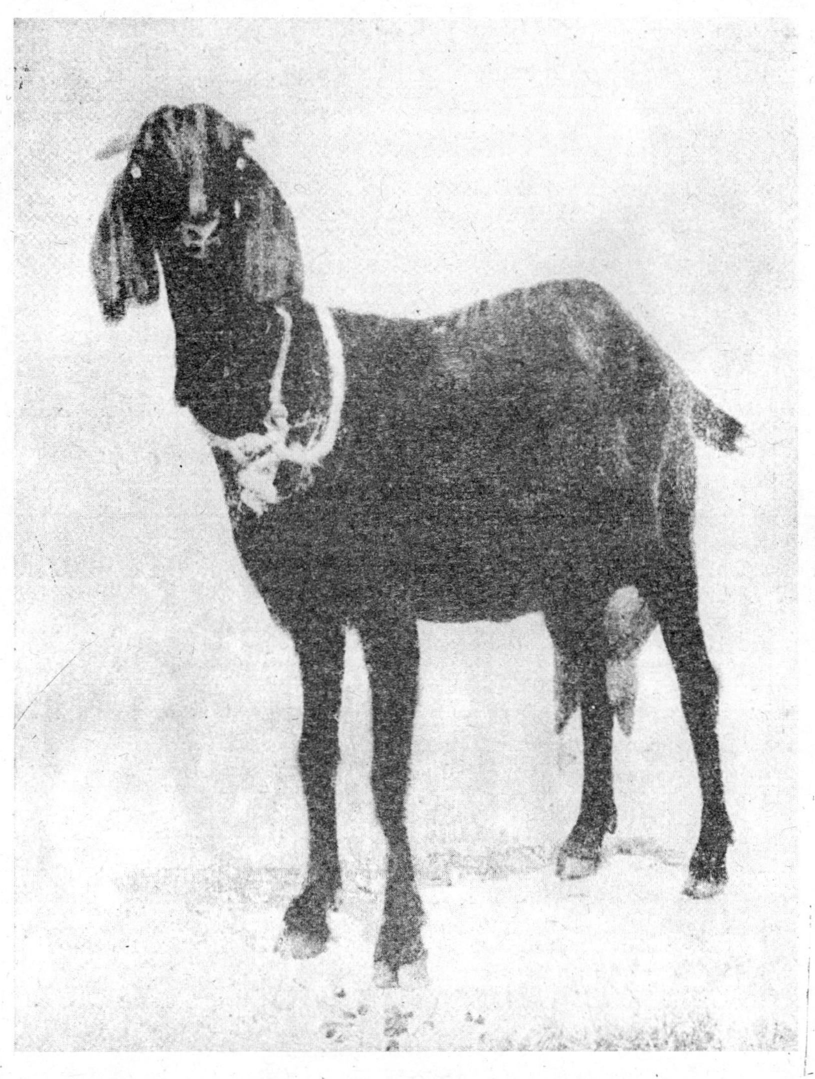

Plate 68. Typical Beetal doe.

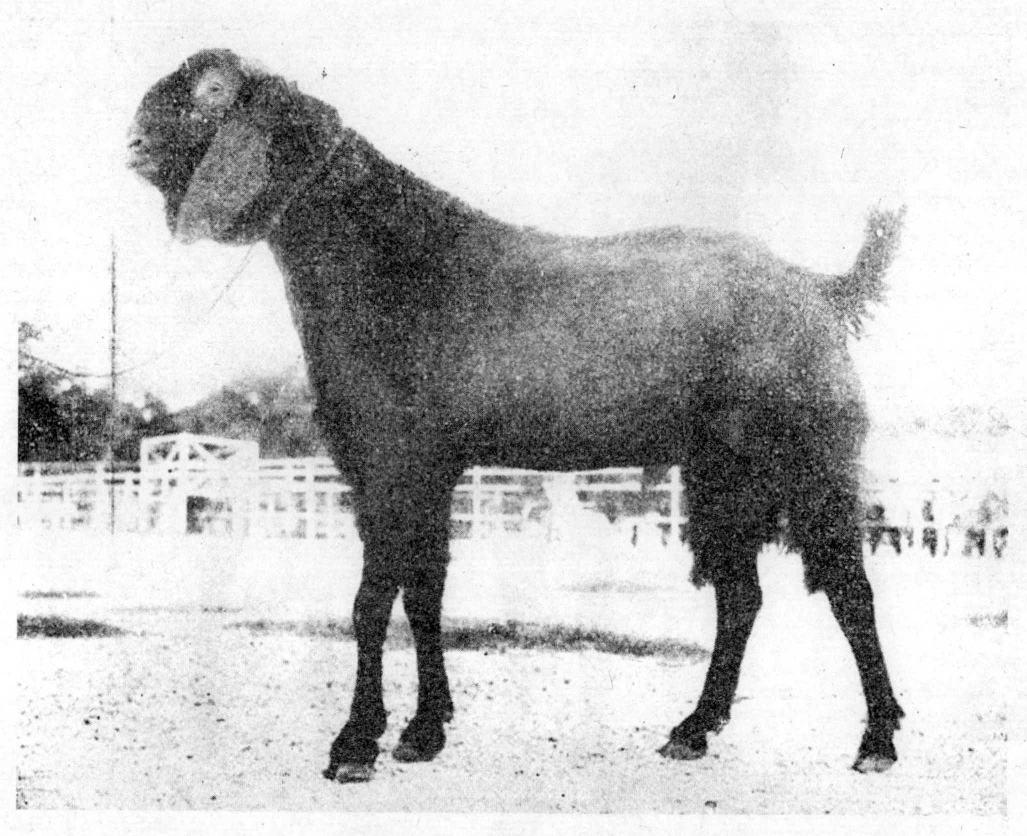

Plate 69. Typical Beetal male.

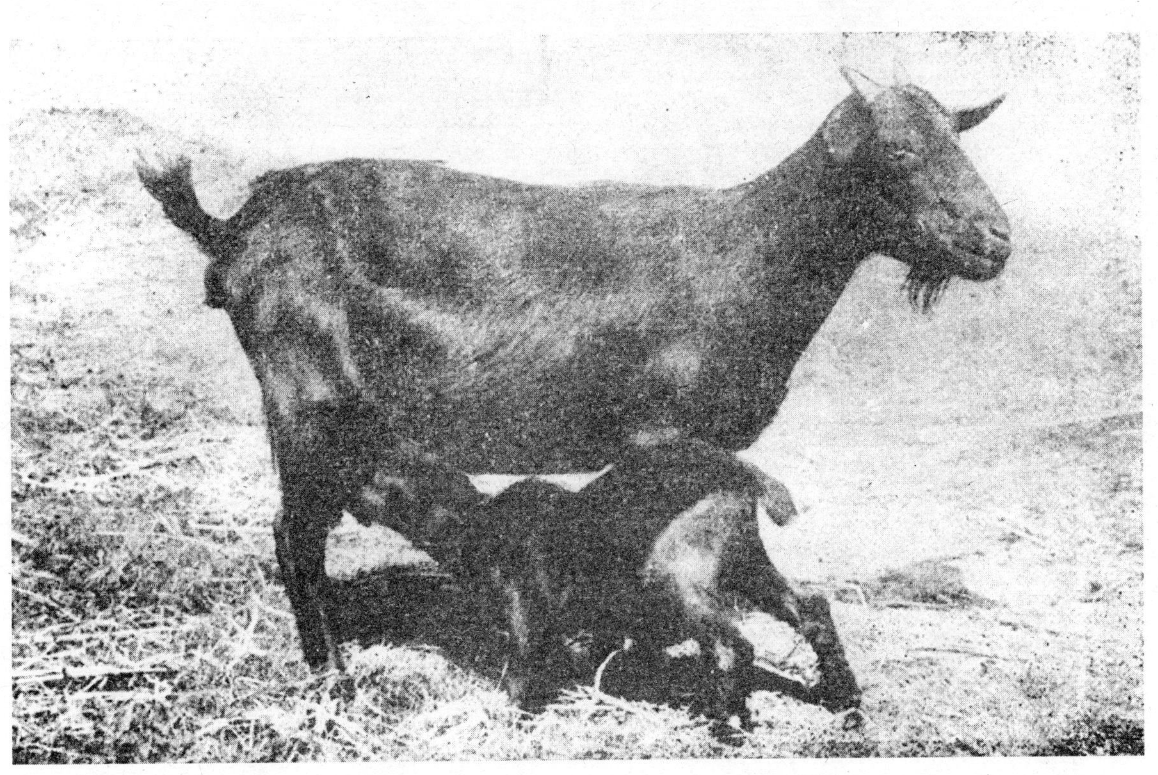

Plate 70. Female Black Bengal goat.

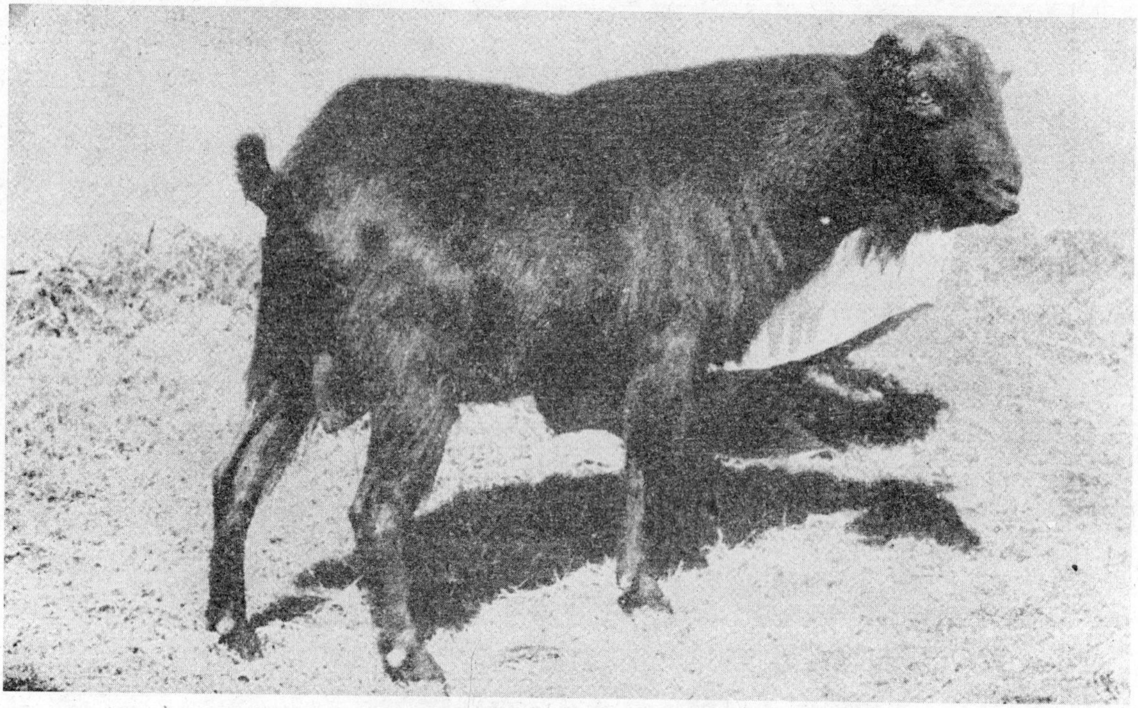

Plate 71. A male Black Bengal goat.

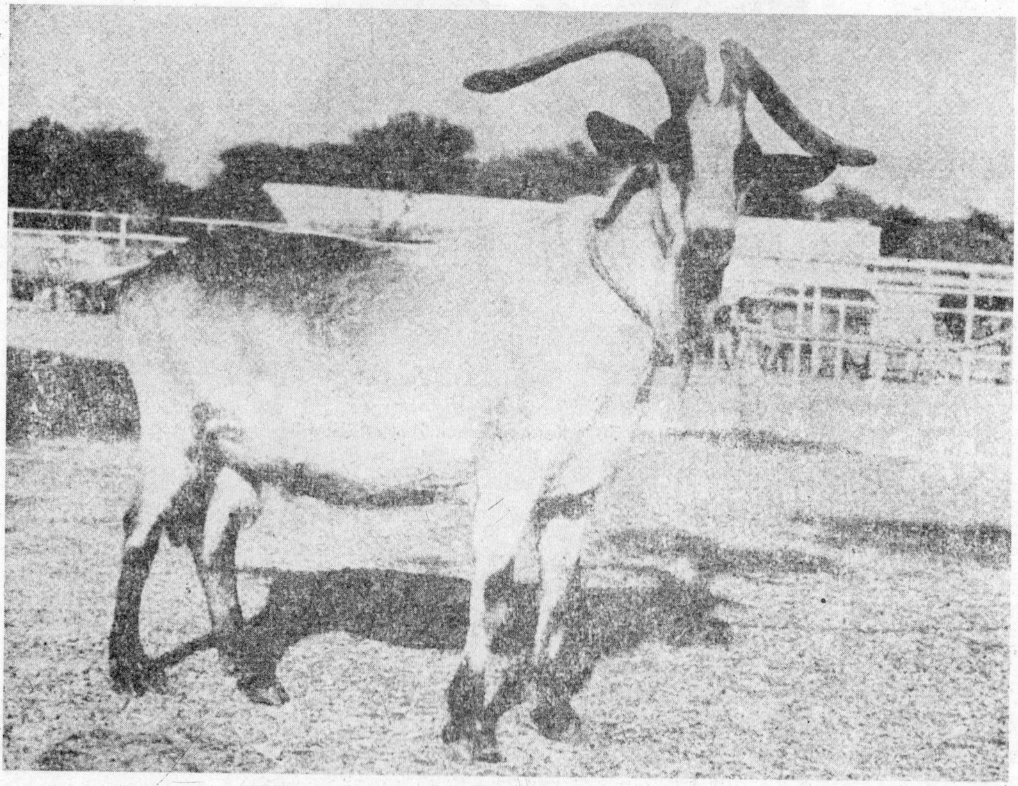

Plate 72. An Alpine male.

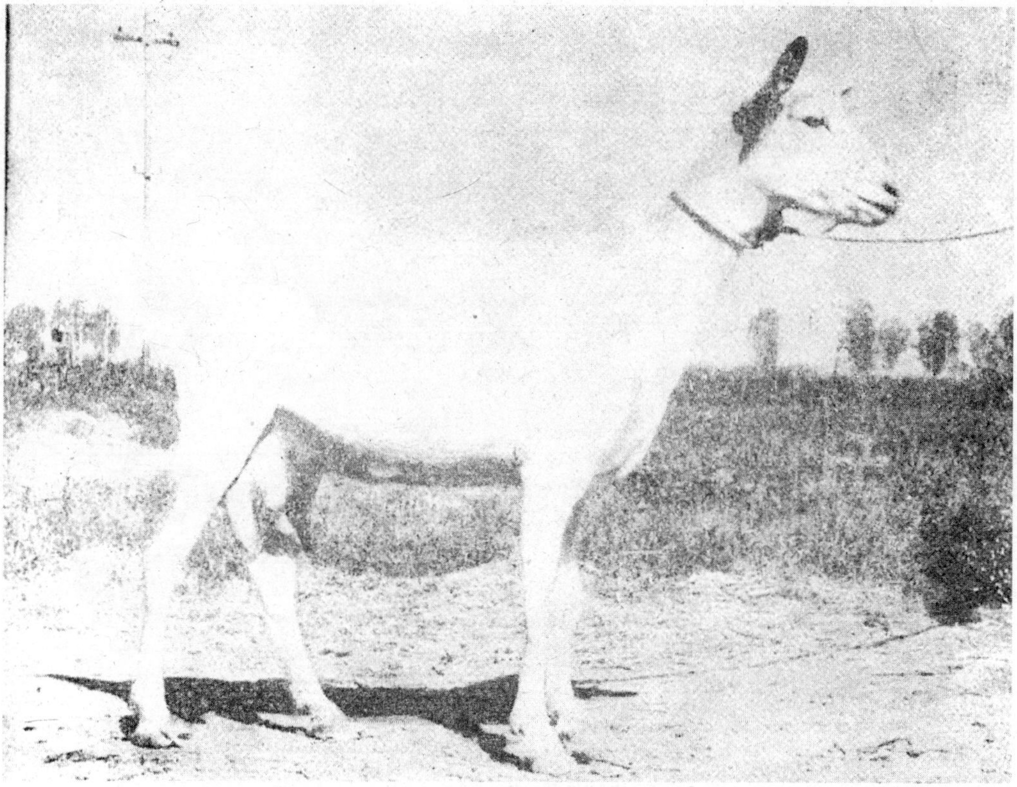

Plate 73. A Saanen female.

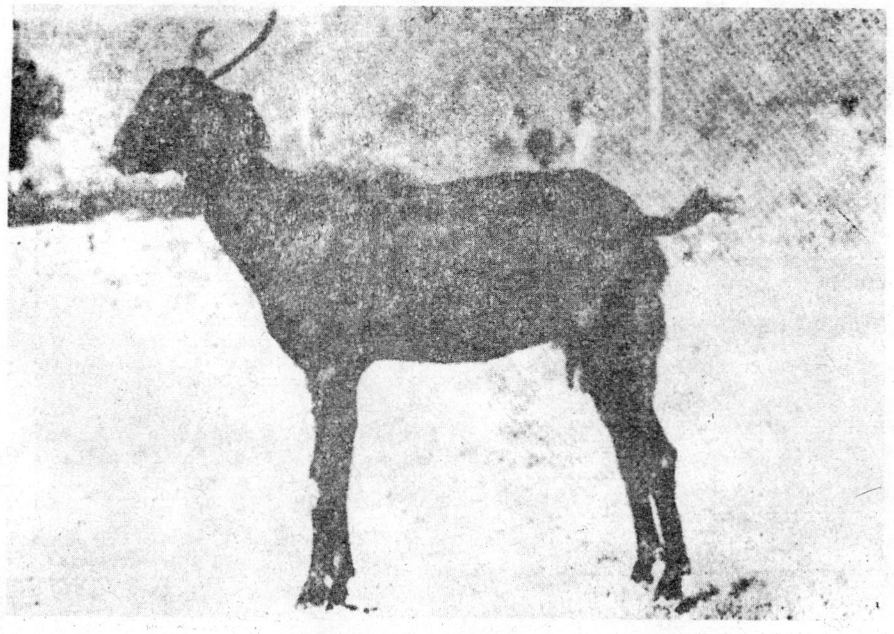

Plate 74. Adult Ganjam female goat.

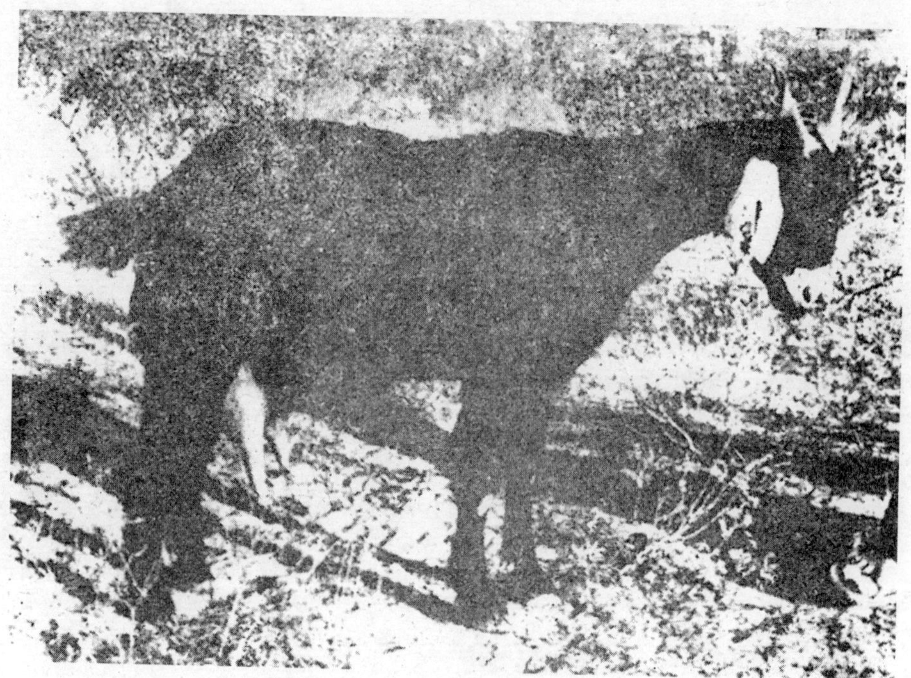

Plate 75. Adult Mehsana female goat.

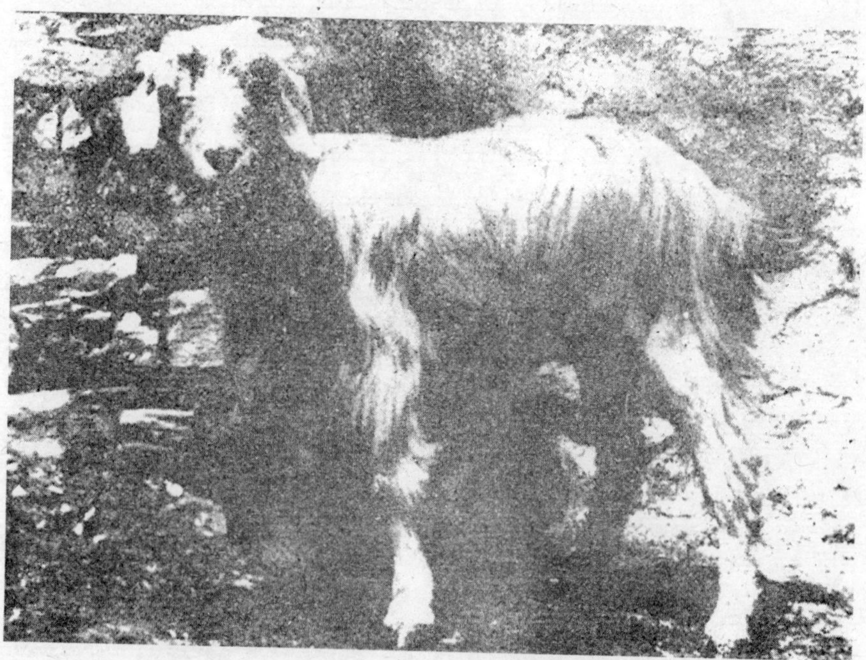

Plate 76. Adult Gaddi male goat.

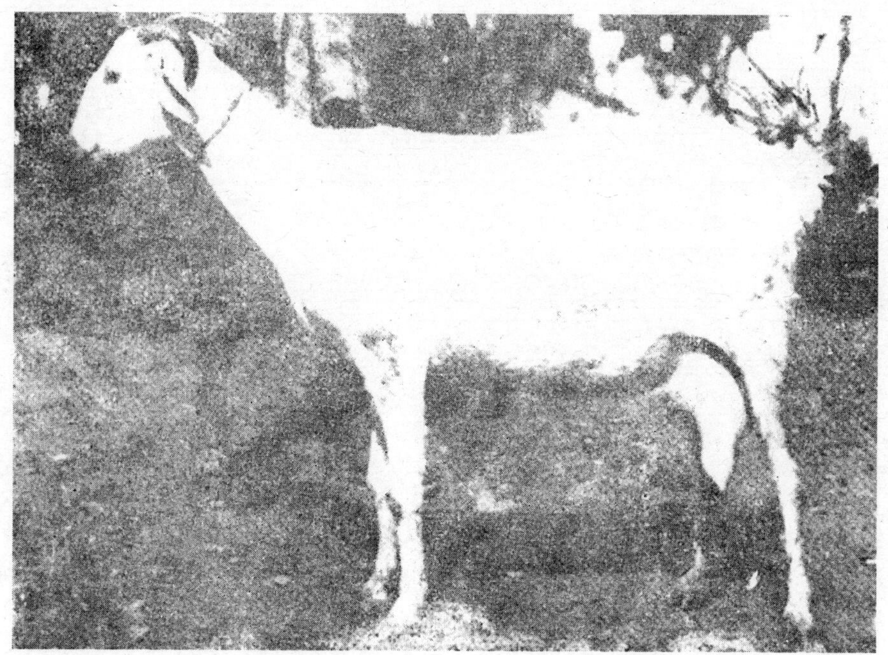

Plate 77. Adult Malabari female goat.

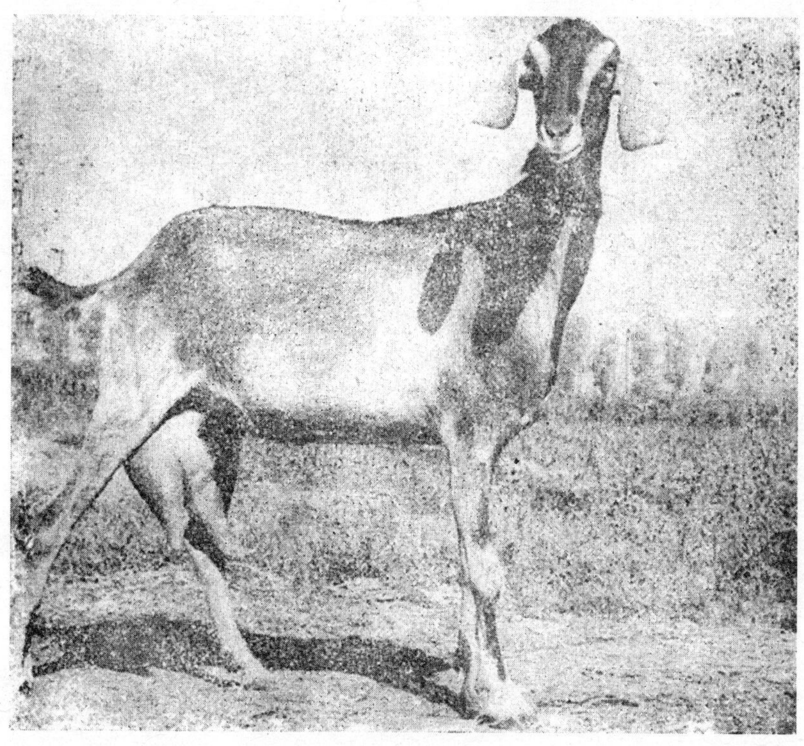

Plate 78. Alpine X Beetal.

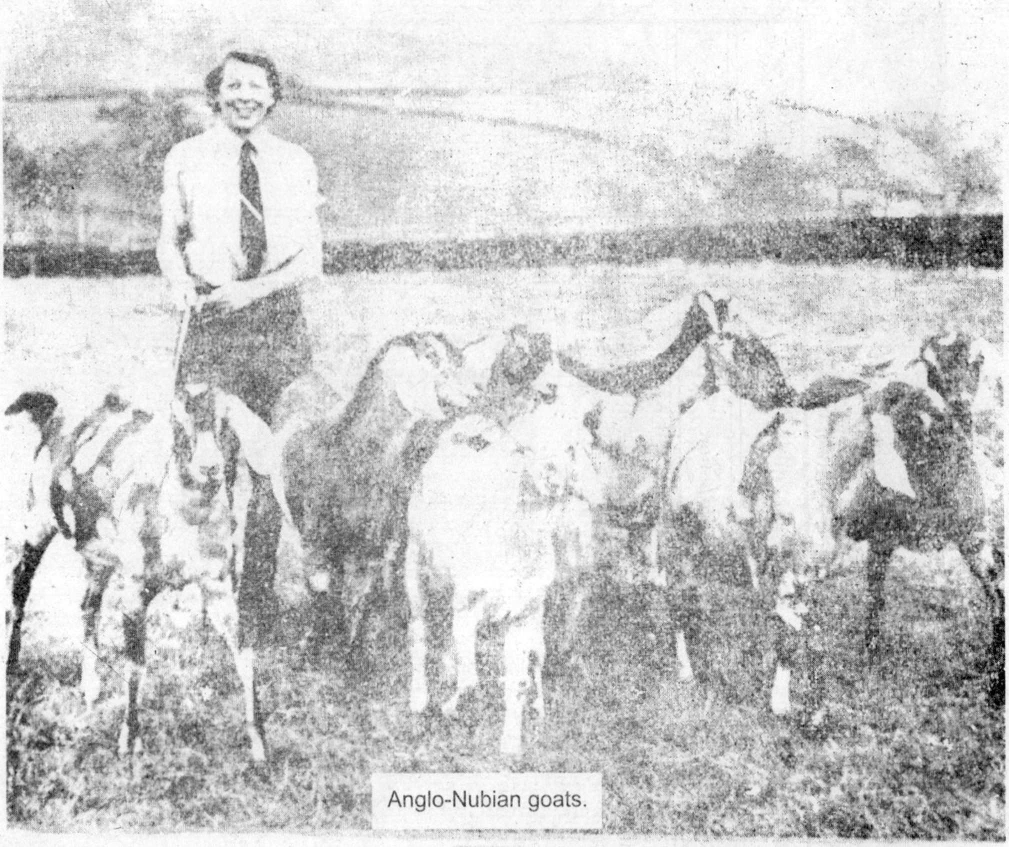

Anglo-Nubian goats.

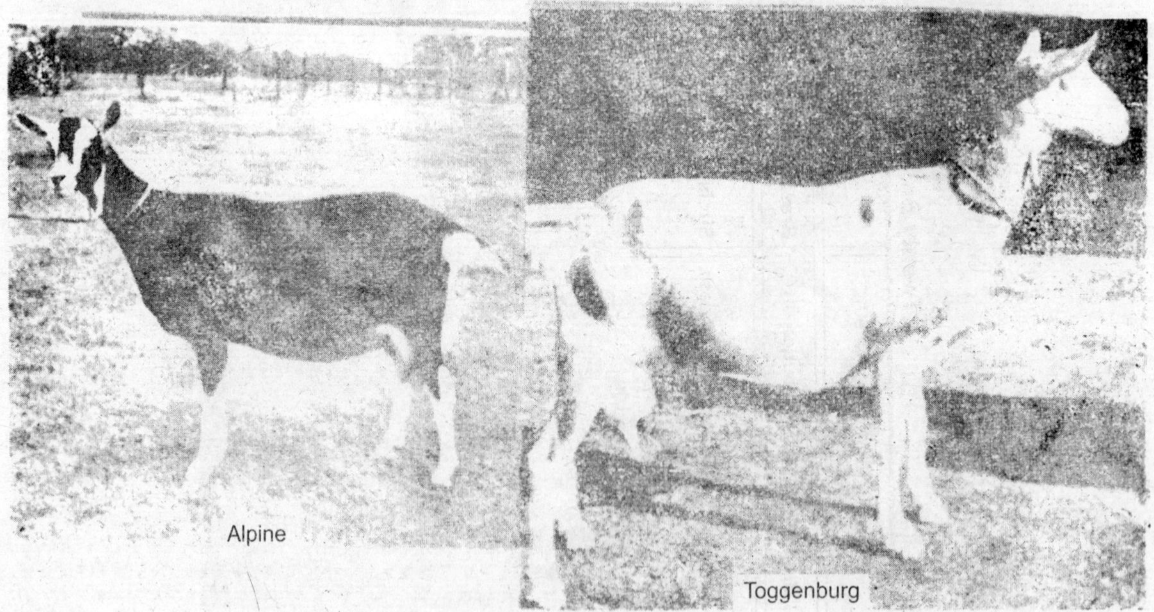

Alpine

Toggenburg

Plate 79. (CHAPTER 16).

Table 16.3

Twenty Breeds of Indian Goats in different Agro-ecological Regions

Northern-temperate		*North-Western Arid & Semi-arid*		*Southern*		*Eastern*	
Breed	**Distribution**	**Breed**	**Distribution**	**Breed**	**Distribution**	**Breed**	**Distribution**
Gaddi	Himachal Pradesh Uttar Pradesh	**Sirohi**	Rajasthan & Gujarat	**Sangamneri**	Maharastra	**Ganjam**	Orissa
Changthangi	Ladakh above 4000 m.	**Marwari**	Rajasthan & Gujarat	**Osmanabadi**	Maharastra	**Bengal**	West Bengal Assam, Manipur, Tripura, Arunachal Pradesh, Meghalaya
Chegu	Himachal Pradesh & Uttar Pradesh	**Jhakrana**	Rajasthan	**Kanni-Adu**	Tamil Nadu		
		Beetal	Punjab & Haryana	**Malabari**	Kerala		
		Barbari	Uttar Pradesh & Rajasthan				
		Jamunapari	Uttar Pradesh				
		Mehsana	Gujarat				
		Gohilwadi	Gujarat				
		Zalawadi	Gujarat				
		Surti	Gujarat				

ii) *Conformation.* There is a great variation in coat colour but they are generally white or light yellowish tan with light brown spots on the neck and face, and occasionally patches of tan or black are found on the body. The typical character of the breed is a highly convex nose line with a tuft of hair known as "Roman nose" or parrot mouth appearance. The ears are very long, flat and drooping. Both sexes are horned with short and thin tail. A thick growth of hair is present on the buttocks, known as feathers. The breed has well developed udder round in shape with large conical teats.

Performance

i) *Milk.* Average daily yield varies from 1.5 to 2.0 kg per day with a total lactation yield of about 200 kg.

ii) *Kidding.* Usually doe kids once a year, giving birth to single in 57% while twins in 43% per cent cases. They kid once a year.

iii) *Meat.* Dressing percentage on pre-slaughter live-weight basis is about 45 per cent at 6 months and 48 per cent at nine months with a bone and meat ratio of 1: 3.9.

BARBARI

Distribution. The breed is a promising dairy type goat which has probably originated in the city of Barbera in British Somali land in East Africa. In India the breed is distributed at Etawah, Agra, Mathura and Aligarh districts of U.P. and Bharatpur district of Rajasthan. In addition to being a good milker it is highly prolific and generally give birth to twin and triplets. It is a dwarf breed highly suited for stall-feeding conditions and hence generally found in the cities.

Breed characteristic.

i) *Size* (Average)	*Adult male*	*Adult female*
Body weight (kg)	40.0	24.0
Body length (cm)	70.5	58.7

ii) *Conformation.* Small animals with compact body. where is wide variation in coat colour, but white with small light brown patches is most common Ears are short, tubular and erect. Both sexes have twisted horns, medium in length and directed upward and backward. Bucks have a large thick beard.

Performance.

i) *Milk.* Daily milk yield averages about 750 ml to 1,000 ml. Average lactation may be 130–200 kgs of milk in a lactation length of 150 days with a fat percentage of about 5.

ii) *Kidding.* It may kid twice in a period of 12–15 months. Litter size; single 25 per cent, twins 65 per cent and triplets 10 per cent.

BEETAL

Distribution. The Beetal is found throughout the state of Punjab and Haryana. True-bred animals are however found in the districts of Gurdaspur, Amritsar and Ferozepur in Punjab. The breed is a good dairy type, second to Jamunapari in size but is superior to it in respect to proliferation and adaptability to various agroclimatic zones and also to stall feeding.

Breed characteristic.

i) *Size* (Average)	*Adult male*	*Adult female*
Body weight (kg)	50–62	35–40
Body length (cm)	86.0	70.5
Chest girth (cm)	86.0	73.5

ii) *Conformation.* The breed is large but slightly smaller than Jamunapari and is good dairy type. Coat colour is variable, predominantly black (about 90%) or brown (10%) having spots of different sizes. The ears are long and flat, curled and drooping. Both sexes have thick, medium-sized horns, carried horizontally with a slight twist directed backward and upward. Roman nose. Male possesses marked beard while females are beardless. The tail is small and thin. The udder is large and developed having big conical teats.

Performance.

Milk & Kidding. Yield per lactation varies from 150–190 kg, averaging daily yield 2.0 kg. The litter size: single 41%, twins 53%, triplets 6%.

SURTI

Distribution. The white goat is distributed in Surat and Baroda. The breed is known to be a good dairy breed and is good for maintenance under complete confinement and stall feeding conditions.

Breed characteristic.

i) *Size* (Average)	*Adult male*	*Adult female*
Body weight (kg)	30.0	32.0
Body length (cm)	65.0	66.0
Chest girth (cm)	70.5	71.5

ii) *Conformation.* Medium sized breed, white in colour with highly developed udder. Ears are medium in size. Both sexes have small horns directed backward. The breed is unable to walk long distnnces and is stall feed. They are most economic to rear as they can live on leaves or on food waste thus brings higher feed efficiency ratio.

Performance.

Milk. The breed is a good milk producer, yields on an average of 2.0 kg per day. By crossing with Sannen it has resulted high potentiality of milk yield.

MARWARI

Distribution. Marwar region of Rajasthan, comprising Jodhpur, Bikaner, Jaisalmer district. It also extends into certain areas of Gujarat.

Breed Characteristics.

i) *Size* (Average)

	Adult male	*Adult female*
Body weight (kg)	33	25
Body length (cm)	70	63
Chest girth (cm)	71	68

ii) *Conformation.* Medium-sized animals. Predominantly jet black colour. The hair covering is lustrous and prominent and grows at the rate of about 10–12 cm annually. The male has a thick beard, but this is absent in females. The ears are small and flat, carried on a small head. Both sexes have short pointed horns, directed upward and backward. Tail is small and thin. The udders are fairly well developed but small and round with small teats placed laterally.

Performance

1) Milk. The average daily milk yield is poor, about 0.8 kg.
2) It is good for meat.

MEHSANA

Distribution. **These are mainly found at Mehsana, Banaskantha, Gandhi Nagar and Ahmedabad districts of Gujarat. The breed is considered as dual purpose, i.e., for meat and milk.**

Breed characteristic.

i) *Size* (Average)

	Adult male	***Adult female***
Body weight (kg)	**36.0**	**32.0**
Body length (cm)	**70.0**	**68.0**
Chest girth (cm)	**76.5**	**72.5**

ii) *Conformation.* The Mehsana is large sized, coat colour is black with white spots at the base of the ear. The hair coat is long and coarse. Ears are always white. Both sexes has twisted horns curved upward and backward. The udder is moderately developed having large and conical teats.

Performance. **Milk yield averages 1.0 kg/day, litter size mostly single. Average yield of hair per goat per year is 200 grams.**

JHAKRANA

Distribution. **The breed is found in Jhakrana and few surrounding villages near Behror, of Alwar district of Rajasthan. The breed is large and also a good dairy type.**

Breed characteristic.

i) *Size* (Average)	*Adult male*	*Adlut female*
Body weight (kg)	55.0	45.0
Body length (cm)	84.0	77.0
Chest girth (cm)	86.0	79.0

ii) *Conformation.* Animals are large and predominantly black with white spots on ears and muzzle. The breed is very similar to Beetal, the main contrast is that Jhakrana is comparatively longer. It has highly developed udder. Forehead is slightly bulging.

Performance.

i) Milk. These goats are used mainly for milk production. Average daily milk yield varies from 2.0–3.0 kg for a lactation length of about 180–200 days.

ii) These are prolific. Kidding is mostly single but in 40% cases twins are given birth. Triplets are not uncommon.

iii) The goats are also useful meat producers, and their skins are popular with the tanning industry.

KUTCHI

Distribution. Kutch district in Gujarat.

Breed Characteristics.

i) *Size* (Average)	*Adult male*	*Adult female*
Body weight (kg)	42–45	30–40
Body length (cm)	76	73
Chest girth (cm)	78	76

ii) *Conformation.* Large animals. The coat is predominantly black, but a few white, brown and spotted animals are also found. Long hair, nose slightly Roman, Cork screw horns painted upwards, ears are long, broad and drooping. The udder is moderately developed with conical shaped teats.

Performance

1) Milk. Average yield varies around 1.5 kg and the lactation length is about 110 days.
2) Hair. Annual yield touches about 500 gm when shorn twice a year.

SIROHI

Distribution. Sirohi district of Rajasthan and Palampur in Gujarat.

Breed Characteristics

i) *Size* (Average)	*Adult male*	*Adult female*
Body weight (kg)	50	40
Body length (cm)	80	60
Chest girth (cm)	80	62

ii) *Conformation.* Compact medium-sized animals. Coat colour predominantly brown with light or dark brown patches; a very few individuals are completely white. The body is covered fairly densely with hair which is short and coarse. The hair grows at the rate of about 2 cm annually. Ears are flat and leaf like, medium-sized and drooping. Both sexes have small horns, curved upward and backward. On average, the birth weight is about 2.0 kg. The age at first kidding is 19–20 months and the litter size is one kid per birth. The breed is well suited to stall feeding.

Performance. The breed is used mainly for meat. The milk yield is relatively small, about 0.5 kg per day, with an average milk yield of 65 kg over a 120-day lactation period.

ZALAWADI

Distribution. Surendranagar and Rajkot districts of Gujarat.

Breed Characteristics

i) *Size* (Average)	*Adult male*	*Adult female*
Body weight (kg)	38	32
Body length (cm)	75	70
Chest girth (cm)	76	74

ii) *Conformation.* Animals are large, black in colour with white marking on ear. Ears are usually long, wide leaf-like and drooping. Both sexes have long twisted horns, pointed upward. Litter size is single.

Performance. The breed is reared primarily for meat. Average daily yield reaches upto 1.5 kg over a lactation period of 195 days.

II. The Southern Peninsular Region

The region comprises the States of Maharashtra, Karnataka, Andhra Pradesh, Tamil Nadu, Kerala and some territories in the Central area. It has about 30% of the total goat population of the country comprising Osmanabadi, Malbari, Sangamneri breeds.

OSMANABADI

Distribution. The goats are mainly distributed at Latur, Tuljapur and Udgir taluks of Osmanabad district of Maharashtra.

Breed characteristic.

i) *Size* (Average)	*Adult males*	*Adult females*
Body weight (kg)	34.0	32.0
Body length (cm)	68.0	66.0
Chest girth (cm)	72.0	71.0

ii) *Conformation.* The goats are large in size. Coat colour varies, but mostly it is black (73%) and the rest are white, brown or spotted. Ninety per cent males are horned; females may be horned or poled.

Performance.

Milk. The breed is considered useful both for meat and milk. Average daily yield varies from 0.5 to 1.5 kg for a lactation length of about 4 months.

The dressing percentage varies from 45 to 50.

In favourable conditions the does will breed regularly twice a year and twinning is common.

MALBARI

Distribution. They are also known as Tellicherry or Cutch mostly reared at Calicut, Cannanore and Malapuram districts of Kerala.

Breed characteristics.

i) *Size* (Average)	*Adult males*	*Adult females*
Body weight (kg)	38.0	31.0
Body length (cm)	70.0	63.0
Chest girth (cm)	73.0	67.0

ii) *Conformation.* The animals are medium in size. They have no uniform colour which varies from completely white to full black. 30% goats are long haired. All males and a small number of females are bearded. Animals are medium sized, head with flat and occasional Roman nose and medium sized ears directed outward and downward.

Performance. The breed is reared mainly for meat purpose and their skin is popular with the tanning industry. Kerala Agricultural University has undertaken cross-breeding programme with Alpine and Saanen for improving reproduction and milk yield. The average milk yield of this breed is 100–190 kg with a lactation period of 180–210 days.

SANGAMNERI

Distribution. The breed is commonly found in Poona and Ahmednagar districts of Maharashtra.

Breed characteristics.

i) *Size* (Average)	*Adult males*	*Adult females*
Body weight (kg)	38.0	29.0
Body length (cm)	69.0	62.5
Body girth (cm)	76.0	71.0

ii) *Conformation.* Medium-sized animals. They have no uniform colour, it varies from white, black or brown, with spots of other colours. Ears are drooping. Both sexes have horns directed backward and upward.

Performance. Milk. Average daily yield varies between 0.5 to 1.0 kgwith an average lactation length of about 165 days.

Meat. Dressing percentage is about 41% at 6 months, 45% at 9 months and 46% at 12 months of age.

III. The Eastern Region

The region comprises the States of Bihar, West Bengal, Orissa, Assam, Meghalaya, Arunachal Pradesh, Mizoram, Manipur, Tripura, Nagaland and Sikkim. The region represents only 25% of the goat population of the country. Major breeds are Bengal (black, brown, white and grey) and Ganjam.

BENGAL

Distribution. The breed is short-legged, compact animal, widely found throughout the eastern regions and also in northern part of Bangladesh.

Breed characteristics.

Size (Average)	*Adult male*	*Adult female*
A. West Bengal, Bihar & Orissa		
Body weight (kg)	32.0	20.0
Body length (cm)	63.0	51.0
Chest girth (cm)	72.0	63.2
B. Assam and other North-eastern States.		
Body weight (kg)	15.0	14.0
Body length (cm)	54.0	55.0
Chest girth (cm)	59.0	59.0

ii) *Conformation.* The breed is known for excellent mutton and skin quality. Animals are small, the predominant colour is black; brown, grey and white are also found. Shoulder and hips are of equal height, chest is wide, ears are nearly upright and pointed. The animal possesses soft but short hair. Multiple births are common, twins or triplets are born in twelve to fourteen months old doe. Both sexes have small to medium size horns directed upward and sometimes backward. Beard is found in both sexes.

Performance. Dressing percentage averages around 45.7%. Its meat is very tender and has a good taste. Skin is of excellent quality and is highly priced. Very poor in milk yield.

GANJAM

Distribution. Ganjam and Koraput districts of southern Orissa is the home land of this breed.

Breed characteristics.

i) *Size* (Average)	*Adult males*	*Adult females*
Body weight (kg)	44.0	31.5
Body length (cm)	76.0	67.5
Chest girth (cm)	83.0	74.5

ii) *Conformation.* Animals are tall, coat colour varies but black predominates over white, brown or spotted. Hairs are short and lustrous. Both sexes have long and straight horns directed upward and slightly backward.

Performance. Very poor in milking aspect, average may be 250 to 300 grams per day.

IV. The Northern Temperate Region

The region comprises Jammu and Kashmir, Himachal Pradesh and hilly tracts of Uttar Pradesh.

The region has only 2.8% of the total goat population of the country including the pashmina producing goats, Changthangi and Chigu. The other important breed of this region is Gaddi.

CHANGTHANGI

Distribution. The breed is also known as Pashmina due to the ability of the breed to produce longer and finer *pashmina* on the sides and shoulders. Pashmina goats are mostly reared in Ladakh, Lahul and Spiti valleys and its neighbouring areas of Himachal Pradesh. Large herds of this breed are found in the Changthang region of Ladakh at an elevation of 4,000 metre.

Breed characteristics.

i) *Size* (Average)	*Adult males*	*Adult females*
Body weight (kg)	20.0	19.8
Body length (cm)	49.0	52.5
Chest girth (cm)	63.0	65.0

ii) *Conformation.* Medium sized animals. Half of the animals are white, the rests are black, grey or brown. Both sexes have large horns, turning outward, upward and inward to form a semi-circle, but a wide variation exists in both shape and size. The breed looks pretty having fast movements and are used for transport in hilly areas. Body is covered with long coarse hair including the facial areas.

Performance. Apart from meat, the breed is highly prized for *pashmina.* The fine costly hair is harvested once a year, generally in June/July, either by shearing or by combing. Average production of pashmina is 215 g with a variation range of 70–500 g per animal. Used for making Kashmir "Rug or Shawl" of high quality.

GADDI

Distribution. The breed is also known as Himalayan and is found in Chamba, Kangra, Kulu, Bilaspur, Simla, Kinnaur, Lahaul and Sipti in Himachal Pradesh and part of Jammu hills. In Uttar Pradesh also the breed is reared at Dehradun, Nainital, Tehrigarhwal and Chamoli hill districts. During winter, the herds graze in the valleys, while in summer they move to higher altitudes where the lush green grass springs up. They are well built, sturdy and can easily move to long distances. Each animal transports about 8 kg of merchandise.

Breed characteristics.

i) *Size* (Average)

	Adult males	*Adult females*
Body weight (kg)	27.0	25.0
Body length (cm)	69.5	65.0
Chest girth (cm)	72.0	69.0

ii) *Conformation.* The animals are medium-sized, coat colour is mostly white but black and brown and combinations of these are also seen. Both sexes have large horns, directed upward and backward and occasionally twisted. Ears are medium, long and drooping. Skin is very tough, covered with coarse long hair measuring 7–10 inches (18–25 cm). The udder is small and rounded with pointed teats.

Performance. Average fleece yield per clip is about 300 g and fibre diameter is 75 micron with medullation per cent of 73.4.

CHIGU

Distribution. Lahaul and Spiti valleys of Himachal Pradesh, Uttar Kashi, Chamoli, and Pithoragarh districts of U.P.

Breed Characteristics

i) *Size* (Average)

	Adult male	*Adult female*
Body weight (kg)	36	25
Body length (cm)	75	69
Chest girth (cm)	80	73

ii) *Conformation.* Medium-sized animals. The coat is usually white, mixed with greyish red. Both sexes have prominent horns, directed upward, backward and outward with one or more twists very similar to Changthangi breed.

Performance. The breed is marked for Pashmina production. Average yearly production is about 120 grams with 5.9 cm. fibre length having 10–12 micron diameter.

Table 16.4

Classification of 20 Indian breeds of Goats according to their major functions

Dairy / Meat	*Meat*	*Fibre*
Jhakrana	Bengal	Gaddi
Beetal	Ganjan	Marwari
Jamunapari	Malabari	Changthani
Barbari	Kannai Adu	Chigu
Surti	Osmanabad	
	Sangamneri	
	Kutchi	
	Zalawadi	
	Gohilwadi	
	Mehsana	
	Sirohi	

Table 16.5 CHARACTERISTICS OF SOME EXOTIC BREEDS OF GOATS INTRODUCED INTO THE TROPICS

Breed	*Country of Origin*	*Height at withers (males & females) (cm.)*	*Av. daily milk yield in the Tropics (kg.)*	*Colour & Horn Character*	*Other Characteristics*
Alpine	Orginated in the Alps, probably from crossing Swiss Alpine breeds with British goats.	75 to 85	0.9 to 1.3 with 3.6% fat.	Colour varies from black to white to black. They may be horned or polled, when present are of the scimitar (curved) type.	The breed is valued first for its milk production. In tropic yield is about 0.9-1.3 kg/day with 3.6% fat. It has erect ears and straight nose. The breed is more adapted to mountanious areas and in tropical environment. Average live weight is 60-65 kg. The breed is not suited in areas of high humidity. There are usually 2 kids in a litter.
Anglo-Nubian	The breed was derived from the Nubian type goat (Jamunapari and Zaraibi) by crossing with English breeds in the UK in the late 19th century.	80 to 100	0.8 to 1.2 with 4.5% fat.	Colour varies but brown and white are usual. Horns when present lie flat over the coat.	It is one of the most outstanding dual purpose (milk and meat) breed. The Anglo-Nubian is usually a big animal with fine skin, glossy coat, long pendulous ears and Roman nose and forehead. The breed has proved to be the most suited to tropical climates and used widely for upgrading indigenous stock for meat and milk in West Indies, Malaysia, Phillipines and India. Average live weight varies between 60-70 kg. There are usually 2 kids in a litter.
Toggenberg	The breed originated from the Toggenberg Valley in north-east Switzerland	65 to 75	1.0 to 3.0 with a fat percentage of 3.5. The lactation period extends upto 10 months	Brown with white stripes on each side of face. Hornless with some exceptions	These are large goats having long thin neck which are kept erect. The skin of the doe is very soft and pliable. The udder is well attached and carried high. Toggenburgs are adaptable to a variety of climates, and have, therefore, been found in West Indies. Venezuela, South Africa, Tanzania and in India. Average live weight is 60-65 kg.
Saanen	Originated in West and North-West Switzerland	75 to 90	1.0 to 3.0 with 3.5% butter fat	White to biscuit in colour with black spots on the nose, ears and udder. The breed is polled.	The goats are large in size with straight nose and erect ears pointed forward and upward. The body has a good dairy conformation and the udder is well developed. It is known as *milk queen* of the goat world. There appears to be a tendency for them to be sensitive to strong sunlight and thus it needed to shade them and provide indoor management. Average live weight 55-70 kg.

In India there is no typical milk and meat breed. The breeds, which have a relatively higher milk production has been known as 'Milch breeds' while others are designated as 'Meat breeds' since these goats are used for meat production only. There is no mohair producing breed in the country. Chegu and Changthangi breeds produce '*pashmina*', other breeds of Northern-temperate region produce medullated fibres only.

Table 16.6 **Means with their standard errors for Pashmina characteristics**

Breed	Annual Pashmina yield (gm)	Staple length (cm)	Fibre diameter (micron)	Medullation %
Chegu	131.66±2.25	6.78±0.32	12.10±0.09	9.40
Changthangi	214.0	4.95±0.11	12.36±0.07	—

Anatomy of the Male Reproductive Tract of Goat and Sheep

The reproductive organs of the ram and buck are essentially similar, though there are noticeable differences in the sizes of the organs. The features of the male reproductive tract are shown in Figure(16.1.) The basic organs are the testes, the scrotum, the epididymides, the different ducts, the accessory or secondary sex glands, and the penis.

The testes

The testes are the male gonads or primary sex organs. They perform two major functions (i) production of male gametes (spermatozoa) and (ii) production of the male sex hormones (androgens). The two functions are related since production of spermatozoa is dependent on androgen production.

The testes of the ram are very large and reach 200–300 grams each in a healthy adult. The testes of the goat buck are somewhat smaller, weighing 100–150 grams each. In both species the size of the testes varies with season, reaching a maximum in the middle of the breeding season. This is important since numbers of spermatozoa produced are correlated with the size of the testes.

Each testis is covered with a tough, fibrous membrane called the *tunica albuginia*, which contains testiculer arteries and veins. Underneath is the main substance of the testis, the yellow-coloured *parenchyma*. The parenchyma consists of several lobules (Fig16.2) Each lobule contains long convoluted tubules, the *seminiferous tubules*, set in *interstitial tissue*. The seminiferous tubules are the site of production of spermatozoa. They drain towards the centre of the testis into straight tubules and from there into a network of ducts called the *rete testis*. The rete testis leads to the head of the epididymis.

The cells which produce spermatozoa, the *spermatogonia*, are located along the basement membrane of the seminiferous tubules where they are supported by specialised cells called *Sertoli cells*. As the sperm cells divide and mature they move from the basement membrane to the lumen of the tubules, and once released into the lumen they are transported to the rete testis.

The interstitial tissue contains blood vessels, nerves, and some specialised cells, the *Leydig cells*, which are principally responsible for androgen production. Although there is some local action of

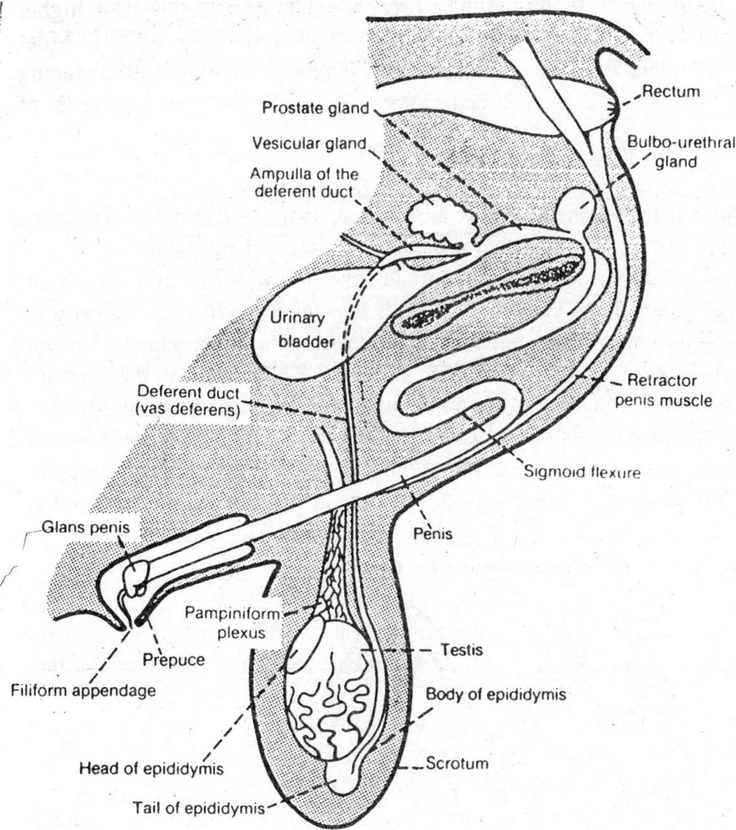

Fig. 16.1 *The reproductive organs of the male*

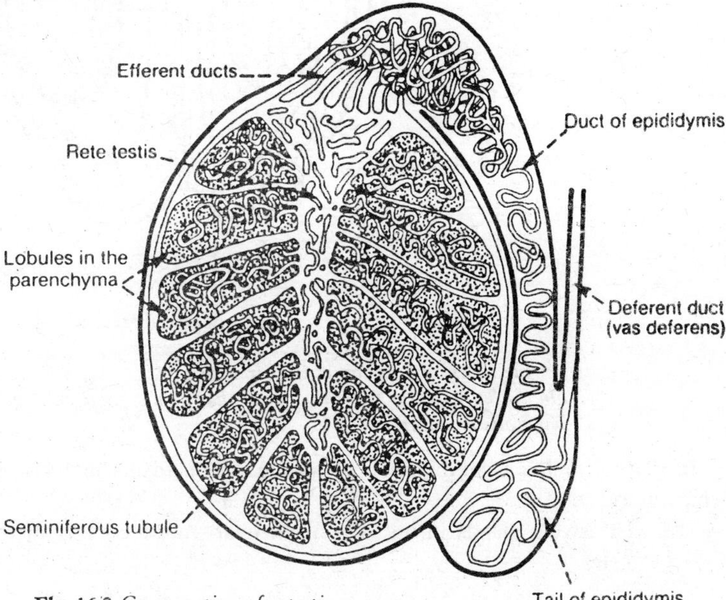

Fig. 16.2 *Cross section of a testis*

androgen within the testes, most of the hormone drains via the blood vessels to the general circulation. Here it acts as a growth promoter, producing the characteristic male body conformation, stimulates the male secondary sex characteristics, and acts on behavioural centres in the brain to promote male sexual behaviour.

The Scrotum

The scrotum is the sac or pouch in which the testes are housed. It has a distinguishable narrowing, or neck, above the testes and a septum which separates the left and right halves.

The wall of the scrotum consists of skin and two membranes, the *tunica dartos* and the *tunica vaginalis* (Fig. 16.3)The outermost layer of the scrotum, the skin, is covered with wool or hair and contains many sweat and sebaceous glands. The tunica dartos provides the main support for the testes. It is closely adhered to the skin and has a muscular structure; it also divides the scrotum into two halves, each containing a testis. A tunica vaginalis encloses each testis and epididymis.

The scrotum not only supports and protects the testes but has an important role in temperature regulation. Production of spermatozoa in the testes occurs normally at 4–7°C below body temperature. Males with undescended testes, that is those with testes kept in or close to the body core, are usually sterile.

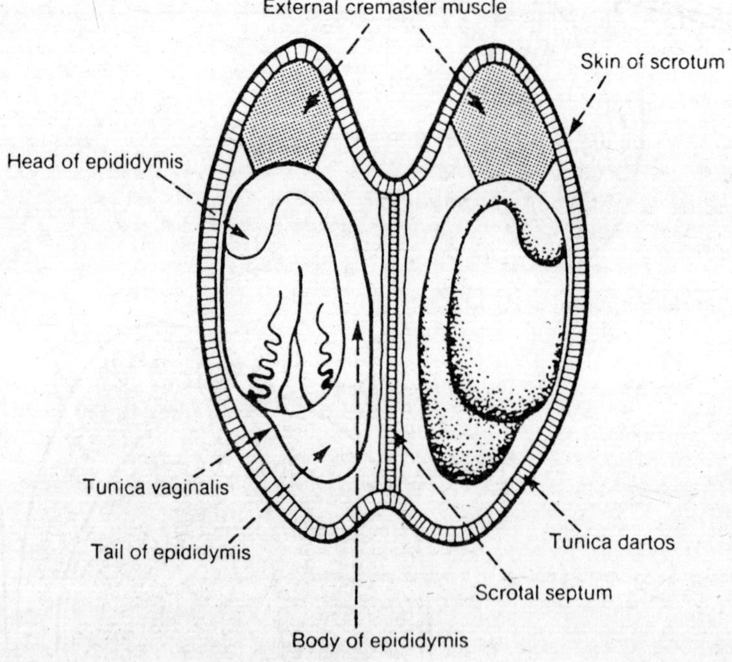

Fig.16.3 *Cross section of the scrotum*
On the left testis the tunica vaginalis has been cut. On the right testis the tunica vaginalis is intact

In normal males a combination of several mechanisms maintain the testes at the appropriate temperature:

(i) The sweat glands in the skin allow evaporative cooling of the scrotum and hence of the testes.

(ii) The tunica dartos muscle contracts or relaxes to regulate suspension of the testes close to or away from the body core according to ambient temperature.
(iii) The *external cremaster muscle*, which connects the tunica vaginalis to the abdomen, also regulates the closeness of the testes to the abdomen.
(iv) The *pampiniform plexus* (Fig.16.1,) an extensive blood vessel system in the neck of the scrotum close to the top of the testis helps to cool the blood supply to the testis.
(v) The wool or hair on the skin of the scrotum helps insulate the testes from the external environment.

In cold conditions the warming mechanisms are usually adequate to maintain proper testicular temperature and production of spermatozoa. However, in extremely hot conditions the cooling mechanisms may not be able to cope ('heat stress'), production of spermatozoa may be affected and temporary sterility may result.

The Epididymides

The two epididymides have an elongated form and are closely associated with the testes Each epididymis has three parts, namely the head (caput), the body (corpus), and the tail (cauda). The head is attached to the top of the testis, and the tail is at the bottom and can be palpated through the wall of the scrotum. There is no precise anatomical distinction between the three parts, though the body is considerably narrower than either the head or the tail. The epididymis comprises, for the main part, only a single convoluted tubule which is about 60 metres long in rams. Several efferent ducts drain the rete testis into this tubule in the head of the epididymis. The tubule increases in diameter towards the tail of the epididymis and the deferent duct, into which it drains.

The epididymides perform the vital functions of transport, maturation and storage of spermatozoa. When spermatozoa are released from the seminiferous tubules they are neither motile nor fertile. They acquire motility and the capacity to fertilise eggs only on passage through the epididymis. A great number of spermatozoa are stored in each epididymal tail (about 20–40 thousand million in rams, 12–16 thousand million in bucks) and are expelled into the deferent duct by contractions of the wall of the epididymal duct.

The Deferent Ducts

The duct which transports spermatozoa from the tail of the epididymis to the *urethra* (the central duct of the penis) is called the deferent duct, or *vas deferens*. One deferent duct is associated with each epididymis, and each one passes close to the body of the epididymis through the inguinal canal into the abdominal cavity. The two ducts meet at the urethra. The last 3–4 cm of each duct (called an *ampulla*) is thick and serves as a storage organ for spermatozoa.

The deferent duct has a strong, thick wall which can be felt through the neck of the scrotum; surgical sectioning of the duct at this point (vasectomy) results in sterility. This operation is used for preparation of teaser males.

The Accessory Sex Glands

This is a group of secondary sex glands in close apposition to the urethra and the junction of the deferent ducts (Fig.16.1)The glands produce fluids which empty into the male tract and mix with spermatozoa to form *semen*.

The accessory sex gland group comprises two *vesicular glands*, one *prostate gland*, and two *bulbo-urethral* glands. In rams and bucks the largest glands of the group are the vesicular glands. They are located close to the junction of the deferent ducts and the urethra. There is muscle present in the connective tissue of the glands, and contraction of this muscle at ejaculation expels the vesicular fluid.

The prostate gland surrounds the urethra behind the vesicular glands. The prostatic fluid drains into the urethra via several small excretory tubules.

The paired bulbo-urethral glands are spherical, compact glands located above the urethra near its exit from the pelvic cavity; secretory ducts release bulbo-urethral fluid during periods of sexual excitement.

The Penis

The penis has two functions, namely deposition of semen in the female reproductive tract and expulsion of urine. Both the semen and urine are voided through the urethra. The urethra is surrounded by a soft cavernous tissue which is well supplied with blood vessels and enclosed within a fibrous outer membrane.

The penis becomes rigid and extended upon sexual excitement. This process, called *erection*, is accomplished in two ways. Upon sexual excitement the vessels which drain the penis become constricted and the spaces in the cavernous tissue become filled with blood, thereby enlarging the penis. On relaxation the blood drains from the cavernous tissue and the penis becomes flaccid again. The penis also has an 'S'-shaped bend, known as the *sigmoid flexure* (Fig.16.1)which enables the penis to be extended (upto 30 cm) during copulation. The penis is normally held in the 'S' position by a retractor muscle; during copulation this muscle extends and the sigmoid flexure straightens out. Only at this time is the bulk of the penis exteriorised from the abdomen, and then only momentarily.

The penis is abundantly innervated with sensory nerve fibres, particularly in the bulbous end to the penis called the *glans penis*. Beyond the glans penis in the ram and the buck there is a narrow extension to the urethra, 3–4 cm long, called the *filiform appendage* (or urethral process). The filiform appendage (or urethral process) rotates rapidly during ejaculation and sprays the semen around the anterior vagina of the female.

The free extremity of the penis is housed in a loose invagination of skin called the *prepuce*, or sheath. Bacteria may accumulate in the *prepuce* and it should be thoroughly cleaned before semen collection. It is also wise to trim the long prepucial hairs.

Anatomy Of The Female Reproductive Tract Of Goat And Sheep

The reproductive organs of the ewe and the goat doe are essentially similar, with minor differences in the sizes and structures of the organs.

The ovaries :

Each female has two ovaries which have two basic functions, (I) production of female gametes, called ova, and (ii) production of the female sex hormones, predominantly

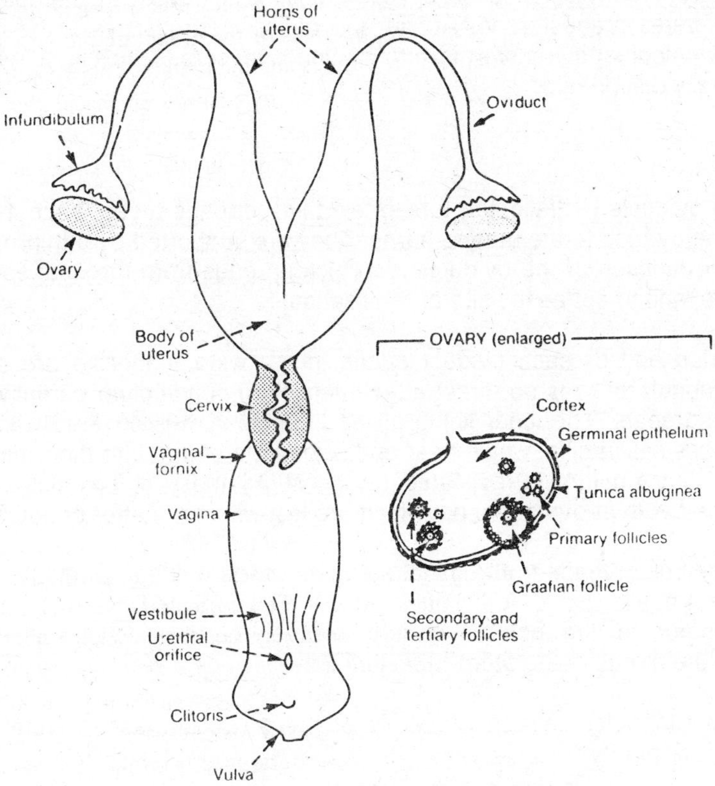

Fig. 16.4 *The reproductive organs of the female*

progesterone and oestrogen, which are essential for the development and maintenance of female characteristices, reproduction, and lactation.

The ovaries are located in the abdominal cavity behind the kindeys, and are supported by the broad utero-ovarian ligament. Each ovary weighs 0.6-3.0 gm, depending on the reproductive state of the female.

The surface of each ovary is covered by a single layer of flattened cells known as the germinal epithelium. Underneath is a layer of tough, dense connective tissue, the tunica albuginea, which surrounds the cortex, which is made up of ovarian stroma, follicles at various stages of development, and corpora lutea or corpora albicantia. The ovaries are well supplied with blood vessels.

Each ovarian follicle contains a single oocyte, which develops into a ripe ovum. A large follicle has an antrum, a fiuid-filled cavity surrounded by the follicle wall. The wall comprises two tissue types separated by a thin membrane, the basement membrane. On the inside of the membrane are the granulosa cells, which are cuboidal and 2 or 3 layers thick; on the outside are the theca cells. The theca and granulosa cells are responsible for follicular hormone production, predominantly oestrogen. After release of the ovum at ovulation, the follicle becomes transformed into a solid yellow body 0.5-1.0 cm in diameter, the corpus luteum, which secretes progesterone. At the end of the oestrous cycle, the corpus luteum becomes pale in colour and transforms into an inactive corpus albicans, resembling scar tissue, and gradually disappears.

The oviducts :

The two oviducts (or fallopian tubes) are thin, tortuous tubes, each 10-20 cm long, extending from the ovaries to the uterine horns. They are supported by a thin membrane (the mesosalpinx). The function of the oviducts is to pick up eggs from the ovaries and transport them to the uterus, and to act as the site of fertilisation.

The ovarian end of each oviduct opens into a wide funnellike process called the infundibulum. Although there is no direct attachment the infundibulum partially encloses the ovary in sheep and goats. The inner lining of the infundibulum is covered with microscopic, finger-like processes called cilia, which bear and sweep the ovum into the tubes. Passage of the ovum to the infundibulum is facilitated by the sticky mass of cumulus oophorus cells which surround the ovum at ovulation, but which are lost within a matter of hours thereafter.

The infundibulum leads to the initial segment of the oviduct, a relatively broad tubal protion called the ampulla. Here fertilisation occurs. The fertilised ovum, then travels down the remaining portion of the tube, which is a relatively narrow section called the isthmus. The oviducts join the uterus at the utero-tubal junction.

There are glandular cells in the walls of the oviduct; these secrete fluids which maintain the ovum or embryo.

The uterus :

The organ consists of two horns and a body. In ewes and does the two uterine horns (9-16 cm long) are joined at the bifurcation. The body of the uterus is short (3-5 cm), and is divided close to the bifurcation by a short septum. Implantation of an embryo and development as a foetus occurs within one of the horns of the uterus. Ovulation occurs randomly between each side. The wall of the uterus consists of three layers, the outer epithelium, the myometrium, and the inner endometrium. Foetal attachment occurs at special sites called caruncles; there are 70-100 of these mushroom-like projections lining the interior surface of the horns.

The cervix :

The cervix is 4-7 cm long and connects the uterus to the anterior vagina. It has a relatively hard structure comprising connective tissue, musculature, and secretory glands on the inner lining. These glands produce cervical mucus and are particularly active at oestrus. The spermatozoa must swim through the cervical mucus to reach the uterus.

The internal wall of the cervix has a number of ridges and crypts which fit together so as to make the cervix directly impassable. This has the effect of sealing off the uterus from the vagina, thereby keeping out infection. In the ewe, the cervical folds fit so closely together that there is only a thin tortuous lumen in the middle of the cervix. In goat does, however, the lumen is much more open, particularlyat oestrus. The posterior end of the cervix projects into the vagina and forms one or more folds or flaps of fibrous tissue which are readily distinguishable from the vaginal wall.

The vagina :

The vagina is the female organ in which semen is deposited during copulation in sheep and goats. It is a common passage for both the urinary and reproductive systems.

The anterior part of the vagina, which contains the entrance to the cervix, forms, a recess, called the vaginal fornix. Posterior to it is the vestibule, a short, narrower portion which closes the vagina off from the exterior. The urethral orifice is located in the lower posterior part of the vestibule. The vestibule also contains secretory glands which produce mucus to lubricate the vagina when the female is in oestrus.

The wall of the vagina is well supplied with blood vessels and nerve cells. Its interior appearance changes depending on the stage of the cycle of the female; during oestrus it is moist and has a red flush. Females with a dry, pale-looking vagina are probably not in oestrus. The external and terminal part of the vagina is the vulva. In the ewe and doe it has a triangular form, with the tip down. The vulva may also have a red flush at oestrus; though this is more pronounced in the goat doe than in the ewe.

REPRODUCTIVITY PERFORMANCE

Reproduction in the Male

The male goats (bucks) have exceptionally high libido (sex desire) except with some European polled breeds particularly of Saanen breed. In this breed the dominant gene which prevents horn growth is closely associated with abnormal sexual development in homozygous polled females. Genetically males, whether polled or horned, are normal like that of heterozygous polled females. With only rare exceptions, all female homozygous polled are intersexes (hermaphrodites), i.e., are phenotypically having more male characters and infertile. Since intersexuality both overt and concealed, can cause severe economic loss, the only safe breeding policy for Saanen will be to mate all polled females to horned males or to use polled males on horned females. In this way the production of homozygous polled females can be avoided, but nearly half the kids will be horned.

A well grown buck-kid may be bred to doe (the female) during his first season at an approximate age of six months. However, the semen was very less in volume and motility score was too low. The age has a significant effect on the semen production.

From records, it appears that semen volume and sperm motility were significantly higher in adults than in 9 month old males. The semen quality of 4-5 months old kids were inadequate for breeding, although, their sexual libido was satisfactory. At the age of 18-24 months bucks may be allowed to serve 25-30 does, and when they attain full maturity 50-60 does in a breeding season may be permitted to serve. Age at puberty differs with the breed. Climatic factors, nutrition along with male reproductive hormones can modify puberty. The electro-ejaculates in bucks have higher ejaculate volume and lower sperm density. Bucks

Table 16.7 **Semen characteristics and other attributes of some Indian small and dwarf bucks**

Attributes	Black Bengal	Barbari	Malabari
1. Reaction time (Secs)	22.7± 1.19	30.60	49.39± 2.5
2. No. of mounts/ejaculate	1.66± 0.053	2.1	—
3. Volume (ml)	0.58± 0.041	0.92± 0.07	0.5± 0.3
4. Initial motility (%)	56.39± 1.279	60.80	71.03
5. Sperm concentration (10^6/ml)	2289± 38.23	2783± 158	3534± 176
6. Abnormal spermatozoa (%)	—	4.5± 0.6	6.12
7. Live spermatozoa (%)	—	68.3± 2.7	63.38± 2.58
8. pH	6.426± 0.031	6.59± 0.01	6.47± 0.16
9. Initial fructose (mg/100 ml)	1062.63± 19.55	1294.5± 15.10	611.94
10. ZO_2 value	16.62± 1.33	—	—

are mostly sexual in winter and spring. During this period they emit a strong odour characteristic to them. The buck when fed, keeps fit for breeding till 8–10 years of age.

B. Reproduction in the Female

The duration of oestrus is usually 24 to 48 hours but in certain breeds, for instance the Indian Beetal, it may be as short as 18 hours on the average. Recurrence of estrus cycle is 18–21 days intervals unless pregnancy occurs. The gestation period is from 145 to 153 days (5 months). Indian goats commonly kid twice in one year and usually three times in two years.

The reproductive activity of goats, like that of sheep, is induced by the shortening length of the day. In India where there is little seasonal difference in the length of the day, the oestrus cycles recur throughout the year. Generally, the incidence of oestrus is highest from May to October. They can be bred in other months also, but during winter the servicings are less effective due to short heat periods. For milch purpose breeds it is better to have one kidding in a year, as the kids keep better health and the lactation period is prolonged.

Sexual desire in female kids have been noticed at an early age of their 14 weeks. Body weight climate, nutrition and even presence of male has been found to modify age of puberty apart

from breed characteristics. In one study at I.V.R.I. (1974) it has been observed that Barbari nannies attain their puberty between 9–10 months whereas Anglo-Nubian takes about 15 months time to reach puberty stage. For getting good results, goats should be bred at the age from 14 to 18 months and should kid for the first time when they are about two years of age.

Does which are shy breeders pass their heat period unnoticed, and do not show any other signs except a slight redness of the genital opening. Bringing the buck near the female for a short time every morning during the breeding season is generally helpful in picking up those in heat.

In does a peculiar behaviour has been noticed where does occasionally accept the male even when they are pregnant. It is not clear why this feature is relatively common in goats and it may well be a species characteristics. It is also not known whether in such cases oestrus occurs and if it does occur whether it is accompanied by any ovulation.

Table 16.8 Characteristics of reproductive cycle and female fertility in some Indian goat breeds

Elements	Barbari	Black Bengal	Malabari
Length of oestrous cycle (days)	19±0.4	20±0.4	20.5
Duration of oestrous (hrs)	38±0.9	40.50	52
Post partum oestrous interval (days)	50.5	61.2	65
Duration of post partum oestrus (hrs)	34	—	52
Doe fertility			
a) No. of inseminations per conception.	—	1.14	2.4
b) Litter size	1.56	2.04	1.6
c) Incidence of multiple births			
Singles (i)	45.6	20.14	47.0
(%) (ii)		22	43.4
Triplets (i)	2.5	25.36	10.6
(%) (ii)		21	6.9
Quadruplets (i)	—	13.43	Occasional
(%) (ii)		3	
d) Kidding interval (days)	238	223.8	289.1
e) Total annual births per 100 does*	239	333	201
References	87, 106 107	29, 72	27, 34

*Calculation based on litter size and kidding interval.

In general, although two kiddings from a doe per year is theoretically feasible but in practice (except Black Bengal goats where yearly two kiddings are common) three kiddings in two years is attained. Meat breeds commonly have a shorter kidding intervals than milk breeds presumably because of the influence of the length of lactation. For example, goats in India and Malayasia the interval between kiddings is 90–120 days but for pure bred and crossbred Anglo-Nubian goats it is 327 and 204 days respectively. The time of ovulation of goat is towards the end of estrus.

Under ordinary conditions, the average life of goat is about 12 years. She should give milk for about 10 lactations. if kidding is taken once a year. A goat is at her prime when 5–7 years of age.

Signs of Heat

1. **The doe (she goat) becomes restless, shakes its tail, dislikes to eat feed properly.**
2. **Sudden drop of milk-yield.**
3. **Swelling and slight redenning of the genital opening.**
4. **Mounting on other goats irrespective of sex.**

Pregnancy diagnosis in goats

A number of tests have been tried for detecting pregnancy in goats at an early stage.

1. *Non-return to Oestrus*

Post breeding/insemination non return to oestrus gives a good idea for detection of pregnancy settling. But at the end of breeding season this is no longer trust-worthy.

2. *Laparotomy*

Gives 90-95% accuracy in goats of 5 weeks gestation.

3. *Laparoscopy / Endoscopy*

Pregnancy can be detected at 40 days of gestation in goats.

4. *Ultrasonic technique*

As it gives immediate results it can be adopted for field use.

5. *Hormonal assay*

With the help of Radio Immuno assay (R I A) and ELISA techniques pregnancy may be diagnosed at a much earlier stage with an accuracy of 95%.

FEEDING HABITS OF GOAT

1. By means of their mobile upper lips and very prehensile tongues, goats are able to graze on very short grass and to browse on foliage not normally eaten by other domestic livestock.

2. Goats have fastidious eating habits. They will accept a wide variety of feed, appreciate it and thrive on it, but what is acceptable to one goat is not always acceptable to others. In general goat will refuse any kind of feed which has been soiled either by himself or by other animals.

3. Goats consumes wide varieties of feeds and vegetation than either sheep or cattle.

4. It has been shown that goats can distinguish between bitter, sweet, salty and sour tastes and that goats have higher tolerance for bitter tastes than cattle.

5. Goats will consume certain species at definite stages of maturity and reject them at other times.

6. The rumen is not developed at birth, but young kids start picking at hay or grass at 2–3 weeks of age and by 3–4 months the rumen is fully functional.

7. Unlike sheep, goats relish eating aromatic herbs in areas of sparse food supply, and hence can penetrate deep into the desert.

8. Browse (by browsing is meant the eating of leaves of bush and trees) forms an important part of the diet of goats. It has been observed that when goats find opportunities to browse for about 8-9 hours a day the goats can take care of their maintenance and slow rate of growth but if goats are to produce large quantities of milk or are to grow quickly and to yield high quality meat, they must have additional leguminous fodders as well as concentrate feeds as per recommendation narrated else where in this chapter.

Table 16.9

Apparent digestibility of various dietary constituents by different ruminant species.

Constituent	*Goat*	*Sheep*	*Cattle*	*Buffaloes*
Dry matter	59.7	59.9	53.5	54.1
Organic matter	64.0	62.6	56.4	56.9
Crude protein	66.4	64.1	49.5	47.5
Ether extract	71.2	73.4	62.9	74.1
Crude fibre	66.9	64.3	61.6	62.0
Nitrogen-free extract	60.9	60.2	52.9	53.2

SOURCE: Jang, S., and B.N. MAJUMDAR, 1962. A Study of Comparative Digestibilities in Different Species of Ruminants, *Ann. Biochem. Med.*, 22: 303–308.

9. The practical rationing of goats should be based on cheap foods such as browse pasture, and agricultural and industrial waste. In rationing goats, it must be firmly borne in mind that they cannot compete with pigs and poultry in efficiency of conversion of concentrates to protein food, nor under most circumstances, can they compete with advanced dairy cattle in utilisation of concentrates for milk production. Full advantage must, therefore, be taken of their remarkably high utilisation of cellulose, which gives them a special ecological niche in tropical farming communities.

10. Despite goats similarity to other livestock in general digestive efficiency, there is considerable evidence that it is exceptionally efficient at digesting crude fibre (cellulose). Jang and Majumdar compared the digestive efficiency of goats, sheep buffaloes and cattle fed on spear grass (*Andropogon-contortus*) in its post-flowering stage and groundnut cake. Crude fibre is exceptionally well-digested by goats. They have also observed that excepting ether extract, goats and sheep utilised the nutrients in the feed better than cattle or buffaloes. Table 159. summarises the comparative digestibilities of the various constituents by the four ruminant species.

11. Paht et al., (1963) reported the species variation in rumen metabolic reactions with reference to NH_3 and total volatile falty acids (TVFA) production at different intervals after feeding.

Table 16.10

Pattern of NH_3 and VFA production in the rumen of different species at various intervals after feeding.

Species	*Time in hours (NH_3 mg/100 ml CRL)*					*TVFA (in eq/L CRL)*
	0	*2*	*4*	*6*	*8*	
Buffalo	16.1± 1.18	28.2± 1.50	22.3± 0.86	15.9± 0.81	13.8± 0.76	62.8± 1.24
Sheep	21.9± 1.7	27.8± 1.54	—	—	17.9± 1.12	65.7± 2.2
Goat	26.1± 0.4	33.1± 1.53	—	—	26.3± 2.5	73.5± 2.08

SOURCE: Pant, H.C., M.D. Pandey, J.S. Rawat and Roy, A. (1963), *Indian Jr. of Dairy Sci.*, Volume 16, page 29-33.

It would be noticed that the concentration of the two important constituents, NH_3 and TVFA is least in buffalo and highest in the goat with sheep occupying the intermediate position. The pattern of appearance and disappearance of NH_3 in the goat was such as to suggest that the synthetic mechanism in this species seems to have less developed.

The factors other than species affecting VFA and NH_3 production in rumen are the solubility of the feed, digestibility, particle size, amino acid composition of the protein, presence of other nitrogenous compounds and the level and nature of the carbohydrate material in the diet also influence the rate of production and utilisation of ammonia.

12. There is evidence that the basal metabolic rate and thyroxine production of goats are higher than in sheep and cattle, which may be why goats appear to require a some what greater maintenance ration than is usually recommended for sheep and cattle.

13. For its size a goat can consume substantially more feed than either cow or sheep. In terms of dry matter (DM) consumption the records even up to 11 per cent of the body weight has been observed compared to only 2.5 to 3 per cent in case of cattle and sheep. Thus there appears to be a distinct difference in intake between meat and dairy type. Meat goats have a DM intake of 3 per cent of their live weight. For dairy goats it has been considered that they should have a DM intake about 5-7 per cent of their live weight. This simply implies that goat can satisfy their requirement both for maintenance and as well as for production out of good fodder and pasture alone. For practical purpose it is desirable to offer concentrates or grain mixtute to all milking and pregnant dry does and also to young stock as they will grow faster. Give more than one cereal grain as it adds variety and palatability.

14. Goats are fond of leguminous fodders. They do not relish fodders like sorghum (*sorghum vulgare*) and maize (*zea mays* L.) silage or straw. They reluctantly eat hay prepared from forest grasses, if cut in early stages, but very much relish hay prepared from leguminous crops.

15. The nutrients conversion efficiency for milk production of a dairy cow is on an average 38 per cent, whereas for goat it ranges between 45 to 71 per cent.

16. Goat has also an outstanding mineral requirement. A small body with a high metabolic rate; a digestive system occupying at least a third of its body, and producing milk richer in minerals than the cows Usually the mineral mixture is added to the concentrate at a 2 per cent level. Salt should also be offered in a separate box for *ad libitum* consumption. The composition of the following mineral mixture is given below as an estimates of the actual requirements.

Table 16.11

The Composition of Mineral Mixture Added at a 2% Level of the Concentrates

1.	Sterilised bone meal	... 35 parts
2.	Finely ground high grade limestone	... 45 ,,
3.	Iodised salt (made by dissolving 14 gms of potassium iodide in water and thoroughly mixing it with 136 kg of salt)	... 20 ,,
4.	Copper sulphate	... 22 gms/ton mineral mixture
5.	Zinc oxide	... 11 gms/ton ,, ,,
6.	Ferrous carbonate	... 11 gms/ton ,, ,,

Calcium and Phosphorus are the minerals needed in largest supply. It is recommended or to feed a mixture of equal parts of iodised salt and dicalcium phosphate at free choice, particularly when non-legume hays are fed. Trace mineral supplements should only be fed on the advice of a competent nutritionists.

17. The energy requirements for maintenance in goats are similar to those of sheep, being 725.8 g starch equivalent (SE) per day per 100 kg live weight. For live weight gain the energy requirement would be 3.0 gm SE per kg live weight gain.

NUTRIENT REQUIREMENTS OF GOAT

Dry Matter

The dry matter (DM) intake is an important consideration since it reflects the capacity in terms of voluntary food intake to utilise the feed. With goats there appears to be distinct difference in intake between meat and dairy types. Meat goats have a DM intake of 3–4 per cent of their liveweight whereas dairy goats have a DM intake of 5–7 per cent of their liveweight. The other factors which affect the DM consumptions are availability of feeds, palatability, moisture content and amount of fibrous material present in feed.

Dry matter requirements as has been observed by ICAR for kids with 10, 15, 20, 25 and 30 kg body and growing at the rate of 50g/day are 425, 600, 700, 800 and 950 g respectively. For maintenance of adult it seems to vary between 66.0 to 70 g/$W^{0.75}$. Variations observed might be due to the size of the species and density of the energy in the feed. However, DM intake of pregnant goat was found to be 2.96 kg/100 kg body weight and 76.30 g/$W^{0.75}$.

Energy

Energy is vital component of goat diets affecting the utilization of other nutrients and overall productivity. The basic maintenance requirement for energy in goat diets is similar to the requirements for sheep. Additional energy is needed in the diet for increased activity, type of terrain, amount of vegetation on range, and distance travelled to get feed. Stall-fed goats with minimum activity need a basic maintenance level in the diet. Light activity requires about 25% more energy. Goats on hilly, semiarid range land need an increase of about 50% above basic maintenance requirements. When vegetation is sparse and goats must travel long distances to graze, the energy requirement is about 75% above the basic maintenance requirements. Wool type goats viz., Angora, Gaddi and Pashmina goats require more energy in the diets after shearing, specially during cold weather.

Energy requirments can be made by good quality roughages in the diet, except for early weaned kids, for does during the last two months of gestation, and lactating dairy goats. Concentrate needs to be added in the diet to meet the energy requirements of these animals. Angora goats will respond to supplemental feeding of grains with higher production of mohair. Goats will also gain weight faster if more energy is provided in the diet.

Energy deficiency will cause growth retardation, delayed puberty, decrease in fertility rate and also lower milk production. With continued deficiency of energy, goats may loose the strength of resistance to infectious and parasitic diseases.

Energy requirement for growth has been found to be 7.25 Kcal ME/g gain, which is equivalent to 4.09 Kcal NE (NRC, 1981). Energy requirement of kids at 10, 15, 20, 25 and 30 kg body weight and growing @ of 50 g/day was found to be 275, 350, 400, 450 and 500 g TDN, respectively (ICAR, 1985). For maintenance average energy requirement has been found to be 105.12 Kcal ME/Kg $W^{0.75}$ per day. For pregnancy energy requirement varies between 194.7 and 228.5 Kcal ME/Kg $W^{0.75}$. The energy value for milk production has been noted to be similar to that of cow i.e., 1218.17 Mcal/Kg of 4% FCM.

Protein

The basic requirement for protein in goat diets is similar to that of sheep and dairy cattle. A minimum level of 6% total protein needs to be provided otherwise feed intake will be reduced. This leads to deficiencies in both energy and protein, which results in reduced rumen activity and lowers the efficiency of feed utilization.

Additional protein is required in the diet for growth, pregnancy, lactation and mohair production. Goats on range need higher levels of protein in the diet than do stall-fed goats because of the increased activity required to get feed. Adding concentrate to the ration will provide the additional protein needed. An excessive amount of protein in the diet of goats with light activity is also undesirable.

Urea may be used to replace part of the protein needed in goat diets. However, urea should never be added to the rations of lactating dairy goats as it will cause toxicities. On the other hand urea has been used successfully upto 1/3 of the total crude protein in forage diets. In concentrate part of the diet upto 1/2 of the protein may be replaced with urea if the goats are fed green forages. Sulphur must be added to urea containing rations generally at a 10:1 ratio of nitrogen to sulphur. It requires about three weeks for the rumen to adapt to the use of urea in the diet.

The most commonly used protein supplements are linseed meal, soyabean meal, brewers' dried grains, and cotton seed meal. One of the most economical sources of protein is good-quality lucerne hay, fed as long hay, chopped hay or pellets.

Protein deficiency symptoms in goats are anorexia, loss of weight, poor hair growth, depressed milk yield and impaired reproduction. Severe deficiencies can lead to digestive disturbances, anaemia and/or edema.

Minerals

Generally, feeds used in goat nutrition provide adequate quantities of the necessary minerals. In some instances, deficiencies may occur, specially of the major minerals. Of the macro minerals that have been shown to be supplemented in goats are salt (sodium and chloride), calcium, phosphorus and sulphur.

Sodium chloride. Lactating does often requires additional salt as milk contains high amounts of sodium. The recommended level is 0.5% of the ration or may be fed at free choice. The mineral helps to maintain pressure in body cells, upon which depends the transfer of nutrients to the cells, the removal of waste materials, in making bile. The chlorine is important for preparing HCl of gastric juice so vital for protein digestion.

Calcium. Must be added to the diets of lactating goats. Milk fever can occur when calcium levels in the blood drop. Apart from this, necessary for bone development, for maintaining the contractability, rhythm, and tonicity of heart muscle etc. The recommended ratio of calcium to phosphorus ranges from 2 : 1 to 4 : 1. If the ratio falls below 2 : 1, urinary calculi may develop in males.

Phosphorus. Deficiency may occur with goats grazing on range lands if the forage is deficient in this mineral. Being essential for sound bones and for the assimilation of carbohydrate and fats, a vital ingredient for protein in all body cells may be provided through defluorinated phosphate, dicalcium phoshate, steamed bone meal and monosodium phosphate.

Vitamins

Goats on range or pasture will usually get enough of the necessary vitamins in the diet. A vitamin supplement may be necessary for goats on high producing lactating stage.

PRACTICAL FEEDING OF GOATS

Despite similarities in sheep and cattle, goats differ markedly from them in grazing habits, sensitivity to sweet, salty, bitter and sour taste in accepting or rejecting the feeds. Goats are more tolerant of eating feeds containing bitter principles and refuse any soiled feed.

In general goat feeding agrees with the expectations based on "universal" formula of feeding ruminants. However, it is noted that (i) a goat generally produces more milk than a cow from the same quantity of nutrients. The nutrients conversion efficiency for milk production of a dairy cow is on an average 38%, whereas for goat it ranges between 45–71%. It has been observed that goats were 4.04% superior to sheep, 7.90% to buffaloes and 8.60% to cows in crude fibre utilization, (ii) a goat uses less feed for its maintenance than a cow and (iii) a goat

Table 16.12

•A Feeding Guide For Goat

Age and Stage of Production	Feed Ingredients	Daily Amount to be fed
Birth to 3 days	Colostrum	Ad libitum
3 days to 3 weeks	Whole milk or replacer	450 c.c.
	Water, salt	Ad libitum
3 weeks to 4 months	Whole milk	450 c.c upto 8 weeks
(Start minimizing milk &	Creep feed	450 g daily
completely stop it when	Lucerne hay	Ad libitum
kids attain 4 mo.)	Water, salt	Ad libitum
4 months to freshening	Conc. Mixture	15–16% C.P. @ 450 g
Dry pregnant	Conc. mixture	15% C.P. @ 400–500 g
	Lucerne hay	Ad libitum
	Water, salt	Ad libitum
Milking doc	Conc. mixture	@ 350 g for each litre of milk
	Trace mineralized salt,	1%
	Molasses	5–7% of conc. mixture
Buck	Only pasture	Non-breeding season
	Conc. mixture	@ 400 g daily at breeding season

uses more fodder for digestion and metabolism than a cow does. No systematic studies have yet been made regarding the requirement of nutrients for various ages and physiological stages of goats in India. However, on the basis of limited work done at Indian Veterinary Research Institute, National Dairy Research Institute, R.B.S. College at Agra, and various other Research Institutes of the country and of the work done in foreign countries including NRC, the following recommendations have been made specially about the nutrient requirements at various ages and physiological conditions of goat.

Feeding Kids

Kids must receive colostrum from the doe within one hour after birth and should continue for 3 days as (i) the total energy reserves of new born kids from well fed does is about 800–900 kcal and kids of under nourished does only 400 kcal. These reserves would be adequate to meet the energy demand in drying the birth coat in a reasonable warm environment, but in winter the heat loss could well approach 150 kcal/hour in kids weighing 3 kg body weight. Thus after the reserves are over and if the suckling is not established, the kids will die, (ii) colostrum is rich in all essential nutrients, (iii) it provides antibodies for protection of many diseases and (iv) it has got laxative properties, cleans from its intestine the accumulated faecal matter known as *meconium*, which is often of a dry, putty-like nature.

In a large herd, the weaning should be practised just after the birth of the kids. If need be in these cases instead of natural suckling, kids may be fed colostrum or dams milk by bottle or pan. (Kids may be weaned as late as six month). After feeding colostrum for 2–3 days, change to whole milk or milk replacer if they are not nursing. Milk replacer are used to save goat milk for human consumption and also to get a faster gain in kids. Feeding replacer may

Table 16.13 **Feeding schedule for kids (Kurar and Mudgal, 1978).**

Body weight (kg)	Milk (ml/day)		Green fodder (kg/day)	Concentrate (g/day)	Composition of kid starter	
	Morning	Evening				
2.5	200	200	-	-	Gram	20.0
3.0	250	250	-	-	Maize	22.0
3.5	300	300	-	-	GN cake	35.0
4.0	300	300	-	-	Min. Mix.	2.5
5.0	300	00	Ad-lib	50	Wheat	
6.0	350	350	-do-	100	bran	20.0
7.0	350	350	-do-	150	Common	
8.0	300	300	-do-	200	Salt	0.5
9.0	250	250	-do-	250		100.0
10.0	100	150	-do-	350		
15.0	100	100	-do-	350		
20.0	-	-	1.5	350		
25.0	-	-	2.0	350		
30.0	-	-	2.5	350		

GN cake - groundnut cake; min. mix. - mineral mixture

be continued till kids are 4 months old. Number of feeding should be thrice daily for one week after birth followed by twice daily. Over feeding of milk may cause loose bowels. The total amount of milk to be fed may gradually be increased by the time kids are six weeks old. Practice mixing of milk replacer with milk. Cows milk may be used in place of goats milk after the kids attain few days of age.

Provide a good legume hay (or fresh green grass) and calf starter along with fresh water at three to four weeks of age. Equal parts of cracked maize, crushed oats, wheat bran and 10% linseed meal may be fed as the concentrate mixture. *Rumen activity will develop quicker and kids will start chewing their cud by the time they are 3 to 4 weeks of age.*

Milk replacer may be fed until kids are four months old. During this time, feed roughages and grains.

From 4 months to breeding, kids may be fed roughages that will provide enough nutrients for normal growth. If low quality roughages are fed supplement the ration with a 12-14% protein ration used for dairy calve at the rate of 350 to 400 g daily. Do not allow growing dairy goats to become too fat. Reduce the intake of energy feeds as neccssary to prevent this.

Always provide clean, fresh water and minerals to kids as they grow. Commercial mineral mixture may be used.

Table 16.14

Feeding schedule for growing and adult stock (Feed per day) followed at N.D.R.I., Karnal

Body weight (kg)	*Milk (g)*		*Concentrate mixture (g) of kid starter (g)*	*Green fodder (kg)*	*Others*
	Morning	*Evening*			
2.5	200	200	—	—	Sulmet 5 ml from 5th day upto 3 days. Benminth 1/2 tab. 10th day. Piparazins 5 g in 2 days at 1 month age. Benminth 1 tab at 1¼ mth. age. Phenovis 5 g in 2 days at 2 months age. Benminth 1 tab at 3 months age. Following deworming at the onset and at the end of monsoon season every year or during flock worm infestation period
3.0	250	250	—	—	
3.5	300	300	—	—	
4.0	300	300	—	—	
5.0	300	300	50	Ab lib	
6.0	350	350	100	,,	
7.0	350	350	350	,,	
8.0	300	300	200	,,	
9.0	250	250	250	,,	
10.0	150	150	350	,,	
15.0	100	100	350	,,	
20.0	—	—	350	1.5	
25.0	—	—	350	2.0	
30.0	—	—	350	2.5	
40.0	—	—	400	4.0	
50.0	—	—	500	5.0	
60.0	—	—	500	5.5	
70.0	—	—	500	6.0	

(Contd.)

Table 16.14 (*Contd.*)

Composition of kid starter (kg)	%	*Composition of concentrate mixture (kg)*	%
Gram	20.0	Gram	15.0
Maize	22.0	Maize	37.0
Ground nut cake	35.0	Ground nut cake	25.0
Wheat bran	20.0	Wheat bran	20.0
Mineral mix.	2.5	Mineral mixture	2.5
Common Salt	0.5	Common Salt	0.5
	100.00		100.00

Green lucerne and berseem are normally preferred for stall fed goats.

Finisher ration

Since goats are slaughtered mostly for lean meat, the ration should be planned to include 30–40% of the dry matter from roughage source and the balance amount from concentrate portion having 12–14% protein and 60–65% TDN. Feeding concentrate more than this amount will yield fat in carcass. In general goat attains slaughtering age by 10–12 months having variable body weights (20 to 30 kg) as specific for various breeds.

Table 16.15

Concentrate mixtures for dairy goats

	(Approx. crude protein content)		
Ingredient	*14%*	*16%*	*18%*
	....	*of mixture*...............	
Ground maize	37.0	35.0	32.0
Crushed oats	37.0	35.0	32.0
Wheat bran	16.0	14.0	15.0
Soybean oil meal (45% CP)	9.0	15.0	20.0
Iodised salt	1.0	1.0	1.0

Table 16.16

Summary of the nutritional requirements of the goat

Nutrient	Requirement
I. Dry matter	2.5–3.0% of liveweight (meat goats): up to 8% of liveweight (milking goats)
II. Energy	
(a) For maintenance	725.8g SE/100 kg live weight/day
(b) for liveweight gain	3.0 g SE/g liveweight gain
(c) for milk production	300 g SE/kg milk
III. Protein	
(a) for maintenance	45–64 g DCP/100 kg liveweight
(b) for milk production	70 g DCP/litre milk
IV. Water	450–680 g/day for a goat weighting 18–20 kg.
V. Dry matter: total water intake ratio	1:4
VI. Minerals	
Calcium	147 mg/kg liveweight
Phosphorus	72 mg/kg liveweight

SOURCE: Devendra L. and M. Burns, (1970), Goat production in the tropics, *Tech. Comw. Bur, Anim. Breed. Genet*, No. 19, *Comw, Agric. Bur.*, Farnham Royal, UK.

Feeding of Pregnant Goats

High quality roughages provide the basic nutrients needed during the last 6 to 8 weeks of gestation when 70 to 80% gain in foetal mass is made. Therefore, liberal feeding of quality leguminous fodder and concentrate having 25% protein should be offered between 400 to 500 g depending upon the condition of doe should be fed. A free choice lick of mineral mixture will take care for the calcium and phosphorus requirement of dam and foetus. Allow good grazing if available and make sure that does get plenty of exercise.

Several days before the does freshen (kidding) reduce the quantum of concentrate ration to one-half and add bran to provide more bulk. After kidding, feed a bran mash for a few days, gradually bringing the doe to the full feed for milk production.

Feeding of Lactating Goat

Nutrient requirements are higher during lactation. The ration for lactating does should contain high quality roughages like lucerne, berseem and other cereal grasses through which it will receive not only fresh nutrients particularly of minerals, vitamins and proteins but also the bulk needed for volatile fatty acids, viz., acetic, propionic and butyric needed for high milk production. To supplement more nutrients particularly of energy, cereal grains at the rate of 350 g for each litre of milk must be provided. The protein per cent may vary from 14 to 16%, the feed may be fed in two lots, at the time of morning and evening milking.

Add 1% trace mineralized salt and 1% calcium-phosphorus mineral mixture to concentrate mixture. Molasses (5 to 7% of concentrate mixture) may be used to increase palatability and to reduce dustiness of feed.

Keep a clean, fresh supply of water available at all times. After two weeks gradually increase the concentrate level to that suggested by milk yield. As soon as the doe leaves some concentrate, reduce the amount until she again cleans it up. The concentrate should be fed on individual requirement basis of each doe. This can be done most easily by feeding the concentrate at milking times.

Table 16.17

Nutrient requirements for lactation in the goat (per kg of milk)

Fat content of milk per cent	*Starch equivalent (SE) (g)*	*Dig. crude proten (DCP) (g)*	*Ca (g)*	*P (g)*
3.5	262	47	0.8	0.7
4.0	280	52	0.9	0.7
4.5	296	59	0.9	0.7
5.0	314	66	1.0	0.7
5.5	331	73	1.1	0.7

SOURCE: Devendra, C. and Burns, M. (1970), Goat production in the tropics, *Tech. Comm. Comw. Bur. Anim. Breed. Genet., No. 19.*

Feeding Breeding Bucks

During the non-breeding season, the buck does not require additional grain if he is on good pasture. During the breeding season, the same concentrate mixture fed to the does may be fed at the rate of 450–900 g (depending on the body weight) daily. Provide roughage free choice along with clean fresh water and minerals. Care must be taken not to allow the buck to get too fat. Reduce the intake of energy feeds as needed to prevent this. Make sure the buck gets plenty of exercise.

ROUTINE OPERATIONS

Handling of Goats

Goats are seldom difficult to handle and frequently learn to come for food and milking when called. They dislike being held by horns and ears and care should be taken not to disturb the nostrils. For an ideal handling it is preferable to hold them with neck or head collars.

Castration

It is done at the age of 2 to 4 weeks although castration at later stage is successful. For this method the Burdizzo's castrator is used. Care should be taken to pass the spermatic chord of each testis in two places, 1/2" apart. At that time testis should be held by hand in such a way that it never reaches near the hinge of the castrator. After castration there may be swelling of the testis which soon becomes normal within 2 or 3 days.

Advantages of castration

1. The palatability of the meat increases.
2. The body weight increases at a rapid rate.
3. The quality of the skin becomes superior.
4. The profit from such castrated goat is always more.

Dehorning

Dehorning is done to avoid keeping horned and polled goats together. It is practised within one week of birth by using caustic potash.

Care of the Feet

Goats frequently suffer from overgrown feet, a condition which causes much unnecessary discomfort and even deformity and arthritis in old age. These conditions can be prevented by pairing the hooves when they become overgrown.

Marking the goats

Three means for marking goats are ear-tattooing, ear-tagging and ear-notching which should be carried out with-in one week after kidding.

Tethering or Staking out the goat :

When there are only one or two goats being raised, tethering can be used. Even with this system goats need to be removed four times a day and given plenty of fresh water particularly in summer. A running tether has a long wire or rope staked at both ends where the tether is attached with some kind of ring. This gives the goat opportunity to forage in a wider area. The goats are tethered along the road side, public pastures and other grounds where there is vegetation. This is the most popular and common system accepted by the goat rearers in India, particularly landless and small dry-land holders and women, children, disabled and old can easily be entrusted with the work of goat keeping.

Exercise Paddock for Stall Fed Goats

When goats are reared in stall under constant confinement either as for research work or for some other reasons, it is of utmost importance to provide the exercise paddock. An enclosure measuring 12 m × 18 m is adequate for 100 to 125 goats. Some shade trees may be planted to provide adequate comfort in summer. The animals should be allowed to roam about in the enclosed area for some fixed period to have sufficient fresh air and exercise.

Goat Shelter or Housing

For efficient production in dairy goats, good health and comfort to the animal is a must. To achieve this, housing of goats is important. The house should protect the goats from sun, rain and cold nights. To prevent water logging the floor of the pen should be raised by about 1 - 1.5 meters from the ground floor. Slotted floors help in easy collection of manure and urine. To protect the goats from cold air a wall of at least 1.5 meter high should be built. If the floor is made of clay it should be compact and slopy towards one corner.

HOUSING

Goats come originally from the open mountains and do not like being closely confined. They like plenty of fresh air and love a clean and dry sleeping place.

Under village conditions, goats generally do not require any special housing. They should, however, be protected against bad weather and wild animals. Under farm and city conditions, it is economical to provide special housing for goats. Each pen may be 5′ in length, 2¼′ wide and 6′ high. This is enough for a pair of goats. Several pens may be made according to the number of goats. In case of milch goats, separate pens for lambs should be constructed at the very adjacent of the dam's pen. The partition between the mother and the kids should be such that both can see each other. The buck should be housed away from the milking goats. The house should have plenty of fresh air, sunshine and well drained. The materials for constructing goat's house may be of anything like bamboo, wooden or *pukka*.

Efficient Goat Shelter for Hot Zones

Scientists at the Central Institute for Research on Goats (CIRG) at Farah near Mathura have designed an effective and low-cost housing for goats. The high-roof shed covered with fire-proof material has been found to be cooler than housings made using conventional reeds, hay thatches and asbestos sheet.

The scientists have established that a shed with its main axis running east-west provides a cooler environment underneath, and it was the best for hot-arid conditions. The open type shed has an advantage over the closed ones. The width and size of the shelter vary with the animal size, and for goats and sheep the optimum has been determined to be five to six metres. The length will depend on the strength of the flock or herd.

The height of the shelter in the hot regions should be between three and five metres, and a height less than this will result in poor ventilation. The heat loss through radiation to cool sky is also curtailed in low roof shelter. The shape of the roof can either be flat, sloped or 'A' shaped. The A-type roof has definite advantages over the rest in the hot region, as one side of the roof will save the other half from direct solar radiation by casting its shadow. This helps in cutting down heat gain from the roof of the shelter.

Of the different materials used for the roof, the fire-proof tar-coated type has been found quite effective. Shelter surroundings should be kept as green as possible to avoid heating up of the shed. For good ventilation and to protect the animals from the direct hit of hot winds, the eastern and western sides of the sheds should be covered up to a metre height. The roof and walls should be white outside and coloured inside. Painting the side-walls white outside reduces the surface temperature inside by 12 to 22°C when compared to unpainted walls in places where temperatures remain above 37°C.

Water can be sprayed on the floor and roof of shelters periodically to reduce heat load on the animals during peak summer. The scientists have also prepared the details of sheds under loose housing system. Adult breeding goats or nannies are to be housed in groups of 60 to 80 goats. Milch goats should not be allowed to run together in their house for getting roughages and concentrates. They should be fed in separate stalls or in a group of eight to ten does.

Goats in an advanced stage of pregnancy, at least four to seven days before kidding, must be housed individually. Kids from one week after birth to sub-adult stages should be kept at the rate of 20 to 25 per shed. By making suitable partitions in a larger shed, unweaned, weaned but immature and near-matured kids can be housed separately. Drought-free small rooms to house 15 to 20 newly born kids are essential to raise a good breeding stock. The bucks should be kept away from the milking goats, in small groups of 10 or 15. Isolation sheds to keep sick and diseased animals must be provided far away from the rest of the sheds.

Besides housing, other facilities to store concentrate feed, medicine, dipping tanks and related material ought to be provided. Feeding and water troughs should be included within the housing shelters and care taken to ensure feed and water supply all the time.

CARE OF KIDS

Almost immediately after birth, the kids, if healthy and strong, are on their legs and make attempts for their mother's teats. Failure to reach the teats, however, is of no consequence, because the kids do not require nourishment for several hours after birth. If more than one kid is born, it may be necessary especially when they are very young, to ensure that the smallest of them gets its due share of milk, because it may be prevented from doing so by the stronger kids. In case the udder is too full, a proportion of the milk should be drawn from as otherwise the weight of the udder will cause discomfort to the animal. As soon as there is free flow of milk. the kids should be put to the teats, and if they do not suck properly, the teats should be held by the hand and pressed into their mouths. Once they have drawn a little of the milk, it will not be long before they take to the normal methods of suckling.

Generally, male kids are heavier than the female kids. At birth, a male kid of the Beetal breed will weigh about 3 kilograms and a female kid about 2-5 kilograms. For the first three or four days after kidding, goats milk like cows milk, is considered unsuitable for human consumption. This milk, the so-called colostrum, is yellowish in appearance and is viscous; it coagulates on boiling. It is nature's first provision of food for the new born and it must be given to the kids whether they are to be reared on the goat or artificially. Colostrum acts as a laxative and, because of its large contents of vitamin A and serum globulin, it confers immunity against certain diseases.

When about two weeks old, kids begin to nibble green food or dry fodder, and it would be well to see that small quantities of these are within their easy reach at this time. It is also important that kids are allowed plenty of open air and sunlight. In the hot weather, this can best be done by keeping them in an enclosure build round a tree so that they may also be provided with shade. The enclosure should be large enough to allow them plenty of exercise.

At the age of 2 to 3 months, the suckling may be practically discontinued and at four months the kids should be completely weaned because by this time they will become fit like the older goats to eat solid food, although they may as well be allowed to suckle a little longer.

Male kids, unless they are required for breeding purposes, should be castrated at the age of 2 to 3 months for it has been proved that castration improved the quality of meat. Otherwise, they should be kept separated from the female kids.

The rearing of kids may be either natural (with mother) or by hand rearing and each has its advantages and disadvantages. In India, it is the natural method that is usually practised and this consists of in leaving the kid to take what amount of milk it can obtain from its mother. Hand rearing is resorted to when weaning is practised or when the goat dies. There are two methods of hand rearing; one consists of feeding the kid with a bottle and the other is feeding it off the pail. Both methods are learned by them easily, but bottle feeding is to be preferred because the saliva that is produced during the process of suckling the milk aids digestion. Kids will also readily take to feeding on a foster mother when they are put on her teats.

As mentioned earlier, kids start nibbling solid food usually two weeks after birth. They become quite fitted for receiving concentrates in their feeds, when they are four months old. The quantity of these to be given will vary with the season but may be approximately 60 grams. Some goat breeders, who keep cattle for ghee production, usually give butter milk to kids at about two months prior to rearing; this is practised in all parts of the erstwhile Kutch state. Hand feeding is also the method commonly used by breeders of Barbari goats, in Etah district.

Male kids for breeding should be fed and handled in much the same way as doe kids, except for the fact that they require a little more milk as well as gram ration than the female kids on account of the larger size they have to attain. Kids with body size below normal should be discarded, as they seldom prove good breeders when mature. They should be fed well at all ages to keep them in good condition, but excessive feeding should be avoided, particularly when they are old because, if fat, they become sluggish and are slow breeders. Where the animal is unduly fat, its grain ration should be cut. At one year, a buck should receive 1.8 kg of grain mixture the allowance being increased by 50 per cent during the breeding season. A liberal amount of fodder should be given. An average of 7 to 8 kg of green fodder per day should be adequate for a full grown Jamunapari buck when entirely stall fed.

In order that the buck may be in good condition and well-suited for breeding it is desirable that it should be on range and graze some two to three miles each day. Bucks often become sluggish and slow breeders for lack of adequate exercise, because they are kept confined in small enclosures. For giving them exercise, they may be yoked to small carriages used for hauling light loads. A buck given plenty of exercise and kept away from does and also allowed company of other bucks will be very active during the breeding season. The buck's hoofs should be regularly attended to as otherwise it may develop foot rot or lameness.

Preventive health care for kids

1. At birth ligature of umbilical cord and application of tincture iodine for two days.

2. Disinfection of kid pens with phenyl (10% solution) or $CuSo_4$ (10% solution).

3. To prevent coccidiosis treatment with amprosol for 5-6 days.

4. Controlling ectoparasites (ticks, flies) by spraying malathion (0.5% solution).

5. Prevention of internal parasites by proper use of antibiotics and antiparasitc drugs.

6. Proper vaccination.

7. Isolation of sick kids from other healthy kids.

8. Check-up by good health specialist.

Table 16.18 Arithmetic mean and S.E. for some important carcass traits of Indian goats

Breed	Age at slaughter (months)	Weight at slaughter (kg)	Hot carcass weight (kg)	Dressing % on wt. at slaughter	Bone (%)
Beetal	5 m	15.64 ± 1.02	6.68 ± 0.46	42.71	—
	9 m	15.42 ± 0.65	7.66 ± 0.30	49.68	—
	12 m	20.33 ± 4.84	9.38 ± 2.74	46.15	23.21
Barbari	—				
	18 m	21.14 ± 0.48	10.55 ± 0.31	49.88	17.72
Jamunapari	6 m	15.56 ± 1.67	7.40 ± 0.92	44.57	—
	9 m	24.00 ± 1.16	11.56 ± 0.65	48.16	—
	12 m	22.92 ± 0.54	10.42 ± 0.23	45.47	21.31
	12 m	22.52 ± 0.97	10.40 ± 0.42	46.16	19.52
	14.5–18.5 m	23.37 ± 2.80	11.06 ± 1.30	47.32	—
Sirohi	6 m	21.80 ± 1.42	10.93 ± 0.84	49.90	13.80
	9 m	37.40 ± 0.62	21.80 ± 0.09	52.10	11.90
Jhakrana	6 m	23.20 ± 0.88	11.32 ± 0.68	48.80	12.82
Marwari	6 m	24.04 ± 1.38	11.76 ± 0.59	49.09	13.83
Kutchi	6 m	21.20 ± 1.20	10.85 ± 0.75	51.14	14.25
Bengal	6 m	10.63 ± 0.63	5.21 ± 0.41	48.82	—
	9 m	12.97 ± 0.91	6.16 ± 0.55	47.11	—
	12 m	11.59 ± 0.84	5.17 ± 0.44	44 62	23.42
	15-24 m	16.62 ± 0.59	7.40 ± 0.46	44.50	—
	24-39 m	22.06 ± 1.86	10.30 ± 1.23	46.60	—

Table 16.19 Age at puberty in males of various breeds

Breed	Age at puberty	Criterion for puberty
Jamunapari	225 days	separation of penis
Beetal	196 days	-do-
Barbari	180 days	-do-
Jamunapari	410 days	1st ejaculation
Beetal	377 days	-do-
Barbari	361 days	-do-
Black Bengal	267 days	-do-

Table 16.20 **Common Diseases of Goat**

Disease	Symptoms	Prevention & Treatment
Mastitis	Enlarged hot, painful udder. Fever. Milk watery with flakes of blood.	Improve hygiene. Application of antibiotics.
Foot rot	Lameness. Hoof will look as if it is rotten and it will smell bad. Signs of pain is seen if pressed.	Trimming, soaking in bath of water with $CuSo_4$
Brucellosis	Abortion in late pregnancy. Retention of placenta and metritis. In bucks infertility, orchitis and swollen joints are seen.	Isolation of infected animals. Vaccination. Blood testing and culling of positive animals.
Internal parasites	Loss of weight. Reduction in milk yield. Diarrhoea. Anemia.	Good quality food and clean water. Proper medication.
External parasites	Restlessness, scratching, loss of weight, reduction in milk yield.	Application of proper chemical as a dust, spray or a dip.
Poisoning	Unsteadiness followed by dullness and unconsciousness. Great pain and vomiting. Convulsion and eventual death.	Keeping goats away from poisonous plants and chemicals Immediate treatment.
Bloat	Distended abdomen on left side, respiratory difficulty, restlessness.	Too much fresh green grass should be avoided. A cup of mineral oil may bring relief. In acute cases removal of gas by making puncture is needed.

Table 16.21 **Vaccination Programme for Goats**

Months	Vaccine	Adult Goat	Kids (above 6 months)
January	Contagious pleuro pneumonia (C.C.P.P.)	0.2 ml I/dermal	0.2 ml I/dermal
March	Haemorrhagic septicaemia (H.S.)	5 ml S/c	2.5 ml S/c
April	Goat Pox	Scrach method	Scrach method
May	Entero toxaemia F.M.D.	5 ml S/c 5 ml s/c	2.5 ml S/c 5 ml S/c
June	Rinderpest	1 ml S/c	1 ml s/c
July	Black quarter	5 ml S/c	2.5 ml S/c
August	F.M.D.	5 ml S/c	0.5 ml S/c
September	Enterotoxaemia	5 ml S/c	2.5 ml S/c

Source: Schultz, R.D. and Scott, F.W. (1978). The Veterinary Clinics. North America. 8:755. W.B. Saunders Co.; Philadelphia, London, Toronto.

Determining the Age of Goats

By just looking at the lower jaw of the goat it will be easy to determine the age of the goat.

Goat is a ruminant and does not have any incisor teeth in the upper jaw but posses hard pad on the top while the lower jaw has eight incisors front teeth. The goats have toward the back of mouth large teeth called molars which help the goat in chewing the grass.

First year of the kid	:	The front teeth are small and sharp in goats with less than one year age.
Second yearling	:	The center pair of teeth fall out and are replaced by two permanent teeth.
Third year	:	Two more large front teeth appear on the side of the centre pair.
Fourth year	:	Six permanent teeth appear.
Fifth year	:	At this age eight permanent teeth appear in the front of lower jaw.

Some information about goat

1.	Birth weight of kid	:	0.94 kg Black Bengal 3.54 kg Jamunapari.
2.	Adult body weight of Indian goats	:	19 to 40 kg
3.	Body temperature	:	39 to 40.5^{0}C
4.	Age of puberty	:	4-5 months.
5.	Breeding season	:	In tropics (all year round) In temperate (Sept to Feb.)
6.	Duration of estrus	:	12 to 48 hrs.
7.	Pregnancy	:	146 to 154 days.

8. Average milk production is 800 gm/day/animal for 150 days.

Comparative Distinguishing Characteristics of Sheep and Goat

	Characteristic	*Sheep*	*Goat*
A.	***General***		
1.	**Chromosome number (2n)**	54	60
2.	**Domestication before to-day**	6,000 - 7000 yrs	8,500-9,000 yrs
3.	**Population x 10^6 (as on 2,000 A.D.)**	1,268.60 (World) 68.20 (India)	588.70 (World) 143.25 (India)
4.	**Annual growth rate (%)**	0.94 (World) 2.34 (India)	1.86 (World) 3.39 (India)
5.	**Number of breeds in India**	40	20
6.	**Position of India in the World's total population**	6th	1st
B.	***Physical Characteristics***		
7.	**Tail**	Generally long, hanging, fairly broad	Short, thin and Upright
8.	**Back and Withers**	Round & well fleshed	Sharp, little flesh
9.	**Thorax**	Barrel-shaped	Flattened laterally
10.	**Radius (shorter & thicker of the two bones on the same side as the thumb)**	1 & 1/4 times length of metacarpus	Twice as long as metacarpus
11.	**Scapula (triangular bone of the shoulder**	Short and broad, superior spine, bent back and thicken	Posseses distinct neck. Spine straight and narrow
12.	**Sacrum (a thick triangular bone situated at the lower end of the spinal column)**	Lateral borders thickened in form of rolls	Lateral borders thin and sharp
13.	**Flesh**	Pale red and fine in structure	Dark red and coarse with goaty odour. Sticky subcutaneous tissue which may have adherent goat hairs
14.	**General appearance**	Fatty and mostly roundish type	Taller, thinner and more angular
15.	**Body covering**	Wool, hair-wool and hair	Hair
16.	**Presence of bear**	No bear or any odoriferous tail gland	Beared and strongly odoriferous tail glands of the male

Characteristic	Sheep	Goat
17. **Face glands**	Present	Absent and no lachrymal pits in the skull
18. **Foot glands in hind feet**	Present	Absent
19. **Nature of horns**	Mostly homonymous	Heteronymous
C. Reproductive behaviour		
20. **Onset of puberty**	4 to 12 months	4 to 8 months
21. **Av. age first service**	12 to 18 months	12 to 18 months
22. **Length estrous cycle**	14 to 20 days	7 to 24 days
23. **Duration of estrous**	24 to 48 hours	16 to 50 hours
24. **Gestation period**	150 days	150 days
25. **Time of ovulation**	12-24 hours before before the end of estrous	25-30 hours after the onset of estrous
26. **Optimum time for service**	18-24 hours after the onset of estrous	12-20 hours after the onset of estrous
27. **Advisable time to breed after parturition**	usually in next winter	80-90 days after parturition
28. **Breeding life span**	5 to 8 years	6 to 10 years
D. Comparative feeding behaviour and digestive physiology		
29. **Activity**	Walk shorter distance	Bipedal stance and walk longer distances
30. **Feeding pattern**	Grazer, less selective	Browser, more selective
31. **Browse and tree leaves**	Less relished, preference is on grazing	Relished and high preference
32. **Variety in feeds**	Preference lesser	Preference greater
33. **Taste sensation**	Less discerning	More discerning
34. **Salivary secretion rate**	Moderate	Greater
35. **Recycling of urea in salvia**	Lesser	Greater
36. **Dry matter intake**		
- **for meat**	3% of B.W.	3% of B.W.
- **for lactation**	3% of B.W.	4-6% of B.W.
37. **Digestive efficiency**	Less efficient	Higher with coarse roughages
38. **Retention time**	Shorter	Longer

Characteristic	Sheep	Goat
39. **Water intake/unit DMI**	Higher	Lower
40. **Rumen NH_3 concentration**	Lower	Higher
41. **Water economy**	Less efficient	More efficient
- Turnover date	Higher	Lower
42. **Fat mobilisation**	Less evident	Increased during periods
43. **Dehydration**		
- Faeces	Relatively higher water loss	Less water loss
- Urine	Less concentrated	More concentrated

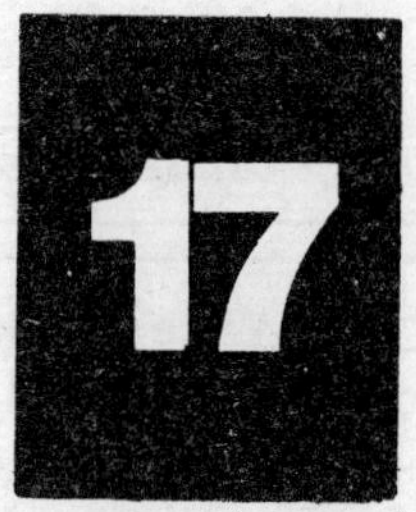

SHEEP

Domestic sheep belong to the phylum *Chordata* (backbone), class *Mammalia* (suckle their young), order *Artiodactyla* (hooved, even-toed), family *Bovidae* (ruminants), genus *Ovis* (domestic and wild sheep), and species *Ovis aries.*

Some common terms in relation to SHEEP

Details		*Expression*	*Details*		*Expression*
Species called as	...	Ovine	Castrated male	...	Wether or Wedder
Group of animals	...	Flock	Castrated female	...	Spayed
Adult male	...	Ram or Tup	Female with its offspring	...	Suckling
Adult female	...	Ewe	Act of parturition	...	Lambing
Young male	...	Ram lamb or Tup lamb	Act of mating	...	Tupping
Young female	...	Ewe lamb or Gimmer lamb	Sound produced	...	Bleating
New-born one	...	Lamb	Pregnancy	...	Gestation

During 1981-82 of the total world sheep population, U.S.S.R. ranked first (17.29 per cent), followed by Australia (16.72 per cent), China (12.79 per cent), New Zealand (8.83 per cent), Turkey (5.92 per cent), India (4.99 per cent), Iran (4.18 per cent) and U.K. (4.01 per cent).

Thus India ranks sixth among the countries of the world in respect to sheep population. The country has by now (1982-83) about 45.03 million sheep.

The Indian sheep population continued to be unaltered much and remained between 40 and 45 million for the past three decades. The production potential of sheep in India is estimated to be between 140 to 145 crores of rupees per annum. This is based on yearly production of about 40 million kg wool, 132 million kg mutton, 16 million pieces of skin and 22 million tonnes of manure.

Among wool producing countries of the world, Australia which has lesser number of sheep in comparison to U.S.S.R., is in top of the list due to high individual yield. Among rest of the countries which lead wool production after Australia are U.S.S.R., New Zealand, Argentina and China (including Taiwan) in decreasing order.

The average annual wool production per sheep is between 3.5 to 5.5 kg of quality wool in Australia, New Zealand and U.S.S.R. whereas in India except Magra (Bikaneri) sheep which annually yields on an average more than 2 kg having staple length of about 5.8 cm, the rest average is less than 1.0 kg per sheep of inferior quality wool.

Table 17.1

Wool Production in India

Year	1977	1982	1983	1984	1985	1986	1987
Production (million kg)	35.00	35.38	37.00	38.00	38.40	39.50	42.00

Instead of raw wool India exports woollen finished products like carpets, garments, shawls, blankets etc., to U.K., U.S.A., Canada, Italy, France, West Germany, U.S.S.R., Japan and Middle East countries. The extent of export withstand a lot of ups and downs.

Table 17.2

Income from Export

Year	1982-83	1983-84	1984-85	1985-86	1986-87
Income (Rs.) in crores	91.02	67.15	88.20	86.75	54.50

To meet various local demands India also imports superior quality wool, mainly to manufacture garments.

Table 17.3

Import of Raw Wool

Year	1979-80	1980-81	1981-82	1982-83	1983-84
Import (Rs.) in crores	31.9	43.1	30.2	28.03	31.03

Advantages of Sheep Farming

1. Sheep do not need expensive buildings to house them and on the other hand require less labour than other kinds of livestock.
2. The foundation stock are relatively cheap and the flock can be multiplied rapidly.
3. Sheep possess a special ability to thrive on natural grasses and, except during certain physiological stages of life, do not need to be given any supplemental feed. In fact there is no substitute for sheep as a class of livestock for utilising waste lands or weeds from the field. No domestic or wild animals are capable of existing on more different sorts of food. Weeds, grasses, shrubs, roots, cereals, leaves, barks and even in times of scarcity, fish and meats all furnish a subsistence to this wonderful animal.
4. Sheep are of economical converter of grass into meat and wool.
5. Sheep will eat more different kinds of plants than any other kind of livestock. This makes them excellent weed destroyer.
6. Unlike goats, sheep hardly damage any tree.
7. The production of wool, meat and manure, provides three different sources of income per year.
8. The structure of their lips helps them to clean grains lost at harvest time, and thus convert waste feed into profitable products.

9. Sheep dung is a valuable fertiliser, and since they are grazed on sub-marginal lands, their droppings are the only means of improving the growth of plants in such areas.

10. Mutton is one kind of meat towards which there is no prejudice by any community in India and further development of superior breeds for mutton production will have a great scope in the developing economy of India.

BREEDS OF SHEEP

Few countries in the world have no sheep. They are found in tropical countries and in the arctic, in hot climates and in cold, on the desert and in humid areas. There are over 800 breeds of sheep in the world, in a variety of sizes, shapes, types and colour.

India's vast genetic resources in sheep is reflected by the presence of 40 breeds of sheep. They are mostly evolved naturally through adaptation to agro-climatic conditions as they are generally been named after their place of origin or on the basis of prominent characteristics.

Broadly speaking, in India there are three main types of sheep, viz., (1) the temperate Himalayan region sheep, yield a mixed fleece of hair and fine wool; (2) the North Western region sheep, produce a wool useful for carpet manufacture, and (3) Southern region sheep have a hairy coat and good for meat and milk. (4) The Eastern region

I. Northern-temperate Region

The region extends from Jammu and Kashmir, Himachal Pradesh, hill districts of Punjab to Garhwal district of Uttar Pradesh. The steep gorgeous hills, rising from the plains, afford grazing facilities at different heights during the year. Rainfall in these areas is scanty. The flocks in the Kangra, Chamba, Kuler and Kashmir valleys when moved to higher altitudes produce wool of better quality. The area mostly comprises with mountains of various altitudes and valleys containing vast forests and pasture lands. The rainfall is moderate to heavy during monsoons and big mountains ranges above 2,500 metres are often subjected to snow falls during winters. Flocks are of migratory type. The region carries 7.6 per cent (3.09 million) of the total sheep population and produces 2.06 million kg or 6 per cent of the total wool produced in the country.

The following are the main breeds of this region.

GADDI

Synonym. Bhadarwah.

Origin and Distribution. It owes its name to the Bhadarwah tehsils in Jammu area of Kashmir State. They are also reared in the Kulu and Kangra Valleys and in the Chamba and Mandi districts of Himachal Pradesh. A class of nomad shepherds called Gaddis rear this breed.

Distinguishing Characters. The sheep are small in size but are very sturdy and very good climbers. They have short tail and ears, horned in the rams but polled in the ewes. They are mostly white, with coloured faces. Flocks graze high mountains during the summer and are moved to lower slopes for the winter.

Production. The fleece is relatively fine and lustrous and can grow to 5 in. length. It is clipped thrice in a year in February, June and October, yet produces a total of only 1 to 1.5 kg fine lustrous wool. The undercoat is used for manufacture of high quality Kulu shawls and blankets.

Table 17.4 Forty Breeds of Indian Sheep in different Agro-ecological Regions

Northern-temperate		*North-Western Arid & Semi-arid*		*Southern*		*Eastern*	
Breed	Distribution	Breed	Distribution	Breed	Distribution	Breed	Distribution
Gaddi	Kashmir Himachal Pradesh	**Chokla**	Rajasthan	**Deccani**	Maharastra Andhra Pradesh Karnataka	**Chottanagpur**	Bihar & W.Bengal
Rampur-Bushair	Himachal Pradesh U.P.	**Nali**	Rajasthan Haryana	**Nellore**	Andhra Pradesh	**Balangar**	Orissa
Bhakarwal	No distinct home	**Marwari**	Rajasthan	**Bellary**	Karnataka	**Ganjam**	Orissa
Karnah	Kashmir	**Jaisalmeri**	Rajasthan	**Hassan**	Karnataka	**Tibetan Sheep**	Arunachal Pradesh
Gurez	Kashmir	**Pugal**	Rajasthan	**Mandya**	Karnataka	**Bonpala**	Sikkim
Kashmir-Merino	—	**Malpura**	Rajasthan	**Mecheri**	Tamil Nadu	**Sahabadi**	Bihar
Changthangi	Kashmir	**Sonadi**	Rajasthan Gujarat	**Kilakarsal**	Tamil Nadu		
Poonchi	Kashmir	**Pattanwadi**	Gujarat	**Vembur**	Tamil Nadu		
		Muzaffarnagri	UP, Delhi, Haryana	**Coimbatore**	Kerala, Karnataka		
		Jalauni	Uttar Pradesh	**Nilgiri**	Tamil Nadu		
		Hissardale	—	**Ramnand White**	Tamil Nadu		
		Magra	Rajasthan	**Madras Red**	Tamil Nadu		
				Tiruchy Black	Tamil Nadu		
				Kenguri	Karnataka		

BHAKARWAL

Synonym. Nil.

Origin and Distribution. The breed originates from lower hills of Himalayas. They are reared by a nomadic tribe called Bhakarwal and hence the name of the breed. In summer flocks are reared over the high ranges of Pirpunchal mountains and in winter they move to the warmer low-lying hills of Jammu and Kashmir.

Distinguishing Characters. Rams are horned, while ewes are hornless with long, broad and drooping ears. The animals are long sized, sturdy and straight backed. In spite of big bulk they are excellent climbers.

Production. The sheep are clipped thrice in a year, March, June and September yielding about 1.5 to 2 kg of long coarse wool.

GUREZ

Synonym. Nil.

Origin and Distribution. The breed comes from Gurez tehsil situated in the high elevated zone of Kashmir State. They graze on nutritious grasses at about 2,500 m. in summer but are stall fed on stored grasses, maize and fodders in winters.

Distinguishing Characters. Biggest among the Kashmir breeds. The majority of these sheep are hornless and have short ears. The rams are virile and active and the ewes are good milkers. The tails are short but broad. Several varieties of colours are common in the breed but white predominates.

Production. The wool is of relatively good quality, being 6 inches long and lacking kemps. Average yield is about 1.5 kg. Mutton is considered to be of superior quality.

RAMPUR BUSHAIR

Origin and Distribution. The region covers Simla, Kinnaur, Nahan, Bilaspur, Solan and Lahaul and Spiti districts of Himachal Pradesh and Dehradun, Rishikesh, Chakrota and Nainital districts of Uttar Pradesh.

Distinguishing Characters. Medium sized animals predominantly white in colour with brown, tan and black are also seen on the fleece in varying proportions. The ears are long and drooping. Nose is Roman type. Males are always horned while females are polled. The fleece is of medium quality. Legs, belly and face are devoid of wool. Adult males weigh about 28 kg while females weigh 25 kg.

Production. Apart from meat the breed also offers annually about 1.0 kg greasy wool of low quality.

POONCHI

Origin and Distribution. Occurring in Poonch, a place situated at a high elevation in the state of Kashmir.

Distinguishing Characters. Majority of the sheep are hornless; tail is short and thick at the base,

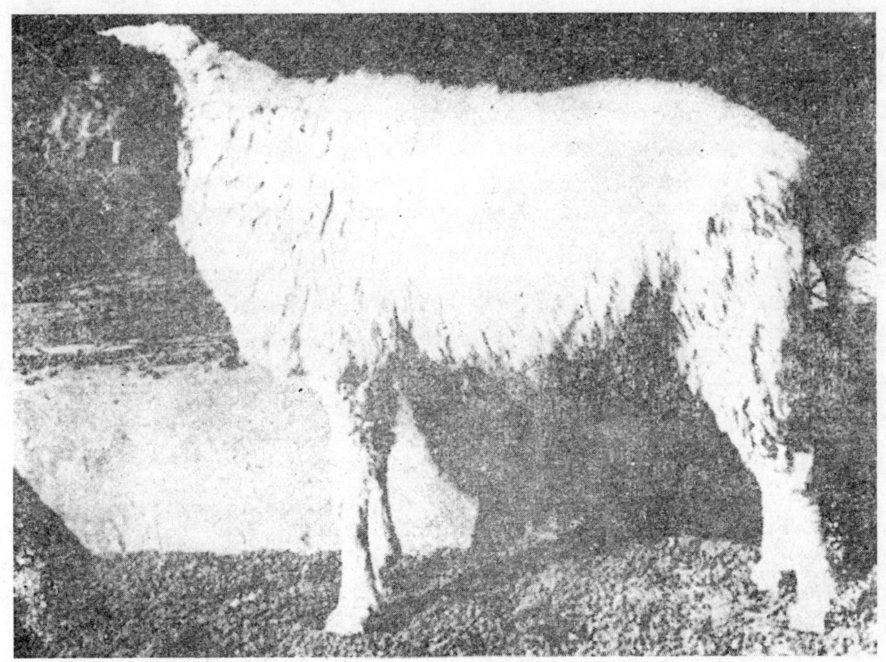

Plate 80. Adult Marwari female sheep.

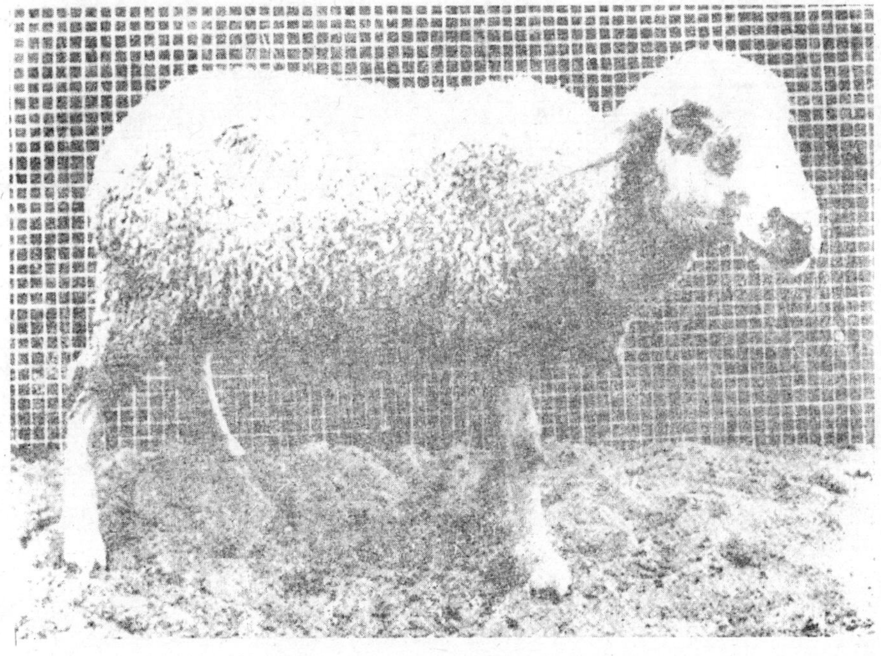

Plate 81. Adult Magna female sheep.

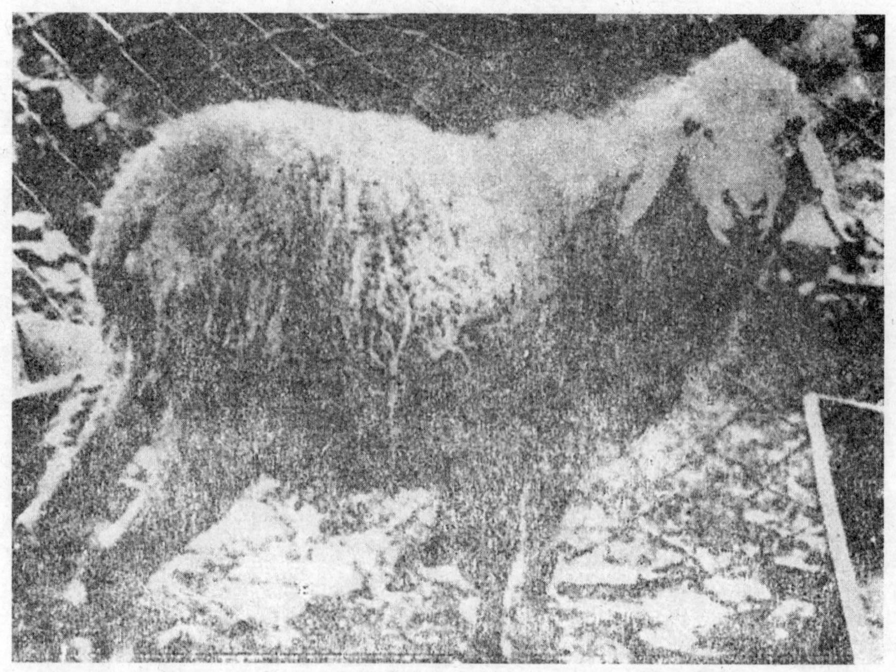

Plate 82. Adult Gaddi female sheep.

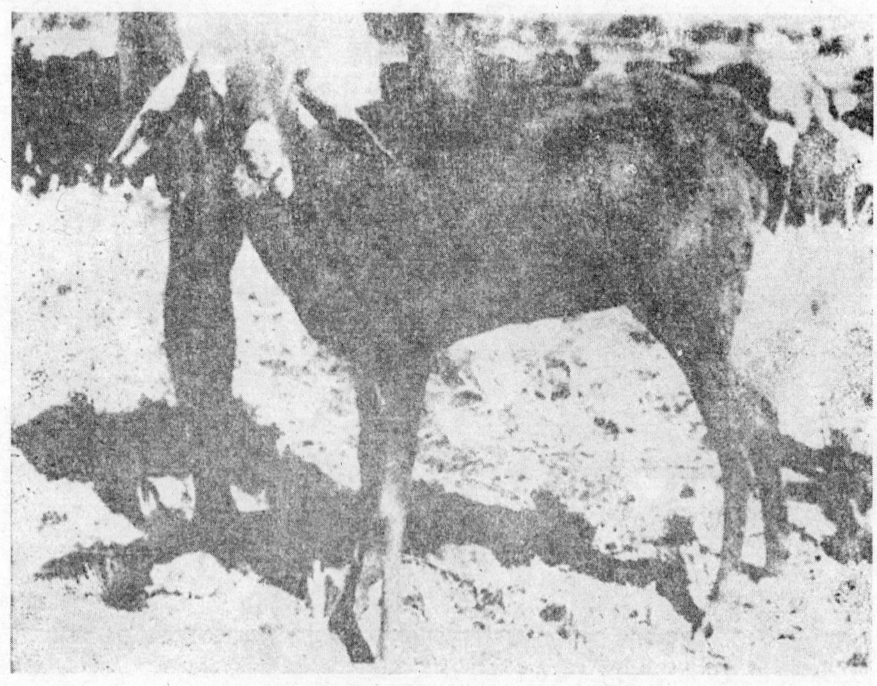

Plate 83. Adult Madras Red female sheep.

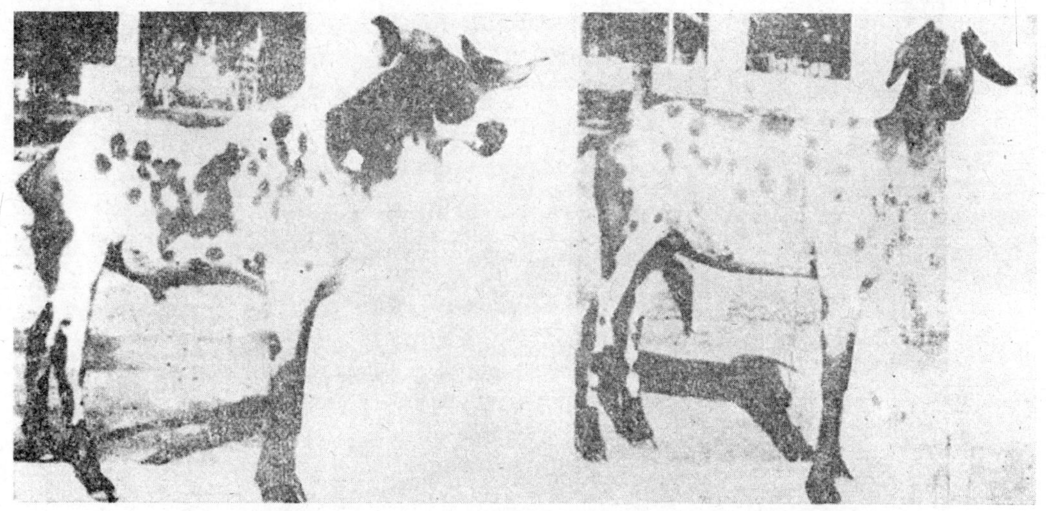

Plate 84. A Vembur Ram (left). A Vembur Ewe (right).

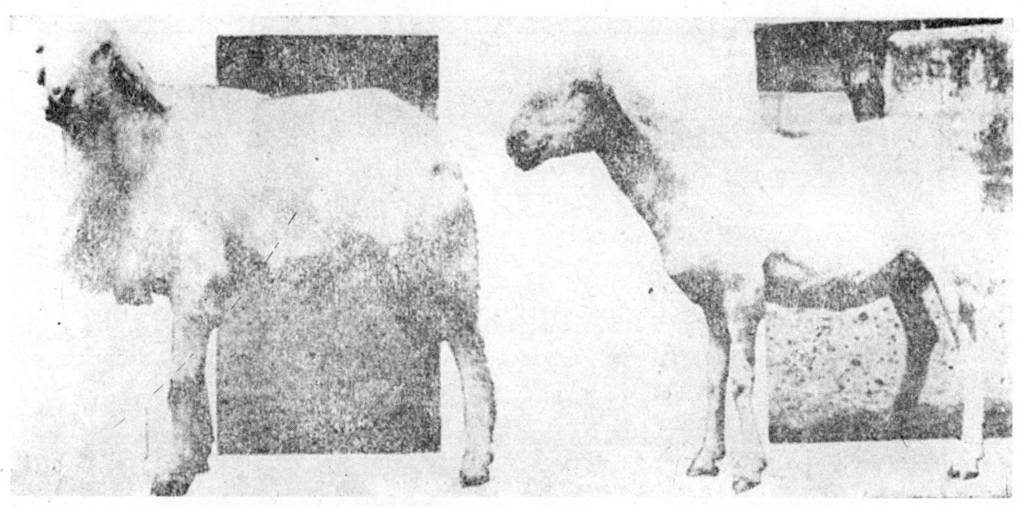

Plate 85. Mecheri Ram (left). A Mechari Ewe (right).

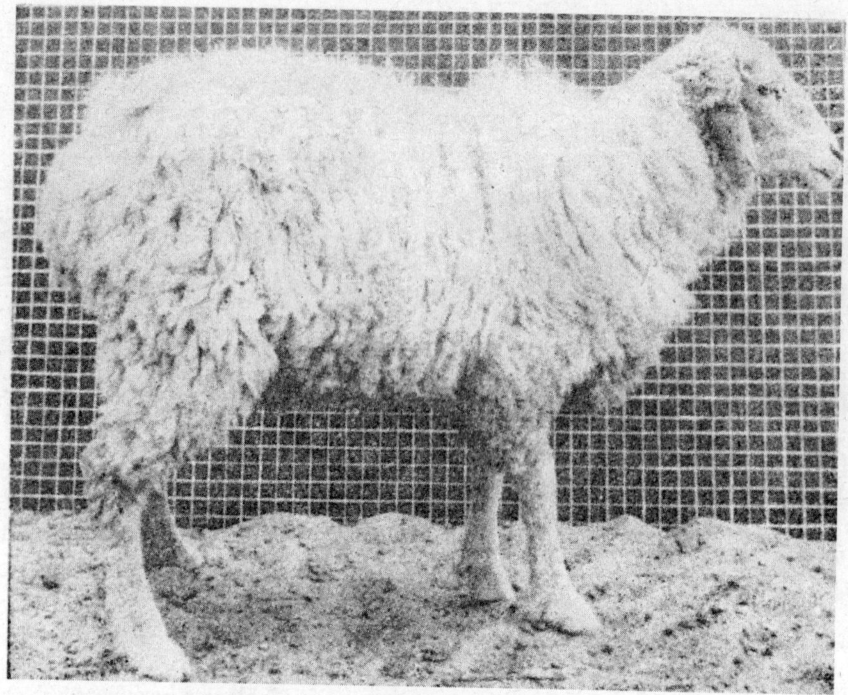

Plate 86. Chokla sheep.

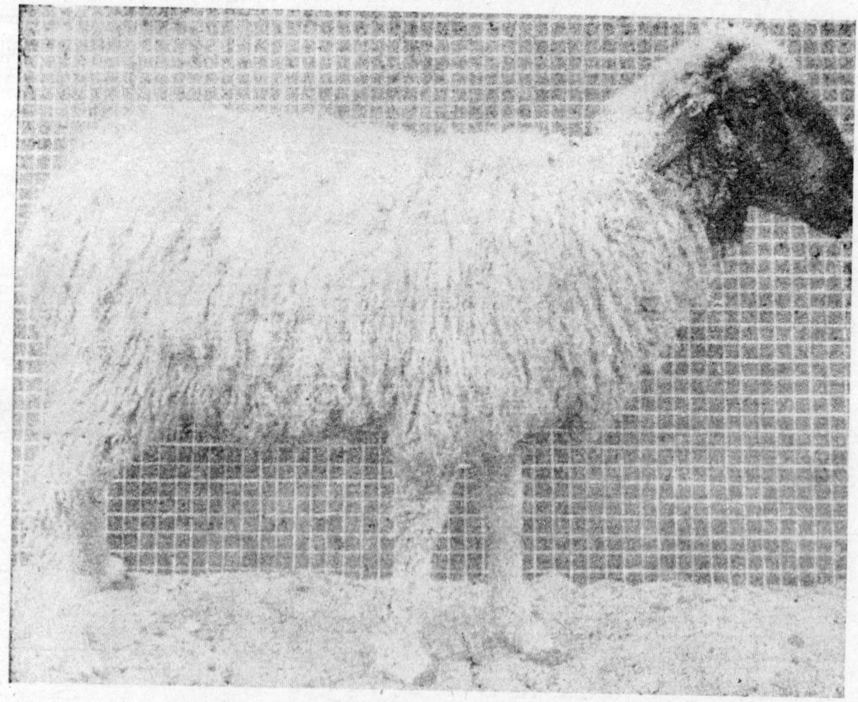

Plate 87. Nali sheep.

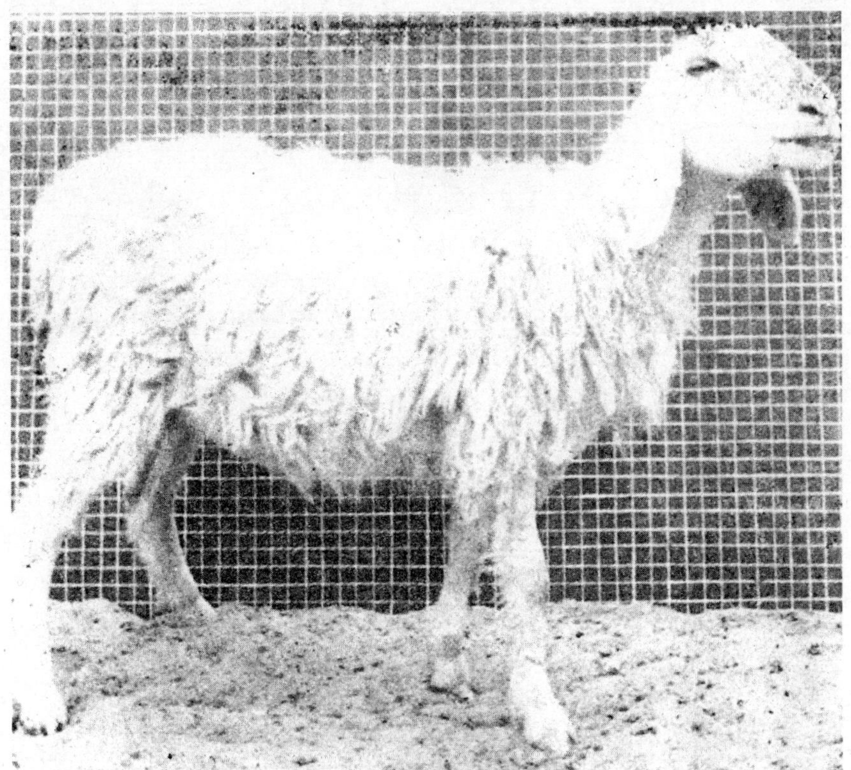

Plate 88(a). Sonadi sheep.

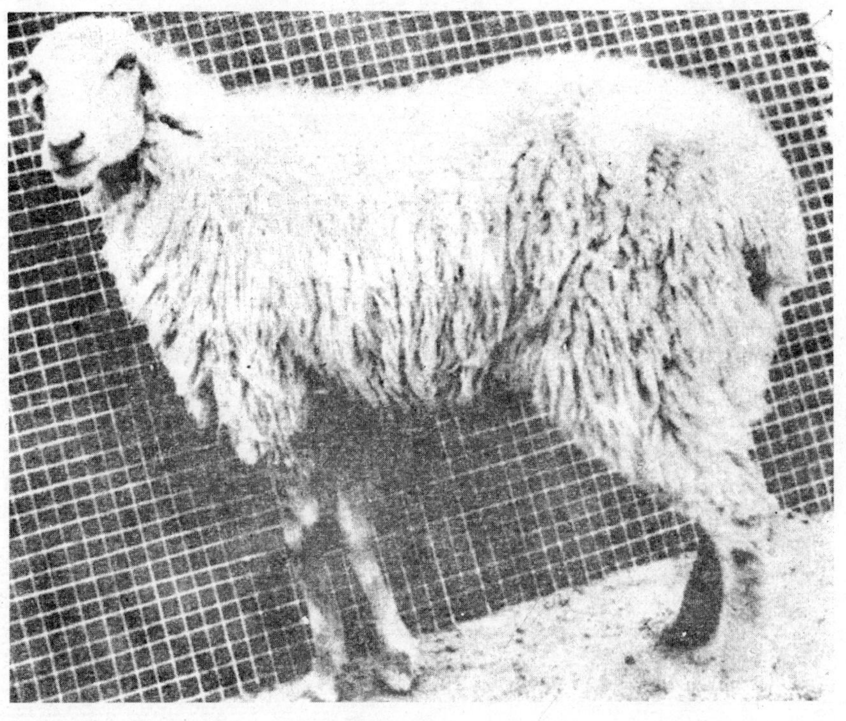

Plate 88(b). Malpura sheep.

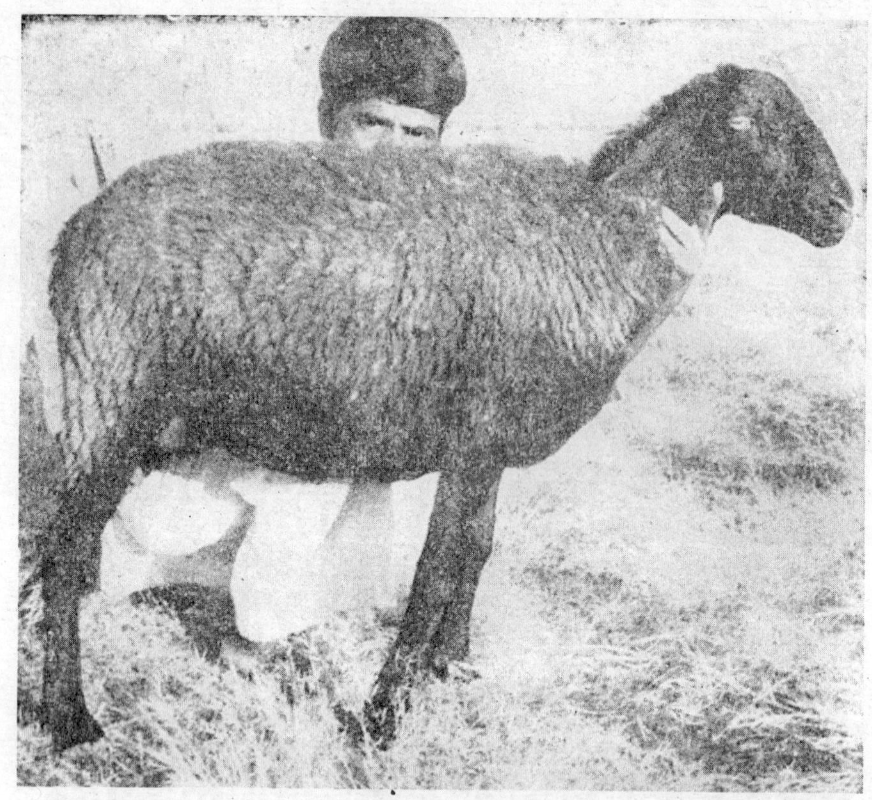

Plate 89. Deccani sheep.

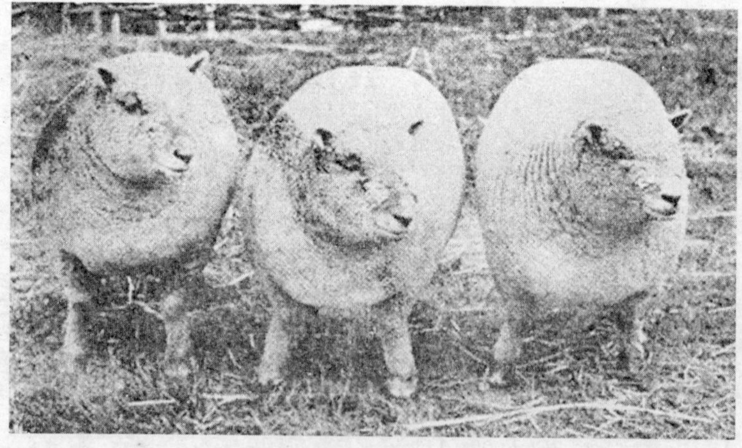

Plate 90. Southdown Shearling Ewe.

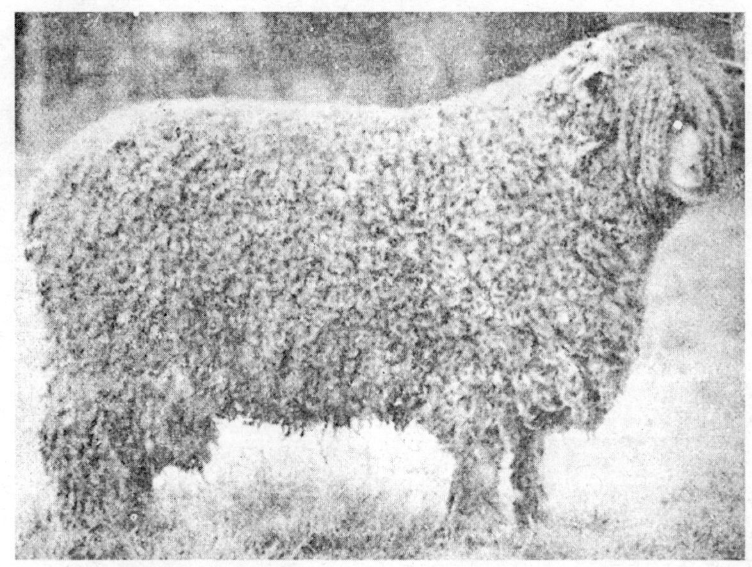

Plate 91. Lincoln Shearling Ram.

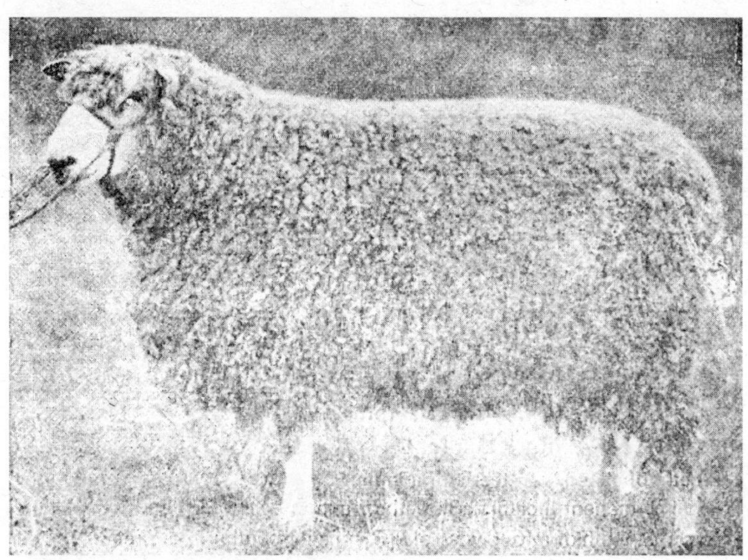

Plate 92. Leicester Shearling Ram.

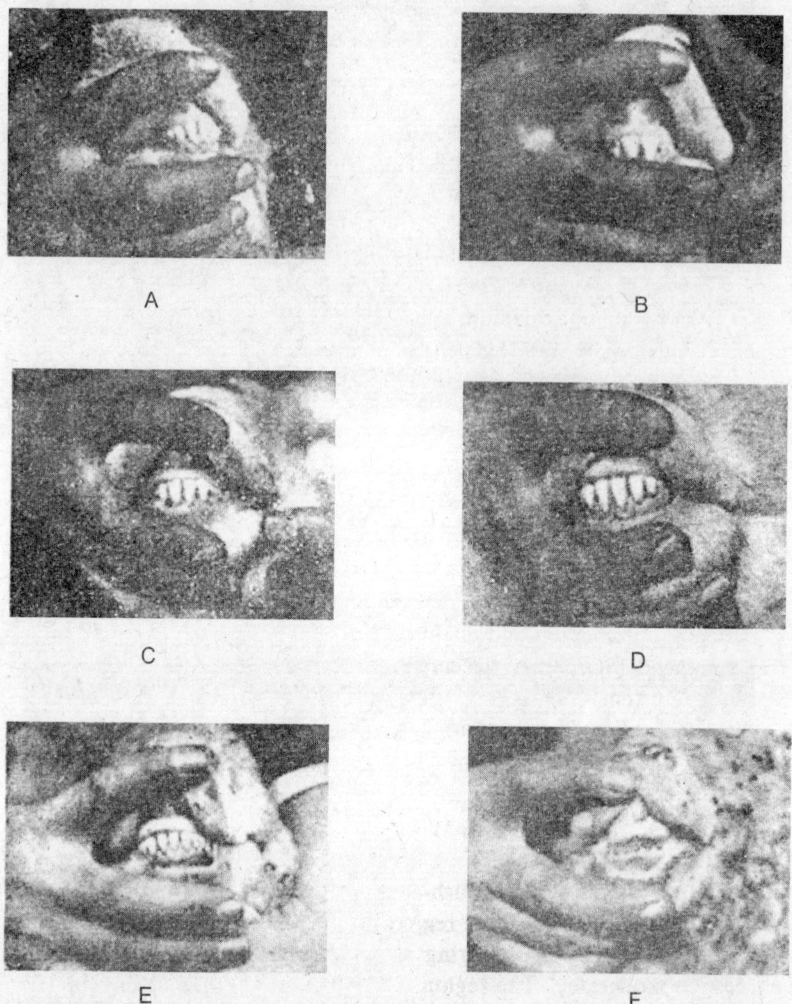

Plate 93. Teeth of sheep. A. teeth of a lamb; B. teeth of a yearling showing the first pair of permanent incisors; C. teeth of a two-year-old; D. teeth of a three-year-old; E. teeth of a four-year-old; F. broken mouth of an old sheep.

ears are generally short and colour is predominantly white including the face, but spotted sheep are also seen, varying brown to light black. Legs are also short, giving a low set conformation.

Production. The breed is best for wool production, average annual yield is 1.6 kg per sheep clipped twice or thrice a year. Flocks are raised on rich summer pastures and are stall-fed during winter on stored grasses and fodders.

KARNAH

Origin and Distribution. Occurring in Karnah tehsil at an altitude of 1,200–4,600 m, best one found in Kel.

Distinguishing Characters. Animals are large. Rams have big curved horns and a prominent nose.

Production. Wool is of fine, medium and short type, free from kemp, and predominantly white; average annual yield is 0.90–1.36 kg per sheep, clipped twice a year. Staple length ranges from 12–15 cm and average fibre diameter between 29 to 32 micron.

KASHMIR MERINO

This breed has originated from crosses of different Merino types (Delaine Merinos and then with Rambouillet and Soviet Merinos) with migratory Indian breeds of Gaddi, Bhakarwal and Poonchi. The animals are thus highly variable because of the involvement of a number of native breeds. It is therefore, very difficult to narrate particular descriptions of Kashmir Merino.

Production. Wool production and quality:

Average 6-monthly greasy fleece weight (kg)	:	1.2
Staple length (cm)	:	15.6
Average fibre diameter (micron)	:	20

II. North-Western Arid and Semi-arid

This region comprises Rajasthan, South-east Punjab, Gujarat and parts of Western Uttar Pradesh. The quality of wool of these regions are not fine and thus used for carpet manufacture. The climate is extremely hot during summer and fairly cold during winter. Rainfall ranges from low to moderate. The region is very receptive to sheep farming and the flocks are of stationary, semi-migratory or migratory types. The region has about 13.1 million sheep (32.4 per cent of the total sheep population) produces 22.1 million kg or 64 per cent of the total wool.

HISSARDALE

Origin and Distribution. Hissardale originated in the earlier part of the century at the Government Livestock Farm, Hissar in Haryana through crossing Australian Merino rams with Bikeneri (Magra) ewes; the exotic inheritance is stabilized at about 75%. The breed is now found in the hilly regions of Kulu, Kangra, etc.

Distinguishing Characteristics. Animals are short in structure. Ears are leaf-like, medium size.

Most animals are polled. Colour is mostly white, although some brown or black patches can be observed.

Production. The wool is fine and good for garments. Annual greasy fleece weighs about 2 kg. per adult animal having fibre length of 6.15 cm with an average fibre diameters of 24 micron.

CHOKLA

Origin and Distribution. The breed is extensively found in the districts of Churu, Jhunjhunu, Sikar and Nagaur of Rajasthan.

Distinguishing Characters. Head is comparatively small with brown in colour. Face is free of wool with broad forehead having prominent Roman nose. The general body structure is of medium size, square and compact. Legs are short with small hard black hooves with rare exceptions of white hooves. The breed is by nature slow maturing and the mutton is lean.

Production. The breed produces the finest wool among all Rajasthan breeds. The average yield is between 1.5 to 2.5 kg per annum.

MAGRA

Origin and Distribution. The breed is widely distributed in Bikaner, Churu and Nagaur districts of Rajasthan.

Distinguishing Characters. Well built body with light pink skin covering. The head is without any wool but covered with white hair, with light brown patches round about the eyes, medium in size, flat forehead, hornless.

Production. The average cut is 2.0 to 2.5 kg soft wool per year. Mature ram weighs about 33 kg while for ewe it is between 25 to 30 kg.

NALI

Origin and Distribution. The breed is abundant in the districts of Ganganagar, Churu and Jhunjhunu districts of Rajasthan.

Distinguishing Characters. Nali sheep is of a large size. It has compact head, large and leafy ears, short legs with amber hooves. The forehead is covered with wool and the face is full of light brown hair.

Production. The animals are clipped twice a year, in the month of March and September and weighs between 2.5 to 3.5 kg per year. Mature ram weighs between 35–40 kg while ewes are between 25–30 kg.

MARWARI

Origin and Distribution. The flock is mostly maintained in Jodhpur, Nagaur, Pali and Barmer districts of Rajasthan.

Distinguishing Characters. Marwari sheep are of black faced, head is also covered with black hair with twisted small ears. Legs are long and thin, body in general sturdy and medium in size.

Production. The animals are clipped twice a year and the yield varies from 1.5 to 2.5 kg per year. The quality of wool is coarse white and contains heterotype hairy fibres and thus is used for rough carpets and blankets. Live weight of rams ranges from 30 to 40 kg while that of ewes varies from 25 to 30 kg.

SONADI

Origin and Distribution. The regions where the breed is extensively found is from Udaipur Division of Rajasthan extending upto Gujarat State.

Distinguishing Characters. Sonadi is considered to have well built bodies with light brown faces. It has got prominent nose and large drooping ears. Mature rams weigh about 30 to 40 kg and the ewes about 25 to 30 kg. The animals have long body and long tails. The belly, legs and head are free from wool.

Production. The quality of wool is coarse and contains a large percentage of kemp. It yields from 0.6 to 1.2 kg of flat white per year. The breed also yields between 1 to 1.5 kg of milk per day.

KATHIWARI

Origin and Distribution. The home of this breed is Kathiwar and the adjoining parts of Kutch, Southern Rajasthan and North Gujarat.

Distinguishing Characters. The animals are medium sized and well built. They are usually of white colour with tan and black hair on the face and legs. The wool is good quality carpet wool and is known as "Joria" wool in Europe after the town from which it is exported.

Production. Wool quality is of long stapled and coarse. The fleece is shorn twice a year in January (0.5 kg) and in September (1 kg).

JAISALMERI

Origin and Distribution. Jaisalmer, Barmer and Jodhpur districts of Rajasthan.

Distinguishing Characters. Tall, well-built animals. Black-coloured, face extends up to the neck. Nose is of 'Roman' type. Ears are long and drooping. Male and female are both hornless. Litter size is usually single.

Production. Fleece (wool covering a sheep) colour is white except that of facial, medium carpet quality and not very dense. Annual greasy fleece weighs about 750 grams with staple length of 6.5 cm.

MALPURA

Origin and Distribution. The breed is very similar to Sonadi but is better in wool production and quality and in body size. It is mostly distributed in Jaipur, Tonk, Swaimadhopur and adjacent areas of Ajmer, Bhilwara districts of Rajasthan.

Distinguishing Characters. Moderately well built animals with long legs and light brown face. Fleece is white, extremely coarse and hairy. Belly and legs are devoid of wool. Both sexes are polled. Single litter size.

Production. Annual yield of fleece is about 1 kg with a staple length of 5.5 cm, medullation (%) is about 70.

III. Southern Region

It includes Maharashtra, Mysore, Andhra Pradesh, Tamil Nadu and parts of Madhya Pradesh. Basically, there are two types of sheep in this zone viz., wool type and meat type. Nearly 50 to 55 per cent of the total sheep population are situated in the region. The climate is warm and humid for a greater part of the year with a small spell of moderate cold during winter. The rainfall is moderate to heavy. It has 21. million or 52 per cent of the sheep of which 10-12 million produce no wool and the rest produce coarse, hairy and coloured fleeces. This region produces 9.68 million kg or 28 per cent of the total wool.

DECCANI

Origin and Distribution. **Mostly found in the South-Eastern parts of Maharashtra and in the neighbouring areas of Andhra Pradesh. In Maharashtra the breed is widely distributed in several districts which include Nasik, Poona, Ahmednagar, Kolhapur, Sholapur and Aurangabad.**

Distinguishing Characters. The animals are small and hardy. The breed has a thin neck, a narrow chest, prominent spinal processes, raised withers, flat ribs, a dropping croup and a poor leg of mutton. Two long fleshy tussels grow under the neck. The rams are usually horned and the ewes polled; it has a Roman nose, lop ears and a short tail. The colour is dominantly black, with some grey and roan.

Production. The fleece consist of a mixture of wool fibres and hairs in varying proportions. The average yield is about 700 grammes annually, usually black and grey in colour, used for the manufacture of rough blankets.

NELLORE

Origin and Distribution. The hometown of this breed is the Nellore district of Andhra Pradesh. At present it is found in Nellore, Cuddapah, Guntur, Nalgonda and surroundings of Andhra Pradesh.

Distinguishing Characters. Tallest breed of sheep in India. It has a short thin tail and the rams have spiral horns like some of the ancient Egyptian sheep. The breed has got a long face and long ears and may show the two appendages of skin hanging from the throat. The average body weight of ewe is about 30 kg and that of ram this is. about 40 kg. Nellore sheep can be sub-classed as (1) red horned, (2) red polled, and (3) horned with white or brownish body colour.

Production. The breed is famous for only mutton and thus their body which is densely covered with short hair are never shorn. Ewes are late maturing and not very prolific.

BELLARY

Origin and Distribution. Large number of these sheep are found in the talukas of Bellary districts in Karnataka State and in the Kilikuntla, Kurnool and Nandikotkur talukas of Karnool districts of Andhra Pradesh.

Distinguishing Characters. The sheep of this breed in South India is similar to "Deccani" in many respects and in fact it is considered by many to be the same breed. The rams are horned and the ewes polled, the colours found are black (most common), white with a black face or black with white patches.

Production. The fleece weight varies from less than 0.5 kg depending on the pasture condition.

MANDYA

Synonym. Baunur.

Origin and Distribution. The breed originated from the village Bannur near Mandya district in Mysore. They are now found in Bangalore, Mandya, Kolar, Mysore and Tumkur.

Distinguishing Characters. A very large breed, the Mandya is set with a fleece devoid of any wool. It has two short wattles hanging near the neck. The brown patch of the neck extends upto the shoulder. Ram weighs about 35 kg while ewe may weighs about 25 kg. The long leafy and drooping ears, short tail, short leg and a Roman nose are all distinguishing characters of the breed.

Production. The breed is reared for milk and meat.

COIMBATORE

Synonym. Karumbai.

Origin and Distribution. Coimbatore and Madurai districts of Tamil Nadu bordering areas of Kerala and Karnataka.

Distinguishing Characters. Animals are of medium in size. Colour is white with black or brown spots. Medium size ears are directed outward and backward. 38% of the males are horned while females are all polled. Fleece is coarse and hairy. Adult males weigh about 25 kg while females attain about 20 kg. Litter size: single.

Production. Dressing percentage on pre-slaughter live weight is about 39%.

MECHERI

Synonyms. Maiylambadi, Thuvaramchambali.

Origin and Distribution. The breed of sheep is found at Mecheri, Kolathoor, Nangavalli, Omalur and Tarmangalam Panchayat Union areas of Salem district and Bhavani taluk of Coimbatore district of Tamil Nadu.

Distinguishing Characteristics. The breed is medium-sized, light brown in colour with occasional white spots on head or in other body parts. Both sexes are polled. Body is covered with very short hairs. First breeding takes place at about 15 months of age. The adult males weigh about 35 kg while female weigh about 21.5 kg.

Production. Dressing percentage on the basis of pre-slaughter live-weight is 54.5%. The skin is of the highest quality of sheep breeds in India and is highly valued.

MADRAS RED

Origin and Distribution. The breed is abundant at Chingalpet and Madras district of Tamil Nadu.

Distinguishing Characteristics. Medium sized animals having body colour predominantly brown, which varies from light tan to dark brown. Some are having white markings on the forehead, inside the thighs and on the lower abdomen. Ears are medium, long and drooping. Rams have strong corrugated and twisted horns while ewes are polled. Body is covered with fine small hairs which are not shorn.

Production. The breed is reared exclusively for meat purpose. It has about 40% dressing percentage. Adult males weigh about 35 kg while for females it is about 23 kg.

VEMBUR

Origin and Distribution. The breed is also known as Karandhai from the name of the village where the breed appears to have originated. At present Vembur sheep are widely distributed in Vembur, Melakkarandhai, Keezhakarandhai, Nagalpuram, Kavundhanapatty and some other villages of Pudur Panchayat Union and Vilathikulam Panchayat areas of Tirunelveli district of Tamil Nadu.

Distinguishing Characteristics. Tall animals. Colour is white with irregular red and fawn patches all over the body. Ears are medium sized and drooping with short and thin tail. Males are having prominent twisted horns while females are polled. Short hairs all over the body are never shorn.

Production. Lambing percentage: 80 per cent, litter size: single. The adult male weighs about 34 kg while the female attains on an average 27 kg.

HASSAN

Origin and Distribution. Hassan district of Karnataka.

Distinguishing Characteristics. Short statured animals. Body colour is white with light brown or black spots. Ears are medium long drooping. Females are always polled while among males one third are horned. Fleece is white, extremely coarse and open. Legs and belly are mostly devoid of wool. Litter size: single.

Production. Mostly used for meat purpose.

TIRUCHY BLACK

Origin and Distribution. The breed is found in many districts of Tamil Nadu.

Distinguishing Characteristics. Short statured animals with black body colour. Males are horned while females are polled. Ears are short and directed downward and forward. The fleece is extremely coarse, hairy and open.

Production. Very good for meat purpose.

IV. Eastern Region

The region comprises the States of Bihar, West Bengal, Orissa, Assam, Meghalaya, Arunachal Pradesh, Mizoram, Manipur, Tripura; Nagaland and Sikkim.

Except for small pockets in Arunachal Pradesh and Sikkim bordering Tibet, where Tibetan sheep yield good carpet wool and medium apparel wool, most sheep in the region produce extremely coarse and hairy fleeces. The important breeds are Shahabadi and Chottanagpuri in

Bihar and part of West Bengal, Ganjam and Balangir in Orissa, Bonapala in Sikkim and Tibetan sheep in parts of Arunachal Pradesh and Sikkim.

It has 3.2 million sheep mostly maintained for meat. The region carries 8 per cent of the total sheep population and produces 0.64 million kg or 2 per cent of the total wool. This region has no distinct breed of its own except in case of Bihar where Sahabadi and Chottanagpuri breeds are found.

CHOTTANAGPURI

Origin and Distribution. Chottanagpur, Ranchi, Palamau, Hazaribagh, Singhbhum, Dhanbad and Santhal parganas of Bihar and Bankura district of West Bengal.

Distinguishing Characters. The common colour of this breed is light grey and brown. The animals are small. Ears are also small and parallel to the head. Both sexes are poled. Fleece is coarse and hairy. Rams and ewes on maturity weigh about 15–20 kg.

Production. The animals are shorn three times a year, in March/April, June/July and October/November and produce a yearly average of 0.18 kg of hairy wool with an average fibre diameter of 52 to 55 micron.

GANJAM

Origin and Distribution. The breed is abundant in Koraput, Phulbani and part of Puri district of Orissa.

Distinguishing Characters. Medium sized animals with coat colour ranging from brown to dark tan; few have white spots on the face and body. Slightly convex nose with medium long tail. Males are horned while females are polled. Fleece is hairy.

Production. Fleece is not shorn. The breed is reared only for meat purpose.

TIBETAN

Origin and Distribution. Mostly found in northern Sikkim and Kameng district of Arunachal Pradesh.

Distinguishing Characteristics. Medium sized animals having white colour with black or brown face. On the body occasionally brown and white spots are observed. Both sexes are horned. Roman nose and small drooping ears. The belly, legs and face are devoid of wool. Males and females on maturity weigh about 25 kg.

Production. Tibetan sheep produce an excellent, lustrous carpet-quality wool. Animals are shorn twice a year, during April/May and October/November. Greasy fleece weigh about 500 g per clip.

SHAHABADI

Origin and Distribution. The breed is abundant in the plains of Bihar particularly in Patna, Gaya, Shahabad and other districts of South Bihar. It is also found in the Purulia districts of West Bengal.

Distinguishing Characters. The usual colour of this breed is white with coloured faces. They have long legs, distinct Roman nose, long tails and in general they are sturdy sheep.

Table 17.5

Average performance of some pure-bred sheep

Name of the breed	Body weight (in kg) at weaning				Mortality (%)			Six monthly production and quality of wool			
	90 days	6 month	9 month	12 month	Dressing (%)	0–3 month	Adult	Greasy fleece (gm)	Staple length (cm)	Average fibre diameter (μ)	Medullation (%)
I. Temperate Himalayan Region											
Gaddi	7.5	10.8	—	14.5	—	20.5	10.7	780	5.7	28.5	26.0
II. North Western Region											
Chokla	11.0	13.5	15.5	18.0	—	25	5.0	1,400	4.8	28.0	24.0
Nali	10.2	13.0	14.5	18.0	48.0	24	10.0	1,500	8.2	35.0	31.0
Marwari	8.0	9.0	14.5	21.0	—	—	3.5	800	6.5	36.5	65.0
Magra	12.0	20.0	22.0	28.0	45.0	29	20.0	1,000	6.0	35.0	48.0
Malpura	9.0	12.5	17.0	21.0	47.0	11	10.0	500	5.6	42.0	72.0
Sonadi	9.2	13.0	16.0	19.0	48.0	13	8.0	450	4.6	53.0	88.0
Muzzafarnagri	10.8	14.5	18.4	25.0	48.5	—	10.0	650	3.8	45.0	70.0
III. Southern Region											
Deccani	13.5	20.9	—	—	49.0	5.3	2.8	359	8.58	52.4	73.7
Nellore	12.0	16.7	—	23.0	47.0	14.0	13.0	—	—	—	—
Bellary	11.0	16.3	—	18.5	—	—	15.0	300	—	59.0	43.4
Mandya	9.8	12.5	—	21.0	45.0	5.3	20.0	375	—	—	—
Coimbatore	7.5	10.8	12.5	14.5	38.0	11.0	7.5	365	5.79	41.0	58.4
Nilgiri	12.0	15.0	19.0	20.0	—	17.0	6.5	600	—	27.5	11.3
IV. Eastern Region											
Sahabadi	—	—	—	—	—	—	—	250	—	50.0	85.0
Chottanagpuri	—	—	—	—	—	—	—	185	—	52.5	84.0

Rams on maturity weighs about 25-30 kg while ewes reach between 20-25 kg.

Production. The fleece is a mixture of coarse wool, hair and kemp. Annual yield is between 500 grammes to 1 kg and obtained in three shearings.

Table 17.6

Classification of 40 Indian breeds of Sheep according to their major functions

Garments Wool (Apparel Woll)	*Carpet Wool*	*Meat & Carpet Wool*	*Meat*
Kashmir Merino	Chokla	Muzzafarnagri	Nellore
Nilgiri	Nali	Jalauni	Mandya
Hissardale	Pattanwadi	Deccani	Hassan
Karnah	Tibetan Sheep	Bellary	Mechari
	Gaddii	Ganjam	Kilakarsal
	Rampur Bushair	Balangir	Vembur
	Bhakarwal	Shahbadi	Ramnad white
	Poonchi	Chottanagpuri	Madras red
	Gurez	Coimbatore	Triuchy Black
	Changthangi	Marwari	Kanguri
	Gaddii	Jaisalmari	
		Pugal	
		Malpura	
		Sonadi	
		Bonpala	

EXOTIC BREEDS OF SHEEP

In order to evolve new breeds of superior quality, a few exotic breeds of sheep have been introduced in India. Merino rams of Australian and German origins and Rambouillet rams of France have been used in large numbers. Southdown breeds of sheep has been imported from California are being used for grading indigenous sheep in the southern region. Recently, Indian Council of Agricultural Research under the All India Co-ordinated Projects on sheep breeding for fine wool and mutton has launched a cross-breeding programme with exotic breeds of sheep.

1. Merinos. It is the most popular fine-wool breed of the world. The breed is a native of Spain and has spread throughout the world. Wrinkles or folds in the skin are qualities of this breed. Ewes are polled, while the rams have rather large, heavy, spirally turned horns. The breed is rather small in size, somewhat upstanding angular than rectangular. Merinos are extremely hardy, being able to survive under adverse weather as well as poor grazing condition.

2. Rambouillet. From Spanish Merino foundations, the French developed a fine wools rain of sheep. the Rambouillet, of much greater size than Merino. It may be considered dual very suitable for range qualities.

3. **Southdown.** These are one of the oldest of the English breeds and have been exported to many countries and used extensively in New Zealand, Australia and U.S.A. The body is small but blocky; the head is distinguished by its "mousey grey face" and short rounded ears. The fleece is of very high quality and second only to Merino; the length is 50 mm-75 mm with an excellent cript, average fleece weight 2 kg.

4. **Lincoln.** The breed is native to England. It is the largest of the British breeds and mature ram may weigh in excess of 152 kg. The wool is long in the staple, reaching 430 mm 480-mm, and is very dense and rather coarse; fleece weight around 4.5 kg 5.4 kg. Ewes are fairly prolific. Lincolns have been very successfully used in cross-breeding and in developing new breeds. In Australia the Lincoln is used chiefly for crossing with large-framed Merino-ewes, producing a good dual purpose sheep.

5. **Leicester.** The breed is one of purest breeds of British long wools. The breed is not so heavy as Lincolns, the average weight of a mature ram being 100 kg and of a ewe 85 kg. They are early matures and fatten readily at an early age under good feeding conditions, producing an excellent type of mutton. Wool is dense, free, even, and lustrous; lock medium width, showing small, well defined wave or cript from skin to tip. The animals are alert, robust showing style and character. The Border Leicester is generally regarded as a cross between the Cheviot and the Leicester.

6. **Corriedale.** The breed is comparatively new. It is a dual purpose breed combining a high class of mutton with a good class of wool. It cuts an average of about 5 kg of wool. The breed is prolific and hardy. The ancestry of this breed is predominantly Lincoln and Merino with the likely addition of some genetic contribution from the Leicester.

RESEARCH AND DEVELOPMENT EFFORT FOR IMPROVING SHEEP PRODUCTION

The sheep research and development activity was taken up as early as in the early 19th century by the East India Company. It imported exotic breeds of sheep for cross-breeding with indigenous breeds. Subsequently with the establishment of Imperial (now Indian) Council of Agricultural Research, research and development programmes were taken up on regional basis. These included selective breeding within indigenous breeds and cross-breeding them with exotic fine wool breeds. These programmes covered almost all important sheep rearing states. Major emphasis on sheep research and development was, however, given after the country attained independence and started its Five Year Development plans. During the Third Five Year Plan, a large number of sheep and wool extension centres were established. Wool grading and marketing programme was initiated in Rajasthan which was subsequently taken up in a number of other states. Realising the importance of sheep in agrarian economy the central Govt. established the Central Sheep & Wool Research Institute (CSWRI) along with its regional stations (added subsequently) in 1962 under an UNDP & GOI Project to undertake fundamental and applied research in sheep production and wool utilisation and imparting post-graduate training in sheep and wool sciences. During the Fourth Plan a large Sheep Breeding Farm in collaboration with the Australian Government was established at Hissar for pure-breeding Corriedale Sheep. Corriedale stud rams are being distributed from this farm to a number of states for cross-breeding for improving wool and mutton production. Another seven large sheep breeding farms were established in Jammu and Kashmir, Uttar Pradesh, Madhya Pradesh, Bihar, Andhra Pradesh and Karnataka for producing exotic pure bred or cross-bred rams. The ICAR started two All India Coordinated Research Projects on Sheep for Fine Wool and Sheep for Mutton with centres for fine wool located at Sheep Breeding Farm, Tal, Hamirpur (H.P.), Sheep Breeding Research Station, Sandynallah (Tamil Nadu), Gujarat Agricultural University, Dentiwada, CSWRI, Avikanagar (Raj.) and mutton centres at Livestock Research Station, APAU, Palamner, National Goat Research Institute, Makhdoom, Mahatma Phule Krishi Vidyapeeth, Rahuri and CSWRI, Avikanagar. These projects aim at evolving (i) new fine wool breeds for different agro-climatic regions capable of producing 2.5 kg of greasy wool annually of 58s to 64s count, (ii) new mutton breeds capable of attaining 30 kg live weight at 6 months under intensive feeding conditions. During the Fifth Five Year Plan, a large number of breeding farms were envisaged to be established in the Central and State Sectors for producing genetically superior breeding stock. Reorganisation and strengthening of the existing sheep breeding farms in the states as well as expansion and reorganisation of sheep and wool extension centres, and organisation of scientific sheep shearing and wool grading programmes were envisaged. A nnmber of sheep development programmes were undertaken under specialised programmes like DPAP, small farmer (SF), marginal farmer (MF) and agricultural labourer (AL) schemes. Setting up of a wool boards in important wool producing states was also envisaged and states of Rajasthan, Gujarat and Karnataka have already set up these boards.

REPRODUCTION

Age of maturity. Sheep normally attain full growth at about 2 years of their age. This age, however, varies from 18 months to 3 years with breeds and localities. The ewes are mated to rams between the ages of 9 to 14 months but is always preferred to wait till ewes attain proper stage of growth to ensure the birth of healthy lambs. Rams are found to be used for breeding purposes as early as one year of their age, but it is desirable to use rams for mating from the age of 2½ till they attain about 7 years of age.

Mating season and oestrus cycle. Sheep are seasonally polyestrus (*poly*—many, *estrus*—heat), meaning that ewes have numerous cycles during which conception can occur but only during a certain season. In India there are three main mating seasons, viz., March to April or summer, June-July, or autumn and September-October, post-monsoon. In general the fertility is high during autumn in the plain whereas in hilly areas fertility is observed in summer.

The cycle is repeated every 16 days on the average (actual range may be 14 to 20 days) until conception occurs. The length of heat averages 30 hours. Unlike females of other species, ewes show few external indications of estrus other than standing to be mounted and that is why heat is generally detected by the help of teaser or of a ram.

It is usual to mate only about 2-3 per cent of the rams with the ewes.

Ovulation and Gestation. The egg is released from the ovary about 24 to 30 hours after the onset of estrus. Therefore, conception is most likely when breeding occurs late in the heat period.

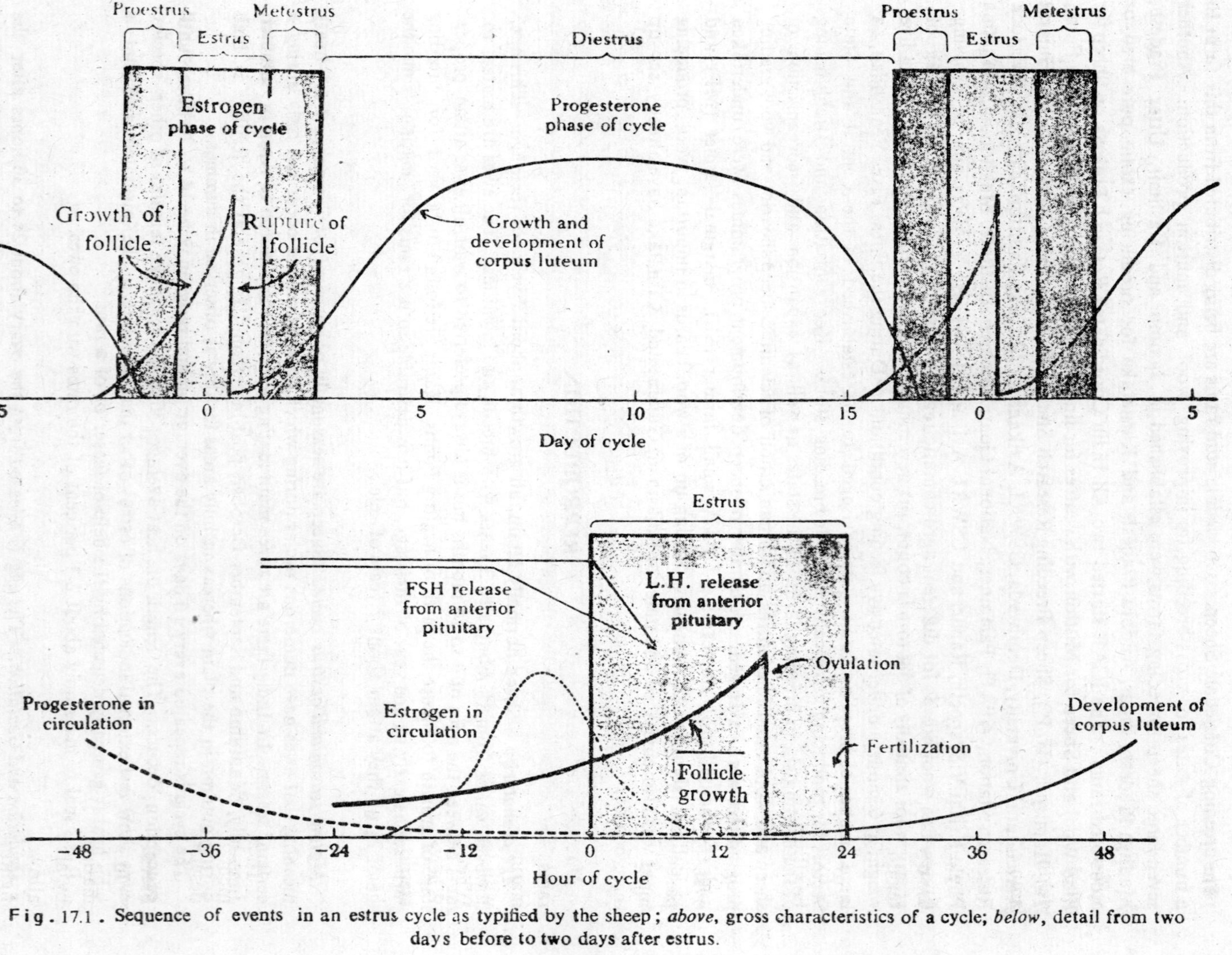

Fig. 17.1. Sequence of events in an estrus cycle as typified by the sheep; *above*, gross characteristics of a cycle; *below*, detail from two days before to two days after estrus.

The length of pregnancy averages 147 days (actual range may be 144 to 152 days).

PREPARING THE EWE FOR BREEDING

Flushing. This is the feeding of extra grain or lush pasture two or three weeks prior to the breeding season for the purpose of increasing the number of ova shed from the ovary for yielding twins. Feeding about 250 gms grains daily to each ewe results an increase in the lamb crop of 10-20 per cent.

Tagging. This refers shearing the locks of wool and dirt from the dock. Ewes sometimes are not bred because wool or tags prevent the ram from making satisfactory connection thus tagging makes service by the ram more certain. The ram is also trimmed around the sheath.

Eyeing. To prevent wool blindness in some breeds the excess wool around the eyes should be clipped away regularly. This process is referred to as eyeing.

Ringing. Before the breeding season starts the wool should be completely removed from all over the body of the ram. He should at least be clipped from the neck and from the belly particularly at the region of the penis. This process is referred to as *ringing*. The process makes it easier for the ram to have proper mating.

Marking the Ram. For the sake of identification of the ewes which have been bred by the rams, it is essential that the rams must have some paints in their breast, which at the time of mating will mark the particular ewe. For this either lamp blacks or venetian red is mixed up with linseed oil to make a paste, which is then applied in the brisket area at least once a week. When the ram mounts the ewe during the course of breeding, she will be marked on the rump. Where ewes are separated into flocks served by one ram, this marking method can detect a sterile male easily because all ewes are repeat breeders.

SYSTEM OF MATING

There are four systems of mating the ewes and some of them are of exclusively for experimental purposes while the others are for commercial purpose. The systems of mating are described below:

Flock System

In this system rams are usually let loose the ewes to serve at will (day and night) during the mating season at the rate of 30–45 ewes per ram. This is the most common practice followed by all commercial flock owners. The only drawback of the system is that when the rams are allowed to run with the ewe flock, the ewes are too much disturbed by the rams pushing and fighting amongst themselves. To avoid this, smaller mating flock of 40–50 with a single ram are the best provided young rams are selected for mating aged ewes while experienced rams for maiden ewes.

Pen System

In this system selected rams are allowed to have mating at night only those ewes which are kept together to make groups after their return in the evening for the grazing land and then the rams alloted are introduced with them. By this system rams are either grazed separately or are stall fed.

Hand Service

By this method the ewes in oestrus are first detected by the vasectomised rams which are then picked up and kept in the breeding pen and served by selected proven sizes. The system is extremely useful for any experimental farm but has got no value in commercial farms.

Artificial Insemination (A.I.)

Artificial Insemination in sheep has played a significant role in improving sheep within a short period of time in Russia and in some European countries. One of the reasons for the success of AI in these countries is the large size of their sheep flocks, which are maintained more or less on a stationary basis on farms. In India this technique, though taken up on an experimental basis for some years, has not yet been extended to the field on a large scale except in Rajasthan. AI in sheep cannot be adopted so easily as in the case of cattle and buffaloes in view of certain problems connected with dilution and preservation of ram semen. The dilution factor of the ram semen is low and its preservability is very poor. Diluted ram semen, not used within 6-8 hours, loses its fertility very rapidly and as such its field use is beset with several technical difficulties.

Inspite of these difficulties, serious attempts should be made to try out this technique in the breeding of sheep in different parts of the country in view of the large scale cross-breeding programmes that have been recommended for rapid increase in wool and mutton production.

CONTROLLING HEAT (SYNCHRONISATION OF HEAT)

It is possible to have all the ewes of the flock coming on heat within a 2-3 day period. The practical advantages of this method are as follows:

(a) The owner may plan the lambing time in such a way, when the climate is most suitable for raising the healthy lambs with least effort.

(b) Breeding programme either by natural processes or by AI becomes easier and economic.

(c) Since most of the ewes are in the same stage of pregnancy, flock management is more effective.

(d) The owner by planning certain period of the year as breeding season may catch the best market time of his animals.

Synchronization of oestrus may be done by various ways but the most common practice is to insert a pessary containing a synthetic hormone called *Cronolone* into the vagina of each ewe using a special instrument. The hormone is then gradually absorbed through the lining of the vagina into the blood stream. The hormone prevents ovulation. The pessary is removed after 15-17 days by pulling on a string attached to it. Most of the ewes come on heat within a few days after the pessary is removed from the vagina and the breeding can then take place.

To prevent strain on the parts of rams while servicing in short period of time, the number of ewes per ram should be reduced to about 20-30.

SIGNS OF PREGNANCY

As discussed earlier in the Reproduction Chapter, the empty follicle after the ovulation froms yellow body, corpus luteum (CL). This secretes the hormone progesterone for making the uterine wall "receptive" to the fertilised egg and to prevent ewes coming from further heat.

A shepherd usually recognises a pregnant ewe by the fact that she has not returned to the ram.

It is comparatively easier to distinguish some weeks before lambing between the ewes, ewes carrying single lambs and those carrying twins. Barren ewes usually put on weight and improve in condition; ewes carrying a single lamb are heavier than at mating time, but leaner when handled; ewes carrying twins are the heaviest and leanest.

Ewes about to lamb will sink away on either side of the rump in front of the hips. The vulva will enlarge, wax will form on the ends of the teats. There will be distension of the udder and the teats will be tight and show signs of filling.

When lambing, an ewe will show a characteristic vertical movement of the tail and will usually lag behind or become separated from the flock. She will scratch the ground with her fore-legs and become fidgety, constantly changing her position by standing and sitting alternately.

Care during Pregnancy

The future productive healthy flock of sheep depends much on the special care regarding feeding and management of pregnant ewes. The following points may be considered as guidelines of the special managemental aspects.

(1) When the flock is large, separate the ewes those are at the verge of lambing.
(2) Ewes should not be subjected to fright.
(3) Pregnant ewes should not be crowded together nor be allowed to jump over hedges or ditches.
(4) They should be protected from inclement weather, specially during severe winter.
(5) They should be provided with shades during midday specially in summer.

About 3-4 weeks before mating the quality of the ewes diet is gradually improved by providing grain ration or by moving them to fresh pasture areas where it is full of green tender grass. This improved feeding is necessary for the following reasons:

1. Provides nourishment for the developing foetus and usually results in a strong lamb at birth.

2. Stimulates udder development and future milk production of the ewe.
3. Builds up body reserves of flesh on the ewe.

LAMBING

The gestation or pregnancy period is 21 weeks or 147 days with a plus and minus variation of 3 days. The onset of birth coincides with the disappearance of the corpus luteum of the ovary and the consequent effects of the release of birth hormone (oxytocin) stored in the posterior pituitary gland. The udder at that time usually becomes red in colour.

An ewe that is about to lamb is restless and usually wanders off to find a sheltered place away from the flock. She lies down, but turns her head in a characteristic manner, looking up almost directly at the sky. As the labour pains increase, she makes a tremendous muscular effort to force the lamb from the uterus to the vaginal passage; that is what we understand by '*strain*". As the ewe continues to strain, she forces, the "*water bag*' (which until now has been used as a cushion to prevent injury to the developing lamb) into the vagina. At first the fluid comes out after bursting of the bag, the next stage is that the lamb's forefeet now appear at the vulva, and then the legs with the head resting on the knees. As soon as the head and shoulders are through the vulva opening, the main difficulty is over and the lamb is quickly born. The navel cord snaps as the lamb drops to the ground, and the ewe will almost immediately stand up and turn round to lick her lamb.

The lamb will shake its head and quickly respond to the massaging effect of the ewe licking its skin. In a few minutes the lamb will rise to its feet, and, provided it is strong and healthy, will be suckling the ewe within a quarter of an hour or so. If the ewe has twins or triplets she will lie down again and deliver the second lamb more quickly and easily than the first born.

If however, difficulty is noticed due to failure of normal birth after an hour's straining, the ewe should be rendered all possible assistance including pulling the lamb downwards slowly provided that the lamb is in the right position. If it fails, the veterinary doctor should immediately be contacted.

Weaning

If the lambs have not been sold by the time they reach 14 weeks old, they must be weaned at this age otherwise big lambs often treat their dams roughly, resulting in damage of teats and udders.

It has been noticed in large flocks that lambs are taken away from the ewes for grazing separately for a few days and then mixed with main flock. In small flocks the shepherd would apply loose fresh cow-dung on the udder of milking ewes before letting them out for grazing with their lambs. The strong smell of the cow-dung on the udder makes the lamb stop suckling and thus they are weaned.

Rest Period

This is one of the important functions of the management processes as it provides a chance to have the time to repair her body tissues in readiness for next season's lambing. The ewe should get her next service approximately one year after the first year is divided as follows:

1st Service	
Pregnancy or gestation	5 months
Suckling lambs	3-3.5 months
Rest period	3.5-4.0 months

This offers an interesting comparison with the dairy cow. Once the cow conceives she never has a rest period; she is always milking and/or feeding a developing foetus. The ewe, on the otherhand, should have a period of actual rest when she neither feeds her lambs nor carries any foetus.

RAISING LAMBS

After lambing as soon as the lamb is breathing, his navel cord should be immersed in tincture of iodine to prevent any navel infection. The shepherd should remove the mucous from the mouth and nostrils. A strong, vigorous lamb usually has no trouble feeding itself soon after birth, but a weak lamb may die if it does not get assistance at this critical period. A weak lamb should be held up to the udder of the ewe and, if necessary, a little milk may be forced into his mouth. In extreme cases it may be necessary to draw a little of the first milk from the udder and to feed it to the lamb with the aid of feeding bottle. Generally, however, if the ewes had been well fed during the gestation period, then milk yield will be sufficient to meet the full requirement of their offsprings which may be judged from growth rates of the lamb. At about 2 weeks of age, the lambs should be trained to eat roughage by placing some hay in a "creep". A creep is a small enclosure in a sheep pen, having opening just wide enough for lambs to pass in but the ewes cannot. The grain trough should be so constructed to prevent the lambs from getting into it and soiling the feed. An excellent concentrate mixture for use in the creep consists of 35 parts of ground maize, 35 parts of crushed oat, 20 parts of wheat bran, 10 parts of linseed meal. After the lambs are 4–5 weeks old it is not necessary to grind or crush any grain except maize. A fresh supply of legume hay, such as lucerne and a new supply of grain should be offered once or twice daily. The feed not eaten by the lambs should be removed and can be fed to the ewes.

Growth rate of lambs mostly depends on yield and quality of the milk of the ewe as they will hardly start grazing until they attain the age of 2–3 weeks. In fact the intake of herbage is not much until they reach about 6 to 8 weeks of their age.

Colostrum has a high level of total solids which drops off rapidly to a rather typical value of about 22%. Colostrum is also characterised by a high level of protein and a low level of lactose. As lactation progress the protein content continued to drop although there was a slight increase (Table 17.7) in sampling collected during 70–90 days of lactation.

The level of feeding lambs during the early months depends on whether the lambs are to be raised for meat or for breeding. In case of meat producers, live weight gain should be between 1 to 2 kg per week and for lambs to be reared for breeding should have the growth rate half of the former case.

At 12 or 14 weeks of age, the lambs should be weaned and separated from their dams. At this stage the ewe can make good body weight gain if the grazing is done on young grasses. If, however, grazing is scanty or the forages are coarse and mature, grain feeding to the ewes will have to be continued. The composition of the mixture may be changed by including 20 parts of oil cake in place of the grains. Ewe lambs which are needed for flock replacement

Table 17.7

Change in composition of ewe's milk during the course of lactation

Time of milk sampled	*Milk composition %*						
	Total solids	*Fat*	*Protein*	*Lactose*	*Ash*	*Ca*	*P*
Colostrum	36.9	14.0	19.4	2.5	1.0	0.181	0.280
3-6 days	22.1	10.5	6.2	4.4	0.91	0.199	0.222

SOURCE: Perrin, D. 1958, *J. Dairy Res.* 25: 70

are to be fed properly for steady gaining in weight. The recommended age for breeding ewes is the first breeding season after the ewes attained one year age, so that they produce their first lamb at about 2 years of age. Ram lambs, which are to be marketed should be castrated when they are 7–14 days old. Wether lambs contain higher proportion of valuable cuts and the meat is better liked than that from ram lambs.

SHEEP NUTRITION

Sheep possess a unique ability to survive on natural grasses, shrubs and farm waste products like residues of the fields. With their small muzzles and split upper lips, they can nibble tiny blades of vegetation which cannot be eaten by bigger animals. Maintaining sheep on concentrates is not the natural methods.

Unfortunately inadequate availability of feeds and forages due to reduction in area and deterioration of grazing lands poses a serious threat to sheep production because of high livestock density. This has been the compelling reason for large scale migration of sheep for the sake of grazing. Today the most important and difficult problem before the sheep industry is to find out ways and means to solve the nutritional problems of the current sheep population. For this it is obligatory to develop arid and semi waste lands into pastures and provide sufficient top feed through plantation of suitable fodder trees as road side plantation or elsewhere, conserve fodders and to increase production of coarse grains for meeting the requirement of sheep.

Nutrients Required by Sheep

Maintenance Needs

1. ENERGY. A deficiency of total energy supply of ewes is the most common nutrient deficiency. This may be due to lack of available feeds, for reasons of drought, low dry matter content of lush, over matured feed or may be due to pastures covered with snow. The effect of low energy intake tells upon the fertility of ewes, lower milk production and shortened lactation period, reduced wool production and more vulnerable to parasitism.

Many environmental factors effect the energy requirement of ewes and rams. They are, air temperature, wind velocity, humidity, wool length and shearing, stress, and distance travelled in grazing. The maintenance of sheep in confinement requires 10–30% less energy than sheep on excellent pasture. The maintenance requirements of mature sheep for energy are calculated as follows:

DE (Digestible energy)	$= 119\ W^{0.75}$
ME (Metabolisable energy)	$= 93\ W^{0.75}$
TDN (Total digestable nutrients)	$= 0.027\ W^{0.75}$

Where W = body weight in kg; DE and ME are kcal and TDN in kg/day (NRC, 1972). The energy requirements for gain would be approximately 15% higher (ARC, 1965). Experiments conducted at Balwant Rajput college, Agra have shown that a low protein and high energy ration produced more wool than as high protein and low energy ration. Energy is, therefore, the prime factor in sheep nutrition. The level of intake of energy can be ensured if the foraging material available in the pasture is of very high quality and sheep are allowed to graze for longer hours. This much of nutrient intake under the present conditions of sheep husbandry is not readily met with, resulting in low wool yield.

The ewe during the first 15 weeks of gestation require energy for maintenance, wool growth and for a 30 gm daily gain. There is little energy required for wool growth in comparison to protein needed. During the last 6 weeks of gestation, increased energy is required. This is because of the rapid development of the foetuses, mammary development and for the prevention of ketosis or pregnancy toxaemia.

2. PROTEIN. Like all other mature ruminants, the quantity of nitrogen or protein in an adult sheep's diet is more important than quality. Although all amino acids are synthesised from either non-protein nitrogenous compounds or from any feed protein, certain amino acids may be limiting, at least for wool production, since protein or amino acids experimentally administered post-ruminally has increased growth markedly. Methionine appears to be the first amino acid to be limited in microbial protein for both wool growth and body gain. Cysteine can replace methionine for wool growth and lysine and threonine are the next most limiting amino acids in microbial protein. The total protein requirements of sheep may be calculated from digestible protein values using the regression,

$Y = 0.929X - 3.48$, where Y = digestible protein and X = crude protein.

A level of 10 per cent protein in the ration has been found to be adequate for wool production since feeding of protein beyond this level does not have any beneficial effect on wool yield. An animal weighing 30 kg needs about 400 grams of TDN and 40 grams of DCP per day for optimum wool production within its genetic potential.

Normally, ewes, even when milking, can obtain sufficient protein from legume or high quality grass, hay, silage and pasture. When silage is the main forage or pasture becomes mature or sparse, protein must be supplemented. Insufficient protein results in reduced appetite, lowered feed intake, poor feed efficiency and weight loss. Reproductive efficiency and wool growth are also reduced. In such cases NPN sources such as urea can be used to provide the necessary nitrogen. Maximum utilisation of urea requires liberal feeding of available carbohydrates. Among minerals S in the ratio of N : S should be 10 : 1.

Table 17.8

Nutrient requirements of sheep* for maintenance

Body weight (kg)	*Dry matter intake (kg)*	*DCP (g)*	*TDN (g)*	*ME (Mcal)*	*Ca (g)*	*P (g)*
20	0.56	25	280	1.03	1.7	1.0
25	0.70	31	350	1.27	2.1	1.6
30	0.83	37	415	1.52	2.4	1.9
35	0.95	42	475	1.72	2.6	2.1
40	1.06	47	530	1.93	2.9	2.3
45	1.17	51	585	2.09	3.2	2.5

*Adult ewes which are non-lactating and are not over 15 weeks of gestation period.

3. MINERALS. In Chapter 10 dealing with minerals, it has already been mentioned that at present twenty one minerals have been found to be most essential for domestic animals but evidence to-date indicates that only fifteen elements can be considered essential for sheep. On the basis of the quantity required, those may be classified as major and trace minerals.

Table 17.9

Estimated requirements for the major minerals and requirements and toxic levels of the trace minerals[a]

Name	*Major minerals requirement, % of diet dry matter*	*Name*	*Trace minerals requirement ppm*	*Toxic level ppm*
Sodium	0.04	Iodine	0.10–0.80	8*
Chlorine	....	Iron	30–50	....
Calcium	0.21–0.52	Copper	5	<25
Phosphorus	0.16–0.37	Molybdenum	>0.5	5–20
Magnesium	0.04–0.08	Cobalt	0.1	100–200
Potassium	0.50	Manganese	20–40	....
Sulphur	0.14–0.26	Zinc	35–50	1000
		Selenium	0.1	5–20
		Fluorine	....	30–200

[a]From NRC (1972)

*High level for pregnancy and lactation in diets not containing goitrogens; increase level if diets contain goitrogens.

The above 15 minerals may again be divided into those that are usually supplied by natural feedstuffs, those that are frequently need to be supplemented and those that cannot be fed lawfully.

The minerals that are normally provided in sufficient amounts in natural feedstuffs include K, Mg, Fe and Mn. As an insurance against deficiency, Fe and Mn are usually added to trace mineralised salt. Trace mineralised salt is frequently offered to sheep as free choice which provides 8 out of 15 essential minerals. These are Na, Cl, I, Co, Fe, Cu, Mn and Zn. Only Ca, P and S are left for possible supplementation in normal situations.

The Zn requirement of sheep has not been researched in this decade, one of the most important clinical signs of Zn deficiency occurs in ram lambs is impaired testicular growth and complete cessation of spermatogenesis. It appears that the requirement of Zn by ram lambs for normal reproduction is greater than for growth.

It is sometimes necessary to supplement S, especially if a NPN source is fed. The most recent NRC recommendation is that S should always be present in the diet of ewes at a ratio of 10 parts N to 1 parts of S.

Consequently providing ewes with minerals under field condition is usually simple, convenient and relatively inexpensive.

From the current research work on minerals as required by sheep it appears that genetically different groups of sheep have got variation in mineral blood concentration. The investigation further revealed that breeds have got significant variation for Ca, P, K, Na, and Cl levels in blood and plasma. It has been estimated that heritability of blood Ca levels to be 0.44 and thus concluded that there is no "normal" blood value range of these minerals for all sheep. Certainly, further work is needed on physiological mechanism of mineral metabolism which are genetically controlled.

Most of the minerals required by sheep are supplied in adequate quantities through the range grasses, shrubs and seeds as normally consumed by them. However, in areas where the soil is deficient in cobalt or copper, these minerals will have to be fed as supplement through fortified mineral mixture. Additional copper is also required in regions where the molybdenum or inorganic sulphate content of the forages is high. In regions where the goitre is more prevalent, iodised salt should be fed to all ewes particularly during the later half of pregnancy. Common salt should always be made available to sheep, as they consume more salt per unit of body weight than the cattle. It is suggested that a box containing common salt may be kept under a small shed in place where the animals spend the night.

The best way to observe whether the non-producing animals are receiving adequate nutrients from their grazing is to weigh them periodically. When the animals either maintain their body weight or gain little weight to the extent of 20 to 30 gms per day, they can be stated to be on maintenance ration.

4. VITAMINS. Ruminants when attain maturity hardly needs any dietary supplementation of extra vitamins. Vitamin A as such is not found in any vegetable source but its precursor, carotene, is present in all green forages. Sheep do not need additional vitamin A if the carotene content is more than 1.5 mg per kg of ration. During summer, when the grass is parched and its carotene content is low some green legume hay or tree leaves may be fed to supplement vitamin A intake. Vitamin D is obtained through irradiation on exposure to sunlight. Sheep with white skin or short wool receive more rays from sunlight than do animals with black skin or long wool. Vitamin C or Ascorbic acid is not at all required as it is synthesised rapidly enough in the tissues to meet daily needs. Also the B vitamins are not required in the diet of

mature sheep as the rumen macroflora synthesise these in adequate amounts. Cobalt is necessary for synthesis of Vitamin B_{12}. Neither Vitamin K_1 nor Vitamin K_2 need to be fed as K_1 occurs in all green leafy materials fresh or dry and Vitamin K_2 is synthesised in the rumen.

Research has failed to relate poor reproductive performance in sheep with vitamin E deficiency. It does not seem to be of practical importance in sheep nutrition except for nursing lambs. A deficiency of Vitamin E and/or Se can cause white muscle disease in lambs 2-8 week of age.

FEEDING OF THE EWE FLOCK

The energy and protein requirements of sheep have already been presented in Table 17.8 but each ewe is not fed separately according to her individual requirements. The ewes are fed as a flock because:

1. It is practically impossible to feed all ewes individually,
2. The bulk of the ewe's energy and protein requirements are provided mostly from daily grazing,
3. The feed requirements of all the ewes in a flock, at any one time are very similar.

The feed requirements of the ewe flock is closely linked with its breeding cycle. This cycle can be divided into three periods:

1. Feeding during resting period,
2. Feeding during gestation period, and
3. Feeding during suckling period.

Feeding during Resting Period

When resting, the requirements of the flock are low. During this period she is kept on a low level of feeding. The flock can be used as scavengers to clear up poor and overgrown pastures, banks stubbles, etc. The practical way to find out whether the non-producing animals are receiving sufficient nutrients from their grazing is to weigh them periodically. If the animals are maintaining their body weight or putting on a little weight, to the extent of about 0.02 to 0.03 kg per day, they can be stated to be on maintenance ration. If they are continually losing body weight, then their grazing will have to be supplemented with additional concentrate mixture. As the breeding season draws near, the ewes will again be put on better pastures, i.e., for flushing. *Flushing* is the practice of increasing the feed intake of the ewe for gaining in weight and also for stimulating ovum production (increasing the number of twins) at the later stage of rest period i.e., usually 3 weeks prior to breeding is followed for increasing 10-20% lambs born. This is usually done either by allowing the ewes to graze excellent pasture or by feeding about 200-300 g of grain per head daily. The results from flushing are variable and may be explained in part, by a number of factors. Yarling ewes do not respond to the same extent as older ewes. Fat ewes are not influenced as favourably as thin ewes. On the other hand, ewes that have been fed to lose weight during their dry period do not respond as well those that were fed to gain very slowly during this time. Most ova are produced during the middle of the breeding season, so flushing at the beginning and at the end tends to give better results than when ovulation rate is at its peak.

Feeding during Gestation Period

The gestation period of ewes wlll range from 144 to 152 days with an average of 148 days. The first half of the gestation period when the developing embryo does not draw heavily on its mother's food supply, is less critical from a nutritional standpoint than the last half. At this stage unless the ewes receive a nutritive ration, weak and dead lambs will be the result. Special feeding care of ewes during the last six weeks of pregnancy will increase the (i) number of viable lambs, (ii) ewes milk yield, (iii) growth rate of lambs, (iv) the quality and quantity of wool clip.

The amounts of nutrients prescribed in Table 17.8 should be increased by 50 per cent to meet the extra requirement of the fast growing foetus. It is to be noted that at advanced stages of gestation the ewe cannot consume excess bulky roughages as the space in the abdomen is reduced due to the growth of the foetus. As such, the ewes on such physiological conditions should be provided with extra concentrates. Normally in addition to grazing, provision of 250 to 300 gms of any concentrate feed having about 25 per cent DCP and 75 per cent of TDN (e.g. gram or mixture of equal parts of crushed cereal grains and bran) is generally fed. Feeding extra feeds to meet heavy demands of the unborn lambs is known as "Steaming-up". If there had been a history of pregnancy disease in the flock, the provision of 100 gms of molasses will be helpful.

A body weight gain of about 100 gms a day for smaller breeds to 150.gms for larger animals is a fair measure of the nutrients intake status at this stage of physiological condition.

Feeding during Suckling Period

Just after lambing, the ewes must produce maximum quantities of milk to nurse the new born at least for about 3 months. To do this, of course, the mother ewes must be properly fed. To avoid udder troubles feed reduced amount of grain mixture for the first ten days but don't forget to provide with all the legume hay she consume. The shephred should at this stage must be cautious to increase the supplemented feed gradually upto 250 to 500 gms either as gram chuni or a mixture of cereal grains and wheat bran in the proportion of 2:1 along with legume hays from 1–2 kg. The mother ewes at this stage can consume dry matter up to 4 per cent of their live weight. Where good pastures are not available all care must be made to provide extra protein and minerals particularly of copper and cobalt other than common salt. The supplemental feeding should have 16–18 per cent crude protein.

Feeding Rams

Generally rams are maintained on the same feeding system as ewes. In case they are overfat they should be thinned by gradual reduction in feed and plenty of exercise. For normal size rams, during breeding time they will require supplementary feeding for a month before as well as during the whole breeding season. At this time an average ram may be offered 250 to 500 grams of the grain mixture consisting of crushed gram 2 parts, wheat bran 1 part and salt 1 part daily according to grazing conditions.

DENTITION

The species has got two sets of teeth i.e., milk teeth which are 20 in number and the permanent teeth numbering 32. These later consist of 8 incisors, 12 premolars and 12 molars. The age of a sheep can easily be determined from its incisors teeth as follows:

8 temporary incisors			about 6–10 months
2 permanent 6 temporary incisors			„ 10–14 months old
4 „	4 „	„	„ 2 years old
6 „	2 „	„	„ 3 years old
8 „	0 „	„	„ 4 years old

The normal lambs has eight (4 pairs) of temporary incisors in the lower jaw. The middle pair is replaced by a larger and permanent pair of incisors when the sheep is about a year old. The next pair is replaced by permanent teeth the following year and so on until the last pair, the fourth or corner pair, are in full wear when the sheep is approximately four years

Determining the Age of Sheep By Their Teeth

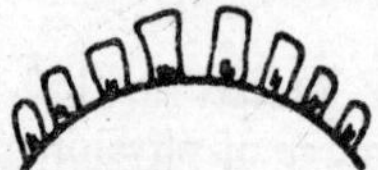

1. Lamb's mouth with 8 incisors; these temporary teeth are called milk teeth.

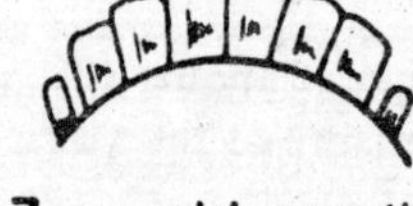

4. 3-yr.-old mouth with 3 pairs of permanent incisors.

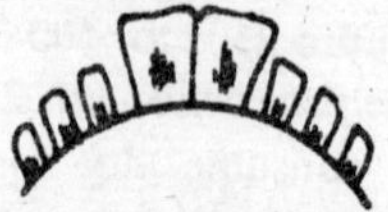

2. Yearling mouth with 1 pair of permanent incisors.

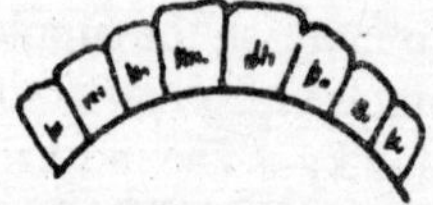

5. 4-yr.-old mouth with 4 pairs of permanent incisors.

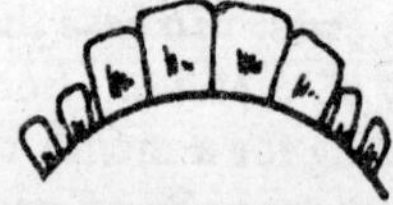

3. 2-yr.-old mouth with 2 pairs of permanent incisors.

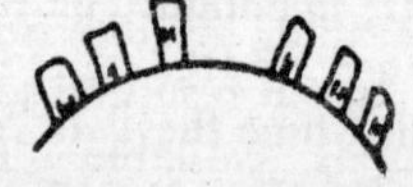

6. Broken mouth condition which may begin to occur about 6 yrs. of age; a sheep that has lost all incisors is called a gummer.

Fig. 17.2 Diagram showing how to determine the age of sheep by the teeth.

old. The time at which these teeth come varies with different breeds, e.g., in Nellore sheep 1st, 2nd, 3rd and 4th incisors erupt on an average, at 1 year 3 months, 1 year 8 months, 2 years 2 months and 2 years 8 months, whereas the corresponding ages for Mandya breed are: 1 year 5 months, 1 year 11 months, 2 years 9 months and 3 years 4 months.

Thus the condition of teeth is an indication of maturity rather than the exact years or months of age.

As the sheep get older, the teeth become long and narrow, and seem to spread apart. Finally they break off, thus producing what is known as broken mouth. When all of the incisors have disappeared, the sheep is known as a gummer. The age at which this condition exists depends to a great extent upon the kind of grazing land on which the sheep are kept. Many sheep have broken mouths by the age of six years if forced to graze pasture grown on heavy soils may have sound mouths at seven or eight years of age.

ESSENTIALS OF SHEEP MANAGEMENT ROUND THE YEAR

Managerial aspects of sheep rearing is vital for efficient production particularly in a state of affairs where raising of sheep is exclusively a pastoral enterprise while other livestock are raised on stall feeding under intensive system of housing.

India is a country of varieties. It has various types of languages, cultures, habits, topography and climate. As mentioned earlier, the country can be divided into four district sheep regions on the basis of topographical and agro-climatic conditions. For the sake of efficient management of sheep all the year round at various regions, all care must be taken to have the recommended managerial practices suited to various climatic conditions round the year.

A. Winter Season (December-January and February)

It is the time when it becomes extremely cold in the temperate and in North Western regions and moderately cold in the Eastern and Southern region. Grazing condition deteriorates due to poor growth of grass.

(1) Provide supplementary feeding to ewes and rams,
(2) Mature animals are now to be prepared to face the strain of coming mating season,
(3) The animals must be protected against cold particularly in temperate regions.

B. Spring Season (March and April)

Mostly the season is mild, heading for the hot season. Occasionally the pasture land will have new grasses coming out resulting scarcity of grazing materials. After the harvest of *Rabi* crops, stabble grazing is available. The sheep show gradual increase in body weight. With the gradual increase in day temperature condition goes in favour of parasitic infestations for which all possible care must be taken. At the same time outbreaks of entero-toxaemia are likely to be experienced. The following operations may be made.

In Dry Northern, Southern and Eastern region: 1. Ewes are then planned for mating. Estrous in ewes range from 20-42 hours, with an average of 30 hours. Ovulation occurs about 24-30 hours after the onset of estrous. If the ewe is not bred, or if she fails to conceive, estrous recurs after an interval of about 17 days.

2. Just prior to breeding season shearing of the flocks make them more active and in many cases, will improve their fertility. Sheep in India are generally shorn immediately after the

end of winter season when warm weather commences and sufficient grazing in the field is available.

3. Dipping at this time of the season is another essential provision for safe-guarding sheep for the following reasons:

(a) To remove excess of falty materials and dung from the fleece prior to clipping;
(b) To cleanse the skin from the products of sweat, shed epithelial scales and other waste materials;
(c) To eradicate the common parasitic agents such as lice, ticks, etc.;
(d) To prevent attack by the sheep-blowflies and consequent infestation with maggots.

The following is a list of dips classified according to disease to be treated.

Maggots	...	Any sulphur dip
Lice	...	DDT, Dieldrin
Ticks	...	BHC, arsenic
Scab	...	Lime sulphur solution

The dip must be carefully made up according to instructions, and fresh dipping powder and fluid added to make up the loss that occurs from the removal of a small amount upon the fleece of each sheep.

In hand bath type of dip, each sheep is lifted individually into the dipping bath, which usually of wood or concrete about 4 ft. long, 3 ft. 6 inches in deep, and 1 ft. 9 inches to 2 ft. wide, and turned over on to its back. They are held in the bath for about 2 minutes, their heads being immersed at least once. Then they are lifted on to a draining board where the excess dip is squeezed from their fleeces and runs back into the bath. Two men are required at the bath and one man is usually engaged catching from the collecting pen.

Precautions

1. For 4 to 5 weeks after service ewes should not be dipped as it might end up with abortion.

2. Sheep should be offered a drink of water before being dipped in hot weather, as there is some risk of thirsty animals drinking the dip, with fatal results if it is a poisonous variety.

3. The dip must be repeated at suitable intervals.

4. Due to Entero-toxaemia 5 to 10 per cent of sheep may die in any season. There are two forms of this acute disease, each caused by a different type of the organism e.g., Clostridium welchei Type C and Type D.

A vaccine is available for preventive purposes and it is advisable to give two doses at an interval of at least 14 days preferably during Spring season.

In temperate regions. In addition to above functions, attention for lambing of ewes followed by care of lambs become additional problems for the sheep owners.

C. Hot Season (May and June)

Day temperature will be gradually on the increasing side. Everywhere the grazing lands will look like barren resulting scarcity of green grasses. However, stubble of rabi harvested crops may provide some feed materials to sheep. Supplementary feeding either as silage or grain mix is necessary.

The picture in the temperate regions will be different, here grasses will continue to grow.

The following operations may suit in Northern, Southern and Eastern regions:

1. *Proper care of pregnant ewes.* When the flock is large, separate the ewes those are close to lambing. At this stage ewes will sink away on either side of the rump in front of the hips, the vulva will enlarge, wax will form on the ends of the teats, udder will distend and the teats will be tight and show signs of filling. Such animals should be protected from inclement weather.

During the first 3 months of pregnancy the ewes should be kept in fairly hard condition, neither gaining nor losing weight. The ewes should act as scavengers, clearing up stubbles. The day to day management involves looking at the pregnant ewes once a day to see that all is well, and checking the feet periodically to see that they are free from any infection.

2. *Steaming up.* As the ewes become heavy in lamb, they will require more nutrients to feed the developing lambs. The feeding of supplementary concentrates during the last two months of pregnancy is strongly recommended. This will lead to stronger and heavier lamb at birth, the ewes will milk better and the risk of pregnancy toxaemia will be considerably reduced. The concentrates should be fed in trough which will need moving daily. Allow at least 0.5 m of trough space per ewe to prevent them knocking each other when feeding.

In practice the effect of steaming up can be achieved by feeding:

8–6 weeks before lambing : 100 g concentrates +usual grazing/head/day
6–4 weaks before lambing : 200 g concentrates +usual grazing/head/day
4–2 weeks before lambing : 300 g concentrates +usual grazing/head/day
2–0 weeks before lambing : 450 g concentrates +usual grazing/head/day

Suitable mixture would be

(1) Cereal grains—40 parts
Wheat bran—30 „
GNC or Linseed cake—20 parts

(2) Barley, Dal or Maize — 46 parts
Sorghum grain — 34 „
Oilcakes — 20 „

(3) Any good dairy concentrate mixture containing 16-18 per cent crude protein.

The feeding of supplemental concentrate mixture can be gradually diminished after 8-10 weeks of lambing.

In temperate regions: Since in this region most of the lambs have already born, the shepherd should remain careful in rearing of lambs scientifically including marking and castration of lambs.

Marking

Marking may be done at the same time the lambs are docked and castrated. Pure bred lambs are marked so that the sires and dams of any lamb could be known. Range sheepmen mark their lambs so that they cannot get mixed up with another's. Apart from these well marked lambs are a precaution against thieves. Marking may be done by any of the following ways:

(1) *Ear notches.* It provides a quick method of marking but the disadvantage is that it makes the ears disfigures and for this reason it is not commonly used by purebred breeders.

(2) *Plastic tags.* Plastic tags having various combinations of letters and numbers may be used. Two tags, one in each ear, may be attached. One tag carries the individual number and the other the flock number. This system will provide identification number of the owner as well as of- the sires and dam of the lamb. Plastic or metal tags are costly for use in large flocks.

(3) *Paint brands.* The method is easy and can be applied with minimum expense and labour. Commercial branding fluids that will remain on sheep for a year, and may be removed from the fleece in the regular scouring process, are now available.

Castration

The three methods of castrating lambs are (1) Elastrator and rubber ring, (2) Burdizzo and (3) Surgical removal.

Elastration and rubber rings. The rings are placed under the scrotum and spermatic cord before the lambs are two days old. Care should be taken to see that both the testicles are below the ring.

Burdizzo or bloodless castrator. By taking the burdizzo in right hand, carefully draw one testicle down with your left hand. Place the spermatic cord between the jaws, then apply pressure. Repeat the second testicle. Lambs are best pinched before they are six weeks old.

Surgical removal. This is a surgical operation and should not be attempted unless accompanied by a veterinary surgeon. The following steps may be followed during surgical removal of the testis:

(i) Wash hands thoroughly,
(ii) Wash the scrotum with warm water and dettol,
(iii) Grasp the end of the scrotum with the left hand and gently force testicles back with the right fingers,
(iv) Pick up sterile scalpel (surgical knife) in right hand and cut off the end of the scrotum,
(v) Grip a testicle between the thumb and first finger. Gently twist, and apply traction to remove the stone,
(vi) Repeat with the second testicle,
(vii) Apply dettol to the wound.

D. **Rainy Season** (July, August and September)

During this season there is abundant growth of pastures. The sheep gains maximum body weight. The early period is ideal for reseeding of pastures, the later period is favourable for lambing. In the temperate region, the rainfall ranges from moderate to heavy, period is not favourable for lambing as the flocks are high up in the alpine pastures with least facility of providing protection.

The managerial practices for the regions at the rainy season may be summarised as below :

Northern, Southern and Eastern region	*Temperate region*
(a) Lambing time, so requires special attention in this regard	(a) Preparation of ewes for breeding
(b) Care of newly born lambs	(b) Deworming of sheep
(c) Deworming of all sheep by feeding anthelmintics	(c) Pairing of overgrown hoofs
(d) Reseeding of pasture lands	(d) Crutching of sheep

E. Autumn Season (October and November)

The condition of grazing land continues to be good. In addition sheep will stubble grazing after harvest of the kharif crops.

Sheep are migrated to remote pastures. Weaning, castration, shearing, dipping and deworming are some of important aspects of sheep farming at this season.

Health Care

Good hygiene and preventive treatments are vital aspects of good production. The signs of good health include general alertness. good movement and absence of lameness, good uniform fleece and absence of rubbing, active feeding and rumination and no wounds, abscesses or injuries.

General Hygiene

Proper cleaning of handling areas and houses. During housing, proper attention should be given to ventilation.

Disinfection

General disinfection of all the equipment used for routine procedures and treatment. Thorough disinfection is required during the lambing season of housed sheep.

Preventive and other treatments

Treatments involve vaccination, dosing (drenching), spraying or dipping, foot bathing and foot treatment. Programme of treatment is usually taken up following consultation with veterinary surgeon.

Control of Parasites

The important parasites of sheep include stomach worms, nodular worms, lung worms, liver flukes, ticks and lice.

Phenothiazine, thiabendazole and tramisol are some of the products that may be used to control stomach and nodular worms. These may be alternated in use to avoid the development of resistant strains of parasites. Each year the ewe flock and rams should receive worming medicines: two weeks before the breeding season. Ticks can be controlled by dipping or spraying with toxaphene, malathion or by dusting with rotenone.

Table 17.10 Vaccination Programme for Sheep

Disease	Vaccine	Age	Dose	Booster	Interval	Season
1. Food andMouth Disease	Foot and Mouth disease vaccine	Adult	5 ml S/c	—	Annual	Preferably Winter/ Autumn
2. Rinderpest	Rinderpest tissue culture vaccine	Adult	1 ml S/c	6 months	Annual	Winter
3. Black disease	Black disease vaccine	Adult	2 ml S/c	—	Annual	All Seasons
4. Lamb dysentry	Lamb dysentry vaccine	Lamb	2 ml S/c	—	Annual	All Seasons
5. Black quarter	Black quarter vaccine (Polyvalent)	Lamb Adult	2 ml S/c 3 ml S/c	—	Annual	All Seasons preferably May/June
6. Enterotoxaemia	Enterotoxaemia vaccine	Lamb Adult	2.5 to 5 ml S/c	7–10 days	Annual	Lambing season
7. Haemorrhagic septicaemia	Haemorrhagic septicaemia adjuvant vaccine	Adult	2ml S/c	—	Annual	March/ June
8. Sheep pox	Sheep pox vaccine	Lamb Sheep	3 ml s/c 5 ml S/c	Repeat at 6 months Repeat annually		December/ March
9. Lung worm	Irradiated lung worm Vaccine	Lamb 3 months age	1000 larvae first dose	One month later 2000 larvae.		

Source: Schultz, R.D. and Scott, F.W. (1978). The Veterinary Clinics. North America. 8:755. W.B. Saunders Co.; Philadelphia, London, Toronto.

Handling Sheep

A sheep should be caught by the nose, flank or by the hind leg (least preferred method). Never catch or hold a sheep by the wool since this will bruise the flesh just under the skin. If the left hand is under the jaw and the right hand on the sheep's rump, the animal can easily be controlled or "nosed" over at will : To mouth a sheep, as in examining the teeth spraddle the neck, raise the head with the left hand under the jaw, and part the lips with the right hand.

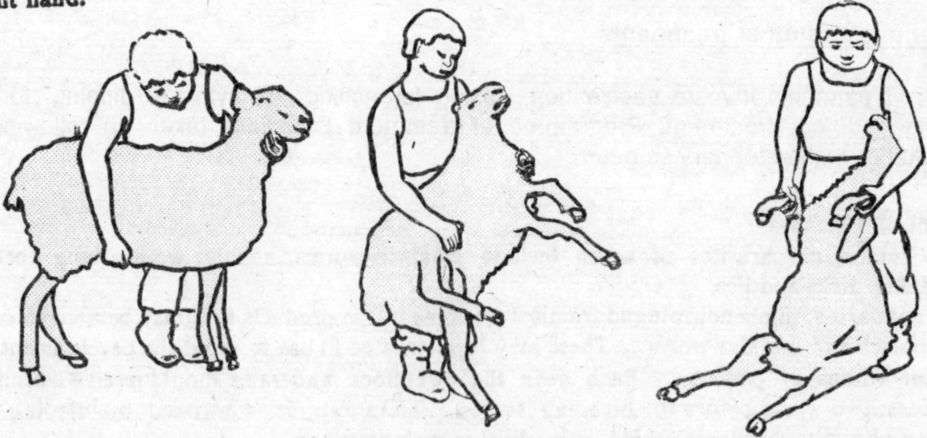

Fig. 17.3. The lift method of casting.

18

CAMEL

Origin

According to geological findings, ancestors of all members of the family Camelidae, viz. Camel, Llama, Alpaca, Guanaco and Vicuna originated in North America. One group migrated to Asia and the other to South America, and that both became extinct in North America probably after the glacial period (ice age) about five million years ago.

The genus *Camelus* has two species, the heavily built, two-humped *Bactrian* camel (*Camelus bactrianus*) which inhabits the deserts of central Asia reaching upto Mongolia and western parts of China. The bactrian camel is very strongly built and copiously covered with long dark brown hair on its humps, neck and shoulders, which is essential to Asiatic mountainous terrains which experience extreme low temperature. In the hot summer it sheds its thick hair for a much lighter and shorter covering. The other species is single-humped Arabian camel (*Camelus dromedarius*) commonly known as *Dromedary* widespread throughout the Middle East, India and North Africa. An adult Bactrian seldom measures more than 7 feet (2 meters) from the ground to the top of the humps—about the height of the shoulder in the taller and more slender Dromedary.

The other two species of the genus *Llama* are Llama (*Llama glama*) and Alpaca (*Llama pacos*), now living in South America lost their hump in the course of evolution. However, they are all hornless ruminants, with elongated neck and longish head, a split upper lip, and feet in the shape of broad pads.

Domestication and Distribution of Dromedary

The dromedary had been domesticated on the borders of Arabia by 1800 B.C. Subsequently the animals were introduced to North Africa, the Nile Valley, and the Middle East as far as north-western India. According to F.A.O. report of 1978-79, in Asia (India, China, Pakistan, Mongolia, Iran, Iraq, Afganisthan, U.S.S.R., Saudi Arabia, Yemen etc.) there are about 5 million camels. In Africa it is about 6.6 millions, in Australia 20,000 and in other countries of the world it is about 230,000 thus comprises about 12 million population in the world.

India possesses about 1.2 million which comprises 10 per cent of the world camels. Rajasthan is number one in the country regarding camel population (753,000) followed by Haryana, Punjab, U.P. and Gujarat having camels 135,000; 115,000; 49,000 and 45,670 respectively.

Zoological Classification

The Camelidae family consists of three genera, (1) the true Camels of Asia (genus:

Camelus); (2) the wild Guanaco and the domesticated Alpaca and Llama of South America (genus; Llama); Vicuna, also of south America (genus: Vicugna).

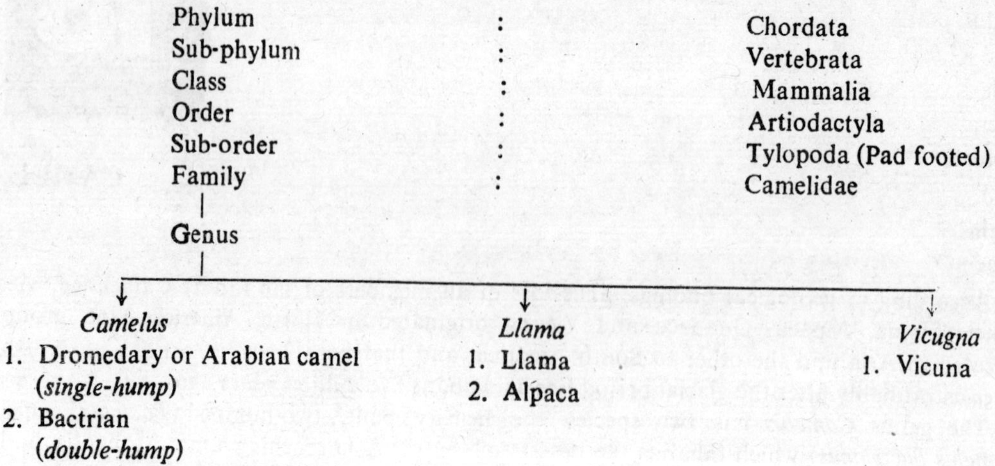

1. Neither the Arabian nor the Bacterian species exist any longer in the wild state, though there are some semi-wild herds, which have escaped from captivity.

2. The Indian Camels are all single humped *C. dromedarius* and as a rule is less heavily built, longer in the hind with soft coat and comparatively thin. Average dromedaries weigh from 454 to 590 kg.

Utility of Camels

Camels are put to a variety of uses in different states in the country depending upon the soil, climate and rainfall. Apart from acting as a significant power source, they are potential suppliers of commercial products such as camel hair, hide, meat, milk, raw bones and manure.

1. A camel can pull a load equivalent to 40 per cent of its body weight. Thus a well built camel can generate about 1.0 horsepower for long periods and can carry 18–20 kg of load for 20 km in 4 hours without showing signs of distress, but when used for speed only they may cover even 150 km a day. They are also used for ploughing lands @ 0.5 to 0.6 ha of land in 8 hours, for pulling carts of 550 kg, drawing water with the help of persian wheels, threshening maize and other grains, crushing sugarcane etc.

2. Camel energy is cost-effective. A recent report shows that more and more people in Rajasthan are seeking loans for buying camels and camel carts. Camels play an important role in the defence of our country. With a long desert border of Rajasthan where BSF and military have to keep constant vigil, camel serves as a valuable means of transport. Camel corps is an important unit of the defence services comprising a crossbred named as *Dogla* breed. During last war between India and Pakistan, Indian Camel Corps repulsed the attacks where Pakistani tanks got stuck in sand. While walking they raise both legs on the same side of the body simultaneously.

3. Milk is another valuable product obtained from camel, a female may yield about 3–5

litres daily. Camel milk on an average consist of 5.1% lactose, 4.8% fat, 3.8% protein and 0.9% ash. The camel female nurses her young for more than a year. The milk composition varies with breed, plain of nutrition, stage of lactation etc,. The milk tastes slightly saline and hard to curdle or to prepare ghee from it. The milk is consumed mostly as liquid milk.

4. It usually gives milk from 10 to 18 months since parturition. Provided that the feeds are made available, in a full lactatian the yield may touch 2,750 litres on twice a day milking. In general the daily yield varies between 5–10 litres. The composition of milk depends upon types of breeds, plain of nutrition, stage of lactation etc. On an average it consists of 5.1% lactose, 4.9% fat, 3.7% protein and 0.8% ash. The composition is very much similar to that of cow's milk except that it has more sugar and is tallowy odour. Acts as a laxative to those who are not used to it. A fermented product *Kumiss* can easily be prepared from it, on the other hand butter preparation is felt difficult. Camel milk is regarded as a cure for diseases of spleen, dropsy and jaundice. The milk is frequently used for infant feeding.

5. Camel hide is used for making suitcases as well as for large skin recepticles (*Kuppas*) used for storing oils and ghee. It does not make good leather.

6. Camel meat is coarse and tough but still is eaten in many countries. Dressing percentage varies between 55 to 65. No attempt has yet been made to develop any specialised meat breed.

7. Camels can halt the desert's advance. Unlike cattle and sheep, which graze on the ground vegetal cover and thus expose the precious topsoil to the action of wind and rain, camels brows on the upper storeys of vegetation; they also range more widely while browsing. Thus bringing more camels into the periphery of desert lands might help slow down the process of desertification.

Indian Camels

(according to region where they are bred)

	Plain Camels		*Hill Camels*
	Desert varieties Mostly found in arid sandy tracts of Bikaner & Jaisalmer in Rajasthan	*Riverine varieties* Mostly found in Western parts of U.P. and Punjab, carry heavy loads. Slow in movement with a speed of about 3 km per hour.	Found mostly in hilly regions of North Punjab. The animals are shorter in stature, compact with muscular body. Short neck, wide chest with short legs, feet are round and hard. Its endurance capacity is good and is therefore employed for loading, riding and ploughing purposes.
Type	Riding	Baggage	Baggage
Breeds	Jaisalmer Bikaner Sindhi	Afgan	Mewati

Breeds of Indian Camel

Indian camels (*Arabian* or *Dromedary*) termed as Plain camels and Hill camels, according to the regions where they are bred. The *Plain Camels* are found in non-hilly areas as against *Hill Camel* which are found in hilly areas.

Plain camels include *Reverine* (animals live in areas where there are provisions of water supply from rivers and canals) and the *Desert* varieties (inhabitants of arid sandy tracts).

Hill camel and the Reverine camels are the *Baggage type* (capable of carrying loads), whereas the Desert camels are *Riding type* (uncapable of carrying significant loads but very good for travelling).

Table 18.1

The Salient Points Regarding Characteristics and Management of Baggage and Riding Camels of India

Riding type	Baggage type
1. Large study animals good for carrying loads both in plain and hilly regions.	1. Good for riding at 3 years of their age.
2. Camels having well developed hump, thick neck, big head, broad chest, strong legs and sound foot-pads.	2. Lighter animal, more active and high on legs with slender limbs. The head is small, chest is broad with well developed muscle. It has small eyes, short ears, thin skin and small feet.
3. A camel may carry from 2 to 3 quintals of load, the maximum load allowed in army is limited to 1.8 quintals	3. Camels can cover 95–115 km at a stretch. Can travel daily about 48 km for days at an average speed of 10 to 11 km per hour. Average adult body weighs between 530 to 560 kg.
4. For the purpose of heavy work, camels of about 6 years of age should only be engaged	4. While riding the tail is tied to one side by a thin rope fastened to the saddle.
5. Marching of camels are always preferable either at night or in the early morning. They should never be standing under load larger than necessary.	5. While riding the camel should never be struck on the neck.
6. All precautions must be taken so that the load is equally shared and balanced on both sides of the hump.	6. A riding camel is first taught to kneel to order and to submit to saddling (a padded leather seat for a rider).

Apart from Desert type camels, viz., Bikaneri, Jaisalmeri, Sindhi, Mahri, other important mixed breeds of camels found in Rajasthan State in sufficient numbers viz., *Marwari, Jalori, Mewari, Shekhawati* or *Bagri, Mewati* and *Kutchi.*

Physical characteristics

Camels have even toed, digitigrade feet (that is, the posterior of the foot is raised). The third and fourth toes are united by thick, fleshy pads and tipped with nail like hooves. Horny

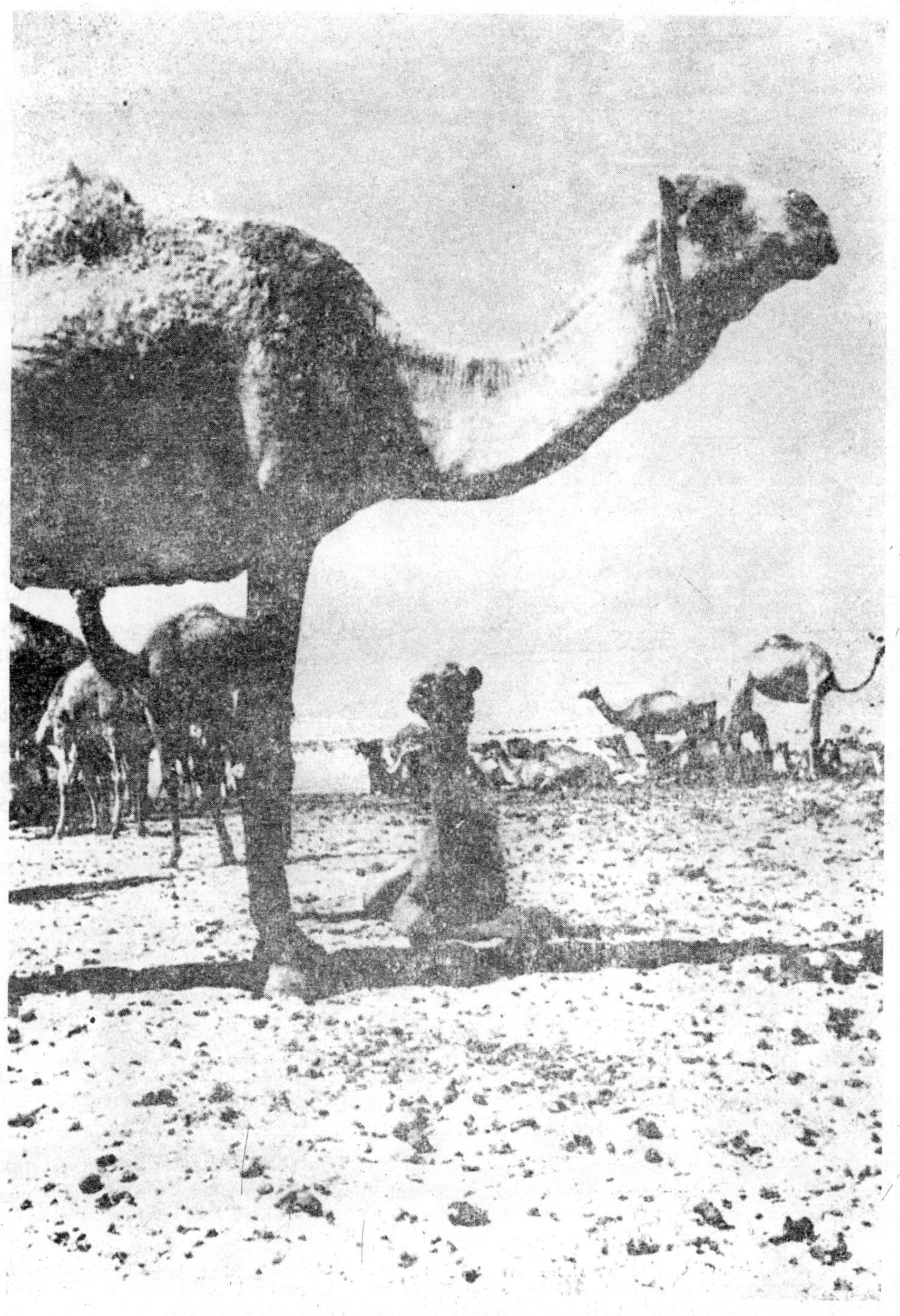

Plate 94. The single-humped Arabian camel, or Dromedary *(Camelus dromedarius)*, ranging in colour from dirty white to dark brown.

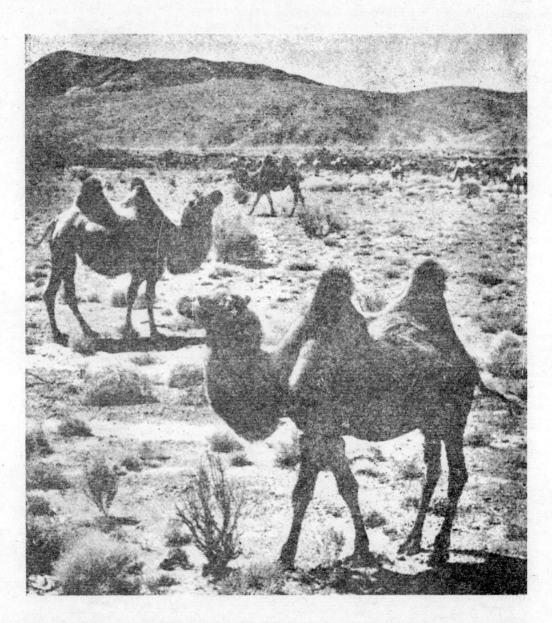

Plate 95. The two-humped Central Asian camel, (*Camelus bactrinaus*) also known as Bactrian, as the species originated from Bactria, the ancient name of Turkistan. In China camal is known as *Fongkyo.*

pads are present on the chest and knees which supports the body at the time camels kneels. They have long arched neck and long legs which give them sufficient height to reach the leaves of trees and tall cacti found in their normal habitat. The muzzle is long with the pendulous upper lip overhanging the lower. These lips are coarse, thick, rubber like prehensile organs well suited for grasping the prickly twigs and thorn bushes which form the only edible vegetation of the barren regions. The ears are small. Adaptations to desert life include broad, flat, thick-soled clover hoofs that do not sink into the sand. As the foot presses on to the ground the broad pads spread out further, giving a greater area of support.

There is one pair of skin glands on the back of the head in both sexes (sexual glands) which serete a black, creamy substance. In adaptation to unfavourable environments, camels have double rows of protective eyelashes, haired ear openings, the abiliy to close the nostrils which is valvuler and lined with hairs and keen senses of sight and smell. It can smell water from miles away and would invariably reach the source if they get lost in the desert. Similarly by instinct it can smell the presence of tiger or lion even from a distance of 2-3 km. The camel's hump is made mostly of fatty tissues. When food is scarce, the camel can draw on this store of fat as it is on oxidation produce metabolic water.

The camel uses mouth for fighting due to its strong teeth. There are on an average 34 teeth with usual variation of 32–38. There are two permanent canine-like teeth on both sides of the lower jaw. These canines reach their full size at 7 years, when they are long and still sharp pointed. As the camel ages all the teeth become worn and blunt, and by 12 years the canines are also gets flattend (stumps).

Behaviour

They are of very low intelligence and this makes their training difficult. The husbandry of camel was never a worthwhile proposition. They require vast areas for pasture and they do not acquaint well with other animals. These are comparatively slow maturing animals. At the age of eight years a camel is in the state of maturity as a horse at five years. That is why camels are put to hard work only after five or six years of their age. On maturity the animals are used for riding, carrying loads, ploughing land, thrashing grains, driving carts, supplying power to Persian waterwheels or to sugarcane or oilseeds crushing mills.

Nature has provided innumerable special features to make it fit to thrive in desert where camel can go without water for a much longer period than any other mammal. Due to its long neck, the camel can have easy access to the branches of high trees.

They possesses superb patience even under conditions of neglect and rough handling but on many occasions stupidity and oostinacy in camel have been noted. The males are quarelsome during the rutting season and bite savagely when they fight.

When water is found in the desert it is drunk in enormous quantities, the excess, being stored in small vessels all round the stomach. This reserve supply allows the camel to survive for about a week without water. Provided with cacti or succulent plants or leaves, it can continue for several months without any liquid.

The camels are slow breeders, producing only one calf every three years, and this takes nearly five years to reach maturity.

The camel consumes all sorts of food, unsuitable for other leaf-eating animals, and can live on leaves of hard, thorny plants like acacia and cactus.

For handling the camel for work, a nose peg made of wood is inserted by piercing one or both the nostrils.

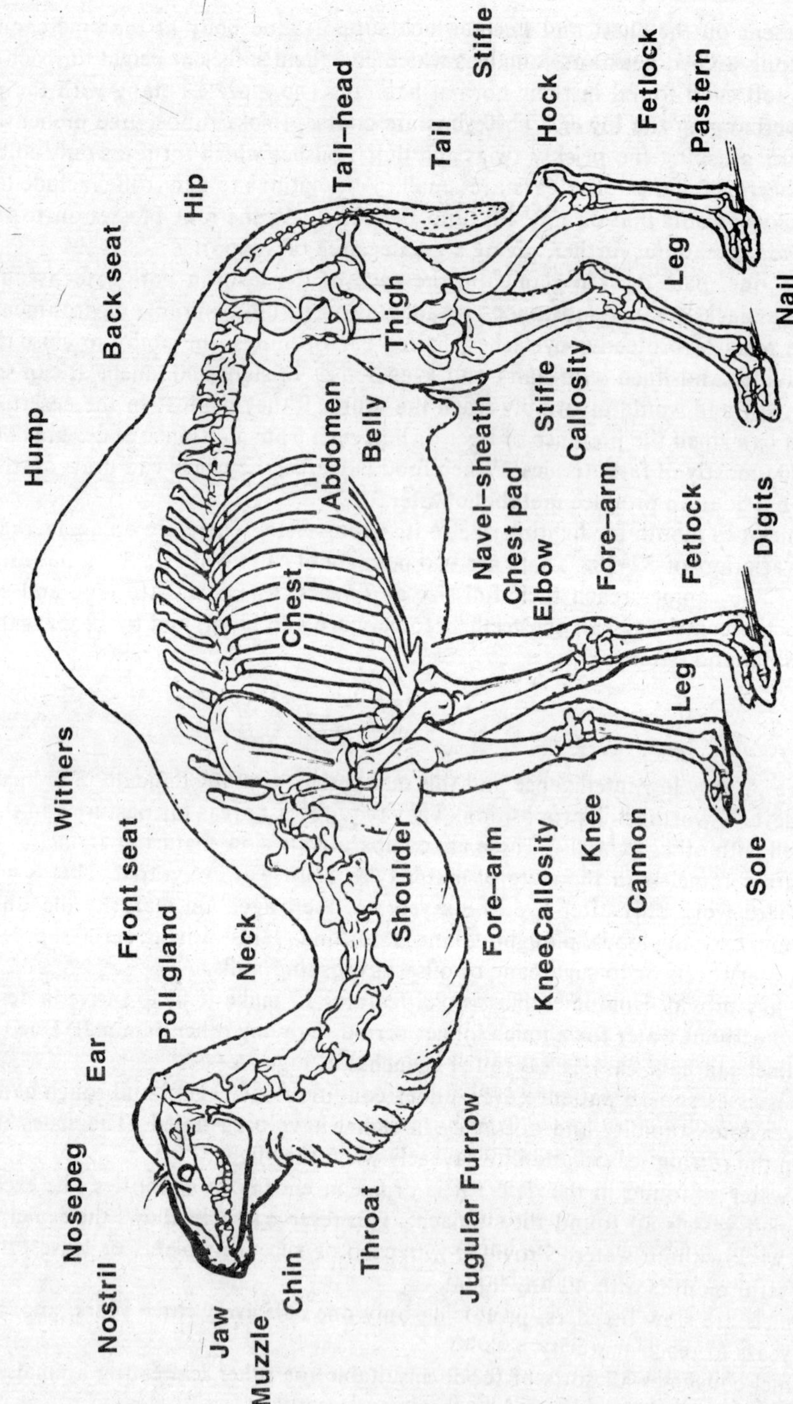

Fig. 18.1 Parts of the camel.

The male camel although shows signs of sexuality as early as two years, but it is felt that they attain full sexual maturity at eight years of age, while cow camel is sexually mature at four to five years of age.

The camel may live to the age of 40 years or more.

Reproduction in the Camels

A. Anatomy of Reproductive Organs

Male

The two small oval shaped testicles are located high up in the perineum behind the thighs. In adult the left testis is slightly heavier than right one. The capsule of the testis is composed of irregularly arranged dense elastic type fibroblastic tissue. During rutting period (the periodic sexual excitement of male camels) the testis becomes turgid while in non-rutting period it is flaccid. Spermatozoa appear pointed and spear shaped in profile and oval when seen on flat surface. In general the camel spermatozoa are smaller than those of other species of domestic animals.

The penis and the urethra have two successive curves i.e., sigmoid flexure as in bull, the first has its convexity forwards and the second has its convexity backwards. The only difference is that in bulls the sigmoid flexure is post-scrotal whereas in the camel it is pre-scrotal. The non-erect penis is directed backwards; otherwise it resembles that of the bull and extension of it at coitus depends mainly on the straightening of the sigmoid flexure. During erection the penis is straightened out to a total length of about 68 cm from the ischial arch. Retraction of the penis is effected by the action of muscles inserted into the second curvature. The penis gradually tapers to its tip which however is not pointed. The tip of the penis is normally 10 cm from the opening of the sheath, which is sufficiently large, flat, pendulous and triangular in shape. The skin over the sheath is black, covered with short hair and bears two rudimentary nipples on its side.

Female

The two ovaries each of 4–5 cm long, 1.5 cm thick, weighing about 15 to 20 grams. The ovaries are situated in the sublumber region under the 6th or 7th vertebra. When matured, the organ appears like a bunch of grapes. Numerous graafian follicles are found in various stages of development on the ovaries in other species. The peculiarity in this species is the presence of graafian follicles at different developmental stages along with the active corpus luteum (CL) of pregnancy. It seems that the presence of a CL in the ovary does not necessarily prevent a graafian follicle from being increased in size. In about 5 per cent cases of pregnancy graafian follicles are seen. Because ovulation is a sequel to coitus, corpora lutea are to be expected only in pregnant camels however, smaller apparently functional corpora lutea occur and probably they are a legacy of early pregnancy failures. The young CL is soft and spherical, brownish on section, with a central blood clot. It can be detached from the ovary by digital pressure exerted at its base. The mature CL is a compact sphere of 2.6 cm diameter and flesh coloured, with a central area of grey connective tissue. Older CL have a greenish or bluish-grey external appearance. Corpora lutea persist throughout pregnancy and the established CL cannot be detached from the ovary by finger pressure.

The left and right ovaries function equally and ovulate alternately. Because ovulation is induced by coitus, the length of oestrous depends on whether and when mating occurs. In the absence of male, oestrous may last for about two weeks, whereas if copulation occurs on the first day of oestrous receptivity may disappear after three days. Twin ovulation occurs in 40% matings.

The uterus is bicornuate, with a well developed uterine body, from which the two horns diverge and taper anteriorly to give a combined uterine shape intermediate between that of the letters Y and T. The left horn is longer than the right, even in the fetus. The endometrium shows irregularly raised mainly longitudinal folds, which are more conspicuous in the right horn. The cervix resembles that of the cow but has five annular mucosal folds. A few centimetres behind the cervix is a concentric fringe-like fold of the anterior vaginal mucosa, which tends to obscure the os uteri externum, and behind it are several progressively less prominent circular folds.

The uterine tubes are 22–24 cm long. Their width increases towards the ovarian end where the tubes are obviously funnel-shaped. The mesosallpinx and the mesovarium together form a very well developed bursa which closely invests the ovary.

The vagina is about 32 cm long and has a number of loose folds behind the cervix. There is no demarcation line between the vulva and vagina. The Gartner's and the Bartholin's glands are well developed in camel.

Mammary glands

The four mammary glands are placed on either side of median plane in prepubic region. The front quarters are comparatively larger than the posterior ones. The teats are short and each has got two orifices. The skin over the udder is blackish.

B. Reproductive Behaviour

Sexual Maturity

She-camel reaches sexual maturity at about 3 years of age but usually they are bred during 4 years of their age, otherwise early breeding will check the growth of the dam and the calf and thereby rarely develops well. The camel breeds only in winter months i.e. during November to March. Normally a she-camel can be bred until 20 years of age and some respond even upto 30 years of their age may be obtained.

Oestrous Cycle

The oestrous cycle in camel of Rajasthan varies from 22 to 24 days with an average of 23 days. Cases have also been recorded with longer intervals between two oestrous cycles. It remains regular between November to March (cold weather). If the cow camel does not conceive upto March, the ovaries become quiescent and inactive but again when the temperature becomes low and the humidity rises up, the she-camel starts coming in heat again and may repeat every 19 days till she conceives within March. The oestrous lasts for 3 to 5 days. As because ovulation is induced by coitus, the length of oestrous depends on whether and when mating occurs. In the absence of male, oestrous may last for two weeks, whereas if copulation occurs on the first day of oestrous, receptivity may disappear in 3 days. Twin ovulation occurs in 14% of matings.

Signs of Oestrous

During oestrous female exhibits typical symptoms of restlessness, excitement, bleating and grunting, frequent micturition and wandering in search of a male. The vulval lips are swollen and there is appearance of slimy discharge. If it is let loose alone there is acute restlessness, animal remains off feed, tries to smell the male urine and homosexual tendency is noticed. The she-Camel moves its tail up and down in rapid succession on the approach of the male or when hearing the gurgling voice of the rutting male.

Vaginal temperature during oestrous is about 99.32 ± 0.09°F while in dioestrous it is 98.56 ± 0.013°F. Similarly the rectal temperature in heat rises to 98.57 ± 0.098°F and in disestrus it comes down to 97.32 ± 0.083°F. Pulse and respiration rate raises to 45.18 ± 0.08 and 7.22 ± 0.13 respectively. The pH of mucus in heat raises to 7.5 ± 0.20 while in dioestrous it becomes 6.77 ± 0.26. The fern pattern of mucus at initiation of oestrous shows a typical pattern which gradually becomes a typical towards the end of heat. This pattern altogether disappears during dioestrum.

Mating Behaviour

The rutting male pursues the oestrous female and on catching up with her, presses his head on her neck and induces her to sit on the ground in a leaning position and the male camel squats like dogs over her with flexed hindlimbs resting on the ground and the forelimbs extended on each side clasping the female. Both male and female face in the same direction. The sexual act takes for about 10–20 minutes and is accompanied by gurgling and frothing by the male and bleating

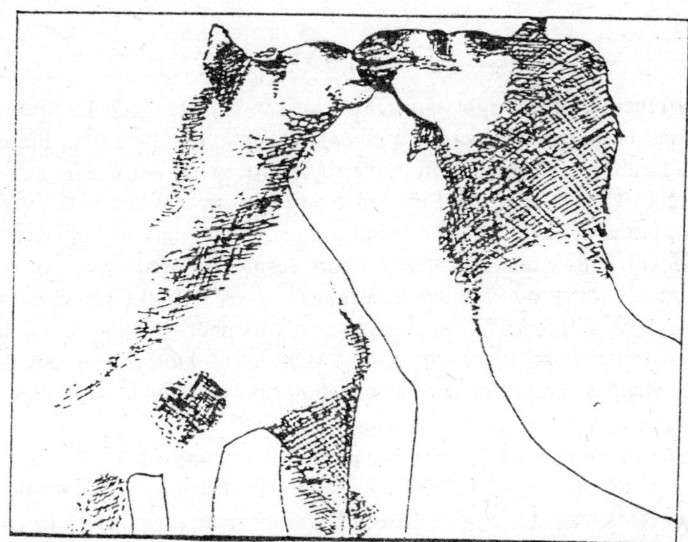

Fig. 18.2 Showing female in oestrus. Starts coming close to male.

by female. If mating takes place in the herd, the other she-camels collect round the conjugating couple to screen them from other animals including human beings. In fact during mating activities, which are interspersed with several bouts of male pelvic thrusting and correspondingly louder vocal responses from the female, the rest of the herd becomes alerted and assembles in a circle round the copulating pair.

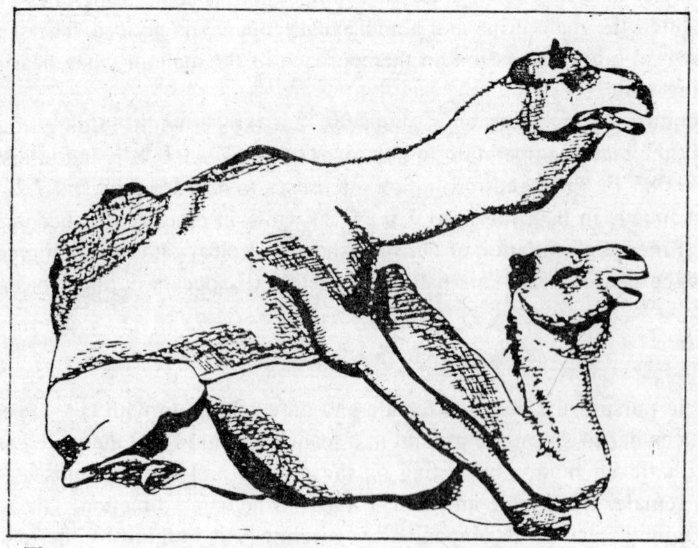

Fig. 18.3 Copulatory action. Male extends fore limbs.

Pregnancy

Despite the equal function of the right and left ovaries, 99% of pregnancies are in the left horn (and uterine body) and although the incidence of twin ovulation is 14% twin births occur to an extent of only 0.4%. Embryonic migration from the right horn to left is frequent and seems always to occur when he right ovary ovulates and the left ovary does not. When both ovaries ovulate at the same oestrous embryos develop initially in both horns but the one in right horn dies when it reaches a size of 2–3 cm. This embryonic death occurs despite the coalescence of the chorions of two embryos. Presumably, allantoic vascular anastomosis does not take place, as in the bovine, and there is no record of a freemartin among the small number of twins born. It is a unique biological curosity that successful placentation of a right-horn embryo does not develop in the corresponding horn, whereas the placenta of a left horn embryo regularly intrudes into the right horn and develops extensively throughout the right horn.

As in the cow, the allantois of the camel elongates quickly and soon protrudes from the left horn into the uterine body and the right horn. Because the uterine body is relatively large, the shape of the whole placenta resembles more closely that of the mare than that of the cow. Moreover, the camel placenta is diffuse type, like the mare's not cotyledonary.

The amount of allantoic fluid increases from about 1.5 litres at a fetal body length 0–10 cm to approximately 5–6 litres at a body length 11–20 cm. This volume is maintained fairly constantly until 90–100 cm when it rises to 6 litres, finally, at a fetal body length of 101–107 cm, the allantoic volume is about 8 litres. The allantoic fluid is like pale urine and sometimes contains yellow-brown hippomanes. The volume of amniotic fluid rises from 13 ml at a fetal body length of 0–10 cm to a final volume of nearly 1 litre, i.e. its amount is always small relative to the allantoic fluid. The amniotic fluid is usually watery but sometimes cloudy and brown with bits of meconium and 'hippomanes'.

Fetal growth is of a linear pattern. Posterior presentations predominate (54–60%) from early pregnancy to a fetal body length 41–50 cm at which point the situation changes to an anterior presentation of 51%. The anterior presentations increase sharply to 93% at a fetal body length of 61–70 cm and then to the final gestation presentation of nearly 100% anterior. There is no tendency in late pregnancy for the amnion to separate from the allantochorion as it may do in the cow.

Gestation Period

The gestation period of a cow camel is comparatively longer than any other domestic ruminant. It varies from 365 to 400 days with an average of 390 days. Usually the first pregnancy is prolonged by 10–20 days. Cow camel gives birth to one calf at a time and breeds once in two years and suckles the offspring for a year. Abortion is common in Indian camels and generally due to either trypanosomiasis or scarcity of food.

Pregnancy Diagnosis in Camel

(a) *Cocking of Tail*

In about 2 to 3 weeks time after the service, the she-camel which has conceived can be distinguished by the way she develops tendency to raise the tail upwards whenever approached by a male or handled by a man. If the tail hangs in the pendulous position, then she is taken as empty and vice versa. However the sign does not prove to be 100 per cent right in every case.

(b) *Rectal Palpation*

The technique of palpation of the genital organs is the same as for the cow but the she-camel needs to be restrained in the sitting position. In connection with early diagnosis it is important to remember four features of camel reproduction:

1. Large corpora lutea are only present in pregnancy.
2. 99% of pregnancies are in the left horn.
3. The empty (or early pregnant) right horn is congenitally shorter than the left.
4. The amount of fetal fluid at all stages of camel pregnancy is less than in the cow.

From the foregoing it is clear that the presence of a palpable corpus luteum in one or both ovaries is a very strong indication of pregnancy. However, a corpus luteum would form after a sterile mating and would be present initially in the cases where embryonic death occurs; but in both these instances the CL would not persist.

The earliest palpable swelling of the pregnant (left) uterine horn is at one month in the bactrian camel. In the dromedary, however, no swelling is palpable until the eighth week when the whole of the left horn is uniformly enlarged. At this time both ovaries (one or both with CLs), together with the uterus, are within the pelvis. It should be noted that because the camel placenta is non-cotyledonary it is not possible to *'slip the fatal membrane'* as in the cow. By the eighth week, vaginal palpation or inspection reveals a plug of adhesive mucus in the os uteri externum.

At the end of the third month the pregnant left horn is clearly larger and softer and in front of the non-pregnant right horn. It is at the pelvic brim and its corresponding ovary is in the abdomen. At the fourth month the uterus is just in front of the pelvic brim but most of it is palpable. A month later the limits of the uterus cannot be defined, although its dorsal surface is still palpable. During the sixth month, and for the remainder of pregnancy, the fetus can be palpated and the ovary on the non-pregnant (right) side can be felt until the tenth or eleventh month. From the seventh month individual parts of the fetus, namely head and legs, can be identified. External observation of the right flank reveals spontaneous fetal movements from the ninth month and the fetus can be ballotted from the tenth month.

In the eleventh month the vulva is slightly swollen and hypertrophy of the udder is first noticed. In the following month there is abdominal enlargement and the camel is lethargic. The caudal part of the uterus now projects backwards and occupies the anterior two-thirds of the pelvis. The sacrosciatic ligaments begin to relax.

In the thirteenth month relaxation of the pelvic ligaments is pronounced, tumefaction of the vulva is marked and hypertrophy of the udder is more evident. The fetus can be balloted from both flanks.

Incidentally, regarding the length of gestation in the camel, almost incredible variations of from 308 to 440 days have been given. The mean duration is probably around 375 days.

(c) *Electronic Pulse Detector*

It is expected that this technique could be successfully used from mid-pregnancy, applying the probe to the right flank or above the uterus per rectum.

(d) *Progesterone test*

Because persistent corpora lutea are said to be present only in pregnancy, a progesterone assay carried out after a suitable interval from copulation should be effective in distinguishing pregnancy from non-pregnancy. Obviously, embryonic death could occur after a positive test result and it remains to be determined in what percentage of instances this would negate the result. Presumably milk, in lactating animals, or blood could be used for this test.

(e) *pH of the Urine*

The urine pH gets alkaline as the stage of pregnancy is advanced. It may touch 8.0 as against pH 7.4 ± 0.08 normally noted in non-pregnant camel.

(f) *Specific Gravity of Urine*

It may vary from 1.038 ± 0.010 to 1.086 ±0.003 in pregnant camels whereas in non-pregnant it is about 1.036.

(g) *Gonadotrophin Test*

The presence of follicle-stimulating hormone in the blood of pregnant camels using immature female mice as in the method devised by Cole Saunders (1935) in the mare. The mouse ovaries showed marked follicular activity when injected with the blood of camels pregnant with fetuses of fetal body lengths between 11 and 58 cm. The source of the gonadotrophic factor in the camel is presumable of placental origin.

Parturition in Camel

The usual signs approaching parturition are swelling of the vulva, enlargement of the udder and sinking of the pelvic ligaments forming a groove on either side of the tall. The premonitory signs of parturition are abdominal distension, mammary hypertrophy, with presence of colostrum, and odema of the vulva. Most camels calve in winter and spring. Almost 100% of presentations are anterior.

First-stage labour lasts 24–48 hours and the period of expulsion is half an hour. If the placenta is retained for more than a day the mother is said to become ill due to the development of endometritis.

During the second stage the she-camel adopts a sitting posture. The allantochorion ruptures before reaching the vulva. There are bouts of straining at intervals of 30–60 seconds and the fetal nose, covered by the amnion, appears first. Later one front foot and then the other are protruded alongside the head and with further straining they are both extended well beyond the head. Maximum straining effort then leads to complete emergence of the head and the rest of the body quickly follows. One's comparative obstetric impression of second-stage labour in the camel is of a rather elegant, untrammelled expulsion of a well-lubricated and beautifully streamlined fetal body. The umbilical cord ruptures as the offspring wriggles away from its mother or when the mother gets up, as she does immediately after the birth. She noses and nibbles at the offspring but does not lick it as do other animals.

During the third stage the she-camel shows intermittent restlessness and may get up and down several times. The after-birth progressively emerges and includes large retention sacs of allantochorion, containing up to 5 litres of allantoic fluid which presumably exerts a gravitational pull on that part of the afterbirth still attached. The fetal membranes may be completely expelled soon after the fetus or, more commonly, within about half-an-hour of birth. They are not eaten by the mother. The young camel can stand, after many unsuccessful attempts, within half an hour. Sufficient care should be taken for nursing the new born including cleaning of mucus from nose, ligature of navel and finally helping the camel calf to stand on its leg within couple of hours (2–4 hrs). Initial unsteadiness is naturally rectified by about a week, but to follow the mother at grazing it takes 3 to 4 weeks.

The she-camel remains lying down (recumbent) after delivery for a maximum of half an hour.

The calf is weaned at about 15 months of age. The camel calf changes its coat of hair when about 2–3 months old but begin to graze between 4–6 weeks.

Infertility

The fertility of camels is good. According to Bedouin breeders, of every 100 she-camels mated, 80–90 bring calves. About 1% are sterile. Poor nutrition in seasons of low rainfall and resultant poor grazing is a cause of reduced sexual activity in both sexes. Abortion is rarely seen. Unthriftiness due to disease leads to infertility and pleuropneumonia is a cause of abortion.

Fertility of she-camels is maintained throughout life; breeding in alternate years, which is the usual practice, a female can yield a total of 12 offspring, although an average of something less than eight seems more likely. One mating per oestrous is usually allowed and it is possible for a male to serve five or six females in a day. It is said that one male can suffice for 200 females, with controlled breeding, but much smaller number is customary.

Male

Both male and female camel have a well defined season of breeding i.e. only during winter months, November to February or March. The male may attain sexual maturity at 3 years of age and serve but his full reproductive capacity is not developed until the ages of 6 years. An adult male may serve 50 females on an average in a year. Unlike in most of the domestic animals where spermatogenesis is a continuous process and the adult male is usually ready for coitus at any time of the year, the males of deer, elephant and camel show their sexual activity in a restricted period of the year viz. November to March known as "rutting period". The average duration of 'Rut' or '*Musth*' in the male is mostly dependent on the plane of nutrition which varies from 3 to 5 months.

During the *musth* condition the male camel emits an offensive odour due to dark reddish secretion of the skin glands (poll-glands or occipital glands) present on the back of the neck, it is rudimentary in female. At this time the male constantly grinds their teeth, foams at the mouth, swallows air and involuntarily belches it out. During the return process, the flap of the mucous membrane attached to the soft palate gets ballooned out (*goulla*) on one side of the mouth like a pink bladder which is withdrawn after a few seconds. Another behavioural peculiarities of the male in rut is the spreading of urine on its back; the back legs are spread apart, penis is rhythmically beaten with the tail and the urine is sporadically deposited first on tail and then it is whisked to the back. It is possible that pheromones are deposited on the back together with the secretion of skin glands to attract a female. *Musth* camels frequently become unmanageable and should be handled very cautiously as at this time the males are quarrelsome and may bite savagely when they fight with other males which show signs of *musth*. Ultimately the weaker males out of fear suppress their *musth* leaving stronger one to take the leading role of breeding. A sexually matured male may serve upto fifty females during single breeding season.

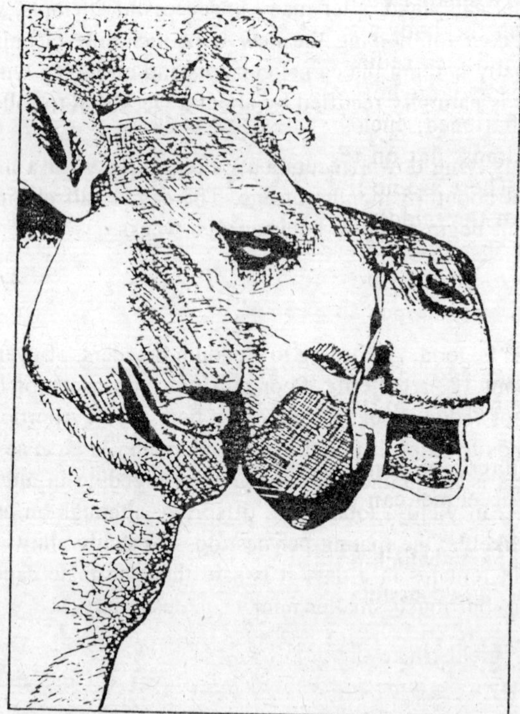

Fig. 18.4 Camel in 'Musth' throwing out the soft palate with tongue on one side.

An additional peculiarity is a profuse secretion of fluid from the poll glands. The rutting peculiarities of male camel are specially marked in the presence of an oestrous female.

To start with, a male in *musth* condition approaches the females. A female which is really in oestrous will not refuse the male otherwise she will cock her tail and the male in that case will approach the next one. A she-camel in oestrous does not cock her tail rather comes closer to '*musth*' and sniffs at his genitals. The male also will reciprocate the same fashion and may go upto gentle biting of each other for generating excitement. During this time *musth* will go on grinding his molar. At maximum point of excitement the male presses his neck against the back of the female to make her sit down for conjugation purposes. During copulation, the bull-camel on an average withdraws and thrusts the penis into the vagina for about 3–4 times and with each forward thrust a fresh ejaculation occurs.

Morphology and Physioloy behind adaptation to hot desert environment

Nature has bestowed on the camel—by virtue of its unique morphological and physiological characteristics—the ability to survive well under hot, dry and harsh desert conditions. These are described as below.

1. Camel has a large body mass. It is of an adaptive advantage as it heats up slowly when exposed to sun, as campared to a smaller body mass.
2. Long limbs help to keep the body away from the ground and thus decrease the chance of heat load in summer due to reflected radiation from the ground.
3. Toes are joined together by large horny sole that confers great advantage on sandy soil. Digital bones are wide and flattened, enclosed in cutaneus pad (sole of the foot). The two protruding digits are spread almost flat on the ground and terminate in short, broad and slightly curved claws or nails. There are no traces of 2nd and 5th toes.
4. The upper lip is cleft in the middle and has a groove which extends the cleft to each nostril. Even smallest amount of moisture from nostril passes to the mouth.
5. The lips are thickened to enable it to browse on thorny plants. Due to long neck it is possible for the camels to browse upper level plants, usually remains untouched by other ruminants.
6. Upper dental pad is tough and horny on the sides of which a pair of lateral incisors are present which enable it to have strong grip, to pull and eat short tough branch or shoot of a tree or shrub.
7. Nostrils contain abundance of hairs which prevents the sand from entering during stormy atmosphere. Further the camel can close the opening of the nostrils voluntarily to prevent entry of sand or dust.
8. Eye lashes are long and heavy which protects the eye from wind blown sand.
9. Large third eyelid also known as nictitating membrane protects the cornea from all foreign objects.
10. Thick extruding brows shields the eye from the rays of the sun.
11. Camels have usually low metabolic rates. They can exist on dry food for two weeks or more.
12. The camel does not lose its appetite during periods of desiccation and can graze over a wide area away from water.
13. A camel may lose about 30% of its weight in body water without ill effects, as compared to about 12% in man.

During the periods of desiccation the blood of most mammals becomes increasingly viscous; it therefore, circulates more and more slowly, until it cannot carry away metabolic body heat to the skin quickly enough, leading to "explosive heat death". This is avoided in camels by a physiological mechanism which ensures that water is lost mostly from the body tissues keeping blood's water content fairly constant.

14. The camel makes use of fat in the hump on its back as it is filled up mostly with fatty substances (not by water as believed by few). These substance when metabolized yields energy as well as water due to reaction of the hydrogen contents with atmospheric oxygen. It has been established that 100 grams of protein on oxidation yields 41 grams of water and 100 grams of fat will yield about 107 grams of water. Thus a 40 kg hump on a dromedary will yield more than 40 litres of water.

15. Because of its ability to lose water from body tissues alone, and because of its relatively small surface area, the camel can afford to sweat. The coarse hair on the back is well ventilated, allowing the evaporation of sweat to occur on the skin and provide maximum cooling.

Sweat glands are similar to other mammals but differ in distribution. Secretion is apocrine. The glands are deeply embeded. In mid body region the distribtion is 200 per cm^2. The glands are functional in summer. Maximum rate of secretion is 280 ml per square meter area. Sweat evaporated directly from the skin rather than from the tips of the hairs like other animals.

Undue water loss from sweating is avoided because the camel's body temperature can vary over a range of 6°C. In summer a camel may have a morning temperature of 34°C (93°F), and on afternoon maximum of 40.7°C (105°F). Sweating does not commence until the higher temperature is reached. The wide variation in the body temperature of camels occurs only during the summer, while in winter it varies much less.

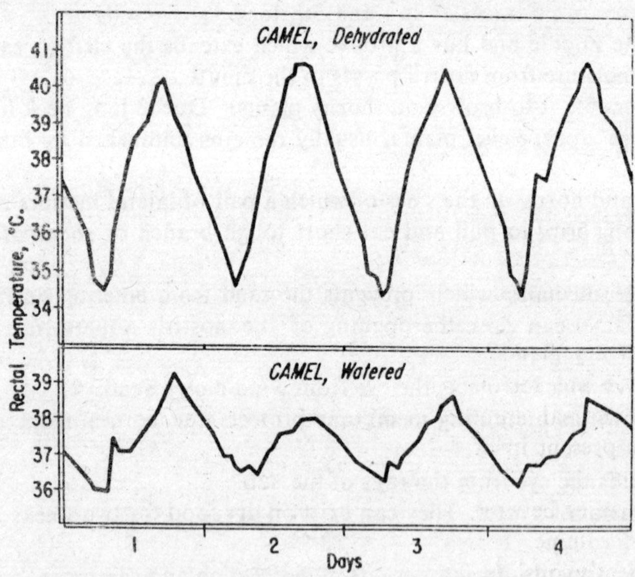

Fig. 18.5: ***Diurnal temperatures in the watered and dehydrated camel.*** The rectal temperature elevations (heat storage) occur during the day and the reductions occur at night. From Schmidt-Nielsen, K.: Osmotic regulation in higher vertebrates. *In* The Harvey Lectures, 1962–1963. Ser. 58. New York, Academic Press, 1963.

16. The long body hair also acts a barrier to the sun's radiation and slows the conduction of heat from the environment.

17. The rate of urine flow is low in camels particularly during water crisis. The amount falls from 5–10 litres (with adequate water supplies) to 0.5 litres.

18. Camels are able to re-absorb the urea in the kidney tubuli to a large extent and thus the excess urea instead of excretion through urine is forced to back in rumen through rumen blood capillaries and also through saliva and thereby utilized by rumen microbes for protein synthesis. In other ruminants the system of re-cycling urea is not so efficient.

19. After a moderate dry period when camels are provided with water, it takes in, at one time, as much water as was lost, may be upto 100 liters. The body fluids rapidly become diluted to an extent that could not be tolerated by other mammals. The red cells in the blood stream swell as much as 240 per cent of their normal size, while in other animals, the cells will burst down causing death if the total volume is increased to more than 130 per cent.

20. The colon has a greater ability to absorb water resulting less loss of water through faeces especially during the scarcity of water period.

Digestive System

The fact that it ruminates and at the same it has distinct morphological and physiological dissimilarities—especially of the polygastric system, distinguishes it from ruminants and thus the camel is classified as a pseudo-ruminant.

The organs are usually grouped under two heads, viz., (i) the accessory organs, comprising teeth, tongue, salivary glands, liver and pancreas and (ii) the alimentary canal, a tube extending from the lips to the anus.

Accessory Organs

1. *Teeth.* A camel in full mouth has 12 molars, 10 premolars, 2 wolfs, 2 canines and 8 incisors as follows:

$$I\frac{2}{6}\ C\frac{1}{1}\ W\frac{1}{1}\ PM\frac{6}{4}\ M\frac{6}{6}=\frac{16\leftarrow\text{Total in upper}}{18\leftarrow\text{Total in lower}}=34 \text{ teeth.}$$

Wolf teeth are not always present. The upper incisors are sometimes absent in females, but when present they are smaller than in males. All the teeth are unusually strong in order to grind down tough vegetation. At birth the incisors are absent. By the second week, the central pair of incisors become visible and by about a month the rest of the incisors appear in the lower jaw.

2. *Salivary glands:* The salivary glands of the camel mostly resemble those of the bovine except that the sublingual glands are relatively small. In total there are the parotid, the maxillary, the sub-lingual, the dorsal and the ventral buccal (molars) and numerous other small salivary glands which are present in the mucosa and submucosa of the tongue, soft palate and the cheek regions.

The total output of saliva varies between 100–180 litres a day, of which parotid secretes nearly one fourth of the total volume. Maximum salivary output takes place during night hours as by nature the camel spends considerable time in rumination at night.

The pH of the saliva is alkaline (pH 8 to 9) which is rich in bicarbonate and phosphate ions.

3. *Liver and Pancreas:* In adult the liver weighs between 8–9 kg, situated on the right side of the median plane. *There is no gall bladder like horse.* The hepatic duct joins the pancreatic

duct before entering the duodenum. The pancreas weighing about 0.5 kg, lies entirely on the right of the median plane.

Alimentary Canal

1. *Stomach*

The camel, llama, alpaca, vicuna chew the cud but are sometimes called pseudoruminants as their stomach is anatomically and physiologically different than that of the true ruminants. The adults retain two incisor teeth in the upper jaw while in true ruminants there are no incisiors.

The forestomach in camelids consists of three distinct compartments. The largest one is compartment 1 (C1). Because of a strong ventral and transversal muscular ridge compartment 1 may be subdivided into a cranial and a caudal portion. In the ventral portion of both sacs there are areas containing oblong, raised, thin walled series of glandular sacs (GS) also known as sacculations or water sacs or acquatic cells or water compartments because of a now discarded theory that camel stores water in them. The sacs are actually glandular regions that secrete mucous and buffers which are rich in carbonates. Its salt content is like that of blood. The story that a person in desert if fails to obtain water from all sources will depend on the water content of these sacs does not hold good since one would really have to be close to death before drinking rotten-testing green soup for satisfying long felt thirst inspite of the fact that the capacity of these sacs estimated to be 5–7 liters while that of the total capacity of compartment 1 is between 30 to 50 litres.

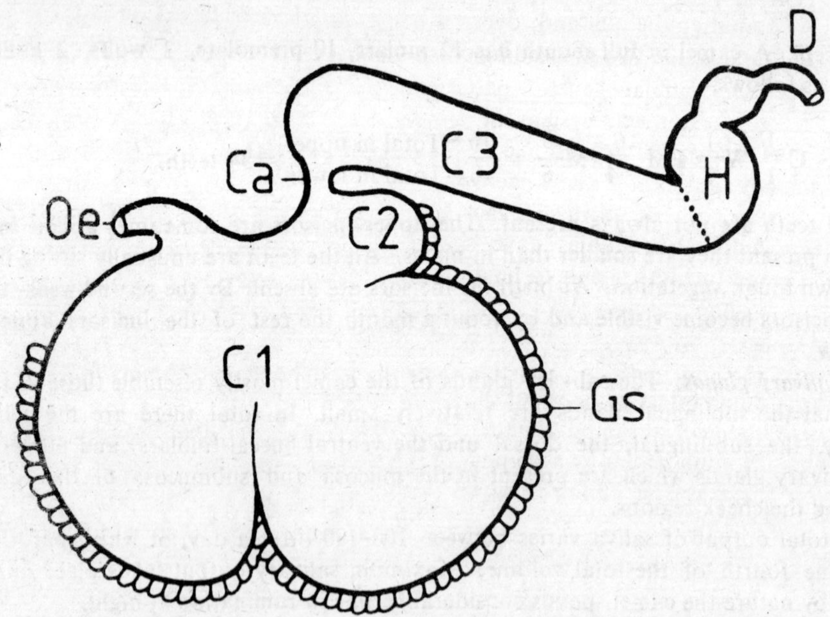

Fig. 18.6. Schematic drawing of the forestomach system of the Camelids. Oe = oesophagus; C1 = compartment 1; C2 = compartment 2; C3 = compartment 3; Ca = canal; H = hindstomach; D = duodenum; Gs = glandular sac.

The relatively small compartment 2 (C2) is incompletely separated from compartment 1 since there is no sphincter between them. Like that of compartment 1, the entire ventral parts of compartment 2 is continuous with the glandular sacs. Unlike the reticulum of ox, it lies on the right of the median plane. The mucous membrane of the compartment forms deep pouches which are separated from each other by muscular bands numbering about ten. Each pouch is divided to form many layers, the deeper ones of which are smaller than the surface ones. The uppermost cells are square or rectangular and arranged in about 12 parallel rows. The mucosa of the pouches are scattered with very small rounded papillae.

These pseudoruminants have a ventricular groove which apparently serves the same function as the reticular groove in the true ruminants. Most of the dorsal parts of C1 and 2 have smooth mucosal membranes without papillae and is covered by unkeratinized stratified squamous epithelium. Ventral aspect of the rumen and reticulum have glandular epithelium that secretes mucous and other material similar in composition to that of saliva.

There are numerous digestive hormonal glands in the epithelium of the camel's forestomachs.

Compartment 3 (C3), which originates from compartment 2, is situated at the right side of compartment 1. C3 is a long tubiform and intestine-like organ formed jointly by the anatomical modification of C3 and HCI producing hindstomach (H) which itself constitutes relatively short terminal part of the tubiform organ. When distended, the compartment may sometimes be felt through the skin on the right side behind the last rib.

The volume of hindstomach is about one-fifth of that of C3. When seen from the outside there is no clear separation from the preceeding compartment 3. Compartment 3 is entirely covered with glandular mucosa arranged in longitudinal folds of different heights. The organ has a simple columnar epithelium and, over its entire length, tubulous glands which basically resemble those found in the two preceeding compartments.

Despite the very similar general patterns of microbial digestion, the morphology and histology of the forestomach system in camelids are quite different from those in true ruminants. Thus many differences exist between the digestive physiology of camels and ruminants, though rumination and anaerobic microbial fermentation in a compartmentalized stomach apply to both of them. In fact both groups have essentially the same digestive requirements. Comparative studies have shown that the basic pattern of motility of the forestomach compartments appears to be quite different.

Intestine and Colon

The camel's small intestine is about 30–40 meters long. The duodenum has a dilation of about 12 cm in diameter at the proximate end. The hepatic and pancreatic ducts join together before opening into duodenum by a common duct.

The colon has a greater ability to absorb water and thus the faeces voided out is dry especially during the summer.

The overall efficiency of the digestive process in this species is superior to cattle, sheep and goat.

Feeds and Feeding

Camels at rest thrive solely on grazing and browsing, but when there are no facilities for sending the animals outside, or under lactation, or under hard work, stall-feeding is resorted to. In summer and rainy season shrubs, bushes and trees provide the maximum required nutrients but in winter supplementary ration including feeding of grain becomes essential.

In general the camels usually prefer to browse (feeding tree leaves, twigs etç.) rather than to graze particularly when grasses are green. It takes about 4 to 6 hours per day for consuming or foraging their feed and another 4 to 6 hours for ruminating. They do not like to forage during intense heat of the day. In some desert areas camels live entirely by browsing on low bush plants such as camel thorn (Alhagimaurorum) and salt worts such as *Haloxylon recurvum*. A certain amount of hand feeding is done with legume straw, millet, chaffed wheat straw, jowar, maize, wheat bran and salt to supplement browsing or grazing. The common tree leaves are of Banyan tree (*Ficus banghalensis*), Peepal (*Ficus religiosa*), Gular (*Ficus glomerata*), White mulberry (*Morus alba*), Sissoo (*Dalbergia sisoo*), Mango (*Mangifera indica*) while common forage crops which are fed are green *Moth* (*Vigma aconitifolius*), *Mung* (*V. aureus*), *Guar* (Cyamopsis psoralioides), *Sainji* (*Melilotus parviflora*), *Taramira* (*Eruca sativa*), *Shaftal* (*Trifloium* sp.) and Sarson (*Brassica campestris*) etc. For bulk diet pea straw (*Missa bhoosa*) is the best dry fodder.

Various types of concentrates consisting of millets, oats, beans, cotton-seed, maize, and bran are fed to Indian camels, but crushed gram is the best of all. Scale of ration per day for stall fed adult working camel in India is:

Millets or grains	1.8 kg
Wheat straw or *bhoose* or	9.0 kg
Dry fodder	13.5 kg
Salt	100 gms

For adults when good grazing is available, the ration per day should include:

Grains or Millets	1.8 kg
Roughages	3.6 kg
Salt	100 gms

The schedule of rationing at Government Camel Breeding Farm, Bikaner in Rajasthan is given below:

Table 18.2

Particulars of the animal	Fodder (kg)	Concentrates (kg)	Salt (gram)
Under 1 year	1.80	0.45	25
1 to 2 years of age	3.60	0.90	50
2 to 3 years of age	5.50	1.40	85
Above 3 years of age	7.25	1.80	100
Stud Camels	8.25	2.25	125

The army camel corps follow the following schedule for feeding their camels as below at the time when the camels are stationed at headquarters.

Gram crushed	1.30 kg
Barley crushed	1.30 kg
Salt	140 gram
Missa (Mixed) *bhoosa*	8–9 kg

Where grazing or browsing is available the quantum of roughage is reduced.

In the army camels are fed once in the morning and again in the afternoon.

It is not recommended to feed the grains all of a sudden in case the camel is not used to it. Grains are always fed in crushed and soaked (6 hours) form. After a long and exhausting journey put it under rest for a while and then provide the camel a drink composed of a small quantity of any flour with molasses along with 1–2 litres of water. Again after a small rest allow him to drink limited quantity of water of about 8–10 litres at a time. The usual feed may now be offered about half an hour or so.

The camels who are not fed at home need at least 8 to 10 hours of grazing and browsing everyday.

The animal is more efficient than the cow in converting coarse vegetation into milk and meat.

Dietary Preference

An important survival strategy of herbivores in a severe environment is the ability to select the more nutritious parts of a plant. There are distinct differences in the forestomach morphology between grazers and browsers. The ability of grazers (cattle) to select plant in a natural pasture is less developed. Browsers (goats and camels) and to a less extent intermediate feeders (sheep) are able to seek herbs, fruits and succulent leaves out of a great variety of plants.

Ruminants that are predominantly grazers have a more voluminous reticulo-rumen and a longer retention of time of feed than browsers or concentrate selectors. Grazers or roughage eaters therefore can utilize fibrous diet more efficiently than concentrate selectors which on the other hand, are able to choose the easily digestible plants from the vegetation in a harsh environment.

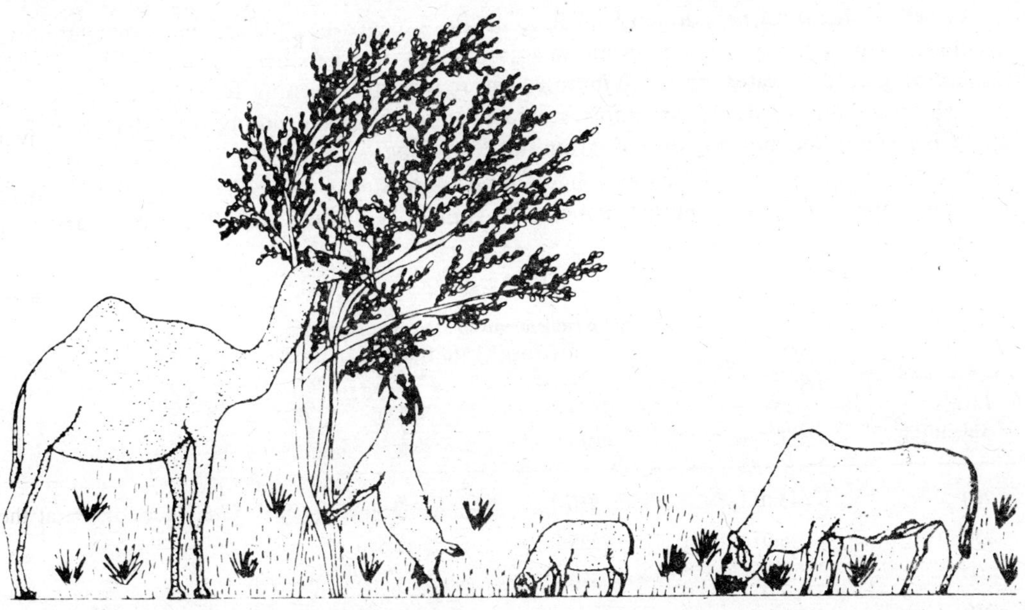

Fig. 18.7. Sketch of dietary preference of Camels, Goat, Sheep and Cattle.

Camels have advantage over both these groups of ruminants. They can live exclusively from a fibrous, low quality diet *due to the long retention of feed particles in the forestomach*; they also eat highly selectively.

Comparative studies on the dietary preferences of goats, sheep and camels showed that sheep spend about 70% of their feeding time in harvesting at the ground level and rarely feed at more than 1 m above the ground, i.e. they depend almost entirely on the herb layer. Goats browse upto 2 m above the ground, with approximately 60% of the feeding time being spent at 0.7 to 1.2 m above ground level. Camels have the highest reach, upto 3 m; although their preferred feeding strata appears to be between 1 and 2 m. above the ground. In such an environment both goats and camels rely to a large extent on deep rooted bushes and trees, which are a more secure feed source during the dry season than the herb layer.

Adaptation to low protein diets

When low protein diets with sufficient available energy for microbial growth are given recycling and utilization of endogenous urea-N is high in camelids, and the renal urea excretion is low. About 90–96% of total urea turnover in camels and llamas was found to be recycled into the gastrointestinal tract.

When feed is fairly available, 6 hours is the minimum time for grazing and browsing and for this another 6 hours are needed for rumination. Camels avoid foraging during the heat of the day. In many parts of the world camels live entirely by browsing on low bush plants such as camelthorn (*Alhagi manrorum*) and salf worts (*Haloxylon recurvum*).

During the scarcity period, camels should be fed supplementary ration consisting of dry and green fodder on twigs etc.

Generally camel owners do not feed concentrates except when the animal is in a run-down condition or is at heavy work or in an advanced stage of pregnancy. Grains should be fed crushed or soaked in water for 15–30 minutes before feeding. Evening feeding of grains is the rule which should not be fed on empty stomach or soon after drinking of water. Salt if fed alone, is given in the morning or with grain in the evening.

Nutrient requirements of camels have been suggested by the I C.A.R. based on the recommendations of the Scientific Panel on Animal Nutrition and Physiology are given below.

Table 18.3

Nutrients Requirement of Growing camels

(Growth rate 100 g/day)

Live weight (kg)	DM (kg)	DCP (g)	TDN (g)	Ca (g)	P (g)
200	5.0	250	2,000	80	30
250	6.0	325	2,500	100	35
300	7.5	350	3,000	120	50
350	9.0	470	3,800	145	60
400	10.0	600	4,700	185	80
450	10.5	650	5,000	200	100

These requirements indicate that the ration containing approximately 4 per cent DCP, 45 per cent TDN, 2 per cent calcium and 1 per cent phosphorus could meet the requirement of adult camel, if fed as per the dry feed requirement per day.

Table 18.4

Nutrient requirements for maintenance of camels

Live weight (kg)	DM (kg)	DCP (g)	TDN (g)	Ca (g)	P (g)
500	12.0	500	5,500	300	100
550	13.0	525	6,000	225	120
600	14.0	550	6,500	250	150
650	15.0	600	7,000	250	150
750	16.5	650	7,500	250	150

Watering of Camels

A camel can tolerate a loss of water at about 30 per cent of its body weight when exposed to severe desert heat, while other mammals under similar situation would die from circulatory failure at a loss of water equivalent to only 12 per cent body weight.

The quantity of water requirement of camel varies according to the type of feed (feeds like bhoosa, salt, high protein etc., will require more water); the climate, (in summer requirement is high); in pregnancy or milking stage water requirement should be high; in diarrhoea or any haemorrhagic condition, the demand rises, during hard work requirement of water is again high. Generally, a camel requires 20–40 liters of water per day which may be offered in two times. In summer, camels should be watered in the morning and evening while in winter they should be watered at mid-day when water gets warmed due to sun rays. Moreover, camels should be given some *bhoosa* or green leaves of trees between the waterings. It may be noted that a thirsty camel if allowed to drink at its choice (*ad lib*), it may drink as high as 130 liters at a time and thereby may suffer from over-distension of its stomach.

As they drink water, the RBC in the blood will start swelling as much as 240 per cent of their normal size thus will retain excess body water for any future emergency. This peculiar character of RBC is not found in other mammals where if their total volume is increased to more than 130 per cent, RBC will burst causing death.

The water given to camels usually on every second day. The water quality is an important factor as polluted one may carry many pathogens sufficient to make the camels sick.

Health and Diseases of Camel

Camel health is important both in terms of the financial loss to the owner resulting from ill health in the herd and in the suffering it may cause to the animals. Financial losses arise from death, culling, reduced work capacity and milk production and from the cost of treatment.

Camel on normal health should have hair coat neither too dull nor too bright. Eyes remain bright without any tears. The animals are without any abnormal discharge from mouth, nostrils or through vagina. The normal temperature of the camel is 36.1°C (97°F) in the morning before the sun gets hot and then rises considerably from dawn to sun set to about 37.9°C (100.3°F). The temperature is taken inside the rectum when the camel is in sitting position in a shade for at least 15 minutes. Young camels at suckling stage usually have one to two degrees higher temperature than the adults. The normal pulse rate varies in the early morning from 32 to 44 beats per minute and in the evening from 35 to 45. The pulse can be felt on the underside of the tail near its root. Respiration in sitting position varies from five to ten per minute. In cold weather it is less and does not go beyond eight.

The common infectious diseases of camels are described as follows:

Trypanosomisasis

Synonyms : Surra, Tibarsa, El-Debab, Mbori

Causative organism : A small single cell parasite found in blood stream and classed under (i) *Trypanosoma brucei* and *Trypanosoma congolense.*

Symptoms : Weakness, body temperature rises to 38 to 39°C in the morning and 40 to 41°C in the evening which usually lasts for few days to few weeks. Loss of appetite, hollow flank and drooping neck are of initial symptoms. The animal stands listlessly with eyes half closed with watery discharged. Pregnant she-camels may abort. Oedema appears under the belly, on hind legs, sheath and scrotum and in advanced stages pneumonia develops. Paralysis, blindness and cold sweats may appear just before death.

Remarks : The disease is common in rainy season and is a serious contagious disease of camels, spread through biting of the parasite and blood sucker flies. About 20% of the camel population suffer from this disease.

Anthrax

Synonyms : Sool

Causative organism: The causative agent is *Bacillus anthracis* relatively large, rod shaped and non-motile bacteria. Spores are highly resistant and are not easily killed by heat, light, and disinfectants.

Symptoms : Sudden death without apparent cause is the most striking symptoms. High temperatures and blood discharges from natural body openings are other symptoms. Swellings may appear on different parts of the body. Spleen enlarges.

Remarks : It appears that infection occurs by way of the mouth and alimentary system. Either the living organism or else the spores are taken in through the feed or with drinking water. The powerful gastric juice probably destroys most of the bacilli, but is unable to harm the spores. These later under the influence of heat and moisture commence to vegetate and by invading the walls of the intestines reach the blood stream.

Preventive measures include segregation of in-contact animals. The carcass of the affected animal should be burnt and the place thoroughly disinfected. No camel should be allowed to graze in the area where anthrax cases have occurred.

Rabies

Synonyms : Nil

Causative organism : Virus disease, present in the saliva of the rabid animal which is transmitted to healthy animals by the bite of a rabid animal. The first symptoms of the disease appear 14 to

90 days after the bite, though an incubation period of 300 days or more has also been recorded.

Symptoms : At the onset the camel cannot eat or drink properly, it looks dull, later there is paralysis of lower jaws with dribbling of saliva. Tongue gets paralysed which hangs down from the mouth. Some camels get vicious and try to bite other animals. Finally the paralytic limbs compel the animals to loose walking power and ultimately dies within 5–8 days.

Remarks : Most common in U.P. Anti-rabic treatment is given to check this disease free of charge by the veterinary department of the State.

Jhooling

Synonyms : Nil

Causative organism : Causal organ is not known, but is suspected to be either fungus or bacteria of streptococci group. Healthy camels when allowed to stay with sick ones contact the disease found only in this species.

Symptoms : The disease which spreads rapidly manifests itself in the form of hot and painful local tumours of a fibrous character usually on the neck, hind quarters and abdomen. After a few days the part begins to itch and the camel rubs it against some hard object which aids in prolifera-tion.

Remarks : It is widely distributed throughout Puñjab and also in Kutch but is seldom found in desert areas. About 20 per cent of the camel population suffer from this disease. Red iodide of murcury is applied over the lesions in the first instance and after 3–4 days redressed with finely powdered potassium permanganate. Three such dressings, at intervals of 4 days each, heal the wound.

Management of Camels

1. At the breeding farms, the practice is to let loose the animals for grazing in the morning till evening when they return. According to age the animals are divided into different groups.
2. Females should never be used to work during the last 2 months of pregnancy rather they should be at liberty on good grazing during this period and for a minimum of 3 weeks after parturition.
3. To avoid camel-calf mortality before they are 3 weeks old, feedings of colostrum (Protein, 17.5%, Lactose, 4.25%, Fat, 0.15% and Ash, 2.60%) high in protein and very low in fat is a must.
4. The newly calved dams with their youngs stay at the farm during the day time for about a month after which they are turned out for grazing.
5. The studs are allowed to move with the non-pregnant group of female during the breeding season from November to March.
6. As the camel reaches 4 years, it is loaded with empty saddle and gradually accustomed to carry more load as well as gets used to the head control and trained to sit and rise at command within next two years, i.e. by the time they attain six years of age.
7. Castration is made between the ages 4 to 6 years which serve better as their work is not interrupted due to rut period nor their attention is drawn by females. Castrates are seldom able to carry heavy loads as the entire male.
8. **Breaking or training of a camel is an art, and it should be practiced between the age of 2½ to 3 years.**
9. **Young camels are brought under control firstly by putting a halter on his head and neck and then tying it with a strong rope for halting purpose. After about a week both**

nostrils are punctured for putting in the nose-pegs to hold the reins (a narrow strap of leather) attached to nose area of the camel. The young camel should be taught as to how to keep to the line of march.

10. Adult males may at any time become violently cruel particularly during breeding season. The she-camels also become excited when her calf is to be handled for restraining. Thus the camels which are by nature docile, gentle and an obedient animal should be handled with all care particularly during breeding season.

11. The best age to break (train) a camel for riding is three years. However, the animal should not be put to any regular work till it attains the age of six years.

12. For baggage animal great care should be taken in properly loading. The load should be equally divided and balanced on both sides of the hump.

13. Clipping is necessary for camels with long hair to keep them cool and healthy from the beginning of March till the end of April. It is done with hand shears. All precautions are taken to avoid any scratch of the skin.

14. Oiling with *taramira* or *sarson* is made after clipping to make the skin softer and free from lice, ticks etc., that may infesting it.

15. Where water is available owners do give a bath to the camel after it has been clipped. Some owners of riding camel give bath once or twice a month in summer for lessening camel odour.

16. The camels are homeotherm but possess remarkable ability to fluctuate body temperature according to ambient environmental conditions. The temperature varies with an individual, season, climate and degree of dehydration. In the early morning, the temperature of a healthy camel is 36°C to 36.5°C rising upto 2°C through the day to the evening. The temperature is taken per rectum.

17. The frequency of pulse in camels varies with time of the day and ambient temperature. The normal pulse rate in the morning is 30–45 per minute rising to 35–50 at evening.

18. The normal respiratory rate in camel ranges from 5–12 per minute. The rate is affected by time of the day, ambient temperature and status of health.

Determination of age

Table 18.5

Age	Incisors	Premolars in lower jaw
Birth	2	–
1 month	4	–
2 months	6	–
1 year	6 crowded and overlapping	–
2 years	6 worn, do not touch	–
3 years	6 well worn	–
4 years	6 very worn, loose	–
5 years	2 permanent	–
6 years	4 permanent	–
7 years	6 permanent	2 appear
8½ years	6 permanent	2 long tushes with sharp points

As camel management depends so much on age it is necessary to be able to estimate this fairly accurately. The camel possesses ten molars and six premolars in the upper jaw and eight molars, four premolars and six incisors in the lower jaw.

Age is estimated from the lower jaw.

After nine years the age is determined by the year of the premolars and incisors. As the camel ages the incisors become blunt and flat, the premolars (tushes) become rounder and gradually become stumps.

Weaning system

On a stud farm weaning is generally carried out at six months, or naturally as the dam dries off between nine and twelve months. The calf will browse with the mother after only a few weeks, giving a gradual transition to solid diet.

Table 18.6

Camelids Compared to Ruminants

Stomach anatomy	very different
Ultrastructure of forestomach mucosa	very different
Forestomach motility	very different
Absorption of solutes in forestomach	faster in camelids
Biochemistry of digestion	similar
Saliva composition and secretion rates	similar
Utilization of endogenous urea when low protein diets are fed	camelids superior
Adaptation to arid regions and to high altitude	camelids often clearly superior

RABBIT

The names "rabbit" and "hare" are often incorrectly used interchangeably. Rabbits and hares have large front teeth, short tails, and large hind legs and feet adapted for running or jumping. In most the length of the ears is considerably greater than the width.

The term 'rabbit' generally refers to small, running animals, with relatively short ears and legs, which give birth to blind, naked young, while 'hare' refers to larger hopping forms, with longer ears and legs whose young are born furred and open-eyed.

Some common terms in relation to RABBIT

Details		Expression	Details		Expression
A mature female rabbit used for breeding	–	DOE	Kits born in a single kindling	–	LITTER
A mature male rabbit used for breeding	–	BUCK	A newly weaned rabbit	–	WEANER
A young rabbit whose eyes are not yet opened	–	KIT	Wool	–	FUR
A young rabbit below 20 weeks age	–	BUNNY	Skin	–	PELT
10 to 12 weeks old rabbits ready for market	–	FRYER	Place where domesticated rabbits are kept	–	RABBITRY
Culled rabbits	–	ROASTER	Consumption of own feceal matter	–	CAECOTROPHY / COPROPHAGY
Act of parturition	–	KINDLING	Rabbits which grow very fast for meat purpose (2 kg. body weight in just 12 weeks)	–	BROILER RABBIT

Rabbits are chiefly nocturnal, although they are sometimes seen in the day time. They have acute senses of smell and hearing. They feed on a wide variety of vegetation. All have large eyes situated on the side of the head and moderately long ears that they frequently move and with which they can detect even faint sounds. They have a keen sense of smell and frequently twitch their nose. Rabbits also have a split in the middle of the upper lip and a pair of chisel like front teeth similar to those of rodents (rats, mice, squirrels, characterized by constantly growing incisors adapted for nibbling). Unlike rodents, rabbits have an extra pair of small teeth behind the front ones for a total of six incisors as opposed to four in rodents. It has also a short and fluffy tail and a thick coat that varies in colour.

Most rabbits live in holes they dig under logs or rocks or in holes made and abandoned by other animals. Hares do not burrow but lie hidden in a depression in the vegetation.

Rabbits can tolerate a wide range of climates from cold and wet to hot and dry. They can withstand temperatures as low as 10°F(–12°C). Usually they avoid very high temperatures by remaining in their burrows (tunnel dug in the ground). Hot humid climate is worst for them.

Rabbits share with rodents (rats, mice, squirrels and guineapigs) the habit of passing food twice through the G.I. tract (*Caecotrophy*). Dried faecal pellets are produced only during the day. At night soft pellets covered with mucus are formed in the caecum and are immediately taken from the anus by the lips. They are stored in the stomach and later mixed with further food taken. This practice is known as *Coprophagy*. The double passage of the food is necessary for the life of the rabbit and rodents. The animals will die in 2–3 weeks if prevented from reaching the anus. The moist pellets probably contain the metabolites that have been produced by breakdown of cellulose by the microbes of caecum, which cannot be absorbed by the organ itself initially.

All species belonging to rabbit are prolific breeders.

Zoological Classification

Rabbits belong to the family *Leporidae*, order *Lagomorpha*. All domestic rabbits originated from the European wild rabbit of the genus *Oryctolagus* and the species *cuniculus*. To-day Europe (USSR, France, Italy, Spain) accounts for 85% of total world output. China comes next to Europe. Rabbits are not reared in most Arab countries.

Taxonomic classification of the rabbit
(Oryctolagus cuniculus)

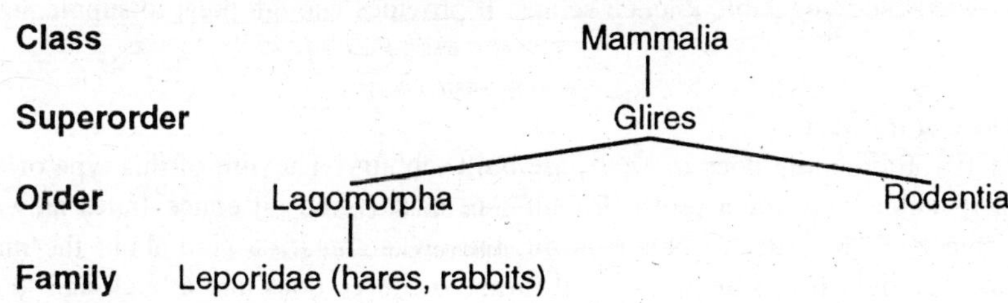

+ Sub-family : Leporinae

– Genus : *Lepus* (hares : numerous species distributed throughout the Old and the New World)

– Genus : *Oryctolagus* (true rabbit, living in Europe and North Africa. One species, *Oryctolagus cuniculus*, with a few sub-species)

– Genus : *Sylvilagus* (American rabbits; numerous species)

– Genus : *Coprolagus* (Asiatic rabbits)

– Genus : *Nesolagus* (Sumatra, one sole species, N. *netscheri*)

– Genus : *Brachylagus* (pygmy rabbit, living in North America)

Purpose of Rabbit farming

Apart from being a good source of white meat which is "Pearly white" and low in fat and cholesterol, can be used for heart patients, rabbits also provide useful wool (fur), skins, manure, toys and novelties. The rabbit is the only farm animal which produces meat @10–15 times or more its own weight in a year through progenies. Being such a prolific multiplier, it is expected to ease the demand of pressure on chicken and mutton.

Advantages of Rabbit rearing

1. Investment on housing and management is less.
2. An efficient producer of meat, feed efficiency is high.
3. Rabbits breed fast (31 days is the average gestation period) and achieve rapid weight gains around 2 kg at 8 weeks of age.
4. They are commonly fed on leafy plants and vegetables with relatively little concentrate feed.
5. Rabbits produce high class protein characterised as lean meat and excellent fur.
6. Rabbit does not have any religious prohibitions, unlike pig and cow meat.

Rabbit Production system

The exact way in which people keep rabbits differs from country to country, but there are three main systems of production.

1. *The Backyard Small Scale Rabbitry*

A few female (does) and one or two male rabbits (buck) are kept in a home-built rabbitry and are fed on greens, weeds and vegetable kitchen scraps. It provides enough meat to supplement the family need.

2. *The Small Commercial Rabbitry*

May have from 10–50 breeding does in a purpose-built rabbitry. The aim of this type of rabbit production is to sell rabbit meat for a profit. Rabbits are usually fed on concentrates as well as bulky leafy vegetable feed. In order to obtain profit, the owner must be sure about the market. New rabbit farmers are advised to start with small farm viz., three does and a buck and to build up gradually after gaining in experiences.

3. *The Large Commercial Rabbitry*

This type of rabbitry is more common in Europe and America. There are some examples of large rabbit units in the tropics, but to support such rabbitries it is necessary to have a reliable market outlet for the carcasses, source of good quality commercial feed, and expert veterinary services.

Breeds

There are many breeds of rabbits in the world which differ in many ways from area to area particularly in their size, breeding ability and adjustment to various climates. Angora breed of rabbits are white, small, weighing from 2.5–3 kg reared exclusively for their excellent wool, quality and quantity. Angora breeds are usually slaughtered very young, after the 2nd or 3rd clipping at most. There are four recognised strains of Angora rabbits namely German, British, Russian and

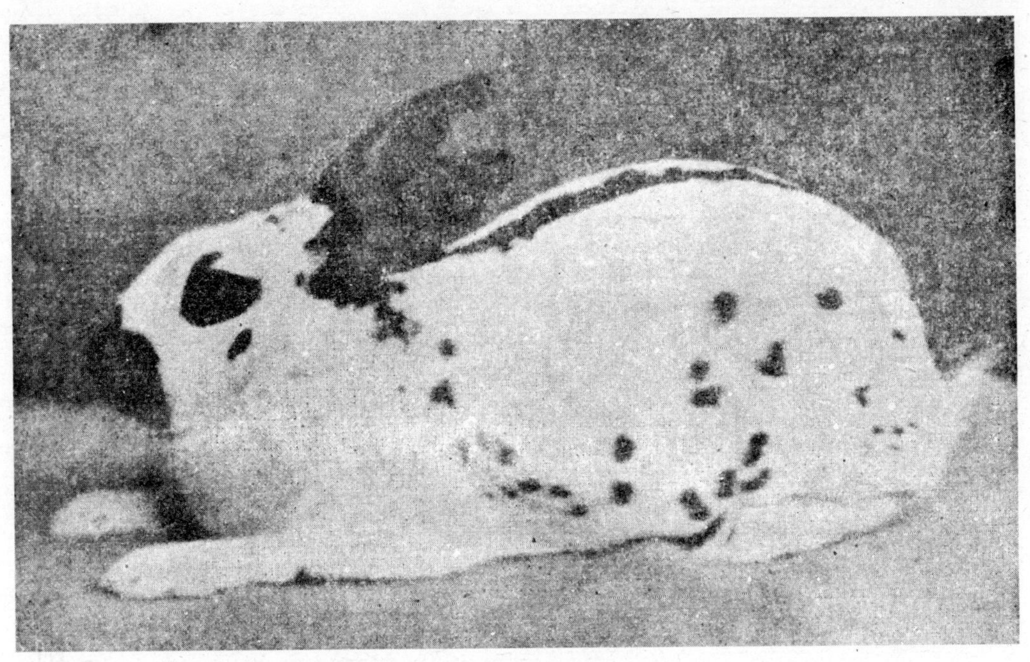

Plate 96. (CHAPTER 19).

British Russian. Among these the German strain is considered the best fur producer in terms of yield, fineness and guard hair content. The fibre is also characterised by very low friction co-efficient which gives the softness to touch and exceptional capacity of slipping. The fibres possess all the properties of keratin, mainly insulation, water absorption and dyeing quality. The coat is 98.5 per cent pure as compared to sheep fleece which is only 50 per cent pure.

The adult female produces the best fibre from 9th month onwards. It produces an average of 1 kg fur per year compared to 700 to 800 gm. by males. It is advisable to maintain fibre producing stock of adult females with reproduction kept at a minimum. Rabbits can be raised in an individual cage to facilitate the production of clean fibre and also to avoid formation of scabs on paws which most often result in reduced production performance. It is preferable to feed them with foodstuffs that are rich in sulphur containing amino acids.

It has been observed that German Angoras produce on an average 1000 gms of fur, fetching about Rs. 800/- in a year, and the Russian Angoras produce about 700 gms per year fetching Rs. 600/- per kg. The maintenance cost may be only around Rs. 400/- per rabbit per year.

The New Zealand white is an example of meat breed. They are large rabbits, with meaty haunches and wide, deep shoulders. An adult buck weighs 4–5 kg, and an adult doe weighs 4.5–5.5 kg. They have white fur. This is the most popular breed in commercial rabbitries and is also widely used in tropical backyard units.

Table 19.1

Breed	*Fur colour*	*Adult weight (kg)*	*Country of origin*
New Zealand white	White	4.5	U.K.
Grey giant	Greyish brown	3.5	Russia
White giant	White	4.0	Russia
Soviet chinchilla	Steel grey	3.5	Russia
Dutch	White/grey	3.0	India
Black brown	Black/Brown	3.5	India
Angora	Usually white	2.5 – 3.0	Europe

Table 19.2

Commercial Characteristics of Rabbits	Backyard producer	Commercial producer
Young born per litter	4 – 9	6 – 12
Young reared per litter	3 – 5	6 – 8
No. of litters per doe per year	3 – 4	5 – 8*
No. of young reared/doe/year	9 – 20	30 – 60*
Weaning weight per litter at 8 weeks	3 – 6 kg	9 – 14 kg
Live weight gain (number of weeks to reach 2 kg body weight)	12 – 24 weeks	8 – 10 weeks
Feed conversion	5 : 1 to 4 : 1	4 : 1 to 3 : 1
Killing out percentage	40 – 50%	50 – 55%
Conformation	Fair	Fair, good

*With *post partum* mating in large commercial rabbitries.

The Division of Fur Animal Breeding, Garsa (Himachal Pradesh) was the first in India to import New Zealand white rabbits from U.K.; followed by imports of Angora (wool type), White Giant, Grey Giant and Soviet Chinchilla (all meat type) from U.S.S.R.

Reproduction and Breeding

At 4 weeks of age gentle pressure on the sides of the reproductive organ with a finger and thumb will first expose the inside mucus membrane where a circular aperture in a male and a slit aperture in a female will confirm about the sex. The testes can always be drawn up out of the scrotum at will.

Bucks (male) and Does (female) mature at about the same age. The small breeds, such as Dutch, reach breeding age at about 5 months, while the larger meat producing breed may take some more time to attain breeding age. In general, does generally reach puberty when they have grown to 70%–75% of their mature weight. It is usually preferable to wait until they reach 80% of their mature weight.

Anatomy of Male Genitals

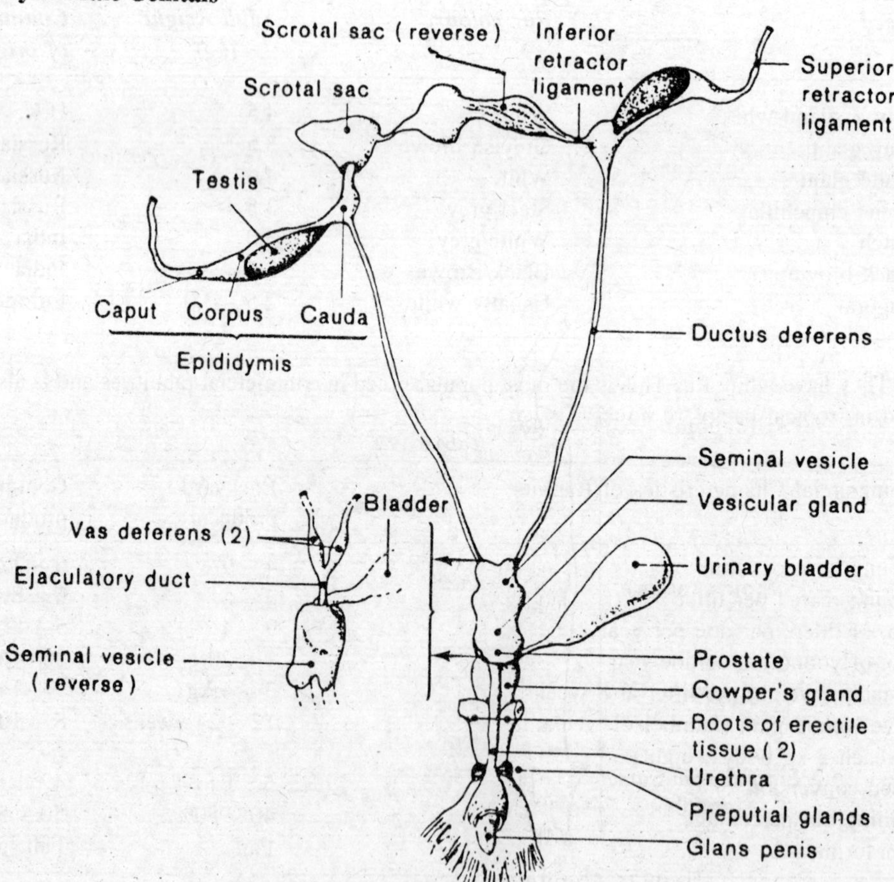

Fig. 19.1 Genital apparatus of male rabbit

In the male, the oval-shaped testes within the scrotum remain in communication with the abdominal cavity, where they were at birth. The rabbit is actually able to withdraw its testes when frightened or fighting with other animals. The testicles descend at about 2 months.

Anatomy of Female Genitals

In the female, ovaries are oval-shaped and do not exceed 1–1.5 cm. Beneath the ovaries is the oviduct, made up of the duct, the ampulla and the isthmus. Though outwardly the uterine horns are joined at the back into a single organ, there are actually two independent uteri of about 7 cm, opening separately through two cervical ducts into the 6–10 cm vaginal. The urethra opens midway along the vagina at the vaginal vestibule.

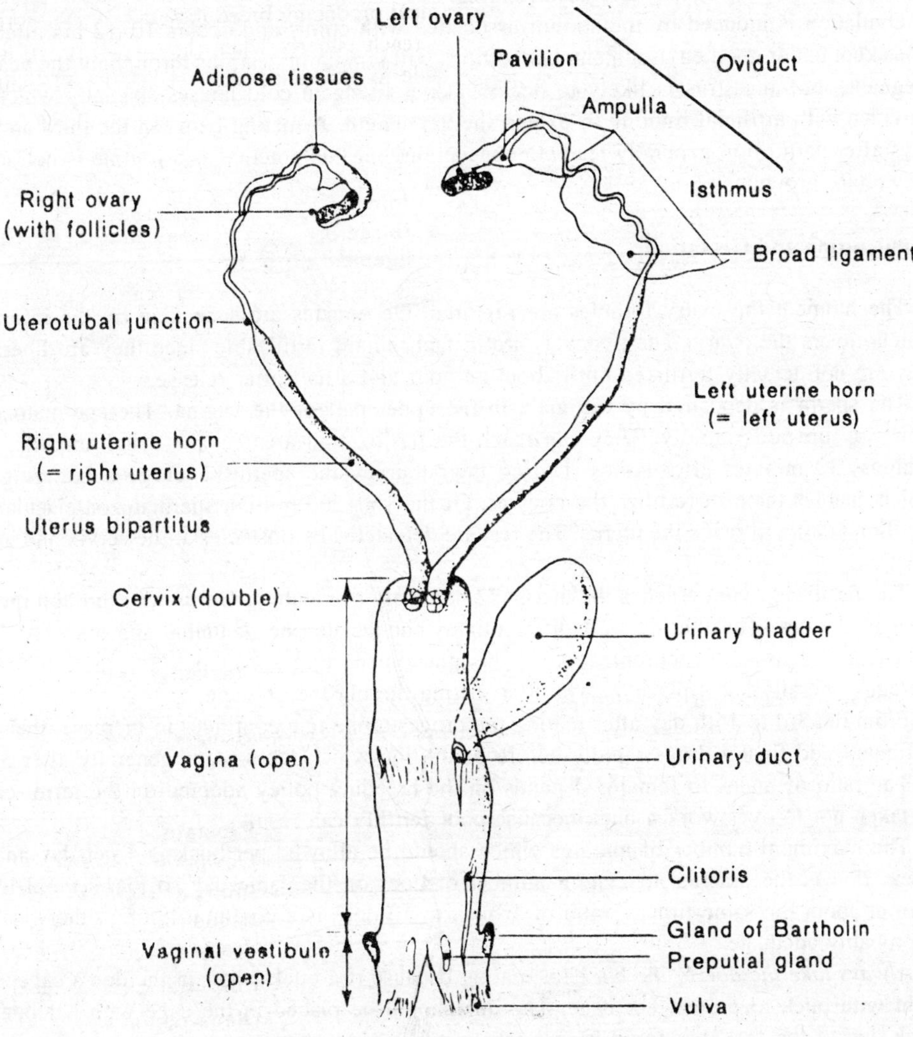

Fig. 19.2 Genital apparatus of female rabbit

Oestrous Cycle

In most domestic mammals ovulation takes place at regular intervals when the female is in heat or oestrous. The interval between two periods of oestrous represents the length of the oestrous cycle (4 days for rats, 17 days for ewes, 21 days for sows, cows mare and buffaloes).

The female rabbit, however, does not have an oestrous cycle with regular periods of heat. Ovulation occurs only after mating. A female rabbit is therefore, considered to be in heat when she accepts service and in dioestrous when she refuses. It has been noted that 90% of the time when a doe has a red vulva she will accept mating and ovulate. A red vulva is therefore a strong indication of oestrous though not a proof as in 10% of the time she does not accept mating in spite of having red vulva. The sexual behaviour of a female rabbit is thus very special. She has no cycle and can stay in heat for several days running.

Ovulation is induced by the stimuli associated with coitus and occurs 10–12 hrs after mating. Does kept under good environmental conditions will remain in oestrous throughout the year (unless pregnant), but anaestrus is likely to occur in does living in cold houses specially which are not provided with artificial lighting to extend the day length. A mating between the third and seventh days after parturition generally leads to conception, but this practice as a routine is not acceptable on welfare grounds.

Fertilization and Gestation

The moment the ovary follicles are ruptured, the oocytes are sucked in by the infundibulum which covers the ovary. The ovocytes are in fact remain fertilizable since they are liberated, but they are not actually fertilized until about an hour and a half after release.

The sperm is deposited by the male in the upper part of the vagina. The spermatozoa make their way upwards rapidly. They can reach the fertilization area (in the distal ampulla, near the isthmus) 30 minutes after coitus. During their journey the sperms undergo a maturing process which enables them to fertilize the oocytes. Of the 150–200 million spermatozoa ejaculated, only 2 billion (1%) will reach the uterus. The rest are defeateted by obstacles at the cervix and uterotubal junction.

The fertilized ovum reaches the uterus 72 hours after ovulation. On its way through the oviduct the egg divides. The uterine wall differentiates but the uterine dentellus appears only 5–8 days after coitus. It is the synchronization of this phenomena that makes possible the implantation of the egg generally takes place 7 days after mating the blastocyst stage.

From the 3rd to 15th day after mating the progesterone rate continues to increase, then remains stationary and finally drops rapidly before parturition which takes place generally after 31 days.

The ratio of males to females depends on the breeding policy adopted on the farm; care must be taken not to over work a buck because poor fertility can result.

The maximum number of matings which should be allowed per buck is 4 per day and 12 per week. If it is the practice to mate a number of does on the same day so that several litters are born at about the same time, a ratio of 1 buck to 10 does is a common figure; otherwise 1 to 15 is probably adequate.

Always take the doe to the buck for mating because if a buck is put in the doe's cage, she may fight with buck to protect her cage. The doe should be placed in the cage with her back to the buck due to the fact that some keen bucks mate at once. A doe, which is anxious to be mated will raise her hind quarters ready for the buck to mount, but some one adopt this position after the buck has started mounting. It may be necessary to hold a young doe during her first mating. One hand should be placed over the ears and shoulders and to support the body, raising the hind quarters so that the doe is in a suitable mating position.

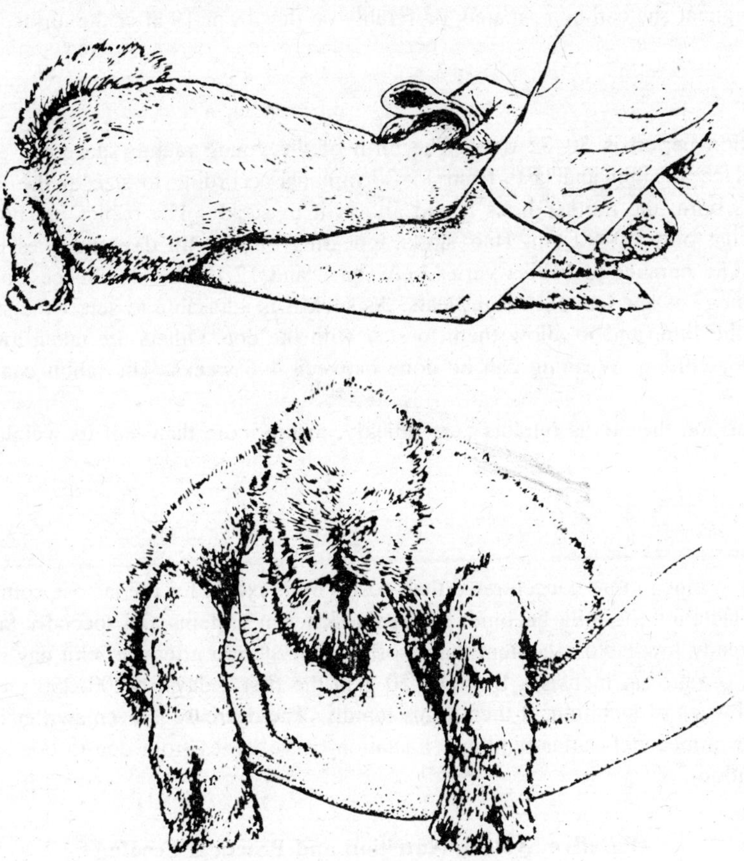

Fig 19.3 Holding the doe for mating

After mating, the buck falls sideways, often emitting a slight scream (to make loud sound). Many breeders allow a buck to mate the doe twice before removing him from the cage. If there is no second mating within a few minutes, the doe should be taken away and re-introduced about 6 hours later. If a doe which is clearly in oestrous fails to accept the buck, she may be placed in a cage previously occupied by a buck and left there. This may stimulate sexual desire.

Although the average number born to does of a commercial strain varies from 8 to 10, litter sizes may range from 2 to 16.

Pregnancy Diagnosis

Pregnancy diagnosis by abdominal palpation should be carried out at between 14 and 16 days after mating. A doe is placed gently on a non-slippery surface so that she is relaxed, because if she is frightened the abdominal muscles will be tensed, making palpation difficult. By placing a hand under the body slightly in front of the hind legs, the embryos can be felt as marble sized ovals slipping between the thumb and fingers on either side of the mid-line of the abdomen. If a doe is not pregnant she can be re-mated, preferably on day 18 or 19 after the unsuccessful mating.

Kindling

The gestation period is 30–32 days. The birth of the young rabbits is known as *kindling.* It often takes place at night and lasts from 15–30 minutes according to size of the litter. As each baby rabbit is born, the mother licks it and allows it to suckle. The babies are born naked and blind and weigh only 30–80 gm. Hair starts appearing on the 4th day and eyes open between 10–14 days. The number of babies varies between 2 and 12. A doe can successfully rear more than eight youngs as she has only eight teats. As such it is advisable to select the strongest eight rabbits from the litter and to allow them to stay with the doe. Others are taken away either for fostering or for culling. Weaning can be done between 4–6 weeks. The rabbit can be bred 4–6 times a year.

After parturition the uterus retracts very quickly, losing more than half its weight in less than 48 hours.

Lactation

Doe's milk is much more concentrated than cow's milk except for the lactose component. After the 3rd week lactation the milk becomes markedly richer in proteins and specially fats (up to 20–22%). The already low lactose content tapers off to almost zero after the 30th day of lactation.

Daily milk production increases from 30–50 g in the first 2 days to 200–250 gm towards the end of the 3rd week of lactation. It then drops rapidly. The decrease is even swifter if the doe has been fertilized immediately after kindling. Lactation curve varies from doe to doe specially with regard to duration.

Digestive System, Nutrition and Practical Feeding

The teeth of a rabbit are designed to cut and grind, and after mastication the feed passes to the single stomach and thence to the intestines. The rabbit, in common with all herbivorous mammals, has a greater relative alimentary tract capacity than have carnivores. In the rabbit this is because of its large caecum and colon, in which there is some microbial digestion of starch and cellulose takes place. The products of this microbial synthesis are utilized by the practice of *Coprophagy.* (Coprophagy means consumption of own faecal matter by the animal). The rabbit passes hard faeces during the day and soft faeces at night. The night faeces are eaten direct from the anus and so undigested components of the diet which have been broken down by micro-organisms in the caecum and colon are passed through the alimentary canal again and utilised. Certain water soluble vitamins, synthesized by bacterial action in the caecum, are absorbed as a result of this process of coprophagy.

Anatomy and Functions of the Rabbit Digestive Tract

The general features of the rabbit digestive tract are shown in Fig 19.4

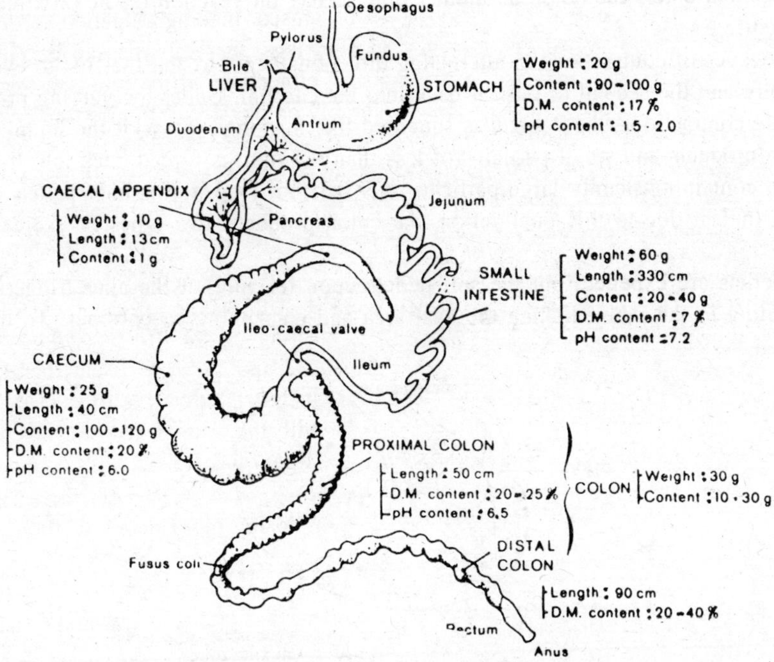

Fig. 19.4 The digestive system of the rabbit

The initiation of the digestive processes occurs when food is consumed. Rabbits masticate their feed very thoroughly, with as many as 120 jaw movements per minute. The material quickly reaches the stomach. The stomach is a thin walled, pouchlike organ. Although in suckling rabbits, the stomach pH ranges from 5 to 6.5 but after weaning it drops to between 2 and 3, and in adult the pH stands to almost 1. The environment effectively kills bacteria and other microorganisms, so that the rabbit stomach and small intestine are essentially sterile. The ingesta remains in the stomach for a few hours (3–6), undergoes little chemical change and are gradually move into small intestine in short interval by strong stomach contractions.

As the contents enter the small intestine they are diluted by the flow of bile and finally with pancreatic juice containing carbohydrate, protein and fat digesting enzyme. The simple nutrients are absorbed and carried by the blood to liver and other body tissues. The particles that are not broken down after a total stay of about $1\frac{1}{2}$ hours in the small intestine enter the caecum.

Here materials have to stay for a certain period (2–12 hrs), while they are attacked by microbial enzymes. The carbohydrate portion like that of rumen fermentation changes into volatile fatty acids (VFA) and absorbed in portal blood stream. The remaining content of the caecum is then evacuated into the colon. The material composed of both large and small food particles (50%) and the rest consists of dead microbes that have developed in caecum, fed on matter from the small intestine.

So far the functioning of the rabbits digestive tract is virtually the same as that of other monogastric animals. Its *uniqueness* lies in the dual function of the *proximal colon*. If the caecum content enters the colon in the early part of the morning, it undergoes few biochemical changes. The colon wall secretes a mucus which gradually envelops the pellets formed by the wall contractions. These pellets gather in elongated clusters and are called soft or night pellets (caecotrophes).

If the caecal content enters the colon at another time of day the reaction of the proximal colon is entirely different.

Successive waves of contractions in alternating directions begin to act; the first to evacuate the content normally and the second to push it back into the caecum. Under the varying pressure and rhythm of these contractions, the content is squeezed like a sponge. Most of the liquid part, containing soluble products and small particles of less than 0.1 mm, is forced back into the caecum. The solid part, containing mainly large particles cver 0.3 mm long, forms hard pellets which are then expelled. In fact due to this dual action, the colon produces two types of excrement: hard and soft.

The hard pellets are expelled, but the soft pellets upon reaching at the anus triggers a neural ıesponse, resulting in the rabbit licking the anal area and consuming caecotropes. To do this the

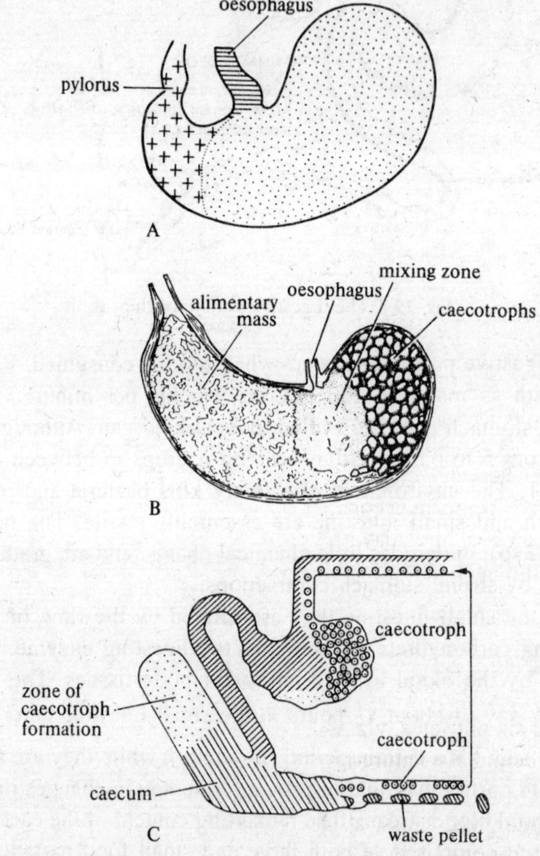

Fig. 19.5 A, Diagram of rabbit stomach. B, Longitudinal section of rabbit stomach. C, Diagram showing the passage of food and caecotrophs traversing the digestive tracts. In the stomach, under the mechanical action of peristalsis the caecotrophs are mixed with the food (mixing zone). In the lowest part of the caecum, the chyme under the action of bacteria is made into caecotrophs, which the animal eats soon after they are expelled from the anus. (B and C after Harder.)

rabbit twists itself round, sucks in the soft faeces as they emerge from the anus, then swallows without chewing them.

By the end of the morning there are large numbers of these pellets inside the stomach.

From then on, the soft pellets follow the same digestive process as normal feed.

The re-ingestion of soft faeces is also known as "*Coprophagy*" (from Greek *copros* = excrement and *phagein* = to eat) is common in rodents including rabbits and hares which are of great nutritional importance.

In rabbits prevention of coprophagy leads to a decrease in the ability to digest food, as well as a decrease in protein utilization and nitrogen retention. When coprophagy is permitted again, there is a corresponding increase in the ability to digest cellulose. In rabbit the soft faeces are not masticated and mixed with other food in the stomach (Fig.); they tend to lodge separately in the fundus of the stomach. The soft faeces are covered by a membrane, and they continue to ferment in the stomach for many hours, one of the fermentation products being lactic acid which aids in further utilization of feed materials to a great extent. The dead microbial content of the soft faeces due to reingestion yields essential amino acids (as in ruminants), the liquid portion of the faeces are rich in vitamins (due to microbial fermentation in caecum) are thus utilized by rabbit. Coprophagy also enhances total yields of energy.

The practice of *coprophagy* or *caecotrophy* has thus a great feed value for rabbits, hares and other rodents.

Feeding of Baby Rabbits

During the first 3 weeks, the only feed for the baby rabbits is the doe's milk. After 2–3 weeks the baby rabbits will start to eat the grass and concentrates, as well as suckling the doe. As they get older, they will adjust themselves to live completely on feed from outside. Till the baby rabbits remain on suckling, it is very important that their mother (does) gets enough good quality feed (concentrates, green roughages and clean water) to sustain lactational demand. A lactating doe while nursing 8 youngs, will consume concentrates more than 250 g/day, while the water consumption may be as high as 3–5 litres/day. All vegetable rations are generally supplemented with salt and a source of calcium, such as bone-meal. Rations must include balanced concentrates mixture.

Feeding of Adult Rabbits

Adult rabbits require all six nutrients, viz. water, carbohydrates, fat, protein, all essential minerals and vitamins like human being. By nature rabbits fulfil their nutrient requirements through:

1. *Green bulky roughages*, viz. grass, all types of green vegetable, leaves and hay.
2. *Concentrates*, which are feed low in crude fibre (under 20%) and high in energy (over 60% TDN). Concentrate mix are prepared by mixing more than one ingredients for enhanching nutritional adequacy of the feed.
3. *Coprophagy* is another important source of nutrients for rabbit which includes partially digested feed, containing protein, energy and vitamins those are needed by the rabbit.
4. *Water* consumption takes place through water content of feeds consumed and directly from drinking of clean water.

Table 19.3

Average Composition of concentrate mixture for Rabbit Feed

Ingredient	% Composition
Bengal gram	25
Wheat	20
Rice bran	20
Groundnut cake	23.5
Meat-cum-bone meal	10
Mineral mixture	1
Common salt	0.5
Total	100.0

Table 19.4

Model Feeding Schedule for Rabbits

	Approximate Body weight (kg)	Quantity to be fed per day	
		Concentrate (g)	Green fodder (g)
Bucks (Male adults)	4 – 5	175	200
Does (Female adults)	4 – 5	150	200
Lactating does	4 – 5	250	250
Weaner (6 weeks)	0.6 – 0.7	50	100

A constant supply of fresh clean water is essential for rabbits.

Rabbits dislike dusty and gritty feeds and selectively eat certain ingredients of mashed feeds. They prefer pelleted feed, which is also the scientific method of feeding rabbits in modern commercial rabbit farming. The advantages of pelleting are that it reduces the rabbits selection of preferred ingredients of the feed and improves growth performance by enhancing the nutrient utilisation. Pellets also require less storage space and are easier to transport.

Rabbits prefer pellets of 4 mm diameter and 10 mm length. Two types of pellets are used for: (1) all-grain pellets, fed with hay or roughage and (2) composite pellets which contain all the elements of a balanced diet, including roughage.

Scientists at the Central Sheep and Wool Research Institute, Avikanagar (Rajasthan) have worked out a technique for pelleting rabbit feed at home or on the farm. After selecting the raw material, thoroughly mix them by hand after sprinkling with molasses and 40 per cent water. Place the mash in a cotton bag and cook in a pressure cooker for 15 minutes. Feed the hot mixture into a meat-mincer and extrude through a 6 mm plate to form pellets. Dry the pellets in the sun, or in an oven at 80°C for four hours. Break up the pellets by hand and pack.

A farmer can prepare 15 kg of pellets per day. The capital costs of the method work out to Rs. 1,000 under present day costing.

Vitamin Requirement In Rabbits Diet

A dietary supply of Vit. A, D, E is necessary. Bacteria in the gut synthesize Vit K and B

Vitamins in adequate quantities, thus dietary supplements are unnecessary. Disease and stress may increase the daily vitamin requirements. Oxidation destroys vitamins A and E more readily than the other vitamin. Feed preparation and storage must be done in a manner that will reduce losses from oxidation. Diets containing > 30% of alfalfa meal generally provides sufficient Vit A level. Levels of vitamins in the diet must be > 5000 I.U/kg and < 75000 I.U/kg. Levels out of this range may cause abortion, resorbed litters and fetal hydrocephalus.

Dietary Fiber Utilization By Rabbits

Rabbits digest fiber poorly because of the selective separation and rapid excretion of large particles in the hind gut. They do need a generous amount of fiber in the diet (15% CF) to promote intestinal motility and minimise intestinal disease. Fiber may also absorb toxins of pathogenic bacteria and eliminate them via the "hard feces". Diets low in fiber promote an increased incidence of intestinal problems e.g. 'Enterotoxemia'. This may be the result of the higher starch content of low fiber diets. Starch is a substrate for the proliferation of pathogenic bacteria such as *Clostridium spiroforme,* which produce a potent toxin High fiber diets (> 20% CF) may result in an increased incidence of cecal impaction and mucoid enteritis. VFA produced in the cecum are important metabolites since they aid in the control of pathogenic organism by helping to maintain a low pH in the cecum.

Low fiber diet usually reduces the growth rate of fryer rabbits and for maximum growth rate a minimum of 10% dietary crude fiber is necessary.
Dietary fiber helps to prevent fur pulling and trichobezoars (hair balls) in the stomach.

Weaning

Weaning means taking away of baby rabbits from their mother at 5–7 weeks old when suckling is stopped. Usually the baby rabbits (litter) are taken away leaving the doe in the hutch (a small cage or pen). Sometimes farmer prefer to leave the litter in the huch and remove the doe so that weaning is less of a shock to the litter.

Management of Rabbits

Determination of Sex of Young Rabbits

This is known as 'sexing' and is usually carried out at the time of weaning when the sexes are fairly easy to distinguish. The young rabbit is balanced on the forearm with the hand under the rump. The thumb and forefinger of the other hand press down gently on either side of the sex organ. In bucks the penis will protrude as a rounded tip, whilst in does the protruding vulva will appear as a slit.

Tatooing

In order to identify individual young rabbits it is necessary to mark them after weaning. Tatooing by ink at inside the ear is the best method. Aluminium ear-tags can be used but these may be torn off by the rabbits with resultant tissue damage.

Weighing

The regular weighing of stock at different stages of their developments is desirable. The weaners can all be weighed together in a basket, or in a small cage.

Castration

Castration is only necessary if male rabbits are to be kept together for a long time such as in the case of Angora rabbits kept for the production of wool.

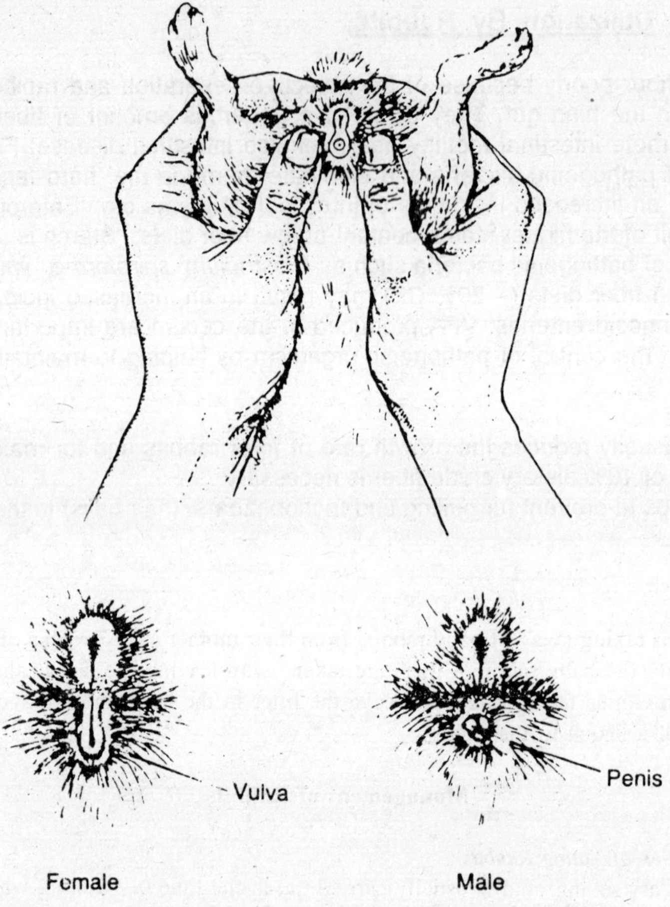

Fig 19.6 Sexing rabbits (female-male)

Breeding Does

One month before the date of their first mating, the does should be separated and put into single hutches (small cages). This will prevent them from having false pregnancies.

Breeding Bucks

Most of the young bucks will be used for meat and skins. Some may be selected for breeding. These bucks should always be kept in single hutches to prevent them from fighting.

Bucks for Meat Production

Rabbits which are kept for meat production can be kept in groups in large hutches. Males and females should be kept apart to avoid fighting. Broiler rabbits are now produced by selection of special breeds, viz., the Soviet chinchilla, grey giant, New Zealand white and New Zealand white grey.

Handling

(a) *Young rabbits:* Upto the age of about eight weeks young rabbits should be picked up and carried in one hand by gently grasping the loin, but the method is no good for rabbits over eight weeks old.

(b) *Medium sized rabbits:* The rabbit may be caught by grasping a loose fold of skin over its shoulders. The other hand should then be placed under the rump to support it before lifting.

(c) *Large rabbits:* Rabbits weighing over 5 kg may be caught in the same manner as above but the other arm should be extended along the side of its body with the hand under the rump for support.

Record Keeping

Accurate records of stock performances must be kept to enable poor producers to be eliminated and good ones used for replacement.

Rabbit Fur/Wool

In order to obtain fur/wool shearing of the rabbit can be done four times a year, when the wool is 6 cm long, shearing should be planned in such a way that it does not fall during the extreme cold of December and January. It can be done with sharp scissors. After shearing, the animal should be protected against adverse climate for 15 days. Good quality wool is long, white, clean and unmated.

Processing of Rabbit Skin

After the slaughter of the rabbit, its skin can be used to make gloves, caps, dolls and other articles. The rabbit skin also can fetch money by selling. The skin can be processed as below:

(a) *Soaking*: The skin should be soaked overnight in clean water having temperature between 20° to 25°C.

(b) *Pickling*: Prepare a solution containing 60–90 g of common salt, 30–40 g of potash alum and 1–3 kg of soda ash per litre of water. Soak the pre-soaked skin again in this solution for about two days. It then can be dried by wringing it in a towel. According to necessity hair may be removed from the skin by scraping with a sharp knife. It is then washed again in clean water and dried in the sun.

Housing

Rabbits need to be housed to protect them and to prevent them from running away. There are several ways of housing rabbits depending largely on the type of rabbit farming, i.e. whether backyard or big commercial type, climate and the availability of finance. Backyard rabbit keepers who usually cannot afford to spend much on materials for his rabbitry, get satisfied with locally available old boxes, offcuts, bamboo, tin cans, etc. The small commercial farmers on the o her hand may be interested to use moderately costly wire cages. Most important features of housing are rabbits not only be protected from extremes of heat, sun and cold, wind, rain and predators, but also should feel comfortable which includes proper space, suitable temperature, dry condition of the cages, proper ventilation along with some room furnitures like feeders, hoppers and hay rack.

On commercial farms as has been said rabbits are kept mostly in wire mesh cages. These can be arranged in a single tier but to make better use of the space in a building, they may be stacked in two, or even three tires. The cages in the upper tires are set back so that no cage is directly above another, to allow the urine and faeces to fall into the pit below. The selected arrangement must permit the staff to handle and feed all the rabbits easily. The cages are made of galvanized wire mesh and the joints must be smooth. An even floor surface is essential to avoid causing abrasions on the under surfaces of the hind feet. A square mesh not exceeding 19 × 19 mm is favoured as this allows faecal pellets to pass through and does not cause foot injuries.

The floor area must allow all the rabbits in the cage to lie comfortably and move around without disturbing the others, and eat and drink without difficulty. For rabbits over 12 weeks of age, the height should be not less than 45 cm. A cage of this height, with a floor space of 0.56 m^2 can accommodate one breeding buck or doe, a doe and litter up to 4 weeks of age, or eight weaners until marketed at 10 weeks old. Many farmers now use cages of this standard size only.

Each cage should have a pellet hopper hooked to the front and if the farmer feeds hay, a hay rack is also fitted outside the cage. For regular drinking water an automatic watering system with a nipple drinker in each cage is an essential provision. To minimize the cost inverted one litter bottles fixed to the side of the cage can be arranged to provide drinking water by any of the following two methods as described below:

(i) The mouth of the bottle is arranged over a shallow tray, most of which is inside the cage. Water passes from the bottle into the tray until stopped by—atmospheric pressure. The rabbits drink from the tray and water flows in to replace what they have drunk.

(ii) A 6 mm glass tube leads from the bottle into the cage. The end of the tube should be previously rounded in a flame so that it is not sharp. Rabbits will soon learn to suck water through the tube. Owing to the narrow diameter of the tube, water will not pass through it without the small amount of suction which the rabbits are able to exert.

Health Care Of Rabbit

Health care is important to make sure that rabbits stay productive. Every rabbit keeper should know how to recognise and if possible, prevent and cure illness which can affect rabbits.

Recognition Of Health & Disease

Sleek and glossy coat without any dull patches, general alertness, bright eyes, free movement, normal appetite, proportionate body, normal growth, no discharges from any parts of body and no swellings and sores, normal pulse rate are all signs of good health. Any signs of abnormality should be immediately noted, investigated and treated.

Table 19.5

Common Rabbit Disease		
Disease	**Clinical signs**	**Prevention and treatment**
Coccidiosis intestinal	Diarrhoea in young. Sudden death.	Wire cage floors. Coccidiostat in food. Sulphamezatine (POM) in water
Hepatic	Often no signs in life but may be loss of condition. At post-mortem white spots on liver.	
Mucoid enteritis	Mucoid material instead of faeces in young	Increase fibre in diet.
Typhlitis	Diarrhoea with mucus. Oedema of caecum on post-mortem	Oxytetracycline (POM) water
Ear canker	Yellowish-brown exudate in ears	Benzene hexachloride (GSL) in ears.
Chronic rhinitis (snuffles)	Sneezing, bilateral nasal discharge	Antibiotics (POM), possibly vaccination
Mastitis	Mammary glands hot and swollen	Improve hygienic, antibiotics (POM)
Sore hocks	Necrosis on underside of hind feet	Avoid rough cage floors. Antiseptic dressing.

POM, requires a veterinary surgeons prescription; GSL, General sale list.

Prevention of disease

Following measures will help to prevent disease -

1. Buy from a reputable breeder.
2. Establishing quarantine quarters for new arrivals and rabbits suspected of having a disease.
3. Proper housing which can prevent the animals from cold, damp, draught and insect attack.
4. Creating hygienic conditions by thorough cleaning and weekly disinfection of hutches, floors and walls of buildings, feeders and drinkers and other equipments.
5. Proper feeding.

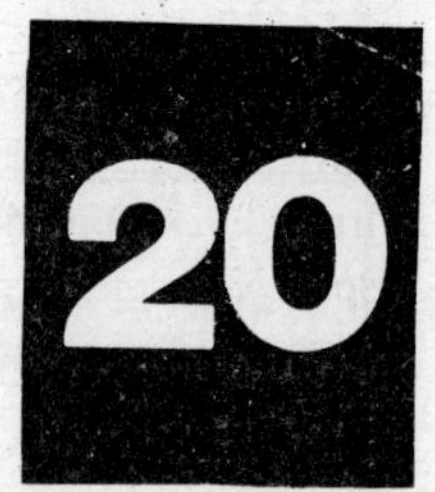

YAK

The yak is the only bovine large animal (ruminant) that dwells in the high hills of the Himalayas even at altitudes of 6,000 metres above the mean sea-level. The normal range of yak is 3,000 to 4,500 metres. Like those of domestic cattle and goat, yak has also chromosome number (2N = 60).

Zoological Name. Poephagus grunniens or *Bos grunniens.*

Zoological Classification

The bovine mammal belongs to the phylum *Chordate* (vertebrates), Class *Mammalia* (milk giving), order *Artiodactyla* (even toed, hoofed animals), family *Bovidae.*

Local Names. Tibetan *dong, brong dong* (wild), *pegu* (domesticated); Hindi *ban chour* (wild), *chour-gau* for domesticated varieties.

Distribution

Northern Ladak, the plateau of Tibet and part of the Kansu Province in China. Within India, Yak predominantly found in Changechenmo valley in Ladak and Spiti valleys of Himachal Pradesh and also in North Eastern States, particularly in Arunachal Pradesh, Sikkim and Nagaland. Small numbers are also found in Garhwal districts of U.P. It is a native of Tibet and surrounding countries in Central Asia. The yak is also found in Pakistan, northern Afghanistan, Bhutan, Mongolia and in Russia.

Population in India

According to 1982 census, the total population of Yak is 1.15 lakhs. A little over 77 per cent of yaks have been reported from Arunachal Pradesh where there are 89,000 yaks of which 59,000 are males and 30,000 are females.

Distinctive Characters

The wild yak is a massively built animal with a drooping head, high humped shoulders, a straight back, and a short sturdy limbs. Shaggy fringes of coarse hair hang from its flanks, cover chest, shoulder, thigh and the lower half of the tail, and form a bushy tuft between its horns and a great mane upon its neck. An adult male weighs about 1000 kg while females are only one third of their weight. In fact the species looks like a heap of black or blackish hair with scarcely any leg visible. *The dewlap is absent.* The back has 14 pairs of ribs instead of the 13 in all other oxen. The withers are formed by an extended spinal process of the vertebra, and since the seventh cervical vertebra is much higher, the line gently slopes to the crops. The skull is bulky, broad and well proportioned because of the considerable length of frontal and nasal bone. The horns are beautifully curved. The size of the base is 50 cm apart. In females the horns are much weaker and more irregularly shaped. The rather long legs have strongly enlarged hoofs (aid in adaptation to life in spongy ground) largely covered by standing water of little depth (swamp) and psuedo-claws which serve as supports when the animals climb in the high mountains. The coat on top of the head, withers and back is rather short but densely matted, while on the shoulders and sides of rump it is longer like a mane. The head hair is curly.

The yak has a thin, hard muzzle, small but dilatable nostrils, enlarged nasal cavity which is highly coiled, large thoracic cavity and well developed lungs. The blood has a high count of red cells. The spongy tissue is well developed in the skeletal system. These features help the animal in having better oxygen-carrying capacity and mechanical economy in movements on the hills. The lengthy tail, which is very hairy from the base, has been exported all over the East as a material for fly-whisks. Massive head is armed with powerful outward-curving horns.

The so-called American Buffalo (which is really a Bison) is a close relation of the Yak, and like it has a humped back.

Wild Yak

The wild yak inhabits the North Tibetan desert which has no trees and bushes, and are located at the lower elevations around 5,000 metres, interspersed with marshes, swamps and lakes. Yak's sense of smell is excellent, although its eye sight is only mediocre. In general they are inhabitant of the coldest, wildest and most desolate mountains, where both arctic and desert conditions prevail. In fact wild yak's existence is one of continuous struggle against the adverse forces of its environment. *It is one of the highest dwelling animals in the world.* In summer time yaks are found at elevations ranging from 4270 to 6100 metre and even in winter they do not descend much below this level.

The colour of a wild yak is a uniform blackish brown with a little white about the muzzle. On the other hand the domestic yaks usually have patches of white on the chest and tail. This tendency to piebald (combination of two colours specially with white and black patches) is never seen in the wild species. Domestic yaks are at times wholly black and, like wild yaks, wander to great heights in search of food.

Usually they live in small herds, except during the spring when the newly sprouting grass attracts large assemblages. In high altitudes where neither man nor wolf go, yaks usually attain the record age of about 25 years when they finally die of old age.

The wild bull's horns are much more massive than those of any domestic yak.

Domestic Yak (Bos mutus grunniens)

The yak had probably been domesticated thousand years (millenium) B.C. by the Tibetans. The yak is much smaller than its wild ancestor. Besides those with the wild black and pure white colour, there are brown, yellow, reddish-grey and piebald domestic yaks. Their coats resemble the wild ones, although in most cases they have an even longer stomach mane. The horns are weaker; even hornless animals are not too rare, at a ratio of 1 : 100. Now the domestic yak has a much wider distribution than the wild original form. Domestic yak makes frequent grunting sounds, in contrast to the wild yak, he is also called "*grunting ox*". The animals can withstand much higher temperature.

Both wild and the domestic yaks rank among the most surefooted mountain animals. They can proceed without stumbling along the worst mountain paths, with a wall of rock on one side and a void on the other but without ever falling.

Yaks for centuries past been domesticated at the Himalayan heights by interbreeding with domestic cattle. Two kinds of hybrids, one horned (ZO) and the other hornless (Zum) are known. Both these hybrids breed true. Yaks also interbreeds with several other members of the genus *Bos*, such as bison, banting, gajal, zebu and European cattle. Interbreeding with buffalo is not possible. *The male offspring of all breeds crossed with yaks are said to be sterile.* More than 90% yaks found in Mangolia lack horns.

Like other bovines yak love to stand or wallow in running water (the icy streams which spring from the snout of a glacier).

Reproduction

The mating (rutting) season begins in September and lasts for one whole month. The old bulls like to live singly or in small groups of 3 to 5 except for mating season when they join the cows for some weeks and have bitter rival fights among themselves during which each animal tries to push his horn into the opponents flank. While such encounters seldom end with the death of one of the animals, serious injuries occur often. However, the wounds heal quickly in the sterile air at these altitudes. Only during the mating season do wild yaks make strange grunting sounds. The rest of the time he is not very vocal. Cows give birth to their calves during April to June after a gestation period of 9 months when the new-grown grass ensures a good feed supply. Calving takes place only during second year because the young are dependent on them for one year. The yak is considered to be fully grown only at 6 to 8 years old.

In case of domestic yak, the oestrous is irregular, cows in contrast to wild form calves every year in April or May.

Utility

The common saying—"What moves in Tibet and Mongolia does so on yaks", highlights the importance of yaks for inhabitants of high altitudes. The utilities are summarised below:

1. Since domestic yak requires little food and is insensitive to cold temperature, it is the best suited domestic animal in Asia at elevations above 2,000 metres.
2. Without the yak, travel and trade in lonely trans-Himalayan regions would be extremely difficult. It easily carries loads of 150 kg over the steepest mountain paths.
3. The milk production is somewhat lower, averages about 500 litres, per year, but the milk has a high nutritious value with a fat content of 7 to 11 per cent (usually the composition found is water 81.85%, Protein 4.06%, Fat 10.9%, total solids 19.25%, Ash 0.98%. The milk is slightly acidic (pH = 6.6). The composition varies from area to area and also on the quantity and quality of feed. In Tibet a milk powder is prepared (besides butter and cheese) by a special process of coagulation.
4. Occasionally, the yak is slaughtered at old age for meat particularly in many parts of hilly tracts. The meat tastes good but is highly rich in fat content. The meat fibres are finer than those of beef and resembles mutton fibres. On analysing shoulder region of the meat it has been found to contain Water 68%, Proteins 20%, Fat 7% and Ash 5.1%, Calcium 1.283% and Phosphorus 1.08%.

5. The yak annually produces 300–600 g of down hair and 1,000–2,000 g of coarse hair. The down hair, similar to pashmina, is used for making garments. The coarse hair is used for preparing bags, ropes, carpets and tents. According to a legend in Hindu mythology, the marriage of Lord Shiva with Parvati was solemnized with a silky–white yak's coat offered by Shiva's mother-in-law.
6. The yak's manure is often the only fuel in the highlands of Tibet which have no trees or bush.
7. Yak bullocks (castrated) are used for ploughing and threshing grains. Crosses between yak and zebu also give more milk and better meat and are excellent work animals for carrying loads at moderate altitudes. *The cross-bred males are always sterile.*

Feeding

Very little is known about the feeding of yaks. They live in small herds, except during the spring when the newly sprouting grass attracts large assemblages. In summer their food consists mainly of wiry tufts of grass and small shrubs which clothes the barren plateau. They also eat much of the 'Salt' encrusted earth, which in spots covers the ground with a white crust. Winter is a time of great privation, when many die of starvation and exposure. Streams and pools are frozen hard, and in lieu of water yak eat the frozen snow, even in summer. When grazing at extreme heights, melting snow is their usual liquid nourishment. When grass is extremely scarce, and cattle and horses cannot survive for long, the yaks are capable of existing by eating up broken and wilted blades of last year's grass which have been blown by the wind and particularly embedded in the soil. In such areas yak may spend upto 8 hours a day licking up dead grass, and thus remain alive and keep on working. For this purpose yaks travel in single file, each animal carefully places its feet in the imprints left by the hoofs of the one preceding it.

In India during June, the yak herdsmen (*bropkas*) move their herds to pastures situated 4,000 – 5,000 metres above the mean sea-level, after making a journey of 3 to 4 days from their villages. At this height the herdsmen live in temporary huts (*chaurigoat*), braving high winds and occasional snowing. The average temperature during this period is 4–5°C. The yaks are allowed to graze from dawn to dusk and milked once in a day. Cash sale is rare, and most transactions are done through barter system. With the onset of winter in October, the herdsmen come down to their villages along with their yaks. The winter pastures of the middle altitudes are very poor both in quantity and nutritive values. Even in summer pasture lands are almost devoid of legumes and are profusely infested with weeds resulting suboptimal production among yaks.

Future Research

The Indian Council of Agriculture Research (ICAR) has established a National Research Centre on Yak in 1989 at Town Hill near Dirang in Arunachal Pradesh to conduct extensive surveys and to study the feeding, breeding management and disease control aspects of this precious animal of hilly regions in India to improve its productivity and utility.

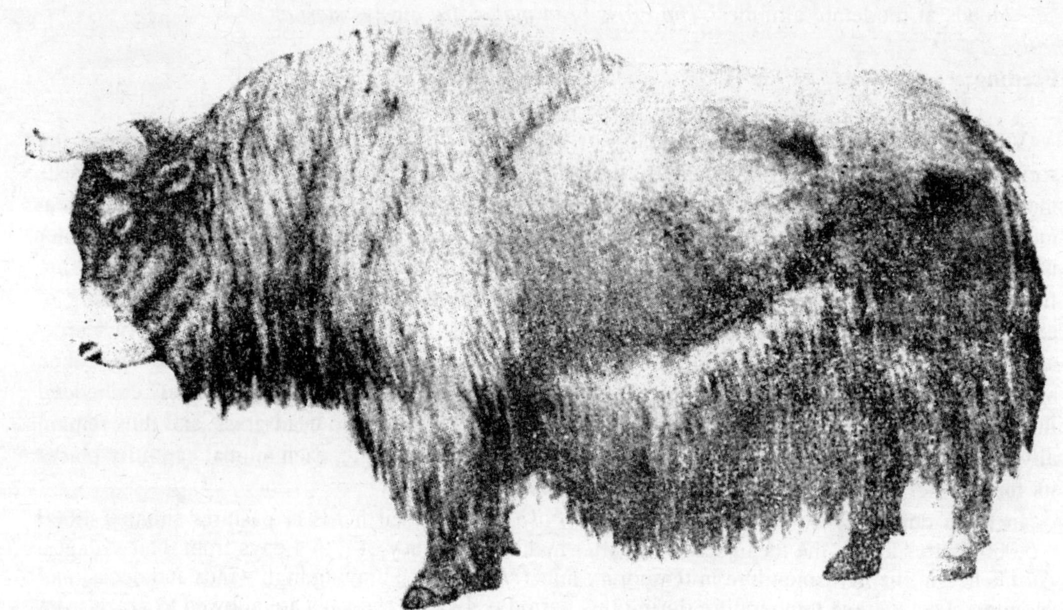

Plate 97. YAK (CHAPTER 20).

Notes on Horse

(*EQUUS CABALLUS*)

Zoological classification

Phylum—Chordata, Class—Mammalia, Order—Perissodactyla Family—Equidae, Genus—Equus, Species—*E. caballus* (horse) *E. asinus* (ass or donkey)

Age of puberty	15—24 months
Breeding life	18 years ± 2 years
Gestation period	336 ± 5 days (average 340 days)
Length of oestrus cycle	21 days ± 5 days
	2 days
Length of oestrus	6 days ± 4 days
Time of ovulation	5th day of heat (1-2 days before end of estrous)
Optimum time for service	2nd--5th day of heat. Repeat 2 days later still on heat.
First heat after parturition	4—14 days
Mammary glands	2
Ejaculate	
Volume (cc)	75—150
Sperm/cc	150 million
Total sperm (billion)	9
Mares allowed to one stallion	30—40
Best breeding season	Early spring
Normal temperature	99.5—101.3°F
Respiration rate/min	8—16
Heart rate/min	32—44
Average productive life (Yrs.)	20—25
Average Milk Composition (%)	Protein—2.7; Fat—1.6; Sugar —6.1; Minerals—0.51; Water —90.00.

Some common terms in relation to HORSE

Expression	*Details*
Stallion	A sexually intact male horse over 3 years old.
Stud	A stallion used for breeding or to the breeding establishment or the form at which the stallion is in service.
Mare	A mature female
Filly	A young female upto 3 years of age
Gelding	A castrated male of any age
Colt	An intact male upto 3 years of age
Foal	Young male or female under one year of age
Weanling	A young horse of either sex just weaned

Important Breeds

Indian : Kathiwari, Marwari, Bhutia, Manipuri and Spiti.
Pakistani : Baluchi, Hirzai, Unmol.

Notes on Elephants

	African elephant (*Loxodonta africans*)	Indian elephant (*Elephas maximus*)
Physical features	Large ears Convex sloping forehead Two finger-like processes on trunk tip Hollow backed with lumbar prominence Tusks in both sexes	Small ears High domed forehead with 2 prominences on top of skull One process on trunk tip Convex backed Tusks in males only, and not always
Mature at	25 years	25 years
Weight at maturity	Male 6000 kg	Male 3000 kg
Geographical distribution	East, Central and West Africa	Ceylon, India, Burma, Thailand, Vietnam, Laos, Malaysia, Indonesia
Uses	Very limited. In small area of Zaire, used for timber transport	Timber extraction and log moving in forested areas
Digestive system	Daily food intake considerable, but only partially digested and utilization low. Mean intake varies from 4·2 to 5·6 of the animal's body weight. Natural food includes bamboo shoots, leaves and various fruits. Working elephants are fed straw, hay and crushed grain as a supplement Daily water consumption of adult 140–230 litres	
Reproduction and breeding	Puberty occurs at between 8 and 12 years. The gestation period is 21–22 months. The calving interval is 4 years. Elephants may live for up to 60–70 years	

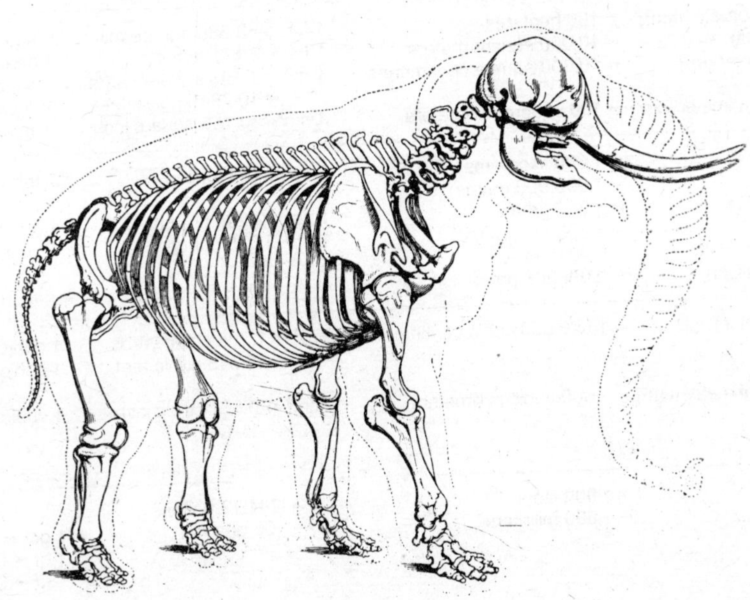

Skeleton of an Indian elephant.

Metric and Temperature Conversion Charts

	Metric Unit (symbol)		Metric to English	English to Metric
LENGTH	kilometer (km)	= 1,000 (10^3) meters	1 km = 0.62 mile	1 mile = 1.609 km
	meter (m)	= 100 centimeters	1 m = 1.09 yards = 3.28 feet	1 yard = 0.914 m 1 foot = 0.305 m
	centimeter (cm)	= 0.01 (10^{-2}) meter	1 cm = 0.394 inch	1 inch = 2.54 cm
	millimeter (mm)	= 0.001 (10^{-3}) meter	1 mm = 0.039 inch	1 inch = 25.4 mm
	micrometer (μm)	= 0.000001 (10^{-6}) meter		
	nanometer (nm)	= 0.000000001 (10^{-9}) meter		
	angstrom (Å)	= 0.0000000001 (10^{-10}) meter		
AREA	square kilometer (km^2)	= 100 hectares	1 km^2 = 0.386 square mile	1 square mile = 2.590 km^2
	hectare (ha)	= 10,000 square meters	1 ha = 2.471 acres	1 acre = 0.405 ha
	square meter (m^2)	= 10,000 square centimeters	1 m^2 = 1.196 square yards = 10.764 square feet	1 square yard = 0.836 m^2 1 square foot = 0.093 m^2
	square centimeter (cm^2)	= 100 square millimeters	1 cm^2 = 0.155 square inch	1 square inch = 6.452 cm^2
MASS	metric ton (t)	= 1,000 kilograms = 1,000,000 grams	1 t = 1.103 tons	1 ton = 0.907 t
	kilogram (kg)	= 1,000 grams	1 kg = 2.205 pounds	1 pound = 0.454 kg
	gram (g)	= 1,000 milligrams	1 g = 0.035 ounce	1 ounce = 28.35 g
	milligram (mg)	= 0.001 gram		
	microgram (μg)	= 0.000001 gram		
VOLUME: SOLIDS	1 cubic meter (m^3)	= 1,000,000 cubic centimeters	1 m^3 = 1.308 cubic yards = 35.315 cubic feet	1 cubic yard = 0.765 m^3 1 cubic foot = 0.028 m^3
	1 cubic centimeter (cm^3)	= 1,000 cubic millimeters	1 cm^3 = 0.061 cubic inch	1 cubic inch = 16.387 cm^3
VOLUME: LIQUIDS	kiloliter (kl)	= 1,000 liters	1 kl = 264.17 gallons	
	liter (l)	= 1,000 milliliters	1 l = 1.06 quarts	1 gal = 3.785 l 1 qt = 0.94 l 1 pt = 0.47 l
	milliliter (ml)	= 0.001 liter	1 ml = 0.034 fluid ounce	1 fluid ounce = 29.57 ml
	microliter (μl)	= 0.000001 liter		

INDEX